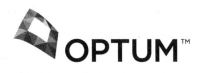

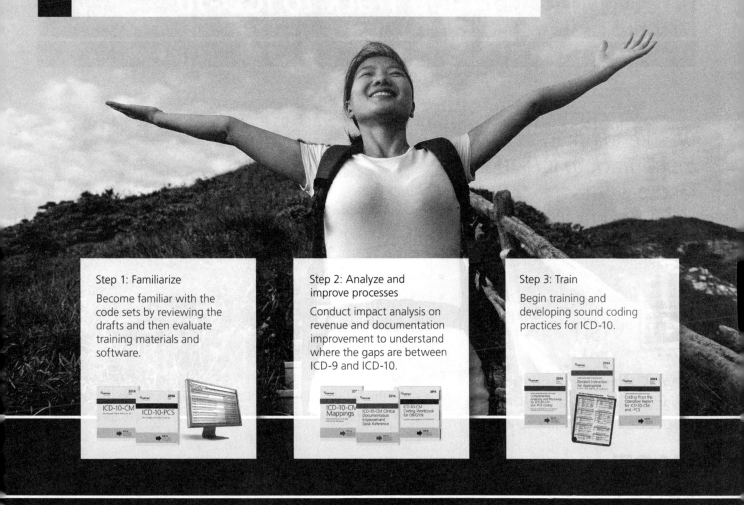

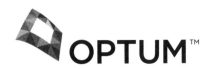

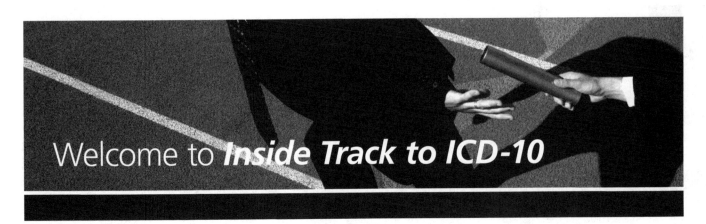

Welcome to *Inside Track to ICD-10*

Be sure to opt in to *Inside Track to ICD-10* (and pass this great benefit along).

VISIT

OptumCoding.com/InsideTrack
to sign up today or scan the QR code below with your smartphone.

Optum *Inside Track to ICD-10,* your new ICD-10 source.

Stay informed with *Inside Track to ICD-10.* Gain exclusive access to ICD-10-CM/PCS training and transition information via email when you purchase an ICD-9-CM, ICD-10-CM or ICD-10-PCS code book or sign up at OptumCoding.com/InsideTrack.

- ICD-10-CM/PCS updates and news
- Monthly eNewsletter
- Exclusive offers

Key features and benefits

For no additional cost, become a member of *Inside Track to ICD-10,* and share this benefit with your colleagues. Gain access to the latest tools and updates, conveniently delivered to your inbox to meet your organization's diagnosis coding needs.

- Stay on top of changing health care, code sets, and regulations with *Inside Track to ICD-10*
- Take advantage of the opportunity to participate in customer surveys and forums to help improve Optum diagnosis coding products
- Learn the latest ICD-10-CM/PCS news, transition updates and tips
- Link right to our online resources through *Inside Track to ICD-10* communications
- Learn about new tools available to help with your ICD-10 transition

13-29438 100-9894

ICD-10 BRINGS BIG CHANGES.
BIGGER OPPORTUNITIES.

ICD-10-CM/PCS
(takes effect Oct.1, 2014)

668%
INCREASE

ICD-9-CM

about **18,000** unique codes

about **140,000** unique codes

 = 1,000 codes

140,000 CODES. ACCESSIBLE IN SECONDS.
Simplify ICD-10 with Optum™ coding and billing solutions.

ICD-10 will have 668% more codes than ICD-9 — but that doesn't mean the transition has to be overwhelming. As an affordable, simplified alternative to coding books, *EncoderPro.com* and *RevenueCyclePro.com* — the industry's leader for web-based coding, billing, and compliance solutions — provides one-click access to ICD-10 codes, data and mapping tools as well as CPT® and HCPCS code sets.

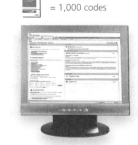

100,000 Users

Rely on Optum coding and billing solutions. Maybe it's time to learn why.

 Call: 1.800.464.3649, option 1

Visit: OptumCoding.com/Transition

Scan this code to register for a custom eSolutions demo.

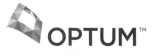 OPTUM™

Order your coding resources and earn rewards at **OptumCoding.com**

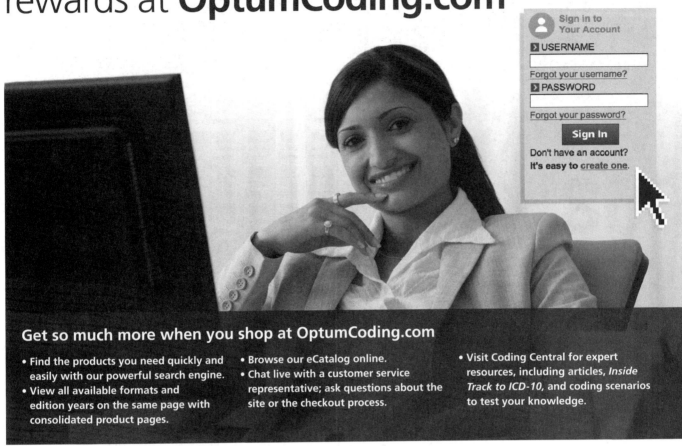

Get so much more when you shop at OptumCoding.com

- Find the products you need quickly and easily with our powerful search engine.
- View all available formats and edition years on the same page with consolidated product pages.

- Browse our eCatalog online.
- Chat live with a customer service representative; ask questions about the site or the checkout process.

- Visit Coding Central for expert resources, including articles, *Inside Track to ICD-10*, and coding scenarios to test your knowledge.

Register on OptumCoding.com for a customized website experience:

- View special website promotions/discounts.
- Get product recommendations based on your order history.
- Research your order history.
- Check on shipment status and tracking.
- View invoices and payment history.
- Pay outstanding invoices online.
- Manage your address book.
- Ship orders to multiple locations.
- Renew your order with a single click.

- Compile a wish list of the products you want and purchase when you're ready.

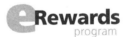Rewards
program

- Register for an account and you are automatically enrolled in our eRewards program! Receive a $50 coupon for every $500 you spend on OptumCoding.com.* When logged in, the eRewards meter keeps track of purchases toward your next reward.

REGISTER NOW: **Visit:** OptumCoding.com/Register **Call:** 800.464.3649, option 1

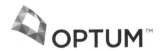

OPTUM™

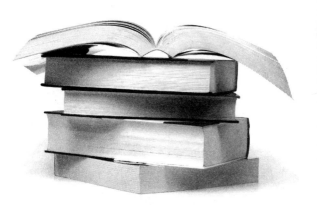

SAVE UP TO 25%

when you renew your coding essentials.

>> Buy 1–2 items, save 15%
Buy 3–5 items, save 20%
Buy 6+ items, save 25%

ITEM #	TITLE INDICATE THE ITEMS YOU WISH TO PURCHASE	QUANTITY	PRICE PER PRODUCT	TOTAL

	Subtotal	
(AK, DE, HI, MT, NH & OR are exempt)	Sales Tax	
1 item $10.95 • 2–4 items $12.95 • 5+ CALL	Shipping & Handling	
	TOTAL AMOUNT ENCLOSED	

Save up to 25% when you renew.

 Visit **www.optumcoding.com** and enter your promo code.

 Call **1.800.464.3649, option 1,** and mention the promo code.

 Fax this order form with purchase order to **801.982.4033.** *Optum no longer accepts credit cards by fax.*

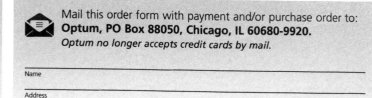 Mail this order form with payment and/or purchase order to:
Optum, PO Box 88050, Chicago, IL 60680-9920.
Optum no longer accepts credit cards by mail.

Name _____

Address _____

_____

Customer Number _____   Contact Number _____

○ CHECK ENCLOSED (PAYABLE TO OPTUM)

○ BILL ME ○ P.O.# _____

(   ) _____
Telephone

(   ) _____
Fax

E-mail _____@_____

PROMO CODE
FOBA14C

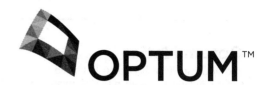

DRG Expert

A comprehensive guidebook to the MS-DRG classification system

Changes effective with discharges on or after October 1, 2013

2014
30th Edition

Optum Notice

Our Commitment to Accuracy

Copyright

Acknowledgments

Ken Kracker, *Product Manager*
Lynn Speirs, *Senior Director, Editorial/Desktop Publishing*
Karen Schmidt, BSN, *Senior Director, Clinical Tehnical Editors*
Stacy Perry, *Manager, Desktop Publishing*
Lisa Singley, *Project Manager*
Kelly Canter, BA, RHIT, CCS, *Technical Editor*
Anita Schmidt, BS, RHIT, *Technical Editor*
Tracy Betzler, *Senior Desktop Publishing Specialist*
Hope M. Dunn, *Senior Desktop Publishing Specialist*
Katie Russell, *Desktop Publishing Specialist*
Kate Holden, *Editor*
Jan Welsh, *Sales Executive,* Optum Data Analytics

About the Technical Editors

Karen Schmidt, BSN

Ms. Schmidt has more than 25 years of health care experience, beginning with a strong clinical background in critical care nursing and later functioning as director of case management, including the components of quality assurance, utilization management, concurrent coding, case-mix analysis, and discharge planning. Her areas of expertise include ICD-9-CM/DRG coding, outpatient observation, billing compliance, implementation of concurrent coding methodology, and physician documentation education. She is an active member of the American Health Information Management Association (AHIMA).

Kelly V. Canter, BA, RHIT, CCS

Ms. Canter has expertise in hospital coding and compliance, specializing in ICD-9-CM and CPT/HCPCS coding and utilization review. Her experience includes conducting coding and medical necessity audits, providing clinician and coding staff education, and managing revenue cycles and hospital quality incentive programs. She has been extensively trained in ICD-10-CM and PCS. Ms. Canter has presented at multiple national conventions on various coding and compliance topics. She is an active member of the American Health Information Management Association (AHIMA) and the Michigan Health Information Management Association (MHIMA).

Anita Schmidt, BS, RHIT

Ms. Schmidt has expertise in level I adult and pediatric trauma hospital coding, specializing in ICD-9-CM, DRG, and CPT coding. Her experience includes analyzing medical record documentation and assigning ICD-9-CM codes and DRGs, and CPT codes for same-day surgery cases. She has conducted coding training and auditing including DRG validation, conducted training in use of the electronic health record, and worked with clinical documentation specialists to identify documentation needs and potential areas for physician education. Ms. Schmidt is an active member of the American Health Information Management Association (AHIMA) and the Minnesota Health Information Management Association (MNHIMA).

Summary of Changes

DRG Expert Website

Optum now maintains a website to accompany *DRG Expert*. Optum will post special reports, Centers for Medicare and Medicaid Services (CMS) information, and updated data files on this website so that the information is available before the next book update. This website address is:

http://www.optumcoding.com/Product/Updates/DRG

This website is available only to customers who purchase the *DRG Expert*. The following password is needed to access this site:

pub14drg

The password will change annually and Optum will supply customers with the new password when it changes.

Available on eBook

The *DRG Expert* is now available as an eBook for your convenience. The eBook version of *DRG Expert* contains a complete copy of this book, including appendixes, and may be purchased separately.

Summary of Changes for FY 2014

The Centers for Medicare and Medicaid Services has issued its final rule on changes to the hospital inpatient prospective payment system (IPPS) and fiscal 2014 rates (*Federal Register,* August 19, 2013). The changes were published in the final rule in August and will be effective October 1, 2013. The Medicare severity diagnosis-related groups (MS-DRGs) are now considered version 31.0 Medicare DRGs and are effective for discharges occurring on or after October 1, 2013.

DRG and Code Changes

- Reassign cases with V45.88 (Status post administration of tPA [rtPA] in a different facility within the last 24 hours prior to admission to current facility) to MS-DRG 065 Intracranial Hemorrhage or Cerebral Infarction with CC from MS-DRG 066 Intracranial Hemorrhage or Cerebral Infarction without CC/MCC.

- Revise the title for MS-DRG 065 to Intracranial Hemorrhage or Cerebral Infarction with CC or tPA in 24 Hours.

- Reassign V64.00–V64.04 and V64.06–V64.09 (Vaccination not carried out), V64.1 (Surgical or other procedure not carried out because of contraindication), V64.2 (Surgical or other procedure not carried out because of patient's decision), and V64.3 (Procedure not carried out for other reasons) to MS-DRG 795 (Normal Newborn) list of Only Secondary Diagnosis from MS-DRG 794 (Neonate with Other Significant Problems).

- Revise the Medicare Code Edit (MCE) by:
  - adding a new discharge status code 69 (Discharged/ transferred to a designated disaster alternative care site) for MS-DRGs 280, 281, and 282 (Acute Myocardial Infarction, Discharged Alive with MCC, CC, without CC/MCC)
  - adding 15 new discharge status codes for MS-DRGs 280, 281, and 282 (Acute Myocardial Infarction, Discharged Alive with MCC, CC, without CC/MCC) to identify discharges and transfers with a planned acute care hospital inpatient readmission
  - adding three patient discharge status codes for MS-DRG 789 (Neonates, Died or Transferred to Another Acute Care Facility) to identify transfers of neonates with a planned acute care hospital inpatient readmission
  - removing codes from the age conflict edit, 751.1(Congenital atresia and stenosis of small intestine), 751.2 (Congenital atresia and stenosis of large intestine, rectum, and anal canal), and 751.61 (Congenital biliary atresia)

- Revise the CC Excludes list by adding 575.0 (Acute cholecystitis) when reported as a secondary diagnosis code with principal diagnosis code 574.00 (Calculus of gallbladder with acute cholecystitis, without mention of obstruction).

- Revise the CC Excludes list by removing 27 diagnosis codes representing atherosclerosis of the extremities and aneurysms, from 440.4 (Chronic total occlusion of artery of the extremities).

- Recalibrate the DRG relative weights as required by the Social Security Act.

ents

Numeric Listing of DRGs

Numeric Listing of DRGs

DRG Listing by Major Diagnostic Category

DRG Listing by Major Diagnostic Category

MDC 8 Diseases And Disorders Of The Musculoskeletal System And Connective Tissue

MDC 9 Diseases And Disorders Of The Skin, Subcutaneous Tissue And Breast

SURGICAL

MEDICAL

MDC 10 Endocrine, Nutritional And Metabolic Diseases And Disorders

SURGICAL

MEDICAL

MDC 11 Diseases And Disorders Of The Kidney And Urinary Tract

SURGICAL

MDC 12   Diseases And Disorders Of The Male Reproductive System

MDC 13   Diseases And Disorders Of The Female Reproductive System

Introduction

The Medicare severity diagnosis-related group (MS-DRG) system organizes ICD-9-CM diagnosis and procedure codes into a complex, comprehensive system based on a few simple principles.

Understanding how the DRG system works enables providers to recover the appropriate payment for inpatient services rendered in an acute care hospital facility, which is consistent with the intent of the federal government when the DRG system was devised. The *DRG Expert* helps providers understand DRGs, thus ensuring appropriate payment.

Note: For information concerning the DRG classification system for long-term acute care hospitals (LTCHs), refer to the section titled "Long Term Acute Care Hospital Prospective Payment System (LTCH PPS)" on page xxii.

Source of Information

Information in the book is taken from the official data published by the Centers for Medicare and Medicaid Services (CMS) in the *Federal Register*, Volume 78, No. 160 August 19, 2013 ("Hospital Inpatient Prospective Payment Systems for Acute Care Hospitals and the Long Term Care Hospital Prospective Payment System Changes and FY2014 Rates; Final Rule"). The information presented is consistent with the fiscal 2014 Grouper, version 31.0.

Basic Characteristics of DRG Classification

A DRG is one of 751 groups that classify patients into clinically cohesive groups that demonstrate similar consumption of hospital resources and length-of-stay patterns. In 1983, Congress mandated a national inpatient prospective payment system (IPPS) for all Medicare inpatients. The following types of hospitals are excluded from the IPPS:

- Psychiatric hospitals and units
- Rehabilitation hospitals and units
- Children's hospitals
- Long-term care hospitals
- Cancer hospitals
- Critical access hospitals

This IPPS uses DRGs to determine hospital reimbursement. CMS administers the IPPS and issues all rules and changes with regard to DRGs.

In addition to calculating reimbursement, DRGs have two major functions. The first is to help evaluate the quality of care. Not only are critical pathways designed around DRGs, but benchmarking and outcomes analysis can be launched using the DRG clinical framework, and quality reviews can be performed to assess coding practices and physician documentation. Ongoing education of physicians, coders, nurses, and utilization review personnel can be guided by the results of DRG analysis.

Second, DRGs assist in evaluating utilization of services. Each DRG represents the average resources needed to treat patients grouped to that DRG relative to the national average of resources used to treat all Medicare patients. The DRG assigned to each hospital inpatient stay also relates to the hospital case mix (i.e., the types of patients the hospital treats). A hospital's Medicare population case complexity is measured by calculation of the case mix index, which is an average of all MS-DRG relative weights for the facility during a given period of time. The higher the case mix index, the more complex the patient population and the higher the required level of resources utilized. Since severity is such an essential component of MS-DRG assignment and case mix index calculation, documentation and code assignment to the highest degree of accuracy and specificity is of utmost importance.

Medicare computes the case-mix adjustment for each fiscal year for all hospitals based upon the case-mix data received. This CMI is then used to adjust the hospital base rate, which is a factor in computing the total hospital payment under IPPS.

The formula for computing the hospital payment for each DRG is as follows:

DRG Relative Weight x Hospital Base Rate = Hospital Payment

The hospital case mix complexity includes the following patient attributes:

- Severity of illness — the level of loss of function or mortality associated with disease
- Prognosis — defined as probable outcome of illness
- Treatment difficulty — patient management problems
- Need for intervention — severity of illness that would result due to lack of immediate or continuing care
- Resource intensity — volume and types of services required for patient management

The DRG system was developed to relate case mix to resource utilization. Reimbursement is adjusted to reflect the resource utilization and does not take into consideration severity of illness, prognosis, treatment difficulty, or need for intervention.

Case mix and complexity can be analyzed and monitored in relation to cost and utilization of services. In addition, high-volume conditions and services can be identified and monitored, and DRG trend analysis can aid in forecasting future staff and facility requirements. One important operating parameter is the CMI, which measures the cost of a hospital's Medicare patient mix in relation to the cost of all Medicare patients. A low case mix may indicate unnecessary revenue loss.

DRG Assignment Process

DRGs are assigned using the principal diagnosis; secondary diagnoses, which include complication/comorbidities; surgical or other invasive procedures; sex of the patient and discharge status. One DRG is assigned to each inpatient stay. Diagnoses and procedures are designated by ICD-9-CM codes. The following describes the typical decision process used to assign a DRG to a case.

A case is assigned to one of 25 major diagnostic categories (MDC), which are mutually exclusive groups based on principal diagnosis. DRG assignment is based upon the following considerations:

- Principal and secondary diagnosis and procedure codes
- Sex of the patient

- Discharge status
- Presence or absence of major complications and comorbidities (MCCs) and/or presence or absence of complications and comorbidities (CCs)
- Birth weight for neonates

Each MDC is organized into one of two sections — surgical or medical. The surgical section classifies all surgical conditions based upon operating room procedures. The medical section classifies all diagnostic conditions based upon diagnosis codes. The majority of MDCs are organized by major body system and/or are associated with a particular medical specialty.

There are two groups of DRGs that are not assigned to MDCs. First, there is the group that may be associated with all MDCs. This group includes DRGs created specifically to report admissions into a facility that have been assigned invalid principal diagnoses (DRG 998), have O.R. procedures unrelated to a principal diagnosis (DRGs 981–983, 984–986, and 987–989), or are ungroupable principal diagnoses (DRG 999). Although the scope is too broad for clinical analysis, the DRGs encompass clinically coherent cases.

Another group not assigned to MDCs is called Pre-MDC DRGs, which consist of cases that are grouped by surgical procedure rather than principal diagnosis. The Pre-MDC DRG group includes bone marrow and organ transplant cases as well as tracheostomy cases.

Further sorting of medical classifications is performed by principal diagnosis type and/or surgical classifications by type of surgery. Finally, the case is analyzed for the presence of MCCs and/or CCs as indicated by ICD-9-CM diagnosis codes, and a DRG is assigned.

Each year, effective October 1 through September 30, DRG assignments are adjusted based on relative weight (RW), arithmetic mean length of stay (AMLOS), and geometric mean length of stay (GMLOS). Annually, new ICD-9-CM codes are also incorporated into the existing DRGs or new DRGs are added for the next fiscal year.

The information contained in this manual reflects the DRG classification system for fiscal 2014, Grouper Version 31.0.

Grouper Version	Effective Time Period
MS 31.0	10/01/2013 – 09/30/2014
MS 30.0	10/01/2012 – 09/30/2013
MS 29.0	10/01/2011 – 09/30/2012
MS 28.0	10/01/2010 – 09/30/2011
MS 27.0	10/01/2009 – 09/30/2010
MS 26.0	10/01/2008 – 09/30/2009
MS 25.0	10/01/2007 – 09/30/2008
CMS 24.0	10/01/2006 – 09/30/2007
CMS 23.0	10/01/2005 – 09/30/2006
CMS 22.0	10/01/2004 – 09/30/2005
CMS 21.0	10/01/2003 – 09/30/2004
CMS 20.0	10/01/2002 – 09/30/2003
CMS 19.0	10/01/2001 – 09/30/2002
CMS 18.0	10/01/2000 – 09/30/2001
CMS 17.0	10/01/1999 – 09/30/2000
CMS 16.0	10/01/1998 – 09/30/1999
CMS 15.0	10/01/1997 – 09/30/1998
CMS 14.0	10/01/1996 – 09/30/1997
CMS 13.0	10/01/1995 – 09/30/1996
CMS 12.0	10/01/1994 – 09/30/1995
CMS 11.0	10/01/1993 – 09/30/1994
CMS 10.0	10/01/1992 – 09/30/1993
CMS 9.0	10/01/1991 – 09/30/1992
CMS 8.0	10/01/1990 – 09/30/1991
CMS 7.0	10/01/1989 – 09/30/1990
CMS 6.0	10/01/1988 – 09/30/1989
CMS 5.0	10/01/1987 – 09/30/1988
CMS 4.0	10/01/1986 – 09/30/1987
CMS 3.0	05/01/1986 – 09/30/1986
CMS 2.0	10/01/1983 – 04/30/1986

Complications and Comorbidities

CMS developed lists of MCC and CC conditions for assignment of hospital cases to appropriate MS-DRGs. When a CC or MCC is present as a secondary diagnosis, it may affect DRG assignment.

The MCC/CC lists are updated annually and can be found in Tables 6I and 6J at http://www.cms.gov/Medicare/Medicare-Fee-for-Service-Payment/AcuteInpatientPPS/FY2014-IPPS-Final-Rule-Home-Page.html.

For certain principal diagnoses, conditions generally considered CCs are not seen as such because a closely related condition deemed a CC would result in duplicative or inconsistent coding. The following parameters determine those secondary diagnoses that are excluded from the CC list:

- Chronic and acute manifestations of the same condition should not be considered CCs for one another.
- Specific and nonspecific diagnosis codes for the same condition should not be considered CCs for one another.
- Conditions that may not coexist such as partial/total, unilateral/bilateral, obstructed/unobstructed, and benign/malignant should not be considered CCs for one another.
- The same condition in anatomically proximal sites should not be considered CCs for one another.
- Closely related conditions should not be considered CCs for one another.

Some conditions are an MCC only if the patient is discharged alive.

Certain MCC/CCs that are considered preventable conditions acquired during the hospital stay, identified as Hospital Acquired Conditions (HAC), with a Present on Admission indicator of "N" and "U" will effect MS-DRG payment. Medicare will not assign the higher paying MS-DRG if the HAC was not present on admission (NPOA) and will be paid as though it was not present. The HAC list can be found at: http://www.cms.gov/Medicare/Medicare-Fee-for-Service-Payment/HospitalAcqCond/Hospital-Acquired_Conditions.html.

Long Term Acute Care Hospital Prospective Payment System (LTCH PPS)

Use of postacute care services has grown rapidly since the implementation of the acute care hospital inpatient prospective payment system. The average length of stay in acute care hospitals has decreased, and patients are increasingly being discharged to postacute care settings such as long term care hospitals (LTCH), skilled nursing facilities (SNF), home health agencies (HHA), and inpatient rehabilitation facilities (IRF) to complete their course of treatment. The increased use of postacute care providers, including hospitals excluded from the acute care hospital inpatient PPS, has resulted in the rapid growth in Medicare payments to these hospitals in recent years.

Under the provisions of the Balanced Budget Refinement Act of 1999 and the Medicare, Medicaid, and SCHIP Benefits Improvement and Protection Act of 2000, over a five-year period LTCHs were transitioned from a blend of reasonable cost-based reimbursement to prospective payment rates beginning October 1, 2002. LTCHs are defined as facilities that have an average length of stay greater than 25 days.

The LTC-DRG system is based on the current DRG system under the acute care hospital inpatient PPS (MS-DRG). The LTC-DRGs model uses the existing hospital inpatient DRG classification system with weights calibrated to account for the difference in resource use by patients exhibiting the case complexity and multiple medical problems characteristic of LTCHs. The existing MS-DRGs were regrouped into classification groups based on patient data called case-mix groups (CMG).

After screening through the Medicare Code Editor, each claim is classified into the appropriate LTC-DRG by the Medicare LTCH Grouper. The LTCH Grouper is specialized computer software based on the Grouper used by the acute care hospital inpatient PPS, which was developed as a means of classifying each case into a DRG on the basis of diagnosis and procedure codes and other demographic information (age and discharge status). Following the LTC-DRG assignment, the Medicare fiscal intermediary determines the prospective payment by using the Medicare Pricer program, which accounts for hospital-specific adjustments.

CMS modified the DRGs for the LTCH PPS by developing LTCH-specific relative weights to account for the fact that LTCHs generally treat patients with multiple medical problems. Therefore, CMS developed a crosswalk of IPPS MS-DRGs to MS-LTC-DRG data, including relative weight (RW), GMLOS, and 5/6 GMLOS for short stay outlier case payment adjustment.

The MS-LTC-DRG is linked to the recalibration and reclassification of the MS-DRGs under the IPPS to be effective with discharges occurring on or after October 1 through September 30 each year.

Appendix C of this manual is the MS-LTC-DRG crosswalk based upon the Grouper Version 31.0.

Keys to a Financially Successful DRG Program

CMS assigns each DRG a relative weight based upon charge data for all Medicare inpatient hospital discharges. Each hospital has a customized base rate that adjusts payment commensurate with the hospital's cost of providing services. The type of hospital and the wage index for the geographic area determines the hospital base rate. DRG relative weights and hospital base rates are adjusted yearly (effective October 1 through September 30) to reflect changes in health care resource consumption as well as economic factors. Payment is determined by multiplying the DRG relative weight by the hospital base rate. The DRG with the highest relative weight is the highest-paying DRG. Regardless of actual costs incurred, the hospital receives only the calculated payment.

The DRG payment system is based on averages. Payment is determined by the resource needs of the average Medicare patient for a given set of diseases or disorders. These resources include the length of stay and the number and intensity of services provided. Therefore, the more efficiently a provider delivers care, the greater the operating margin will be.

The keys to a financially successful DRG program are:

- Decreased length of stay
- Decreased resource utilization (tests and procedures)
- Increased intensity of case-management services resulting in optimal length of stay for the patient and facility
- Increased preadmission testing
- Improved medical record documentation

The Physician's Role

Proper DRG assignment requires a complete and thorough accounting of the following:

- Principal diagnosis
- Procedures
- Complications
- Comorbidities (all relevant pre-existing conditions)
- Signs and symptoms when diagnoses are not established
- Discharge status

Because DRG assignment is based on documentation in the medical record, the record should:

- Be comprehensive and complete
- Include all diagnoses, procedures, complications, and comorbidities, as well as abnormal test results documented by the physician. It should also include any suspected conditions and what was done to investigate or evaluate them.
- Be timely

All dictation, signatures, etc., should be completed in the medical record as patient care is provided and must be:

- Legible
- Well documented

The information should be documented properly. With complete information in the medical record, coders can effectively analyze, code, and report the required information. This ensures that proper payment is received. For example, if the physician documents that a patient with a skull fracture was in a coma for less than one hour, DRGs 085–087 may be assigned. If the physician documents that the coma lasted for more than one hour, DRGs 082–084 may be assigned, with a resulting payment difference.

Physicians must be actively involved in the query process. They should respond to a query in a timely fashion and document their response, as established by the process, to ensure it meets regulatory requirements and is maintained in some form on the permanent medical record.

DRG Expert Organization

Summary of Changes
As a special feature, a summary of all the important changes in the DRG system for the current year is presented in this section.

Numeric DRG Listing
This section is a numeric listing of all DRGs with MDC, and page reference.

DRG Listing by Major Diagnostic Category
The "MDC List" section is a numerical listing of the MDCs with the category title. Each MDC then is separated into a surgical DRG list and medical DRG list for the MDC. Also, the page reference for each DRG is noted.

Introduction
The introduction addresses the basic characteristics of DRG classification, a brief overview of the DRG assignment process inclusive of complications and comorbidities, Long Term Acute Care Hospital Prospective Payment System, keys to a financially successful DRG program, and the physician's role in proper DRG assignment.

Glossary of DRG Terms
This section of the introduction contains definitions of terms associated with the DRG classification system.

Definitions of the DRGs
The book contains a list of the 25 MDCs. Preceding each MDC is a list of all ICD-9-CM diagnosis codes that are assigned to each MDC. They are listed in numeric order, beginning with MDC 1. Please note that there are no diagnosis codes for the Pre-MDC DRGs, since they are grouped according to procedure code. Each MDC is divided into surgical and medical sections (when appropriate). Listed in each section are the applicable DRGs and their associated diagnosis and/or procedure codes. Beside each DRG title is its GMLOS, AMLOS, and RW. Under each DRG is a list of diagnosis and/or procedure codes that determine assignment of the case to that DRG.

Indexes
Your *DRG Expert* allows you to locate a DRG by searching alphabetically (code narrative) or numerically (ICD-9-CM codes) by either disease or procedure.

The indexes are arranged in the following order at the back of the book:

- Alphabetic Index to Diseases
- Numeric Index to Diseases
- Alphabetic Index to Procedures
- Numeric Index to Procedures

Appendix A, Lists of CCs and MCCs
CMS conducted a review of over 13,500 diagnosis codes to determine which codes should be classified as CCs as part of their process to develop MS-DRGs. CMS then did an additional analysis to further refine secondary diagnoses into what will now be known as Major CCs (MCCs). The lists in this section represent diagnosis codes designated as CCs and MCCs under the MS-DRGs.

Appendix B, MS-DRG Surgical Hierarchy Table
Since patients may be assigned to only one DRG per admission, a tool was necessary to enable the evaluation of the relative resource consumption for cases involving multiple surgeries that individually group to different surgical DRGs within an MDC. The surgical hierarchy table in this section reflects the relative resource requirements of the various surgical procedures of each MDC. Arranging the surgical DRGs in this manner helps you assign the DRG that accurately reflects the resource utilization for multiple surgery cases and, thereby, assign the case to the highest surgical DRG.

Appendix C, MS-LTC-DRG Crosswalk
CMS modified the DRGs for the LTCH PPS by developing LTCH-specific relative weights to account for the fact that LTCHs generally treat patients with multiple medical problems. Therefore, CMS developed a crosswalk of IPPS MS-DRG to MS-LTC-DRG data, including RW, GMLOS, and short stay outlier thresholds. Appendix C of this manual is the MS-LTC-DRG crosswalk based upon the Grouper Version 31.0.

Appendix D, National Average Payment Table
This section lists all DRGs in numerical order. Each DRG is listed with the DRG title, the symbol ⊤ indicating that the DRG was selected as a qualified discharge that may be paid as a transfer case, the symbol 𝖲𝖯 indicating that the DRG is subject to the special payment methodology, the GMLOS, the ALMOS, the relative weight, and the average national payment.

CMS established a postacute care transfer policy effective October 1, 1998. The purpose of the IPPS postacute care transfer payment policy is to avoid providing an incentive for a hospital to transfer patients to another hospital early in the patients' stay in order to minimize costs while still receiving the full DRG payment. The transfer policy adjusts the payments to approximate the reduced costs of transfer cases. CMS adopted new criteria to expand the postacute care transfer policy beginning with the FY 2006 IPPS. The new criteria to determine which DRGs should be included are as follows:

- The DRG has at least 2,050 postacute care transfer cases;
- At least 5.5 percent of the cases in the DRG are discharged to postacute care prior to the geometric mean length of stay for the DRG;
- The DRG has a geometric mean length of stay of at least 3.0 days; and,
- If the DRG is one of a paired set of DRGs based on the presence or absence of a comorbidity or complication, both paired DRGs are included if either one meets the first three criteria.

If a DRG is included on the list of Post-Acute Transfer or Special Payment DRGs and has one of the following discharge disposition (patient status) codes assigned, it is subject to the reimbursement policy:

02	Discharged/Transferred to a Short-Term General Hospital for Inpatient Care (both participating and non-participating hospitals are included in the transfer policy)
03	Discharged/Transferred to SNF with Medicare Certification in Anticipation of Covered Skilled Care
05	Discharged/Transferred to a Designated Cancer Center or Children's Hospital
06	Discharged/Transferred to Home Under Care of Organized Home Health Service Organization in Anticipation of Covered Skilled Care

07   Left against medical advice

62   Discharged/Transferred to an Inpatient Rehabilitation Facility (IRF) Including Rehabilitation Distinct Part Units of a Hospital

63   Discharged/Transferred to a Medicare Certified Long-term Care Hospital

65   Discharged/Transferred to a Psychiatric Hospital or Psychiatric Distinct Part Unit of a Hospital

66   Discharged/Transferred to a Critical Access Hospital

CMS conformed the previous postacute care transfer policy to the new MS-DRGs. Consistent with policy under which both DRGs in a CC/non CC pair are qualifying DRGs if one of the pair qualifies, each MS-DRG that shares a base MS-DRG will be a qualifying DRG if one of the MS-DRGs in the subgroup qualifies.

The same rationale will apply to MS-DRGs subject to special payment methodology. An MS-DRG will be subject to the special payment methodology if it shares a base MS-DRG with an MS-DRG that meets criteria for receiving the special payment methodology.

This section identifies the MS-DRGs that meet the postacute care transfer criteria and the MS-DRGs that meet the special payment criteria.

The national average payment for each DRG is calculated by multiplying the current RW of the DRG and national average hospital Medicare base rate. The national average hospital Medicare base rate is the sum of the full update labor-related and nonlabor-related amounts published in the *Federal Register*, FY 2014 Final Rule, Table 1A. National Adjusted Operating Standardized Amounts; Labor/Nonlabor (if wage index greater than 1) or Table 1B. National Adjusted Operating Standardized Amounts; Labor/Nonlabor (if wage index less than or equal to 1).

Appendix E, 2012 MedPAR National Data Table

The MedPAR Benchmarking Data represents Inpatient Medicare 2012 MedPAR benchmarking data designed to provide a high-level benchmark of discharges, length of stay, age, total charges, and total reimbursement on a DRG basis at a national level for hospitals. In order to provide data in the format presented, the data from the MedPAR dataset requires manipulation. Listed below is a definition of each data element as well as other terms used in the section. Any required calculations used to derive calculated amounts are also described below.

Weighted Average - Aggregated results for the selected peer group are reported as weighted averages. To calculate a weighted average for the peer group amounts, we multiply the volume by the individual item to get the hospital's total. For example, if a hospital had 100 cases of DRG 127 with an average charge of $10,000, we'd multiply 100 times $10,000 to get $1,000,000. We then sum these amounts (charge, cost, length of stay etc) for all of the hospitals in the peer group. Next, we divide those sums by the total number of admissions for that DRG. This produces a weighted average result for the group.

Average Length of Stay - The sum of all days reported by a hospital or peer group for a DRG divided by the number of times the DRG was reported. Peer groups are weighted averages.

Charge Per Admit - The average charge for all times the service was supplied by the facility. Average charge is the sum of all charges for the reported DRG divided by the number of discharges for that DRG.

Discharges - The total number of times this DRG was reported by the provider. Because of privacy rules, no information is shown where a provider or peer group's volume is less than 11 cases. When this happens, all corresponding fields will be blank and the case mix index will be shown as a 0. Note: Some reports use the term "admissions" to identify the number of patients receiving care under a specific DRG. This report uses the term discharges, which can be used interchangeably with the term admissions.

Average Allowed - The average amount allowed for the claim from all sources. The average allowed is the sum of the outlier payments, disproportionate share, indirect medical education, capital total, copayments and deductibles and bill total per diem.

Average Age - The average age is calculated using the Census Bureau's Middle Population Projection Series to assign specific ages to claims based on the age range reported and the weighted distribution within the range for that population group. In total, the age ranges will match the distribution reported by the Census Bureau. These assigned ages are then averaged by DRG and by severity to produce the average age in the report.

Appendix F, Medicare Case Mix Index Table

The Medicare Case Mix Index (CMI) is a ratio calculated from publicly available data from the 2014 Medicare IPPS Impact File using acute care hospitals where CMI > 0.0. The formula to calculate this ratio is as follows, add all the Medicare relative weights and then divide that number by the total number of Medicare discharges. The CMI data is important benchmark information that allows organizations to set goals based on best practices in the industry. It is an indicator that shows the increase or decrease in severity to Medicare patients at a facility. It can also reflect issues with documentation and proper code assignment. If the documentation is not as comprehensive as it should be it is difficult to assign a code at the greatest level of specificity, determine the principal diagnosis or primary procedure, and identify secondary conditions that may have impact on the proper DRG assignment therefore impacting reimbursement. Also included is average daily census and average daily beds.

For questions or additional information specific to Appendixes E and F contact,

Jan Welsh, Data Analytics
Optum
1.800.859.2447, option 2, or
614.410.7637.

Instructions for Using *DRG Expert*

If the DRG is known, use the "Numeric DRG Listing." The DRGs are numerically ordered in this section. Locate the designated DRG and check the DRG title, the MDC into which the DRG falls, and the reference page number. Turn to the referenced page for a complete list of codes that group to the DRG, as well as the reimbursement data for the DRG. Scan the list for codes with an asterisk (*). The asterisk indicates a sequence or range of codes, and all codes within that code category or subcategory are represented. See an ICD-9-CM code book for specific codes.

If the MDC to which the case groups is known but the specific DRG is not, use the "DRG Listed by Major Diagnostic Category" to locate potential DRG selections. Find the MDC, determine whether the case is surgical or medical, scan the DRG and title list, and then turn to the referenced page for further information.

If the DRG is not known, follow the steps below to determine DRG assignment:

1. Determine whether the case had an operating room procedure (certain operating room procedures do not qualify and do not appear in this book). If so, refer to either the alphabetic or numeric procedure index to locate all potential DRG assignments.

   Look for the specific code or search by main term with qualifier, then body site and qualifier. Main terms are listed as specific operative procedures.

   Example:

   57.85 Cystourethroplasty and plastic repair of bladder neck

   Use the main term "Operation" when the procedure is unspecified.

   Example:

   07.5* Operations on pineal gland

   To locate a diagnostic procedure, look for the specific code under "Diagnostic procedure," and the body site, in that order.

   Example:

   67.1* Diagnostic procedures on cervix

   Note: An asterisk denotes an incomplete code that represents a sequence or range of codes. Refer to the ICD-9-CM code book for the specific codes.

2. If the case lacks an operating room procedure, look up the diagnosis by using either the alphabetic or numeric diagnosis index.

   To locate a diagnosis, look for the specific code or the condition, qualifier, then body site and qualifier, in that order.

   Example:

   805* Fracture of vertebral column without mention of spinal cord injury

3. In some cases it is necessary to scan the list of codes in the index for both the category code (three-digit code) and the subcategory (four-digit code) level of the code, listed in the index with an asterisk. Note the pages referenced for the DRG to which the category code and the subcategory code ranges are assigned. Turn to the page or pages and review the DRG descriptions to determine the correct DRG to assign to the case.

   Example:

   In the index, code 263.0 Malnutrition, degree, moderate, directs the coder to DRG 791 Prematurity with Major Problems. Code 263.0 is listed as a secondary diagnosis of major problem. However, this DRG assignment is appropriate only for newborns and other neonates. The category level, 263*, refers the coder to DRGs 640 Miscellaneous Disorders of Nutrition, Metabolism, and Fluids and Electrolytes with MCC, and to DRG 977 HIV With or Without Other Related Condition. The coder must make the final determination of the correct DRG assignment using these DRG choices.

4. Turn to the page(s) and review the DRG descriptions. Determine which is the correct DRG.

   Often a diagnosis or procedure code is assigned to more than one DRG. Not every DRG entry has a full list of the codes that group to the particular DRG, but refers to a DRG entry that does contain the full list. As in the example above for 263* Other and unspecified protein-calorie malnutrition, the index refers the coder to DRG 640 Miscellaneous Disorders of Nutrition, Metabolism, and Fluids and Electrolytes with MCC. However, DRG 640 and 641 are considered DRGs in a subgroup. The only difference in the assignment of either of the DRGs is the presence or absence of an MCC. In the guidebook a note appears under DRG 641 that says "Select principal diagnosis listed under DRG 640." That means that code 263* groups to

DRGs 640 & 641 depending on the presence or absence of an MCC. Be careful to examine all possible potential DRG assignments when the DRG title includes qualifiers such as "with MCC" versus "without MCC," "with CC" versus "without CC," and "with CC/MCC" versus "without CC/MCC." These qualifiers are highlighted in the title as an alert to the coder.

Also note those codes listed with an asterisk (*). The asterisk indicates a sequence or range of codes, and all codes within that code category or subcategory are represented. See an ICD-9-CM code book for specific codes.

5. Examine the medical record closely for the following considerations: the patient's principal diagnosis, secondary diagnoses, which include complication/comorbidities; surgical or other invasive procedures; sex of the patient and discharge status; and birth weight for neonates. Documentation must support selection of the final DRG.

6. Know and follow the Official Coding Guidelines for Coding and Reporting. The rules for selection of principal diagnosis are essential in DRG assignment, especially those related to admission to inpatient status from outpatient observation and outpatient ambulatory surgery

Important Protocols of *DRG Expert*

More than one DRG: Many diagnosis and procedure codes group to more than one DRG. Be sure to check every DRG referenced.

Asterisks: Some codes are followed by an asterisk, which indicates that the ICD-9-CM code is incomplete and represents a sequence or range of codes. Refer to the ICD-9-CM code book for the specific codes included in the code range.

A complete DRG title is necessary to understand the nature of the cases the DRG comprises.

Example:

DRG 698   Other Kidney and Urinary Tract Diagnoses with MCC

DRG 699   Other Kidney and Urinary Tract Diagnoses with CC

DRG 700   Other Kidney and Urinary Tract Diagnoses without CC/MCC

A complete review of the DRG title is necessary to understand that correct DRG assignment depends on two factors — the presence/absence of a MCC and/or CC and patient disposition. Review DRGs that precede or follow the target DRG, and determine how their narrative descriptions differ. It is possible another DRG with a higher relative weight may be assigned appropriately.

The symbol ● indicates a new MS-DRG.

The symbol ▲ indicates a revised MS-DRG title.

The symbol ⊺ indicates a DRG selected as a qualified discharge that may be paid as a transfer case.

The symbol ▤ indicates a DRG that is subject to the special payment methodology.

The symbol ▽ indicates that the DRG is one of the targeted subgroups of DRGs identified as a DRG having the potential for "upcoding" or "DRG creep." These DRGs should be considered as probable targets of an audit. The symbol reminds the coder to carefully consider the documentation that supports the DRG assignment.

The symbol ☑ indicates that there is the potential for assigning a more appropriate, higher-paying DRG. The coder should review the medical documentation to identify all the major factors that might justify assigning the case to a higher-paying DRG.

A **red color bar** indicates a surgical DRG.

A **blue color bar** indicates a medical DRG.

A **pink color bar** indicates an MCC.

A **gray color bar** indicates a CC.

A **yellow color bar** indicates a procedure proxy, whereby the inclusion of a specific procedure code acts as a proxy for the MCC or CC for the case. If the procedure code is assigned, the MCC or CC code typically required would not be necessary for DRG grouping.

The terms principal or secondary diagnosis indicates DRGs that are based on specific principal or secondary diagnosis requirements.

Bold text **OR, AND, WITH,** and **WITHOUT** alerts the user to those complex DRGs that have additional diagnosis or procedure qualifications.

SURGICAL

DRG 001 **Heart Transplant or Implant of Heart Assist System with MCC**

GMLOS 28.3 AMLOS 35.9 RW 25.3518

Operating Room Procedures
33.6 Combined heart-lung transplantation
37.51 Heart transplantation
37.52 Implantation of total internal biventricular heart replacement system
37.66 Insertion of implantable heart assist system
OR
37.60 Implantation or insertion of biventricular external heart assist system
OR
37.63 Repair of heart assist system
OR
37.65 Implant of single ventricular (extracorporeal) external heart assist system
AND
37.64 Removal of external heart assist system(s) or device(s)

DRG 002 **Heart Transplant or Implant of Heart Assist System without MCC**

GMLOS 15.9 AMLOS 18.6 RW 15.2738 ☑

Select operating room procedure OR any procedure combinations listed under DRG 001

DRG 003 **ECMO or Tracheostomy with Mechanical Ventilation 96+ Hours or Principal Diagnosis Except Face, Mouth and Neck with Major O.R.**

GMLOS 27.2 AMLOS 33.2 RW 17.6369 ⊺

Operating Room Procedure
39.65 Extracorporeal membrane oxygenation (ECMO)
OR

Nonoperating Room Procedure
31.1 Temporary tracheostomy
OR

Operating Room Procedures
31.21 Mediastinal tracheostomy
31.29 Other permanent tracheostomy
AND EITHER

Principal Diagnosis

Any diagnosis EXCEPT mouth, larynx and pharynx disorders listed under DRG 011
OR

Nonoperating Room Procedure
96.72 Continuous invasive mechanical ventilation for 96 consecutive hours or more

WITH

Operating Room Procedures

Any O.R. procedure not listed in DRGs 984-989

DRG 004 **Tracheostomy with Mechanical Ventilation 96+ Hours or Principal Diagnosis Except Face, Mouth and Neck without Major O.R.**

GMLOS 20.3 AMLOS 24.7 RW 10.9288 ☑⊺

Nonoperating Room Procedure
31.1 Temporary tracheostomy
OR

Operating Room Procedures
31.21 Mediastinal tracheostomy
31.29 Other permanent tracheostomy
AND EITHER

Principal Diagnosis

Any diagnosis EXCEPT mouth, larynx and pharynx disorders listed under DRG 011
OR

Nonoperating Room Procedure
96.72 Continuous invasive mechanical ventilation for 96 consecutive hours or more

DRG 005 **Liver Transplant with MCC or Intestinal Transplant**

GMLOS 15.1 AMLOS 20.1 RW 10.4214

Operating Room Procedures
46.97 Transplant of intestine
50.51 Auxiliary liver transplant
50.59 Other transplant of liver

DRG 006 **Liver Transplant without MCC**

GMLOS 7.9 AMLOS 9.0 RW 4.7639 ☑

Operating Room Procedures
50.51 Auxiliary liver transplant
50.59 Other transplant of liver

DRG 007 **Lung Transplant**

GMLOS 15.4 AMLOS 17.9 RW 9.1929 ☑

Operating Room Procedures
33.5* Lung transplant

DRG 008 **Simultaneous Pancreas/Kidney Transplant**

GMLOS 9.5 AMLOS 11.0 RW 5.1527

Principal or Secondary Diagnosis
249* Secondary diabetes mellitus
250.0* Diabetes mellitus without mention of complication
250.1* Diabetes with ketoacidosis
250.2* Diabetes with hyperosmolarity
250.3* Diabetes with other coma
250.4* Diabetes with renal manifestations
250.5* Diabetes with ophthalmic manifestations
250.6* Diabetes with neurological manifestations
250.7* Diabetes with peripheral circulatory disorders
250.8* Diabetes with other specified manifestations

| 250.9* | Diabetes with unspecified complication |
| 251.3 | Postsurgical hypoinsulinemia |

AND

Principal or Secondary Diagnosis

403.01	Hypertensive chronic kidney disease, malignant, with chronic kidney disease stage V or end stage renal disease
403.11	Hypertensive chronic kidney disease, benign, with chronic kidney disease stage V or end stage renal disease
403.91	Hypertensive chronic kidney disease, unspecified, with chronic kidney disease stage V or end stage renal disease
404.02	Hypertensive heart and chronic kidney disease, malignant, without heart failure and with chronic kidney disease stage V or end stage renal disease
404.03	Hypertensive heart and chronic kidney disease, malignant, with heart failure and with chronic kidney disease stage V or end stage renal disease
404.12	Hypertensive heart and chronic kidney disease, benign, without heart failure and with chronic kidney disease stage V or end stage renal disease
404.13	Hypertensive heart and chronic kidney disease, benign, with heart failure and chronic kidney disease stage V or end stage renal disease
404.92	Hypertensive heart and chronic kidney disease, unspecified, without heart failure and with chronic kidney disease stage V or end stage renal disease
404.93	Hypertensive heart and chronic kidney disease, unspecified, with heart failure and chronic kidney disease stage V or end stage renal disease
585*	Chronic kidney disease (CKD)
V42.0	Kidney replaced by transplant
V43.89	Other organ or tissue replaced by other means

AND

Any of the following procedure combinations

| 52.80 | Pancreatic transplant, not otherwise specified |

AND

| 55.69 | Other kidney transplantation |

OR

| 52.82 | Homotransplant of pancreas |

AND

| 55.69 | Other kidney transplantation |

DRG 009   Bone Marrow Transplant
GMLOS 0.0   AMLOS 0.0   RW 0.0000

Omitted in October 2011 grouper version

DRG 010   Pancreas Transplant
GMLOS 8.8   AMLOS 10.3   RW 4.1554   ☑

Principal or Secondary Diagnosis

249*	Secondary diabetes mellitus
250.0*	Diabetes mellitus without mention of complication
250.1*	Diabetes with ketoacidosis
250.2*	Diabetes with hyperosmolarity
250.3*	Diabetes with other coma
250.4*	Diabetes with renal manifestations
250.5*	Diabetes with ophthalmic manifestations
250.6*	Diabetes with neurological manifestations
250.7*	Diabetes with peripheral circulatory disorders
250.8*	Diabetes with other specified manifestations
250.9*	Diabetes with unspecified complication
251.3	Postsurgical hypoinsulinemia

AND

Operating Room Procedures

| 52.80 | Pancreatic transplant, not otherwise specified |
| 52.82 | Homotransplant of pancreas |

DRG 011   Tracheostomy for Face, Mouth, and Neck Diagnoses with MCC
GMLOS 11.4   AMLOS 14.0   RW 4.7246   ☑

Operating Room Procedures

| 30.3 | Complete laryngectomy |
| 30.4 | Radical laryngectomy |

OR

Principal Diagnosis

012.3*	Tuberculous laryngitis
032.0	Faucial diphtheria
032.1	Nasopharyngeal diphtheria
032.2	Anterior nasal diphtheria
032.3	Laryngeal diphtheria
034.0	Streptococcal sore throat
054.2	Herpetic gingivostomatitis
074.0	Herpangina
098.6	Gonococcal infection of pharynx
099.51	Chlamydia trachomatis infection of pharynx
101	Vincent's angina
102.5	Gangosa due to yaws
112.0	Candidiasis of mouth
140*	Malignant neoplasm of lip
141*	Malignant neoplasm of tongue
142*	Malignant neoplasm of major salivary glands
143*	Malignant neoplasm of gum
144*	Malignant neoplasm of floor of mouth
145*	Malignant neoplasm of other and unspecified parts of mouth
146*	Malignant neoplasm of oropharynx
147*	Malignant neoplasm of nasopharynx
148*	Malignant neoplasm of hypopharynx
149*	Malignant neoplasm of other and ill-defined sites within the lip, oral cavity, and pharynx
160*	Malignant neoplasm of nasal cavities, middle ear, and accessory sinuses
161*	Malignant neoplasm of larynx
165.0	Malignant neoplasm of upper respiratory tract, part unspecified
170.1	Malignant neoplasm of mandible
173.0*	Other and unspecified malignant neoplasm of skin of lip
176.2	Kaposi's sarcoma of palate
193	Malignant neoplasm of thyroid gland
195.0	Malignant neoplasm of head, face, and neck
196.0	Secondary and unspecified malignant neoplasm of lymph nodes of head, face, and neck
200.01	Reticulosarcoma of lymph nodes of head, face, and neck
200.11	Lymphosarcoma of lymph nodes of head, face, and neck
200.21	Burkitt's tumor or lymphoma of lymph nodes of head, face, and neck
200.81	Other named variants of lymphosarcoma and reticulosarcoma of lymph nodes of head, face, and neck
201.01	Hodgkin's paragranuloma of lymph nodes of head, face, and neck
201.11	Hodgkin's granuloma of lymph nodes of head, face, and neck
201.21	Hodgkin's sarcoma of lymph nodes of head, face, and neck
201.41	Hodgkin's disease, lymphocytic-histiocytic predominance of lymph nodes of head, face, and neck
201.51	Hodgkin's disease, nodular sclerosis, of lymph nodes of head, face, and neck
201.61	Hodgkin's disease, mixed cellularity, involving lymph nodes of head, face, and neck
201.71	Hodgkin's disease, lymphocytic depletion, of lymph nodes of head, face, and neck
201.91	Hodgkin's disease, unspecified type, of lymph nodes of head, face, and neck
202.01	Nodular lymphoma of lymph nodes of head, face, and neck
202.11	Mycosis fungoides of lymph nodes of head, face, and neck

Pre MDC—SURGICAL *(side tab)*

202.21	Sezary's disease of lymph nodes of head, face, and neck
202.31	Malignant histiocytosis of lymph nodes of head, face, and neck
202.41	Leukemic reticuloendotheliosis of lymph nodes of head, face, and neck
202.51	Letterer-Siwe disease of lymph nodes of head, face, and neck
202.61	Malignant mast cell tumors of lymph nodes of head, face, and neck
202.81	Other malignant lymphomas of lymph nodes of head, face, and neck
202.91	Other and unspecified malignant neoplasms of lymphoid and histiocytic tissue of lymph nodes of head, face, and neck
210*	Benign neoplasm of lip, oral cavity, and pharynx
212.0	Benign neoplasm of nasal cavities, middle ear, and accessory sinuses
212.1	Benign neoplasm of larynx
213.0	Benign neoplasm of bones of skull and face
213.1	Benign neoplasm of lower jaw bone
226	Benign neoplasm of thyroid glands
228.00	Hemangioma of unspecified site
228.01	Hemangioma of skin and subcutaneous tissue
228.09	Hemangioma of other sites
230.0	Carcinoma in situ of lip, oral cavity, and pharynx
231.0	Carcinoma in situ of larynx
235.0	Neoplasm of uncertain behavior of major salivary glands
235.1	Neoplasm of uncertain behavior of lip, oral cavity, and pharynx
235.6	Neoplasm of uncertain behavior of larynx
242*	Thyrotoxicosis with or without goiter
245*	Thyroiditis
246.2	Cyst of thyroid
246.3	Hemorrhage and infarction of thyroid
246.8	Other specified disorders of thyroid
246.9	Unspecified disorder of thyroid
327.2*	Organic sleep apnea
327.3*	Circadian rhythm sleep disorder
327.4*	Organic parasomnia
327.5*	Organic sleep related movement disorders
327.8	Other organic sleep disorders
460	Acute nasopharyngitis (common cold)
462	Acute pharyngitis
463	Acute tonsillitis
464.00	Acute laryngitis, without mention of obstruction
464.01	Acute laryngitis, with obstruction
464.2*	Acute laryngotracheitis
464.3*	Acute epiglottitis
464.4	Croup
464.50	Unspecified supraglottis, without mention of obstruction
464.51	Unspecified supraglottis, with obstruction
465*	Acute upper respiratory infections of multiple or unspecified sites
470	Deviated nasal septum
472.1	Chronic pharyngitis
472.2	Chronic nasopharyngitis
474*	Chronic disease of tonsils and adenoids
475	Peritonsillar abscess
476.0	Chronic laryngitis
476.1	Chronic laryngotracheitis
478.2*	Other diseases of pharynx, not elsewhere classified
478.3*	Paralysis of vocal cords or larynx
478.4	Polyp of vocal cord or larynx
478.5	Other diseases of vocal cords
478.6	Edema of larynx
478.7*	Other diseases of larynx, not elsewhere classified
478.8	Upper respiratory tract hypersensitivity reaction, site unspecified
478.9	Other and unspecified diseases of upper respiratory tract
519.0*	Tracheostomy complications
519.11	Acute bronchospasm
519.19	Other diseases of trachea and bronchus
520*	Disorders of tooth development and eruption
521*	Diseases of hard tissues of teeth
522*	Diseases of pulp and periapical tissues
523*	Gingival and periodontal diseases
524*	Dentofacial anomalies, including malocclusion
525*	Other diseases and conditions of the teeth and supporting structures
526*	Diseases of the jaws
527*	Diseases of the salivary glands
528*	Diseases of the oral soft tissues, excluding lesions specific for gingiva and tongue
529*	Diseases and other conditions of the tongue
682.0	Cellulitis and abscess of face
682.1	Cellulitis and abscess of neck
748.2	Congenital web of larynx
748.3	Other congenital anomaly of larynx, trachea, and bronchus
749.0*	Cleft palate
749.1*	Cleft lip
749.2*	Cleft palate with cleft lip
750.0	Tongue tie
750.1*	Other congenital anomalies of tongue
750.21	Congenital absence of salivary gland
750.22	Congenital accessory salivary gland
750.23	Congenital atresia, salivary duct
750.24	Congenital fistula of salivary gland
750.25	Congenital fistula of lip
750.26	Other specified congenital anomalies of mouth
750.27	Congenital diverticulum of pharynx
750.29	Other specified congenital anomaly of pharynx
780.51	Insomnia with sleep apnea, unspecified
780.53	Hypersomnia with sleep apnea, unspecified
780.57	Unspecified sleep apnea
784.8	Hemorrhage from throat
784.92	Jaw pain
802.2*	Mandible, closed fracture
802.3*	Mandible, open fracture
802.4	Malar and maxillary bones, closed fracture
802.5	Malar and maxillary bones, open fracture
802.6	Orbital floor (blow-out), closed fracture
802.7	Orbital floor (blow-out), open fracture
802.8	Other facial bones, closed fracture
802.9	Other facial bones, open fracture
807.5	Closed fracture of larynx and trachea
807.6	Open fracture of larynx and trachea
830*	Dislocation of jaw
873.2*	Open wound of nose, without mention of complication
873.3*	Open wound of nose, complicated
873.40	Open wound of face, unspecified site, without mention of complication
873.41	Open wound of cheek, without mention of complication
873.43	Open wound of lip, without mention of complication
873.44	Open wound of jaw, without mention of complication
873.50	Open wound of face, unspecified site, complicated
873.51	Open wound of cheek, complicated
873.53	Open wound of lip, complicated
873.54	Open wound of jaw, complicated
873.60	Open wound of mouth, unspecified site, without mention of complication
873.61	Open wound of buccal mucosa, without mention of complication
873.62	Open wound of gum (alveolar process), without mention of complication
873.64	Open wound of tongue and floor of mouth, without mention of complication
873.65	Open wound of palate, without mention of complication
873.69	Open wound of mouth, other and multiple sites, without mention of complication
873.70	Open wound of mouth, unspecified site, complicated
873.71	Open wound of buccal mucosa, complicated

Pre MDC—SURGICAL

Surgical	Medical	CC Indicator	MCC Indicator	Procedure Proxy

873.72	Open wound of gum (alveolar process), complicated
873.74	Open wound of tongue and floor of mouth, complicated
873.75	Open wound of palate, complicated
873.79	Open wound of mouth, other and multiple sites, complicated
874.00	Open wound of larynx with trachea, without mention of complication
874.01	Open wound of larynx, without mention of complication
874.02	Open wound of trachea, without mention of complication
874.10	Open wound of larynx with trachea, complicated
874.11	Open wound of larynx, complicated
874.12	Open wound of trachea, complicated
874.2	Open wound of thyroid gland, without mention of complication
874.3	Open wound of thyroid gland, complicated
874.4	Open wound of pharynx, without mention of complication
874.5	Open wound of pharynx, complicated
874.8	Open wound of other and unspecified parts of neck, without mention of complication
874.9	Open wound of other and unspecified parts of neck, complicated
900.82	Injury to multiple blood vessels of head and neck
900.89	Injury to other specified blood vessels of head and neck
900.9	Injury to unspecified blood vessel of head and neck
925*	Crushing injury of face, scalp, and neck
933*	Foreign body in pharynx and larynx
935.0	Foreign body in mouth
947.0	Burn of mouth and pharynx
959.0*	Injury, other and unspecified, head, face, and neck
V10.01	Personal history of malignant neoplasm of tongue
V10.02	Personal history of malignant neoplasm of other and unspecified parts of oral cavity and pharynx
V10.21	Personal history of malignant neoplasm of larynx

AND EITHER

Nonoperating Room Procedure

31.1	Temporary tracheostomy

OR

Operating Room Procedures

31.21	Mediastinal tracheostomy
31.29	Other permanent tracheostomy

DRG 012 Tracheostomy for Face, Mouth, and Neck Diagnoses with CC
GMLOS 8.3   AMLOS 9.8   RW 3.2291   ☑

Select principal diagnosis and operating and nonoperating room procedures listed under DRG 011

DRG 013 Tracheostomy for Face, Mouth, and Neck Diagnoses without CC/MCC
GMLOS 5.7   AMLOS 6.5   RW 2.1647   ☑

Select principal diagnosis and operating and nonoperating room procedures listed under DRG 011

DRG 014 Allogeneic Bone Marrow Transplant
GMLOS 20.7   AMLOS 26.2   RW 10.6157

Operating Room Procedures

41.02	Allogeneic bone marrow transplant with purging
41.03	Allogeneic bone marrow transplant without purging
41.05	Allogeneic hematopoietic stem cell transplant without purging
41.06	Cord blood stem cell transplant
41.08	Allogeneic hematopoietic stem cell transplant with purging

DRG 015 Autologous Bone Marrow Transplant
GMLOS 0.0   AMLOS 0.0   RW 0.0000

Omitted in October 2012 grouper version

DRG 016 Autologous Bone Marrow Transplant with CC/MCC
GMLOS 18.1   AMLOS 19.5   RW 6.0304   ☑

Operating Room Procedures

41.00	Bone marrow transplant, not otherwise specified
41.01	Autologous bone marrow transplant without purging
41.04	Autologous hematopoietic stem cell transplant without purging
41.07	Autologous hematopoietic stem cell transplant with purging
41.09	Autologous bone marrow transplant with purging

DRG 017 Autologous Bone Marrow Transplant without CC/MCC
GMLOS 9.9   AMLOS 13.2   RW 4.2906   ☑

Operating Room Procedures

41.00	Bone marrow transplant, not otherwise specified
41.01	Autologous bone marrow transplant without purging
41.04	Autologous hematopoietic stem cell transplant without purging
41.07	Autologous hematopoietic stem cell transplant with purging
41.09	Autologous bone marrow transplant with purging

Pre MDC—SURGICAL

Ⓣ *Transfer DRG*   ⓈⓅ *Special Payment*   ☑ *Optimization Potential*   ▽ *Targeted Potential*   * *Code Range*   ● *New DRG*   ▲ *Revised DRG Title*

Diseases And Disorders Of The Nervous System

003.21	045.02	090.42	249.61	327.52	337.00	344.02	346.82	355.71
006.5	045.03	090.49	250.60	330.0	337.01	344.03	346.83	355.79
013.00	045.10	091.81	250.61	330.1	337.09	344.04	346.90	355.8
013.01	045.11	094.0	250.62	330.2	337.1	344.09	346.91	355.9
013.02	045.12	094.1	250.63	330.3	337.20	344.1	346.92	356.0
013.03	045.13	094.2	307.20	330.8	337.21	344.2	346.93	356.1
013.04	045.90	094.3	307.21	330.9	337.22	344.30	347.00	356.2
013.05	045.91	094.81	307.22	331.0	337.29	344.31	347.01	356.3
013.06	045.92	094.82	307.23	331.11	337.3	344.32	347.10	356.4
013.10	045.93	094.85	307.81	331.19	337.9	344.40	347.11	356.8
013.11	046.0	094.87	310.2	331.2	338.0	344.41	348.0	356.9
013.12	046.11	094.89	310.81	331.3	338.21	344.42	348.1	357.0
013.13	046.19	094.9	310.89	331.4	338.22	344.5	348.2	357.1
013.14	046.2	098.82	315.35	331.5	338.28	344.60	348.30	357.2
013.15	046.3	100.81	320.0	331.6	338.29	344.81	348.31	357.3
013.16	046.71	100.89	320.1	331.7	338.4	344.89	348.39	357.4
013.20	046.72	112.83	320.2	331.81	339.00	344.9	348.4	357.5
013.21	046.79	114.2	320.3	331.82	339.01	345.00	348.5	357.6
013.22	046.8	115.01	320.7	331.83	339.02	345.01	348.81	357.7
013.23	046.9	115.11	320.81	331.89	339.03	345.10	348.82	357.81
013.24	047.0	115.91	320.82	331.9	339.04	345.11	348.89	357.82
013.25	047.1	130.0	320.89	332.0	339.05	345.2	348.9	357.89
013.26	047.8	137.1	320.9	332.1	339.09	345.3	349.0	357.9
013.30	047.9	138	321.0	333.0	339.10	345.40	349.1	358.00
013.31	048	139.0	321.1	333.1	339.11	345.41	349.2	358.01
013.32	049.0	191.0	321.2	333.2	339.12	345.50	349.81	358.1
013.33	049.1	191.1	321.3	333.3	339.20	345.51	349.82	358.2
013.34	049.8	191.2	321.4	333.4	339.21	345.60	349.89	358.30
013.35	049.9	191.3	321.8	333.5	339.22	345.61	349.9	358.31
013.36	052.0	191.4	322.0	333.6	339.3	345.70	350.1	358.39
013.40	052.2	191.5	322.1	333.71	339.41	345.71	350.2	358.8
013.41	053.0	191.6	322.2	333.72	339.42	345.80	350.8	358.9
013.42	053.10	191.7	322.9	333.79	339.43	345.81	350.9	359.0
013.43	053.11	191.8	323.01	333.82	339.44	345.90	351.0	359.1
013.44	053.12	191.9	323.02	333.83	339.81	345.91	351.1	359.21
013.45	053.13	192.0	323.1	333.84	339.82	346.00	351.8	359.22
013.46	053.14	192.1	323.2	333.85	339.83	346.01	351.9	359.23
013.50	053.19	192.2	323.41	333.89	339.84	346.02	352.0	359.24
013.51	054.3	192.3	323.42	333.90	339.85	346.03	352.1	359.29
013.52	054.72	192.8	323.51	333.91	339.89	346.10	352.2	359.3
013.53	054.74	192.9	323.52	333.92	340	346.11	352.3	359.4
013.54	055.0	194.4	323.61	333.93	341.0	346.12	352.4	359.5
013.55	056.00	194.5	323.62	333.94	341.1	346.13	352.5	359.6
013.56	056.01	194.6	323.63	333.99	341.20	346.20	352.6	359.81
013.60	056.09	198.3	323.71	334.0	341.21	346.21	352.9	359.89
013.61	058.21	198.4	323.72	334.1	341.22	346.22	353.0	359.9
013.62	058.29	225.0	323.81	334.2	341.8	346.23	353.1	377.00
013.63	062.0	225.1	323.82	334.3	341.9	346.30	353.2	377.01
013.64	062.1	225.2	323.9	334.4	342.00	346.31	353.3	377.04
013.65	062.2	225.3	324.0	334.8	342.01	346.32	353.4	377.51
013.66	062.3	225.4	324.1	334.9	342.02	346.33	353.5	377.52
013.80	062.4	225.8	324.9	335.0	342.10	346.40	353.6	377.53
013.81	062.5	225.9	325	335.10	342.11	346.41	353.8	377.54
013.82	062.8	227.4	326	335.11	342.12	346.42	353.9	377.61
013.83	062.9	227.5	327.21	335.19	342.80	346.43	354.0	377.62
013.84	063.0	227.6	327.25	335.20	342.81	346.50	354.1	377.63
013.85	063.1	228.02	327.27	335.21	342.82	346.51	354.2	377.71
013.86	063.2	237.1	327.30	335.22	342.90	346.52	354.3	377.72
013.90	063.8	237.3	327.31	335.23	342.91	346.53	354.4	377.73
013.91	063.9	237.5	327.32	335.24	342.92	346.60	354.5	377.75
013.92	064	237.6	327.33	335.29	343.0	346.61	354.8	377.9
013.93	066.2	237.70	327.34	335.8	343.1	346.62	354.9	378.86
013.94	071	237.71	327.35	335.9	343.2	346.63	355.0	379.45
013.95	072.1	237.72	327.36	336.0	343.3	346.70	355.1	388.61
013.96	072.2	237.73	327.37	336.1	343.4	346.71	355.2	430
036.0	072.72	237.79	327.39	336.2	343.8	346.72	355.3	431
036.1	078.81	237.9	327.41	336.3	343.9	346.73	355.4	432.0
045.00	090.40	239.6	327.43	336.8	344.00	346.80	355.5	432.1
045.01	090.41	249.60	327.51	336.9	344.01	346.81	355.6	432.9

433.00	740.2	800.16	801.10	803.02	803.94	804.86	851.04	851.96
433.01	741.00	800.19	801.11	803.03	803.95	804.89	851.05	851.99
433.10	741.01	800.20	801.12	803.04	803.96	804.90	851.06	852.00
433.11	741.02	800.21	801.13	803.05	803.99	804.91	851.09	852.01
433.20	741.03	800.22	801.14	803.06	804.00	804.92	851.10	852.02
433.21	741.90	800.23	801.15	803.09	804.01	804.93	851.11	852.03
433.30	741.91	800.24	801.16	803.10	804.02	804.94	851.12	852.04
433.31	741.92	800.25	801.19	803.11	804.03	804.95	851.13	852.05
433.80	741.93	800.26	801.20	803.12	804.04	804.96	851.14	852.06
433.81	742.0	800.29	801.21	803.13	804.05	804.99	851.15	852.09
433.90	742.1	800.30	801.22	803.14	804.06	806.00	851.16	852.10
433.91	742.2	800.31	801.23	803.15	804.09	806.01	851.19	852.11
434.00	742.3	800.32	801.24	803.16	804.10	806.02	851.20	852.12
434.01	742.4	800.33	801.25	803.19	804.11	806.03	851.21	852.13
434.10	742.51	800.34	801.26	803.20	804.12	806.04	851.22	852.14
434.11	742.53	800.35	801.29	803.21	804.13	806.05	851.23	-852.15
434.90	742.59	800.36	801.30	803.22	804.14	806.06	851.24	852.16
434.91	742.8	800.39	801.31	803.23	804.15	806.07	851.25	852.19
435.0	742.9	800.40	801.32	803.24	804.16	806.08	851.26	852.20
435.1	747.81	800.41	801.33	803.25	804.19	806.09	851.29	852.21
435.2	747.82	800.42	801.34	803.26	804.20	806.10	851.30	852.22
435.3	756.17	800.43	801.35	803.29	804.21	806.11	851.31	852.23
435.8	759.5	800.44	801.36	803.30	804.22	806.12	851.32	852.24
435.9	779.7	800.45	801.39	803.31	804.23	806.13	851.33	852.25
436	780.01	800.46	801.40	803.32	804.24	806.14	851.34	852.26
437.0	780.03	800.49	801.41	803.33	804.25	806.15	851.35	852.29
437.1	780.09	800.50	801.42	803.34	804.26	806.16	851.36	852.30
437.2	780.31	800.51	801.43	803.35	804.29	806.17	851.39	852.31
437.3	780.32	800.52	801.44	803.36	804.30	806.18	851.40	852.32
437.4	780.33	800.53	801.45	803.39	804.31	806.19	851.41	852.33
437.5	780.39	800.54	801.46	803.40	804.32	806.20	851.42	852.34
437.6	780.72	800.55	801.49	803.41	804.33	806.21	851.43	852.35
437.7	781.0	800.56	801.50	803.42	804.34	806.22	851.44	852.36
437.8	781.1	800.59	801.51	803.43	804.35	806.23	851.45	852.39
437.9	781.2	800.60	801.52	803.44	804.36	806.24	851.46	852.40
438.0	781.3	800.61	801.53	803.45	804.39	806.25	851.49	852.41
438.10	781.4	800.62	801.54	803.46	804.40	806.26	851.50	852.42
438.11	781.6	800.63	801.55	803.49	804.41	806.27	851.51	852.43
438.12	781.8	800.64	801.56	803.50	804.42	806.28	851.52	852.44
438.13	781.91	800.65	801.59	803.51	804.43	806.29	851.53	852.45
438.14	781.92	800.66	801.60	803.52	804.44	806.30	851.54	852.49
438.19	781.94	800.69	801.61	803.53	804.45	806.31	851.55	852.50
438.20	781.99	800.70	801.62	803.54	804.46	806.32	851.56	852.51
438.21	782.0	800.71	801.63	803.55	804.49	806.33	851.59	852.52
438.22	784.0	800.72	801.64	803.56	804.50	806.34	851.60	852.53
438.30	784.3	800.73	801.65	803.59	804.51	806.35	851.61	852.54
438.31	784.51	800.74	801.66	803.60	804.52	806.36	851.62	852.55
438.32	784.52	800.75	801.69	803.61	804.53	806.37	851.63	852.56
438.40	784.59	800.76	801.70	803.62	804.54	806.38	851.64	852.59
438.41	792.0	800.79	801.71	803.63	804.55	806.39	851.65	853.00
438.42	793.0	800.80	801.72	803.64	804.56	806.4	851.66	853.01
438.50	794.00	800.81	801.73	803.65	804.59	806.5	851.69	853.02
438.51	794.01	800.82	801.74	803.66	804.60	806.60	851.70	853.03
438.52	794.02	800.83	801.75	803.69	804.61	806.61	851.71	853.04
438.53	794.09	800.84	801.76	803.70	804.62	806.62	851.72	853.05
438.6	794.10	800.85	801.79	803.71	804.63	806.69	851.73	853.06
438.7	794.19	800.86	801.80	803.72	804.64	806.70	851.74	853.09
438.81	796.1	800.89	801.81	803.73	804.65	806.71	851.75	853.10
438.82	798.0	800.90	801.82	803.74	804.66	806.72	851.76	853.11
438.83	799.53	800.91	801.83	803.75	804.69	806.79	851.79	853.12
438.84	800.00	800.92	801.84	803.76	804.70	806.8	851.80	853.13
438.85	800.01	800.93	801.85	803.79	804.71	806.9	851.81	853.14
438.89	800.02	800.94	801.86	803.80	804.72	850.0	851.82	853.15
438.9	800.03	800.95	801.89	803.81	804.73	850.11	851.83	853.16
723.2	800.04	800.96	801.90	803.82	804.74	850.12	851.84	853.19
723.3	800.05	800.99	801.91	803.83	804.75	850.2	851.85	854.00
723.4	800.06	801.00	801.92	803.84	804.76	850.3	851.86	854.01
729.2	800.09	801.01	801.93	803.85	804.79	850.4	851.89	854.02
736.05	800.10	801.02	801.94	803.86	804.80	850.5	851.90	854.03
736.06	800.11	801.03	801.95	803.89	804.81	850.9	851.91	854.04
736.07	800.12	801.04	801.96	803.90	804.82	851.00	851.92	854.05
736.74	800.13	801.05	801.99	803.91	804.83	851.01	851.93	854.06
740.0	800.14	801.06	803.00	803.92	804.84	851.02	851.94	854.09
740.1	800.15	801.09	803.01	803.93	804.85	851.03	851.95	

854.10	907.2	951.2	952.04	952.15	953.1	955.0	956.1	996.2
854.11	907.3	951.3	952.05	952.16	953.2	955.1	956.2	996.63
854.12	907.4	951.4	952.06	952.17	953.3	955.2	956.3	996.75
854.13	907.5	951.6	952.07	952.18	953.4	955.3	956.4	997.00
854.14	907.9	951.7	952.08	952.19	953.5	955.4	956.5	997.01
854.15	950.1	951.8	952.09	952.2	953.8	955.5	956.8	997.02
854.16	950.2	951.9	952.10	952.3	953.9	955.6	956.9	997.09
854.19	950.3	952.00	952.11	952.4	954.0	955.7	957.0	V53.01
905.0	950.9	952.01	952.12	952.8	954.1	955.8	957.1	V53.02
907.0	951.0	952.02	952.13	952.9	954.8	955.9	957.8	V53.09
907.1	951.1	952.03	952.14	953.0	954.9	956.0	957.9	

SURGICAL

DRG 020	**Intracranial Vascular Procedures with Principal Diagnosis of Hemorrhage with MCC**	
	GMLOS 14.3 AMLOS 17.4 RW 9.3897	

Principal Diagnosis
094.87	Syphilitic ruptured cerebral aneurysm
430	Subarachnoid hemorrhage
431	Intracerebral hemorrhage
432*	Other and unspecified intracranial hemorrhage

Operating Room Procedures
02.13	Ligation of meningeal vessel
38.01	Incision of intracranial vessels
38.11	Endarterectomy of intracranial vessels
38.31	Resection of intracranial vessels with anastomosis
38.41	Resection of intracranial vessels with replacement
38.51	Ligation and stripping of varicose veins of intracranial vessels
38.61	Other excision of intracranial vessels
38.81	Other surgical occlusion of intracranial vessels
39.28	Extracranial-intracranial (EC-IC) vascular bypass
39.51	Clipping of aneurysm
39.52	Other repair of aneurysm
39.53	Repair of arteriovenous fistula
39.72	Endovascular (total) embolization or occlusion of head and neck vessels
39.75	Endovascular embolization or occlusion of vessel(s) of head or neck using bare coils
39.76	Endovascular embolization or occlusion of vessel(s) of head or neck using bioactive coils
39.79	Other endovascular procedures on other vessels

DRG 021	**Intracranial Vascular Procedures with Principal Diagnosis of Hemorrhage with CC**	
	GMLOS 11.9 AMLOS 13.4 RW 6.4458	☑

Select principal diagnosis and operating room procedures listed under DRG 020

DRG 022	**Intracranial Vascular Procedures with Principal Diagnosis of Hemorrhage without CC/MCC**	
	GMLOS 5.5 AMLOS 7.3 RW 4.7113	☑

Select principal diagnosis and operating room procedures listed under DRG 020

DRG 023	**Craniotomy with Major Device Implant/Acute Complex Central Nervous System Principal Diagnosis with MCC or Chemo Implant**	
	GMLOS 8.0 AMLOS 11.2 RW 5.1587	T

Operating Room Procedures
00.62	Percutaneous angioplasty of intracranial vessel(s)
01.12	Open biopsy of cerebral meninges
01.14	Open biopsy of brain
01.15	Biopsy of skull
01.18	Other diagnostic procedures on brain and cerebral meninges
01.19	Other diagnostic procedures on skull
01.21	Incision and drainage of cranial sinus
01.22	Removal of intracranial neurostimulator lead(s)
01.23	Reopening of craniotomy site
01.24	Other craniotomy
01.25	Other craniectomy
01.28	Placement of intracerebral catheter(s) via burr hole(s)
01.31	Incision of cerebral meninges

01.32	Lobotomy and tractotomy
01.39	Other incision of brain
01.41	Operations on thalamus
01.42	Operations on globus pallidus
01.51	Excision of lesion or tissue of cerebral meninges
01.52	Hemispherectomy
01.53	Lobectomy of brain
01.59	Other excision or destruction of lesion or tissue of brain
01.6	Excision of lesion of skull
02.0*	Cranioplasty
02.1*	Repair of cerebral meninges
02.2*	Ventriculostomy
02.91	Lysis of cortical adhesions
02.92	Repair of brain
02.93	Implantation or replacement of intracranial neurostimulator lead(s)
02.94	Insertion or replacement of skull tongs or halo traction device
02.99	Other operations on skull, brain, and cerebral meninges
04.01	Excision of acoustic neuroma
04.41	Decompression of trigeminal nerve root
07.13	Biopsy of pituitary gland, transfrontal approach
07.14	Biopsy of pituitary gland, transsphenoidal approach
07.15	Biopsy of pituitary gland, unspecified approach
07.17	Biopsy of pineal gland
07.5*	Operations on pineal gland
07.6*	Hypophysectomy
07.7*	Other operations on hypophysis
17.54	Percutaneous atherectomy of intracranial vessel(s)
17.61	Laser interstitial thermal therapy [LITT] of lesion or tissue of brain under guidance
29.92	Division of glossopharyngeal nerve
38.01	Incision of intracranial vessels
38.11	Endarterectomy of intracranial vessels
38.31	Resection of intracranial vessels with anastomosis
38.41	Resection of intracranial vessels with replacement
38.51	Ligation and stripping of varicose veins of intracranial vessels
38.61	Other excision of intracranial vessels
38.81	Other surgical occlusion of intracranial vessels
39.28	Extracranial-intracranial (EC-IC) vascular bypass
39.51	Clipping of aneurysm
39.52	Other repair of aneurysm
39.53	Repair of arteriovenous fistula
39.72	Endovascular (total) embolization or occlusion of head and neck vessels
39.74	Endovascular removal of obstruction from head and neck vessel(s)
39.75	Endovascular embolization or occlusion of vessel(s) of head or neck using bare coils
39.76	Endovascular embolization or occlusion of vessel(s) of head or neck using bioactive coils
39.79	Other endovascular procedures on other vessels
AND	

Any of the following

Acute Complex CNS Principal Diagnosis
003.21	Salmonella meningitis
006.5	Amebic brain abscess
013*	Tuberculosis of meninges and central nervous system
036.0	Meningococcal meningitis
036.1	Meningococcal encephalitis
045.0*	Acute paralytic poliomyelitis specified as bulbar
045.1*	Acute poliomyelitis with other paralysis
045.9*	Acute unspecified poliomyelitis
052.2	Postvaricella myelitis
053.14	Herpes zoster myelitis
054.3	Herpetic meningoencephalitis
054.72	Herpes simplex meningitis
054.74	Herpes simplex myelitis

T *Transfer DRG*   SP *Special Payment*   ☑ *Optimization Potential*   ᵀᴾᵍ *Targeted Potential*   * *Code Range*   ● *New DRG*   ▲ *Revised DRG Title*

055.0	Postmeasles encephalitis
058.21	Human herpesvirus 6 encephalitis
058.29	Other human herpesvirus encephalitis
062*	Mosquito-borne viral encephalitis
063*	Tick-borne viral encephalitis
064	Viral encephalitis transmitted by other and unspecified arthropods
066.2	Venezuelan equine fever
071	Rabies
072.1	Mumps meningitis
072.2	Mumps encephalitis
091.81	Early syphilis, acute syphilitic meningitis (secondary)
094.2	Syphilitic meningitis
094.81	Syphilitic encephalitis
098.82	Gonococcal meningitis
100.8*	Other specified leptospiral infections
112.83	Candidal meningitis
114.2	Coccidioidal meningitis
115.01	Histoplasma capsulatum meningitis
115.11	Histoplasma duboisii meningitis
115.91	Unspecified Histoplasmosis meningitis
130.0	Meningoencephalitis due to toxoplasmosis
320*	Bacterial meningitis
321.0	Cryptococcal meningitis
321.1	Meningitis in other fungal diseases
321.2	Meningitis due to viruses not elsewhere classified
321.3	Meningitis due to trypanosomiasis
323.0*	Encephalitis, myelitis, and encephalomyelitis in viral diseases classified elsewhere
323.1	Encephalitis, myelitis, and encephalomyelitis in rickettsial diseases classified elsewhere
323.2	Encephalitis, myelitis, and encephalomyelitis in protozoal diseases classified elsewhere
323.4*	Other encephalitis, myelitis, and encephalomyelitis due to other infections classified elsewhere
323.5*	Encephalitis, myelitis, and encephalomyelitis following immunization procedures
323.6*	Postinfectious encephalitis, myelitis, and encephalomyelitis
323.7*	Toxic encephalitis, myelitis, and encephalomyelitis
323.8*	Other causes of encephalitis, myelitis, and encephalomyelitis
323.9	Unspecified causes of encephalitis, myelitis, and encephalomyelitis
324*	Intracranial and intraspinal abscess
325	Phlebitis and thrombophlebitis of intracranial venous sinuses
341.2*	Acute (transverse) myelitis
430	Subarachnoid hemorrhage
431	Intracerebral hemorrhage
432.9	Unspecified intracranial hemorrhage
433.01	Occlusion and stenosis of basilar artery with cerebral infarction
433.11	Occlusion and stenosis of carotid artery with cerebral infarction
433.21	Occlusion and stenosis of vertebral artery with cerebral infarction
433.31	Occlusion and stenosis of multiple and bilateral precerebral arteries with cerebral infarction
433.81	Occlusion and stenosis of other specified precerebral artery with cerebral infarction
433.91	Occlusion and stenosis of unspecified precerebral artery with cerebral infarction
434.01	Cerebral thrombosis with cerebral infarction
434.11	Cerebral embolism with cerebral infarction
434.91	Unspecified cerebral artery occlusion with cerebral infarction
851.1*	Cortex (cerebral) contusion with open intracranial wound
851.2*	Cortex (cerebral) laceration without mention of open intracranial wound
851.3*	Cortex (cerebral) laceration with open intracranial wound

851.5*	Cerebellar or brain stem contusion with open intracranial wound
851.6*	Cerebellar or brain stem laceration without mention of open intracranial wound
851.7*	Cerebellar or brain stem laceration with open intracranial wound
851.8*	Other and unspecified cerebral laceration and contusion, without mention of open intracranial wound
851.9*	Other and unspecified cerebral laceration and contusion, with open intracranial wound
852.0*	Subarachnoid hemorrhage following injury without mention of open intracranial wound
852.1*	Subarachnoid hemorrhage following injury, with open intracranial wound
852.3*	Subdural hemorrhage following injury, with open intracranial wound
853.0*	Other and unspecified intracranial hemorrhage following injury, without mention of open intracranial wound
853.1*	Other and unspecified intracranial hemorrhage following injury with open intracranial wound
854.1*	Intracranial injury of other and unspecified nature with open intracranial wound

OR

The following procedure combination

02.93	Implantation or replacement of intracranial neurostimulator lead(s)
	AND
01.20	Cranial implantation or replacement of neurostimulator pulse generator

OR

02.93	Implantation or replacement of intracranial neurostimulator lead(s)
	AND
86.95	Insertion or replacement of multiple array neurostimulator pulse generator, not specified as rechargeable

OR

02.93	Implantation or replacement of intracranial neurostimulator lead(s)
	AND
86.98	Insertion or replacement of multiple array (two or more) rechargeable neurostimulator pulse generator

OR

Nonoperating Room Procedure

00.10	Implantation of chemotherapeutic agent

DRG 024　Craniotomy with Major Device Implant/Acute Complex Central Nervous System Principal Diagnosis without MCC

GMLOS 4.5　　　　AMLOS 6.6　　　　RW 3.7121　　☑Ⓣ

Operating Room Procedures

00.62	Percutaneous angioplasty of intracranial vessel(s)
01.12	Open biopsy of cerebral meninges
01.14	Open biopsy of brain
01.15	Biopsy of skull
01.18	Other diagnostic procedures on brain and cerebral meninges
01.19	Other diagnostic procedures on skull
01.21	Incision and drainage of cranial sinus
01.22	Removal of intracranial neurostimulator lead(s)
01.23	Reopening of craniotomy site
01.24	Other craniotomy
01.25	Other craniectomy
01.28	Placement of intracerebral catheter(s) via burr hole(s)
01.31	Incision of cerebral meninges
01.32	Lobotomy and tractotomy
01.39	Other incision of brain
01.41	Operations on thalamus

01.42	Operations on globus pallidus	062*	Mosquito-borne viral encephalitis
01.51	Excision of lesion or tissue of cerebral meninges	063*	Tick-borne viral encephalitis
01.52	Hemispherectomy	064	Viral encephalitis transmitted by other and unspecified arthropods
01.53	Lobectomy of brain	066.2	Venezuelan equine fever
01.59	Other excision or destruction of lesion or tissue of brain	071	Rabies
01.6	Excision of lesion of skull	072.1	Mumps meningitis
02.0*	Cranioplasty	072.2	Mumps encephalitis
02.1*	Repair of cerebral meninges	091.81	Early syphilis, acute syphilitic meningitis (secondary)
02.2*	Ventriculostomy	094.2	Syphilitic meningitis
02.91	Lysis of cortical adhesions	094.81	Syphilitic encephalitis
02.92	Repair of brain	098.82	Gonococcal meningitis
02.93	Implantation or replacement of intracranial neurostimulator lead(s)	100.8*	Other specified leptospiral infections
02.94	Insertion or replacement of skull tongs or halo traction device	112.83	Candidal meningitis
		114.2	Coccidioidal meningitis
02.99	Other operations on skull, brain, and cerebral meninges	115.01	Histoplasma capsulatum meningitis
04.01	Excision of acoustic neuroma	115.11	Histoplasma duboisii meningitis
04.41	Decompression of trigeminal nerve root	115.91	Unspecified Histoplasmosis meningitis
07.13	Biopsy of pituitary gland, transfrontal approach	130.0	Meningoencephalitis due to toxoplasmosis
07.14	Biopsy of pituitary gland, transsphenoidal approach	320*	Bacterial meningitis
07.15	Biopsy of pituitary gland, unspecified approach	321.0	Cryptococcal meningitis
07.17	Biopsy of pineal gland	321.1	Meningitis in other fungal diseases
07.5*	Operations on pineal gland	321.2	Meningitis due to viruses not elsewhere classified
07.6*	Hypophysectomy	321.3	Meningitis due to trypanosomiasis
07.7*	Other operations on hypophysis	323.01	Encephalitis and encephalomyelitis in viral diseases classified elsewhere
17.54	Percutaneous atherectomy of intracranial vessel(s)	323.02	Myelitis in viral diseases classified elsewhere
17.61	Laser interstitial thermal therapy [LITT] of lesion or tissue of brain under guidance	323.1	Encephalitis, myelitis, and encephalomyelitis in rickettsial diseases classified elsewhere
29.92	Division of glossopharyngeal nerve	323.2	Encephalitis, myelitis, and encephalomyelitis in protozoal diseases classified elsewhere
38.01	Incision of intracranial vessels		
38.11	Endarterectomy of intracranial vessels	323.41	Other encephalitis and encephalomyelitis due to other infections classified elsewhere
38.31	Resection of intracranial vessels with anastomosis	323.42	Other myelitis due to other infections classified elsewhere
38.41	Resection of intracranial vessels with replacement	323.51	Encephalitis and encephalomyelitis following immunization procedures
38.51	Ligation and stripping of varicose veins of intracranial vessels	323.52	Myelitis following immunization procedures
38.61	Other excision of intracranial vessels	323.61	Infectious acute disseminated encephalomyelitis [ADEM]
38.81	Other surgical occlusion of intracranial vessels	323.62	Other postinfectious encephalitis and encephalomyelitis
39.28	Extracranial-intracranial (EC-IC) vascular bypass	323.63	Postinfectious myelitis
39.51	Clipping of aneurysm	323.71	Toxic encephalitis and encephalomyelitis
39.52	Other repair of aneurysm	323.72	Toxic myelitis
39.53	Repair of arteriovenous fistula	323.81	Other causes of encephalitis and encephalomyelitis
39.72	Endovascular (total) embolization or occlusion of head and neck vessels	323.82	Other causes of myelitis
39.74	Endovascular removal of obstruction from head and neck vessel(s)	323.9	Unspecified causes of encephalitis, myelitis, and encephalomyelitis
39.75	Endovascular embolization or occlusion of vessel(s) of head or neck using bare coils	324*	Intracranial and intraspinal abscess
		325	Phlebitis and thrombophlebitis of intracranial venous sinuses
39.76	Endovascular embolization or occlusion of vessel(s) of head or neck using bioactive coils	341.20	Acute (transverse) myelitis NOS
39.79	Other endovascular procedures on other vessels	341.21	Acute (transverse) myelitis in conditions classified elsewhere
		341.22	Idiopathic transverse myelitis

AND

Any of the following

Acute Complex CNS Principal Diagnosis

003.21	Salmonella meningitis	430	Subarachnoid hemorrhage
006.5	Amebic brain abscess	431	Intracerebral hemorrhage
013*	Tuberculosis of meninges and central nervous system	432.9	Unspecified intracranial hemorrhage
036.0	Meningococcal meningitis	433.01	Occlusion and stenosis of basilar artery with cerebral infarction
036.1	Meningococcal encephalitis	433.11	Occlusion and stenosis of carotid artery with cerebral infarction
045.0*	Acute paralytic poliomyelitis specified as bulbar		
045.1*	Acute poliomyelitis with other paralysis	433.21	Occlusion and stenosis of vertebral artery with cerebral infarction
045.9*	Acute unspecified poliomyelitis	433.31	Occlusion and stenosis of multiple and bilateral precerebral arteries with cerebral infarction
052.2	Postvaricella myelitis		
053.14	Herpes zoster myelitis	433.81	Occlusion and stenosis of other specified precerebral artery with cerebral infarction
054.3	Herpetic meningoencephalitis		
054.72	Herpes simplex meningitis	433.91	Occlusion and stenosis of unspecified precerebral artery with cerebral infarction
054.74	Herpes simplex myelitis		
055.0	Postmeasles encephalitis	434.01	Cerebral thrombosis with cerebral infarction
058.21	Human herpesvirus 6 encephalitis	434.11	Cerebral embolism with cerebral infarction
058.29	Other human herpesvirus encephalitis		

Ⓣ Transfer DRG   ⓢⓟ Special Payment   ☑ Optimization Potential   ▽TGT Targeted Potential   * Code Range   ● New DRG   ▲ Revised DRG Title

10   Valid 10/01/2013-09/30/2014   © 2013 OptumInsight, Inc.

434.91	Unspecified cerebral artery occlusion with cerebral infarction
851.1*	Cortex (cerebral) contusion with open intracranial wound
851.2*	Cortex (cerebral) laceration without mention of open intracranial wound
851.3*	Cortex (cerebral) laceration with open intracranial wound
851.5*	Cerebellar or brain stem contusion with open intracranial wound
851.6*	Cerebellar or brain stem laceration without mention of open intracranial wound
851.7*	Cerebellar or brain stem laceration with open intracranial wound
851.8*	Other and unspecified cerebral laceration and contusion, without mention of open intracranial wound
851.9*	Other and unspecified cerebral laceration and contusion, with open intracranial wound
852.0*	Subarachnoid hemorrhage following injury without mention of open intracranial wound
852.1*	Subarachnoid hemorrhage following injury, with open intracranial wound
852.3*	Subdural hemorrhage following injury, with open intracranial wound
853.0*	Other and unspecified intracranial hemorrhage following injury, without mention of open intracranial wound
853.1*	Other and unspecified intracranial hemorrhage following injury with open intracranial wound
854.1*	Intracranial injury of other and unspecified nature with open intracranial wound

OR

The following procedure combination

02.93	Implantation or replacement of intracranial neurostimulator lead(s)
	AND
01.20	Cranial implantation or replacement of neurostimulator pulse generator

OR

02.93	Implantation or replacement of intracranial neurostimulator lead(s)
	AND
86.95	Insertion or replacement of multiple array neurostimulator pulse generator, not specified as rechargeable

OR

02.93	Implantation or replacement of intracranial neurostimulator lead(s)
	AND
86.98	Insertion or replacement of multiple array (two or more) rechargeable neurostimulator pulse generator

DRG 025 Craniotomy and Endovascular Intracranial Procedures with MCC

GMLOS 7.8	AMLOS 10.1	RW 4.4422	☑ Ⓣ

Operating Room Procedures

00.62	Percutaneous angioplasty of intracranial vessel(s)
01.12	Open biopsy of cerebral meninges
01.14	Open biopsy of brain
01.15	Biopsy of skull
01.18	Other diagnostic procedures on brain and cerebral meninges
01.19	Other diagnostic procedures on skull
01.21	Incision and drainage of cranial sinus
01.22	Removal of intracranial neurostimulator lead(s)
01.23	Reopening of craniotomy site
01.24	Other craniotomy
01.25	Other craniectomy
01.28	Placement of intracerebral catheter(s) via burr hole(s)
01.31	Incision of cerebral meninges
01.32	Lobotomy and tractotomy

01.39	Other incision of brain
01.41	Operations on thalamus
01.42	Operations on globus pallidus
01.51	Excision of lesion or tissue of cerebral meninges
01.52	Hemispherectomy
01.53	Lobectomy of brain
01.59	Other excision or destruction of lesion or tissue of brain
01.6	Excision of lesion of skull
02.01	Opening of cranial suture
02.02	Elevation of skull fracture fragments
02.03	Formation of cranial bone flap
02.04	Bone graft to skull
02.05	Insertion of skull plate
02.06	Other cranial osteoplasty
02.07	Removal of skull plate
02.1*	Repair of cerebral meninges
02.2*	Ventriculostomy
02.91	Lysis of cortical adhesions
02.92	Repair of brain
02.93	Implantation or replacement of intracranial neurostimulator lead(s)
02.94	Insertion or replacement of skull tongs or halo traction device
02.99	Other operations on skull, brain, and cerebral meninges
04.01	Excision of acoustic neuroma
04.41	Decompression of trigeminal nerve root
07.13	Biopsy of pituitary gland, transfrontal approach
07.14	Biopsy of pituitary gland, transsphenoidal approach
07.15	Biopsy of pituitary gland, unspecified approach
07.17	Biopsy of pineal gland
07.5*	Operations on pineal gland
07.6*	Hypophysectomy
07.7*	Other operations on hypophysis
17.54	Percutaneous atherectomy of intracranial vessel(s)
17.61	Laser interstitial thermal therapy [LITT] of lesion or tissue of brain under guidance
29.92	Division of glossopharyngeal nerve
38.01	Incision of intracranial vessels
38.11	Endarterectomy of intracranial vessels
38.31	Resection of intracranial vessels with anastomosis
38.41	Resection of intracranial vessels with replacement
38.51	Ligation and stripping of varicose veins of intracranial vessels
38.61	Other excision of intracranial vessels
38.81	Other surgical occlusion of intracranial vessels
39.28	Extracranial-intracranial (EC-IC) vascular bypass
39.51	Clipping of aneurysm
39.52	Other repair of aneurysm
39.53	Repair of arteriovenous fistula
39.72	Endovascular (total) embolization or occlusion of head and neck vessels
39.74	Endovascular removal of obstruction from head and neck vessel(s)
39.75	Endovascular embolization or occlusion of vessel(s) of head or neck using bare coils
39.76	Endovascular embolization or occlusion of vessel(s) of head or neck using bioactive coils
39.79	Other endovascular procedures on other vessels

MDC 1: Diseases And Disorders Of The Nervous System—SURGICAL

DRG 026   Craniotomy and Endovascular Intracranial Procedures with CC

GMLOS 5.0	AMLOS 6.5	RW 2.9842	☑ T

Select operating room procedures listed under DRG 025

DRG 027   Craniotomy and Endovascular Intracranial Procedures without CC/MCC

GMLOS 2.6	AMLOS 3.4	RW 2.2505	☑ T

Select operating room procedures listed under DRG 025

DRG 028   Spinal Procedures with MCC

GMLOS 9.6	AMLOS 12.3	RW 5.4339	☑ SP

Operating Room Procedures
- 03.0*   Exploration and decompression of spinal canal structures
- 03.1   Division of intraspinal nerve root
- 03.2*   Chordotomy
- 03.32   Biopsy of spinal cord or spinal meninges
- 03.39   Other diagnostic procedures on spinal cord and spinal canal structures
- 03.4   Excision or destruction of lesion of spinal cord or spinal meninges
- 03.5*   Plastic operations on spinal cord structures
- 03.6   Lysis of adhesions of spinal cord and nerve roots
- 03.7*   Shunt of spinal theca
- 03.93   Implantation or replacement of spinal neurostimulator lead(s)
- 03.94   Removal of spinal neurostimulator lead(s)
- 03.97   Revision of spinal thecal shunt
- 03.98   Removal of spinal thecal shunt
- 03.99   Other operations on spinal cord and spinal canal structures
- 77.81   Other partial ostectomy of scapula, clavicle, and thorax (ribs and sternum)
- 77.91   Total ostectomy of scapula, clavicle, and thorax (ribs and sternum)
- 80.50   Excision or destruction of intervertebral disc, unspecified
- 80.51   Excision of intervertebral disc
- 80.53   Repair of the anulus fibrosus with graft or prosthesis
- 80.54   Other and unspecified repair of the anulus fibrosus
- 80.59   Other destruction of intervertebral disc
- 81.00   Spinal fusion, not otherwise specified
- 81.01   Atlas-axis spinal fusion
- 81.02   Other cervical fusion of the anterior column, anterior technique
- 81.03   Other cervical fusion of the posterior column, posterior technique
- 81.04   Dorsal and dorsolumbar fusion of the anterior column, anterior technique
- 81.05   Dorsal and dorsolumbar fusion of the posterior column, posterior technique
- 81.06   Lumbar and lumbosacral fusion of the anterior column, anterior technique
- 81.07   Lumbar and lumbosacral fusion of the posterior column, posterior technique
- 81.08   Lumbar and lumbosacral fusion of the anterior column, posterior technique
- 81.3*   Refusion of spine
- 84.59   Insertion of other spinal devices
- 84.6*   Replacement of spinal disc
- 84.80   Insertion or replacement of interspinous process device(s)
- 84.82   Insertion or replacement of pedicle-based dynamic stabilization device(s)
- 84.84   Insertion or replacement of facet replacement device(s)

DRG 029   Spinal Procedures with CC or Spinal Neurostimulator

GMLOS 4.6	AMLOS 6.2	RW 3.0782	☑ SP

Operating Room Procedures
- 03.0*   Exploration and decompression of spinal canal structures
- 03.1   Division of intraspinal nerve root
- 03.2*   Chordotomy
- 03.32   Biopsy of spinal cord or spinal meninges
- 03.39   Other diagnostic procedures on spinal cord and spinal canal structures
- 03.4   Excision or destruction of lesion of spinal cord or spinal meninges
- 03.5*   Plastic operations on spinal cord structures
- 03.6   Lysis of adhesions of spinal cord and nerve roots
- 03.7*   Shunt of spinal theca
- 03.93   Implantation or replacement of spinal neurostimulator lead(s)
- 03.94   Removal of spinal neurostimulator lead(s)
- 03.97   Revision of spinal thecal shunt
- 03.98   Removal of spinal thecal shunt
- 03.99   Other operations on spinal cord and spinal canal structures
- 77.81   Other partial ostectomy of scapula, clavicle, and thorax (ribs and sternum)
- 77.91   Total ostectomy of scapula, clavicle, and thorax (ribs and sternum)
- 80.50   Excision or destruction of intervertebral disc, unspecified
- 80.51   Excision of intervertebral disc
- 80.53   Repair of the anulus fibrosus with graft or prosthesis
- 80.54   Other and unspecified repair of the anulus fibrosus
- 80.59   Other destruction of intervertebral disc
- 81.00   Spinal fusion, not otherwise specified
- 81.01   Atlas-axis spinal fusion
- 81.02   Other cervical fusion of the anterior column, anterior technique
- 81.03   Other cervical fusion of the posterior column, posterior technique
- 81.04   Dorsal and dorsolumbar fusion of the anterior column, anterior technique
- 81.05   Dorsal and dorsolumbar fusion of the posterior column, posterior technique
- 81.06   Lumbar and lumbosacral fusion of the anterior column, anterior technique
- 81.07   Lumbar and lumbosacral fusion of the posterior column, posterior technique
- 81.08   Lumbar and lumbosacral fusion of the anterior column, posterior technique
- 81.3*   Refusion of spine
- 84.59   Insertion of other spinal devices
- 84.6*   Replacement of spinal disc
- 84.80   Insertion or replacement of interspinous process device(s)
- 84.82   Insertion or replacement of pedicle-based dynamic stabilization device(s)
- 84.84   Insertion or replacement of facet replacement device(s)

OR

Any of the following procedure combinations
- 03.93   Implantation or replacement of spinal neurostimulator lead(s)
  AND
- 86.94   Insertion or replacement of single array neurostimulator pulse generator, not specified as rechargeable

OR

- 03.93   Implantation or replacement of spinal neurostimulator lead(s)
  AND
- 86.95   Insertion or replacement of multiple array neurostimulator pulse generator, not specified as rechargeable

---

☑ *Transfer DRG*   SP *Special Payment*   ☑ *Optimization Potential*   ▽ *Targeted Potential*   * *Code Range*   ● *New DRG*   ▲ *Revised DRG Title*

12   Valid 10/01/2013-09/30/2014   © 2013 OptumInsight, Inc.

OR

03.93   Implantation or replacement of spinal neurostimulator lead(s)

AND

86.97   Insertion or replacement of single array rechargeable neurostimulator pulse generator

OR

03.93   Implantation or replacement of spinal neurostimulator lead(s)

AND

86.98   Insertion or replacement of multiple array (two or more) rechargeable neurostimulator pulse generator

DRG 030   Spinal Procedures without CC/MCC
GMLOS 2.5   **AMLOS 3.3**   **RW 1.8091**   ☑ 🅿

Operating Room Procedures

03.0*	Exploration and decompression of spinal canal structures
03.1	Division of intraspinal nerve root
03.2*	Chordotomy
03.32	Biopsy of spinal cord or spinal meninges
03.39	Other diagnostic procedures on spinal cord and spinal canal structures
03.4	Excision or destruction of lesion of spinal cord or spinal meninges
03.5*	Plastic operations on spinal cord structures
03.6	Lysis of adhesions of spinal cord and nerve roots
03.7*	Shunt of spinal theca
03.93	Implantation or replacement of spinal neurostimulator lead(s)
03.94	Removal of spinal neurostimulator lead(s)
03.97	Revision of spinal thecal shunt
03.98	Removal of spinal thecal shunt
03.99	Other operations on spinal cord and spinal canal structures
77.81	Other partial ostectomy of scapula, clavicle, and thorax (ribs and sternum)
77.91	Total ostectomy of scapula, clavicle, and thorax (ribs and sternum)
80.50	Excision or destruction of intervertebral disc, unspecified
80.51	Excision of intervertebral disc
80.53	Repair of the anulus fibrosus with graft or prosthesis
80.54	Other and unspecified repair of the anulus fibrosus
80.59	Other destruction of intervertebral disc
81.00	Spinal fusion, not otherwise specified
81.01	Atlas-axis spinal fusion
81.02	Other cervical fusion of the anterior column, anterior technique
81.03	Other cervical fusion of the posterior column, posterior technique
81.04	Dorsal and dorsolumbar fusion of the anterior column, anterior technique
81.05	Dorsal and dorsolumbar fusion of the posterior column, posterior technique
81.06	Lumbar and lumbosacral fusion of the anterior column, anterior technique
81.07	Lumbar and lumbosacral fusion of the posterior column, posterior technique
81.08	Lumbar and lumbosacral fusion of the anterior column, posterior technique
81.3*	Refusion of spine
84.59	Insertion of other spinal devices
84.6*	Replacement of spinal disc
84.80	Insertion or replacement of interspinous process device(s)
84.82	Insertion or replacement of pedicle-based dynamic stabilization device(s)
84.84	Insertion or replacement of facet replacement device(s)

DRG 031   Ventricular Shunt Procedures with MCC
GMLOS 7.7   **AMLOS 11.0**   **RW 3.9460**   ☑🆃

Operating Room Procedures

02.3*	Extracranial ventricular shunt
02.42	Replacement of ventricular shunt
02.43	Removal of ventricular shunt

DRG 032   Ventricular Shunt Procedures with CC
GMLOS 3.4   **AMLOS 4.9**   **RW 1.9780**   ☑🆃

Select operating room procedures listed under DRG 031

DRG 033   Ventricular Shunt Procedures without CC/MCC
GMLOS 2.0   **AMLOS 2.5**   **RW 1.5226**   ☑🆃

Select operating room procedures listed under DRG 031

DRG 034   Carotid Artery Stent Procedure with MCC
GMLOS 4.7   **AMLOS 6.9**   **RW 3.4145**

Operating Room Procedures

00.61	Percutaneous angioplasty of extracranial vessel(s)
17.53	Percutaneous atherectomy of extracranial vessel(s)

AND

Nonoperating Room Procedure

00.63	Percutaneous insertion of carotid artery stent(s)

DRG 035   Carotid Artery Stent Procedure with CC
GMLOS 2.1   **AMLOS 3.1**   **RW 2.1781**   ☑

Select operating and nonoperating room procedures listed under DRG 034

DRG 036   Carotid Artery Stent Procedure without CC/MCC
GMLOS 1.3   **AMLOS 1.5**   **RW 1.7224**   ☑

Select operating and nonoperating room procedures listed under DRG 034

DRG 037   Extracranial Procedures with MCC
GMLOS 5.5   **AMLOS 7.9**   **RW 3.0641**   ☑

Operating Room Procedures

00.61	Percutaneous angioplasty of extracranial vessel(s)
17.53	Percutaneous atherectomy of extracranial vessel(s)
17.56	Atherectomy of other non-coronary vessel(s)
38.10	Endarterectomy, unspecified site
38.12	Endarterectomy of other vessels of head and neck
38.32	Resection of other vessels of head and neck with anastomosis
38.62	Other excision of other vessels of head and neck
39.22	Aorta-subclavian-carotid bypass
39.29	Other (peripheral) vascular shunt or bypass
39.3*	Suture of vessel
39.50	Angioplasty of other non-coronary vessel(s)
39.56	Repair of blood vessel with tissue patch graft
39.57	Repair of blood vessel with synthetic patch graft
39.58	Repair of blood vessel with unspecified type of patch graft
39.59	Other repair of vessel
39.77	Temporary (partial) therapeutic endovascular occlusion of vessel
39.92	Injection of sclerosing agent into vein

Surgical   Medical   CC Indicator   MCC Indicator   Procedure Proxy

<table>
<tr><td>

DRG 038 **Extracranial Procedures with CC**
    GMLOS 2.4   AMLOS 3.5   RW 1.5958   ☑

Select operating room procedures listed under DRG 037

DRG 039 **Extracranial Procedures without CC/MCC**
    GMLOS 1.4   AMLOS 1.6   RW 1.0452   ☑

Select operating room procedures listed under DRG 037

DRG 040 **Peripheral/Cranial Nerve and Other Nervous System Procedures with MCC**
    GMLOS 8.3   AMLOS 11.0   RW 3.7851   ☑ SP

Operating Room Procedures

01.20	Cranial implantation or replacement of neurostimulator pulse generator
01.29	Removal of cranial neurostimulator pulse generator
04.02	Division of trigeminal nerve
04.03	Division or crushing of other cranial and peripheral nerves
04.04	Other incision of cranial and peripheral nerves
04.05	Gasserian ganglionectomy
04.06	Other cranial or peripheral ganglionectomy
04.07	Other excision or avulsion of cranial and peripheral nerves
04.12	Open biopsy of cranial or peripheral nerve or ganglion
04.19	Other diagnostic procedures on cranial and peripheral nerves and ganglia
04.3	Suture of cranial and peripheral nerves
04.42	Other cranial nerve decompression
04.43	Release of carpal tunnel
04.44	Release of tarsal tunnel
04.49	Other peripheral nerve or ganglion decompression or lysis of adhesions
04.5	Cranial or peripheral nerve graft
04.6	Transposition of cranial and peripheral nerves
04.7*	Other cranial or peripheral neuroplasty
04.91	Neurectasis
04.92	Implantation or replacement of peripheral neurostimulator lead(s)
04.93	Removal of peripheral neurostimulator lead(s)
04.99	Other operations on cranial and peripheral nerves
05.0	Division of sympathetic nerve or ganglion
05.1*	Diagnostic procedures on sympathetic nerves or ganglia
05.2*	Sympathectomy
05.8*	Other operations on sympathetic nerves or ganglia
05.9	Other operations on nervous system
07.19	Other diagnostic procedures on adrenal glands, pituitary gland, pineal gland, and thymus
07.8*	Thymectomy
07.95	Thoracoscopic incision of thymus
07.98	Other and unspecified thoracoscopic operations on thymus
08.5*	Other adjustment of lid position
27.62	Correction of cleft palate
27.69	Other plastic repair of palate
29.4	Plastic operation on pharynx
29.59	Other repair of pharynx
37.74	Insertion or replacement of epicardial lead (electrode) into epicardium
37.75	Revision of lead (electrode)
37.76	Replacement of transvenous atrial and/or ventricular lead(s) (electrode(s))
37.77	Removal of lead(s) (electrodes) without replacement
37.79	Revision or relocation of cardiac device pocket
37.80	Insertion of permanent pacemaker, initial or replacement, type of device not specified
37.85	Replacement of any type of pacemaker device with single-chamber device, not specified as rate responsive
37.86	Replacement of any type of pacemaker device with single-chamber device, rate responsive

</td><td>

37.87	Replacement of any type of pacemaker device with dual-chamber device
37.89	Revision or removal of pacemaker device
38.02	Incision of other vessels of head and neck
38.21	Biopsy of blood vessel
38.42	Resection of other vessels of head and neck with replacement
38.7	Interruption of the vena cava
38.82	Other surgical occlusion of other vessels of head and neck
40.11	Biopsy of lymphatic structure
44.00	Vagotomy, not otherwise specified
54.95	Incision of peritoneum
81.71	Arthroplasty of metacarpophalangeal and interphalangeal joint with implant
81.72	Arthroplasty of metacarpophalangeal and interphalangeal joint without implant
81.74	Arthroplasty of carpocarpal or carpometacarpal joint with implant
81.75	Arthroplasty of carpocarpal or carpometacarpal joint without implant
81.79	Other repair of hand, fingers, and wrist
82.5*	Transplantation of muscle and tendon of hand
82.6*	Reconstruction of thumb
82.7*	Plastic operation on hand with graft or implant
82.8*	Other plastic operations on hand
83.13	Other tenotomy
83.14	Fasciotomy
83.19	Other division of soft tissue
83.21	Open biopsy of soft tissue
83.41	Excision of tendon for graft
83.43	Excision of muscle or fascia for graft
83.45	Other myectomy
83.49	Other excision of soft tissue
83.7*	Reconstruction of muscle and tendon
83.81	Tendon graft
83.82	Graft of muscle or fascia
83.83	Tendon pulley reconstruction on muscle, tendon, and fascia
83.85	Other change in muscle or tendon length
83.87	Other plastic operations on muscle
83.88	Other plastic operations on tendon
83.89	Other plastic operations on fascia
83.92	Insertion or replacement of skeletal muscle stimulator
83.93	Removal of skeletal muscle stimulator
84.11	Amputation of toe
84.12	Amputation through foot
84.13	Disarticulation of ankle
84.14	Amputation of ankle through malleoli of tibia and fibula
84.15	Other amputation below knee
84.16	Disarticulation of knee
84.17	Amputation above knee
86.06	Insertion of totally implantable infusion pump
86.22	Excisional debridement of wound, infection, or burn
86.4	Radical excision of skin lesion
86.60	Free skin graft, not otherwise specified
86.61	Full-thickness skin graft to hand
86.62	Other skin graft to hand
86.63	Full-thickness skin graft to other sites
86.65	Heterograft to skin
86.66	Homograft to skin
86.67	Dermal regenerative graft
86.69	Other skin graft to other sites
86.70	Pedicle or flap graft, not otherwise specified
86.71	Cutting and preparation of pedicle grafts or flaps
86.72	Advancement of pedicle graft
86.74	Attachment of pedicle or flap graft to other sites
86.75	Revision of pedicle or flap graft
86.81	Repair for facial weakness
86.91	Excision of skin for graft
86.93	Insertion of tissue expander

</td></tr>
</table>

Ⓣ *Transfer DRG*   SP *Special Payment*   ☑ *Optimization Potential*   ᵀᴬᴿ *Targeted Potential*   * *Code Range*   ● *New DRG*   ▲ *Revised DRG Title*

86.94   Insertion or replacement of single array neurostimulator pulse generator, not specified as rechargeable

86.95   Insertion or replacement of multiple array neurostimulator pulse generator, not specified as rechargeable

86.96   Insertion or replacement of other neurostimulator pulse generator

86.97   Insertion or replacement of single array rechargeable neurostimulator pulse generator

86.98   Insertion or replacement of multiple array (two or more) rechargeable neurostimulator pulse generator

92.27   Implantation or insertion of radioactive elements

OR

Any of the following procedure combinations

37.70   Initial insertion of lead (electrode), not otherwise specified
AND
37.80   Insertion of permanent pacemaker, initial or replacement, type of device not specified

OR

37.70   Initial insertion of lead (electrode), not otherwise specified
AND
37.81   Initial insertion of single-chamber device, not specified as rate responsive

OR

37.70   Initial insertion of lead (electrode), not otherwise specified
AND
37.82   Initial insertion of single-chamber device, rate responsive

OR

37.70   Initial insertion of lead (electrode), not otherwise specified
AND
37.85   Replacement of any type of pacemaker device with single-chamber device, not specified as rate responsive

OR

37.70   Initial insertion of lead (electrode), not otherwise specified
AND
37.86   Replacement of any type of pacemaker device with single-chamber device, rate responsive

OR

37.70   Initial insertion of lead (electrode), not otherwise specified
AND
37.87   Replacement of any type of pacemaker device with dual-chamber device

OR

37.71   Initial insertion of transvenous lead (electrode) into ventricle
AND
37.80   Insertion of permanent pacemaker, initial or replacement, type of device not specified

OR

37.71   Initial insertion of transvenous lead (electrode) into ventricle
AND
37.81   Initial insertion of single-chamber device, not specified as rate responsive

OR

37.71   Initial insertion of transvenous lead (electrode) into ventricle
AND
37.82   Initial insertion of single-chamber device, rate responsive

OR

37.71   Initial insertion of transvenous lead (electrode) into ventricle
AND
37.85   Replacement of any type of pacemaker device with single-chamber device, not specified as rate responsive

OR

37.71   Initial insertion of transvenous lead (electrode) into ventricle

AND

37.86   Replacement of any type of pacemaker device with single-chamber device, rate responsive

OR

37.71   Initial insertion of transvenous lead (electrode) into ventricle
AND
37.87   Replacement of any type of pacemaker device with dual-chamber device

OR

37.72   Initial insertion of transvenous leads (electrodes) into atrium and ventricle
AND
37.80   Insertion of permanent pacemaker, initial or replacement, type of device not specified

OR

37.72   Initial insertion of transvenous leads (electrodes) into atrium and ventricle
AND
37.83   Initial insertion of dual-chamber device

OR

37.73   Initial insertion of transvenous lead (electrode) into atrium
AND
37.80   Insertion of permanent pacemaker, initial or replacement, type of device not specified

OR

37.73   Initial insertion of transvenous lead (electrode) into atrium
AND
37.81   Initial insertion of single-chamber device, not specified as rate responsive

OR

37.73   Initial insertion of transvenous lead (electrode) into atrium
AND
37.82   Initial insertion of single-chamber device, rate responsive

OR

37.73   Initial insertion of transvenous lead (electrode) into atrium
AND
37.85   Replacement of any type of pacemaker device with single-chamber device, not specified as rate responsive

OR

37.73   Initial insertion of transvenous lead (electrode) into atrium
AND
37.86   Replacement of any type of pacemaker device with single-chamber device, rate responsive

OR

37.73   Initial insertion of transvenous lead (electrode) into atrium
AND
37.87   Replacement of any type of pacemaker device with dual-chamber device

OR

37.74   Insertion or replacement of epicardial lead (electrode) into epicardium
AND
37.80   Insertion of permanent pacemaker, initial or replacement, type of device not specified

OR

37.74   Insertion or replacement of epicardial lead (electrode) into epicardium
AND
37.81   Initial insertion of single-chamber device, not specified as rate responsive

OR

37.74   Insertion or replacement of epicardial lead (electrode) into epicardium

---

Surgical   *Medical*   *CC Indicator*   *MCC Indicator*   *Procedure Proxy*

AND

37.82 Initial insertion of single-chamber device, rate responsive

OR

37.74 Insertion or replacement of epicardial lead (electrode) into epicardium
AND
37.83 Initial insertion of dual-chamber device

OR

37.74 Insertion or replacement of epicardial lead (electrode) into epicardium
AND
37.85 Replacement of any type of pacemaker device with single-chamber device, not specified as rate responsive

OR

37.74 Insertion or replacement of epicardial lead (electrode) into epicardium
AND
37.86 Replacement of any type of pacemaker device with single-chamber device, rate responsive

OR

37.74 Insertion or replacement of epicardial lead (electrode) into epicardium
AND
37.87 Replacement of any type of pacemaker device with dual-chamber device

OR

37.76 Replacement of transvenous atrial and/or ventricular lead(s) (electrode(s))
AND
37.80 Insertion of permanent pacemaker, initial or replacement, type of device not specified

OR

37.76 Replacement of transvenous atrial and/or ventricular lead(s) (electrode(s))
AND
37.85 Replacement of any type of pacemaker device with single-chamber device, not specified as rate responsive

OR

37.76 Replacement of transvenous atrial and/or ventricular lead(s) (electrode(s))
AND
37.86 Replacement of any type of pacemaker device with single-chamber device, rate responsive

OR

37.76 Replacement of transvenous atrial and/or ventricular lead(s) (electrode(s))
AND
37.87 Replacement of any type of pacemaker device with dual-chamber device

OR

Nonoperating Room Procedures
92.3* Stereotactic radiosurgery

DRG 041 Peripheral/Cranial Nerve and Other Nervous System Procedures with CC or Peripheral Neurostimulator
GMLOS 5.0   AMLOS 6.4   RW 2.1731   ☑ SP

Operating Room Procedures
01.20 Cranial implantation or replacement of neurostimulator pulse generator
01.29 Removal of cranial neurostimulator pulse generator
04.02 Division of trigeminal nerve
04.03 Division or crushing of other cranial and peripheral nerves
04.04 Other incision of cranial and peripheral nerves
04.05 Gasserian ganglionectomy

04.06 Other cranial or peripheral ganglionectomy
04.07 Other excision or avulsion of cranial and peripheral nerves
04.12 Open biopsy of cranial or peripheral nerve or ganglion
04.19 Other diagnostic procedures on cranial and peripheral nerves and ganglia
04.3 Suture of cranial and peripheral nerves
04.42 Other cranial nerve decompression
04.43 Release of carpal tunnel
04.44 Release of tarsal tunnel
04.49 Other peripheral nerve or ganglion decompression or lysis of adhesions
04.5 Cranial or peripheral nerve graft
04.6 Transposition of cranial and peripheral nerves
04.7* Other cranial or peripheral neuroplasty
04.91 Neurectasis
04.92 Implantation or replacement of peripheral neurostimulator lead(s)
04.93 Removal of peripheral neurostimulator lead(s)
04.99 Other operations on cranial and peripheral nerves
05.0 Division of sympathetic nerve or ganglion
05.1* Diagnostic procedures on sympathetic nerves or ganglia
05.2* Sympathectomy
05.8* Other operations on sympathetic nerves or ganglia
05.9 Other operations on nervous system
07.19 Other diagnostic procedures on adrenal glands, pituitary gland, pineal gland, and thymus
07.8* Thymectomy
07.95 Thoracoscopic incision of thymus
07.98 Other and unspecified thoracoscopic operations on thymus
08.5* Other adjustment of lid position
27.62 Correction of cleft palate
27.69 Other plastic repair of palate
29.4 Plastic operation on pharynx
29.59 Other repair of pharynx
37.74 Insertion or replacement of epicardial lead (electrode) into epicardium
37.75 Revision of lead (electrode)
37.76 Replacement of transvenous atrial and/or ventricular lead(s) (electrode(s))
37.77 Removal of lead(s) (electrodes) without replacement
37.79 Revision or relocation of cardiac device pocket
37.80 Insertion of permanent pacemaker, initial or replacement, type of device not specified
37.85 Replacement of any type of pacemaker device with single-chamber device, not specified as rate responsive
37.86 Replacement of any type of pacemaker device with single-chamber device, rate responsive
37.87 Replacement of any type of pacemaker device with dual-chamber device
37.89 Revision or removal of pacemaker device
38.02 Incision of other vessels of head and neck
38.21 Biopsy of blood vessel
38.42 Resection of other vessels of head and neck with replacement
38.7 Interruption of the vena cava
38.82 Other surgical occlusion of other vessels of head and neck
40.11 Biopsy of lymphatic structure
44.00 Vagotomy, not otherwise specified
54.95 Incision of peritoneum
81.71 Arthroplasty of metacarpophalangeal and interphalangeal joint with implant
81.72 Arthroplasty of metacarpophalangeal and interphalangeal joint without implant
81.74 Arthroplasty of carpocarpal or carpometacarpal joint with implant
81.75 Arthroplasty of carpocarpal or carpometacarpal joint without implant
81.79 Other repair of hand, fingers, and wrist
82.5* Transplantation of muscle and tendon of hand
82.6* Reconstruction of thumb

82.7*	Plastic operation on hand with graft or implant
82.8*	Other plastic operations on hand
83.13	Other tenotomy
83.14	Fasciotomy
83.19	Other division of soft tissue
83.21	Open biopsy of soft tissue
83.41	Excision of tendon for graft
83.43	Excision of muscle or fascia for graft
83.45	Other myectomy
83.49	Other excision of soft tissue
83.7*	Reconstruction of muscle and tendon
83.81	Tendon graft
83.82	Graft of muscle or fascia
83.83	Tendon pulley reconstruction on muscle, tendon, and fascia
83.85	Other change in muscle or tendon length
83.87	Other plastic operations on muscle
83.88	Other plastic operations on tendon
83.89	Other plastic operations on fascia
83.92	Insertion or replacement of skeletal muscle stimulator
83.93	Removal of skeletal muscle stimulator
84.11	Amputation of toe
84.12	Amputation through foot
84.13	Disarticulation of ankle
84.14	Amputation of ankle through malleoli of tibia and fibula
84.15	Other amputation below knee
84.16	Disarticulation of knee
84.17	Amputation above knee
86.06	Insertion of totally implantable infusion pump
86.22	Excisional debridement of wound, infection, or burn
86.4	Radical excision of skin lesion
86.60	Free skin graft, not otherwise specified
86.61	Full-thickness skin graft to hand
86.62	Other skin graft to hand
86.63	Full-thickness skin graft to other sites
86.65	Heterograft to skin
86.66	Homograft to skin
86.67	Dermal regenerative graft
86.69	Other skin graft to other sites
86.70	Pedicle or flap graft, not otherwise specified
86.71	Cutting and preparation of pedicle grafts or flaps
86.72	Advancement of pedicle graft
86.74	Attachment of pedicle or flap graft to other sites
86.75	Revision of pedicle or flap graft
86.81	Repair for facial weakness
86.91	Excision of skin for graft
86.93	Insertion of tissue expander
86.94	Insertion or replacement of single array neurostimulator pulse generator, not specified as rechargeable
86.95	Insertion or replacement of multiple array neurostimulator pulse generator, not specified as rechargeable
86.96	Insertion or replacement of other neurostimulator pulse generator
86.97	Insertion or replacement of single array rechargeable neurostimulator pulse generator
86.98	Insertion or replacement of multiple array (two or more) rechargeable neurostimulator pulse generator
92.27	Implantation or insertion of radioactive elements

OR

Any of the following procedure combinations

37.70	Initial insertion of lead (electrode), not otherwise specified
	AND
37.80	Insertion of permanent pacemaker, initial or replacement, type of device not specified

OR

37.70	Initial insertion of lead (electrode), not otherwise specified
	AND
37.81	Initial insertion of single-chamber device, not specified as rate responsive

OR

37.70	Initial insertion of lead (electrode), not otherwise specified
	AND
37.82	Initial insertion of single-chamber device, rate responsive

OR

37.70	Initial insertion of lead (electrode), not otherwise specified
	AND
37.85	Replacement of any type of pacemaker device with single-chamber device, not specified as rate responsive

OR

37.70	Initial insertion of lead (electrode), not otherwise specified
	AND
37.86	Replacement of any type of pacemaker device with single-chamber device, rate responsive

OR

37.70	Initial insertion of lead (electrode), not otherwise specified
	AND
37.87	Replacement of any type of pacemaker device with dual-chamber device

OR

37.71	Initial insertion of transvenous lead (electrode) into ventricle
	AND
37.80	Insertion of permanent pacemaker, initial or replacement, type of device not specified

OR

37.71	Initial insertion of transvenous lead (electrode) into ventricle
	AND
37.81	Initial insertion of single-chamber device, not specified as rate responsive

OR

37.71	Initial insertion of transvenous lead (electrode) into ventricle
	AND
37.82	Initial insertion of single-chamber device, rate responsive

OR

37.71	Initial insertion of transvenous lead (electrode) into ventricle
	AND
37.85	Replacement of any type of pacemaker device with single-chamber device, not specified as rate responsive

OR

37.71	Initial insertion of transvenous lead (electrode) into ventricle
	AND
37.86	Replacement of any type of pacemaker device with single-chamber device, rate responsive

OR

37.71	Initial insertion of transvenous lead (electrode) into ventricle
	AND
37.87	Replacement of any type of pacemaker device with dual-chamber device

OR

37.72	Initial insertion of transvenous leads (electrodes) into atrium and ventricle
	AND
37.80	Insertion of permanent pacemaker, initial or replacement, type of device not specified

OR

37.72	Initial insertion of transvenous leads (electrodes) into atrium and ventricle
	AND
37.83	Initial insertion of dual-chamber device

OR

37.73	Initial insertion of transvenous lead (electrode) into atrium
	AND
37.80	Insertion of permanent pacemaker, initial or replacement, type of device not specified

MDC 1: Diseases And Disorders Of The Nervous System—SURGICAL

MDC 1: Diseases And Disorders Of The Nervous System—SURGICAL

OR

37.73	Initial insertion of transvenous lead (electrode) into atrium

AND

37.81	Initial insertion of single-chamber device, not specified as rate responsive

OR

37.73 Initial insertion of transvenous lead (electrode) into atrium

AND

37.82 Initial insertion of single-chamber device, rate responsive

OR

37.73 Initial insertion of transvenous lead (electrode) into atrium

AND

37.85 Replacement of any type of pacemaker device with single-chamber device, not specified as rate responsive

OR

37.73 Initial insertion of transvenous lead (electrode) into atrium

AND

37.86 Replacement of any type of pacemaker device with single-chamber device, rate responsive

OR

37.73 Initial insertion of transvenous lead (electrode) into atrium

AND

37.87 Replacement of any type of pacemaker device with dual-chamber device

OR

37.74 Insertion or replacement of epicardial lead (electrode) into epicardium

AND

37.80 Insertion of permanent pacemaker, initial or replacement, type of device not specified

OR

37.74 Insertion or replacement of epicardial lead (electrode) into epicardium

AND

37.81 Initial insertion of single-chamber device, not specified as rate responsive

OR

37.74 Insertion or replacement of epicardial lead (electrode) into epicardium

AND

37.82 Initial insertion of single-chamber device, rate responsive

OR

37.74 Insertion or replacement of epicardial lead (electrode) into epicardium

AND

37.83 Initial insertion of dual-chamber device

OR

37.74 Insertion or replacement of epicardial lead (electrode) into epicardium

AND

37.85 Replacement of any type of pacemaker device with single-chamber device, not specified as rate responsive

OR

37.74 Insertion or replacement of epicardial lead (electrode) into epicardium

AND

37.86 Replacement of any type of pacemaker device with single-chamber device, rate responsive

OR

37.74 Insertion or replacement of epicardial lead (electrode) into epicardium

AND

37.87 Replacement of any type of pacemaker device with dual-chamber device

OR

37.76 Replacement of transvenous atrial and/or ventricular lead(s) (electrode(s))

AND

37.80 Insertion of permanent pacemaker, initial or replacement, type of device not specified

OR

37.76 Replacement of transvenous atrial and/or ventricular lead(s) (electrode(s))

AND

37.85 Replacement of any type of pacemaker device with single-chamber device, not specified as rate responsive

OR

37.76 Replacement of transvenous atrial and/or ventricular lead(s) (electrode(s))

AND

37.86 Replacement of any type of pacemaker device with single-chamber device, rate responsive

OR

37.76 Replacement of transvenous atrial and/or ventricular lead(s) (electrode(s))

AND

37.87 Replacement of any type of pacemaker device with dual-chamber device

OR

Nonoperating Room Procedures

92.3* Stereotactic radiosurgery

OR

Any of the following procedure combinations

04.92 Implantation or replacement of peripheral neurostimulator lead(s)

AND

86.94 Insertion or replacement of single array neurostimulator pulse generator, not specified as rechargeable

OR

04.92 Implantation or replacement of peripheral neurostimulator lead(s)

AND

86.95 Insertion or replacement of multiple array neurostimulator pulse generator, not specified as rechargeable

OR

04.92 Implantation or replacement of peripheral neurostimulator lead(s)

AND

86.97 Insertion or replacement of single array rechargeable neurostimulator pulse generator

OR

04.92 Implantation or replacement of peripheral neurostimulator lead(s)

AND

86.98 Insertion or replacement of multiple array (two or more) rechargeable neurostimulator pulse generator

DRG 042 **Peripheral/Cranial Nerve and Other Nervous System Procedures without CC/MCC**

GMLOS 2.6 AMLOS 3.4 RW 1.8616 ☑ SP

Select operating room procedures or procedure combinations listed under DRG 040

Ⓣ *Transfer DRG* Ⓢ *Special Payment* ☑ *Optimization Potential* ⓉⒼ *Targeted Potential* * *Code Range* ● *New DRG* ▲ *Revised DRG Title*

18 Valid 10/01/2013–09/30/2014 © 2013 OptumInsight, Inc.

MEDICAL

DRG 052   Spinal Disorders and Injuries with CC/MCC
        GMLOS 4.0   AMLOS 5.3   RW 1.4102   ☑

Principal Diagnosis
343.0	Diplegic infantile cerebral palsy
343.1	Hemiplegic infantile cerebral palsy
343.2	Quadriplegic infantile cerebral palsy
343.4	Infantile hemiplegia
344.0*	Quadriplegia and quadriparesis
344.1	Paraplegia
344.2	Diplegia of upper limbs
780.72	Functional quadriplegia
806*	Fracture of vertebral column with spinal cord injury
907.2	Late effect of spinal cord injury
952*	Spinal cord injury without evidence of spinal bone injury

DRG 053   Spinal Disorders and Injuries without CC/MCC
        GMLOS 2.7   AMLOS 3.3   RW 0.8746   ☑

Select principal diagnosis listed under DRG 052

DRG 054   Nervous System Neoplasms with MCC
        GMLOS 4.1   AMLOS 5.5   RW 1.3195   ☑Ⓣ

Principal Diagnosis
191*	Malignant neoplasm of brain
192*	Malignant neoplasm of other and unspecified parts of nervous system
194.4	Malignant neoplasm of pineal gland
194.5	Malignant neoplasm of carotid body
194.6	Malignant neoplasm of aortic body and other paraganglia
198.3	Secondary malignant neoplasm of brain and spinal cord
198.4	Secondary malignant neoplasm of other parts of nervous system
225*	Benign neoplasm of brain and other parts of nervous system
227.4	Benign neoplasm of pineal gland
227.5	Benign neoplasm of carotid body
227.6	Benign neoplasm of aortic body and other paraganglia
237.1	Neoplasm of uncertain behavior of pineal gland
237.3	Neoplasm of uncertain behavior of paraganglia
237.5	Neoplasm of uncertain behavior of brain and spinal cord
237.6	Neoplasm of uncertain behavior of meninges
237.9	Neoplasm of uncertain behavior of other and unspecified parts of nervous system
239.6	Neoplasm of unspecified nature of brain

DRG 055   Nervous System Neoplasms without MCC
        GMLOS 3.1   AMLOS 4.2   RW 1.0100   ☑Ⓣ

Select principal diagnosis listed under DRG 054

DRG 056   Degenerative Nervous System Disorders with MCC
        GMLOS 5.3   AMLOS 7.1   RW 1.7368   ☑Ⓣ

Principal Diagnosis
046*	Slow virus infections and prion diseases of central nervous system
094.0	Tabes dorsalis
094.1	General paresis
094.82	Syphilitic Parkinsonism
094.85	Syphilitic retrobulbar neuritis
094.89	Other specified neurosyphilis
094.9	Unspecified neurosyphilis
310.8*	Other specified nonpsychotic mental disorder following organic brain damage
330*	Cerebral degenerations usually manifest in childhood
331.0	Alzheimer's disease
331.1*	Frontotemporal dementia
331.2	Senile degeneration of brain
331.3	Communicating hydrocephalus
331.4	Obstructive hydrocephalus
331.5	Idiopathic normal pressure hydrocephalus [INPH]
331.6	Corticobasal degeneration
331.7	Cerebral degeneration in diseases classified elsewhere
331.82	Dementia with Lewy bodies
331.83	Mild cognitive impairment, so stated
331.89	Other cerebral degeneration
331.9	Unspecified cerebral degeneration
332*	Parkinson's disease
333.0	Other degenerative diseases of the basal ganglia
333.4	Huntington's chorea
333.5	Other choreas
333.6	Genetic torsion dystonia
333.71	Athetoid cerebral palsy
333.90	Unspecified extrapyramidal disease and abnormal movement disorder
333.94	Restless legs syndrome [RLS]
333.99	Other extrapyramidal disease and abnormal movement disorder
335*	Anterior horn cell disease
336.0	Syringomyelia and syringobulbia
342*	Hemiplegia and hemiparesis
358.0*	Myasthenia gravis
358.1	Myasthenic syndromes in diseases classified elsewhere
358.3*	Lambert-Eaton syndrome
379.45	Argyll Robertson pupil, atypical
438*	Late effects of cerebrovascular disease

DRG 057   Degenerative Nervous System Disorders without MCC
        GMLOS 3.6   AMLOS 4.7   RW 0.9841   ☑Ⓣ

Select principal diagnosis listed under DRG 056

DRG 058   Multiple Sclerosis and Cerebellar Ataxia with MCC
        GMLOS 5.4   AMLOS 7.1   RW 1.6027   ☑

Principal Diagnosis
334*	Spinocerebellar disease
340	Multiple sclerosis
341.0	Neuromyelitis optica
341.1	Schilder's disease
341.8	Other demyelinating diseases of central nervous system
341.9	Unspecified demyelinating disease of central nervous system

DRG 059   Multiple Sclerosis and Cerebellar Ataxia with CC
        GMLOS 4.0   AMLOS 4.9   RW 1.0399   ☑

Select principal diagnosis listed under DRG 058

DRG 060   Multiple Sclerosis and Cerebellar Ataxia without CC/MCC
        GMLOS 3.1   AMLOS 3.7   RW 0.7899   ☑

Select principal diagnosis listed under DRG 058

DRG 061   Acute Ischemic Stroke with Use of Thrombolytic Agent with MCC
        GMLOS 5.8   AMLOS 7.5   RW 2.7316

Principal Diagnosis
433.01	Occlusion and stenosis of basilar artery with cerebral infarction
433.11	Occlusion and stenosis of carotid artery with cerebral infarction
433.21	Occlusion and stenosis of vertebral artery with cerebral infarction

Surgical	Medical	CC Indicator	MCC Indicator	Procedure Proxy

433.31   Occlusion and stenosis of multiple and bilateral precerebral arteries with cerebral infarction
433.81   Occlusion and stenosis of other specified precerebral artery with cerebral infarction
433.91   Occlusion and stenosis of unspecified precerebral artery with cerebral infarction
434.01   Cerebral thrombosis with cerebral infarction
434.11   Cerebral embolism with cerebral infarction
434.91   Unspecified cerebral artery occlusion with cerebral infarction

AND

Nonoperating Room Procedure
99.10   Injection or infusion of thrombolytic agent

DRG 062   Acute Ischemic Stroke with Use of Thrombolytic Agent with CC
GMLOS 4.2   AMLOS 4.9   RW 1.8561   ☑

Select principal diagnosis AND nonoperating room procedure listed under DRG 061

DRG 063   Acute Ischemic Stroke with Use of Thrombolytic Agent without CC/MCC
GMLOS 3.0   AMLOS 3.4   RW 1.4685   ☑

Select principal diagnosis AND nonoperating room procedure listed under DRG 061

DRG 064   Intracranial Hemorrhage or Cerebral Infarction with MCC
GMLOS 4.7   AMLOS 6.3   RW 1.7417   ☑ ▽ T

Principal Diagnosis
430   Subarachnoid hemorrhage
431   Intracerebral hemorrhage
432*   Other and unspecified intracranial hemorrhage
433.01   Occlusion and stenosis of basilar artery with cerebral infarction
433.11   Occlusion and stenosis of carotid artery with cerebral infarction
433.21   Occlusion and stenosis of vertebral artery with cerebral infarction
433.31   Occlusion and stenosis of multiple and bilateral precerebral arteries with cerebral infarction
433.81   Occlusion and stenosis of other specified precerebral artery with cerebral infarction
433.91   Occlusion and stenosis of unspecified precerebral artery with cerebral infarction
434.01   Cerebral thrombosis with cerebral infarction
434.11   Cerebral embolism with cerebral infarction
434.91   Unspecified cerebral artery occlusion with cerebral infarction

▲ DRG 065 Intracranial Hemorrhage or Cerebral Infarction with CC or tPA in 24 Hours
GMLOS 3.5   AMLOS 4.3   RW 1.0776   ☑ ▽ T

Principal Diagnosis
430   Subarachnoid hemorrhage
431   Intracerebral hemorrhage
432*   Other and unspecified intracranial hemorrhage
433.01   Occlusion and stenosis of basilar artery with cerebral infarction
433.11   Occlusion and stenosis of carotid artery with cerebral infarction
433.21   Occlusion and stenosis of vertebral artery with cerebral infarction

433.31   Occlusion and stenosis of multiple and bilateral precerebral arteries with cerebral infarction
433.81   Occlusion and stenosis of other specified precerebral artery with cerebral infarction
433.91   Occlusion and stenosis of unspecified precerebral artery with cerebral infarction
434.01   Cerebral thrombosis with cerebral infarction
434.11   Cerebral embolism with cerebral infarction
434.91   Unspecified cerebral artery occlusion with cerebral infarction

AND

Secondary Diagnosis
V45.88   Status post administration of tPA (rtPA) in a different facility within the last 24 hours prior to admission to current facility

DRG 066   Intracranial Hemorrhage or Cerebral Infarction without CC/MCC
GMLOS 2.5   AMLOS 2.9   RW 0.7566   ☑ ▽ T

Select principal diagnosis listed under DRG 064

DRG 067   Nonspecific Cerebrovascular Accident and Precerebral Occlusion without Infarction with MCC
GMLOS 4.1   AMLOS 5.3   RW 1.4172   ☑ ▽

Principal Diagnosis
433.00   Occlusion and stenosis of basilar artery without mention of cerebral infarction
433.10   Occlusion and stenosis of carotid artery without mention of cerebral infarction
433.20   Occlusion and stenosis of vertebral artery without mention of cerebral infarction
433.30   Occlusion and stenosis of multiple and bilateral precerebral arteries without mention of cerebral infarction
433.80   Occlusion and stenosis of other specified precerebral artery without mention of cerebral infarction
433.90   Occlusion and stenosis of unspecified precerebral artery without mention of cerebral infarction
434.00   Cerebral thrombosis without mention of cerebral infarction
434.10   Cerebral embolism without mention of cerebral infarction
434.90   Unspecified cerebral artery occlusion without mention of cerebral infarction
436   Acute, but ill-defined, cerebrovascular disease

DRG 068   Nonspecific Cerebrovascular Accident and Precerebral Occlusion without Infarction without MCC
GMLOS 2.5   AMLOS 3.1   RW 0.8582   ☑ ▽

Select principal diagnosis listed under DRG 067

DRG 069   Transient Ischemia
GMLOS 2.2   AMLOS 2.6   RW 0.6948   ☑ ▽

Principal Diagnosis
435*   Transient cerebral ischemia
437.1   Other generalized ischemic cerebrovascular disease

DRG 070   Nonspecific Cerebrovascular Disorders with MCC
GMLOS 4.9   AMLOS 6.6   RW 1.6593   ☑ T

Principal Diagnosis
348.3*   Encephalopathy, not elsewhere classified
348.81   Temporal sclerosis
348.89   Other conditions of brain
348.9   Unspecified condition of brain
349.89   Other specified disorder of nervous system
349.9   Unspecified disorders of nervous system
437.0   Cerebral atherosclerosis

T Transfer DRG   SP Special Payment   ☑ Optimization Potential   ▽ Targeted Potential   * Code Range   ● New DRG   ▲ Revised DRG Title

20   Valid 10/01/2013–09/30/2014   © 2013 OptumInsight, Inc.

437.7	Transient global amnesia
437.8	Other ill-defined cerebrovascular disease
437.9	Unspecified cerebrovascular disease

DRG 071   Nonspecific Cerebrovascular Disorders with CC
GMLOS 3.6   AMLOS 4.6   RW 0.9796   ☑Ⓣ

Select principal diagnosis listed under DRG 070

DRG 072   Nonspecific Cerebrovascular Disorders without CC/MCC
GMLOS 2.3   AMLOS 2.9   RW 0.6919   ☑Ⓣ

Select principal diagnosis listed under DRG 070

DRG 073   Cranial and Peripheral Nerve Disorders with MCC
GMLOS 3.9   AMLOS 5.3   RW 1.3014   ☑

Principal Diagnosis

053.10	Herpes zoster with unspecified nervous system complication
053.11	Geniculate herpes zoster
053.12	Postherpetic trigeminal neuralgia
053.13	Postherpetic polyneuropathy
053.19	Other herpes zoster with nervous system complications
056.00	Unspecified rubella neurological complication
072.72	Mumps polyneuropathy
249.6*	Secondary diabetes mellitus with neurological manifestations
250.6*	Diabetes with neurological manifestations
337*	Disorders of the autonomic nervous system
344.60	Cauda equina syndrome without mention of neurogenic bladder
350*	Trigeminal nerve disorders
351*	Facial nerve disorders
352*	Disorders of other cranial nerves
353*	Nerve root and plexus disorders
354*	Mononeuritis of upper limb and mononeuritis multiplex
355*	Mononeuritis of lower limb and unspecified site
356.0	Hereditary peripheral neuropathy
356.1	Peroneal muscular atrophy
356.2	Hereditary sensory neuropathy
356.4	Idiopathic progressive polyneuropathy
356.8	Other specified idiopathic peripheral neuropathy
356.9	Unspecified hereditary and idiopathic peripheral neuropathy
357.1	Polyneuropathy in collagen vascular disease
357.2	Polyneuropathy in diabetes
357.3	Polyneuropathy in malignant disease
357.4	Polyneuropathy in other diseases classified elsewhere
357.5	Alcoholic polyneuropathy
357.6	Polyneuropathy due to drugs
357.7	Polyneuropathy due to other toxic agents
357.8*	Other inflammatory and toxic neuropathy
357.9	Unspecified inflammatory and toxic neuropathy
358.2	Toxic myoneural disorders
358.8	Other specified myoneural disorders
358.9	Unspecified myoneural disorders
723.2	Cervicocranial syndrome
723.3	Cervicobrachial syndrome (diffuse)
723.4	Brachial neuritis or radiculitis NOS
729.2	Unspecified neuralgia, neuritis, and radiculitis
736.05	Wrist drop (acquired)
736.06	Claw hand (acquired)
736.07	Club hand, acquired
736.74	Claw foot, acquired
951.0	Injury to oculomotor nerve
951.1	Injury to trochlear nerve
951.2	Injury to trigeminal nerve
951.3	Injury to abducens nerve
951.4	Injury to facial nerve
951.6	Injury to accessory nerve
951.7	Injury to hypoglossal nerve
951.8	Injury to other specified cranial nerves
951.9	Injury to unspecified cranial nerve
953*	Injury to nerve roots and spinal plexus
954*	Injury to other nerve(s) of trunk, excluding shoulder and pelvic girdles
955*	Injury to peripheral nerve(s) of shoulder girdle and upper limb
956*	Injury to peripheral nerve(s) of pelvic girdle and lower limb
957*	Injury to other and unspecified nerves

DRG 074   Cranial and Peripheral Nerve Disorders without MCC
GMLOS 3.1   AMLOS 3.9   RW 0.8786   ☑

Select principal diagnosis listed under DRG 073

DRG 075   Viral Meningitis with CC/MCC
GMLOS 5.2   AMLOS 6.5   RW 1.5918   ☑

Principal Diagnosis

047*	Meningitis due to enterovirus
048	Other enterovirus diseases of central nervous system
049.0	Lymphocytic choriomeningitis
049.1	Meningitis due to adenovirus
053.0	Herpes zoster with meningitis
054.72	Herpes simplex meningitis
072.1	Mumps meningitis

DRG 076   Viral Meningitis without CC/MCC
GMLOS 3.2   AMLOS 3.7   RW 0.8425   ☑

Select principal diagnosis listed under DRG 075

DRG 077   Hypertensive Encephalopathy with MCC
GMLOS 4.6   AMLOS 6.0   RW 1.6290   ☑

Principal Diagnosis

437.2	Hypertensive encephalopathy

DRG 078   Hypertensive Encephalopathy with CC
GMLOS 3.1   AMLOS 3.9   RW 0.9467   ☑

Select principal diagnosis listed under DRG 077

DRG 079   Hypertensive Encephalopathy without CC/MCC
GMLOS 2.3   AMLOS 2.8   RW 0.7118   ☑

Select principal diagnosis listed under DRG 077

DRG 080   Nontraumatic Stupor and Coma with MCC
GMLOS 3.7   AMLOS 5.1   RW 1.2252   ☑

Principal Diagnosis

348.4	Compression of brain
348.5	Cerebral edema
348.82	Brain death
780.01	Coma
780.03	Persistent vegetative state
780.09	Other alteration of consciousness

MDC 1: Diseases And Disorders Of The Nervous System—MEDICAL

Surgical	Medical	CC Indicator	MCC Indicator	Procedure Proxy

MDC 1: Diseases And Disorders Of The Nervous System—MEDICAL

DRG 081	**Nontraumatic Stupor and Coma without MCC**

GMLOS 2.6   AMLOS 3.4   RW 0.7455   ☑

Select principal diagnosis listed under DRG 080

DRG 082	**Traumatic Stupor and Coma, Coma Greater Than One Hour with MCC**

GMLOS 3.4   AMLOS 5.7   RW 1.9463   ☑

Principal Diagnosis of Traumatic Stupor and Coma > 1 Hour

800.03   Closed fracture of vault of skull without mention of intracranial injury, moderate (1-24 hours) loss of consciousness

800.04   Closed fracture of vault of skull without mention of intracranial injury, prolonged (more than 24 hours) loss of consciousness and return to pre-existing conscious level

800.05   Closed fracture of vault of skull without mention of intracranial injury, prolonged (more than 24 hours) loss of consciousness, without return to pre-existing conscious level

800.06   Closed fracture of vault of skull without mention of intracranial injury, loss of consciousness of unspecified duration

800.13   Closed fracture of vault of skull with cerebral laceration and contusion, moderate (1-24 hours) loss of consciousness

800.14   Closed fracture of vault of skull with cerebral laceration and contusion, prolonged (more than 24 hours) loss of consciousness and return to pre-existing conscious level

800.15   Closed fracture of vault of skull with cerebral laceration and contusion, prolonged (more than 24 hours) loss of consciousness, without return to pre-existing conscious level

800.16   Closed fracture of vault of skull with cerebral laceration and contusion, loss of consciousness of unspecified duration

800.23   Closed fracture of vault of skull with subarachnoid, subdural, and extradural hemorrhage, moderate (1-24 hours) loss of consciousness

800.24   Closed fracture of vault of skull with subarachnoid, subdural, and extradural hemorrhage, prolonged (more than 24 hours) loss of consciousness and return to pre-existing conscious level

800.25   Closed fracture of vault of skull with subarachnoid, subdural, and extradural hemorrhage, prolonged (more than 24 hours) loss of consciousness, without return to pre-existing conscious level

800.26   Closed fracture of vault of skull with subarachnoid, subdural, and extradural hemorrhage, loss of consciousness of unspecified duration

800.33   Closed fracture of vault of skull with other and unspecified intracranial hemorrhage, moderate (1-24 hours) loss of consciousness

800.34   Closed fracture of vault of skull with other and unspecified intracranial hemorrhage, prolonged (more than 24 hours) loss of consciousness and return to pre-existing conscious level

800.35   Closed fracture of vault of skull with other and unspecified intracranial hemorrhage, prolonged (more than 24 hours) loss of consciousness, without return to pre-existing conscious level

800.36   Closed fracture of vault of skull with other and unspecified intracranial hemorrhage, loss of consciousness of unspecified duration

800.43   Closed fracture of vault of skull with intracranial injury of other and unspecified nature, moderate (1-24 hours) loss of consciousness

800.44   Closed fracture of vault of skull with intracranial injury of other and unspecified nature, prolonged (more than 24 hours) loss of consciousness and return to pre-existing conscious level

800.45   Closed fracture of vault of skull with intracranial injury of other and unspecified nature, prolonged (more than 24 hours) loss of consciousness, without return to pre-existing conscious level

800.46   Closed fracture of vault of skull with intracranial injury of other and unspecified nature, loss of consciousness of unspecified duration

800.53   Open fracture of vault of skull without mention of intracranial injury, moderate (1-24 hours) loss of consciousness

800.54   Open fracture of vault of skull without mention of intracranial injury, prolonged (more than 24 hours) loss of consciousness and return to pre-existing conscious level

800.55   Open fracture of vault of skull without mention of intracranial injury, prolonged (more than 24 hours) loss of consciousness, without return to pre-existing conscious level

800.56   Open fracture of vault of skull without mention of intracranial injury, loss of consciousness of unspecified duration

800.63   Open fracture of vault of skull with cerebral laceration and contusion, moderate (1-24 hours) loss of consciousness

800.64   Open fracture of vault of skull with cerebral laceration and contusion, prolonged (more than 24 hours) loss of consciousness and return to pre-existing conscious level

800.65   Open fracture of vault of skull with cerebral laceration and contusion, prolonged (more than 24 hours) loss of consciousness, without return to pre-existing conscious level

800.66   Open fracture of vault of skull with cerebral laceration and contusion, loss of consciousness of unspecified duration

800.73   Open fracture of vault of skull with subarachnoid, subdural, and extradural hemorrhage, moderate (1-24 hours) loss of consciousness

800.74   Open fracture of vault of skull with subarachnoid, subdural, and extradural hemorrhage, prolonged (more than 24 hours) loss of consciousness and return to pre-existing conscious level

800.75   Open fracture of vault of skull with subarachnoid, subdural, and extradural hemorrhage, prolonged (more than 24 hours) loss of consciousness, without return to pre-existing conscious level

800.76   Open fracture of vault of skull with subarachnoid, subdural, and extradural hemorrhage, loss of consciousness of unspecified duration

800.83   Open fracture of vault of skull with other and unspecified intracranial hemorrhage, moderate (1-24 hours) loss of consciousness

800.84   Open fracture of vault of skull with other and unspecified intracranial hemorrhage, prolonged (more than 24 hours) loss of consciousness and return to pre-existing conscious level

800.85   Open fracture of vault of skull with other and unspecified intracranial hemorrhage, prolonged (more than 24 hours) loss of consciousness, without return to pre-existing conscious level

800.86   Open fracture of vault of skull with other and unspecified intracranial hemorrhage, loss of consciousness of unspecified duration

800.93   Open fracture of vault of skull with intracranial injury of other and unspecified nature, moderate (1-24 hours) loss of consciousness

800.94   Open fracture of vault of skull with intracranial injury of other and unspecified nature, prolonged (more than 24 hours) loss of consciousness and return to pre-existing conscious level

800.95   Open fracture of vault of skull with intracranial injury of other and unspecified nature, prolonged (more than 24 hours) loss of consciousness, without return to pre-existing conscious level

---

Ⓣ *Transfer DRG*   ⓈⓅ *Special Payment*   ☑ *Optimization Potential*   ⓋⒾ *Targeted Potential*   * *Code Range*   ● *New DRG*   ▲ *Revised DRG Title*

Code	Description
800.96	Open fracture of vault of skull with intracranial injury of other and unspecified nature, loss of consciousness of unspecified duration
801.03	Closed fracture of base of skull without mention of intracranial injury, moderate (1-24 hours) loss of consciousness
801.04	Closed fracture of base of skull without mention of intracranial injury, prolonged (more than 24 hours) loss of consciousness and return to pre-existing conscious level
801.05	Closed fracture of base of skull without mention of intracranial injury, prolonged (more than 24 hours) loss of consciousness, without return to pre-existing conscious level
801.06	Closed fracture of base of skull without mention of intracranial injury, loss of consciousness of unspecified duration
801.13	Closed fracture of base of skull with cerebral laceration and contusion, moderate (1-24 hours) loss of consciousness
801.14	Closed fracture of base of skull with cerebral laceration and contusion, prolonged (more than 24 hours) loss of consciousness and return to pre-existing conscious level
801.15	Closed fracture of base of skull with cerebral laceration and contusion, prolonged (more than 24 hours) loss of consciousness, without return to pre-existing conscious level
801.16	Closed fracture of base of skull with cerebral laceration and contusion, loss of consciousness of unspecified duration
801.23	Closed fracture of base of skull with subarachnoid, subdural, and extradural hemorrhage, moderate (1-24 hours) loss of consciousness
801.24	Closed fracture of base of skull with subarachnoid, subdural, and extradural hemorrhage, prolonged (more than 24 hours) loss of consciousness and return to pre-existing conscious level
801.25	Closed fracture of base of skull with subarachnoid, subdural, and extradural hemorrhage, prolonged (more than 24 hours) loss of consciousness, without return to pre-existing conscious level
801.26	Closed fracture of base of skull with subarachnoid, subdural, and extradural hemorrhage, loss of consciousness of unspecified duration
801.33	Closed fracture of base of skull with other and unspecified intracranial hemorrhage, moderate (1-24 hours) loss of consciousness
801.34	Closed fracture of base of skull with other and unspecified intracranial hemorrhage, prolonged (more than 24 hours) loss of consciousness and return to pre-existing conscious level
801.35	Closed fracture of base of skull with other and unspecified intracranial hemorrhage, prolonged (more than 24 hours) loss of consciousness, without return to pre-existing conscious level
801.36	Closed fracture of base of skull with other and unspecified intracranial hemorrhage, loss of consciousness of unspecified duration
801.43	Closed fracture of base of skull with intracranial injury of other and unspecified nature, moderate (1-24 hours) loss of consciousness
801.44	Closed fracture of base of skull with intracranial injury of other and unspecified nature, prolonged (more than 24 hours) loss of consciousness and return to pre-existing conscious level
801.45	Closed fracture of base of skull with intracranial injury of other and unspecified nature, prolonged (more than 24 hours) loss of consciousness, without return to pre-existing conscious level
801.46	Closed fracture of base of skull with intracranial injury of other and unspecified nature, loss of consciousness of unspecified duration
801.53	Open fracture of base of skull without mention of intracranial injury, moderate (1-24 hours) loss of consciousness
801.54	Open fracture of base of skull without mention of intracranial injury, prolonged (more than 24 hours) loss of consciousness and return to pre-existing conscious level
801.55	Open fracture of base of skull without mention of intracranial injury, prolonged (more than 24 hours) loss of consciousness, without return to pre-existing conscious level
801.56	Open fracture of base of skull without mention of intracranial injury, loss of consciousness of unspecified duration
801.63	Open fracture of base of skull with cerebral laceration and contusion, moderate (1-24 hours) loss of consciousness
801.64	Open fracture of base of skull with cerebral laceration and contusion, prolonged (more than 24 hours) loss of consciousness and return to pre-existing conscious level
801.65	Open fracture of base of skull with cerebral laceration and contusion, prolonged (more than 24 hours) loss of consciousness, without return to pre-existing conscious level
801.66	Open fracture of base of skull with cerebral laceration and contusion, loss of consciousness of unspecified duration
801.73	Open fracture of base of skull with subarachnoid, subdural, and extradural hemorrhage, moderate (1-24 hours) loss of consciousness
801.74	Open fracture of base of skull with subarachnoid, subdural, and extradural hemorrhage, prolonged (more than 24 hours) loss of consciousness and return to pre-existing conscious level
801.75	Open fracture of base of skull with subarachnoid, subdural, and extradural hemorrhage, prolonged (more than 24 hours) loss of consciousness, without return to pre-existing conscious level
801.76	Open fracture of base of skull with subarachnoid, subdural, and extradural hemorrhage, loss of consciousness of unspecified duration
801.83	Open fracture of base of skull with other and unspecified intracranial hemorrhage, moderate (1-24 hours) loss of consciousness
801.84	Open fracture of base of skull with other and unspecified intracranial hemorrhage, prolonged (more than 24 hours) loss of consciousness and return to pre-existing conscious level
801.85	Open fracture of base of skull with other and unspecified intracranial hemorrhage, prolonged (more than 24 hours) loss of consciousness, without return to pre-existing conscious level
801.86	Open fracture of base of skull with other and unspecified intracranial hemorrhage, loss of consciousness of unspecified duration
801.93	Open fracture of base of skull with intracranial injury of other and unspecified nature, moderate (1-24 hours) loss of consciousness
801.94	Open fracture of base of skull with intracranial injury of other and unspecified nature, prolonged (more than 24 hours) loss of consciousness and return to pre-existing conscious level
801.95	Open fracture of base of skull with intracranial injury of other and unspecified nature, prolonged (more than 24 hours) loss of consciousness, without return to pre-existing conscious level
801.96	Open fracture of base of skull with intracranial injury of other and unspecified nature, loss of consciousness of unspecified duration
803.03	Other closed skull fracture without mention of intracranial injury, moderate (1-24 hours) loss of consciousness

Surgical	Medical	CC Indicator	MCC Indicator	Procedure Proxy

MDC 1: Diseases And Disorders Of The Nervous System—MEDICAL

803.04 Other closed skull fracture without mention of intracranial injury, prolonged (more than 24 hours) loss of consciousness and return to pre-existing conscious level

803.05 Other closed skull fracture without mention of intracranial injury, prolonged (more than 24 hours) loss of consciousness, without return to pre-existing conscious level

803.06 Other closed skull fracture without mention of intracranial injury, loss of consciousness of unspecified duration

803.13 Other closed skull fracture with cerebral laceration and contusion, moderate (1-24 hours) loss of consciousness

803.14 Other closed skull fracture with cerebral laceration and contusion, prolonged (more than 24 hours) loss of consciousness and return to pre-existing conscious level

803.15 Other closed skull fracture with cerebral laceration and contusion, prolonged (more than 24 hours) loss of consciousness, without return to pre-existing conscious level

803.16 Other closed skull fracture with cerebral laceration and contusion, loss of consciousness of unspecified duration

803.23 Other closed skull fracture with subarachnoid, subdural, and extradural hemorrhage, moderate (1-24 hours) loss of consciousness

803.24 Other closed skull fracture with subarachnoid, subdural, and extradural hemorrhage, prolonged (more than 24 hours) loss of consciousness and return to pre-existing conscious level

803.25 Other closed skull fracture with subarachnoid, subdural, and extradural hemorrhage, prolonged (more than 24 hours) loss of consciousness, without return to pre-existing conscious level

803.26 Other closed skull fracture with subarachnoid, subdural, and extradural hemorrhage, loss of consciousness of unspecified duration

803.33 Other closed skull fracture with other and unspecified intracranial hemorrhage, moderate (1-24 hours) loss of consciousness

803.34 Other closed skull fracture with other and unspecified intracranial hemorrhage, prolonged (more than 24 hours) loss of consciousness and return to pre-existing conscious level

803.35 Other closed skull fracture with other and unspecified intracranial hemorrhage, prolonged (more than 24 hours) loss of consciousness, without return to pre-existing conscious level

803.36 Other closed skull fracture with other and unspecified intracranial hemorrhage, loss of consciousness of unspecified duration

803.43 Other closed skull fracture with intracranial injury of other and unspecified nature, moderate (1-24 hours) loss of consciousness

803.44 Other closed skull fracture with intracranial injury of other and unspecified nature, prolonged (more than 24 hours) loss of consciousness and return to pre-existing conscious level

803.45 Other closed skull fracture with intracranial injury of other and unspecified nature, prolonged (more than 24 hours) loss of consciousness, without return to pre-existing conscious level

803.46 Other closed skull fracture with intracranial injury of other and unspecified nature, loss of consciousness of unspecified duration

803.53 Other open skull fracture without mention of intracranial injury, moderate (1-24 hours) loss of consciousness

803.54 Other open skull fracture without mention of intracranial injury, prolonged (more than 24 hours) loss of consciousness and return to pre-existing conscious level

803.55 Other open skull fracture without mention of intracranial injury, prolonged (more than 24 hours) loss of consciousness, without return to pre-existing conscious level

803.56 Other open skull fracture without mention of intracranial injury, loss of consciousness of unspecified duration

803.63 Other open skull fracture with cerebral laceration and contusion, moderate (1-24 hours) loss of consciousness

803.64 Other open skull fracture with cerebral laceration and contusion, prolonged (more than 24 hours) loss of consciousness and return to pre-existing conscious level

803.65 Other open skull fracture with cerebral laceration and contusion, prolonged (more than 24 hours) loss of consciousness, without return to pre-existing conscious level

803.66 Other open skull fracture with cerebral laceration and contusion, loss of consciousness of unspecified duration

803.73 Other open skull fracture with subarachnoid, subdural, and extradural hemorrhage, moderate (1-24 hours) loss of consciousness

803.74 Other open skull fracture with subarachnoid, subdural, and extradural hemorrhage, prolonged (more than 24 hours) loss of consciousness and return to pre-existing conscious level

803.75 Other open skull fracture with subarachnoid, subdural, and extradural hemorrhage, prolonged (more than 24 hours) loss of consciousness, without return to pre-existing conscious level

803.76 Other open skull fracture with subarachnoid, subdural, and extradural hemorrhage, loss of consciousness of unspecified duration

803.83 Other open skull fracture with other and unspecified intracranial hemorrhage, moderate (1-24 hours) loss of consciousness

803.84 Other open skull fracture with other and unspecified intracranial hemorrhage, prolonged (more than 24 hours) loss of consciousness and return to pre-existing conscious level

803.85 Other open skull fracture with other and unspecified intracranial hemorrhage, prolonged (more than 24 hours) loss of consciousness, without return to pre-existing conscious level

803.86 Other open skull fracture with other and unspecified intracranial hemorrhage, loss of consciousness of unspecified duration

803.93 Other open skull fracture with intracranial injury of other and unspecified nature, moderate (1-24 hours) loss of consciousness

803.94 Other open skull fracture with intracranial injury of other and unspecified nature, prolonged (more than 24 hours) loss of consciousness and return to pre-existing conscious level

803.95 Other open skull fracture with intracranial injury of other and unspecified nature, prolonged (more than 24 hours) loss of consciousness, without return to pre-existing conscious level

803.96 Other open skull fracture with intracranial injury of other and unspecified nature, loss of consciousness of unspecified duration

804.03 Closed fractures involving skull or face with other bones, without mention of intracranial injury, moderate (1-24 hours) loss of consciousness

804.04 Closed fractures involving skull or face with other bones, without mention or intracranial injury, prolonged (more than 24 hours) loss of consciousness and return to pre-existing conscious level

804.05 Closed fractures involving skull or face with other bones, without mention of intracranial injury, prolonged (more than 24 hours) loss of consciousness, without return to pre-existing conscious level

804.06 Closed fractures involving skull of face with other bones, without mention of intracranial injury, loss of consciousness of unspecified duration

---

Ⓣ *Transfer DRG*   ⓈⓅ *Special Payment*   ☑ *Optimization Potential*   ▽ *Targeted Potential*   * *Code Range*   ● *New DRG*   ▲ *Revised DRG Title*

804.13	Closed fractures involving skull or face with other bones, with cerebral laceration and contusion, moderate (1-24 hours) loss of consciousness
804.14	Closed fractures involving skull or face with other bones, with cerebral laceration and contusion, prolonged (more than 24 hours) loss of consciousness and return to pre-existing conscious level
804.15	Closed fractures involving skull or face with other bones, with cerebral laceration and contusion, prolonged (more than 24 hours) loss of consciousness, without return to pre-existing conscious level
804.16	Closed fractures involving skull or face with other bones, with cerebral laceration and contusion, loss of consciousness of unspecified duration
804.23	Closed fractures involving skull or face with other bones with subarachnoid, subdural, and extradural hemorrhage, moderate (1-24 hours) loss of consciousness
804.24	Closed fractures involving skull or face with other bones with subarachnoid, subdural, and extradural hemorrhage, prolonged (more than 24 hours) loss of consciousness and return to pre-existing conscious level
804.25	Closed fractures involving skull or face with other bones with subarachnoid, subdural, and extradural hemorrhage, prolonged (more than 24 hours) loss of consciousness, without return to pre-existing conscious level
804.26	Closed fractures involving skull or face with other bones with subarachnoid, subdural, and extradural hemorrhage, loss of consciousness of unspecified duration
804.33	Closed fractures involving skull or face with other bones, with other and unspecified intracranial hemorrhage, moderate (1-24 hours) loss of consciousness
804.34	Closed fractures involving skull or face with other bones, with other and unspecified intracranial hemorrhage, prolonged (more than 24 hours) loss of consciousness and return to preexisting conscious level
804.35	Closed fractures involving skull or face with other bones, with other and unspecified intracranial hemorrhage, prolonged (more than 24 hours) loss of consciousness, without return to pre-existing conscious level
804.36	Closed fractures involving skull or face with other bones, with other and unspecified intracranial hemorrhage, loss of consciousness of unspecified duration
804.43	Closed fractures involving skull or face with other bones, with intracranial injury of other and unspecified nature, moderate (1-24 hours) loss of consciousness
804.44	Closed fractures involving skull or face with other bones, with intracranial injury of other and unspecified nature, prolonged (more than 24 hours) loss of consciousness and return to pre-existing conscious level
804.45	Closed fractures involving skull or face with other bones, with intracranial injury of other and unspecified nature, prolonged (more than 24 hours) loss of consciousness, without return to pre-existing conscious level
804.46	Closed fractures involving skull or face with other bones, with intracranial injury of other and unspecified nature, loss of consciousness of unspecified duration
804.53	Open fractures involving skull or face with other bones, without mention of intracranial injury, moderate (1-24 hours) loss of consciousness
804.54	Open fractures involving skull or face with other bones, without mention of intracranial injury, prolonged (more than 24 hours) loss of consciousness and return to pre-existing conscious level
804.55	Open fractures involving skull or face with other bones, without mention of intracranial injury, prolonged (more than 24 hours) loss of consciousness, without return to pre-existing conscious level
804.56	Open fractures involving skull or face with other bones, without mention of intracranial injury, loss of consciousness of unspecified duration
804.63	Open fractures involving skull or face with other bones, with cerebral laceration and contusion, moderate (1-24 hours) loss of consciousness
804.64	Open fractures involving skull or face with other bones, with cerebral laceration and contusion, prolonged (more than 24 hours) loss of consciousness and return to pre-existing conscious level
804.65	Open fractures involving skull or face with other bones, with cerebral laceration and contusion, prolonged (more than 24 hours) loss of consciousness, without return to pre-existing conscious level
804.66	Open fractures involving skull or face with other bones, with cerebral laceration and contusion, loss of consciousness of unspecified duration
804.73	Open fractures involving skull or face with other bones with subarachnoid, subdural, and extradural hemorrhage, moderate (1-24 hours) loss of consciousness
804.74	Open fractures involving skull or face with other bones with subarachnoid, subdural, and extradural hemorrhage, prolonged (more than 24 hours) loss of consciousness and return to pre-existing conscious level
804.75	Open fractures involving skull or face with other bones with subarachnoid, subdural, and extradural hemorrhage, prolonged (more than 24 hours) loss of consciousness, without return to pre-existing conscious level
804.76	Open fractures involving skull or face with other bones with subarachnoid, subdural, and extradural hemorrhage, loss of consciousness of unspecified duration
804.83	Open fractures involving skull or face with other bones, with other and unspecified intracranial hemorrhage, moderate (1-24 hours) loss of consciousness
804.84	Open fractures involving skull or face with other bones, with other and unspecified intracranial hemorrhage, prolonged (more than 24 hours) loss of consciousness and return to pre-existing conscious level
804.85	Open fractures involving skull or face with other bones, with other and unspecified intracranial hemorrhage, prolonged (more than 24 hours) loss of consciousness, without return to pre-existing conscious level
804.86	Open fractures involving skull or face with other bones, with other and unspecified intracranial hemorrhage, loss of consciousness of unspecified duration
804.93	Open fractures involving skull or face with other bones, with intracranial injury of other and unspecified nature, moderate (1-24 hours) loss of consciousness
804.94	Open fractures involving skull or face with other bones, with intracranial injury of other and unspecified nature, prolonged (more than 24 hours) loss of consciousness and return to pre-existing conscious level
804.95	Open fractures involving skull or face with other bones, with intracranial injury of other and unspecified nature, prolonged (more than 24 hours) loss of consciousness, without return to pre-existing conscious level
804.96	Open fractures involving skull or face with other bones, with intracranial injury of other and unspecified nature, loss of consciousness of unspecified duration
851.03	Cortex (cerebral) contusion without mention of open intracranial wound, moderate (1-24 hours) loss of consciousness
851.04	Cortex (cerebral) contusion without mention of open intracranial wound, prolonged (more than 24 hours) loss of consciousness and return to pre-existing conscious level
851.05	Cortex (cerebral) contusion without mention of open intracranial wound, prolonged (more than 24 hours) loss of consciousness, without return to pre-existing conscious level
851.06	Cortex (cerebral) contusion without mention of open intracranial wound, loss of consciousness of unspecified duration

MDC 1: Diseases And Disorders Of The Nervous System—MEDICAL

| Surgical | Medical | CC Indicator | MCC Indicator | Procedure Proxy |

851.13	Cortex (cerebral) contusion with open intracranial wound, moderate (1-24 hours) loss of consciousness	851.73	Cerebellar or brain stem laceration with open intracranial wound, moderate (1-24 hours) loss of consciousness
851.14	Cortex (cerebral) contusion with open intracranial wound, prolonged (more than 24 hours) loss of consciousness and return to pre-existing conscious level	851.74	Cerebellar or brain stem laceration with open intracranial wound, prolonged (more than 24 hours) loss of consciousness and return to pre-existing conscious level
851.15	Cortex (cerebral) contusion with open intracranial wound, prolonged (more than 24 hours) loss of consciousness, without return to pre-existing conscious level	851.75	Cerebellar or brain stem laceration with open intracranial wound, prolonged (more than 24 hours) loss of consciousness, without return to pre-existing conscious level
851.16	Cortex (cerebral) contusion with open intracranial wound, loss of consciousness of unspecified duration	851.76	Cerebellar or brain stem laceration with open intracranial wound, loss of consciousness of unspecified duration
851.23	Cortex (cerebral) laceration without mention of open intracranial wound, moderate (1-24 hours) loss of consciousness	851.83	Other and unspecified cerebral laceration and contusion, without mention of open intracranial wound, moderate (1-24 hours) loss of consciousness
851.24	Cortex (cerebral) laceration without mention of open intracranial wound, prolonged (more than 24 hours) loss of consciousness and return to pre-existing conscious level	851.84	Other and unspecified cerebral laceration and contusion, without mention of open intracranial wound, prolonged (more than 24 hours) loss of consciousness and return to preexisting conscious level
851.25	Cortex (cerebral) laceration without mention of open intracranial wound, prolonged (more than 24 hours) loss of consciousness, without return to pre-existing conscious level	851.85	Other and unspecified cerebral laceration and contusion, without mention of open intracranial wound, prolonged (more than 24 hours) loss of consciousness, without return to pre-existing conscious level
851.26	Cortex (cerebral) laceration without mention of open intracranial wound, loss of consciousness of unspecified duration	851.86	Other and unspecified cerebral laceration and contusion, without mention of open intracranial wound, loss of consciousness of unspecified duration
851.33	Cortex (cerebral) laceration with open intracranial wound, moderate (1-24 hours) loss of consciousness	851.93	Other and unspecified cerebral laceration and contusion, with open intracranial wound, moderate (1-24 hours) loss of consciousness
851.34	Cortex (cerebral) laceration with open intracranial wound, prolonged (more than 24 hours) loss of consciousness and return to pre-existing conscious level	851.94	Other and unspecified cerebral laceration and contusion, with open intracranial wound, prolonged (more than 24 hours) loss of consciousness and return to pre-existing conscious level
851.35	Cortex (cerebral) laceration with open intracranial wound, prolonged (more than 24 hours) loss of consciousness, without return to pre-existing conscious level	851.95	Other and unspecified cerebral laceration and contusion, with open intracranial wound, prolonged (more than 24 hours) loss of consciousness, without return to pre-existing conscious level
851.36	Cortex (cerebral) laceration with open intracranial wound, loss of consciousness of unspecified duration	851.96	Other and unspecified cerebral laceration and contusion, with open intracranial wound, loss of consciousness of unspecified duration
851.43	Cerebellar or brain stem contusion without mention of open intracranial wound, moderate (1-24 hours) loss of consciousness	852.03	Subarachnoid hemorrhage following injury, without mention of open intracranial wound, moderate (1-24 hours) loss of consciousness
851.44	Cerebellar or brain stem contusion without mention of open intracranial wound, prolonged (more than 24 hours) loss consciousness and return to pre-existing conscious level	852.04	Subarachnoid hemorrhage following injury, without mention of open intracranial wound, prolonged (more than 24 hours) loss of consciousness and return to pre-existing conscious level
851.45	Cerebellar or brain stem contusion without mention of open intracranial wound, prolonged (more than 24 hours) loss of consciousness, without return to pre-existing conscious level	852.05	Subarachnoid hemorrhage following injury, without mention of open intracranial wound, prolonged (more than 24 hours) loss of consciousness, without return to pre-existing conscious level
851.46	Cerebellar or brain stem contusion without mention of open intracranial wound, loss of consciousness of unspecified duration	852.06	Subarachnoid hemorrhage following injury, without mention of open intracranial wound, loss of consciousness of unspecified duration
851.53	Cerebellar or brain stem contusion with open intracranial wound, moderate (1-24 hours) loss of consciousness	852.13	Subarachnoid hemorrhage following injury, with open intracranial wound, moderate (1-24 hours) loss of consciousness
851.54	Cerebellar or brain stem contusion with open intracranial wound, prolonged (more than 24 hours) loss of consciousness and return to pre-existing conscious level	852.14	Subarachnoid hemorrhage following injury, with open intracranial wound, prolonged (more than 24 hours) loss of consciousness and return to pre-existing conscious level
851.55	Cerebellar or brain stem contusion with open intracranial wound, prolonged (more than 24 hours) loss of consciousness, without return to pre-existing conscious level	852.15	Subarachnoid hemorrhage following injury, with open intracranial wound, prolonged (more than 24 hours) loss of consciousness, without return to pre-existing conscious level
851.56	Cerebellar or brain stem contusion with open intracranial wound, loss of consciousness of unspecified duration	852.16	Subarachnoid hemorrhage following injury, with open intracranial wound, loss of consciousness of unspecified duration
851.63	Cerebellar or brain stem laceration without mention of open intracranial wound, moderate (1-24 hours) loss of consciousness	852.23	Subdural hemorrhage following injury, without mention of open intracranial wound, moderate (1-24 hours) loss of consciousness
851.64	Cerebellar or brain stem laceration without mention of open intracranial wound, prolonged (more than 24 hours) loss of consciousness and return to pre-existing conscious level		
851.65	Cerebellar or brain stem laceration without mention of open intracranial wound, prolonged (more than 24 hours) loss of consciousness, without return to pre-existing conscious level		
851.66	Cerebellar or brain stem laceration without mention of open intracranial wound, loss of consciousness of unspecified duration		

MDC 1: Diseases And Disorders Of The Nervous System—MEDICAL

T Transfer DRG   SP Special Payment   ☑ Optimization Potential   ▽ Targeted Potential   * Code Range   ● New DRG   ▲ Revised DRG Title

26   Valid 10/01/2013-09/30/2014   © 2013 OptumInsight, Inc.

852.24   Subdural hemorrhage following injury, without mention of open intracranial wound, prolonged (more than 24 hours) loss of consciousness and return to pre-existing conscious level

852.25   Subdural hemorrhage following injury, without mention of open intracranial wound, prolonged (more than 24 hours) loss of consciousness, without return to pre-existing conscious level

852.26   Subdural hemorrhage following injury, without mention of open intracranial wound, loss of consciousness of unspecified duration

852.33   Subdural hemorrhage following injury, with open intracranial wound, moderate (1-24 hours) loss of consciousness

852.34   Subdural hemorrhage following injury, with open intracranial wound, prolonged (more than 24 hours) loss of consciousness and return to pre-existing conscious level

852.35   Subdural hemorrhage following injury, with open intracranial wound, prolonged (more than 24 hours) loss of consciousness, without return to pre-existing conscious level

852.36   Subdural hemorrhage following injury, with open intracranial wound, loss of consciousness of unspecified duration

852.43   Extradural hemorrhage following injury, without mention of open intracranial wound, moderate (1-24 hours) loss of consciousness

852.44   Extradural hemorrhage following injury, without mention of open intracranial wound, prolonged (more than 24 hours) loss of consciousness and return to pre-existing conscious level

852.45   Extradural hemorrhage following injury, without mention of open intracranial wound, prolonged (more than 24 hours) loss of consciousness, without return to pre-existing conscious level

852.46   Extradural hemorrhage following injury, without mention of open intracranial wound, loss of consciousness of unspecified duration

852.53   Extradural hemorrhage following injury, with open intracranial wound, moderate (1-24 hours) loss of consciousness

852.54   Extradural hemorrhage following injury, with open intracranial wound, prolonged (more than 24 hours) loss of consciousness and return to pre-existing conscious level

852.55   Extradural hemorrhage following injury, with open intracranial wound, prolonged (more than 24 hours) loss of consciousness, without return to pre-existing conscious level

852.56   Extradural hemorrhage following injury, with open intracranial wound, loss of consciousness of unspecified duration

853.03   Other and unspecified intracranial hemorrhage following injury, without mention of open intracranial wound, moderate (1-24 hours) loss of consciousness

853.04   Other and unspecified intracranial hemorrhage following injury, without mention of open intracranial wound, prolonged (more than 24 hours) loss of consciousness and return to preexisting conscious level

853.05   Other and unspecified intracranial hemorrhage following injury. Without mention of open intracranial wound, prolonged (more than 24 hours) loss of consciousness, without return to pre-existing conscious level

853.06   Other and unspecified intracranial hemorrhage following injury, without mention of open intracranial wound, loss of consciousness of unspecified duration

853.13   Other and unspecified intracranial hemorrhage following injury, with open intracranial wound, moderate (1-24 hours) loss of consciousness

853.14   Other and unspecified intracranial hemorrhage following injury, with open intracranial wound, prolonged (more than 24 hours) loss of consciousness and return to pre-existing conscious level

853.15   Other and unspecified intracranial hemorrhage following injury, with open intracranial wound, prolonged (more than 24 hours) loss of consciousness, without return to pre-existing conscious level

853.16   Other and unspecified intracranial hemorrhage following injury, with open intracranial wound, loss of consciousness of unspecified duration

854.03   Intracranial injury of other and unspecified nature, without mention of open intracranial wound, moderate (1-24 hours) loss of consciousness

854.04   Intracranial injury of other and unspecified nature, without mention of open intracranial wound, prolonged (more than 24 hours) loss of consciousness and return to pre-existing conscious level

854.05   Intracranial injury of other and unspecified nature, without mention of open intracranial wound, prolonged (more than 24 hours) loss of consciousness, without return to pre-existing conscious level

854.06   Intracranial injury of other and unspecified nature, without mention of open intracranial wound, loss of consciousness of unspecified duration

854.13   Intracranial injury of other and unspecified nature, with open intracranial wound, moderate (1-24 hours) loss of consciousness

854.14   Intracranial injury of other and unspecified nature, with open intracranial wound, prolonged (more than 24 hours) loss of consciousness and return to pre-existing conscious level

854.15   Intracranial injury of other and unspecified nature, with open intracranial wound, prolonged (more than 24 hours) loss of consciousness, without return to pre-existing conscious level

854.16   Intracranial injury of other and unspecified nature, with open intracranial wound, loss of consciousness of unspecified duration

OR

Principal Diagnosis of Traumatic Stupor and Coma

800.00   Closed fracture of vault of skull without mention of intracranial injury, unspecified state of consciousness

800.01   Closed fracture of vault of skull without mention of intracranial injury, no loss of consciousness

800.02   Closed fracture of vault of skull without mention of intracranial injury, brief (less than one hour) loss of consciousness

800.09   Closed fracture of vault of skull without mention of intracranial injury, unspecified concussion

800.10   Closed fracture of vault of skull with cerebral laceration and contusion, unspecified state of consciousness

800.11   Closed fracture of vault of skull with cerebral laceration and contusion, no loss of consciousness

800.12   Closed fracture of vault of skull with cerebral laceration and contusion, brief (less than one hour) loss of consciousness

800.19   Closed fracture of vault of skull with cerebral laceration and contusion, unspecified concussion

800.20   Closed fracture of vault of skull with subarachnoid, subdural, and extradural hemorrhage, unspecified state of consciousness

800.21   Closed fracture of vault of skull with subarachnoid, subdural, and extradural hemorrhage, no loss of consciousness

800.22   Closed fracture of vault of skull with subarachnoid, subdural, and extradural hemorrhage, brief (less than one hour) loss of consciousness

800.29   Closed fracture of vault of skull with subarachnoid, subdural, and extradural hemorrhage, unspecified concussion

Surgical	Medical	CC Indicator	MCC Indicator	Procedure Proxy

MDC 1: Diseases And Disorders Of The Nervous System—MEDICAL

800.30	Closed fracture of vault of skull with other and unspecified intracranial hemorrhage, unspecified state of consciousness
800.31	Closed fracture of vault of skull with other and unspecified intracranial hemorrhage, no loss of consciousness
800.32	Closed fracture of vault of skull with other and unspecified intracranial hemorrhage, brief (less than one hour) loss of consciousness
800.39	Closed fracture of vault of skull with other and unspecified intracranial hemorrhage, unspecified concussion
800.40	Closed fracture of vault of skull with intracranial injury of other and unspecified nature, unspecified state of consciousness
800.41	Closed fracture of vault of skull with intracranial injury of other and unspecified nature, no loss of consciousness
800.42	Closed fracture of vault of skull with intracranial injury of other and unspecified nature, brief (less than one hour) loss of consciousness
800.49	Closed fracture of vault of skull with intracranial injury of other and unspecified nature, unspecified concussion
800.50	Open fracture of vault of skull without mention of intracranial injury, unspecified state of consciousness
800.51	Open fracture of vault of skull without mention of intracranial injury, no loss of consciousness
800.52	Open fracture of vault of skull without mention of intracranial injury, brief (less than one hour) loss of consciousness
800.59	Open fracture of vault of skull without mention of intracranial injury, unspecified concussion
800.60	Open fracture of vault of skull with cerebral laceration and contusion, unspecified state of consciousness
800.61	Open fracture of vault of skull with cerebral laceration and contusion, no loss of consciousness
800.62	Open fracture of vault of skull with cerebral laceration and contusion, brief (less than one hour) loss of consciousness
800.69	Open fracture of vault of skull with cerebral laceration and contusion, unspecified concussion
800.70	Open fracture of vault of skull with subarachnoid, subdural, and extradural hemorrhage, unspecified state of consciousness
800.71	Open fracture of vault of skull with subarachnoid, subdural, and extradural hemorrhage, no loss of consciousness
800.72	Open fracture of vault of skull with subarachnoid, subdural, and extradural hemorrhage, brief (less than one hour) loss of consciousness
800.79	Open fracture of vault of skull with subarachnoid, subdural, and extradural hemorrhage, unspecified concussion
800.80	Open fracture of vault of skull with other and unspecified intracranial hemorrhage, unspecified state of consciousness
800.81	Open fracture of vault of skull with other and unspecified intracranial hemorrhage, no loss of consciousness
800.82	Open fracture of vault of skull with other and unspecified intracranial hemorrhage, brief (less than one hour) loss of consciousness
800.89	Open fracture of vault of skull with other and unspecified intracranial hemorrhage, unspecified concussion
800.90	Open fracture of vault of skull with intracranial injury of other and unspecified nature, unspecified state of consciousness
800.91	Open fracture of vault of skull with intracranial injury of other and unspecified nature, no loss of consciousness
800.92	Open fracture of vault of skull with intracranial injury of other and unspecified nature, brief (less than one hour) loss of consciousness
800.99	Open fracture of vault of skull with intracranial injury of other and unspecified nature, unspecified concussion
801.00	Closed fracture of base of skull without mention of intracranial injury, unspecified state of consciousness
801.01	Closed fracture of base of skull without mention of intracranial injury, no loss of consciousness
801.02	Closed fracture of base of skull without mention of intracranial injury, brief (less than one hour) loss of consciousness
801.09	Closed fracture of base of skull without mention of intracranial injury, unspecified concussion
801.10	Closed fracture of base of skull with cerebral laceration and contusion, unspecified state of consciousness
801.11	Closed fracture of base of skull with cerebral laceration and contusion, no loss of consciousness
801.12	Closed fracture of base of skull with cerebral laceration and contusion, brief (less than one hour) loss of consciousness
801.19	Closed fracture of base of skull with cerebral laceration and contusion, unspecified concussion
801.20	Closed fracture of base of skull with subarachnoid, subdural, and extradural hemorrhage, unspecified state of consciousness
801.21	Closed fracture of base of skull with subarachnoid, subdural, and extradural hemorrhage, no loss of consciousness
801.22	Closed fracture of base of skull with subarachnoid, subdural, and extradural hemorrhage, brief (less than one hour) loss of consciousness
801.29	Closed fracture of base of skull with subarachnoid, subdural, and extradural hemorrhage, unspecified concussion
801.30	Closed fracture of base of skull with other and unspecified intracranial hemorrhage, unspecified state of consciousness
801.31	Closed fracture of base of skull with other and unspecified intracranial hemorrhage, no loss of consciousness
801.32	Closed fracture of base of skull with other and unspecified intracranial hemorrhage, brief (less than one hour) loss of consciousness
801.39	Closed fracture of base of skull with other and unspecified intracranial hemorrhage, unspecified concussion
801.40	Closed fracture of base of skull with intracranial injury of other and unspecified nature, unspecified state of consciousness
801.41	Closed fracture of base of skull with intracranial injury of other and unspecified nature, no loss of consciousness
801.42	Closed fracture of base of skull with intracranial injury of other and unspecified nature, brief (less than one hour) loss of consciousness
801.49	Closed fracture of base of skull with intracranial injury of other and unspecified nature, unspecified concussion
801.50	Open fracture of base of skull without mention of intracranial injury, unspecified state of consciousness
801.51	Open fracture of base of skull without mention of intracranial injury, no loss of consciousness
801.52	Open fracture of base of skull without mention of intracranial injury, brief (less than one hour) loss of consciousness
801.59	Open fracture of base of skull without mention of intracranial injury, unspecified concussion
801.60	Open fracture of base of skull with cerebral laceration and contusion, unspecified state of consciousness
801.61	Open fracture of base of skull with cerebral laceration and contusion, no loss of consciousness
801.62	Open fracture of base of skull with cerebral laceration and contusion, brief (less than one hour) loss of consciousness
801.69	Open fracture of base of skull with cerebral laceration and contusion, unspecified concussion
801.70	Open fracture of base of skull with subarachnoid, subdural, and extradural hemorrhage, unspecified state of consciousness
801.71	Open fracture of base of skull with subarachnoid, subdural, and extradural hemorrhage, no loss of consciousness
801.72	Open fracture of base of skull with subarachnoid, subdural, and extradural hemorrhage, brief (less than one hour) loss of consciousness
801.79	Open fracture of base of skull with subarachnoid, subdural, and extradural hemorrhage, unspecified concussion

Ⓣ *Transfer DRG*   ⑤ *Special Payment*   ☑ *Optimization Potential*   ▽ *Targeted Potential*   * *Code Range*   ● *New DRG*   ▲ *Revised DRG Title*

28   Valid 10/01/2013-09/30/2014   © 2013 OptumInsight, Inc.

801.80   Open fracture of base of skull with other and unspecified intracranial hemorrhage, unspecified state of consciousness

801.81   Open fracture of base of skull with other and unspecified intracranial hemorrhage, no loss of consciousness

801.82   Open fracture of base of skull with other and unspecified intracranial hemorrhage, brief (less than one hour) loss of consciousness

801.89   Open fracture of base of skull with other and unspecified intracranial hemorrhage, unspecified concussion

801.90   Open fracture of base of skull with intracranial injury of other and unspecified nature, unspecified state of consciousness

801.91   Open fracture of base of skull with intracranial injury of other and unspecified nature, no loss of consciousness

801.92   Open fracture of base of skull with intracranial injury of other and unspecified nature, brief (less than one hour) loss of consciousness

801.99   Open fracture of base of skull with intracranial injury of other and unspecified nature, unspecified concussion

803.00   Other closed skull fracture without mention of intracranial injury, unspecified state of consciousness

803.01   Other closed skull fracture without mention of intracranial injury, no loss of consciousness

803.02   Other closed skull fracture without mention of intracranial injury, brief (less than one hour) loss of consciousness

803.09   Other closed skull fracture without mention of intracranial injury, unspecified concussion

803.10   Other closed skull fracture with cerebral laceration and contusion, unspecified state of consciousness

803.11   Other closed skull fracture with cerebral laceration and contusion, no loss of consciousness

803.12   Other closed skull fracture with cerebral laceration and contusion, brief (less than one hour) loss of consciousness

803.19   Other closed skull fracture with cerebral laceration and contusion, unspecified concussion

803.20   Other closed skull fracture with subarachnoid, subdural, and extradural hemorrhage, unspecified state of consciousness

803.21   Other closed skull fracture with subarachnoid, subdural, and extradural hemorrhage, no loss of consciousness

803.22   Other closed skull fracture with subarachnoid, subdural, and extradural hemorrhage, brief (less than one hour) loss of consciousness

803.29   Other closed skull fracture with subarachnoid, subdural, and extradural hemorrhage, unspecified concussion

803.30   Other closed skull fracture with other and unspecified intracranial hemorrhage, unspecified state of unconsciousness

803.31   Other closed skull fracture with other and unspecified intracranial hemorrhage, no loss of consciousness

803.32   Other closed skull fracture with other and unspecified intracranial hemorrhage, brief (less than one hour) loss of consciousness

803.39   Other closed skull fracture with other and unspecified intracranial hemorrhage, unspecified concussion

803.40   Other closed skull fracture with intracranial injury of other and unspecified nature, unspecified state of consciousness

803.41   Other closed skull fracture with intracranial injury of other and unspecified nature, no loss of consciousness

803.42   Other closed skull fracture with intracranial injury of other and unspecified nature, brief (less than one hour) loss of consciousness

803.49   Other closed skull fracture with intracranial injury of other and unspecified nature, unspecified concussion

803.50   Other open skull fracture without mention of injury, state of consciousness unspecified

803.51   Other open skull fracture without mention of intracranial injury, no loss of consciousness

803.52   Other open skull fracture without mention of intracranial injury, brief (less than one hour) loss of consciousness

803.59   Other open skull fracture without mention of intracranial injury, unspecified concussion

803.60   Other open skull fracture with cerebral laceration and contusion, unspecified state of consciousness

803.61   Other open skull fracture with cerebral laceration and contusion, no loss of consciousness

803.62   Other open skull fracture with cerebral laceration and contusion, brief (less than one hour) loss of consciousness

803.69   Other open skull fracture with cerebral laceration and contusion, unspecified concussion

803.70   Other open skull fracture with subarachnoid, subdural, and extradural hemorrhage, unspecified state of consciousness

803.71   Other open skull fracture with subarachnoid, subdural, and extradural hemorrhage, no loss of consciousness

803.72   Other open skull fracture with subarachnoid, subdural, and extradural hemorrhage, brief (less than one hour) loss of consciousness

803.79   Other open skull fracture with subarachnoid, subdural, and extradural hemorrhage, unspecified concussion

803.80   Other open skull fracture with other and unspecified intracranial hemorrhage, unspecified state of consciousness

803.81   Other open skull fracture with other and unspecified intracranial hemorrhage, no loss of consciousness

803.82   Other open skull fracture with other and unspecified intracranial hemorrhage, brief (less than one hour) loss of consciousness

803.89   Other open skull fracture with other and unspecified intracranial hemorrhage, unspecified concussion

803.90   Other open skull fracture with intracranial injury of other and unspecified nature, unspecified state of consciousness

803.91   Other open skull fracture with intracranial injury of other and unspecified nature, no loss of consciousness

803.92   Other open skull fracture with intracranial injury of other and unspecified nature, brief (less than one hour) loss of consciousness

803.99   Other open skull fracture with intracranial injury of other and unspecified nature, unspecified concussion

804.00   Closed fractures involving skull or face with other bones, without mention of intracranial injury, unspecified state of consciousness

804.01   Closed fractures involving skull or face with other bones, without mention of intracranial injury, no loss of consciousness

804.02   Closed fractures involving skull or face with other bones, without mention of intracranial injury, brief (less than one hour) loss of consciousness

804.09   Closed fractures involving skull of face with other bones, without mention of intracranial injury, unspecified concussion

804.10   Closed fractures involving skull or face with other bones, with cerebral laceration and contusion, unspecified state of consciousness

804.11   Closed fractures involving skull or face with other bones, with cerebral laceration and contusion, no loss of consciousness

804.12   Closed fractures involving skull or face with other bones, with cerebral laceration and contusion, brief (less than one hour) loss of consciousness

804.19   Closed fractures involving skull or face with other bones, with cerebral laceration and contusion, unspecified concussion

804.20   Closed fractures involving skull or face with other bones with subarachnoid, subdural, and extradural hemorrhage, unspecified state of consciousness

804.21   Closed fractures involving skull or face with other bones with subarachnoid, subdural, and extradural hemorrhage, no loss of consciousness

804.22   Closed fractures involving skull or face with other bones with subarachnoid, subdural, and extradural hemorrhage, brief (less than one hour) loss of consciousness

Surgical	Medical	CC Indicator	MCC Indicator	Procedure Proxy

804.29 Closed fractures involving skull or face with other bones with subarachnoid, subdural, and extradural hemorrhage, unspecified concussion

804.30 Closed fractures involving skull or face with other bones, with other and unspecified intracranial hemorrhage, unspecified state of consciousness

804.31 Closed fractures involving skull or face with other bones, with other and unspecified intracranial hemorrhage, no loss of consciousness

804.32 Closed fractures involving skull or face with other bones, with other and unspecified intracranial hemorrhage, brief (less than one hour) loss of consciousness

804.39 Closed fractures involving skull or face with other bones, with other and unspecified intracranial hemorrhage, unspecified concussion

804.40 Closed fractures involving skull or face with other bones, with intracranial injury of other and unspecified nature, unspecified state of consciousness

804.41 Closed fractures involving skull or face with other bones, with intracranial injury of other and unspecified nature, no loss of consciousness

804.42 Closed fractures involving skull or face with other bones, with intracranial injury of other and unspecified nature, brief (less than one hour) loss of consciousness

804.49 Closed fractures involving skull or face with other bones, with intracranial injury of other and unspecified nature, unspecified concussion

804.50 Open fractures involving skull or face with other bones, without mention of intracranial injury, unspecified state of consciousness

804.51 Open fractures involving skull or face with other bones, without mention of intracranial injury, no loss of consciousness

804.52 Open fractures involving skull or face with other bones, without mention of intracranial injury, brief (less than one hour) loss of consciousness

804.59 Open fractures involving skull or face with other bones, without mention of intracranial injury, unspecified concussion

804.60 Open fractures involving skull or face with other bones, with cerebral laceration and contusion, unspecified state of consciousness

804.61 Open fractures involving skull or face with other bones, with cerebral laceration and contusion, no loss of consciousness

804.62 Open fractures involving skull or face with other bones, with cerebral laceration and contusion, brief (less than one hour) loss of consciousness

804.69 Open fractures involving skull or face with other bones, with cerebral laceration and contusion, unspecified concussion

804.70 Open fractures involving skull or face with other bones with subarachnoid, subdural, and extradural hemorrhage, unspecified state of consciousness

804.71 Open fractures involving skull or face with other bones with subarachnoid, subdural, and extradural hemorrhage, no loss of consciousness

804.72 Open fractures involving skull or face with other bones with subarachnoid, subdural, and extradural hemorrhage, brief (less than one hour) loss of consciousness

804.79 Open fractures involving skull or face with other bones with subarachnoid, subdural, and extradural hemorrhage, unspecified concussion

804.80 Open fractures involving skull or face with other bones, with other and unspecified intracranial hemorrhage, unspecified state of consciousness

804.81 Open fractures involving skull or face with other bones, with other and unspecified intracranial hemorrhage, no loss of consciousness

804.82 Open fractures involving skull or face with other bones, with other and unspecified intracranial hemorrhage, brief (less than one hour) loss of consciousness

804.89 Open fractures involving skull or face with other bones, with other and unspecified intracranial hemorrhage, unspecified concussion

804.90 Open fractures involving skull or face with other bones, with intracranial injury of other and unspecified nature, unspecified state of consciousness

804.91 Open fractures involving skull or face with other bones, with intracranial injury of other and unspecified nature, no loss of consciousness

804.92 Open fractures involving skull or face with other bones, with intracranial injury of other and unspecified nature, brief (less than one hour) loss of consciousness

804.99 Open fractures involving skull or face with other bones, with intracranial injury of other and unspecified nature, unspecified concussion

851.00 Cortex (cerebral) contusion without mention of open intracranial wound, state of consciousness unspecified

851.01 Cortex (cerebral) contusion without mention of open intracranial wound, no loss of consciousness

851.02 Cortex (cerebral) contusion without mention of open intracranial wound, brief (less than 1 hour) loss of consciousness

851.09 Cortex (cerebral) contusion without mention of open intracranial wound, unspecified concussion

851.10 Cortex (cerebral) contusion with open intracranial wound, unspecified state of consciousness

851.11 Cortex (cerebral) contusion with open intracranial wound, no loss of consciousness

851.12 Cortex (cerebral) contusion with open intracranial wound, brief (less than 1 hour) loss of consciousness

851.19 Cortex (cerebral) contusion with open intracranial wound, unspecified concussion

851.20 Cortex (cerebral) laceration without mention of open intracranial wound, unspecified state of consciousness

851.21 Cortex (cerebral) laceration without mention of open intracranial wound, no loss of consciousness

851.22 Cortex (cerebral) laceration without mention of open intracranial wound, brief (less than 1 hour) loss of consciousness

851.29 Cortex (cerebral) laceration without mention of open intracranial wound, unspecified concussion

851.30 Cortex (cerebral) laceration with open intracranial wound, unspecified state of consciousness

851.31 Cortex (cerebral) laceration with open intracranial wound, no loss of consciousness

851.32 Cortex (cerebral) laceration with open intracranial wound, brief (less than 1 hour) loss of consciousness

851.39 Cortex (cerebral) laceration with open intracranial wound, unspecified concussion

851.40 Cerebellar or brain stem contusion without mention of open intracranial wound, unspecified state of consciousness

851.41 Cerebellar or brain stem contusion without mention of open intracranial wound, no loss of consciousness

851.42 Cerebellar or brain stem contusion without mention of open intracranial wound, brief (less than 1 hour) loss of consciousness

851.49 Cerebellar or brain stem contusion without mention of open intracranial wound, unspecified concussion

851.50 Cerebellar or brain stem contusion with open intracranial wound, unspecified state of consciousness

851.51 Cerebellar or brain stem contusion with open intracranial wound, no loss of consciousness

851.52 Cerebellar or brain stem contusion with open intracranial wound, brief (less than 1 hour) loss of consciousness

851.59 Cerebellar or brain stem contusion with open intracranial wound, unspecified concussion

851.60 Cerebellar or brain stem laceration without mention of open intracranial wound, unspecified state of consciousness

851.61 Cerebellar or brain stem laceration without mention of open intracranial wound, no loss of consciousness

Ⓣ *Transfer DRG*   ⓈⓅ *Special Payment*   ☑ *Optimization Potential*   ▽ *Targeted Potential*   * *Code Range*   ● *New DRG*   ▲ *Revised DRG Title*

30   Valid 10/01/2013-09/30/2014   © 2013 OptumInsight, Inc.

MDC 1: Diseases And Disorders Of The Nervous System—MEDICAL

851.62 Cerebellar or brain stem laceration without mention of open intracranial wound, brief (less than 1 hour) loss of consciousness

851.69 Cerebellar or brain stem laceration without mention of open intracranial wound, unspecified concussion

851.70 Cerebellar or brain stem laceration with open intracranial wound, state of consciousness unspecified

851.71 Cerebellar or brain stem laceration with open intracranial wound, no loss of consciousness

851.72 Cerebellar or brain stem laceration with open intracranial wound, brief (less than one hour) loss of consciousness

851.79 Cerebellar or brain stem laceration with open intracranial wound, unspecified concussion

851.80 Other and unspecified cerebral laceration and contusion, without mention of open intracranial wound, unspecified state of consciousness

851.81 Other and unspecified cerebral laceration and contusion, without mention of open intracranial wound, no loss of consciousness

851.82 Other and unspecified cerebral laceration and contusion, without mention of open intracranial wound, brief (less than 1 hour) loss of consciousness

851.89 Other and unspecified cerebral laceration and contusion, without mention of open intracranial wound, unspecified concussion

851.90 Other and unspecified cerebral laceration and contusion, with open intracranial wound, unspecified state of consciousness

851.91 Other and unspecified cerebral laceration and contusion, with open intracranial wound, no loss of consciousness

851.92 Other and unspecified cerebral laceration and contusion, with open intracranial wound, brief (less than 1 hour) loss of consciousness

851.99 Other and unspecified cerebral laceration and contusion, with open intracranial wound, unspecified concussion

852.00 Subarachnoid hemorrhage following injury, without mention of open intracranial wound, unspecified state of consciousness

852.01 Subarachnoid hemorrhage following injury, without mention of open intracranial wound, no loss of consciousness

852.02 Subarachnoid hemorrhage following injury, without mention of open intracranial wound, brief (less than 1 hour) loss of consciousness

852.09 Subarachnoid hemorrhage following injury, without mention of open intracranial wound, unspecified concussion

852.10 Subarachnoid hemorrhage following injury, with open intracranial wound, unspecified state of consciousness

852.11 Subarachnoid hemorrhage following injury, with open intracranial wound, no loss of consciousness

852.12 Subarachnoid hemorrhage following injury, with open intracranial wound, brief (less than 1 hour) loss of consciousness

852.19 Subarachnoid hemorrhage following injury, with open intracranial wound, unspecified concussion

852.20 Subdural hemorrhage following injury, without mention of open intracranial wound, unspecified state of consciousness

852.21 Subdural hemorrhage following injury, without mention of open intracranial wound, no loss of consciousness

852.22 Subdural hemorrhage following injury, without mention of open intracranial wound, brief (less than one hour) loss of consciousness

852.29 Subdural hemorrhage following injury, without mention of open intracranial wound, unspecified concussion

852.30 Subdural hemorrhage following injury, with open intracranial wound, state of consciousness unspecified

852.31 Subdural hemorrhage following injury, with open intracranial wound, no loss of consciousness

852.32 Subdural hemorrhage following injury, with open intracranial wound, brief (less than 1 hour) loss of consciousness

852.39 Subdural hemorrhage following injury, with open intracranial wound, unspecified concussion

852.40 Extradural hemorrhage following injury, without mention of open intracranial wound, unspecified state of consciousness

852.41 Extradural hemorrhage following injury, without mention of open intracranial wound, no loss of consciousness

852.42 Extradural hemorrhage following injury, without mention of open intracranial wound, brief (less than 1 hour) loss of consciousness

852.49 Extradural hemorrhage following injury, without mention of open intracranial wound, unspecified concussion

852.50 Extradural hemorrhage following injury, with open intracranial wound, state of consciousness unspecified

852.51 Extradural hemorrhage following injury, with open intracranial wound, no loss of consciousness

852.52 Extradural hemorrhage following injury, with open intracranial wound, brief (less than 1 hour) loss of consciousness

852.59 Extradural hemorrhage following injury, with open intracranial wound, unspecified concussion

853.00 Other and unspecified intracranial hemorrhage following injury, without mention of open intracranial wound, unspecified state of consciousness

853.01 Other and unspecified intracranial hemorrhage following injury, without mention of open intracranial wound, no loss of consciousness

853.02 Other and unspecified intracranial hemorrhage following injury, without mention of open intracranial wound, brief (less than 1 hour) loss of consciousness

853.09 Other and unspecified intracranial hemorrhage following injury, without mention of open intracranial wound, unspecified concussion

853.10 Other and unspecified intracranial hemorrhage following injury, with open intracranial wound, unspecified state of consciousness

853.11 Other and unspecified intracranial hemorrhage following injury, with open intracranial wound, no loss of consciousness

853.12 Other and unspecified intracranial hemorrhage following injury, with open intracranial wound, brief (less than 1 hour) loss of consciousness

853.19 Other and unspecified intracranial hemorrhage following injury, with open intracranial wound, unspecified concussion

854.00 Intracranial injury of other and unspecified nature, without mention of open intracranial wound, unspecified state of consciousness

854.01 Intracranial injury of other and unspecified nature, without mention of open intracranial wound, no loss of consciousness

854.02 Intracranial injury of other and unspecified nature, without mention of open intracranial wound, brief (less than 1 hour) loss of consciousness

854.09 Intracranial injury of other and unspecified nature, without mention of open intracranial wound, unspecified concussion

854.10 Intracranial injury of other and unspecified nature, with open intracranial wound, unspecified state of consciousness

854.11 Intracranial injury of other and unspecified nature, with open intracranial wound, no loss of consciousness

854.12 Intracranial injury of other and unspecified nature, with open intracranial wound, brief (less than 1 hour) loss of consciousness

854.19 Intracranial injury of other and unspecified nature, with open intracranial wound, with unspecified concussion

AND

Secondary Diagnosis of Traumatic Stupor and Coma > 1 Hour

Above listed diagnoses with description of loss of consciousness greater than one hour or of unspecified duration

DRG 083   Traumatic Stupor and Coma, Coma Greater Than One Hour with CC

GMLOS 3.4   AMLOS 4.4   RW 1.2643   ☑

Select principal diagnosis of coma greater than one hour OR principal diagnosis of traumatic stupor AND a secondary diagnosis of coma greater than one hour listed under DRG 082

DRG 084   Traumatic Stupor and Coma, Coma Greater Than One Hour without CC/MCC

GMLOS 2.1   AMLOS 2.7   RW 0.8491   ☑

Select principal diagnosis of coma greater than one hour OR principal diagnosis of traumatic stupor AND a secondary diagnosis of coma greater than one hour listed under DRG 082

DRG 085   Traumatic Stupor and Coma, Coma Less Than One Hour with MCC

GMLOS 4.9   AMLOS 6.7   RW 1.9733   ☑ⓣ

Select principal diagnosis listed under DRG 082 excluding those with loss of consciousness of greater than one hour or of unspecified duration

DRG 086   Traumatic Stupor and Coma, Coma Less Than One Hour with CC

GMLOS 3.3   AMLOS 4.2   RW 1.1105   ☑ⓣ

Select principal diagnosis listed under DRG 082 excluding those with loss of consciousness of greater than one hour or of unspecified duration

DRG 087   Traumatic Stupor and Coma, Coma Less Than One Hour without CC/MCC

GMLOS 2.2   AMLOS 2.7   RW 0.7345   ☑ⓣ

Select principal diagnosis listed under DRG 082 excluding those with loss of consciousness of greater than one hour or of unspecified duration

DRG 088   Concussion with MCC

GMLOS 3.9   AMLOS 5.1   RW 1.5029   ☑

Principal Diagnosis
850*   Concussion

DRG 089   Concussion with CC

GMLOS 2.7   AMLOS 3.3   RW 0.9406   ☑

Select principal diagnosis listed under DRG 088

DRG 090   Concussion without CC/MCC

GMLOS 1.9   AMLOS 2.3   RW 0.7140   ☑

Select principal diagnosis under DRG 088

DRG 091   Other Disorders of Nervous System with MCC

GMLOS 4.3   AMLOS 5.9   RW 1.5851   ☑ⓣ

Principal Diagnosis
078.81   Epidemic vertigo
094.87   Syphilitic ruptured cerebral aneurysm
137.1   Late effects of central nervous system tuberculosis

138   Late effects of acute poliomyelitis
139.0   Late effects of viral encephalitis
228.02   Hemangioma of intracranial structures
237.7*   Neurofibromatosis
307.2*   Tics
315.35   Childhood onset fluency disorder
323.71   Toxic encephalitis and encephalomyelitis
323.72   Toxic myelitis
325   Phlebitis and thrombophlebitis of intracranial venous sinuses
326   Late effects of intracranial abscess or pyogenic infection
327.21   Primary central sleep apnea
327.25   Congenital central alveolar hypoventilation syndrome
327.27   Central sleep apnea in conditions classified elsewhere
327.3*   Circadian rhythm sleep disorder
327.41   Confusional arousals
327.43   Recurrent isolated sleep paralysis
327.51   Periodic limb movement disorder
327.52   Sleep related leg cramps
331.81   Reye's syndrome
333.1   Essential and other specified forms of tremor
333.2   Myoclonus
333.3   Tics of organic origin
333.72   Acute dystonia due to drugs
333.79   Other acquired torsion dystonia
333.82   Orofacial dyskinesia
333.83   Spasmodic torticollis
333.84   Organic writers' cramp
333.85   Subacute dyskinesia due to drugs
333.89   Other fragments of torsion dystonia
333.91   Stiff-man syndrome
333.92   Neuroleptic malignant syndrome
333.93   Benign shuddering attacks
336.1   Vascular myelopathies
336.2   Subacute combined degeneration of spinal cord in diseases classified elsewhere
336.3   Myelopathy in other diseases classified elsewhere
336.8   Other myelopathy
336.9   Unspecified disease of spinal cord
338.0   Central pain syndrome
338.2*   Chronic pain
338.4   Chronic pain syndrome
343.3   Monoplegic infantile cerebral palsy
343.8   Other specified infantile cerebral palsy
343.9   Unspecified infantile cerebral palsy
344.3*   Monoplegia of lower limb
344.4*   Monoplegia of upper limb
344.5   Unspecified monoplegia
344.8*   Other specified paralytic syndromes
344.9   Unspecified paralysis
347*   Cataplexy and narcolepsy
348.0   Cerebral cysts
348.1   Anoxic brain damage
349.1   Nervous system complications from surgically implanted device
349.2   Disorders of meninges, not elsewhere classified
349.81   Cerebrospinal fluid rhinorrhea
349.82   Toxic encephalopathy
356.3   Refsum's disease
359.0   Congenital hereditary muscular dystrophy
359.1   Hereditary progressive muscular dystrophy
359.21   Myotonic muscular dystrophy
359.22   Myotonia congenita
359.23   Myotonic chondrodystrophy
359.24   Drug-induced myotonia
359.29   Other specified myotonic disorder
359.3   Periodic paralysis
359.4   Toxic myopathy
359.5   Myopathy in endocrine diseases classified elsewhere

359.6	Symptomatic inflammatory myopathy in diseases classified elsewhere
359.81	Critical illness myopathy
359.89	Other myopathies
359.9	Unspecified myopathy
377.00	Unspecified papilledema
377.01	Papilledema associated with increased intracranial pressure
377.04	Foster-Kennedy syndrome
377.5*	Disorders of optic chiasm
377.6*	Disorders of other visual pathways
377.7*	Disorders of visual cortex
377.9	Unspecified disorder of optic nerve and visual pathways
378.86	Internuclear ophthalmoplegia
388.61	Cerebrospinal fluid otorrhea
437.3	Cerebral aneurysm, nonruptured
437.5	Moyamoya disease
437.6	Nonpyogenic thrombosis of intracranial venous sinus
740*	Anencephalus and similar anomalies
741*	Spina bifida
742*	Other congenital anomalies of nervous system
747.81	Congenital anomaly of cerebrovascular system
747.82	Congenital spinal vessel anomaly
756.17	Spina bifida occulta
759.5	Tuberous sclerosis
779.7	Periventricular leukomalacia
781.0	Abnormal involuntary movements
781.1	Disturbances of sensation of smell and taste
781.2	Abnormality of gait
781.3	Lack of coordination
781.4	Transient paralysis of limb
781.6	Meningismus
781.8	Neurological neglect syndrome
781.91	Loss of height
781.92	Abnormal posture
781.94	Facial weakness
781.99	Other symptoms involving nervous and musculoskeletal systems
782.0	Disturbance of skin sensation
784.3	Aphasia
784.5*	Other speech disturbance
792.0	Nonspecific abnormal finding in cerebrospinal fluid
793.0	Nonspecific (abnormal) findings on radiological and other examination of skull and head
794.0*	Nonspecific abnormal results of function study of brain and central nervous system
794.10	Nonspecific abnormal response to unspecified nerve stimulation
794.19	Other nonspecific abnormal result of function study of peripheral nervous system and special senses
796.1	Abnormal reflex
798.0	Sudden infant death syndrome
799.53	Visuospatial deficit
905.0	Late effect of fracture of skull and face bones
907.0	Late effect of intracranial injury without mention of skull fracture
907.1	Late effect of injury to cranial nerve
907.3	Late effect of injury to nerve root(s), spinal plexus(es), and other nerves of trunk
907.4	Late effect of injury to peripheral nerve of shoulder girdle and upper limb
907.5	Late effect of injury to peripheral nerve of pelvic girdle and lower limb
907.9	Late effect of injury to other and unspecified nerve
950.1	Injury to optic chiasm
950.2	Injury to optic pathways
950.3	Injury to visual cortex
950.9	Injury to unspecified optic nerve and pathways
996.2	Mechanical complication of nervous system device, implant, and graft

996.63	Infection and inflammatory reaction due to nervous system device, implant, and graft
996.75	Other complications due to nervous system device, implant, and graft
997.0*	Nervous system complications
V53.0*	Fitting and adjustment of devices related to nervous system and special senses

DRG 092 Other Disorders of Nervous System with CC
GMLOS 3.1   AMLOS 3.9   RW 0.8918   ☑ⓣ

Select principal diagnosis listed under DRG 091

DRG 093 Other Disorders of Nervous System without CC/MCC
GMLOS 2.2   AMLOS 2.7   RW 0.6614   ☑ⓣ

Select principal diagnosis listed under DRG 091

DRG 094 Bacterial and Tuberculous Infections of Nervous System with MCC
GMLOS 8.3   AMLOS 10.8   RW 3.4974

Principal Diagnosis

003.21	Salmonella meningitis
013*	Tuberculosis of meninges and central nervous system
036.0	Meningococcal meningitis
036.1	Meningococcal encephalitis
098.82	Gonococcal meningitis
320*	Bacterial meningitis
324*	Intracranial and intraspinal abscess
357.0	Acute infective polyneuritis

DRG 095 Bacterial and Tuberculous Infections of Nervous System with CC
GMLOS 6.2   AMLOS 7.7   RW 2.2787   ☑

Select principal diagnosis listed under DRG 094

DRG 096 Bacterial and Tuberculous Infections of Nervous System without CC/MCC
GMLOS 4.5   AMLOS 5.4   RW 1.9694   ☑

Select principal diagnosis listed under DRG 094

DRG 097 Nonbacterial Infections of Nervous System Except Viral Meningitis with MCC
GMLOS 8.5   AMLOS 11.0   RW 3.1963   ☑

Principal Diagnosis

006.5	Amebic brain abscess
045.0*	Acute paralytic poliomyelitis specified as bulbar
045.1*	Acute poliomyelitis with other paralysis
045.9*	Acute unspecified poliomyelitis
049.8	Other specified non-arthropod-borne viral diseases of central nervous system
049.9	Unspecified non-arthropod-borne viral disease of central nervous system
052.0	Postvaricella encephalitis
052.2	Postvaricella myelitis
053.14	Herpes zoster myelitis
054.3	Herpetic meningoencephalitis
054.74	Herpes simplex myelitis
055.0	Postmeasles encephalitis
056.01	Encephalomyelitis due to rubella
056.09	Other neurological rubella complications
058.21	Human herpesvirus 6 encephalitis
058.29	Other human herpesvirus encephalitis
062*	Mosquito-borne viral encephalitis
063*	Tick-borne viral encephalitis

MDC 1: Diseases And Disorders Of The Nervous System—MEDICAL

064	Viral encephalitis transmitted by other and unspecified arthropods	
066.2	Venezuelan equine fever	
071	Rabies	
072.2	Mumps encephalitis	
090.4*	Juvenile neurosyphilis	
091.81	Early syphilis, acute syphilitic meningitis (secondary)	
094.2	Syphilitic meningitis	
094.3	Asymptomatic neurosyphilis	
094.81	Syphilitic encephalitis	
100.8*	Other specified leptospiral infections	
112.83	Candidal meningitis	
114.2	Coccidioidal meningitis	
115.01	Histoplasma capsulatum meningitis	
115.11	Histoplasma duboisii meningitis	
115.91	Unspecified Histoplasmosis meningitis	
130.0	Meningoencephalitis due to toxoplasmosis	
321*	Meningitis due to other organisms	
322*	Meningitis of unspecified cause	
323.0*	Encephalitis, myelitis, and encephalomyelitis in viral diseases classified elsewhere	
323.1	Encephalitis, myelitis, and encephalomyelitis in rickettsial diseases classified elsewhere	
323.2	Encephalitis, myelitis, and encephalomyelitis in protozoal diseases classified elsewhere	
323.4*	Other encephalitis, myelitis, and encephalomyelitis due to other infections classified elsewhere	
323.5*	Encephalitis, myelitis, and encephalomyelitis following immunization procedures	
323.6*	Postinfectious encephalitis, myelitis, and encephalomyelitis	
323.8*	Other causes of encephalitis, myelitis, and encephalomyelitis	
323.9	Unspecified causes of encephalitis, myelitis, and encephalomyelitis	
341.2*	Acute (transverse) myelitis	

DRG 098 **Nonbacterial Infections of Nervous System Except Viral Meningitis with CC**

GMLOS 5.8   AMLOS 7.4   RW 1.7657   ☑

Select principal diagnosis listed under DRG 097

DRG 099 **Nonbacterial Infections of Nervous System Except Viral Meningitis without CC/MCC**

GMLOS 4.1   AMLOS 5.0   RW 1.1835   ☑

Select principal diagnosis listed under DRG 097

DRG 100 **Seizures with MCC**

GMLOS 4.2   AMLOS 5.7   RW 1.5185   ☑ⓣ

Principal Diagnosis
345*	Epilepsy and recurrent seizures
780.3*	Convulsions

DRG 101 **Seizures without MCC**

GMLOS 2.6   AMLOS 3.3   RW 0.7569   ☑ⓣ

Select principal diagnosis listed under DRG 100

DRG 102 **Headaches with MCC**

GMLOS 3.1   AMLOS 4.2   RW 1.0430   ☑

Principal Diagnosis
307.81	Tension headache
310.2	Postconcussion syndrome
339*	Other headache syndromes
346*	Migraine
348.2	Benign intracranial hypertension

349.0	Reaction to spinal or lumbar puncture
437.4	Cerebral arteritis
784.0	Headache

DRG 103 **Headaches without MCC**

GMLOS 2.3   AMLOS 2.9   RW 0.6663   ☑

Select principal diagnosis listed under DRG 102

ⓣ *Transfer DRG*   ⓢ *Special Payment*   ☑ *Optimization Potential*   ⓦ *Targeted Potential*   * *Code Range*   ● *New DRG*   ▲ *Revised DRG Title*

MDC 2
Diseases And Disorders Of The Eye

017.30	224.3	361.02	362.64	364.21	365.74	368.30	369.8	371.53
017.31	224.4	361.03	362.65	364.22	365.81	368.31	369.9	371.54
017.32	224.5	361.04	362.66	364.23	365.82	368.32	370.00	371.55
017.33	224.6	361.05	362.70	364.24	365.83	368.33	370.01	371.56
017.34	224.7	361.06	362.71	364.3	365.89	368.34	370.02	371.57
017.35	224.8	361.07	362.72	364.41	365.9	368.40	370.03	371.58
017.36	224.9	361.10	362.73	364.42	366.00	368.41	370.04	371.60
032.81	228.03	361.11	362.74	364.51	366.01	368.42	370.05	371.61
036.81	232.1	361.12	362.75	364.52	366.02	368.43	370.06	371.62
053.20	234.0	361.13	362.76	364.53	366.03	368.44	370.07	371.70
053.21	249.50	361.14	362.77	364.54	366.04	368.45	370.20	371.71
053.22	249.51	361.19	362.81	364.55	366.09	368.46	370.21	371.72
053.29	250.50	361.2	362.82	364.56	366.10	368.47	370.22	371.73
054.40	250.51	361.30	362.83	364.57	366.11	368.51	370.23	371.81
054.41	250.52	361.31	362.84	364.59	366.12	368.52	370.24	371.82
054.42	250.53	361.32	362.85	364.60	366.13	368.53	370.31	371.89
054.43	264.0	361.33	362.89	364.61	366.14	368.54	370.32	371.9
054.44	264.1	361.81	362.9	364.62	366.15	368.55	370.33	372.00
054.49	264.2	361.89	363.00	364.63	366.16	368.59	370.34	372.01
055.71	264.3	361.9	363.01	364.64	366.17	368.60	370.35	372.02
076.0	264.4	362.01	363.03	364.70	366.18	368.61	370.40	372.03
076.1	264.5	362.02	363.04	364.71	366.19	368.62	370.44	372.04
076.9	264.6	362.03	363.05	364.72	366.20	368.63	370.49	372.05
077.0	264.7	362.04	363.06	364.73	366.21	368.69	370.50	372.06
077.1	333.81	362.05	363.07	364.74	366.22	368.8	370.52	372.10
077.2	360.00	362.06	363.08	364.75	366.23	368.9	370.54	372.11
077.3	360.01	362.07	363.10	364.76	366.30	369.00	370.55	372.12
077.4	360.02	362.10	363.11	364.77	366.31	369.01	370.59	372.13
077.8	360.03	362.11	363.12	364.81	366.32	369.02	370.60	372.14
077.98	360.04	362.12	363.13	364.82	366.33	369.03	370.61	372.15
077.99	360.11	362.13	363.14	364.89	366.34	369.04	370.62	372.20
090.3	360.12	362.14	363.15	364.9	366.41	369.05	370.63	372.21
091.50	360.13	362.15	363.20	365.00	366.42	369.06	370.64	372.22
091.51	360.14	362.16	363.21	365.01	366.43	369.07	370.8	372.30
091.52	360.19	362.17	363.22	365.02	366.44	369.08	370.9	372.31
094.83	360.20	362.18	363.30	365.03	366.45	369.10	371.00	372.33
094.84	360.21	362.20	363.31	365.04	366.46	369.11	371.01	372.34
095.0	360.23	362.21	363.32	365.05	366.50	369.12	371.02	372.39
098.40	360.24	362.22	363.33	365.06	366.51	369.13	371.03	372.40
098.41	360.29	362.23	363.34	365.10	366.52	369.14	371.04	372.41
098.42	360.30	362.24	363.35	365.11	366.53	369.15	371.05	372.42
098.43	360.31	362.25	363.40	365.12	366.8	369.16	371.10	372.43
098.49	360.32	362.26	363.41	365.13	366.9	369.17	371.11	372.44
098.81	360.33	362.27	363.42	365.14	367.0	369.18	371.12	372.45
115.02	360.34	362.29	363.43	365.15	367.1	369.20	371.13	372.50
115.12	360.40	362.30	363.50	365.20	367.20	369.21	371.14	372.51
115.92	360.41	362.31	363.51	365.21	367.21	369.22	371.15	372.52
130.1	360.42	362.32	363.52	365.22	367.22	369.23	371.16	372.53
130.2	360.43	362.33	363.53	365.23	367.31	369.24	371.20	372.54
139.1	360.44	362.34	363.54	365.24	367.32	369.25	371.21	372.55
172.1	360.50	362.35	363.55	365.31	367.4	369.3	371.22	372.56
173.10	360.51	362.36	363.56	365.32	367.51	369.4	371.23	372.61
173.11	360.52	362.37	363.57	365.41	367.52	369.60	371.24	372.62
173.12	360.53	362.40	363.61	365.42	367.53	369.61	371.30	372.63
173.19	360.54	362.41	363.62	365.43	367.81	369.62	371.31	372.64
190.0	360.55	362.42	363.63	365.44	367.89	369.63	371.32	372.71
190.1	360.59	362.43	363.70	365.51	367.9	369.64	371.33	372.72
190.2	360.60	362.50	363.71	365.52	368.00	369.65	371.40	372.73
190.3	360.61	362.51	363.72	365.59	368.01	369.66	371.41	372.74
190.4	360.62	362.52	363.8	365.60	368.02	369.67	371.42	372.75
190.5	360.63	362.53	363.9	365.61	368.03	369.68	371.43	372.81
190.6	360.64	362.54	364.00	365.62	368.10	369.69	371.44	372.89
190.7	360.65	362.55	364.01	365.63	368.11	369.70	371.45	372.9
190.8	360.69	362.56	364.02	365.64	368.12	369.71	371.46	373.00
190.9	360.81	362.57	364.03	365.65	368.13	369.72	371.48	373.01
216.1	360.89	362.60	364.04	365.70	368.14	369.73	371.49	373.02
224.0	360.9	362.61	364.05	365.71	368.15	369.74	371.50	373.11
224.1	361.00	362.62	364.10	365.72	368.16	369.75	371.51	373.12
224.2	361.01	362.63	364.11	365.73	368.2	369.76	371.52	373.13

373.2	374.56	375.89	377.12	378.23	379.05	379.60	743.53	918.2
373.31	374.81	375.9	377.13	378.24	379.06	379.61	743.54	918.9
373.32	374.82	376.00	377.14	378.30	379.07	379.62	743.55	921.0
373.33	374.83	376.01	377.15	378.31	379.09	379.63	743.56	921.1
373.34	374.84	376.02	377.16	378.32	379.11	379.8	743.57	921.2
373.4	374.85	376.03	377.21	378.33	379.12	379.90	743.58	921.3
373.5	374.86	376.04	377.22	378.34	379.13	379.91	743.59	921.9
373.6	374.87	376.10	377.23	378.35	379.14	379.92	743.61	930.0
373.8	374.89	376.11	377.24	378.40	379.15	379.93	743.62	930.1
373.9	374.9	376.12	377.30	378.41	379.16	379.99	743.63	930.2
374.00	375.00	376.13	377.31	378.42	379.19	694.61	743.64	930.8
374.01	375.01	376.21	377.32	378.43	379.21	743.00	743.65	930.9
374.02	375.02	376.22	377.33	378.44	379.22	743.03	743.66	940.0
374.03	375.03	376.30	377.34	378.45	379.23	743.06	743.69	940.1
374.04	375.11	376.31	377.39	378.50	379.24	743.10	743.8	940.2
374.05	375.12	376.32	377.41	378.51	379.25	743.11	743.9	940.3
374.10	375.13	376.33	377.42	378.52	379.26	743.12	794.11	940.4
374.11	375.14	376.34	377.43	378.53	379.27	743.20	794.12	940.5
374.12	375.15	376.35	377.49	378.54	379.29	743.21	794.13	940.9
374.13	375.16	376.36	378.00	378.55	379.31	743.22	794.14	941.02
374.14	375.20	376.40	378.01	378.56	379.32	743.30	802.6	941.12
374.20	375.21	376.41	378.02	378.60	379.33	743.31	802.7	941.22
374.21	375.22	376.42	378.03	378.61	379.34	743.32	870.0	941.32
374.22	375.30	376.43	378.04	378.62	379.39	743.33	870.1	941.42
374.23	375.31	376.44	378.05	378.63	379.40	743.34	870.2	941.52
374.30	375.32	376.45	378.06	378.71	379.41	743.35	870.3	950.0
374.31	375.33	376.46	378.07	378.72	379.42	743.36	870.4	976.5
374.32	375.41	376.47	378.08	378.73	379.43	743.37	870.8	996.51
374.33	375.42	376.50	378.10	378.81	379.46	743.39	870.9	996.53
374.34	375.43	376.51	378.11	378.82	379.49	743.41	871.0	998.82
374.41	375.51	376.52	378.12	378.83	379.50	743.42	871.1	V42.5
374.43	375.52	376.6	378.13	378.84	379.51	743.43	871.2	V43.0
374.44	375.53	376.81	378.14	378.85	379.52	743.44	871.3	V43.1
374.45	375.54	376.82	378.15	378.87	379.53	743.45	871.4	V45.78
374.46	375.55	376.89	378.16	378.9	379.54	743.46	871.5	
374.50	375.56	376.9	378.17	379.00	379.55	743.47	871.6	
374.52	375.57	377.02	378.18	379.01	379.56	743.48	871.7	
374.53	375.61	377.03	378.20	379.02	379.57	743.49	871.9	
374.54	375.69	377.10	378.21	379.03	379.58	743.51	918.0	
374.55	375.81	377.11	378.22	379.04	379.59	743.52	918.1	

SURGICAL

DRG 113   Orbital Procedures with CC/MCC
GMLOS 4.0   AMLOS 5.6   RW 1.8998

Operating Room Procedures
16.0*	Orbitotomy
16.22	Diagnostic aspiration of orbit
16.23	Biopsy of eyeball and orbit
16.29	Other diagnostic procedures on orbit and eyeball
16.3*	Evisceration of eyeball
16.4*	Enucleation of eyeball
16.5*	Exenteration of orbital contents
16.6*	Secondary procedures after removal of eyeball
16.7*	Removal of ocular or orbital implant
16.8*	Repair of injury of eyeball and orbit
16.92	Excision of lesion of orbit
16.98	Other operations on orbit
76.46	Other reconstruction of other facial bone
76.79	Other open reduction of facial fracture
76.91	Bone graft to facial bone
76.92	Insertion of synthetic implant in facial bone

DRG 114   Orbital Procedures without CC/MCC
GMLOS 2.3   AMLOS 2.9   RW 1.0216   ☑

Select operating room procedures listed under DRG 113

DRG 115   Extraocular Procedures Except Orbit
GMLOS 3.2   AMLOS 4.3   RW 1.2543   ☑

Operating Room Procedures
08.11	Biopsy of eyelid
08.2*	Excision or destruction of lesion or tissue of eyelid
08.3*	Repair of blepharoptosis and lid retraction
08.4*	Repair of entropion or ectropion
08.5*	Other adjustment of lid position
08.6*	Reconstruction of eyelid with flaps or grafts
08.7*	Other reconstruction of eyelid
08.9*	Other operations on eyelids
09*	Operations on lacrimal system
10*	Operations on conjunctiva
11.0	Magnetic removal of embedded foreign body from cornea
11.2*	Diagnostic procedures on cornea
11.3*	Excision of pterygium
11.4*	Excision or destruction of tissue or other lesion of cornea
11.61	Lamellar keratoplasty with autograft
11.62	Other lamellar keratoplasty
11.71	Keratomileusis
11.72	Keratophakia
11.74	Thermokeratoplasty
11.76	Epikeratophakia
11.91	Tattooing of cornea
12.84	Excision or destruction of lesion of sclera
12.87	Scleral reinforcement with graft
12.88	Other scleral reinforcement
12.89	Other operations on sclera
14.6	Removal of surgically implanted material from posterior segment of eye
15*	Operations on extraocular muscles
16.93	Excision of lesion of eye, unspecified structure
16.99	Other operations on eyeball
38.21	Biopsy of blood vessel
86.22	Excisional debridement of wound, infection, or burn
86.4	Radical excision of skin lesion
95.04	Eye examination under anesthesia

DRG 116   Intraocular Procedures with CC/MCC
GMLOS 3.2   AMLOS 4.8   RW 1.4806

Operating Room Procedures
11.1	Incision of cornea
11.5*	Repair of cornea
11.60	Corneal transplant, not otherwise specified
11.63	Penetrating keratoplasty with autograft
11.64	Other penetrating keratoplasty
11.69	Other corneal transplant
11.73	Keratoprosthesis
11.75	Radial keratotomy
11.79	Other reconstructive surgery on cornea
11.92	Removal of artificial implant from cornea
11.99	Other operations on cornea
12.0*	Removal of intraocular foreign body from anterior segment of eye
12.1*	Iridotomy and simple iridectomy
12.21	Diagnostic aspiration of anterior chamber of eye
12.22	Biopsy of iris
12.29	Other diagnostic procedures on iris, ciliary body, sclera, and anterior chamber
12.31	Lysis of goniosynechiae
12.32	Lysis of other anterior synechiae
12.33	Lysis of posterior synechiae
12.34	Lysis of corneovitreal adhesions
12.35	Coreoplasty
12.39	Other iridoplasty
12.40	Removal of lesion of anterior segment of eye, not otherwise specified
12.41	Destruction of lesion of iris, nonexcisional
12.42	Excision of lesion of iris
12.43	Destruction of lesion of ciliary body, nonexcisional
12.44	Excision of lesion of ciliary body
12.51	Goniopuncture without goniotomy
12.52	Goniotomy without goniopuncture
12.53	Goniotomy with goniopuncture
12.54	Trabeculotomy ab externo
12.55	Cyclodialysis
12.59	Other facilitation of intraocular circulation
12.6*	Scleral fistulization
12.7*	Other procedures for relief of elevated intraocular pressure
12.81	Suture of laceration of sclera
12.82	Repair of scleral fistula
12.83	Revision of operative wound of anterior segment, not elsewhere classified
12.85	Repair of scleral staphyloma with graft
12.86	Other repair of scleral staphyloma
12.91	Therapeutic evacuation of anterior chamber
12.92	Injection into anterior chamber
12.93	Removal or destruction of epithelial downgrowth from anterior chamber
12.97	Other operations on iris
12.98	Other operations on ciliary body
12.99	Other operations on anterior chamber
13*	Operations on lens
14.0*	Removal of foreign body from posterior segment of eye
14.1*	Diagnostic procedures on retina, choroid, vitreous, and posterior chamber
14.21	Destruction of chorioretinal lesion by diathermy
14.22	Destruction of chorioretinal lesion by cryotherapy
14.26	Destruction of chorioretinal lesion by radiation therapy
14.27	Destruction of chorioretinal lesion by implantation of radiation source
14.29	Other destruction of chorioretinal lesion
14.31	Repair of retinal tear by diathermy
14.32	Repair of retinal tear by cryotherapy
14.39	Other repair of retinal tear
14.4*	Repair of retinal detachment with scleral buckling and implant

14.5*	Other repair of retinal detachment
14.7*	Operations on vitreous
14.8*	Implantation of epiretinal visual prosthesis
14.9	Other operations on retina, choroid, and posterior chamber
16.1	Removal of penetrating foreign body from eye, not otherwise specified

DRG 117 Intraocular Procedures without CC/MCC
GMLOS 1.8   **AMLOS 2.4**   **RW 0.8211**   ☑

Select operating room procedures listed under DRG 116

MEDICAL

DRG 121 Acute Major Eye Infections with CC/MCC
GMLOS 3.9   **AMLOS 4.8**   **RW 1.0215**   ☑

Principal Diagnosis

360.00	Unspecified purulent endophthalmitis
360.01	Acute endophthalmitis
360.02	Panophthalmitis
360.04	Vitreous abscess
360.13	Parasitic endophthalmitis NOS
360.19	Other endophthalmitis
370.00	Unspecified corneal ulcer
370.03	Central corneal ulcer
370.04	Hypopyon ulcer
370.05	Mycotic corneal ulcer
370.06	Perforated corneal ulcer
370.55	Corneal abscess
375.01	Acute dacryoadenitis
375.31	Acute canaliculitis, lacrimal
375.32	Acute dacryocystitis
376.01	Orbital cellulitis
376.02	Orbital periostitis
376.03	Orbital osteomyelitis
376.04	Orbital tenonitis

DRG 122 Acute Major Eye Infections without CC/MCC
GMLOS 2.9   **AMLOS 3.5**   **RW 0.6147**   ☑

Select principal diagnosis listed under DRG 121

DRG 123 Neurological Eye Disorders
GMLOS 2.2   **AMLOS 2.7**   **RW 0.6963**   ☑

Principal Diagnosis

036.81	Meningococcal optic neuritis
362.3*	Retinal vascular occlusion
365.12	Low tension open-angle glaucoma
367.52	Total or complete internal ophthalmoplegia
368.11	Sudden visual loss
368.12	Transient visual loss
368.2	Diplopia
368.40	Unspecified visual field defect
368.41	Scotoma involving central area in visual field
368.43	Sector or arcuate defects in visual field
368.44	Other localized visual field defect
368.45	Generalized contraction or constriction in visual field
368.46	Homonymous bilateral field defects in visual field
368.47	Heteronymous bilateral field defects in visual field
368.55	Acquired color vision deficiencies
374.30	Unspecified ptosis of eyelid
374.31	Paralytic ptosis
374.32	Myogenic ptosis
374.45	Other sensorimotor disorders of eyelid
376.34	Intermittent exophthalmos

376.35	Pulsating exophthalmos
376.36	Lateral displacement of globe of eye
376.82	Myopathy of extraocular muscles
377.10	Unspecified optic atrophy
377.11	Primary optic atrophy
377.12	Postinflammatory optic atrophy
377.15	Partial optic atrophy
377.16	Hereditary optic atrophy
377.21	Drusen of optic disc
377.24	Pseudopapilledema
377.3*	Optic neuritis
377.4*	Other disorders of optic nerve
378.5*	Paralytic strabismus
378.72	Progressive external ophthalmoplegia
378.73	Strabismus in other neuromuscular disorders
378.87	Other dissociated deviation of eye movements
379.40	Unspecified abnormal pupillary function
379.41	Anisocoria
379.42	Miosis (persistent), not due to miotics
379.43	Mydriasis (persistent), not due to mydriatics
379.46	Tonic pupillary reaction
379.49	Other anomaly of pupillary function
379.50	Unspecified nystagmus
379.52	Latent nystagmus
379.54	Nystagmus associated with disorders of the vestibular system
379.55	Dissociated nystagmus
379.57	Nystagmus with deficiencies of saccadic eye movements
379.58	Nystagmus with deficiencies of smooth pursuit movements

DRG 124 Other Disorders of the Eye with MCC
GMLOS 3.7   **AMLOS 5.1**   **RW 1.1990**

Principal Diagnosis

017.3*	Tuberculosis of eye
032.81	Conjunctival diphtheria
053.2*	Herpes zoster with ophthalmic complications
054.4*	Herpes simplex with ophthalmic complications
055.71	Measles keratoconjunctivitis
076*	Trachoma
077*	Other diseases of conjunctiva due to viruses and Chlamydiae
090.3	Syphilitic interstitial keratitis
091.5*	Early syphilis, uveitis due to secondary syphilis
094.83	Syphilitic disseminated retinochoroiditis
094.84	Syphilitic optic atrophy
095.0	Syphilitic episcleritis
098.4*	Gonococcal infection of eye
098.81	Gonococcal keratosis (blennorrhagica)
115.02	Histoplasma capsulatum retinitis
115.12	Histoplasma duboisii retinitis
115.92	Unspecified Histoplasmosis retinitis
130.1	Conjunctivitis due to toxoplasmosis
130.2	Chorioretinitis due to toxoplasmosis
139.1	Late effects of trachoma
172.1	Malignant melanoma of skin of eyelid, including canthus
173.1*	Other and unspecified malignant neoplasm of eyelid, including canthus
190*	Malignant neoplasm of eye
216.1	Benign neoplasm of eyelid, including canthus
224*	Benign neoplasm of eye
228.03	Hemangioma of retina
232.1	Carcinoma in situ of eyelid, including canthus
234.0	Carcinoma in situ of eye
249.5*	Secondary diabetes mellitus with ophthalmic manifestations
250.5*	Diabetes with ophthalmic manifestations
264.0	Vitamin A deficiency with conjunctival xerosis
264.1	Vitamin A deficiency with conjunctival xerosis and Bitot's spot
264.2	Vitamin A deficiency with corneal xerosis

MDC 2: Diseases And Disorders Of The Eye—MEDICAL

Ⓣ *Transfer DRG*   ⓈⓅ *Special Payment*   ☑ *Optimization Potential*   ⓋⓅ *Targeted Potential*   * *Code Range*   ● *New DRG*   ▲ *Revised DRG Title*

264.3	Vitamin A deficiency with corneal ulceration and xerosis
264.4	Vitamin A deficiency with keratomalacia
264.5	Vitamin A deficiency with night blindness
264.6	Vitamin A deficiency with xerophthalmic scars of cornea
264.7	Other ocular manifestations of vitamin A deficiency
333.81	Blepharospasm
360.03	Chronic endophthalmitis
360.11	Sympathetic uveitis
360.12	Panuveitis
360.14	Ophthalmia nodosa
360.2*	Degenerative disorders of globe
360.3*	Hypotony of eye
360.4*	Degenerated conditions of globe
360.5*	Retained (old) intraocular foreign body, magnetic
360.6*	Retained (old) intraocular foreign body, nonmagnetic
360.8*	Other disorders of globe
360.9	Unspecified disorder of globe
361.0*	Retinal detachment with retinal defect
361.1*	Retinoschisis and retinal cysts
361.2	Serous retinal detachment
361.3*	Retinal defects without detachment
361.8*	Other forms of retinal detachment
361.9	Unspecified retinal detachment
362.0*	Diabetic retinopathy
362.1*	Other background retinopathy and retinal vascular changes
362.2*	Other proliferative retinopathy
362.4*	Separation of retinal layers
362.5*	Degeneration of macula and posterior pole of retina
362.6*	Peripheral retinal degenerations
362.7*	Hereditary retinal dystrophies
362.8*	Other retinal disorders
362.9	Unspecified retinal disorder
363*	Chorioretinal inflammations, scars, and other disorders of choroid
364.0*	Acute and subacute iridocyclitis
364.1*	Chronic iridocyclitis
364.2*	Certain types of iridocyclitis
364.3	Unspecified iridocyclitis
364.41	Hyphema
364.42	Rubeosis iridis
364.5*	Degenerations of iris and ciliary body
364.6*	Cysts of iris, ciliary body, and anterior chamber
364.7*	Adhesions and disruptions of iris and ciliary body
364.8*	Other disorders of iris and ciliary body
364.9	Unspecified disorder of iris and ciliary body
365.0*	Borderline glaucoma (glaucoma suspect)
365.10	Unspecified open-angle glaucoma
365.11	Primary open-angle glaucoma
365.13	Pigmentary open-angle glaucoma
365.14	Open-angle glaucoma of childhood
365.15	Residual stage of open angle glaucoma
365.2*	Primary angle-closure glaucoma
365.3*	Corticosteroid-induced glaucoma
365.4*	Glaucoma associated with congenital anomalies, dystrophies, and systemic syndromes
365.5*	Glaucoma associated with disorders of the lens
365.6*	Glaucoma associated with other ocular disorders
365.7*	Glaucoma stage
365.8*	Other specified forms of glaucoma
365.9	Unspecified glaucoma
366*	Cataract
367.0	Hypermetropia
367.1	Myopia
367.2*	Astigmatism
367.3*	Anisometropia and aniseikonia
367.4	Presbyopia
367.51	Paresis of accommodation
367.53	Spasm of accommodation
367.8*	Other disorders of refraction and accommodation
367.9	Unspecified disorder of refraction and accommodation
368.0*	Amblyopia ex anopsia
368.10	Unspecified subjective visual disturbance
368.13	Visual discomfort
368.14	Visual distortions of shape and size
368.15	Other visual distortions and entoptic phenomena
368.16	Psychophysical visual disturbances
368.3*	Other disorders of binocular vision
368.42	Scotoma of blind spot area in visual field
368.51	Protan defect in color vision
368.52	Deutan defect in color vision
368.53	Tritan defect in color vision
368.54	Achromatopsia
368.59	Other color vision deficiencies
368.6*	Night blindness
368.8	Other specified visual disturbances
368.9	Unspecified visual disturbance
369*	Blindness and low vision
370.01	Marginal corneal ulcer
370.02	Ring corneal ulcer
370.07	Mooren's ulcer
370.2*	Superficial keratitis without conjunctivitis
370.3*	Certain types of keratoconjunctivitis
370.4*	Other and unspecified keratoconjunctivitis
370.50	Unspecified interstitial keratitis
370.52	Diffuse interstitial keratitis
370.54	Sclerosing keratitis
370.59	Other interstitial and deep keratitis
370.6*	Corneal neovascularization
370.8	Other forms of keratitis
370.9	Unspecified keratitis
371*	Corneal opacity and other disorders of cornea
372*	Disorders of conjunctiva
373*	Inflammation of eyelids
374.0*	Entropion and trichiasis of eyelid
374.1*	Ectropion
374.2*	Lagophthalmos
374.33	Mechanical ptosis
374.34	Blepharochalasis
374.41	Eyelid retraction or lag
374.43	Abnormal innervation syndrome of eyelid
374.44	Sensory disorders of eyelid
374.46	Blepharophimosis
374.50	Unspecified degenerative disorder of eyelid
374.52	Hyperpigmentation of eyelid
374.53	Hypopigmentation of eyelid
374.54	Hypertrichosis of eyelid
374.55	Hypotrichosis of eyelid
374.56	Other degenerative disorders of skin affecting eyelid
374.8*	Other disorders of eyelid
374.9	Unspecified disorder of eyelid
375.00	Unspecified dacryoadenitis
375.02	Chronic dacryoadenitis
375.03	Chronic enlargement of lacrimal gland
375.1*	Other disorders of lacrimal gland
375.2*	Epiphora
375.30	Unspecified dacryocystitis
375.33	Phlegmonous dacryocystitis
375.4*	Chronic inflammation of lacrimal passages
375.5*	Stenosis and insufficiency of lacrimal passages
375.6*	Other changes of lacrimal passages
375.8*	Other disorders of lacrimal system
375.9	Unspecified disorder of lacrimal system
376.00	Unspecified acute inflammation of orbit
376.1*	Chronic inflammatory disorders of orbit
376.2*	Endocrine exophthalmos
376.30	Unspecified exophthalmos
376.31	Constant exophthalmos
376.32	Orbital hemorrhage
376.33	Orbital edema or congestion
376.4*	Deformity of orbit

Surgical ◢	Medical ◢	CC Indicator ◢	MCC Indicator ◢	Procedure Proxy ◢

MDC 2: Diseases And Disorders Of The Eye—MEDICAL

MDC 2: Diseases And Disorders Of The Eye—MEDICAL

376.5*	Enophthalmos
376.6	Retained (old) foreign body following penetrating wound of orbit
376.81	Orbital cysts
376.89	Other orbital disorder
376.9	Unspecified disorder of orbit
377.02	Papilledema associated with decreased ocular pressure
377.03	Papilledema associated with retinal disorder
377.13	Optic atrophy associated with retinal dystrophies
377.14	Glaucomatous atrophy (cupping) of optic disc
377.22	Crater-like holes of optic disc
377.23	Coloboma of optic disc
378.0*	Esotropia
378.1*	Exotropia
378.2*	Intermittent heterotropia
378.3*	Other and unspecified heterotropia
378.4*	Heterophoria
378.6*	Mechanical strabismus
378.71	Duane's syndrome
378.81	Palsy of conjugate gaze
378.82	Spasm of conjugate gaze
378.83	Convergence insufficiency or palsy in binocular eye movement
378.84	Convergence excess or spasm in binocular eye movement
378.85	Anomalies of divergence in binocular eye movement
378.9	Unspecified disorder of eye movements
379.0*	Scleritis and episcleritis
379.1*	Other disorders of sclera
379.2*	Disorders of vitreous body
379.3*	Aphakia and other disorders of lens
379.51	Congenital nystagmus
379.53	Visual deprivation nystagmus
379.56	Other forms of nystagmus
379.59	Other irregularities of eye movements
379.6*	Inflammation (infection) of postprocedural bleb
379.8	Other specified disorders of eye and adnexa
379.9*	Unspecified disorder of eye and adnexa
694.61	Benign mucous membrane pemphigoid with ocular involvement
743*	Congenital anomalies of eye
794.11	Nonspecific abnormal retinal function studies
794.12	Nonspecific abnormal electro-oculogram (EOG)
794.13	Nonspecific abnormal visually evoked potential
794.14	Nonspecific abnormal oculomotor studies
802.6	Orbital floor (blow-out), closed fracture
802.7	Orbital floor (blow-out), open fracture
870*	Open wound of ocular adnexa
871*	Open wound of eyeball
918*	Superficial injury of eye and adnexa
921.0	Black eye, not otherwise specified
921.1	Contusion of eyelids and periocular area
921.2	Contusion of orbital tissues
921.3	Contusion of eyeball
921.9	Unspecified contusion of eye
930*	Foreign body on external eye
940*	Burn confined to eye and adnexa
941.02	Burn of unspecified degree of eye (with other parts of face, head, and neck)
941.12	Erythema due to burn (first degree) of eye (with other parts face, head, and neck)
941.22	Blisters, with epidermal loss due to burn (second degree) of eye (with other parts of face, head, and neck)
941.32	Full-thickness skin loss due to burn (third degree NOS) of eye (with other parts of face, head, and neck)
941.42	Deep necrosis of underlying tissues due to burn (deep third degree) of eye (with other parts of face, head, and neck), without mention of loss of a body part
941.52	Deep necrosis of underlying tissues due to burn (deep third degree) of eye (with other parts of face, head, and neck), with loss of a body part

950.0	Optic nerve injury
976.5	Poisoning by eye anti-infectives and other eye drugs
996.51	Mechanical complication due to corneal graft
996.53	Mechanical complication due to ocular lens prosthesis
998.82	Cataract fragments in eye following surgery
V42.5	Cornea replaced by transplant
V43.0	Eye globe replaced by other means
V43.1	Lens replaced by other means
V45.78	Acquired absence of organ, eye

DRG 125   **Other Disorders of the Eye without MCC**

          GMLOS 2.5   **AMLOS 3.1**   **RW 0.6812**   ☑

Select principal diagnosis listed under DRG 124

☐ *Transfer DRG*   ☐ *Special Payment*   ☑ *Optimization Potential*   ☐ *Targeted Potential*   * *Code Range*   ● *New DRG*   ▲ *Revised DRG Title*

012.30	144.9	231.0	382.2	386.33	389.8	478.33	522.6	524.60
012.31	145.0	235.0	382.3	386.34	389.9	478.34	522.7	524.61
012.32	145.1	235.1	382.4	386.35	460	478.4	522.8	524.62
012.33	145.2	235.6	382.9	386.40	461.0	478.5	522.9	524.63
012.34	145.3	327.20	383.00	386.41	461.1	478.6	523.00	524.64
012.35	145.4	327.23	383.01	386.42	461.2	478.70	523.01	524.69
012.36	145.5	327.24	383.02	386.43	461.3	478.71	523.10	524.70
015.60	145.6	327.26	383.1	386.48	461.8	478.74	523.11	524.71
015.61	145.8	327.29	383.20	386.50	461.9	478.75	523.20	524.72
015.62	145.9	327.40	383.21	386.51	462	478.79	523.21	524.73
015.63	146.0	327.42	383.22	386.52	463	478.8	523.22	524.74
015.64	146.1	327.44	383.30	386.53	464.00	478.9	523.23	524.75
015.65	146.2	327.49	383.31	386.54	464.01	487.1	523.24	524.76
015.66	146.3	327.53	383.32	386.55	464.20	520.0	523.25	524.79
017.40	146.4	327.59	383.33	386.56	464.21	520.1	523.30	524.81
017.41	146.5	327.8	383.81	386.58	464.30	520.2	523.31	524.82
017.42	146.6	380.00	383.89	386.8	464.31	520.3	523.32	524.89
017.43	146.7	380.10	383.9	386.9	464.4	520.4	523.33	524.9
017.44	146.8	380.11	384.00	387.0	464.50	520.5	523.40	525.0
017.45	146.9	380.12	384.01	387.1	464.51	520.6	523.41	525.10
017.46	147.0	380.13	384.09	387.2	465.0	520.7	523.42	525.11
032.0	147.1	380.14	384.1	387.8	465.8	520.8	523.5	525.12
032.1	147.2	380.15	384.20	387.9	465.9	520.9	523.6	525.13
032.2	147.3	380.16	384.21	388.00	470	521.00	523.8	525.19
032.3	147.8	380.21	384.22	388.01	471.0	521.01	523.9	525.20
034.0	147.9	380.22	384.23	388.02	471.1	521.02	524.00	525.21
053.71	148.0	380.23	384.24	388.10	471.8	521.03	524.01	525.22
054.2	148.1	380.30	384.25	388.11	471.9	521.04	524.02	525.23
054.73	148.2	380.31	384.81	388.12	472.0	521.05	524.03	525.24
055.2	148.3	380.32	384.82	388.2	472.1	521.06	524.04	525.25
074.0	148.8	380.39	384.9	388.30	472.2	521.07	524.05	525.26
094.86	148.9	380.4	385.00	388.31	473.0	521.08	524.06	525.3
098.6	149.0	380.50	385.01	388.32	473.1	521.09	524.07	525.40
099.51	149.1	380.51	385.02	388.40	473.2	521.10	524.09	525.41
101	149.8	380.52	385.03	388.41	473.3	521.11	524.10	525.42
102.5	149.9	380.53	385.09	388.42	473.8	521.12	524.11	525.43
112.0	160.0	380.81	385.10	388.43	473.9	521.13	524.12	525.44
112.82	160.1	380.89	385.11	388.44	474.00	521.14	524.19	525.50
140.0	160.2	380.9	385.12	388.5	474.01	521.15	524.20	525.51
140.1	160.3	381.00	385.13	388.60	474.02	521.20	524.21	525.52
140.3	160.4	381.01	385.19	388.69	474.10	521.21	524.22	525.53
140.4	160.5	381.02	385.21	388.70	474.11	521.22	524.23	525.54
140.5	160.8	381.03	385.22	388.71	474.12	521.23	524.24	525.60
140.6	160.9	381.04	385.23	388.72	474.2	521.24	524.25	525.61
140.8	161.0	381.05	385.24	388.8	474.8	521.25	524.26	525.62
140.9	161.1	381.06	385.30	388.9	474.9	521.30	524.27	525.63
141.0	161.2	381.10	385.31	389.00	475	521.31	524.28	525.64
141.1	161.3	381.19	385.32	389.01	476.0	521.32	524.29	525.65
141.2	161.8	381.20	385.33	389.02	476.1	521.33	524.30	525.66
141.3	161.9	381.29	385.35	389.03	477.0	521.34	524.31	525.67
141.4	165.0	381.3	385.82	389.04	477.1	521.35	524.32	525.69
141.5	176.2	381.4	385.83	389.05	477.2	521.40	524.33	525.71
141.6	195.0	381.50	385.89	389.06	477.8	521.41	524.34	525.72
141.8	210.0	381.51	385.9	389.08	477.9	521.42	524.35	525.73
141.9	210.1	381.52	386.00	389.10	478.0	521.49	524.36	525.79
142.0	210.2	381.60	386.01	389.11	478.11	521.5	524.37	525.8
142.1	210.3	381.61	386.02	389.12	478.19	521.6	524.39	525.9
142.2	210.4	381.62	386.03	389.13	478.20	521.7	524.4	526.0
142.8	210.5	381.63	386.04	389.14	478.21	521.81	524.50	526.1
142.9	210.6	381.7	386.10	389.15	478.22	521.89	524.51	526.2
143.0	210.7	381.81	386.11	389.16	478.24	521.9	524.52	526.3
143.1	210.8	381.89	386.12	389.17	478.25	522.0	524.53	526.4
143.8	210.9	381.9	386.19	389.18	478.26	522.1	524.54	526.5
143.9	212.0	382.00	386.2	389.20	478.29	522.2	524.55	526.61
144.0	212.1	382.01	386.30	389.21	478.30	522.3	524.56	526.62
144.1	213.1	382.02	386.31	389.22	478.31	522.4	524.57	526.63
144.8	230.0	382.1	386.32	389.7	478.32	522.5	524.59	526.69

526.81	528.72	744.22	749.04	750.25	802.1	807.6	873.22	873.75
526.89	528.79	744.23	749.10	750.26	802.20	830.0	873.23	873.79
526.9	528.8	744.24	749.11	750.27	802.21	830.1	873.29	874.00
527.0	528.9	744.29	749.12	750.29	802.22	848.1	873.30	874.01
527.1	529.0	744.3	749.13	780.4	802.23	872.00	873.31	874.10
527.2	529.1	744.41	749.14	780.51	802.24	872.01	873.32	874.11
527.3	529.2	744.42	749.20	780.53	802.25	872.02	873.33	874.4
527.4	529.3	744.43	749.21	780.57	802.26	872.10	873.39	874.5
527.5	529.4	744.46	749.22	784.1	802.27	872.11	873.43	931
527.6	529.5	744.47	749.23	784.40	802.28	872.12	873.44	932
527.7	529.6	744.49	749.24	784.41	802.29	872.61	873.53	933.0
527.8	529.8	744.81	749.25	784.42	802.30	872.62	873.54	933.1
527.9	529.9	744.82	750.0	784.43	802.31	872.63	873.60	935.0
528.00	738.0	744.83	750.10	784.44	802.32	872.64	873.61	947.0
528.01	738.7	744.84	750.11	784.49	802.33	872.69	873.62	951.5
528.02	744.00	744.89	750.12	784.7	802.34	872.71	873.63	993.0
528.09	744.01	748.0	750.13	784.8	802.35	872.72	873.64	993.1
528.1	744.02	748.1	750.15	784.91	802.36	872.73	873.65	994.6
528.2	744.03	748.2	750.16	784.92	802.37	872.74	873.69	
528.3	744.04	748.3	750.19	784.99	802.38	872.79	873.70	
528.4	744.05	749.00	750.21	792.4	802.39	872.8	873.71	
528.5	744.09	749.01	750.22	794.15	802.4	872.9	873.72	
528.6	744.1	749.02	750.23	794.16	802.5	873.20	873.73	
528.71	744.21	749.03	750.24	802.0	807.5	873.21	873.74	

And Disorders Of The Ear, Nose, Mouth And Throat

SURGICAL

DRG 129 Major Head and Neck Procedures with CC/MCC or Major Device

GMLOS 3.6   AMLOS 5.1   RW 2.1925   ☑

Operating Room Procedures

20.96	Implantation or replacement of cochlear prosthetic device, not otherwise specified
20.97	Implantation or replacement of cochlear prosthetic device, single channel
20.98	Implantation or replacement of cochlear prosthetic device, multiple channel
25.3	Complete glossectomy
25.4	Radical glossectomy
27.32	Wide excision or destruction of lesion or tissue of bony palate
30.1	Hemilaryngectomy
30.29	Other partial laryngectomy
40.40	Radical neck dissection, not otherwise specified
40.41	Radical neck dissection, unilateral
40.42	Radical neck dissection, bilateral
40.50	Radical excision of lymph nodes, not otherwise specified
40.59	Radical excision of other lymph nodes
76.31	Partial mandibulectomy
76.41	Total mandibulectomy with synchronous reconstruction
76.42	Other total mandibulectomy

DRG 130 Major Head and Neck Procedures without CC/MCC

GMLOS 2.1   AMLOS 2.6   RW 1.2687   ☑

Operating Room Procedures

25.3	Complete glossectomy
25.4	Radical glossectomy
27.32	Wide excision or destruction of lesion or tissue of bony palate
30.1	Hemilaryngectomy
30.29	Other partial laryngectomy
40.40	Radical neck dissection, not otherwise specified
40.41	Radical neck dissection, unilateral
40.42	Radical neck dissection, bilateral
40.50	Radical excision of lymph nodes, not otherwise specified
40.59	Radical excision of other lymph nodes
76.31	Partial mandibulectomy
76.41	Total mandibulectomy with synchronous reconstruction
76.42	Other total mandibulectomy

DRG 131 Cranial/Facial Procedures with CC/MCC

GMLOS 3.9   AMLOS 5.4   RW 2.2038   ☑

Operating Room Procedures

01.23	Reopening of craniotomy site
01.24	Other craniotomy
01.25	Other craniectomy
01.6	Excision of lesion of skull
02.01	Opening of cranial suture
02.02	Elevation of skull fracture fragments
02.03	Formation of cranial bone flap
02.04	Bone graft to skull
02.05	Insertion of skull plate
02.06	Other cranial osteoplasty
02.07	Removal of skull plate
02.99	Other operations on skull, brain, and cerebral meninges
16.01	Orbitotomy with bone flap
16.02	Orbitotomy with insertion of orbital implant
16.09	Other orbitotomy
16.51	Exenteration of orbit with removal of adjacent structures
16.52	Exenteration of orbit with therapeutic removal of orbital bone
16.59	Other exenteration of orbit
16.63	Revision of enucleation socket with graft
16.64	Other revision of enucleation socket
16.89	Other repair of injury of eyeball or orbit
16.92	Excision of lesion of orbit
16.98	Other operations on orbit
21.4	Resection of nose
21.72	Open reduction of nasal fracture
76.01	Sequestrectomy of facial bone
76.19	Other diagnostic procedures on facial bones and joints
76.2	Local excision or destruction of lesion of facial bone
76.39	Partial ostectomy of other facial bone
76.43	Other reconstruction of mandible
76.44	Total ostectomy of other facial bone with synchronous reconstruction
76.45	Other total ostectomy of other facial bone
76.46	Other reconstruction of other facial bone
76.6*	Other facial bone repair and orthognathic surgery
76.70	Reduction of facial fracture, not otherwise specified
76.72	Open reduction of malar and zygomatic fracture
76.74	Open reduction of maxillary fracture
76.76	Open reduction of mandibular fracture
76.77	Open reduction of alveolar fracture
76.79	Other open reduction of facial fracture
76.91	Bone graft to facial bone
76.92	Insertion of synthetic implant in facial bone
76.94	Open reduction of temporomandibular dislocation
76.97	Removal of internal fixation device from facial bone
76.99	Other operations on facial bones and joints

DRG 132 Cranial/Facial Procedures without CC/MCC

GMLOS 2.0   AMLOS 2.6   RW 1.2855   ☑

Select operating room procedures listed under DRG 131

DRG 133 Other Ear, Nose, Mouth and Throat O.R. Procedures with CC/MCC

GMLOS 3.6   AMLOS 5.3   RW 1.7824   ☑

Operating Room Procedures

04.01	Excision of acoustic neuroma
04.02	Division of trigeminal nerve
04.03	Division or crushing of other cranial and peripheral nerves
04.04	Other incision of cranial and peripheral nerves
04.05	Gasserian ganglionectomy
04.06	Other cranial or peripheral ganglionectomy
04.07	Other excision or avulsion of cranial and peripheral nerves
04.12	Open biopsy of cranial or peripheral nerve or ganglion
04.19	Other diagnostic procedures on cranial and peripheral nerves and ganglia
04.41	Decompression of trigeminal nerve root
04.42	Other cranial nerve decompression
04.49	Other peripheral nerve or ganglion decompression or lysis of adhesions
04.71	Hypoglossal-facial anastomosis
04.72	Accessory-facial anastomosis
04.73	Accessory-hypoglossal anastomosis
04.74	Other anastomosis of cranial or peripheral nerve
04.75	Revision of previous repair of cranial and peripheral nerves
04.76	Repair of old traumatic injury of cranial and peripheral nerves
04.92	Implantation or replacement of peripheral neurostimulator lead(s)
04.93	Removal of peripheral neurostimulator lead(s)
04.99	Other operations on cranial and peripheral nerves
05.21	Sphenopalatine ganglionectomy
05.22	Cervical sympathectomy
06.09	Other incision of thyroid field

MDC 3: Diseases And Disorders Of The Ear, Nose, Mouth And Throat—SURGICAL

06.6	Excision of lingual thyroid
06.7	Excision of thyroglossal duct or tract
09.12	Biopsy of lacrimal sac
09.19	Other diagnostic procedures on lacrimal system
09.43	Probing of nasolacrimal duct
09.44	Intubation of nasolacrimal duct
09.81	Dacryocystorhinostomy (DCR)
09.99	Other operations on lacrimal system
16.65	Secondary graft to exenteration cavity
16.66	Other revision of exenteration cavity
18.21	Excision of preauricular sinus
18.3*	Other excision of external ear
18.5	Surgical correction of prominent ear
18.6	Reconstruction of external auditory canal
18.7*	Other plastic repair of external ear
18.9	Other operations on external ear
19*	Reconstructive operations on middle ear
20.01	Myringotomy with insertion of tube
20.23	Incision of middle ear
20.32	Biopsy of middle and inner ear
20.39	Other diagnostic procedures on middle and inner ear
20.5*	Other excision of middle ear
20.6*	Fenestration of inner ear
20.7*	Incision, excision, and destruction of inner ear
20.91	Tympanosympathectomy
20.93	Repair of oval and round windows
20.95	Implantation of electromagnetic hearing device
20.99	Other operations on middle and inner ear
21.04	Control of epistaxis by ligation of ethmoidal arteries
21.05	Control of epistaxis by (transantral) ligation of the maxillary artery
21.06	Control of epistaxis by ligation of the external carotid artery
21.07	Control of epistaxis by excision of nasal mucosa and skin grafting of septum and lateral nasal wall
21.09	Control of epistaxis by other means
21.5	Submucous resection of nasal septum
21.6*	Turbinectomy
21.82	Closure of nasal fistula
21.83	Total nasal reconstruction
21.84	Revision rhinoplasty
21.85	Augmentation rhinoplasty
21.86	Limited rhinoplasty
21.87	Other rhinoplasty
21.88	Other septoplasty
21.89	Other repair and plastic operations on nose
21.99	Other operations on nose
27.54	Repair of cleft lip
27.62	Correction of cleft palate
27.63	Revision of cleft palate repair
27.69	Other plastic repair of palate
28.0	Incision and drainage of tonsil and peritonsillar structures
28.11	Biopsy of tonsils and adenoids
28.19	Other diagnostic procedures on tonsils and adenoids
28.2	Tonsillectomy without adenoidectomy
28.3	Tonsillectomy with adenoidectomy
28.4	Excision of tonsil tag
28.5	Excision of lingual tonsil
28.6	Adenoidectomy without tonsillectomy
28.7	Control of hemorrhage after tonsillectomy and adenoidectomy
28.91	Removal of foreign body from tonsil and adenoid by incision
28.92	Excision of lesion of tonsil and adenoid
28.99	Other operations on tonsils and adenoids
29.0	Pharyngotomy
29.2	Excision of branchial cleft cyst or vestige
29.31	Cricopharyngeal myotomy
29.32	Pharyngeal diverticulectomy
29.33	Pharyngectomy (partial)
29.39	Other excision or destruction of lesion or tissue of pharynx
29.4	Plastic operation on pharynx
29.51	Suture of laceration of pharynx
29.52	Closure of branchial cleft fistula
29.53	Closure of other fistula of pharynx
29.54	Lysis of pharyngeal adhesions
29.59	Other repair of pharynx
29.92	Division of glossopharyngeal nerve
29.99	Other operations on pharynx
30.0*	Excision or destruction of lesion or tissue of larynx
30.21	Epiglottidectomy
30.22	Vocal cordectomy
31.3	Other incision of larynx or trachea
31.45	Open biopsy of larynx or trachea
31.5	Local excision or destruction of lesion or tissue of trachea
31.6*	Repair of larynx
31.71	Suture of laceration of trachea
31.72	Closure of external fistula of trachea
31.73	Closure of other fistula of trachea
31.74	Revision of tracheostomy
31.75	Reconstruction of trachea and construction of artificial larynx
31.79	Other repair and plastic operations on trachea
31.91	Division of laryngeal nerve
31.92	Lysis of adhesions of trachea or larynx
31.98	Other operations on larynx
31.99	Other operations on trachea
34.22	Mediastinoscopy
38.00	Incision of vessel, unspecified site
38.02	Incision of other vessels of head and neck
38.12	Endarterectomy of other vessels of head and neck
38.21	Biopsy of blood vessel
38.32	Resection of other vessels of head and neck with anastomosis
38.42	Resection of other vessels of head and neck with replacement
38.62	Other excision of other vessels of head and neck
38.82	Other surgical occlusion of other vessels of head and neck
39.98	Control of hemorrhage, not otherwise specified
39.99	Other operations on vessels
40.11	Biopsy of lymphatic structure
40.19	Other diagnostic procedures on lymphatic structures
40.21	Excision of deep cervical lymph node
40.23	Excision of axillary lymph node
40.29	Simple excision of other lymphatic structure
40.3	Regional lymph node excision
40.9	Other operations on lymphatic structures
42.01	Incision of esophageal web
42.09	Other incision of esophagus
42.10	Esophagostomy, not otherwise specified
42.11	Cervical esophagostomy
42.12	Exteriorization of esophageal pouch
42.19	Other external fistulization of esophagus
42.21	Operative esophagoscopy by incision
42.25	Open biopsy of esophagus
42.31	Local excision of esophageal diverticulum
42.32	Local excision of other lesion or tissue of esophagus
42.39	Other destruction of lesion or tissue of esophagus
42.40	Esophagectomy, not otherwise specified
42.41	Partial esophagectomy
42.42	Total esophagectomy
42.51	Intrathoracic esophagoesophagostomy
42.52	Intrathoracic esophagogastrostomy
42.53	Intrathoracic esophageal anastomosis with interposition of small bowel
42.54	Other intrathoracic esophagoenterostomy
42.55	Intrathoracic esophageal anastomosis with interposition of colon
42.56	Other intrathoracic esophagocolostomy
42.58	Intrathoracic esophageal anastomosis with other interposition
42.59	Other intrathoracic anastomosis of esophagus

Ⓣ *Transfer DRG*   Ⓢ *Special Payment*   ☑ *Optimization Potential*   ◱ *Targeted Potential*   ** Code Range*   ● *New DRG*   ▲ *Revised DRG Title*

Valid 10/01/2013–09/30/2014   © 2013 OptumInsight, Inc.

42.61	Antesternal esophagoesophagostomy
42.62	Antesternal esophagogastrostomy
42.63	Antesternal esophageal anastomosis with interposition of small bowel
42.64	Other antesternal esophagoenterostomy
42.65	Antesternal esophageal anastomosis with interposition of colon
42.66	Other antesternal esophagocolostomy
42.68	Other antesternal esophageal anastomosis with interposition
42.69	Other antesternal anastomosis of esophagus
42.7	Esophagomyotomy
42.82	Suture of laceration of esophagus
42.83	Closure of esophagostomy
42.84	Repair of esophageal fistula, not elsewhere classified
42.86	Production of subcutaneous tunnel without esophageal anastomosis
42.87	Other graft of esophagus
42.89	Other repair of esophagus
50.12	Open biopsy of liver
76.09	Other incision of facial bone
76.11	Biopsy of facial bone
76.5	Temporomandibular arthroplasty
77.19	Other incision of other bone, except facial bones, without division
77.30	Other division of bone, unspecified site
77.40	Biopsy of bone, unspecified site
77.49	Biopsy of other bone, except facial bones
77.69	Local excision of lesion or tissue of other bone, except facial bones
77.79	Excision of other bone for graft, except facial bones
77.89	Other partial ostectomy of other bone, except facial bones
77.99	Total ostectomy of other bone, except facial bones
79.29	Open reduction of fracture of other specified bone, except facial bones, without internal fixation
79.39	Open reduction of fracture of other specified bone, except facial bones, with internal fixation
79.69	Debridement of open fracture of other specified bone, except facial bones
83.02	Myotomy
83.39	Excision of lesion of other soft tissue
83.49	Other excision of soft tissue
86.22	Excisional debridement of wound, infection, or burn
86.4	Radical excision of skin lesion
86.63	Full-thickness skin graft to other sites
86.66	Homograft to skin
86.67	Dermal regenerative graft
86.69	Other skin graft to other sites
86.70	Pedicle or flap graft, not otherwise specified
86.71	Cutting and preparation of pedicle grafts or flaps
86.72	Advancement of pedicle graft
86.74	Attachment of pedicle or flap graft to other sites
86.75	Revision of pedicle or flap graft
86.81	Repair for facial weakness
86.82	Facial rhytidectomy
86.84	Relaxation of scar or web contracture of skin
86.87	Fat graft of skin and subcutaneous tissue
86.89	Other repair and reconstruction of skin and subcutaneous tissue
86.91	Excision of skin for graft
86.93	Insertion of tissue expander
92.27	Implantation or insertion of radioactive elements

DRG 134　Other Ear, Nose, Mouth and Throat O.R. Procedures without CC/MCC

GMLOS 1.8　　　AMLOS 2.4　　　RW 0.9584　　☑

Select operating room procedures listed under DRG 133

DRG 135　Sinus and Mastoid Procedures with CC/MCC

GMLOS 4.1　　　AMLOS 5.9　　　RW 2.0110

Operating Room Procedures

20.21	Incision of mastoid
20.22	Incision of petrous pyramid air cells
20.4*	Mastoidectomy
20.92	Revision of mastoidectomy
22.12	Open biopsy of nasal sinus
22.3*	External maxillary antrotomy
22.4*	Frontal sinusotomy and sinusectomy
22.5*	Other nasal sinusotomy
22.6*	Other nasal sinusectomy
22.7*	Repair of nasal sinus
22.9	Other operations on nasal sinuses

DRG 136　Sinus and Mastoid Procedures without CC/MCC

GMLOS 1.8　　　AMLOS 2.4　　　RW 0.9709　　☑

Select operating room procedures listed under DRG 135

DRG 137　Mouth Procedures with CC/MCC

GMLOS 3.7　　　AMLOS 5.0　　　RW 1.3477　　☑

Operating Room Procedures

24.2	Gingivoplasty
24.4	Excision of dental lesion of jaw
24.5	Alveoloplasty
25.02	Open biopsy of tongue
25.1	Excision or destruction of lesion or tissue of tongue
25.2	Partial glossectomy
25.59	Other repair and plastic operations on tongue
25.94	Other glossotomy
25.99	Other operations on tongue
27.0	Drainage of face and floor of mouth
27.1	Incision of palate
27.21	Biopsy of bony palate
27.22	Biopsy of uvula and soft palate
27.31	Local excision or destruction of lesion or tissue of bony palate
27.42	Wide excision of lesion of lip
27.43	Other excision of lesion or tissue of lip
27.49	Other excision of mouth
27.53	Closure of fistula of mouth
27.55	Full-thickness skin graft to lip and mouth
27.56	Other skin graft to lip and mouth
27.57	Attachment of pedicle or flap graft to lip and mouth
27.59	Other plastic repair of mouth
27.61	Suture of laceration of palate
27.7*	Operations on uvula
27.92	Incision of mouth, unspecified structure
27.99	Other operations on oral cavity

DRG 138　Mouth Procedures without CC/MCC

GMLOS 2.0　　　AMLOS 2.5　　　RW 0.8304　　☑

Select operating room procedures listed under DRG 137

Surgical　　　　　_Medical_　　　　　CC Indicator　　　　　MCC Indicator　　　　　_Procedure Proxy_

DRG 139   Salivary Gland Procedures
GMLOS 1.5   AMLOS 2.0   RW 0.9169   ☑

Operating Room Procedures
26.12   Open biopsy of salivary gland or duct
26.2*   Excision of lesion of salivary gland
26.3*   Sialoadenectomy
26.4*   Repair of salivary gland or duct
26.99   Other operations on salivary gland or duct

MEDICAL

DRG 146   Ear, Nose, Mouth and Throat Malignancy with MCC
GMLOS 5.6   AMLOS 8.2   RW 2.0402   ☑

Principal Diagnosis
140*   Malignant neoplasm of lip
141*   Malignant neoplasm of tongue
142*   Malignant neoplasm of major salivary glands
143*   Malignant neoplasm of gum
144*   Malignant neoplasm of floor of mouth
145*   Malignant neoplasm of other and unspecified parts of mouth
146*   Malignant neoplasm of oropharynx
147*   Malignant neoplasm of nasopharynx
148*   Malignant neoplasm of hypopharynx
149*   Malignant neoplasm of other and ill-defined sites within the lip, oral cavity, and pharynx
160*   Malignant neoplasm of nasal cavities, middle ear, and accessory sinuses
161*   Malignant neoplasm of larynx
165.0   Malignant neoplasm of upper respiratory tract, part unspecified
176.2   Kaposi's sarcoma of palate
195.0   Malignant neoplasm of head, face, and neck
230.0   Carcinoma in situ of lip, oral cavity, and pharynx
231.0   Carcinoma in situ of larynx
235.0   Neoplasm of uncertain behavior of major salivary glands
235.1   Neoplasm of uncertain behavior of lip, oral cavity, and pharynx
235.6   Neoplasm of uncertain behavior of larynx

DRG 147   Ear, Nose, Mouth and Throat Malignancy with CC
GMLOS 3.9   AMLOS 5.4   RW 1.2317   ☑

Select principal diagnosis listed under DRG 146

DRG 148   Ear, Nose, Mouth and Throat Malignancy without CC/MCC
GMLOS 2.3   AMLOS 3.0   RW 0.7688   ☑

Select principal diagnosis listed under DRG 146

DRG 149   Dysequilibrium
GMLOS 2.1   AMLOS 2.5   RW 0.6184   ☑

Principal Diagnosis
386.0* Meniere's disease
386.1* Other and unspecified peripheral vertigo
386.2   Vertigo of central origin
386.3* Labyrinthitis
386.5* Labyrinthine dysfunction
386.8   Other disorders of labyrinth
386.9   Unspecified vertiginous syndromes and labyrinthine disorders
780.4   Dizziness and giddiness
994.6   Motion sickness

DRG 150   Epistaxis with MCC
GMLOS 3.7   AMLOS 4.9   RW 1.3298   ☑

Principal Diagnosis
784.7   Epistaxis

DRG 151   Epistaxis without MCC
GMLOS 2.2   AMLOS 2.8   RW 0.6557   ☑

Select principal diagnosis listed under DRG 150

DRG 152   Otitis Media and Upper Respiratory Infection with MCC
GMLOS 3.3   AMLOS 4.3   RW 1.0042   ☑

Principal Diagnosis
034.0   Streptococcal sore throat
055.2   Postmeasles otitis media
074.0   Herpangina
098.6   Gonococcal infection of pharynx
099.51 Chlamydia trachomatis infection of pharynx
101   Vincent's angina
380.00 Unspecified perichondritis of pinna
381.0* Acute nonsuppurative otitis media
381.1* Chronic serous otitis media
381.2* Chronic mucoid otitis media
381.3   Other and unspecified chronic nonsuppurative otitis media
381.4   Nonsuppurative otitis media, not specified as acute or chronic
381.5* Eustachian salpingitis
382*   Suppurative and unspecified otitis media
383.0* Acute mastoiditis
383.1   Chronic mastoiditis
383.2* Petrositis
383.9   Unspecified mastoiditis
384.0* Acute myringitis without mention of otitis media
384.1   Chronic myringitis without mention of otitis media
460   Acute nasopharyngitis (common cold)
461*   Acute sinusitis
462   Acute pharyngitis
463   Acute tonsillitis
464.00 Acute laryngitis, without mention of obstruction
464.01 Acute laryngitis, with obstruction
464.2* Acute laryngotracheitis
464.3* Acute epiglottitis
464.4   Croup
464.50 Unspecified supraglottis, without mention of obstruction
464.51 Unspecified supraglottis, with obstruction
465*   Acute upper respiratory infections of multiple or unspecified sites
472*   Chronic pharyngitis and nasopharyngitis
473*   Chronic sinusitis
474.00 Chronic tonsillitis
474.01 Chronic adenoiditis
474.02 Chronic tonsillitis and adenoiditis
475   Peritonsillar abscess
476*   Chronic laryngitis and laryngotracheitis
477*   Allergic rhinitis
478.21 Cellulitis of pharynx or nasopharynx
478.22 Parapharyngeal abscess
478.24 Retropharyngeal abscess
478.71 Cellulitis and perichondritis of larynx
478.8   Upper respiratory tract hypersensitivity reaction, site unspecified
478.9   Other and unspecified diseases of upper respiratory tract
487.1   Influenza with other respiratory manifestations
993.0   Barotrauma, otitic
993.1   Barotrauma, sinus

Ⓣ *Transfer DRG*   🆂🅿 *Special Payment*   ☑ *Optimization Potential*   🆈🅴🆂 *Targeted Potential*   * *Code Range*   ● *New DRG*   ▲ *Revised DRG Title*

DRG 153　Otitis Media and Upper Respiratory Infection without MCC
　　　GMLOS 2.4　　　AMLOS 2.9　　　RW 0.6439　　☑

Select principal diagnosis listed under DRG 152

DRG 154　Other Ear, Nose, Mouth and Throat Diagnoses with MCC
　　　GMLOS 4.1　　　AMLOS 5.5　　　RW 1.3785　　☑

Principal Diagnosis

012.3*	Tuberculous laryngitis
015.6*	Tuberculosis of mastoid
017.4*	Tuberculosis of ear
032.0	Faucial diphtheria
032.1	Nasopharyngeal diphtheria
032.2	Anterior nasal diphtheria
032.3	Laryngeal diphtheria
053.71	Otitis externa due to herpes zoster
054.73	Herpes simplex otitis externa
094.86	Syphilitic acoustic neuritis
102.5	Gangosa due to yaws
112.82	Candidal otitis externa
210.2	Benign neoplasm of major salivary glands
210.5	Benign neoplasm of tonsil
210.6	Benign neoplasm of other parts of oropharynx
210.7	Benign neoplasm of nasopharynx
210.8	Benign neoplasm of hypopharynx
210.9	Benign neoplasm of pharynx, unspecified
212.0	Benign neoplasm of nasal cavities, middle ear, and accessory sinuses
212.1	Benign neoplasm of larynx
327.20	Organic sleep apnea, unspecified
327.23	Obstructive sleep apnea (adult) (pediatric)
327.24	Idiopathic sleep related nonobstructive alveolar hypoventilation
327.26	Sleep related hypoventilation/hypoxemia in conditions classifiable elsewhere
327.29	Other organic sleep apnea
327.40	Organic parasomnia, unspecified
327.42	REM sleep behavior disorder
327.44	Parasomnia in conditions classified elsewhere
327.49	Other organic parasomnia
327.53	Sleep related bruxism
327.59	Other organic sleep related movement disorders
327.8	Other organic sleep disorders
380.1*	Infective otitis externa
380.2*	Other otitis externa
380.3*	Noninfectious disorders of pinna
380.4	Impacted cerumen
380.5*	Acquired stenosis of external ear canal
380.8*	Other disorders of external ear
380.9	Unspecified disorder of external ear
381.6*	Obstruction of Eustachian tube
381.7	Patulous Eustachian tube
381.8*	Other disorders of Eustachian tube
381.9	Unspecified Eustachian tube disorder
383.3*	Complications following mastoidectomy
383.8*	Other disorders of mastoid
384.2*	Perforation of tympanic membrane
384.8*	Other specified disorders of tympanic membrane
384.9	Unspecified disorder of tympanic membrane
385*	Other disorders of middle ear and mastoid
386.4*	Labyrinthine fistula
387*	Otosclerosis
388.0*	Degenerative and vascular disorders of ear
388.1*	Noise effects on inner ear
388.2	Unspecified sudden hearing loss
388.3*	Tinnitus
388.40	Unspecified abnormal auditory perception
388.41	Diplacusis
388.42	Hyperacusis

388.43	Impairment of auditory discrimination
388.44	Other abnormal auditory perception, recruitment
388.5	Disorders of acoustic nerve
388.60	Unspecified otorrhea
388.69	Other otorrhea
388.7*	Otalgia
388.8	Other disorders of ear
388.9	Unspecified disorder of ear
389*	Hearing loss
470	Deviated nasal septum
471*	Nasal polyps
474.1*	Hypertrophy of tonsils and adenoids
474.2	Adenoid vegetations
474.8	Other chronic disease of tonsils and adenoids
474.9	Unspecified chronic disease of tonsils and adenoids
478.0	Hypertrophy of nasal turbinates
478.1*	Other diseases of nasal cavity and sinuses
478.20	Unspecified disease of pharynx
478.25	Edema of pharynx or nasopharynx
478.26	Cyst of pharynx or nasopharynx
478.29	Other disease of pharynx or nasopharynx
478.3*	Paralysis of vocal cords or larynx
478.4	Polyp of vocal cord or larynx
478.5	Other diseases of vocal cords
478.6	Edema of larynx
478.70	Unspecified disease of larynx
478.74	Stenosis of larynx
478.75	Laryngeal spasm
478.79	Other diseases of larynx
527*	Diseases of the salivary glands
738.0	Acquired deformity of nose
738.7	Cauliflower ear
744.0*	Congenital anomalies of ear causing impairment of hearing
744.1	Congenital anomalies of accessory auricle
744.2*	Other specified congenital anomalies of ear
744.3	Unspecified congenital anomaly of ear
744.4*	Congenital branchial cleft cyst or fistula; preauricular sinus
744.89	Other specified congenital anomaly of face and neck
748.0	Congenital choanal atresia
748.1	Other congenital anomaly of nose
748.2	Congenital web of larynx
748.3	Other congenital anomaly of larynx, trachea, and bronchus
750.21	Congenital absence of salivary gland
750.22	Congenital accessory salivary gland
750.23	Congenital atresia, salivary duct
750.24	Congenital fistula of salivary gland
750.27	Congenital diverticulum of pharynx
750.29	Other specified congenital anomaly of pharynx
780.51	Insomnia with sleep apnea, unspecified
780.53	Hypersomnia with sleep apnea, unspecified
780.57	Unspecified sleep apnea
784.1	Throat pain
784.4*	Voice and resonance disorders
784.8	Hemorrhage from throat
784.91	Postnasal drip
784.99	Other symptoms involving head and neck
792.4	Nonspecific abnormal finding in saliva
794.15	Nonspecific abnormal auditory function studies
794.16	Nonspecific abnormal vestibular function studies
802.0	Nasal bones, closed fracture
802.1	Nasal bones, open fracture
807.5	Closed fracture of larynx and trachea
807.6	Open fracture of larynx and trachea
872*	Open wound of ear
873.20	Open wound of nose, unspecified site, without mention of complication
873.21	Open wound of nasal septum, without mention of complication
873.22	Open wound of nasal cavity, without mention of complication

873.23	Open wound of nasal sinus, without mention of complication
873.29	Open wound of nose, multiple sites, without mention of complication
873.3*	Open wound of nose, complicated
874.00	Open wound of larynx with trachea, without mention of complication
874.01	Open wound of larynx, without mention of complication
874.10	Open wound of larynx with trachea, complicated
874.11	Open wound of larynx, complicated
874.4	Open wound of pharynx, without mention of complication
874.5	Open wound of pharynx, complicated
931	Foreign body in ear
932	Foreign body in nose
933*	Foreign body in pharynx and larynx
947.0	Burn of mouth and pharynx
951.5	Injury to acoustic nerve

DRG 155 **Other Ear, Nose, Mouth and Throat Diagnoses with CC**

GMLOS 3.1   AMLOS 3.9   RW 0.8610   ☑

Select principal diagnosis listed under DRG 154

DRG 156 **Other Ear, Nose, Mouth and Throat Diagnoses without CC/MCC**

GMLOS 2.3   AMLOS 2.8   RW 0.6160   ☑

Select principal diagnosis listed under DRG 154

DRG 157 **Dental and Oral Diseases with MCC**

GMLOS 4.5   AMLOS 6.1   RW 1.5380   ☑

Principal Diagnosis

054.2	Herpetic gingivostomatitis
112.0	Candidiasis of mouth
210.0	Benign neoplasm of lip
210.1	Benign neoplasm of tongue
210.3	Benign neoplasm of floor of mouth
210.4	Benign neoplasm of other and unspecified parts of mouth
213.1	Benign neoplasm of lower jaw bone
520*	Disorders of tooth development and eruption
521*	Diseases of hard tissues of teeth
522*	Diseases of pulp and periapical tissues
523*	Gingival and periodontal diseases
524*	Dentofacial anomalies, including malocclusion
525*	Other diseases and conditions of the teeth and supporting structures
526*	Diseases of the jaws
528*	Diseases of the oral soft tissues, excluding lesions specific for gingiva and tongue
529*	Diseases and other conditions of the tongue
744.81	Macrocheilia
744.82	Microcheilia
744.83	Macrostomia
744.84	Microstomia
749*	Cleft palate and cleft lip
750.0	Tongue tie
750.1*	Other congenital anomalies of tongue
750.25	Congenital fistula of lip
750.26	Other specified congenital anomalies of mouth
784.92	Jaw pain
802.2*	Mandible, closed fracture
802.3*	Mandible, open fracture
802.4	Malar and maxillary bones, closed fracture
802.5	Malar and maxillary bones, open fracture
830*	Dislocation of jaw
848.1	Sprain and strain of jaw
873.43	Open wound of lip, without mention of complication
873.44	Open wound of jaw, without mention of complication
873.53	Open wound of lip, complicated

873.54	Open wound of jaw, complicated
873.6*	Open wound of internal structures of mouth, without mention of complication
873.7*	Open wound of internal structure of mouth, complicated
935.0	Foreign body in mouth

DRG 158 **Dental and Oral Diseases with CC**

GMLOS 3.1   AMLOS 3.9   RW 0.8525   ☑

Select principal diagnosis listed under DRG 157

DRG 159 **Dental and Oral Diseases without CC/MCC**

GMLOS 2.1   AMLOS 2.6   RW 0.6100   ☑

Select principal diagnosis listed under DRG 157

Ⓣ *Transfer DRG*   ⓢⓟ *Special Payment*   ☑ *Optimization Potential*   ᵀᴳ *Targeted Potential*   * *Code Range*   ● *New DRG*   ▲ *Revised DRG Title*

48   Valid 10/01/2013–09/30/2014   © 2013 OptumInsight, Inc.

MDC 3: Diseases And Disorders Of The Ear, Nose, Mouth And Throat—MEDICAL

Diseases And Disorders Of The Respiratory System

003.22	011.34	012.13	163.1	482.1	493.90	516.0	748.60	807.16
006.4	011.35	012.14	163.8	482.2	493.91	516.1	748.61	807.17
010.00	011.36	012.15	163.9	482.30	493.92	516.2	748.69	807.18
010.01	011.40	012.16	164.2	482.31	494.0	516.30	748.8	807.19
010.02	011.41	012.20	164.3	482.32	494.1	516.31	748.9	807.2
010.03	011.42	012.21	164.8	482.39	495.0	516.32	754.81	807.3
010.04	011.43	012.22	164.9	482.40	495.1	516.33	754.82	807.4
010.05	011.44	012.23	165.8	482.41	495.2	516.34	756.3	839.61
010.06	011.45	012.24	165.9	482.42	495.3	516.35	756.6	839.71
010.10	011.46	012.25	176.4	482.49	495.4	516.36	770.7	848.3
010.11	011.50	012.26	195.1	482.81	495.5	516.37	781.5	848.40
010.12	011.51	012.80	197.0	482.82	495.6	516.4	786.00	848.41
010.13	011.52	012.81	197.1	482.83	495.7	516.5	786.01	848.42
010.14	011.53	012.82	197.2	482.84	495.8	516.61	786.02	848.49
010.15	011.54	012.83	197.3	482.89	495.9	516.62	786.03	860.0
010.16	011.55	012.84	209.21	482.9	496	516.63	786.04	860.1
010.80	011.56	012.85	209.61	483.0	500	516.64	786.05	860.2
010.81	011.60	012.86	212.2	483.1	501	516.69	786.06	860.3
010.82	011.61	020.3	212.3	483.8	502	516.8	786.07	860.4
010.83	011.62	020.4	212.4	484.1	503	516.9	786.09	860.5
010.84	011.63	020.5	212.5	484.3	504	517.1	786.1	861.20
010.85	011.64	021.2	212.8	484.5	505	517.2	786.2	861.21
010.86	011.65	022.1	212.9	484.6	506.0	517.3	786.30	861.22
010.90	011.66	031.0	213.3	484.7	506.1	517.8	786.31	861.30
010.91	011.70	033.0	214.2	484.8	506.2	518.0	786.39	861.31
010.92	011.71	033.1	231.1	485	506.3	518.1	786.4	861.32
010.93	011.72	033.8	231.2	486	506.4	518.2	786.52	862.0
010.94	011.73	033.9	231.8	487.0	506.9	518.3	786.6	862.1
010.95	011.74	039.1	231.9	488.01	507.0	518.4	786.7	862.21
010.96	011.75	052.1	235.7	488.02	507.1	518.51	786.8	862.29
011.00	011.76	055.1	235.8	488.11	507.8	518.52	786.9	862.31
011.01	011.80	073.0	235.9	488.12	508.0	518.53	793.11	862.39
011.02	011.81	074.1	239.1	488.81	508.1	518.6	793.19	874.02
011.03	011.82	095.1	277.02	488.82	508.2	518.7	794.2	874.12
011.04	011.83	112.4	278.03	490	508.8	518.81	795.51	908.0
011.05	011.84	114.0	306.1	491.0	508.9	518.82	795.52	934.0
011.06	011.85	114.4	327.22	491.1	510.0	518.83	799.01	934.1
011.10	011.86	114.5	415.11	491.20	510.9	518.84	799.02	934.8
011.11	011.90	115.05	415.12	491.21	511.0	518.89	799.1	934.9
011.12	011.91	115.15	415.13	491.22	511.1	519.00	807.00	947.1
011.13	011.92	115.95	415.19	491.8	511.81	519.01	807.01	958.0
011.14	011.93	121.2	416.2	491.9	511.89	519.02	807.02	958.1
011.15	011.94	122.1	464.10	492.0	511.9	519.09	807.03	958.7
011.16	011.95	130.4	464.11	492.8	512.0	519.11	807.04	996.84
011.20	011.96	135	466.0	493.00	512.1	519.19	807.05	997.31
011.21	012.00	136.3	466.11	493.01	512.2	519.2	807.06	997.32
011.22	012.01	137.0	466.19	493.02	512.81	519.3	807.07	997.39
011.23	012.02	162.0	480.0	493.10	512.82	519.4	807.08	999.1
011.24	012.03	162.2	480.1	493.11	512.83	519.8	807.09	V42.6
011.25	012.04	162.3	480.2	493.12	512.84	519.9	807.10	V45.76
011.26	012.05	162.4	480.3	493.20	512.89	573.5	807.11	V55.0
011.30	012.06	162.5	480.8	493.21	513.0	714.81	807.12	V71.2
011.31	012.10	162.8	480.9	493.22	513.1	733.6	807.13	
011.32	012.11	162.9	481	493.81	514	748.4	807.14	
011.33	012.12	163.0	482.0	493.82	515	748.5	807.15	

SURGICAL

DRG 163 Major Chest Procedures with MCC
GMLOS 11.0   AMLOS 13.4   RW 5.0952   ☑T

Operating Room Procedures

07.16	Biopsy of thymus
07.8*	Thymectomy
07.9*	Other operations on thymus
17.69	Laser interstitial thermal therapy [LITT] of lesion or tissue of other and unspecified site under guidance
31.73	Closure of other fistula of trachea
31.75	Reconstruction of trachea and construction of artificial larynx
31.79	Other repair and plastic operations on trachea
32.09	Other local excision or destruction of lesion or tissue of bronchus
32.1	Other excision of bronchus
32.20	Thoracoscopic excision of lesion or tissue of lung
32.21	Plication of emphysematous bleb
32.22	Lung volume reduction surgery
32.23	Open ablation of lung lesion or tissue
32.25	Thoracoscopic ablation of lung lesion or tissue
32.26	Other and unspecified ablation of lung lesion or tissue
32.27	Bronchoscopic bronchial thermoplasty, ablation of airway smooth muscle
32.29	Other local excision or destruction of lesion or tissue of lung
32.3*	Segmental resection of lung
32.4*	Lobectomy of lung
32.5*	Pneumonectomy
32.6	Radical dissection of thoracic structures
32.9	Other excision of lung
33.0	Incision of bronchus
33.1	Incision of lung
33.25	Open biopsy of bronchus
33.28	Open biopsy of lung
33.34	Thoracoplasty
33.39	Other surgical collapse of lung
33.4*	Repair and plastic operation on lung and bronchus
33.92	Ligation of bronchus
33.98	Other operations on bronchus
33.99	Other operations on lung
34.02	Exploratory thoracotomy
34.03	Reopening of recent thoracotomy site
34.27	Biopsy of diaphragm
34.3	Excision or destruction of lesion or tissue of mediastinum
34.5*	Pleurectomy
34.6	Scarification of pleura
34.73	Closure of other fistula of thorax
34.74	Repair of pectus deformity
34.8*	Operations on diaphragm
34.93	Repair of pleura
37.12	Pericardiotomy
37.24	Biopsy of pericardium
37.31	Pericardiectomy
37.91	Open chest cardiac massage
38.05	Incision of other thoracic vessels
38.15	Endarterectomy of other thoracic vessels
38.35	Resection of other thoracic vessels with anastomosis
38.45	Resection of other thoracic vessels with replacement
38.55	Ligation and stripping of varicose veins of other thoracic vessel
38.65	Other excision of other thoracic vessel
38.85	Other surgical occlusion of other thoracic vessel
39.54	Re-entry operation (aorta)
39.98	Control of hemorrhage, not otherwise specified
40.22	Excision of internal mammary lymph node
40.52	Radical excision of periaortic lymph nodes
40.6*	Operations on thoracic duct

53.7*	Repair of diaphragmatic hernia, abdominal approach
53.8*	Repair of diaphragmatic hernia, thoracic approach

DRG 164 Major Chest Procedures with CC
GMLOS 5.6   AMLOS 6.7   RW 2.6086   ☑T

Select operating room procedures listed under DRG 163

DRG 165 Major Chest Procedures without CC/MCC
GMLOS 3.3   AMLOS 4.0   RW 1.7943   ☑T

Select operating room procedures listed under DRG 163

DRG 166 Other Respiratory System O.R. Procedures with MCC
GMLOS 8.8   AMLOS 11.2   RW 3.6741   ☑T

Operating Room Procedures

17.56	Atherectomy of other non-coronary vessel(s)
30.01	Marsupialization of laryngeal cyst
30.09	Other excision or destruction of lesion or tissue of larynx
30.1	Hemilaryngectomy
30.2*	Other partial laryngectomy
31.3	Other incision of larynx or trachea
31.45	Open biopsy of larynx or trachea
31.5	Local excision or destruction of lesion or tissue of trachea
31.6*	Repair of larynx
31.71	Suture of laceration of trachea
31.72	Closure of external fistula of trachea
31.74	Revision of tracheostomy
31.91	Division of laryngeal nerve
31.92	Lysis of adhesions of trachea or larynx
31.98	Other operations on larynx
31.99	Other operations on trachea
32.24	Percutaneous ablation of lung lesion or tissue
33.20	Thoracoscopic lung biopsy
33.27	Closed endoscopic biopsy of lung
33.29	Other diagnostic procedures on lung or bronchus
33.93	Puncture of lung
34.06	Thoracoscopic drainage of pleural cavity
34.1	Incision of mediastinum
34.20	Thoracoscopic pleural biopsy
34.21	Transpleural thoracoscopy
34.22	Mediastinoscopy
34.26	Open biopsy of mediastinum
34.28	Other diagnostic procedures on chest wall, pleura, and diaphragm
34.29	Other diagnostic procedures on mediastinum
34.4	Excision or destruction of lesion of chest wall
34.79	Other repair of chest wall
34.99	Other operations on thorax
38.21	Biopsy of blood vessel
38.7	Interruption of the vena cava
39.29	Other (peripheral) vascular shunt or bypass
39.31	Suture of artery
39.50	Angioplasty of other non-coronary vessel(s)
39.99	Other operations on vessels
40.11	Biopsy of lymphatic structure
40.19	Other diagnostic procedures on lymphatic structures
40.21	Excision of deep cervical lymph node
40.23	Excision of axillary lymph node
40.24	Excision of inguinal lymph node
40.29	Simple excision of other lymphatic structure
40.3	Regional lymph node excision
40.4*	Radical excision of cervical lymph nodes
40.50	Radical excision of lymph nodes, not otherwise specified
40.59	Radical excision of other lymph nodes
50.12	Open biopsy of liver
54.11	Exploratory laparotomy
77.01	Sequestrectomy of scapula, clavicle, and thorax (ribs and sternum)

T Transfer DRG   SP Special Payment   ☑ Optimization Potential   Targeted Potential   * Code Range   ● New DRG   ▲ Revised DRG Title

77.11	Other incision of scapula, clavicle, and thorax (ribs and sternum) without division
77.21	Wedge osteotomy of scapula, clavicle, and thorax (ribs and sternum)
77.31	Other division of scapula, clavicle, and thorax (ribs and sternum)
77.41	Biopsy of scapula, clavicle, and thorax (ribs and sternum)
77.49	Biopsy of other bone, except facial bones
77.61	Local excision of lesion or tissue of scapula, clavicle, and thorax (ribs and sternum)
77.71	Excision of scapula, clavicle, and thorax (ribs and sternum) for graft
77.81	Other partial ostectomy of scapula, clavicle, and thorax (ribs and sternum)
77.91	Total ostectomy of scapula, clavicle, and thorax (ribs and sternum)
78.01	Bone graft of scapula, clavicle, and thorax (ribs and sternum)
78.11	Application of external fixator device, scapula, clavicle, and thorax [ribs and sternum]
78.41	Other repair or plastic operations on scapula, clavicle, and thorax (ribs and sternum)
78.51	Internal fixation of scapula, clavicle, and thorax (ribs and sternum) without fracture reduction
78.61	Removal of implanted device from scapula, clavicle, and thorax (ribs and sternum)
78.71	Osteoclasis of scapula, clavicle, and thorax (ribs and sternum)
78.81	Diagnostic procedures on scapula, clavicle, and thorax (ribs and sternum) not elsewhere classified
78.91	Insertion of bone growth stimulator into scapula, clavicle and thorax (ribs and sternum)
83.21	Open biopsy of soft tissue
84.94	Insertion of sternal fixation device with rigid plates
86.06	Insertion of totally implantable infusion pump
86.22	Excisional debridement of wound, infection, or burn
86.69	Other skin graft to other sites
92.27	Implantation or insertion of radioactive elements

DRG 167 **Other Respiratory System O.R. Procedures with CC**
GMLOS 5.2 AMLOS 6.6 RW 1.9860 ☑ T

Select operating room procedures listed under DRG 166

DRG 168 **Other Respiratory System O.R. Procedures without CC/MCC**
GMLOS 3.0 AMLOS 3.9 RW 1.3101 ☑ T

Select operating room procedures listed under DRG 166

MEDICAL

DRG 175 **Pulmonary Embolism with MCC**
GMLOS 5.3 AMLOS 6.4 RW 1.5346 ☑ T

Principal Diagnosis
415.1*	Pulmonary embolism and infarction
416.2	Chronic pulmonary embolism
958.0	Air embolism as an early complication of trauma
958.1	Fat embolism as an early complication of trauma
999.1	Air embolism as complication of medical care, not elsewhere classified

DRG 176 **Pulmonary Embolism without MCC**
GMLOS 3.7 AMLOS 4.4 RW 0.9891 ☑ T

Select principal diagnosis listed under DRG 175

DRG 177 **Respiratory Infections and Inflammations with MCC**
GMLOS 6.4 AMLOS 7.9 RW 1.9934 ☑ ▽ T

Principal Diagnosis
003.22	Salmonella pneumonia
006.4	Amebic lung abscess
010*	Primary tuberculous infection
011*	Pulmonary tuberculosis
012.0*	Tuberculous pleurisy
012.1*	Tuberculosis of intrathoracic lymph nodes
012.2*	Isolated tracheal or bronchial tuberculosis
012.8*	Other specified respiratory tuberculosis
020.3	Primary pneumonic plague
020.4	Secondary pneumonic plague
020.5	Pneumonic plague, unspecified
021.2	Pulmonary tularemia
022.1	Pulmonary anthrax
031.0	Pulmonary diseases due to other mycobacteria
039.1	Pulmonary actinomycotic infection
052.1	Varicella (hemorrhagic) pneumonitis
055.1	Postmeasles pneumonia
073.0	Ornithosis with pneumonia
095.1	Syphilis of lung
112.4	Candidiasis of lung
114.0	Primary coccidioidomycosis (pulmonary)
114.4	Chronic pulmonary coccidioidomycosis
114.5	Unspecified pulmonary coccidioidomycosis
115.05	Histoplasma capsulatum pneumonia
115.15	Histoplasma duboisii pneumonia
115.95	Unspecified Histoplasmosis pneumonia
121.2	Paragonimiasis
122.1	Echinococcus granulosus infection of lung
130.4	Pneumonitis due to toxoplasmosis
136.3	Pneumocystosis
277.02	Cystic fibrosis with pulmonary manifestations
482.0	Pneumonia due to Klebsiella pneumoniae
482.1	Pneumonia due to Pseudomonas
482.4*	Pneumonia due to Staphylococcus
482.8*	Pneumonia due to other specified bacteria
484*	Pneumonia in infectious diseases classified elsewhere
507*	Pneumonitis due to solids and liquids
510*	Empyema
511.1	Pleurisy with effusion, with mention of bacterial cause other than tuberculosis
513*	Abscess of lung and mediastinum
519.2	Mediastinitis
795.5*	Nonspecific reaction to test for tuberculosis
V71.2	Observation for suspected tuberculosis

OR

Principal Diagnosis
487.0	Influenza with pneumonia

AND

Secondary Diagnosis
482.0	Pneumonia due to Klebsiella pneumoniae
482.1	Pneumonia due to Pseudomonas
482.40	Pneumonia due to Staphylococcus, unspecified
482.41	Methicillin susceptible pneumonia due to Staphylococcus aureus
482.42	Methicillin resistant pneumonia due to Staphylococcus aureus
482.49	Other Staphylococcus pneumonia
482.81	Pneumonia due to anaerobes
482.82	Pneumonia due to Escherichia coli (E. coli)
482.83	Pneumonia due to other gram-negative bacteria
482.84	Legionnaires' disease
482.89	Pneumonia due to other specified bacteria

Surgical	Medical	CC Indicator	MCC Indicator	Procedure Proxy

DRG 178 Respiratory Infections and Inflammations with CC
GMLOS 5.1   AMLOS 6.1   RW 1.3955   ☑ ⚐ T

Select principal diagnosis listed under DRG 177

DRG 179 Respiratory Infections and Inflammations without CC/MCC
GMLOS 3.7   AMLOS 4.5   RW 0.9741   ☑ ⚐ T

Select principal diagnosis listed under DRG 177

DRG 180 Respiratory Neoplasms with MCC
GMLOS 5.4   AMLOS 7.1   RW 1.7026   ☑

Principal Diagnosis

162*	Malignant neoplasm of trachea, bronchus, and lung
163*	Malignant neoplasm of pleura
164.2	Malignant neoplasm of anterior mediastinum
164.3	Malignant neoplasm of posterior mediastinum
164.8	Malignant neoplasm of other parts of mediastinum
164.9	Malignant neoplasm of mediastinum, part unspecified
165.8	Malignant neoplasm of other sites within the respiratory system and intrathoracic organs
165.9	Malignant neoplasm of ill-defined sites within the respiratory system
176.4	Kaposi's sarcoma of lung
195.1	Malignant neoplasm of thorax
197.0	Secondary malignant neoplasm of lung
197.1	Secondary malignant neoplasm of mediastinum
197.2	Secondary malignant neoplasm of pleura
197.3	Secondary malignant neoplasm of other respiratory organs
209.21	Malignant carcinoid tumor of the bronchus and lung
209.61	Benign carcinoid tumor of the bronchus and lung
212.2	Benign neoplasm of trachea
212.3	Benign neoplasm of bronchus and lung
212.4	Benign neoplasm of pleura
212.5	Benign neoplasm of mediastinum
212.8	Benign neoplasm of other specified sites of respiratory and intrathoracic organs
212.9	Benign neoplasm of respiratory and intrathoracic organs, site unspecified
213.3	Benign neoplasm of ribs, sternum, and clavicle
214.2	Lipoma of intrathoracic organs
231.1	Carcinoma in situ of trachea
231.2	Carcinoma in situ of bronchus and lung
231.8	Carcinoma in situ of other specified parts of respiratory system
231.9	Carcinoma in situ of respiratory system, part unspecified
235.7	Neoplasm of uncertain behavior of trachea, bronchus, and lung
235.8	Neoplasm of uncertain behavior of pleura, thymus, and mediastinum
235.9	Neoplasm of uncertain behavior of other and unspecified respiratory organs
239.1	Neoplasm of unspecified nature of respiratory system
511.81	Malignant pleural effusion

DRG 181 Respiratory Neoplasms with CC
GMLOS 3.8   AMLOS 5.0   RW 1.1725   ☑

Select principal diagnosis listed under DRG 180

DRG 182 Respiratory Neoplasms without CC/MCC
GMLOS 2.6   AMLOS 3.3   RW 0.7905   ☑

Select principal diagnosis listed under DRG 180

DRG 183 Major Chest Trauma with MCC
GMLOS 4.8   AMLOS 5.9   RW 1.4649   ☑

Principal Diagnosis

807.03	Closed fracture of three ribs
807.04	Closed fracture of four ribs
807.05	Closed fracture of five ribs
807.06	Closed fracture of six ribs
807.07	Closed fracture of seven ribs
807.08	Closed fracture of eight or more ribs
807.09	Closed fracture of multiple ribs, unspecified
807.1*	Open fracture of rib(s)
807.2	Closed fracture of sternum
807.3	Open fracture of sternum
807.4	Flail chest
839.61	Closed dislocation, sternum
839.71	Open dislocation, sternum
861.22	Lung laceration without mention of open wound into thorax
861.32	Lung laceration with open wound into thorax
862.0	Diaphragm injury without mention of open wound into cavity
862.1	Diaphragm injury with open wound into cavity
862.21	Bronchus injury without mention of open wound into cavity
862.31	Bronchus injury with open wound into cavity
874.02	Open wound of trachea, without mention of complication
874.12	Open wound of trachea, complicated

DRG 184 Major Chest Trauma with CC
GMLOS 3.4   AMLOS 4.1   RW 0.9832   ☑

Select principal diagnosis listed under DRG 183

DRG 185 Major Chest Trauma without CC/MCC
GMLOS 2.5   AMLOS 2.9   RW 0.6907   ☑

Select principal diagnosis listed under DRG 183

DRG 186 Pleural Effusion with MCC
GMLOS 4.9   AMLOS 6.3   RW 1.5727   ☑ T

Principal Diagnosis

511.89	Other specified forms of effusion, except tuberculous
511.9	Unspecified pleural effusion

DRG 187 Pleural Effusion with CC
GMLOS 3.6   AMLOS 4.5   RW 1.0808   ☑ T

Select principal diagnosis listed under DRG 186

DRG 188 Pleural Effusion without CC/MCC
GMLOS 2.6   AMLOS 3.3   RW 0.7468   ☑ T

Select principal diagnosis listed under DRG 186

DRG 189 Pulmonary Edema and Respiratory Failure
GMLOS 3.9   AMLOS 5.0   RW 1.2184   ☑ ⚐

Principal Diagnosis

506.1	Acute pulmonary edema due to fumes and vapors
514	Pulmonary congestion and hypostasis
518.4	Unspecified acute edema of lung
518.5*	Pulmonary insufficiency following trauma and surgery
518.81	Acute respiratory failure
518.83	Chronic respiratory failure
518.84	Acute and chronic respiratory failure

T Transfer DRG   SP Special Payment   ☑ Optimization Potential   ⚐ Targeted Potential   * Code Range   ● New DRG   ▲ Revised DRG Title

DRG 190   Chronic Obstructive Pulmonary Disease with MCC
GMLOS 4.2   AMLOS 5.1   RW 1.1708   ☑ ▽ T

Principal Diagnosis
491.1   Mucopurulent chronic bronchitis
491.2*   Obstructive chronic bronchitis
491.8   Other chronic bronchitis
491.9   Unspecified chronic bronchitis
492.0   Emphysematous bleb
492.8   Other emphysema
493.20   Chronic obstructive asthma, unspecified
493.21   Chronic obstructive asthma with status asthmaticus
493.22   Chronic obstructive asthma, with (acute) exacerbation
494*   Bronchiectasis
496   Chronic airway obstruction, not elsewhere classified
506.4   Chronic respiratory conditions due to fumes and vapors
506.9   Unspecified respiratory conditions due to fumes and vapors
748.61   Congenital bronchiectasis

DRG 191   Chronic Obstructive Pulmonary Disease with CC
GMLOS 3.5   AMLOS 4.2   RW 0.9343   ☑ ▽ T

Select principal diagnosis listed under DRG 190

DRG 192   Chronic Obstructive Pulmonary Disease without CC/MCC
GMLOS 2.8   AMLOS 3.3   RW 0.7120   ☑ ▽ T

Select principal diagnosis listed under DRG 190

DRG 193   Simple Pneumonia and Pleurisy with MCC
GMLOS 5.0   AMLOS 6.1   RW 1.4550   ☑ ▽ T

Principal Diagnosis
074.1   Epidemic pleurodynia
480*   Viral pneumonia
481   Pneumococcal pneumonia (streptococcus pneumoniae pneumonia)
482.2   Pneumonia due to Hemophilus influenzae (H. influenzae)
482.3*   Pneumonia due to Streptococcus
482.9   Unspecified bacterial pneumonia
483*   Pneumonia due to other specified organism
485   Bronchopneumonia, organism unspecified
486   Pneumonia, organism unspecified
487.0   Influenza with pneumonia
488.01   Influenza due to identified avian influenza virus with pneumonia
488.02   Influenza due to identified avian influenza virus with other respiratory manifestations
488.11   Influenza due to identified 2009 H1N1 influenza virus with pneumonia
488.12   Influenza due to identified 2009 H1N1 influenza virus with other respiratory manifestations
488.81   Influenza due to identified novel influenza A virus with pneumonia
488.82   Influenza due to identified novel influenza A virus with other respiratory manifestations
511.0   Pleurisy without mention of effusion or current tuberculosis

DRG 194   Simple Pneumonia and Pleurisy with CC
GMLOS 3.8   AMLOS 4.6   RW 0.9771   ☑ ▽ T

Select principal diagnosis listed under DRG 193

DRG 195   Simple Pneumonia and Pleurisy without CC/MCC
GMLOS 2.9   AMLOS 3.4   RW 0.6997   ☑ T

Select principal diagnosis listed under DRG 193

DRG 196   Interstitial Lung Disease with MCC
GMLOS 5.4   AMLOS 6.8   RW 1.6686   ☑ T

Principal Diagnosis
135   Sarcoidosis
137.0   Late effects of respiratory or unspecified tuberculosis
495*   Extrinsic allergic alveolitis
500   Coal workers' pneumoconiosis
501   Asbestosis
502   Pneumoconiosis due to other silica or silicates
503   Pneumoconiosis due to other inorganic dust
504   Pneumonopathy due to inhalation of other dust
505   Unspecified pneumoconiosis
508.1   Chronic and other pulmonary manifestations due to radiation
515   Postinflammatory pulmonary fibrosis
516*   Other alveolar and parietoalveolar pneumonopathy
517.1   Rheumatic pneumonia
517.2   Lung involvement in systemic sclerosis
517.3   Acute chest syndrome
517.8   Lung involvement in other diseases classified elsewhere
518.3   Pulmonary eosinophilia
518.6   Allergic bronchopulmonary aspergillosis
714.81   Rheumatoid lung
770.7   Chronic respiratory disease arising in the perinatal period

DRG 197   Interstitial Lung Disease with CC
GMLOS 3.8   AMLOS 4.7   RW 1.0627   ☑ T

Select principal diagnosis listed under DRG 196

DRG 198   Interstitial Lung Disease without CC/MCC
GMLOS 2.9   AMLOS 3.6   RW 0.7958   ☑ T

Select principal diagnosis listed under DRG 196

DRG 199   Pneumothorax with MCC
GMLOS 5.9   AMLOS 7.6   RW 1.8127   ☑

Principal Diagnosis
512.0   Spontaneous tension pneumothorax
512.1   Iatrogenic pneumothorax
512.2   Postoperative air leak
512.8*   Other pneumothorax and air leak
518.1   Interstitial emphysema
860*   Traumatic pneumothorax and hemothorax
958.7   Traumatic subcutaneous emphysema

DRG 200   Pneumothorax with CC
GMLOS 3.3   AMLOS 4.3   RW 0.9692   ☑ ▽

Select principal diagnosis listed under DRG 199

DRG 201   Pneumothorax without CC/MCC
GMLOS 2.6   AMLOS 3.3   RW 0.7053   ☑

Select principal diagnosis listed under DRG 199

DRG 202   Bronchitis and Asthma with CC/MCC
GMLOS 3.2   AMLOS 3.9   RW 0.8678   ☑ ▽

Principal Diagnosis
033*   Whooping cough
464.1*   Acute tracheitis
466*   Acute bronchitis and bronchiolitis
490   Bronchitis, not specified as acute or chronic
491.0   Simple chronic bronchitis
493.0*   Extrinsic asthma
493.1*   Intrinsic asthma
493.8*   Other forms of asthma

Surgical ▨   Medical ▨   CC Indicator ▨   MCC Indicator ▨   Procedure Proxy ▨

493.9*   Unspecified asthma
519.1*   Other diseases of trachea and bronchus, not elsewhere classified

DRG 203   Bronchitis and Asthma without CC/MCC
GMLOS 2.5   AMLOS 3.0   RW 0.6391   ☑ ▽

Select principal diagnosis listed under DRG 202

DRG 204   Respiratory Signs and Symptoms
GMLOS 2.1   AMLOS 2.7   RW 0.6780   ☑

Principal Diagnosis
327.22   High altitude periodic breathing
518.82   Other pulmonary insufficiency, not elsewhere classified
786.0*   Dyspnea and respiratory abnormalities
786.1   Stridor
786.2   Cough
786.3*   Hemoptysis
786.4   Abnormal sputum
786.52   Painful respiration
786.6   Swelling, mass, or lump in chest
786.7   Abnormal chest sounds
786.8   Hiccough
786.9   Other symptoms involving respiratory system and chest
793.19   Other nonspecific abnormal finding of lung field

DRG 205   Other Respiratory System Diagnoses with MCC
GMLOS 4.0   AMLOS 5.4   RW 1.3935   ☑ T

Principal Diagnosis
278.03   Obesity hypoventilation syndrome
306.1   Respiratory malfunction arising from mental factors
506.0   Bronchitis and pneumonitis due to fumes and vapors
506.2   Upper respiratory inflammation due to fumes and vapors
506.3   Other acute and subacute respiratory conditions due to fumes and vapors
508.0   Acute pulmonary manifestations due to radiation
508.2   Respiratory conditions due to smoke inhalation
508.8   Respiratory conditions due to other specified external agents
508.9   Respiratory conditions due to unspecified external agent
518.0   Pulmonary collapse
518.2   Compensatory emphysema
518.7   Transfusion related acute lung injury [TRALI]
518.89   Other diseases of lung, not elsewhere classified
519.0*   Tracheostomy complications
519.3   Other diseases of mediastinum, not elsewhere classified
519.4   Disorders of diaphragm
519.8   Other diseases of respiratory system, not elsewhere classified
519.9   Unspecified disease of respiratory system
573.5   Hepatopulmonary syndrome
733.6   Tietze's disease
748.4   Congenital cystic lung
748.5   Congenital agenesis, hypoplasia, and dysplasia of lung
748.60   Unspecified congenital anomaly of lung
748.69   Other congenital anomaly of lung
748.8   Other specified congenital anomaly of respiratory system
748.9   Unspecified congenital anomaly of respiratory system
754.81   Pectus excavatum
754.82   Pectus carinatum
756.3   Other congenital anomaly of ribs and sternum
756.6   Congenital anomaly of diaphragm
781.5   Clubbing of fingers
793.11   Solitary pulmonary nodule
794.2   Nonspecific abnormal results of pulmonary system function study
799.0*   Asphyxia and hypoxemia
799.1   Respiratory arrest

807.00   Closed fracture of rib(s), unspecified
807.01   Closed fracture of one rib
807.02   Closed fracture of two ribs
848.3   Sprain and strain of ribs
848.4*   Sprain and strain of sternum
861.20   Unspecified lung injury without mention of open wound into thorax
861.21   Lung contusion without mention of open wound into thorax
861.30   Unspecified lung injury with open wound into thorax
861.31   Lung contusion with open wound into thorax
862.29   Injury to other specified intrathoracic organs without mention of open wound into cavity
862.39   Injury to other specified intrathoracic organs with open wound into cavity
908.0   Late effect of internal injury to chest
934.0   Foreign body in trachea
934.1   Foreign body in main bronchus
934.8   Foreign body in other specified parts of trachea, bronchus, and lung
934.9   Foreign body in respiratory tree, unspecified
947.1   Burn of larynx, trachea, and lung
996.84   Complications of transplanted lung
997.3*   Respiratory complications
V42.6   Lung replaced by transplant
V45.76   Acquired absence of organ, lung
V55.0   Attention to tracheostomy

DRG 206   Other Respiratory System Diagnoses without MCC
GMLOS 2.5   AMLOS 3.2   RW 0.7911   ☑ T

Select principal diagnosis listed under DRG 205

DRG 207   Respiratory System Diagnosis with Ventilator Support 96+ Hours
GMLOS 12.1   AMLOS 14.1   RW 5.2556   ☑ ▽ T

Select principal diagnosis from MDC 4
AND

Nonoperating Room Procedure
96.72   Continuous invasive mechanical ventilation for 96 consecutive hours or more

DRG 208   Respiratory System Diagnosis with Ventilator Support <96 Hours
GMLOS 5.0   AMLOS 6.8   RW 2.2871   ☑ ▽

Select principal diagnosis from MDC 4
AND

Nonoperating Room Procedures
96.70   Continuous invasive mechanical ventilation of unspecified duration
96.71   Continuous invasive mechanical ventilation for less than 96 consecutive hours

---

T Transfer DRG   SP Special Payment   ☑ Optimization Potential   ▽ Targeted Potential   * Code Range   ● New DRG   ▲ Revised DRG Title

MDC 5
Diseases And Disorders Of The Circulatory System

032.82	395.2	410.60	422.93	427.9	442.3	453.52	74	
036.40	395.9	410.61	422.99	428.0	442.81	453.6	745.	
036.41	396.0	410.62	423.0	428.1	442.82	453.71	745	
036.42	396.1	410.70	423.1	428.20	442.83	453.72	745.	
036.43	396.2	410.71	423.2	428.21	442.84	453.73	745.9	
074.20	396.3	410.72	423.3	428.22	442.89	453.74	746.00	
074.21	396.8	410.80	423.8	428.23	442.9	453.75	746.01	
074.22	396.9	410.81	423.9	428.30	443.1	453.76	746.02	
074.23	397.0	410.82	424.0	428.31	443.21	453.77	746.09	
086.0	397.1	410.90	424.1	428.32	443.22	453.79	746.1	796.3
093.0	397.9	410.91	424.2	428.33	443.24	453.81	746.2	798.1
093.1	398.0	410.92	424.3	428.40	443.29	453.82	746.3	798.2
093.20	398.90	411.0	424.90	428.41	443.81	453.83	746.4	861.00
093.21	398.91	411.1	424.91	428.42	443.82	453.84	746.5	861.01
093.22	398.99	411.81	424.99	428.43	443.89	453.85	746.6	861.02
093.23	401.0	411.89	425.0	428.9	443.9	453.86	746.7	861.03
093.24	401.1	412	425.11	429.0	444.01	453.87	746.81	861.10
093.81	401.9	413.0	425.18	429.1	444.09	453.89	746.82	861.11
093.82	402.00	413.1	425.2	429.2	444.1	453.9	746.83	861.12
093.89	402.01	413.9	425.3	429.3	444.21	454.0	746.84	861.13
093.9	402.10	414.00	425.4	429.4	444.22	454.1	746.85	908.3
098.83	402.11	414.01	425.5	429.5	444.81	454.2	746.86	908.4
098.84	402.90	414.02	425.7	429.6	444.89	454.8	746.87	996.00
098.85	402.91	414.03	425.8	429.71	444.9	454.9	746.89	996.01
112.81	404.00	414.04	425.9	429.79	445.01	456.3	746.9	996.02
115.03	404.01	414.05	426.0	429.81	445.02	456.8	747.0	996.03
115.04	404.03	414.06	426.10	429.82	445.89	458.0	747.10	996.04
115.13	404.10	414.07	426.11	429.83	447.0	458.1	747.11	996.09
115.14	404.11	414.10	426.12	429.89	447.1	458.21	747.20	996.1
115.93	404.13	414.11	426.13	429.9	447.2	458.29	747.21	996.61
115.94	404.90	414.12	426.2	440.0	447.5	458.8	747.22	996.62
130.3	404.91	414.19	426.3	440.20	447.70	458.9	747.29	996.71
164.1	404.93	414.2	426.4	440.21	447.71	459.0	747.31	996.72
212.7	405.01	414.3	426.50	440.22	447.72	459.10	747.32	996.73
228.00	405.09	414.4	426.51	440.23	447.73	459.11	747.39	996.74
228.09	405.11	414.8	426.52	440.24	447.8	459.12	747.40	996.83
249.70	405.19	414.9	426.53	440.29	447.9	459.13	747.41	997.1
249.71	405.91	415.0	426.54	440.30	448.0	459.19	747.42	997.2
250.70	405.99	416.0	426.6	440.31	448.9	459.2	747.49	997.79
250.71	410.00	416.1	426.7	440.32	449	459.30	747.5	999.2
250.72	410.01	416.8	426.81	440.4	451.0	459.31	747.60	999.31
250.73	410.02	416.9	426.82	440.8	451.11	459.32	747.61	999.32
306.2	410.10	417.0	426.89	440.9	451.19	459.33	747.62	999.33
391.0	410.11	417.1	426.9	441.00	451.2	459.39	747.63	999.81
391.1	410.12	417.8	427.0	441.01	451.81	459.81	747.64	999.82
391.2	410.20	417.9	427.1	441.02	451.82	459.89	747.69	999.88
391.8	410.21	420.0	427.2	441.03	451.83	459.9	747.89	V42.1
391.9	410.22	420.90	427.31	441.1	451.84	745.0	747.9	V42.2
392.0	410.30	420.91	427.32	441.2	451.89	745.10	759.82	V43.21
392.9	410.31	420.99	427.41	441.3	451.9	745.11	780.2	V43.22
393	410.32	421.0	427.42	441.4	453.1	745.12	785.0	V43.3
394.0	410.40	421.1	427.5	441.5	453.2	745.19	785.1	V43.4
394.1	410.41	421.9	427.60	441.6	453.40	745.2	785.2	V53.31
394.2	410.42	422.0	427.61	441.7	453.41	745.3	785.3	V53.32
394.9	410.50	422.90	427.69	441.9	453.42	745.4	785.4	V53.39
395.0	410.51	422.91	427.81	442.0	453.50	745.5	785.50	V71.7
395.1	410.52	422.92	427.89	442.2	453.51	745.60	785.51	

MDC 5: Diseases And Disorders Of The Circulatory System—SURGICAL

SURGICAL

DRG 215 Other Heart Assist System Implant
GMLOS 10.0   **AMLOS 16.7**   **RW 14.7790**   ☑

Operating Room Procedures
37.53	Replacement or repair of thoracic unit of (total) replacement heart system
37.54	Replacement or repair of other implantable component of (total) replacement heart system
37.60	Implantation or insertion of biventricular external heart assist system
37.62	Insertion of temporary non-implantable extracorporeal circulatory assist device
37.63	Repair of heart assist system
37.65	Implant of single ventricular (extracorporeal) external heart assist system

DRG 216 Cardiac Valve and Other Major Cardiothoracic Procedures with Cardiac Catheterization with MCC
GMLOS 13.1   **AMLOS 15.8**   **RW 9.4801**   SP

Operating Room Procedures
35.05	Endovascular replacement of aortic valve
35.06	Transapical replacement of aortic valve
35.07	Endovascular replacement of pulmonary valve
35.08	Transapical replacement of pulmonary valve
35.09	Endovascular replacement of unspecified heart valve
35.1*	Open heart valvuloplasty without replacement
35.2*	Open and other replacement of heart valve
35.33	Annuloplasty
37.68	Insertion of percutaneous external heart assist device
38.45	Resection of other thoracic vessels with replacement
39.73	Endovascular implantation of graft in thoracic aorta

AND

Nonoperating Room Procedures
37.21	Right heart cardiac catheterization
37.22	Left heart cardiac catheterization
37.23	Combined right and left heart cardiac catheterization
37.26	Catheter based invasive electrophysiologic testing
88.52	Angiocardiography of right heart structures
88.53	Angiocardiography of left heart structures
88.54	Combined right and left heart angiocardiography
88.55	Coronary arteriography using single catheter
88.56	Coronary arteriography using two catheters
88.57	Other and unspecified coronary arteriography
88.58	Negative-contrast cardiac roentgenography

DRG 217 Cardiac Valve and Other Major Cardiothoracic Procedures with Cardiac Catheterization with CC
GMLOS 8.4   **AMLOS 9.7**   **RW 6.2835**   ☑ SP

Select operating room procedure AND nonoperating room procedure listed under DRG 216

DRG 218 Cardiac Valve and Other Major Cardiothoracic Procedures with Cardiac Catheterization without CC/MCC
GMLOS 6.1   **AMLOS 7.2**   **RW 5.4262**   ☑ SP

Select operating room procedure AND nonoperating room procedure listed under DRG 216

DRG 219 Cardiac Valve and Other Major Cardiothoracic Procedures without Cardiac Catheterization with MCC
GMLOS 10.0   **AMLOS 12.1**   **RW 7.9191**   ☑ SP

Operating Room Procedures
35.05	Endovascular replacement of aortic valve
35.06	Transapical replacement of aortic valve
35.07	Endovascular replacement of pulmonary valve
35.08	Transapical replacement of pulmonary valve
35.09	Endovascular replacement of unspecified heart valve
35.1*	Open heart valvuloplasty without replacement
35.2*	Open and other replacement of heart valve
35.33	Annuloplasty
37.68	Insertion of percutaneous external heart assist device
38.45	Resection of other thoracic vessels with replacement
39.73	Endovascular implantation of graft in thoracic aorta

DRG 220 Cardiac Valve and Other Major Cardiothoracic Procedures without Cardiac Catheterization with CC
GMLOS 6.6   **AMLOS 7.3**   **RW 5.2917**   ☑ SP

Select operating room procedures listed under DRG 219

DRG 221 Cardiac Valve and Other Major Cardiothoracic Procedures without Cardiac Catheterization without CC/MCC
GMLOS 4.9   **AMLOS 5.5**   **RW 4.6424**   ☑ SP

Select operating room procedures listed under DRG 219

DRG 222 Cardiac Defibrillator Implant with Cardiac Catheterization with Acute Myocardial Infarction/Heart Failure/Shock with MCC
GMLOS 9.6   **AMLOS 11.9**   **RW 8.8167**   ☑

Principal Diagnosis
398.91	Rheumatic heart failure (congestive)
402.01	Malignant hypertensive heart disease with heart failure
402.11	Benign hypertensive heart disease with heart failure
402.91	Hypertensive heart disease, unspecified, with heart failure
404.01	Hypertensive heart and chronic kidney disease, malignant, with heart failure and with chronic kidney disease stage I through stage IV, or unspecified
404.03	Hypertensive heart and chronic kidney disease, malignant, with heart failure and with chronic kidney disease stage V or end stage renal disease
404.11	Hypertensive heart and chronic kidney disease, benign, with heart failure and with chronic kidney disease stage I through stage IV, or unspecified
404.13	Hypertensive heart and chronic kidney disease, benign, with heart failure and chronic kidney disease stage V or end stage renal disease
404.91	Hypertensive heart and chronic kidney disease, unspecified, with heart failure and with chronic kidney disease stage I through stage IV, or unspecified
404.93	Hypertensive heart and chronic kidney disease, unspecified, with heart failure and chronic kidney disease stage V or end stage renal disease
410.01	Acute myocardial infarction of anterolateral wall, initial episode of care
410.11	Acute myocardial infarction of other anterior wall, initial episode of care
410.21	Acute myocardial infarction of inferolateral wall, initial episode of care
410.31	Acute myocardial infarction of inferoposterior wall, initial episode of care
410.41	Acute myocardial infarction of other inferior wall, initial episode of care
410.51	Acute myocardial infarction of other lateral wall, initial episode of care

---

Ⓣ *Transfer DRG*   SP *Special Payment*   ☑ *Optimization Potential*   ▽ *Targeted Potential*   * *Code Range*   ● *New DRG*   ▲ *Revised DRG Title*

Valid 10/01/2013-09/30/2014

410.61	Acute myocardial infarction, true posterior wall infarction, initial episode of care
410.71	Acute myocardial infarction, subendocardial infarction, initial episode of care
410.81	Acute myocardial infarction of other specified sites, initial episode of care
410.91	Acute myocardial infarction, unspecified site, initial episode of care
428.0	Congestive heart failure, unspecified
428.1	Left heart failure
428.2*	Systolic heart failure
428.3*	Diastolic heart failure
428.4*	Combined systolic and diastolic heart failure
428.9	Unspecified heart failure
785.50	Unspecified shock
785.51	Cardiogenic shock

AND

Operating Room Procedures

00.51	Implantation of cardiac resynchronization defibrillator, total system (CRT-D)
17.51	Implantation of rechargeable cardiac contractility modulation [CCM], total system
37.94	Implantation or replacement of automatic cardioverter/defibrillator, total system (AICD)

OR

Any of the following procedure combinations

00.52	Implantation or replacement of transvenous lead (electrode) into left ventricular coronary venous system
	AND
00.54	Implantation or replacement of cardiac resynchronization defibrillator pulse generator device only (CRT-D)

OR

37.74	Insertion or replacement of epicardial lead (electrode) into epicardium
	AND
00.54	Implantation or replacement of cardiac resynchronization defibrillator pulse generator device only (CRT-D)

OR

37.74	Insertion or replacement of epicardial lead (electrode) into epicardium
	AND
37.96	Implantation of automatic cardioverter/defibrillator pulse generator only

OR

37.74	Insertion or replacement of epicardial lead (electrode) into epicardium
	AND
37.98	Replacement of automatic cardioverter/defibrillator pulse generator only

OR

37.95	Implantation of automatic cardioverter/defibrillator leads(s) only
	AND
00.54	Implantation or replacement of cardiac resynchronization defibrillator pulse generator device only (CRT-D)

OR

37.95	Implantation of automatic cardioverter/defibrillator leads(s) only
	AND
37.96	Implantation of automatic cardioverter/defibrillator pulse generator only

OR

| 37.97 | Replacement of automatic cardioverter/defibrillator leads(s) only |

AND

| 00.54 | Implantation or replacement of cardiac resynchronization defibrillator pulse generator device only (CRT-D) |

OR

37.97	Replacement of automatic cardioverter/defibrillator leads(s) only
	AND
37.98	Replacement of automatic cardioverter/defibrillator pulse generator only

AND

Nonoperating Room Procedures

37.21	Right heart cardiac catheterization
37.22	Left heart cardiac catheterization
37.23	Combined right and left heart cardiac catheterization
88.52	Angiocardiography of right heart structures
88.53	Angiocardiography of left heart structures
88.54	Combined right and left heart angiocardiography
88.55	Coronary arteriography using single catheter
88.56	Coronary arteriography using two catheters
88.57	Other and unspecified coronary arteriography
88.58	Negative-contrast cardiac roentgenography

DRG 223 Cardiac Defibrillator Implant with Cardiac Catheterization with Acute Myocardial Infarction/Heart Failure/Shock without MCC

| GMLOS 4.6 | AMLOS 6.2 | RW 6.4257 | ☑ |

Select principal diagnosis AND operating room procedure OR procedure combinations AND nonoperating room procedure listed under DRG 222

DRG 224 Cardiac Defibrillator Implant with Cardiac Catheterization without Acute Myocardial Infarction/Heart Failure/Shock with MCC

| GMLOS 8.1 | AMLOS 10.0 | RW 7.7224 | ☑ |

Select any principal diagnosis listed under MDC 5 excluding acute myocardial infarction, heart failure and shock

Select any operating room procedure OR procedure combination AND nonoperating room procedure listed under DRG 222

DRG 225 Cardiac Defibrillator Implant with Cardiac Catheterization without Acute Myocardial Infarction/Heart Failure/Shock without MCC

| GMLOS 4.1 | AMLOS 4.9 | RW 5.9206 | ☑ |

Select any principal diagnosis listed under MDC 5 excluding acute myocardial infarction, heart failure and shock

Select any operating room procedure OR procedure combination AND nonoperating room procedure listed under DRG 222

DRG 226 Cardiac Defibrillator Implant without Cardiac Catheterization with MCC

| GMLOS 6.0 | AMLOS 8.4 | RW 7.0099 | ☑ |

Operating Room Procedures

00.51	Implantation of cardiac resynchronization defibrillator, total system (CRT-D)
17.51	Implantation of rechargeable cardiac contractility modulation [CCM], total system
37.94	Implantation or replacement of automatic cardioverter/defibrillator, total system (AICD)

OR

Any of the following procedure combinations

| 00.52 | Implantation or replacement of transvenous lead (electrode) into left ventricular coronary venous system |

MDC 5: Diseases And Disorders Of The Circulatory System—SURGICAL

AND

00.54   Implantation or replacement of cardiac resynchronization defibrillator pulse generator device only (CRT-D)

OR

37.74   Insertion or replacement of epicardial lead (electrode) into epicardium

AND

00.54   Implantation or replacement of cardiac resynchronization defibrillator pulse generator device only (CRT-D)

OR

37.74   Insertion or replacement of epicardial lead (electrode) into epicardium

AND

37.96   Implantation of automatic cardioverter/defibrillator pulse generator only

OR

37.74   Insertion or replacement of epicardial lead (electrode) into epicardium

AND

37.98   Replacement of automatic cardioverter/defibrillator pulse generator only

OR

37.95   Implantation of automatic cardioverter/defibrillator leads(s) only

AND

00.54   Implantation or replacement of cardiac resynchronization defibrillator pulse generator device only (CRT-D)

OR

37.95   Implantation of automatic cardioverter/defibrillator leads(s) only

AND

37.96   Implantation of automatic cardioverter/defibrillator pulse generator only

OR

37.97   Replacement of automatic cardioverter/defibrillator leads(s) only

AND

00.54   Implantation or replacement of cardiac resynchronization defibrillator pulse generator device only (CRT-D)

OR

37.97   Replacement of automatic cardioverter/defibrillator leads(s) only

AND

37.98   Replacement of automatic cardioverter/defibrillator pulse generator only

DRG 227   Cardiac Defibrillator Implant without Cardiac Catheterization without MCC

GMLOS 2.2   AMLOS 3.2   RW 5.5397   ☑

Select operating room procedure OR procedure combination listed under DRG 226

DRG 228   Other Cardiothoracic Procedures with MCC

GMLOS 11.1   AMLOS 13.2   RW 6.8682   ☑

Operating Room Procedures

35.31   Operations on papillary muscle
35.32   Operations on chordae tendineae
35.34   Infundibulectomy
35.35   Operations on trabeculae carneae cordis
35.39   Operations on other structures adjacent to valves of heart
35.42   Creation of septal defect in heart
35.50   Repair of unspecified septal defect of heart with prosthesis
35.51   Repair of atrial septal defect with prosthesis, open technique

35.53   Repair of ventricular septal defect with prosthesis, open technique
35.54   Repair of endocardial cushion defect with prosthesis
35.55   Repair of ventricular septal defect with prosthesis, closed technique
35.6*   Repair of atrial and ventricular septa with tissue graft
35.7*   Other and unspecified repair of atrial and ventricular septa
35.8*   Total repair of certain congenital cardiac anomalies
35.91   Interatrial transposition of venous return
35.92   Creation of conduit between right ventricle and pulmonary artery
35.93   Creation of conduit between left ventricle and aorta
35.94   Creation of conduit between atrium and pulmonary artery
35.95   Revision of corrective procedure on heart
35.98   Other operations on septa of heart
35.99   Other operations on valves of heart
36.03   Open chest coronary artery angioplasty
36.2   Heart revascularization by arterial implant
36.3*   Other heart revascularization
36.9*   Other operations on vessels of heart
37.10   Incision of heart, not otherwise specified
37.11   Cardiotomy
37.32   Excision of aneurysm of heart
37.33   Excision or destruction of other lesion or tissue of heart, open approach
37.35   Partial ventriculectomy
37.37   Excision or destruction of other lesion or tissue of heart, thoracoscopic approach

DRG 229   Other Cardiothoracic Procedures with CC

GMLOS 6.9   AMLOS 7.8   RW 4.4413   ☑

Select operating room procedure OR procedure combination listed under DRG 228

DRG 230   Other Cardiothoracic Procedures without CC/MCC

GMLOS 4.4   AMLOS 5.1   RW 3.6669   ☑

Select operating room procedure OR procedure combination listed under DRG 228

DRG 231   Coronary Bypass with PTCA with MCC

GMLOS 10.7   AMLOS 12.4   RW 7.8158

Operating Room Procedures

36.1*   Bypass anastomosis for heart revascularization

AND

Operating Room Procedures

00.66   Percutaneous transluminal coronary angioplasty [PTCA]
17.55   Transluminal coronary atherectomy
35.96   Percutaneous balloon valvuloplasty
35.97   Percutaneous mitral valve repair with implant

DRG 232   Coronary Bypass with PTCA without MCC

GMLOS 8.1   AMLOS 8.9   RW 5.6145   ☑

Select operating room procedures listed under DRG 231

DRG 233   Coronary Bypass with Cardiac Catheterization with MCC

GMLOS 11.9   AMLOS 13.4   RW 7.3887   ☑ T

Operating Room Procedures

36.1*   Bypass anastomosis for heart revascularization

AND

Nonoperating Room Procedures

37.21   Right heart cardiac catheterization
37.22   Left heart cardiac catheterization
37.23   Combined right and left heart cardiac catheterization

---

88.52	Angiocardiography of right heart structures
88.53	Angiocardiography of left heart structures
88.54	Combined right and left heart angiocardiography
88.55	Coronary arteriography using single catheter
88.56	Coronary arteriography using two catheters
88.57	Other and unspecified coronary arteriography
88.58	Negative-contrast cardiac roentgenography

DRG 234   **Coronary Bypass with Cardiac Catheterization without MCC**

GMLOS 8.0   AMLOS 8.6   RW 4.8270   ☑Ⓣ

Select operating room procedure AND nonoperating room procedure listed under DRG 233

DRG 235   **Coronary Bypass without Cardiac Catheterization with MCC**

GMLOS 9.2   AMLOS 10.6   RW 5.8478   ☑Ⓣ

Operating Room Procedures

36.1*	Bypass anastomosis for heart revascularization

DRG 236   **Coronary Bypass without Cardiac Catheterization without MCC**

GMLOS 6.0   AMLOS 6.5   RW 3.8011   ☑Ⓣ

Select operating room procedure listed under DRG 235

DRG 237   **Major Cardiovascular Procedures with MCC**

GMLOS 6.9   AMLOS 9.8   RW 5.0962   ☑

Operating Room Procedures

35.0*	Closed heart valvotomy or transcatheter replacement of heart valve
37.12	Pericardiotomy
37.24	Biopsy of pericardium
37.31	Pericardiectomy
37.4*	Repair of heart and pericardium
37.55	Removal of internal biventricular heart replacement system
37.61	Implant of pulsation balloon
37.64	Removal of external heart assist system(s) or device(s)
37.67	Implantation of cardiomyostimulation system
37.91	Open chest cardiac massage
37.99	Other operations on heart and pericardium
38.04	Incision of aorta
38.05	Incision of other thoracic vessels
38.06	Incision of abdominal arteries
38.07	Incision of abdominal veins
38.14	Endarterectomy of aorta
38.15	Endarterectomy of other thoracic vessels
38.16	Endarterectomy of abdominal arteries
38.34	Resection of aorta with anastomosis
38.35	Resection of other thoracic vessels with anastomosis
38.36	Resection of abdominal arteries with anastomosis
38.37	Resection of abdominal veins with anastomosis
38.44	Resection of abdominal aorta with replacement
38.46	Resection of abdominal arteries with replacement
38.47	Resection of abdominal veins with replacement
38.55	Ligation and stripping of varicose veins of other thoracic vessel
38.64	Other excision of abdominal aorta
38.65	Other excision of other thoracic vessel
38.66	Other excision of abdominal arteries
38.67	Other excision of abdominal veins
38.84	Other surgical occlusion of abdominal aorta
38.85	Other surgical occlusion of other thoracic vessel
38.86	Other surgical occlusion of abdominal arteries
38.87	Other surgical occlusion of abdominal veins
39.0	Systemic to pulmonary artery shunt

39.1	Intra-abdominal venous shunt
39.21	Caval-pulmonary artery anastomosis
39.22	Aorta-subclavian-carotid bypass
39.23	Other intrathoracic vascular shunt or bypass
39.24	Aorta-renal bypass
39.25	Aorta-iliac-femoral bypass
39.26	Other intra-abdominal vascular shunt or bypass
39.52	Other repair of aneurysm
39.54	Re-entry operation (aorta)
39.71	Endovascular implantation of other graft in abdominal aorta
39.72	Endovascular (total) embolization or occlusion of head and neck vessels
39.75	Endovascular embolization or occlusion of vessel(s) of head or neck using bare coils
39.76	Endovascular embolization or occlusion of vessel(s) of head or neck using bioactive coils
39.78	Endovascular implantation of branching or fenestrated graft(s) in aorta
39.79	Other endovascular procedures on other vessels

DRG 238   **Major Cardiovascular Procedures without MCC**

GMLOS 2.6   AMLOS 3.8   RW 3.3576   ☑

Operating Room Procedures

35.0*	Closed heart valvotomy or transcatheter replacement of heart valve
37.12	Pericardiotomy
37.24	Biopsy of pericardium
37.31	Pericardiectomy
37.4*	Repair of heart and pericardium
37.55	Removal of internal biventricular heart replacement system
37.61	Implant of pulsation balloon
37.64	Removal of external heart assist system(s) or device(s)
37.67	Implantation of cardiomyostimulation system
37.91	Open chest cardiac massage
37.99	Other operations on heart and pericardium
38.04	Incision of aorta
38.05	Incision of other thoracic vessels
38.06	Incision of abdominal arteries
38.07	Incision of abdominal veins
38.14	Endarterectomy of aorta
38.15	Endarterectomy of other thoracic vessels
38.16	Endarterectomy of abdominal arteries
38.34	Resection of aorta with anastomosis
38.35	Resection of other thoracic vessels with anastomosis
38.36	Resection of abdominal arteries with anastomosis
38.37	Resection of abdominal veins with anastomosis
38.44	Resection of abdominal aorta with replacement
38.46	Resection of abdominal arteries with replacement
38.47	Resection of abdominal veins with replacement
38.55	Ligation and stripping of varicose veins of other thoracic vessel
38.64	Other excision of abdominal aorta
38.65	Other excision of other thoracic vessel
38.66	Other excision of abdominal arteries
38.67	Other excision of abdominal veins
38.84	Other surgical occlusion of abdominal aorta
38.85	Other surgical occlusion of other thoracic vessel
38.86	Other surgical occlusion of abdominal arteries
38.87	Other surgical occlusion of abdominal veins
39.0	Systemic to pulmonary artery shunt
39.1	Intra-abdominal venous shunt
39.21	Caval-pulmonary artery anastomosis
39.22	Aorta-subclavian-carotid bypass
39.23	Other intrathoracic vascular shunt or bypass
39.24	Aorta-renal bypass
39.25	Aorta-iliac-femoral bypass
39.26	Other intra-abdominal vascular shunt or bypass
39.52	Other repair of aneurysm
39.54	Re-entry operation (aorta)

MDC 5: Diseases And Disorders Of The Circulatory System—SURGICAL

Surgical	Medical	CC Indicator	MCC Indicator	Procedure Proxy

39.71	Endovascular implantation of other graft in abdominal aorta
39.72	Endovascular (total) embolization or occlusion of head and neck vessels
39.75	Endovascular embolization or occlusion of vessel(s) of head or neck using bare coils
39.76	Endovascular embolization or occlusion of vessel(s) of head or neck using bioactive coils
39.78	Endovascular implantation of branching or fenestrated graft(s) in aorta
39.79	Other endovascular procedures on other vessels

DRG 239 Amputation for Circulatory System Disorders Except Upper Limb and Toe with MCC

GMLOS 10.9 **AMLOS 13.9** **RW 4.8601** [T]

Operating Room Procedures

84.10	Lower limb amputation, not otherwise specified
84.12	Amputation through foot
84.13	Disarticulation of ankle
84.14	Amputation of ankle through malleoli of tibia and fibula
84.15	Other amputation below knee
84.16	Disarticulation of knee
84.17	Amputation above knee
84.18	Disarticulation of hip
84.19	Abdominopelvic amputation
84.91	Amputation, not otherwise specified

DRG 240 Amputation for Circulatory System Disorders Except Upper Limb and Toe with CC

GMLOS 7.2 **AMLOS 8.8** **RW 2.6789** ☑[T]

Select operating room procedures listed under DRG 239

DRG 241 Amputation for Circulatory System Disorders Except Upper Limb and Toe without CC/MCC

GMLOS 4.6 **AMLOS 5.5** **RW 1.4226** ☑[T]

Select operating room procedures listed under DRG 239

DRG 242 Permanent Cardiac Pacemaker Implant with MCC

GMLOS 5.9 **AMLOS 7.6** **RW 3.7491** ☑[T]

Operating Room Procedure

| 00.50 | Implantation of cardiac resynchronization pacemaker without mention of defibrillation, total system (CRT-P) |

OR

Any of the following procedure combinations

00.52	Implantation or replacement of transvenous lead (electrode) into left ventricular coronary venous system
	AND
00.53	Implantation or replacement of cardiac resynchronization pacemaker pulse generator only (CRT-P)

OR

37.70	Initial insertion of lead (electrode), not otherwise specified
	AND
00.53	Implantation or replacement of cardiac resynchronization pacemaker pulse generator only (CRT-P)

OR

37.70	Initial insertion of lead (electrode), not otherwise specified
	AND
37.80	Insertion of permanent pacemaker, initial or replacement, type of device not specified

OR

37.70	Initial insertion of lead (electrode), not otherwise specified
	AND
37.81	Initial insertion of single-chamber device, not specified as rate responsive

OR

37.70	Initial insertion of lead (electrode), not otherwise specified
	AND
37.82	Initial insertion of single-chamber device, rate responsive

OR

37.70	Initial insertion of lead (electrode), not otherwise specified
	AND
37.85	Replacement of any type of pacemaker device with single-chamber device, not specified as rate responsive

OR

37.70	Initial insertion of lead (electrode), not otherwise specified
	AND
37.86	Replacement of any type of pacemaker device with single-chamber device, rate responsive

OR

37.70	Initial insertion of lead (electrode), not otherwise specified
	AND
37.87	Replacement of any type of pacemaker device with dual-chamber device

OR

37.71	Initial insertion of transvenous lead (electrode) into ventricle
	AND
00.53	Implantation or replacement of cardiac resynchronization pacemaker pulse generator only (CRT-P)

OR

37.71	Initial insertion of transvenous lead (electrode) into ventricle
	AND
37.80	Insertion of permanent pacemaker, initial or replacement, type of device not specified

OR

37.71	Initial insertion of transvenous lead (electrode) into ventricle
	AND
37.81	Initial insertion of single-chamber device, not specified as rate responsive

OR

37.71	Initial insertion of transvenous lead (electrode) into ventricle
	AND
37.82	Initial insertion of single-chamber device, rate responsive

OR

37.71	Initial insertion of transvenous lead (electrode) into ventricle
	AND
37.85	Replacement of any type of pacemaker device with single-chamber device, not specified as rate responsive

OR

37.71	Initial insertion of transvenous lead (electrode) into ventricle
	AND
37.86	Replacement of any type of pacemaker device with single-chamber device, rate responsive

OR

37.71	Initial insertion of transvenous lead (electrode) into ventricle
	AND
37.87	Replacement of any type of pacemaker device with dual-chamber device

OR

37.72	Initial insertion of transvenous leads (electrodes) into atrium and ventricle
	AND
00.53	Implantation or replacement of cardiac resynchronization pacemaker pulse generator only (CRT-P)

OR

| 37.72 | Initial insertion of transvenous leads (electrodes) into atrium and ventricle |

[T] *Transfer DRG* [S] *Special Payment* ☑ *Optimization Potential* ▽ *Targeted Potential* *Code Range* ● *New DRG* ▲ *Revised DRG Title*

60   Valid 10/01/2013-09/30/2014   © 2013 OptumInsight, Inc.

AND

37.80   Insertion of permanent pacemaker, initial or replacement, type of device not specified

OR

37.72   Initial insertion of transvenous leads (electrodes) into atrium and ventricle
     AND

37.83   Initial insertion of dual-chamber device

OR

37.73   Initial insertion of transvenous lead (electrode) into atrium
     AND

00.53   Implantation or replacement of cardiac resynchronization pacemaker pulse generator only (CRT-P)

OR

37.73   Initial insertion of transvenous lead (electrode) into atrium
     AND

37.80   Insertion of permanent pacemaker, initial or replacement, type of device not specified

OR

37.73   Initial insertion of transvenous lead (electrode) into atrium
     AND

37.81   Initial insertion of single-chamber device, not specified as rate responsive

OR

37.73   Initial insertion of transvenous lead (electrode) into atrium
     AND

37.82   Initial insertion of single-chamber device, rate responsive

OR

37.73   Initial insertion of transvenous lead (electrode) into atrium
     AND

37.85   Replacement of any type of pacemaker device with single-chamber device, not specified as rate responsive

OR

37.73   Initial insertion of transvenous lead (electrode) into atrium
     AND

37.86   Replacement of any type of pacemaker device with single-chamber device, rate responsive

OR

37.73   Initial insertion of transvenous lead (electrode) into atrium
     AND

37.87   Replacement of any type of pacemaker device with dual-chamber device

OR

37.74   Insertion or replacement of epicardial lead (electrode) into epicardium
     AND

00.53   Implantation or replacement of cardiac resynchronization pacemaker pulse generator only (CRT-P)

OR

37.74   Insertion or replacement of epicardial lead (electrode) into epicardium
     AND

37.80   Insertion of permanent pacemaker, initial or replacement, type of device not specified

OR

37.74   Insertion or replacement of epicardial lead (electrode) into epicardium
     AND

37.81   Initial insertion of single-chamber device, not specified as rate responsive

OR

37.74   Insertion or replacement of epicardial lead (electrode) into epicardium

AND

37.82   Initial insertion of single-chamber device, rate responsive

OR

37.74   Insertion or replacement of epicardial lead (electrode) into epicardium
     AND

37.83   Initial insertion of dual-chamber device

OR

37.74   Insertion or replacement of epicardial lead (electrode) into epicardium
     AND

37.85   Replacement of any type of pacemaker device with single-chamber device, not specified as rate responsive

OR

37.74   Insertion or replacement of epicardial lead (electrode) into epicardium
     AND

37.86   Replacement of any type of pacemaker device with single-chamber device, rate responsive

OR

37.74   Insertion or replacement of epicardial lead (electrode) into epicardium
     AND

37.87   Replacement of any type of pacemaker device with dual-chamber device

OR

37.76   Replacement of transvenous atrial and/or ventricular lead(s) (electrode(s))
     AND

00.53   Implantation or replacement of cardiac resynchronization pacemaker pulse generator only (CRT-P)

OR

37.76   Replacement of transvenous atrial and/or ventricular lead(s) (electrode(s))
     AND

37.80   Insertion of permanent pacemaker, initial or replacement, type of device not specified

OR

37.76   Replacement of transvenous atrial and/or ventricular lead(s) (electrode(s))
     AND

37.85   Replacement of any type of pacemaker device with single-chamber device, not specified as rate responsive

OR

37.76   Replacement of transvenous atrial and/or ventricular lead(s) (electrode(s))
     AND

37.86   Replacement of any type of pacemaker device with single-chamber device, rate responsive

OR

37.76   Replacement of transvenous atrial and/or ventricular lead(s) (electrode(s))
     AND

37.87   Replacement of any type of pacemaker device with dual-chamber device

DRG 243   **Permanent Cardiac Pacemaker Implant with CC**
     GMLOS 3.7   AMLOS 4.6   RW 2.6716   ☑Ⓣ

Select operating room procedure or combinations listed under DRG 242

Surgical   *Medical*   *CC Indicator*   *MCC Indicator*   *Procedure Proxy*

MDC 5: Diseases And Disorders Of The Circulatory System—SURGICAL

MDC 5: Diseases And Disorders Of The Circulatory System—SURGICAL

DRG 244   Permanent Cardiac Pacemaker Implant without CC/MCC

GMLOS 2.4   AMLOS 2.9   RW 2.1608   ☑ⓣ

Select operating room procedure or combinations listed under DRG 242

DRG 245   AICD Generator Procedures

GMLOS 3.3   AMLOS 4.7   RW 4.7022   ☑

Operating Room Procedures

00.54	Implantation or replacement of cardiac resynchronization defibrillator pulse generator device only (CRT-D)
17.52	Implantation or replacement of cardiac contractility modulation [CCM] rechargeable pulse generator only
37.96	Implantation of automatic cardioverter/defibrillator pulse generator only
37.98	Replacement of automatic cardioverter/defibrillator pulse generator only

DRG 246   Percutaneous Cardiovascular Procedure with Drug-Eluting Stent with MCC or 4+ Vessels/Stents

GMLOS 3.9   AMLOS 5.2   RW 3.1830   ☑

Operating Room Procedures

00.66	Percutaneous transluminal coronary angioplasty [PTCA]
17.55	Transluminal coronary atherectomy
35.96	Percutaneous balloon valvuloplasty
35.97	Percutaneous mitral valve repair with implant
36.09	Other removal of coronary artery obstruction
37.34	Excision or destruction of other lesion or tissue of heart, endovascular approach

OR

Nonoperating Room Procedures

37.26	Catheter based invasive electrophysiologic testing
37.27	Cardiac mapping

AND

Nonoperating Room Procedure

36.07	Insertion of drug-eluting coronary artery stent(s)

OR

Any of the following procedure combinations:

00.43	Procedure on four or more vessels
	AND
00.66	Percutaneous transluminal coronary angioplasty [PTCA]
OR	
00.48	Insertion of four or more vascular stents
	AND
00.66	Percutaneous transluminal coronary angioplasty [PTCA]

DRG 247   Percutaneous Cardiovascular Procedure with Drug-Eluting Stent without MCC

GMLOS 2.1   AMLOS 2.5   RW 2.0408   ☑

Operating Room Procedures

00.66	Percutaneous transluminal coronary angioplasty [PTCA]
17.55	Transluminal coronary atherectomy
35.96	Percutaneous balloon valvuloplasty
35.97	Percutaneous mitral valve repair with implant
36.09	Other removal of coronary artery obstruction
37.34	Excision or destruction of other lesion or tissue of heart, endovascular approach

OR

Nonoperating Room Procedures

37.26	Catheter based invasive electrophysiologic testing
37.27	Cardiac mapping

AND

Nonoperating Room Procedure

36.07	Insertion of drug-eluting coronary artery stent(s)

DRG 248   Percutaneous Cardiovascular Procedure with Non Drug-Eluting Stent with MCC or 4+ Vessels/Stents

GMLOS 4.6   AMLOS 6.2   RW 2.9479   ☑

Operating Room Procedures

00.66	Percutaneous transluminal coronary angioplasty [PTCA]
17.55	Transluminal coronary atherectomy
35.96	Percutaneous balloon valvuloplasty
35.97	Percutaneous mitral valve repair with implant
36.09	Other removal of coronary artery obstruction
37.34	Excision or destruction of other lesion or tissue of heart, endovascular approach

OR

Nonoperating Room Procedures

37.26	Catheter based invasive electrophysiologic testing
37.27	Cardiac mapping

AND

Nonoperating Room Procedure

36.06	Insertion of non-drug-eluting coronary artery stent(s)

OR

Operating Room Procedure

92.27	Implantation or insertion of radioactive elements

OR

Any of the following procedure combinations:

00.43	Procedure on four or more vessels
	AND
00.66	Percutaneous transluminal coronary angioplasty [PTCA]
OR	
00.48	Insertion of four or more vascular stents
	AND
00.66	Percutaneous transluminal coronary angioplasty [PTCA]

DRG 249   Percutaneous Cardiovascular Procedure with Non Drug-Eluting Stent without MCC

GMLOS 2.4   AMLOS 3.0   RW 1.8245   ☑

Operating Room Procedures

00.66	Percutaneous transluminal coronary angioplasty [PTCA]
17.55	Transluminal coronary atherectomy
35.96	Percutaneous balloon valvuloplasty
35.97	Percutaneous mitral valve repair with implant
36.09	Other removal of coronary artery obstruction
37.34	Excision or destruction of other lesion or tissue of heart, endovascular approach

OR

Nonoperating Room Procedures

37.26	Catheter based invasive electrophysiologic testing
37.27	Cardiac mapping

AND

Operating Room Procedure

92.27	Implantation or insertion of radioactive elements

OR

Nonoperating Room Procedure

36.06	Insertion of non-drug-eluting coronary artery stent(s)

ⓣ Transfer DRG   ⓢ Special Payment   ☑ Optimization Potential   Ⓣ Targeted Potential   * Code Range   ● New DRG   ▲ Revised DRG Title

62   Valid 10/01/2013-09/30/2014   © 2013 OptumInsight, Inc.

DRG 250   Percutaneous Cardiovascular Procedure without Coronary Artery Stent with MCC

GMLOS 5.1   **AMLOS 7.0**   **RW 2.9881**   ☑

Operating Room Procedures
00.66	Percutaneous transluminal coronary angioplasty [PTCA]
17.55	Transluminal coronary atherectomy
35.52	Repair of atrial septal defect with prosthesis, closed technique
35.96	Percutaneous balloon valvuloplasty
35.97	Percutaneous mitral valve repair with implant
36.09	Other removal of coronary artery obstruction
37.34	Excision or destruction of other lesion or tissue of heart, endovascular approach

OR

Nonoperating Room Procedures
37.26	Catheter based invasive electrophysiologic testing
37.27	Cardiac mapping
37.90	Insertion of left atrial appendage device

DRG 251   Percutaneous Cardiovascular Procedure without Coronary Artery Stent without MCC

GMLOS 2.4   **AMLOS 3.1**   **RW 1.9737**   ☑

Select operating procedures OR nonoperating room procedures listed under DRG 250

DRG 252   Other Vascular Procedures with MCC

GMLOS 5.3   **AMLOS 7.7**   **RW 3.1477**   ☑

Operating Room Procedures
00.61	Percutaneous angioplasty of extracranial vessel(s)
00.62	Percutaneous angioplasty of intracranial vessel(s)
04.92	Implantation or replacement of peripheral neurostimulator lead(s)
17.53	Percutaneous atherectomy of extracranial vessel(s)
17.54	Percutaneous atherectomy of intracranial vessel(s)
17.56	Atherectomy of other non-coronary vessel(s)
38.00	Incision of vessel, unspecified site
38.02	Incision of other vessels of head and neck
38.03	Incision of upper limb vessels
38.08	Incision of lower limb arteries
38.10	Endarterectomy, unspecified site
38.12	Endarterectomy of other vessels of head and neck
38.13	Endarterectomy of upper limb vessels
38.18	Endarterectomy of lower limb arteries
38.21	Biopsy of blood vessel
38.29	Other diagnostic procedures on blood vessels
38.30	Resection of vessel with anastomosis, unspecified site
38.32	Resection of other vessels of head and neck with anastomosis
38.33	Resection of upper limb vessels with anastomosis
38.38	Resection of lower limb arteries with anastomosis
38.40	Resection of vessel with replacement, unspecified site
38.42	Resection of other vessels of head and neck with replacement
38.43	Resection of upper limb vessels with replacement
38.48	Resection of lower limb arteries with replacement
38.52	Ligation and stripping of varicose veins of other vessels of head and neck
38.57	Ligation and stripping of abdominal varicose veins
38.60	Other excision of vessels, unspecified site
38.62	Other excision of other vessels of head and neck
38.63	Other excision of upper limb vessels
38.68	Other excision of lower limb arteries
38.7	Interruption of the vena cava
38.80	Other surgical occlusion of vessels, unspecified site
38.82	Other surgical occlusion of other vessels of head and neck
38.83	Other surgical occlusion of upper limb vessels
38.88	Other surgical occlusion of lower limb arteries
39.29	Other (peripheral) vascular shunt or bypass
39.30	Suture of unspecified blood vessel
39.31	Suture of artery
39.41	Control of hemorrhage following vascular surgery
39.49	Other revision of vascular procedure
39.50	Angioplasty of other non-coronary vessel(s)
39.51	Clipping of aneurysm
39.53	Repair of arteriovenous fistula
39.55	Reimplantation of aberrant renal vessel
39.56	Repair of blood vessel with tissue patch graft
39.57	Repair of blood vessel with synthetic patch graft
39.58	Repair of blood vessel with unspecified type of patch graft
39.59	Other repair of vessel
39.77	Temporary (partial) therapeutic endovascular occlusion of vessel
39.8*	Operations on carotid body, carotid sinus and other vascular bodies
39.91	Freeing of vessel
39.94	Replacement of vessel-to-vessel cannula
39.99	Other operations on vessels
86.96	Insertion or replacement of other neurostimulator pulse generator

DRG 253   Other Vascular Procedures with CC

GMLOS 4.1   **AMLOS 5.5**   **RW 2.5172**   ☑

Select operating room procedures listed under DRG 252

DRG 254   Other Vascular Procedures without CC/MCC

GMLOS 2.2   **AMLOS 2.9**   **RW 1.7012**   ☑

Select operating room procedures listed under DRG 252

DRG 255   Upper Limb and Toe Amputation for Circulatory System Disorders with MCC

GMLOS 6.8   **AMLOS 8.8**   **RW 2.6404**   ☑ T

Operating Room Procedures
84.0*	Amputation of upper limb
84.11	Amputation of toe
84.3	Revision of amputation stump

DRG 256   Upper Limb and Toe Amputation for Circulatory System Disorders with CC

GMLOS 5.3   **AMLOS 6.5**   **RW 1.5973**   ☑ T

Select operating room procedures listed under DRG 255

DRG 257   Upper Limb and Toe Amputation for Circulatory System Disorders without CC/MCC

GMLOS 3.0   **AMLOS 3.7**   **RW 0.9017**   ☑ T

Select operating room procedures listed under DRG 255

DRG 258   Cardiac Pacemaker Device Replacement with MCC

GMLOS 4.9   **AMLOS 6.2**   **RW 2.7229**   ☑

Operating Room Procedures
00.53	Implantation or replacement of cardiac resynchronization pacemaker pulse generator only (CRT-P)
00.57	Implantation or replacement of subcutaneous device for intracardiac or great vessel hemodynamic monitoring
37.80	Insertion of permanent pacemaker, initial or replacement, type of device not specified
37.85	Replacement of any type of pacemaker device with single-chamber device, not specified as rate responsive
37.86	Replacement of any type of pacemaker device with single-chamber device, rate responsive

MDC 5: Diseases And Disorders Of The Circulatory System—SURGICAL

37.87	Replacement of any type of pacemaker device with dual-chamber device

DRG 259   Cardiac Pacemaker Device Replacement without MCC

GMLOS 2.7   AMLOS 3.4   RW 1.9462   ☑

Select operating room procedures listed under DRG 258

DRG 260   Cardiac Pacemaker Revision Except Device Replacement with MCC

GMLOS 7.7   AMLOS 10.5   RW 3.7238   ☑

Operating Room Procedures

00.56	Insertion or replacement of implantable pressure sensor with lead for intracardiac or great vessel hemodynamic monitoring
37.74	Insertion or replacement of epicardial lead (electrode) into epicardium
37.75	Revision of lead (electrode)
37.76	Replacement of transvenous atrial and/or ventricular lead(s) (electrode(s))
37.77	Removal of lead(s) (electrodes) without replacement
37.79	Revision or relocation of cardiac device pocket
37.89	Revision or removal of pacemaker device

DRG 261   Cardiac Pacemaker Revision Except Device Replacement with CC

GMLOS 3.2   AMLOS 4.3   RW 1.7284   ☑

Select operating room procedures listed under DRG 260

DRG 262   Cardiac Pacemaker Revision Except Device Replacement without CC/MCC

GMLOS 2.3   AMLOS 2.9   RW 1.3866   ☑

Select operating room procedures listed under DRG 260

DRG 263   Vein Ligation and Stripping

GMLOS 3.6   AMLOS 5.2   RW 1.8888   ☑

Operating Room Procedures

38.09	Incision of lower limb veins
38.39	Resection of lower limb veins with anastomosis
38.49	Resection of lower limb veins with replacement
38.50	Ligation and stripping of varicose veins, unspecified site
38.53	Ligation and stripping of varicose veins of upper limb vessels
38.59	Ligation and stripping of lower limb varicose veins
38.69	Other excision of lower limb veins
38.89	Other surgical occlusion of lower limb veins
39.32	Suture of vein
39.92	Injection of sclerosing agent into vein

DRG 264   Other Circulatory System O.R. Procedures

GMLOS 5.6   AMLOS 8.2   RW 2.7138   ☑Ⓣ

Operating Room Procedures

05.0	Division of sympathetic nerve or ganglion
05.2*	Sympathectomy
05.89	Other operations on sympathetic nerves or ganglia
17.32	Laparoscopic cecectomy
17.33	Laparoscopic right hemicolectomy
17.34	Laparoscopic resection of transverse colon
17.35	Laparoscopic left hemicolectomy
17.39	Other laparoscopic partial excision of large intestine
21.04	Control of epistaxis by ligation of ethmoidal arteries
21.05	Control of epistaxis by (transantral) ligation of the maxillary artery
21.06	Control of epistaxis by ligation of the external carotid artery
21.07	Control of epistaxis by excision of nasal mucosa and skin grafting of septum and lateral nasal wall
21.09	Control of epistaxis by other means
25.1	Excision or destruction of lesion or tissue of tongue
31.72	Closure of external fistula of trachea
31.74	Revision of tracheostomy
33.20	Thoracoscopic lung biopsy
33.27	Closed endoscopic biopsy of lung
33.28	Open biopsy of lung
34.02	Exploratory thoracotomy
34.03	Reopening of recent thoracotomy site
34.1	Incision of mediastinum
34.21	Transpleural thoracoscopy
34.22	Mediastinoscopy
34.26	Open biopsy of mediastinum
34.29	Other diagnostic procedures on mediastinum
38.26	Insertion of implantable pressure sensor without lead for intracardiac or great vessel hemodynamic monitoring
39.27	Arteriovenostomy for renal dialysis
39.42	Revision of arteriovenous shunt for renal dialysis
39.43	Removal of arteriovenous shunt for renal dialysis
39.93	Insertion of vessel-to-vessel cannula
39.98	Control of hemorrhage, not otherwise specified
40.1*	Diagnostic procedures on lymphatic structures
40.21	Excision of deep cervical lymph node
40.23	Excision of axillary lymph node
40.24	Excision of inguinal lymph node
40.29	Simple excision of other lymphatic structure
40.3	Regional lymph node excision
41.5	Total splenectomy
43.6	Partial gastrectomy with anastomosis to duodenum
43.7	Partial gastrectomy with anastomosis to jejunum
43.82	Laparoscopic vertical (sleeve) gastrectomy
43.89	Open and other partial gastrectomy
43.99	Other total gastrectomy
44.38	Laparoscopic gastroenterostomy
44.39	Other gastroenterostomy without gastrectomy
45.61	Multiple segmental resection of small intestine
45.62	Other partial resection of small intestine
45.72	Open and other cecectomy
45.73	Open and other right hemicolectomy
45.74	Open and other resection of transverse colon
45.75	Open and other left hemicolectomy
45.79	Other and unspecified partial excision of large intestine
45.8*	Total intra-abdominal colectomy
45.93	Other small-to-large intestinal anastomosis
46.03	Exteriorization of large intestine
46.13	Permanent colostomy
47.09	Other appendectomy
48.25	Open biopsy of rectum
48.35	Local excision of rectal lesion or tissue
48.62	Anterior resection of rectum with synchronous colostomy
48.63	Other anterior resection of rectum
48.69	Other resection of rectum
50.12	Open biopsy of liver
54.0	Incision of abdominal wall
54.11	Exploratory laparotomy
54.19	Other laparotomy
54.93	Creation of cutaneoperitoneal fistula
54.95	Incision of peritoneum
55.91	Decapsulation of kidney
84.94	Insertion of sternal fixation device with rigid plates
86.06	Insertion of totally implantable infusion pump
86.22	Excisional debridement of wound, infection, or burn
86.4	Radical excision of skin lesion
86.60	Free skin graft, not otherwise specified
86.61	Full-thickness skin graft to hand
86.62	Other skin graft to hand
86.63	Full-thickness skin graft to other sites
86.65	Heterograft to skin

Ⓣ *Transfer DRG*   ⓢⓅ *Special Payment*   ☑ *Optimization Potential*   🆃 *Targeted Potential*   * *Code Range*   ● *New DRG*   ▲ *Revised DRG Title*

86.66	Homograft to skin	
86.67	Dermal regenerative graft	
86.69	Other skin graft to other sites	
86.70	Pedicle or flap graft, not otherwise specified	
86.71	Cutting and preparation of pedicle grafts or flaps	
86.72	Advancement of pedicle graft	
86.74	Attachment of pedicle or flap graft to other sites	
86.75	Revision of pedicle or flap graft	
86.91	Excision of skin for graft	
86.93	Insertion of tissue expander	
92.27	Implantation or insertion of radioactive elements	

OR

The following procedure combination

00.56	Insertion or replacement of implantable pressure sensor with lead for intracardiac or great vessel hemodynamic monitoring
	AND
00.57	Implantation or replacement of subcutaneous device for intracardiac or great vessel hemodynamic monitoring

DRG 265 AICD Lead Procedures
GMLOS 2.5   AMLOS 3.6   RW 2.6890   ☑

Operating Room Procedures

00.52	Implantation or replacement of transvenous lead (electrode) into left ventricular coronary venous system
37.95	Implantation of automatic cardioverter/defibrillator leads(s) only
37.97	Replacement of automatic cardioverter/defibrillator leads(s) only

---

MEDICAL

DRG 280 Acute Myocardial Infarction, Discharged Alive with MCC
GMLOS 4.7   AMLOS 6.0   RW 1.7431   ☑ ▽ T

Principal or Secondary Diagnosis

410.01	Acute myocardial infarction of anterolateral wall, initial episode of care
410.11	Acute myocardial infarction of other anterior wall, initial episode of care
410.21	Acute myocardial infarction of inferolateral wall, initial episode of care
410.31	Acute myocardial infarction of inferoposterior wall, initial episode of care
410.41	Acute myocardial infarction of other inferior wall, initial episode of care
410.51	Acute myocardial infarction of other lateral wall, initial episode of care
410.61	Acute myocardial infarction, true posterior wall infarction, initial episode of care
410.71	Acute myocardial infarction, subendocardial infarction, initial episode of care
410.81	Acute myocardial infarction of other specified sites, initial episode of care
410.91	Acute myocardial infarction, unspecified site, initial episode of care

DRG 281 Acute Myocardial Infarction, Discharged Alive with CC
GMLOS 3.1   AMLOS 3.8   RW 1.0568   ☑ ▽ T

Select principal or secondary diagnoses listed under DRG 280

DRG 282 Acute Myocardial Infarction, Discharged Alive without CC/MCC
GMLOS 2.1   AMLOS 2.5   RW 0.7551   ☑ ▽ T

Select principal or secondary diagnoses listed under DRG 280

DRG 283 Acute Myocardial Infarction, Expired with MCC
GMLOS 3.0   AMLOS 4.7   RW 1.6885   ☑

Select principal or secondary diagnoses listed under DRG 280

DRG 284 Acute Myocardial Infarction, Expired with CC
GMLOS 1.8   AMLOS 2.5   RW 0.7614   ☑

Select principal or secondary diagnosis listed under DRG 280

DRG 285 Acute Myocardial Infarction, Expired without CC/MCC
GMLOS 1.4   AMLOS 1.7   RW 0.5227   ☑

Select principal or secondary diagnosis listed under DRG 280

DRG 286 Circulatory Disorders Except Acute Myocardial Infarction, with Cardiac Catheterization with MCC
GMLOS 4.9   AMLOS 6.7   RW 2.1058   ☑ ▽

Select any principal diagnosis listed under MDC 5 excluding AMI

Nonoperating Room Procedures

37.21	Right heart cardiac catheterization
37.22	Left heart cardiac catheterization
37.23	Combined right and left heart cardiac catheterization
88.52	Angiocardiography of right heart structures
88.53	Angiocardiography of left heart structures
88.54	Combined right and left heart angiocardiography
88.55	Coronary arteriography using single catheter
88.56	Coronary arteriography using two catheters
88.57	Other and unspecified coronary arteriography
88.58	Negative-contrast cardiac roentgenography

DRG 287 Circulatory Disorders Except Acute Myocardial Infarction, with Cardiac Catheterization without MCC
GMLOS 2.4   AMLOS 3.1   RW 1.0866   ☑ ▽

Select any principal diagnosis listed under MDC 5 excluding AMI

Select nonoperating room procedure listed under DRG 286

DRG 288 Acute and Subacute Endocarditis with MCC
GMLOS 7.8   AMLOS 9.9   RW 2.7956   T

Principal Diagnosis

036.42	Meningococcal endocarditis
093.20	Unspecified syphilitic endocarditis of valve
098.84	Gonococcal endocarditis
112.81	Candidal endocarditis
115.04	Histoplasma capsulatum endocarditis
115.14	Histoplasma duboisii endocarditis
115.94	Unspecified Histoplasmosis endocarditis
421.0	Acute and subacute bacterial endocarditis
421.1	Acute and subacute infective endocarditis in diseases classified elsewhere
421.9	Unspecified acute endocarditis

Surgical   *Medical*   *CC Indicator*   *MCC Indicator*   *Procedure Proxy*

DRG 289   Acute and Subacute Endocarditis with CC
GMLOS 5.7   AMLOS 7.0   RW 1.7891   ☑ T

Select principal diagnosis listed under DRG 288

DRG 290   Acute and Subacute Endocarditis without CC/MCC
GMLOS 3.9   AMLOS 4.8   RW 1.2359   ☑ T

Select principal diagnosis listed under DRG 288

DRG 291   Heart Failure and Shock with MCC
GMLOS 4.6   AMLOS 5.9   RW 1.5031   ☑ ᵀᵃʳ T

Principal Diagnosis

398.91	Rheumatic heart failure (congestive)
402.01	Malignant hypertensive heart disease with heart failure
402.11	Benign hypertensive heart disease with heart failure
402.91	Hypertensive heart disease, unspecified, with heart failure
404.01	Hypertensive heart and chronic kidney disease, malignant, with heart failure and with chronic kidney disease stage I through stage IV, or unspecified
404.03	Hypertensive heart and chronic kidney disease, malignant, with heart failure and with chronic kidney disease stage V or end stage renal disease
404.11	Hypertensive heart and chronic kidney disease, benign, with heart failure and with chronic kidney disease stage I through stage IV, or unspecified
404.13	Hypertensive heart and chronic kidney disease, benign, with heart failure and chronic kidney disease stage V or end stage renal disease
404.91	Hypertensive heart and chronic kidney disease, unspecified, with heart failure and with chronic kidney disease stage I through stage IV, or unspecified
404.93	Hypertensive heart and chronic kidney disease, unspecified, with heart failure and chronic kidney disease stage V or end stage renal disease
428*	Heart failure
785.50	Unspecified shock
785.51	Cardiogenic shock

DRG 292   Heart Failure and Shock with CC
GMLOS 3.7   AMLOS 4.5   RW 0.9938   ☑ ᵀᵃʳ T

Select principal diagnosis listed under DRG 291

DRG 293   Heart Failure and Shock without CC/MCC
GMLOS 2.6   AMLOS 3.1   RW 0.6723   ☑ ᵀᵃʳ T

Select principal diagnosis listed under DRG 291

DRG 294   Deep Vein Thrombophlebitis with CC/MCC
GMLOS 4.0   AMLOS 4.9   RW 0.9439   ☑ ᵀᵃʳ

Principal Diagnosis

451.1*	Phlebitis and thrombophlebitis of deep veins of lower extremities
451.2	Phlebitis and thrombophlebitis of lower extremities, unspecified
451.81	Phlebitis and thrombophlebitis of iliac vein
453.2	Other venous embolism and thrombosis, of inferior vena cava

DRG 295   Deep Vein Thrombophlebitis without CC/MCC
GMLOS 3.1   AMLOS 3.6   RW 0.6287   ☑ ᵀᵃʳ

Select principal diagnosis listed under DRG 294

DRG 296   Cardiac Arrest, Unexplained with MCC
GMLOS 1.9   AMLOS 2.9   RW 1.3013   ☑

Principal Diagnosis

427.5	Cardiac arrest
798.1	Instantaneous death
798.2	Death occurring in less than 24 hours from onset of symptoms, not otherwise explained

DRG 297   Cardiac Arrest, Unexplained with CC
GMLOS 1.2   AMLOS 1.5   RW 0.6063   ☑

Select principal diagnosis listed under DRG 296

DRG 298   Cardiac Arrest, Unexplained without CC/MCC
GMLOS 1.0   AMLOS 1.1   RW 0.4260   ☑

Select principal diagnosis listed under DRG 296

DRG 299   Peripheral Vascular Disorders with MCC
GMLOS 4.4   AMLOS 5.6   RW 1.3647   ☑ ᵀᵃʳ T

Principal Diagnosis

249.7*	Secondary diabetes mellitus with peripheral circulatory disorders
250.7*	Diabetes with peripheral circulatory disorders
440.0	Atherosclerosis of aorta
440.2*	Atherosclerosis of native arteries of the extremities
440.3*	Atherosclerosis of bypass graft of extremities
440.4	Chronic total occlusion of artery of the extremities
440.8	Atherosclerosis of other specified arteries
440.9	Generalized and unspecified atherosclerosis
441.0*	Dissection of aorta
441.1	Thoracic aneurysm, ruptured
441.2	Thoracic aneurysm without mention of rupture
441.3	Abdominal aneurysm, ruptured
441.4	Abdominal aneurysm without mention of rupture
441.5	Aortic aneurysm of unspecified site, ruptured
441.6	Thoracoabdominal aneurysm, ruptured
441.7	Thoracoabdominal aneurysm without mention of rupture
441.9	Aortic aneurysm of unspecified site without mention of rupture
442.0	Aneurysm of artery of upper extremity
442.2	Aneurysm of iliac artery
442.3	Aneurysm of artery of lower extremity
442.8*	Aneurysm of other specified artery
442.9	Other aneurysm of unspecified site
443.1	Thromboangiitis obliterans (Buerger's disease)
443.21	Dissection of carotid artery
443.22	Dissection of iliac artery
443.24	Dissection of vertebral artery
443.29	Dissection of other artery
443.8*	Other specified peripheral vascular diseases
443.9	Unspecified peripheral vascular disease
444.0*	Arterial embolism and thrombosis of abdominal aorta
444.1	Embolism and thrombosis of thoracic aorta
444.2*	Embolism and thrombosis of arteries of the extremities
444.8*	Embolism and thrombosis of other specified artery
444.9	Embolism and thrombosis of unspecified artery
445.0*	Atheroembolism of extremities
445.89	Atheroembolism of other site
447.0	Arteriovenous fistula, acquired
447.1	Stricture of artery
447.2	Rupture of artery
447.5	Necrosis of artery
447.7*	Aortic ectasia
447.8	Other specified disorders of arteries and arterioles
447.9	Unspecified disorders of arteries and arterioles
448.0	Hereditary hemorrhagic telangiectasia
448.9	Other and unspecified capillary diseases

MDC 5: Diseases And Disorders Of The Circulatory System—MEDICAL

T Transfer DRG   SP Special Payment   ☑ Optimization Potential   ᵀᵃʳ Targeted Potential   * Code Range   ● New DRG   ▲ Revised DRG Title

449	Septic arterial embolism	
451.0	Phlebitis and thrombophlebitis of superficial vessels of lower extremities	
451.82	Phlebitis and thrombophlebitis of superficial veins of upper extremities	
451.83	Phlebitis and thrombophlebitis of deep veins of upper extremities	
451.84	Phlebitis and thrombophlebitis of upper extremities, unspecified	
451.89	Phlebitis and thrombophlebitis of other site	
451.9	Phlebitis and thrombophlebitis of unspecified site	
453.1	Thrombophlebitis migrans	
453.4*	Acute venous embolism and thrombosis of deep vessels of lower extremity	
453.5*	Chronic venous embolism and thrombosis of deep vessels of lower extremity	
453.6	Venous embolism and thrombosis of superficial vessels of lower extremity	
453.7*	Chronic venous embolism and thrombosis of other specified vessels	
453.8*	Acute venous embolism and thrombosis of other specified veins	
453.9	Embolism and thrombosis of unspecified site	
454.0	Varicose veins of lower extremities with ulcer	
454.1	Varicose veins of lower extremities with inflammation	
454.2	Varicose veins of lower extremities with ulcer and inflammation	
454.8	Varicose veins of the lower extremities with other complications	
454.9	Asymptomatic varicose veins	
456.3	Sublingual varices	
456.8	Varices of other sites	
459.1*	Postphlebitic syndrome	
459.2	Compression of vein	
459.3*	Chronic venous hypertension	
459.81	Unspecified venous (peripheral) insufficiency	
747.5	Congenital absence or hypoplasia of umbilical artery	
747.6*	Other congenital anomaly of peripheral vascular system	
747.89	Other specified congenital anomaly of circulatory system	
747.9	Unspecified congenital anomaly of circulatory system	
785.4	Gangrene	
908.3	Late effect of injury to blood vessel of head, neck, and extremities	
908.4	Late effect of injury to blood vessel of thorax, abdomen, and pelvis	
997.2	Peripheral vascular complications	
997.79	Vascular complications of other vessels	

DRG 300   Peripheral Vascular Disorders with CC
GMLOS 3.6   AMLOS 4.5   RW 0.9666   ☑ ▽ T

Select principal diagnosis listed under DRG 299

DRG 301   Peripheral Vascular Disorders without CC/MCC
GMLOS 2.7   AMLOS 3.3   RW 0.6681   ☑ ▽ T

Select principal diagnosis listed under DRG 299

DRG 302   Atherosclerosis with MCC
GMLOS 2.9   AMLOS 3.9   RW 1.0287   ☑ ▽

Principal Diagnosis
412	Old myocardial infarction
414.0*	Coronary atherosclerosis
414.2	Chronic total occlusion of coronary artery
414.3	Coronary atherosclerosis due to lipid rich plaque
414.4	Coronary atherosclerosis due to calcified coronary lesion
414.8	Other specified forms of chronic ischemic heart disease
414.9	Unspecified chronic ischemic heart disease
429.2	Unspecified cardiovascular disease

429.3	Cardiomegaly
429.89	Other ill-defined heart disease
429.9	Unspecified heart disease
459.89	Other specified circulatory system disorders
459.9	Unspecified circulatory system disorder
793.2	Nonspecific (abnormal) findings on radiological and other examination of other intrathoracic organs

DRG 303   Atherosclerosis without MCC
GMLOS 1.9   AMLOS 2.3   RW 0.6034   ☑ ▽

Select principal diagnosis listed under DRG 302

DRG 304   Hypertension with MCC
GMLOS 3.3   AMLOS 4.4   RW 1.0268   ☑

Principal Diagnosis
401.0	Essential hypertension, malignant
401.1	Essential hypertension, benign
401.9	Unspecified essential hypertension
402.00	Malignant hypertensive heart disease without heart failure
402.10	Benign hypertensive heart disease without heart failure
402.90	Unspecified hypertensive heart disease without heart failure
404.00	Hypertensive heart and chronic kidney disease, malignant, without heart failure and with chronic kidney disease stage I through stage IV, or unspecified
404.10	Hypertensive heart and chronic kidney disease, benign, without heart failure and with chronic kidney disease stage I through stage IV, or unspecified
404.90	Hypertensive heart and chronic kidney disease, unspecified, without heart failure and with chronic kidney disease stage I through stage IV, or unspecified
405*	Secondary hypertension

DRG 305   Hypertension without MCC
GMLOS 2.1   AMLOS 2.6   RW 0.6176   ☑

Select principal diagnosis listed under DRG 304

DRG 306   Cardiac Congenital and Valvular Disorders with MCC
GMLOS 3.9   AMLOS 5.3   RW 1.3659   ☑

Principal Diagnosis
074.22	Coxsackie endocarditis
093.0	Aneurysm of aorta, specified as syphilitic
093.1	Syphilitic aortitis
093.21	Syphilitic endocarditis, mitral valve
093.22	Syphilitic endocarditis, aortic valve
093.23	Syphilitic endocarditis, tricuspid valve
093.24	Syphilitic endocarditis, pulmonary valve
391.1	Acute rheumatic endocarditis
394*	Diseases of mitral valve
395*	Diseases of aortic valve
396*	Diseases of mitral and aortic valves
397*	Diseases of other endocardial structures
424*	Other diseases of endocardium
429.5	Rupture of chordae tendineae
429.6	Rupture of papillary muscle
429.81	Other disorders of papillary muscle
745.0	Bulbus cordis anomalies and anomalies of cardiac septal closure, common truncus
745.1*	Transposition of great vessels
745.2	Tetralogy of Fallot
745.3	Bulbus cordis anomalies and anomalies of cardiac septal closure, common ventricle
745.4	Ventricular septal defect
745.5	Ostium secundum type atrial septal defect
745.60	Unspecified type congenital endocardial cushion defect
745.61	Ostium primum defect
745.69	Other congenital endocardial cushion defect

Surgical   *Medical*   CC Indicator   MCC Indicator   Procedure Proxy

745.7	Cor biloculare
745.8	Other bulbus cordis anomalies and anomalies of cardiac septal closure
745.9	Unspecified congenital defect of septal closure
746.0*	Congenital anomalies of pulmonary valve
746.1	Congenital tricuspid atresia and stenosis
746.2	Ebstein's anomaly
746.3	Congenital stenosis of aortic valve
746.4	Congenital insufficiency of aortic valve
746.5	Congenital mitral stenosis
746.6	Congenital mitral insufficiency
746.7	Hypoplastic left heart syndrome
746.81	Congenital subaortic stenosis
746.82	Cor triatriatum
746.83	Congenital infundibular pulmonic stenosis
746.84	Congenital obstructive anomalies of heart, not elsewhere classified
746.85	Congenital coronary artery anomaly
746.87	Congenital malposition of heart and cardiac apex
746.89	Other specified congenital anomaly of heart
746.9	Unspecified congenital anomaly of heart
747.0	Patent ductus arteriosus
747.1*	Coarctation of aorta
747.2*	Other congenital anomaly of aorta
747.3*	Anomalies of pulmonary artery
747.4*	Congenital anomalies of great veins
759.82	Marfan's syndrome
785.2	Undiagnosed cardiac murmurs
996.02	Mechanical complication due to heart valve prosthesis

DRG 307   Cardiac Congenital and Valvular Disorders without MCC

| GMLOS 2.6 | AMLOS 3.3 | RW 0.7917 | ☑ |

Select principal diagnosis listed under DRG 306

DRG 308   Cardiac Arrhythmia and Conduction Disorders with MCC

| GMLOS 3.8 | AMLOS 4.9 | RW 1.2088 | ☑ ▽ |

Principal Diagnosis

426*	Conduction disorders
427.0	Paroxysmal supraventricular tachycardia
427.1	Paroxysmal ventricular tachycardia
427.2	Unspecified paroxysmal tachycardia
427.3*	Atrial fibrillation and flutter
427.4*	Ventricular fibrillation and flutter
427.6*	Premature beats
427.8*	Other specified cardiac dysrhythmias
427.9	Unspecified cardiac dysrhythmia
746.86	Congenital heart block
785.0	Unspecified tachycardia
785.1	Palpitations
996.01	Mechanical complication due to cardiac pacemaker (electrode)
996.04	Mechanical complication due to automatic implantable cardiac defibrillator

DRG 309   Cardiac Arrhythmia and Conduction Disorders with CC

| GMLOS 2.7 | AMLOS 3.3 | RW 0.7867 | ☑ ▽ |

Select principal diagnosis listed under DRG 308

DRG 310   Cardiac Arrhythmia and Conduction Disorders without CC/MCC

| GMLOS 1.9 | AMLOS 2.3 | RW 0.5512 | ☑ ▽ |

Select principal diagnosis listed under DRG 308

DRG 311   Angina Pectoris

| GMLOS 1.8 | AMLOS 2.2 | RW 0.5649 | ☑ ▽ |

Principal Diagnosis

411.1	Intermediate coronary syndrome
411.81	Acute coronary occlusion without myocardial infarction
411.89	Other acute and subacute form of ischemic heart disease
413.0	Angina decubitus
413.1	Prinzmetal angina
413.9	Other and unspecified angina pectoris

DRG 312   Syncope and Collapse

| GMLOS 2.4 | AMLOS 3.0 | RW 0.7228 | ☑ |

Principal Diagnosis

458.0	Orthostatic hypotension
458.2*	Iatrogenic hypotension
780.2	Syncope and collapse

DRG 313   Chest Pain

| GMLOS 1.8 | AMLOS 2.1 | RW 0.5992 | ☑ ▽ |

Principal Diagnosis

786.50	Chest pain, unspecified
786.51	Precordial pain
786.59	Chest pain, other
V71.7	Observation for suspected cardiovascular disease

DRG 314   Other Circulatory System Diagnoses with MCC

| GMLOS 4.9 | AMLOS 6.7 | RW 1.8941 | ☑ T |

Principal Diagnosis

032.82	Diphtheritic myocarditis
036.40	Meningococcal carditis, unspecified
036.41	Meningococcal pericarditis
036.43	Meningococcal myocarditis
074.20	Coxsackie carditis, unspecified
074.21	Coxsackie pericarditis
074.23	Coxsackie myocarditis
086.0	Chagas' disease with heart involvement
093.8*	Other specified cardiovascular syphilis
093.9	Unspecified cardiovascular syphilis
098.83	Gonococcal pericarditis
098.85	Other gonococcal heart disease
115.03	Histoplasma capsulatum pericarditis
115.13	Histoplasma duboisii pericarditis
115.93	Unspecified Histoplasmosis pericarditis
130.3	Myocarditis due to toxoplasmosis
164.1	Malignant neoplasm of heart
212.7	Benign neoplasm of heart
228.00	Hemangioma of unspecified site
228.09	Hemangioma of other sites
306.2	Cardiovascular malfunction arising from mental factors
391.0	Acute rheumatic pericarditis
391.2	Acute rheumatic myocarditis
391.8	Other acute rheumatic heart disease
391.9	Unspecified acute rheumatic heart disease
392*	Rheumatic chorea
393	Chronic rheumatic pericarditis
398.0	Rheumatic myocarditis
398.90	Unspecified rheumatic heart disease
398.99	Other and unspecified rheumatic heart diseases
410.00	Acute myocardial infarction of anterolateral wall, episode of care unspecified
410.02	Acute myocardial infarction of anterolateral wall, subsequent episode of care
410.10	Acute myocardial infarction of other anterior wall, episode of care unspecified
410.12	Acute myocardial infarction of other anterior wall, subsequent episode of care

---

T *Transfer DRG*   S *Special Payment*   ☑ *Optimization Potential*   ▽ *Targeted Potential*   * *Code Range*   ● *New DRG*   ▲ *Revised DRG Title*

410.20	Acute myocardial infarction of inferolateral wall, episode of care unspecified
410.22	Acute myocardial infarction of inferolateral wall, subsequent episode of care
410.30	Acute myocardial infarction of inferoposterior wall, episode of care unspecified
410.32	Acute myocardial infarction of inferoposterior wall, subsequent episode of care
410.40	Acute myocardial infarction of other inferior wall, episode of care unspecified
410.42	Acute myocardial infarction of other inferior wall, subsequent episode of care
410.50	Acute myocardial infarction of other lateral wall, episode of care unspecified
410.52	Acute myocardial infarction of other lateral wall, subsequent episode of care
410.60	Acute myocardial infarction, true posterior wall infarction, episode of care unspecified
410.62	Acute myocardial infarction, true posterior wall infarction, subsequent episode of care
410.70	Acute myocardial infarction, subendocardial infarction, episode of care unspecified
410.72	Acute myocardial infarction, subendocardial infarction, subsequent episode of care
410.80	Acute myocardial infarction of other specified sites, episode of care unspecified
410.82	Acute myocardial infarction of other specified sites, subsequent episode of care
410.90	Acute myocardial infarction, unspecified site, episode of care unspecified
410.92	Acute myocardial infarction, unspecified site, subsequent episode of care
411.0	Postmyocardial infarction syndrome
414.1*	Aneurysm and dissection of heart
415.0	Acute cor pulmonale
416.0	Primary pulmonary hypertension
416.1	Kyphoscoliotic heart disease
416.8	Other chronic pulmonary heart diseases
416.9	Unspecified chronic pulmonary heart disease
417*	Other diseases of pulmonary circulation
420*	Acute pericarditis
422*	Acute myocarditis
423*	Other diseases of pericardium
425*	Cardiomyopathy
429.0	Unspecified myocarditis
429.1	Myocardial degeneration
429.4	Functional disturbances following cardiac surgery
429.71	Acquired cardiac septal defect
429.79	Other certain sequelae of myocardial infarction, not elsewhere classified
429.82	Hyperkinetic heart disease
429.83	Takotsubo syndrome
458.1	Chronic hypotension
458.8	Other specified hypotension
458.9	Unspecified hypotension
459.0	Unspecified hemorrhage
785.3	Other abnormal heart sounds
785.9	Other symptoms involving cardiovascular system
794.30	Nonspecific abnormal unspecified cardiovascular function study
794.31	Nonspecific abnormal electrocardiogram (ECG) (EKG)
794.39	Other nonspecific abnormal cardiovascular system function study
796.2	Elevated blood pressure reading without diagnosis of hypertension
796.3	Nonspecific low blood pressure reading
861.0*	Heart injury, without mention of open wound into thorax
861.1*	Heart injury, with open wound into thorax
996.00	Mechanical complication of unspecified cardiac device, implant, and graft

996.03	Mechanical complication due to coronary bypass graft
996.09	Mechanical complication of cardiac device, implant, and graft, other
996.1	Mechanical complication of other vascular device, implant, and graft
996.61	Infection and inflammatory reaction due to cardiac device, implant, and graft
996.62	Infection and inflammatory reaction due to other vascular device, implant, and graft
996.71	Other complications due to heart valve prosthesis
996.72	Other complications due to other cardiac device, implant, and graft
996.73	Other complications due to renal dialysis device, implant, and graft
996.74	Other complications due to other vascular device, implant, and graft
996.83	Complications of transplanted heart
997.1	Cardiac complications
999.2	Other vascular complications of medical care, not elsewhere classified
999.31	Other and unspecified infection due to central venous catheter
999.32	Bloodstream infection due to central venous catheter
999.33	Local infection due to central venous catheter
999.81	Extravasation of vesicant chemotherapy
999.82	Extravasation of other vesicant agent
999.88	Other infusion reaction
V42.1	Heart replaced by transplant
V42.2	Heart valve replaced by transplant
V43.2*	Heart replaced by other means
V43.3	Heart valve replaced by other means
V43.4	Blood vessel replaced by other means
V53.3*	Fitting and adjustment of cardiac device

DRG 315 Other Circulatory System Diagnoses with CC
GMLOS 3.1   AMLOS 4.0   RW 0.9534   ☑Ⓣ

Select principal diagnosis listed under DRG 314

DRG 316 Other Circulatory System Diagnoses without CC/MCC
GMLOS 2.0   AMLOS 2.5   RW 0.6358   ☑Ⓣ

Select principal diagnosis listed under DRG 314

Diseases And Disorders Of The Digestive System

001.0	014.83	152.0	211.4	531.41	535.30	552.01	564.5	750.8
001.1	014.84	152.1	211.8	531.50	535.31	552.02	564.6	750.9
001.9	014.85	152.2	211.9	531.51	535.40	552.03	564.7	751.0
003.0	014.86	152.3	214.3	531.60	535.41	552.1	564.81	751.1
004.0	017.80	152.8	228.04	531.61	535.50	552.20	564.89	751.2
004.1	017.81	152.9	230.1	531.70	535.51	552.21	564.9	751.3
004.2	017.82	153.0	230.2	531.71	535.60	552.29	565.0	751.4
004.3	017.83	153.1	230.3	531.90	535.61	552.3	565.1	751.5
004.8	017.84	153.2	230.4	531.91	535.70	552.8	566	751.8
004.9	017.85	153.3	230.5	532.00	535.71	552.9	567.0	751.9
005.0	017.86	153.4	230.6	532.01	536.0	553.00	567.1	756.70
005.2	021.1	153.5	230.7	532.10	536.1	553.01	567.21	756.71
005.3	022.2	153.6	230.9	532.11	536.2	553.02	567.22	756.72
005.4	032.83	153.7	235.2	532.20	536.3	553.03	567.23	756.73
005.81	039.2	153.8	235.4	532.21	536.40	553.1	567.29	756.79
005.89	040.2	153.9	235.5	532.30	536.41	553.20	567.31	759.3
005.9	054.71	154.0	239.0	532.31	536.42	553.21	567.38	759.4
006.0	078.82	154.1	251.5	532.40	536.49	553.29	567.39	787.01
006.1	091.1	154.2	271.2	532.41	536.8	553.3	567.81	787.02
006.2	091.69	154.3	271.3	532.50	536.9	553.8	567.82	787.03
007.0	095.2	154.8	277.03	532.51	537.0	553.9	567.89	787.04
007.1	098.7	158.8	289.2	532.60	537.1	555.0	567.9	787.1
007.2	098.86	158.9	306.4	532.61	537.2	555.1	568.0	787.20
007.3	099.52	159.0	447.4	532.70	537.3	555.2	568.81	787.21
007.4	099.56	159.8	455.0	532.71	537.4	555.9	568.82	787.22
007.5	112.84	159.9	455.1	532.90	537.5	556.0	568.89	787.23
007.8	112.85	176.3	455.2	532.91	537.6	556.1	568.9	787.24
007.9	123.0	195.2	455.3	533.00	537.81	556.2	569.0	787.29
008.00	123.1	197.4	455.4	533.01	537.82	556.3	569.1	787.3
008.01	123.2	197.5	455.5	533.10	537.83	556.4	569.2	787.4
008.02	123.3	197.6	455.6	533.11	537.84	556.5	569.3	787.5
008.03	123.4	197.8	455.7	533.20	537.89	556.6	569.41	787.60
008.04	123.5	209.00	455.8	533.21	537.9	556.8	569.42	787.61
008.09	123.6	209.01	455.9	533.30	538	556.9	569.43	787.62
008.1	123.8	209.02	456.0	533.31	539.01	557.0	569.44	787.63
008.2	123.9	209.03	456.1	533.40	539.09	557.1	569.49	787.7
008.3	126.0	209.10	456.20	533.41	539.81	557.9	569.5	787.91
008.41	126.1	209.11	456.21	533.50	539.89	558.1	569.60	787.99
008.42	126.2	209.12	530.0	533.51	540.0	558.2	569.61	789.00
008.43	126.3	209.13	530.10	533.60	540.1	558.3	569.62	789.01
008.44	126.8	209.14	530.11	533.61	540.9	558.41	569.69	789.02
008.45	126.9	209.15	530.12	533.70	541	558.42	569.71	789.03
008.46	127.0	209.16	530.13	533.71	542	558.9	569.79	789.04
008.47	127.1	209.17	530.19	533.90	543.0	560.0	569.81	789.05
008.49	127.2	209.23	530.20	533.91	543.9	560.1	569.82	789.06
008.5	127.3	209.25	530.21	534.00	550.00	560.2	569.83	789.07
008.61	127.4	209.26	530.3	534.01	550.01	560.30	569.84	789.09
008.62	127.5	209.27	530.4	534.10	550.02	560.31	569.85	789.30
008.63	127.6	209.40	530.5	534.11	550.03	560.32	569.86	789.31
008.64	127.7	209.41	530.6	534.20	550.10	560.39	569.87	789.32
008.65	127.9	209.42	530.7	534.21	550.11	560.81	569.89	789.33
008.66	129	209.43	530.81	534.30	550.12	560.89	569.9	789.34
008.67	150.0	209.50	530.82	534.31	550.13	560.9	578.0	789.35
008.69	150.1	209.51	530.83	534.40	550.90	562.00	578.1	789.36
008.8	150.2	209.52	530.84	534.41	550.91	562.01	578.9	789.37
009.0	150.3	209.53	530.85	534.50	550.92	562.02	579.0	789.39
009.1	150.4	209.54	530.86	534.51	550.93	562.03	579.1	789.40
009.2	150.5	209.55	530.87	534.60	551.00	562.10	579.2	789.41
009.3	150.8	209.56	530.89	534.61	551.01	562.11	579.3	789.42
014.00	150.9	209.57	530.9	534.70	551.02	562.12	579.4	789.43
014.01	151.0	209.63	531.00	534.71	551.03	562.13	579.8	789.44
014.02	151.1	209.65	531.01	534.90	551.1	564.00	579.9	789.45
014.03	151.2	209.66	531.10	534.91	551.20	564.01	617.5	789.46
014.04	151.3	209.67	531.11	535.00	551.21	564.02	619.1	789.47
014.05	151.4	209.74	531.20	535.01	551.29	564.09	750.3	789.49
014.06	151.5	211.0	531.21	535.10	551.3	564.1	750.4	789.60
014.80	151.6	211.1	531.30	535.11	551.8	564.2	750.5	789.61
014.81	151.8	211.2	531.31	535.20	551.9	564.3	750.6	789.62
014.82	151.9	211.3	531.40	535.21	552.00	564.4	750.7	789.63

789.64	793.6	796.78	863.30	863.46	863.59	868.10	947.3	V55.3
789.65	796.70	796.79	863.31	863.49	863.80	868.13	997.41	V55.4
789.66	796.71	862.22	863.39	863.50	863.85	908.1	997.49	
789.67	796.72	862.32	863.40	863.51	863.89	935.1	997.71	
789.69	796.73	863.0	863.41	863.52	863.90	935.2	V53.50	
789.7	796.74	863.1	863.42	863.53	863.95	936	V53.51	
789.9	796.75	863.20	863.43	863.54	863.99	937	V53.59	
792.1	796.76	863.21	863.44	863.55	868.00	938	V55.1	
793.4	796.77	863.29	863.45	863.56	868.03	947.2	V55.2	

SURGICAL

DRG 326 Stomach, Esophageal and Duodenal Procedures with MCC
GMLOS 11.6   AMLOS 14.9   RW 5.6013   T

Operating Room Procedures

29.3*	Excision or destruction of lesion or tissue of pharynx
31.73	Closure of other fistula of trachea
38.05	Incision of other thoracic vessels
38.35	Resection of other thoracic vessels with anastomosis
38.45	Resection of other thoracic vessels with replacement
38.65	Other excision of other thoracic vessel
38.85	Other surgical occlusion of other thoracic vessel
39.1	Intra-abdominal venous shunt
42.01	Incision of esophageal web
42.09	Other incision of esophagus
42.1*	Esophagostomy
42.21	Operative esophagoscopy by incision
42.25	Open biopsy of esophagus
42.31	Local excision of esophageal diverticulum
42.32	Local excision of other lesion or tissue of esophagus
42.39	Other destruction of lesion or tissue of esophagus
42.4*	Excision of esophagus
42.5*	Intrathoracic anastomosis of esophagus
42.6*	Antesternal anastomosis of esophagus
42.7	Esophagomyotomy
42.82	Suture of laceration of esophagus
42.83	Closure of esophagostomy
42.84	Repair of esophageal fistula, not elsewhere classified
42.85	Repair of esophageal stricture
42.86	Production of subcutaneous tunnel without esophageal anastomosis
42.87	Other graft of esophagus
42.89	Other repair of esophagus
42.91	Ligation of esophageal varices
43.0	Gastrotomy
43.3	Pyloromyotomy
43.42	Local excision of other lesion or tissue of stomach
43.49	Other destruction of lesion or tissue of stomach
43.5	Partial gastrectomy with anastomosis to esophagus
43.6	Partial gastrectomy with anastomosis to duodenum
43.7	Partial gastrectomy with anastomosis to jejunum
43.8*	Other partial gastrectomy
43.9*	Total gastrectomy
44.0*	Vagotomy
44.11	Transabdominal gastroscopy
44.15	Open biopsy of stomach
44.21	Dilation of pylorus by incision
44.29	Other pyloroplasty
44.3*	Gastroenterostomy without gastrectomy
44.40	Suture of peptic ulcer, not otherwise specified
44.41	Suture of gastric ulcer site
44.42	Suture of duodenal ulcer site
44.5	Revision of gastric anastomosis
44.61	Suture of laceration of stomach
44.63	Closure of other gastric fistula
44.64	Gastropexy
44.65	Esophagogastroplasty
44.66	Other procedures for creation of esophagogastric sphincteric competence
44.67	Laparoscopic procedures for creation of esophagogastric sphincteric competence
44.68	Laparoscopic gastroplasty
44.69	Other repair of stomach
44.91	Ligation of gastric varices
44.92	Intraoperative manipulation of stomach
44.99	Other operations on stomach
45.01	Incision of duodenum
45.31	Other local excision of lesion of duodenum
45.32	Other destruction of lesion of duodenum
46.71	Suture of laceration of duodenum
46.72	Closure of fistula of duodenum
51.82	Pancreatic sphincterotomy
51.83	Pancreatic sphincteroplasty
52.7	Radical pancreaticoduodenectomy
53.7*	Repair of diaphragmatic hernia, abdominal approach
53.8*	Repair of diaphragmatic hernia, thoracic approach

DRG 327 Stomach, Esophageal and Duodenal Procedures with CC
GMLOS 6.1   AMLOS 8.0   RW 2.6598   ☑ T

Select operating room procedures listed under DRG 326

DRG 328 Stomach, Esophageal and Duodenal Procedures without CC/MCC
GMLOS 2.6   AMLOS 3.4   RW 1.4765   ☑ T

Select operating room procedures listed under DRG 326

DRG 329 Major Small and Large Bowel Procedures with MCC
GMLOS 11.9   AMLOS 14.6   RW 5.1272   ☑ T

Operating Room Procedures

17.3*	Laparoscopic partial excision of large intestine
45.5*	Isolation of intestinal segment
45.6*	Other excision of small intestine
45.7*	Open and other partial excision of large intestine
45.8*	Total intra-abdominal colectomy
45.9*	Intestinal anastomosis
46.0*	Exteriorization of intestine
46.10	Colostomy, not otherwise specified
46.11	Temporary colostomy
46.13	Permanent colostomy
46.20	Ileostomy, not otherwise specified
46.21	Temporary ileostomy
46.22	Continent ileostomy
46.23	Other permanent ileostomy
46.73	Suture of laceration of small intestine, except duodenum
46.74	Closure of fistula of small intestine, except duodenum
46.75	Suture of laceration of large intestine
46.76	Closure of fistula of large intestine
46.79	Other repair of intestine
46.80	Intra-abdominal manipulation of intestine, not otherwise specified
46.81	Intra-abdominal manipulation of small intestine
46.82	Intra-abdominal manipulation of large intestine
46.91	Myotomy of sigmoid colon
46.92	Myotomy of other parts of colon
46.93	Revision of anastomosis of small intestine
46.94	Revision of anastomosis of large intestine
46.99	Other operations on intestines
47.92	Closure of appendiceal fistula
48.1	Proctostomy
48.71	Suture of laceration of rectum
48.72	Closure of proctostomy
48.74	Rectorectostomy
48.75	Abdominal proctopexy
48.76	Other proctopexy
70.52	Repair of rectocele
70.53	Repair of cystocele and rectocele with graft or prosthesis
70.55	Repair of rectocele with graft or prosthesis
70.72	Repair of colovaginal fistula
70.73	Repair of rectovaginal fistula
70.74	Repair of other vaginoenteric fistula

Valid 10/01/2013-09/30/2014

DRG 330 **Major Small and Large Bowel Procedures with CC**
GMLOS 7.3   AMLOS 8.5   RW 2.5609   ☑🅃

Select operating room procedures listed under DRG 329

DRG 331 **Major Small and Large Bowel Procedures without CC/MCC**
GMLOS 4.4   AMLOS 4.9   RW 1.6380   ☑🅃

Select operating room procedures listed under DRG 329

DRG 332 **Rectal Resection with MCC**
GMLOS 10.9   AMLOS 13.2   RW 4.7072   ☑🅃

Operating Room Procedures
48.4*   Pull-through resection of rectum
48.5*   Abdominoperineal resection of rectum
48.6*   Other resection of rectum
49.75   Implantation or revision of artificial anal sphincter
49.76   Removal of artificial anal sphincter
68.8   Pelvic evisceration

DRG 333 **Rectal Resection with CC**
GMLOS 6.4   AMLOS 7.4   RW 2.4466   ☑🅃

Select operating room procedures listed under DRG 332

DRG 334 **Rectal Resection without CC/MCC**
GMLOS 3.7   AMLOS 4.3   RW 1.5849   ☑🅃

Select operating room procedures listed under DRG 332

DRG 335 **Peritoneal Adhesiolysis with MCC**
GMLOS 10.7   AMLOS 13.0   RW 4.1615   🅃

Operating Room Procedures
54.5*   Lysis of peritoneal adhesions

DRG 336 **Peritoneal Adhesiolysis with CC**
GMLOS 7.0   AMLOS 8.4   RW 2.3513   ☑🅃

Select operating room procedures listed under DRG 335

DRG 337 **Peritoneal Adhesiolysis without CC/MCC**
GMLOS 4.1   AMLOS 5.0   RW 1.5742   ☑🅃

Select operating room procedures listed under DRG 335

DRG 338 **Appendectomy with Complicated Principal Diagnosis with MCC**
GMLOS 7.8   AMLOS 9.5   RW 3.1217   ☑

Principal Diagnosis
153.5   Malignant neoplasm of appendix
209.11   Malignant carcinoid tumor of the appendix
540.0   Acute appendicitis with generalized peritonitis
540.1   Acute appendicitis with peritoneal abscess

Operating Room Procedures
47.0*   Appendectomy
47.2   Drainage of appendiceal abscess
47.99   Other operations on appendix

DRG 339 **Appendectomy with Complicated Principal Diagnosis with CC**
GMLOS 5.1   AMLOS 6.0   RW 1.7117   ☑

Select principal diagnosis and operating room procedure listed under DRG 338

DRG 340 **Appendectomy with Complicated Principal Diagnosis without CC/MCC**
GMLOS 3.0   AMLOS 3.5   RW 1.1741   ☑

Select principal diagnosis and operating room procedure listed under DRG 338

DRG 341 **Appendectomy without Complicated Principal Diagnosis with MCC**
GMLOS 4.6   AMLOS 6.3   RW 2.1821   ☑

Operating Room Procedures
47.0*   Appendectomy
47.2   Drainage of appendiceal abscess
47.99   Other operations on appendix

DRG 342 **Appendectomy without Complicated Principal Diagnosis with CC**
GMLOS 2.8   AMLOS 3.5   RW 1.2968   ☑

Select operating room procedures listed under DRG 341

DRG 343 **Appendectomy without Complicated Principal Diagnosis without CC/MCC**
GMLOS 1.6   AMLOS 1.9   RW 0.9358   ☑

Select operating room procedures listed under DRG 341

DRG 344 **Minor Small and Large Bowel Procedures with MCC**
GMLOS 8.9   AMLOS 11.3   RW 3.5966   ☑

Operating Room Procedures
45.00   Incision of intestine, not otherwise specified
45.02   Other incision of small intestine
45.03   Incision of large intestine
45.11   Transabdominal endoscopy of small intestine
45.15   Open biopsy of small intestine
45.21   Transabdominal endoscopy of large intestine
45.26   Open biopsy of large intestine
45.34   Other destruction of lesion of small intestine, except duodenum
45.49   Other destruction of lesion of large intestine
46.5*   Closure of intestinal stoma
46.6*   Fixation of intestine
47.91   Appendicostomy
48.0   Proctotomy
48.21   Transabdominal proctosigmoidoscopy
48.25   Open biopsy of rectum
56.84   Closure of other fistula of ureter
57.83   Repair of fistula involving bladder and intestine
69.42   Closure of fistula of uterus
70.75   Repair of other fistula of vagina
71.72   Repair of fistula of vulva or perineum

DRG 345 **Minor Small and Large Bowel Procedures with CC**
GMLOS 5.5   AMLOS 6.5   RW 1.6865   ☑

Select operating room procedures listed under DRG 344

DRG 346 **Minor Small and Large Bowel Procedures without CC/MCC**
GMLOS 4.0   AMLOS 4.4   RW 1.2174   ☑

Select operating room procedures listed under DRG 344

Surgical	Medical	CC Indicator	MCC Indicator	Procedure Proxy

MDC 6: Diseases And Disorders Of The Digestive System—SURGICAL

DRG 347 Anal and Stomal Procedures with MCC
GMLOS 6.3   AMLOS 8.5   RW 2.5182   ☑

Operating Room Procedures

45.33	Local excision of lesion or tissue of small intestine, except duodenum
45.41	Excision of lesion or tissue of large intestine
46.4*	Revision of intestinal stoma
48.35	Local excision of rectal lesion or tissue
48.73	Closure of other rectal fistula
48.79	Other repair of rectum
48.8*	Incision or excision of perirectal tissue or lesion
48.9*	Other operations on rectum and perirectal tissue
49.01	Incision of perianal abscess
49.02	Other incision of perianal tissue
49.04	Other excision of perianal tissue
49.1*	Incision or excision of anal fistula
49.39	Other local excision or destruction of lesion or tissue of anus
49.44	Destruction of hemorrhoids by cryotherapy
49.45	Ligation of hemorrhoids
49.46	Excision of hemorrhoids
49.49	Other procedures on hemorrhoids
49.5*	Division of anal sphincter
49.6	Excision of anus
49.71	Suture of laceration of anus
49.72	Anal cerclage
49.73	Closure of anal fistula
49.79	Other repair of anal sphincter
49.9*	Other operations on anus

DRG 348 Anal and Stomal Procedures with CC
GMLOS 4.0   AMLOS 5.1   RW 1.3585   ☑

Select operating room procedures listed under DRG 347

DRG 349 Anal and Stomal Procedures without CC/MCC
GMLOS 2.4   AMLOS 3.0   RW 0.8834   ☑

Select operating room procedures listed under DRG 347

DRG 350 Inguinal and Femoral Hernia Procedures with MCC
GMLOS 5.8   AMLOS 7.8   RW 2.4598   ☑

Operating Room Procedures

17.1*	Laparoscopic unilateral repair of inguinal hernia
17.2*	Laparoscopic bilateral repair of inguinal hernia
53.0*	Other unilateral repair of inguinal hernia
53.1*	Other bilateral repair of inguinal hernia
53.2*	Unilateral repair of femoral hernia
53.3*	Bilateral repair of femoral hernia

DRG 351 Inguinal and Femoral Hernia Procedures with CC
GMLOS 3.5   AMLOS 4.5   RW 1.3761   ☑

Select operating room procedures listed under DRG 350

DRG 352 Inguinal and Femoral Hernia Procedures without CC/MCC
GMLOS 2.0   AMLOS 2.5   RW 0.9239   ☑

Select operating room procedures listed under DRG 350

DRG 353 Hernia Procedures Except Inguinal and Femoral with MCC
GMLOS 6.2   AMLOS 8.0   RW 2.7885   ☑

Operating Room Procedures

53.4*	Repair of umbilical hernia
53.5*	Repair of other hernia of anterior abdominal wall (without graft or prosthesis)
53.6*	Repair of other hernia of anterior abdominal wall with graft or prosthesis

53.9	Other hernia repair
54.71	Repair of gastroschisis
54.72	Other repair of abdominal wall

DRG 354 Hernia Procedures Except Inguinal and Femoral with CC
GMLOS 4.0   AMLOS 5.0   RW 1.6401   ☑

Select operating room procedures listed under DRG 353

DRG 355 Hernia Procedures Except Inguinal and Femoral without CC/MCC
GMLOS 2.5   AMLOS 3.0   RW 1.1783   ☑

Select operating room procedures listed under DRG 353

DRG 356 Other Digestive System O.R. Procedures with MCC
GMLOS 8.6   AMLOS 11.5   RW 3.8388   ☑ⓣ

Operating Room Procedures

17.56	Atherectomy of other non-coronary vessel(s)
17.63	Laser interstitial thermal therapy [LITT] of lesion or tissue of liver under guidance
38.04	Incision of aorta
38.06	Incision of abdominal arteries
38.07	Incision of abdominal veins
38.14	Endarterectomy of aorta
38.16	Endarterectomy of abdominal arteries
38.34	Resection of aorta with anastomosis
38.36	Resection of abdominal arteries with anastomosis
38.37	Resection of abdominal veins with anastomosis
38.46	Resection of abdominal arteries with replacement
38.47	Resection of abdominal veins with replacement
38.57	Ligation and stripping of abdominal varicose veins
38.64	Other excision of abdominal aorta
38.66	Other excision of abdominal arteries
38.67	Other excision of abdominal veins
38.7	Interruption of the vena cava
38.84	Other surgical occlusion of abdominal aorta
38.86	Other surgical occlusion of abdominal arteries
38.87	Other surgical occlusion of abdominal veins
39.26	Other intra-abdominal vascular shunt or bypass
39.27	Arteriovenostomy for renal dialysis
39.49	Other revision of vascular procedure
39.50	Angioplasty of other non-coronary vessel(s)
39.91	Freeing of vessel
39.98	Control of hemorrhage, not otherwise specified
39.99	Other operations on vessels
40.1*	Diagnostic procedures on lymphatic structures
40.21	Excision of deep cervical lymph node
40.23	Excision of axillary lymph node
40.24	Excision of inguinal lymph node
40.29	Simple excision of other lymphatic structure
40.3	Regional lymph node excision
40.5*	Radical excision of other lymph nodes
40.9	Other operations on lymphatic structures
41.5	Total splenectomy
49.74	Gracilis muscle transplant for anal incontinence
50.12	Open biopsy of liver
50.14	Laparoscopic liver biopsy
50.19	Other diagnostic procedures on liver
50.23	Open ablation of liver lesion or tissue
50.24	Percutaneous ablation of liver lesion or tissue
50.25	Laparoscopic ablation of liver lesion or tissue
50.26	Other and unspecified ablation of liver lesion or tissue
50.29	Other destruction of lesion of liver
51.03	Other cholecystostomy
51.13	Open biopsy of gallbladder or bile ducts
51.19	Other diagnostic procedures on biliary tract
51.22	Cholecystectomy
51.23	Laparoscopic cholecystectomy

ⓣ *Transfer DRG*   ⓢᴾ *Special Payment*   ☑ *Optimization Potential*   � *Targeted Potential*   * *Code Range*   ● *New DRG*   ▲ *Revised DRG Title*

74   Valid 10/01/2013–09/30/2014   © 2013 OptumInsight, Inc.

51.32	Anastomosis of gallbladder to intestine
51.36	Choledochoenterostomy
51.37	Anastomosis of hepatic duct to gastrointestinal tract
51.59	Incision of other bile duct
51.62	Excision of ampulla of Vater (with reimplantation of common duct)
51.63	Other excision of common duct
51.69	Excision of other bile duct
51.81	Dilation of sphincter of Oddi
52.12	Open biopsy of pancreas
52.19	Other diagnostic procedures on pancreas
52.92	Cannulation of pancreatic duct
52.99	Other operations on pancreas
54.0	Incision of abdominal wall
54.1*	Laparotomy
54.21	Laparoscopy
54.22	Biopsy of abdominal wall or umbilicus
54.23	Biopsy of peritoneum
54.29	Other diagnostic procedures on abdominal region
54.3	Excision or destruction of lesion or tissue of abdominal wall or umbilicus
54.4	Excision or destruction of peritoneal tissue
54.6*	Suture of abdominal wall and peritoneum
54.73	Other repair of peritoneum
54.74	Other repair of omentum
54.75	Other repair of mesentery
54.92	Removal of foreign body from peritoneal cavity
54.93	Creation of cutaneoperitoneal fistula
54.94	Creation of peritoneovascular shunt
54.95	Incision of peritoneum
70.50	Repair of cystocele and rectocele
86.06	Insertion of totally implantable infusion pump
86.22	Excisional debridement of wound, infection, or burn
86.60	Free skin graft, not otherwise specified
86.63	Full-thickness skin graft to other sites
86.65	Heterograft to skin
86.66	Homograft to skin
86.67	Dermal regenerative graft
86.69	Other skin graft to other sites
86.70	Pedicle or flap graft, not otherwise specified
86.71	Cutting and preparation of pedicle grafts or flaps
86.72	Advancement of pedicle graft
86.74	Attachment of pedicle or flap graft to other sites
86.75	Revision of pedicle or flap graft
86.93	Insertion of tissue expander
92.27	Implantation or insertion of radioactive elements

DRG 357 **Other Digestive System O.R. Procedures with CC**
GMLOS 5.4   AMLOS 6.9   RW 2.1448   ☑ⓣ

Select operating room procedures listed under DRG 356

DRG 358 **Other Digestive System O.R. Procedures without CC/MCC**
GMLOS 3.2   AMLOS 4.1   RW 1.3942   ☑ⓣ

Select operating room procedures listed under DRG 356

MEDICAL

DRG 368 **Major Esophageal Disorders with MCC**
GMLOS 5.0   AMLOS 6.6   RW 1.8779   ☑

Principal Diagnosis
017.8*	Tuberculosis of esophagus
112.84	Candidiasis of the esophagus
456.0	Esophageal varices with bleeding
456.1	Esophageal varices without mention of bleeding

456.20	Esophageal varices with bleeding in diseases classified elsewhere
530.4	Perforation of esophagus
530.7	Gastroesophageal laceration-hemorrhage syndrome
530.82	Esophageal hemorrhage
530.84	Tracheoesophageal fistula
750.3	Congenital tracheoesophageal fistula, esophageal atresia and stenosis
750.4	Other specified congenital anomaly of esophagus
862.22	Esophagus injury without mention of open wound into cavity
947.2	Burn of esophagus

DRG 369 **Major Esophageal Disorders with CC**
GMLOS 3.5   AMLOS 4.2   RW 1.0660   ☑

Select principal diagnosis listed under DRG 368

DRG 370 **Major Esophageal Disorders without CC/MCC**
GMLOS 2.5   AMLOS 3.0   RW 0.7486   ☑

Select principal diagnosis listed under DRG 368

DRG 371 **Major Gastrointestinal Disorders and Peritoneal Infections with MCC**
GMLOS 6.2   AMLOS 7.9   RW 1.9027   ☑ⓣ

Principal Diagnosis
001*	Cholera
003.0	Salmonella gastroenteritis
004*	Shigellosis
005.0	Staphylococcal food poisoning
005.2	Food poisoning due to Clostridium perfringens (C. welchii)
005.3	Food poisoning due to other Clostridia
005.4	Food poisoning due to Vibrio parahaemolyticus
005.8*	Other bacterial food poisoning
006.0	Acute amebic dysentery without mention of abscess
006.1	Chronic intestinal amebiasis without mention of abscess
006.2	Amebic nondysenteric colitis
007*	Other protozoal intestinal diseases
008.00	Intestinal infection due to unspecified E. coli
008.01	Intestinal infection due to enteropathogenic E. coli
008.02	Intestinal infection due to enterotoxigenic E. coli
008.03	Intestinal infection due to enteroinvasive E. coli
008.04	Intestinal infection due to enterohemorrhagic E. coli
008.09	Intestinal infection due to other intestinal E. coli infections
008.1	Intestinal infection due to Arizona group of paracolon bacilli
008.2	Intestinal infection due to aerobacter aerogenes
008.3	Intestinal infections due to proteus (mirabilis) (morganii)
008.41	Intestinal infections due to staphylococcus
008.42	Intestinal infections due to pseudomonas
008.43	Intestinal infections due to campylobacter
008.44	Intestinal infections due to yersinia enterocolitica
008.45	Intestinal infections due to clostridium difficile
008.46	Intestinal infections due to other anaerobes
008.47	Intestinal infections due to other gram-negative bacteria
008.49	Intestinal infection due to other organisms
008.5	Intestinal infection due to unspecified bacterial enteritis
014*	Tuberculosis of intestines, peritoneum, and mesenteric glands
021.1	Enteric tularemia
022.2	Gastrointestinal anthrax
032.83	Diphtheritic peritonitis
039.2	Abdominal actinomycotic infection
095.2	Syphilitic peritonitis
098.86	Gonococcal peritonitis
123.1	Cysticercosis
123.5	Sparganosis (larval diphyllobothriasis)
123.6	Hymenolepiasis
123.8	Other specified cestode infection

Surgical	Medical	CC Indicator	MCC Indicator	Procedure Proxy

123.9	Unspecified cestode infection
126*	Ancylostomiasis and necatoriasis
540.0	Acute appendicitis with generalized peritonitis
540.1	Acute appendicitis with peritoneal abscess
567.0	Peritonitis in infectious diseases classified elsewhere
567.1	Pneumococcal peritonitis
567.2*	Other suppurative peritonitis
567.3*	Retroperitoneal infections
567.89	Other specified peritonitis
567.9	Unspecified peritonitis
569.5	Abscess of intestine

DRG 372 Major Gastrointestinal Disorders and Peritoneal Infections with CC
GMLOS 4.8   AMLOS 5.8   RW 1.1733   ☑Ⓣ

Select principal diagnosis listed under DRG 371

DRG 373 Major Gastrointestinal Disorders and Peritoneal Infections without CC/MCC
GMLOS 3.6   AMLOS 4.2   RW 0.8103   ☑Ⓣ

Select principal diagnosis listed under DRG 371

DRG 374 Digestive Malignancy with MCC
GMLOS 6.2   AMLOS 8.4   RW 2.1051   ☑Ⓣ

Principal Diagnosis

150*	Malignant neoplasm of esophagus
151*	Malignant neoplasm of stomach
152*	Malignant neoplasm of small intestine, including duodenum
153*	Malignant neoplasm of colon
154*	Malignant neoplasm of rectum, rectosigmoid junction, and anus
158.8	Malignant neoplasm of specified parts of peritoneum
158.9	Malignant neoplasm of peritoneum, unspecified
159.0	Malignant neoplasm of intestinal tract, part unspecified
159.8	Malignant neoplasm of other sites of digestive system and intra-abdominal organs
159.9	Malignant neoplasm of ill-defined sites of digestive organs and peritoneum
176.3	Kaposi's sarcoma of gastrointestinal sites
195.2	Malignant neoplasm of abdomen
197.4	Secondary malignant neoplasm of small intestine including duodenum
197.5	Secondary malignant neoplasm of large intestine and rectum
197.6	Secondary malignant neoplasm of retroperitoneum and peritoneum
197.8	Secondary malignant neoplasm of other digestive organs and spleen
209.0*	Malignant carcinoid tumors of the small intestine
209.1*	Malignant carcinoid tumors of the appendix, large intestine, and rectum
209.23	Malignant carcinoid tumor of the stomach
209.25	Malignant carcinoid tumor of foregut, not otherwise specified
209.26	Malignant carcinoid tumor of midgut, not otherwise specified
209.27	Malignant carcinoid tumor of hindgut, not otherwise specified
209.74	Secondary neuroendocrine tumor of peritoneum
230.1	Carcinoma in situ of esophagus
230.2	Carcinoma in situ of stomach
230.3	Carcinoma in situ of colon
230.4	Carcinoma in situ of rectum
230.5	Carcinoma in situ of anal canal
230.6	Carcinoma in situ of anus, unspecified
230.7	Carcinoma in situ of other and unspecified parts of intestine
230.9	Carcinoma in situ of other and unspecified digestive organs

235.2	Neoplasm of uncertain behavior of stomach, intestines, and rectum
235.4	Neoplasm of uncertain behavior of retroperitoneum and peritoneum
235.5	Neoplasm of uncertain behavior of other and unspecified digestive organs
239.0	Neoplasm of unspecified nature of digestive system

DRG 375 Digestive Malignancy with CC
GMLOS 4.2   AMLOS 5.4   RW 1.2561   ☑Ⓣ

Select principal diagnosis listed under DRG 374

DRG 376 Digestive Malignancy without CC/MCC
GMLOS 2.7   AMLOS 3.5   RW 0.8738   ☑Ⓣ

Select principal diagnosis listed under DRG 374

DRG 377 GI Hemorrhage with MCC
GMLOS 4.8   AMLOS 6.1   RW 1.7629   ☑ⓋⓉ

Principal Diagnosis

531.0*	Acute gastric ulcer with hemorrhage
531.2*	Acute gastric ulcer with hemorrhage and perforation
531.4*	Chronic or unspecified gastric ulcer with hemorrhage
531.6*	Chronic or unspecified gastric ulcer with hemorrhage and perforation
532.0*	Acute duodenal ulcer with hemorrhage
532.2*	Acute duodenal ulcer with hemorrhage and perforation
532.4*	Chronic or unspecified duodenal ulcer with hemorrhage
532.6*	Chronic or unspecified duodenal ulcer with hemorrhage and perforation
533.0*	Acute peptic ulcer, unspecified site, with hemorrhage
533.2*	Acute peptic ulcer, unspecified site, with hemorrhage and perforation
533.4*	Chronic or unspecified peptic ulcer, unspecified site, with hemorrhage
533.6*	Chronic or unspecified peptic ulcer, unspecified site, with hemorrhage and perforation
534.0*	Acute gastrojejunal ulcer with hemorrhage
534.2*	Acute gastrojejunal ulcer with hemorrhage and perforation
534.4*	Chronic or unspecified gastrojejunal ulcer with hemorrhage
534.6*	Chronic or unspecified gastrojejunal ulcer with hemorrhage and perforation
535.01	Acute gastritis with hemorrhage
535.11	Atrophic gastritis with hemorrhage
535.21	Gastric mucosal hypertrophy with hemorrhage
535.31	Alcoholic gastritis with hemorrhage
535.41	Other specified gastritis with hemorrhage
535.51	Unspecified gastritis and gastroduodenitis with hemorrhage
535.61	Duodenitis with hemorrhage
535.71	Eosinophilic gastritis with hemorrhage
537.83	Angiodysplasia of stomach and duodenum with hemorrhage
537.84	Dieulafoy lesion (hemorrhagic) of stomach and duodenum
562.02	Diverticulosis of small intestine with hemorrhage
562.03	Diverticulitis of small intestine with hemorrhage
562.12	Diverticulosis of colon with hemorrhage
562.13	Diverticulitis of colon with hemorrhage
569.3	Hemorrhage of rectum and anus
569.85	Angiodysplasia of intestine with hemorrhage
578*	Gastrointestinal hemorrhage

DRG 378 GI Hemorrhage with CC
GMLOS 3.3   AMLOS 3.9   RW 1.0029   ☑ⓋⓉ

Select principal diagnosis listed under DRG 377

Ⓣ *Transfer DRG*   🅢 *Special Payment*   ☑ *Optimization Potential*   Ⓥ *Targeted Potential*   * *Code Range*   ● *New DRG*   ▲ *Revised DRG Title*

Valid 10/01/2013–09/30/2014
© 2013 OptumInsight, Inc.

MDC 6: Diseases And Disorders Of The Digestive System—MEDICAL

DRG 379   **GI Hemorrhage without CC/MCC**
GMLOS 2.4   AMLOS 2.8   RW 0.6937   ☑🔽Ⓣ

Select principal diagnosis listed under DRG 377

DRG 380   **Complicated Peptic Ulcer with MCC**
GMLOS 5.5   AMLOS 7.2   RW 1.9223   ☑Ⓣ

Principal Diagnosis
251.5   Abnormality of secretion of gastrin
530.2*   Ulcer of esophagus
530.85   Barrett's esophagus
531.1*   Acute gastric ulcer with perforation
531.31   Acute gastric ulcer without mention of hemorrhage or perforation, with obstruction
531.5*   Chronic or unspecified gastric ulcer with perforation
531.71   Chronic gastric ulcer without mention of hemorrhage or perforation, with obstruction
531.91   Gastric ulcer, unspecified as acute or chronic, without mention of hemorrhage or perforation, with obstruction
532.1*   Acute duodenal ulcer with perforation
532.31   Acute duodenal ulcer without mention of hemorrhage or perforation, with obstruction
532.5*   Chronic or unspecified duodenal ulcer with perforation
532.71   Chronic duodenal ulcer without mention of hemorrhage or perforation, with obstruction
532.91   Duodenal ulcer, unspecified as acute or chronic, without mention of hemorrhage or perforation, with obstruction
533.1*   Acute peptic ulcer, unspecified site, with perforation
533.31   Acute peptic ulcer, unspecified site, without mention of hemorrhage and perforation, with obstruction
533.5*   Chronic or unspecified peptic ulcer, unspecified site, with perforation
533.71   Chronic peptic ulcer of unspecified site without mention of hemorrhage or perforation, with obstruction
533.91   Peptic ulcer, unspecified site, unspecified as acute or chronic, without mention of hemorrhage or perforation, with obstruction
534.1*   Acute gastrojejunal ulcer with perforation
534.3*   Acute gastrojejunal ulcer without mention of hemorrhage or perforation
534.5*   Chronic or unspecified gastrojejunal ulcer with perforation
534.7*   Chronic gastrojejunal ulcer without mention of hemorrhage or perforation
534.9*   Gastrojejunal ulcer, unspecified as acute or chronic, without mention of hemorrhage or perforation
537.0   Acquired hypertrophic pyloric stenosis
537.3   Other obstruction of duodenum
751.0   Meckel's diverticulum

DRG 381   **Complicated Peptic Ulcer with CC**
GMLOS 3.8   AMLOS 4.6   RW 1.1199   ☑Ⓣ

Select principal diagnosis listed under DRG 380

DRG 382   **Complicated Peptic Ulcer without CC/MCC**
GMLOS 2.7   AMLOS 3.3   RW 0.7784   ☑Ⓣ

Select principal diagnosis listed under DRG 380

DRG 383   **Uncomplicated Peptic Ulcer with MCC**
GMLOS 4.4   AMLOS 5.5   RW 1.3850   ☑

Principal Diagnosis
531.30   Acute gastric ulcer without mention of hemorrhage, perforation, or obstruction
531.70   Chronic gastric ulcer without mention of hemorrhage, perforation, without mention of obstruction
531.90   Gastric ulcer, unspecified as acute or chronic, without mention of hemorrhage, perforation, or obstruction

532.30   Acute duodenal ulcer without mention of hemorrhage, perforation, or obstruction
532.70   Chronic duodenal ulcer without mention of hemorrhage, perforation, or obstruction
532.90   Duodenal ulcer, unspecified as acute or chronic, without hemorrhage, perforation, or obstruction
533.30   Acute peptic ulcer, unspecified site, without mention of hemorrhage, perforation, or obstruction
533.70   Chronic peptic ulcer, unspecified site, without mention of hemorrhage, perforation, or obstruction
533.90   Peptic ulcer, unspecified site, unspecified as acute or chronic, without mention of hemorrhage, perforation, or obstruction

DRG 384   **Uncomplicated Peptic Ulcer without MCC**
GMLOS 3.0   AMLOS 3.6   RW 0.8501   ☑

Select principal diagnosis listed under DRG 383

DRG 385   **Inflammatory Bowel Disease with MCC**
GMLOS 6.0   AMLOS 7.8   RW 1.7973   ☑

Principal Diagnosis
555*   Regional enteritis
556*   Ulcerative colitis

DRG 386   **Inflammatory Bowel Disease with CC**
GMLOS 4.0   AMLOS 5.0   RW 1.0097   ☑

Select principal diagnosis listed under DRG 385

DRG 387   **Inflammatory Bowel Disease without CC/MCC**
GMLOS 3.1   AMLOS 3.8   RW 0.7533   ☑

Select principal diagnosis listed under DRG 385

DRG 388   **GI Obstruction with MCC**
GMLOS 5.3   AMLOS 7.0   RW 1.6170   ☑🔽Ⓣ

Principal Diagnosis
560*   Intestinal obstruction without mention of hernia

DRG 389   **GI Obstruction with CC**
GMLOS 3.6   AMLOS 4.5   RW 0.8853   ☑🔽Ⓣ

Select principal diagnosis listed under DRG 388

DRG 390   **GI Obstruction without CC/MCC**
GMLOS 2.7   AMLOS 3.2   RW 0.6046   ☑🔽Ⓣ

Select principal diagnosis listed under DRG 388

DRG 391   **Esophagitis, Gastroenteritis and Miscellaneous Digestive Disorders with MCC**
GMLOS 3.9   AMLOS 5.1   RW 1.1903   ☑🔽

Principal Diagnosis
005.9   Unspecified food poisoning
008.6*   Intestinal infection, enteritis due to specified virus
008.8   Intestinal infection due to other organism, NEC
009*   Ill-defined intestinal infections
078.82   Epidemic vomiting syndrome
112.85   Candidiasis of the intestine
123.0   Taenia solium infection, intestinal form
123.2   Taenia saginata infection
123.3   Taeniasis, unspecified
123.4   Diphyllobothriasis, intestinal
127.0   Ascariasis
127.1   Anisakiasis

| Surgical | Medical | CC Indicator | MCC Indicator | Procedure Proxy |

127.2	Strongyloidiasis
127.3	Trichuriasis
127.4	Enterobiasis
127.5	Capillariasis
127.6	Trichostrongyliasis
127.7	Other specified intestinal helminthiasis
127.9	Unspecified intestinal helminthiasis
129	Unspecified intestinal parasitism
228.04	Hemangioma of intra-abdominal structures
271.2	Hereditary fructose intolerance
271.3	Intestinal disaccharidase deficiencies and disaccharide malabsorption
306.4	Gastrointestinal malfunction arising from mental factors
447.4	Celiac artery compression syndrome
530.0	Achalasia and cardiospasm
530.1*	Esophagitis
530.3	Stricture and stenosis of esophagus
530.5	Dyskinesia of esophagus
530.6	Diverticulum of esophagus, acquired
530.81	Esophageal reflux
530.83	Esophageal leukoplakia
530.89	Other specified disorder of the esophagus
530.9	Unspecified disorder of esophagus
535.00	Acute gastritis without mention of hemorrhage
535.10	Atrophic gastritis without mention of hemorrhage
535.20	Gastric mucosal hypertrophy without mention of hemorrhage
535.30	Alcoholic gastritis without mention of hemorrhage
535.40	Other specified gastritis without mention of hemorrhage
535.50	Unspecified gastritis and gastroduodenitis without mention of hemorrhage
535.60	Duodenitis without mention of hemorrhage
535.70	Eosinophilic gastritis without mention of hemorrhage
536.0	Achlorhydria
536.1	Acute dilatation of stomach
536.2	Persistent vomiting
536.3	Gastroparesis
536.8	Dyspepsia and other specified disorders of function of stomach
536.9	Unspecified functional disorder of stomach
537.1	Gastric diverticulum
537.2	Chronic duodenal ileus
537.4	Fistula of stomach or duodenum
537.5	Gastroptosis
537.6	Hourglass stricture or stenosis of stomach
537.81	Pylorospasm
537.82	Angiodysplasia of stomach and duodenum (without mention of hemorrhage)
537.89	Other specified disorder of stomach and duodenum
537.9	Unspecified disorder of stomach and duodenum
538	Gastrointestinal mucositis (ulcerative)
552.3	Diaphragmatic hernia with obstruction
553.3	Diaphragmatic hernia without mention of obstruction or gangrene
558.3	Gastroenteritis and colitis, allergic
558.4*	Eosinophilic gastroenteritis and colitis
558.9	Other and unspecified noninfectious gastroenteritis and colitis
562.00	Diverticulosis of small intestine (without mention of hemorrhage)
562.01	Diverticulitis of small intestine (without mention of hemorrhage)
562.10	Diverticulosis of colon (without mention of hemorrhage)
562.11	Diverticulitis of colon (without mention of hemorrhage)
564.0*	Constipation
564.1	Irritable bowel syndrome
564.2	Postgastric surgery syndromes
564.3	Vomiting following gastrointestinal surgery
564.4	Other postoperative functional disorders
564.5	Functional diarrhea

564.6	Anal spasm
564.8*	Other specified functional disorders of intestine
564.9	Unspecified functional disorder of intestine
579*	Intestinal malabsorption
617.5	Endometriosis of intestine
787*	Symptoms involving digestive system
789.0*	Abdominal pain
789.3*	Abdominal or pelvic swelling, mass, or lump
789.6*	Abdominal tenderness
789.7	Colic
789.9	Other symptoms involving abdomen and pelvis
792.1	Nonspecific abnormal finding in stool contents
793.4	Nonspecific (abnormal) findings on radiological and other examination of gastrointestinal tract
793.6	Nonspecific (abnormal) findings on radiological and other examination of abdominal area, including retroperitoneum

DRG 392　Esophagitis, Gastroenteritis and Miscellaneous Digestive Disorders without MCC

GMLOS 2.9　　　**AMLOS 3.5**　　　**RW 0.7395**　☑ 🅥

Select principal diagnosis listed under DRG 391

DRG 393　Other Digestive System Diagnoses with MCC

GMLOS 4.7　　　**AMLOS 6.5**　　　**RW 1.6563**　☑ 🅥

Principal Diagnosis

040.2	Whipple's disease
054.71	Visceral herpes simplex
091.1	Primary anal syphilis
091.69	Early syphilis, secondary syphilis of other viscera
098.7	Gonococcal infection of anus and rectum
099.52	Chlamydia trachomatis infection of anus and rectum
099.56	Chlamydia trachomatis infection of peritoneum
209.4*	Benign carcinoid tumors of the small intestine
209.5*	Benign carcinoid tumors of the appendix, large intestine, and rectum
209.63	Benign carcinoid tumor of the stomach
209.65	Benign carcinoid tumor of foregut, not otherwise specified
209.66	Benign carcinoid tumor of midgut, not otherwise specified
209.67	Benign carcinoid tumor of hindgut, not otherwise specified
211.0	Benign neoplasm of esophagus
211.1	Benign neoplasm of stomach
211.2	Benign neoplasm of duodenum, jejunum, and ileum
211.3	Benign neoplasm of colon
211.4	Benign neoplasm of rectum and anal canal
211.8	Benign neoplasm of retroperitoneum and peritoneum
211.9	Benign neoplasm of other and unspecified site of the digestive system
214.3	Lipoma of intra-abdominal organs
277.03	Cystic fibrosis with gastrointestinal manifestations
289.2	Nonspecific mesenteric lymphadenitis
455*	Hemorrhoids
456.21	Esophageal varices without mention of bleeding in diseases classified elsewhere
530.86	Infection of esophagostomy
530.87	Mechanical complication of esophagostomy
536.4*	Gastrostomy complications
539*	Complications of bariatric procedures
540.9	Acute appendicitis without mention of peritonitis
541	Appendicitis, unqualified
542	Other appendicitis
543*	Other diseases of appendix
550*	Inguinal hernia
551*	Other hernia of abdominal cavity, with gangrene
552.0*	Femoral hernia with obstruction
552.1	Umbilical hernia with obstruction
552.2*	Ventral hernia with obstruction
552.8	Hernia of other specified site, with obstruction
552.9	Hernia of unspecified site, with obstruction

553.0*	Femoral hernia without mention of obstruction or gangrene
553.1	Umbilical hernia without mention of obstruction or gangrene
553.2*	Ventral hernia without mention of obstruction or gangrene
553.8	Hernia of other specified sites of abdominal cavity without mention of obstruction or gangrene
553.9	Hernia of unspecified site of abdominal cavity without mention of obstruction or gangrene
557*	Vascular insufficiency of intestine
558.1	Gastroenteritis and colitis due to radiation
558.2	Toxic gastroenteritis and colitis
564.7	Megacolon, other than Hirschsprung's
565*	Anal fissure and fistula
566	Abscess of anal and rectal regions
567.81	Choleperitonitis
567.82	Sclerosing mesenteritis
568*	Other disorders of peritoneum
569.0	Anal and rectal polyp
569.1	Rectal prolapse
569.2	Stenosis of rectum and anus
569.4*	Other specified disorders of rectum and anus
569.6*	Colostomy and enterostomy complications
569.7*	Complications of intestinal pouch
569.81	Fistula of intestine, excluding rectum and anus
569.82	Ulceration of intestine
569.83	Perforation of intestine
569.84	Angiodysplasia of intestine (without mention of hemorrhage)
569.86	Dieulafoy lesion (hemorrhagic) of intestine
569.87	Vomiting of fecal matter
569.89	Other specified disorder of intestines
569.9	Unspecified disorder of intestine
619.1	Digestive-genital tract fistula, female
750.5	Congenital hypertrophic pyloric stenosis
750.6	Congenital hiatus hernia
750.7	Other specified congenital anomalies of stomach
750.8	Other specified congenital anomalies of upper alimentary tract
750.9	Unspecified congenital anomaly of upper alimentary tract
751.1	Congenital atresia and stenosis of small intestine
751.2	Congenital atresia and stenosis of large intestine, rectum, and anal canal
751.3	Hirschsprung's disease and other congenital functional disorders of colon
751.4	Congenital anomalies of intestinal fixation
751.5	Other congenital anomalies of intestine
751.8	Other specified congenital anomalies of digestive system
751.9	Unspecified congenital anomaly of digestive system
756.7*	Congenital anomaly of abdominal wall
759.3	Situs inversus
759.4	Conjoined twins
789.4*	Abdominal rigidity
796.7*	Abnormal cytologic smear of anus and anal HPV
862.32	Esophagus injury with open wound into cavity
863.0	Stomach injury without mention of open wound into cavity
863.1	Stomach injury with open wound into cavity
863.2*	Small intestine injury without mention of open wound into cavity
863.3*	Small intestine injury with open wound into cavity
863.4*	Colon or rectal injury without mention of open wound into cavity
863.5*	Injury to colon or rectum with open wound into cavity
863.80	Gastrointestinal tract injury, unspecified site, without mention of open wound into cavity
863.85	Appendix injury without mention of open wound into cavity
863.89	Injury to other and unspecified gastrointestinal sites without mention of open wound into cavity
863.90	Gastrointestinal tract injury, unspecified site, with open wound into cavity
863.95	Appendix injury with open wound into cavity
863.99	Injury to other and unspecified gastrointestinal sites with open wound into cavity
868.00	Injury to unspecified intra-abdominal organ without mention of open wound into cavity
868.03	Peritoneum injury without mention of open wound into cavity
868.10	Injury to unspecified intra-abdominal organ, with open wound into cavity
868.13	Peritoneum injury with open wound into cavity
908.1	Late effect of internal injury to intra-abdominal organs
935.1	Foreign body in esophagus
935.2	Foreign body in stomach
936	Foreign body in intestine and colon
937	Foreign body in anus and rectum
938	Foreign body in digestive system, unspecified
947.3	Burn of gastrointestinal tract
997.4*	Digestive system complications, not elsewhere classified
997.71	Vascular complications of mesenteric artery
V53.5*	Fitting and adjustment of other gastrointestinal appliance and device
V55.1	Attention to gastrostomy
V55.2	Attention to ileostomy
V55.3	Attention to colostomy
V55.4	Attention to other artificial opening of digestive tract

DRG 394 **Other Digestive System Diagnoses with CC**

GMLOS 3.5	AMLOS 4.4	RW 0.9653	☑ ▽

Select principal diagnosis listed under DRG 393

DRG 395 **Other Digestive System Diagnoses without CC/MCC**

GMLOS 2.4	AMLOS 3.0	RW 0.6669	☑ ▽

Select principal diagnosis listed under DRG 393

MDC 6: Diseases And Disorders Of The Digestive System—MEDICAL

Surgical	Medical	CC Indicator	MCC Indicator	Procedure Proxy

006.3	070.59	155.2	452	572.8	574.60	576.1	793.3	864.13
070.0	070.6	156.0	453.0	573.0	574.61	576.2	794.8	864.14
070.1	070.70	156.1	570	573.1	574.70	576.3	863.81	864.15
070.20	070.71	156.2	571.0	573.2	574.71	576.4	863.82	864.19
070.21	070.9	156.8	571.1	573.3	574.80	576.5	863.83	868.02
070.22	072.3	156.9	571.2	573.4	574.81	576.8	863.84	868.12
070.23	072.71	157.0	571.3	573.8	574.90	576.9	863.91	996.82
070.30	091.62	157.1	571.40	573.9	574.91	577.0	863.92	996.86
070.31	095.3	157.2	571.41	574.00	575.0	577.1	863.93	V02.60
070.32	120.1	157.3	571.42	574.01	575.10	577.2	863.94	V02.61
070.33	121.0	157.4	571.49	574.10	575.11	577.8	864.00	V02.62
070.41	121.1	157.8	571.5	574.11	575.12	577.9	864.01	V02.69
070.42	121.3	157.9	571.6	574.20	575.2	751.60	864.02	V42.7
070.43	121.4	197.7	571.8	574.21	575.3	751.61	864.03	V42.83
070.44	122.0	209.72	571.9	574.30	575.4	751.62	864.04	V59.6
070.49	122.5	211.5	572.0	574.31	575.5	751.69	864.05	
070.51	122.8	211.6	572.1	574.40	575.6	751.7	864.09	
070.52	130.5	230.8	572.2	574.41	575.8	782.4	864.10	
070.53	155.0	235.3	572.3	574.50	575.9	789.1	864.11	
070.54	155.1	277.4	572.4	574.51	576.0	791.4	864.12	

SURGICAL

DRG 405   Pancreas, Liver and Shunt Procedures with MCC
GMLOS 11.0   AMLOS 14.5   RW 5.4333   T

Operating Room Procedures

17.63	Laser interstitial thermal therapy [LITT] of lesion or tissue of liver under guidance
39.1	Intra-abdominal venous shunt
50.0	Hepatotomy
50.21	Marsupialization of lesion of liver
50.22	Partial hepatectomy
50.23	Open ablation of liver lesion or tissue
50.24	Percutaneous ablation of liver lesion or tissue
50.25	Laparoscopic ablation of liver lesion or tissue
50.26	Other and unspecified ablation of liver lesion or tissue
50.29	Other destruction of lesion of liver
50.3	Lobectomy of liver
50.4	Total hepatectomy
50.61	Closure of laceration of liver
50.69	Other repair of liver
51.43	Insertion of choledochohepatic tube for decompression
51.82	Pancreatic sphincterotomy
51.83	Pancreatic sphincteroplasty
52.0*	Pancreatotomy
52.22	Other excision or destruction of lesion or tissue of pancreas or pancreatic duct
52.3	Marsupialization of pancreatic cyst
52.4	Internal drainage of pancreatic cyst
52.5*	Partial pancreatectomy
52.6	Total pancreatectomy
52.7	Radical pancreaticoduodenectomy
52.80	Pancreatic transplant, not otherwise specified
52.81	Reimplantation of pancreatic tissue
52.82	Homotransplant of pancreas
52.83	Heterotransplant of pancreas
52.92	Cannulation of pancreatic duct
52.95	Other repair of pancreas
52.96	Anastomosis of pancreas
52.99	Other operations on pancreas
54.94	Creation of peritoneovascular shunt

DRG 406   Pancreas, Liver and Shunt Procedures with CC
GMLOS 6.0   AMLOS 7.6   RW 2.7667   ☑ T

Select operating room procedures listed under DRG 405

DRG 407   Pancreas, Liver and Shunt Procedures without CC/MCC
GMLOS 4.2   AMLOS 5.1   RW 1.9139   ☑ T

Select operating room procedures listed under DRG 405

DRG 408   Biliary Tract Procedures Except Only Cholecystectomy with or without C.D.E. with MCC
GMLOS 10.6   AMLOS 13.2   RW 4.1182

Operating Room Procedures

51.02	Trocar cholecystostomy
51.03	Other cholecystostomy
51.04	Other cholecystotomy
51.3*	Anastomosis of gallbladder or bile duct
51.49	Incision of other bile ducts for relief of obstruction
51.59	Incision of other bile duct
51.61	Excision of cystic duct remnant
51.62	Excision of ampulla of Vater (with reimplantation of common duct)
51.63	Other excision of common duct
51.69	Excision of other bile duct
51.7*	Repair of bile ducts
51.81	Dilation of sphincter of Oddi
51.89	Other operations on sphincter of Oddi
51.91	Repair of laceration of gallbladder
51.92	Closure of cholecystostomy
51.93	Closure of other biliary fistula
51.94	Revision of anastomosis of biliary tract
51.95	Removal of prosthetic device from bile duct
51.99	Other operations on biliary tract

WITH OR WITHOUT

Operating Room Procedures

51.41	Common duct exploration for removal of calculus
51.42	Common duct exploration for relief of other obstruction
51.51	Exploration of common bile duct

DRG 409   Biliary Tract Procedures Except Only Cholecystectomy with or without C.D.E. with CC
GMLOS 6.7   AMLOS 7.9   RW 2.4337   ☑

Select operating room procedures listed under DRG 408

DRG 410   Biliary Tract Procedures Except Only Cholecystectomy with or without C.D.E. without CC/MCC
GMLOS 4.3   AMLOS 5.0   RW 1.5123   ☑

Select operating room procedures listed under DRG 408

DRG 411   Cholecystectomy with C.D.E. with MCC
GMLOS 9.3   AMLOS 11.3   RW 3.5968   ☑

Operating Room Procedures

51.41	Common duct exploration for removal of calculus
51.42	Common duct exploration for relief of other obstruction
51.51	Exploration of common bile duct

AND

Operating Room Procedures

51.2*	Cholecystectomy

DRG 412   Cholecystectomy with C.D.E. with CC
GMLOS 6.5   AMLOS 7.6   RW 2.3659   ☑

Select operating room procedures listed under DRG 411

DRG 413   Cholecystectomy with C.D.E. without CC/MCC
GMLOS 4.2   AMLOS 5.0   RW 1.7220   ☑

Select operating room procedures listed under DRG 411

DRG 414   Cholecystectomy Except by Laparoscope without C.D.E. with MCC
GMLOS 8.8   AMLOS 10.6   RW 3.6208   ☑ T

Operating Room Procedures

51.21	Other partial cholecystectomy
51.22	Cholecystectomy

DRG 415   Cholecystectomy Except by Laparoscope without C.D.E. with CC
GMLOS 5.8   AMLOS 6.7   RW 2.0173   ☑ T

Select operating room procedures listed under DRG 414

DRG 416   Cholecystectomy Except by Laparoscope without C.D.E. without CC/MCC
GMLOS 3.5   AMLOS 4.1   RW 1.3268   ☑ T

Select operating room procedures listed under DRG 414

Surgical	Medical	CC Indicator	MCC Indicator	Procedure Proxy

System And Pancreas—MEDICAL

MDC 7: Diseases And Disord

DRG 417 **Laparoscopic Cholecystectomy without C.D.E. with MCC**
GMLOS 6.0   AMLOS 7.5   RW 2.4784   ☑

Operating room procedures
51.23   Laparoscopic cholecystectomy
51.24   Laparoscopic partial cholecystectomy

DRG 418 **Laparoscopic Cholecystectomy without C.D.E. with CC**
GMLOS 4.1   AMLOS 5.0   RW 1.6536   ☑

Select operating room procedures listed under DRG 417

DRG 419 **Laparoscopic Cholecystectomy without C.D.E. without CC/MCC**
GMLOS 2.6   AMLOS 3.1   RW 1.2239   ☑

Select operating room procedures listed under DRG 417

DRG 420 **Hepatobiliary Diagnostic Procedures with MCC**
GMLOS 8.7   AMLOS 12.3   RW 3.6786   ☑

Operating Room Procedures
44.11   Transabdominal gastroscopy
50.12   Open biopsy of liver
50.14   Laparoscopic liver biopsy
50.19   Other diagnostic procedures on liver
51.13   Open biopsy of gallbladder or bile ducts
51.19   Other diagnostic procedures on biliary tract
52.12   Open biopsy of pancreas
52.19   Other diagnostic procedures on pancreas
54.11   Exploratory laparotomy
54.19   Other laparotomy
54.21   Laparoscopy
54.23   Biopsy of peritoneum
54.29   Other diagnostic procedures on abdominal region
87.53   Intraoperative cholangiogram

DRG 421 **Hepatobiliary Diagnostic Procedures with CC**
GMLOS 4.6   AMLOS 6.3   RW 1.7714   ☑

Select operating room procedures listed under DRG 420

DRG 422 **Hepatobiliary Diagnostic Procedures without CC/MCC**
GMLOS 3.1   AMLOS 3.9   RW 1.2175   ☑

Select operating room procedures listed under DRG 420

DRG 423 **Other Hepatobiliary or Pancreas O.R. Procedures with MCC**
GMLOS 9.6   AMLOS 13.0   RW 4.2183   ☑

Operating Room Procedures
03.2*   Chordotomy
17.56   Atherectomy of other non-coronary vessel(s)
38.7   Interruption of the vena cava
39.26   Other intra-abdominal vascular shunt or bypass
39.29   Other (peripheral) vascular shunt or bypass
39.49   Other revision of vascular procedure
39.50   Angioplasty of other non-coronary vessel(s)
39.98   Control of hemorrhage, not otherwise specified
40.11   Biopsy of lymphatic structure
42.91   Ligation of esophageal varices
43.0   Gastrotomy
43.42   Local excision of other lesion or tissue of stomach
44.32   Percutaneous [endoscopic] gastrojejunostomy
44.38   Laparoscopic gastroenterostomy
44.39   Other gastroenterostomy without gastrectomy
44.63   Closure of other gastric fistula
44.91   Ligation of gastric varices
44.92   Intraoperative manipulation of stomach
45.01   Incision of duodenum

45.31   Other local excision of lesion of duodenum
45.32   Other destruction of lesion of duodenum
46.80   Intra-abdominal manipulation of intestine, not otherwise specified
46.81   Intra-abdominal manipulation of small intestine
46.82   Intra-abdominal manipulation of large intestine
46.99   Other operations on intestines
54.0   Incision of abdominal wall
54.12   Reopening of recent laparotomy site
54.4   Excision or destruction of peritoneal tissue
54.5*   Lysis of peritoneal adhesions
54.61   Reclosure of postoperative disruption of abdominal wall
54.62   Delayed closure of granulating abdominal wound
54.64   Suture of peritoneum
54.72   Other repair of abdominal wall
54.73   Other repair of peritoneum
54.74   Other repair of omentum
54.75   Other repair of mesentery
54.93   Creation of cutaneoperitoneal fistula
54.95   Incision of peritoneum
86.06   Insertion of totally implantable infusion pump
86.22   Excisional debridement of wound, infection, or burn

DRG 424 **Other Hepatobiliary or Pancreas O.R. Procedures with CC**
GMLOS 6.3   AMLOS 8.2   RW 2.3149   ☑

Select operating room procedures listed under DRG 423

DRG 425 **Other Hepatobiliary or Pancreas O.R. Procedures without CC/MCC**
GMLOS 3.8   AMLOS 4.9   RW 1.6396   ☑

Select operating room procedures listed under DRG 423

MEDICAL

DRG 432 **Cirrhosis and Alcoholic Hepatitis with MCC**
GMLOS 4.7   AMLOS 6.3   RW 1.7150   ☑

Principal Diagnosis
571.1   Acute alcoholic hepatitis
571.2   Alcoholic cirrhosis of liver
571.3   Unspecified alcoholic liver damage
571.5   Cirrhosis of liver without mention of alcohol
571.6   Biliary cirrhosis

DRG 433 **Cirrhosis and Alcoholic Hepatitis with CC**
GMLOS 3.3   AMLOS 4.1   RW 0.9249   ☑

Select principal diagnosis listed under DRG 432

DRG 434 **Cirrhosis and Alcoholic Hepatitis without CC/MCC**
GMLOS 2.4   AMLOS 3.0   RW 0.6156   ☑

Select principal diagnosis listed under DRG 432

DRG 435 **Malignancy of Hepatobiliary System or Pancreas with MCC**
GMLOS 5.2   AMLOS 6.9   RW 1.7356   ☑

Principal Diagnosis
155*   Malignant neoplasm of liver and intrahepatic bile ducts
156*   Malignant neoplasm of gallbladder and extrahepatic bile ducts
157*   Malignant neoplasm of pancreas
197.7   Secondary malignant neoplasm of liver
209.72   Secondary neuroendocrine tumor of liver

Ⓣ *Transfer DRG*   🆂🅿 *Special Payment*   ☑ *Optimization Potential*   ᵛ *Targeted Potential*   * *Code Range*   ● *New DRG*   ▲ *Revised DRG Title*

230.8	Carcinoma in situ of liver and biliary system
235.3	Neoplasm of uncertain behavior of liver and biliary passages

DRG 436   Malignancy of Hepatobiliary System or Pancreas with CC
GMLOS 3.9   AMLOS 5.0   RW 1.1548   ☑

Select principal diagnosis listed under DRG 435

DRG 437   Malignancy of Hepatobiliary System or Pancreas without CC/MCC
GMLOS 2.8   AMLOS 3.6   RW 0.9282   ☑

Select principal diagnosis listed under DRG 435

DRG 438   Disorders of Pancreas Except Malignancy with MCC
GMLOS 5.1   AMLOS 7.0   RW 1.7210   ☑

Principal Diagnosis

072.3	Mumps pancreatitis
211.6	Benign neoplasm of pancreas, except islets of Langerhans
577*	Diseases of pancreas
751.7	Congenital anomalies of pancreas
863.81	Pancreas head injury without mention of open wound into cavity
863.82	Pancreas body injury without mention of open wound into cavity
863.83	Pancreas tail injury without mention of open wound into cavity
863.84	Pancreas injury, multiple and unspecified sites, without mention of open wound into cavity
863.91	Pancreas head injury with open wound into cavity
863.92	Pancreas body injury with open wound into cavity
863.93	Pancreas tail injury with open wound into cavity
863.94	Pancreas injury, multiple and unspecified sites, with open wound into cavity
996.86	Complications of transplanted pancreas
V42.83	Pancreas replaced by transplant

DRG 439   Disorders of Pancreas Except Malignancy with CC
GMLOS 3.6   AMLOS 4.5   RW 0.9162   ☑

Select principal diagnosis listed under DRG 438

DRG 440   Disorders of Pancreas Except Malignancy without CC/MCC
GMLOS 2.7   AMLOS 3.2   RW 0.6452   ☑

Select principal diagnosis listed under DRG 438

DRG 441   Disorders of Liver Except Malignancy, Cirrhosis, Alcoholic Hepatitis with MCC
GMLOS 5.0   AMLOS 6.8   RW 1.8534   ☑Ⓣ

Principal Diagnosis

006.3	Amebic liver abscess
070*	Viral hepatitis
072.71	Mumps hepatitis
091.62	Early syphilis, secondary syphilitic hepatitis
095.3	Syphilis of liver
120.1	Schistosomiasis due to schistosoma mansoni
121.0	Opisthorchiasis
121.1	Clonorchiasis
121.3	Fascioliasis
121.4	Fasciolopsiasis
122.0	Echinococcus granulosus infection of liver
122.5	Echinococcus multilocularis infection of liver
122.8	Unspecified echinococcus of liver
130.5	Hepatitis due to toxoplasmosis
211.5	Benign neoplasm of liver and biliary passages
277.4	Disorders of bilirubin excretion

452	Portal vein thrombosis
453.0	Budd-Chiari syndrome
570	Acute and subacute necrosis of liver
571.0	Alcoholic fatty liver
571.4*	Chronic hepatitis
571.8	Other chronic nonalcoholic liver disease
571.9	Unspecified chronic liver disease without mention of alcohol
572*	Liver abscess and sequelae of chronic liver disease
573.0	Chronic passive congestion of liver
573.1	Hepatitis in viral diseases classified elsewhere
573.2	Hepatitis in other infectious diseases classified elsewhere
573.3	Unspecified hepatitis
573.4	Hepatic infarction
573.8	Other specified disorders of liver
573.9	Unspecified disorder of liver
751.62	Congenital cystic disease of liver
751.69	Other congenital anomaly of gallbladder, bile ducts, and liver
782.4	Jaundice, unspecified, not of newborn
789.1	Hepatomegaly
791.4	Biliuria
794.8	Nonspecific abnormal results of liver function study
864*	Injury to liver
996.82	Complications of transplanted liver
V02.6*	Carrier or suspected carrier of viral hepatitis
V42.7	Liver replaced by transplant
V59.6	Liver donor

DRG 442   Disorders of Liver Except Malignancy, Cirrhosis, Alcoholic Hepatitis with CC
GMLOS 3.4   AMLOS 4.3   RW 0.9280   ☑Ⓣ

Select principal diagnosis listed under DRG 441

DRG 443   Disorders of Liver Except Malignancy, Cirrhosis, Alcoholic Hepatitis without CC/MCC
GMLOS 2.6   AMLOS 3.2   RW 0.6418   ☑Ⓣ

Select principal diagnosis listed under DRG 441

DRG 444   Disorders of the Biliary Tract with MCC
GMLOS 4.7   AMLOS 6.1   RW 1.6060   ☑

Principal Diagnosis

574*	Cholelithiasis
575*	Other disorders of gallbladder
576*	Other disorders of biliary tract
751.60	Unspecified congenital anomaly of gallbladder, bile ducts, and liver
751.61	Congenital biliary atresia
793.3	Nonspecific (abnormal) findings on radiological and other examination of biliary tract
868.02	Bile duct and gallbladder injury without mention of open wound into cavity
868.12	Bile duct and gallbladder injury, with open wound into cavity

DRG 445   Disorders of the Biliary Tract with CC
GMLOS 3.4   AMLOS 4.2   RW 1.0476   ☑

Select principal diagnosis listed under DRG 444

DRG 446   Disorders of the Biliary Tract without CC/MCC
GMLOS 2.4   AMLOS 2.9   RW 0.7499   ☑

Select principal diagnosis listed under DRG 444

MDC 7: Diseases And Disorders Of The Hepatobiliary System And Pancreas—MEDICAL

Surgical   Medical   CC Indicator   MCC Indicator   Procedure Proxy

MDC 8
Diseases And Disorders Of The Musculoskeletal System And Connective Tissue

003.23	170.0	446.20	711.49	712.26	715.22	716.40	717.9	718.77
003.24	170.1	446.21	711.50	712.27	715.23	716.41	718.00	718.78
015.00	170.2	446.29	711.51	712.28	715.24	716.42	718.01	718.79
015.01	170.3	446.3	711.52	712.29	715.25	716.43	718.02	718.80
015.02	170.4	446.4	711.53	712.30	715.26	716.44	718.03	718.81
015.03	170.5	446.5	711.54	712.31	715.27	716.45	718.04	718.82
015.04	170.6	446.6	711.55	712.32	715.28	716.46	718.05	718.83
015.05	170.7	446.7	711.56	712.33	715.30	716.47	718.07	718.84
015.06	170.8	447.6	711.57	712.34	715.31	716.48	718.08	718.85
015.10	170.9	696.0	711.58	712.35	715.32	716.49	718.09	718.86
015.11	171.0	710.0	711.59	712.36	715.33	716.50	718.10	718.87
015.12	171.2	710.1	711.60	712.37	715.34	716.51	718.11	718.88
015.13	171.3	710.2	711.61	712.38	715.35	716.52	718.12	718.89
015.14	171.4	710.3	711.62	712.39	715.36	716.53	718.13	718.90
015.15	171.5	710.4	711.63	712.80	715.37	716.54	718.14	718.91
015.16	171.6	710.5	711.64	712.81	715.38	716.55	718.15	718.92
015.20	171.7	710.8	711.65	712.82	715.80	716.56	718.17	718.93
015.21	171.8	710.9	711.66	712.83	715.89	716.57	718.18	718.94
015.22	171.9	711.00	711.67	712.84	715.90	716.58	718.19	718.95
015.23	198.5	711.01	711.68	712.85	715.91	716.59	718.20	718.97
015.24	209.73	711.02	711.69	712.86	715.92	716.60	718.21	718.98
015.25	213.0	711.03	711.70	712.87	715.93	716.61	718.22	718.99
015.26	213.2	711.04	711.71	712.88	715.94	716.62	718.23	719.00
015.50	213.4	711.05	711.72	712.89	715.95	716.63	718.24	719.01
015.51	213.5	711.06	711.73	712.90	715.96	716.64	718.25	719.02
015.52	213.6	711.07	711.74	712.91	715.97	716.65	718.26	719.03
015.53	213.7	711.08	711.75	712.92	715.98	716.66	718.27	719.04
015.54	213.8	711.09	711.76	712.93	716.00	716.67	718.28	719.05
015.55	213.9	711.10	711.77	712.94	716.01	716.68	718.29	719.06
015.56	215.0	711.11	711.78	712.95	716.02	716.80	718.30	719.07
015.70	215.2	711.12	711.79	712.96	716.03	716.81	718.31	719.08
015.71	215.3	711.13	711.80	712.97	716.04	716.82	718.32	719.09
015.72	215.4	711.14	711.81	712.98	716.05	716.83	718.33	719.10
015.73	215.5	711.15	711.82	712.99	716.06	716.84	718.34	719.11
015.74	215.6	711.16	711.83	713.0	716.07	716.85	718.35	719.12
015.75	215.7	711.17	711.84	713.1	716.08	716.86	718.36	719.13
015.76	215.8	711.18	711.85	713.2	716.09	716.87	718.37	719.14
015.80	215.9	711.19	711.86	713.3	716.10	716.88	718.38	719.15
015.81	238.0	711.20	711.87	713.4	716.11	716.89	718.39	719.16
015.82	238.1	711.21	711.88	713.5	716.12	716.90	718.40	719.17
015.83	239.2	711.22	711.89	713.6	716.13	716.91	718.41	719.18
015.84	268.0	711.23	711.90	713.7	716.14	716.92	718.42	719.19
015.85	268.1	711.24	711.91	713.8	716.15	716.93	718.43	719.20
015.86	268.2	711.25	711.92	714.0	716.16	716.94	718.44	719.21
015.90	274.00	711.26	711.93	714.1	716.17	716.95	718.45	719.22
015.91	274.01	711.27	711.94	714.2	716.18	716.96	718.46	719.23
015.92	274.02	711.28	711.95	714.30	716.19	716.97	718.47	719.24
015.93	274.03	711.29	711.96	714.31	716.20	716.98	718.48	719.25
015.94	274.81	711.30	711.97	714.32	716.21	716.99	718.49	719.26
015.95	274.82	711.31	711.98	714.33	716.22	717.0	718.50	719.27
015.96	274.89	711.32	711.99	714.4	716.23	717.1	718.51	719.28
036.82	274.9	711.33	712.10	714.89	716.24	717.2	718.52	719.29
040.81	277.30	711.34	712.11	714.9	716.25	717.3	718.53	719.30
056.71	277.31	711.35	712.12	715.00	716.26	717.40	718.54	719.31
091.61	277.39	711.36	712.13	715.04	716.27	717.41	718.55	719.32
095.5	279.41	711.37	712.14	715.09	716.28	717.42	718.56	719.33
095.6	279.49	711.38	712.15	715.10	716.29	717.43	718.57	719.34
095.7	306.0	711.39	712.16	715.11	716.30	717.49	718.58	719.35
098.50	359.71	711.40	712.17	715.12	716.31	717.5	718.59	719.36
098.51	359.79	711.41	712.18	715.13	716.32	717.6	718.65	719.37
098.52	380.01	711.42	712.19	715.14	716.33	717.7	718.70	719.38
098.53	380.02	711.43	712.20	715.15	716.34	717.81	718.71	719.39
098.59	380.03	711.44	712.21	715.16	716.35	717.82	718.72	719.40
099.3	390	711.45	712.22	715.17	716.36	717.83	718.73	719.41
102.6	443.0	711.46	712.23	715.18	716.37	717.84	718.74	719.42
136.1	446.0	711.47	712.24	715.20	716.38	717.85	718.75	719.43
137.3	446.1	711.48	712.25	715.21	716.39	717.89	718.76	719.44

719.45	722.52	727.1	730.09	732.8	736.76	755.01	759.81	812.09
719.46	722.6	727.2	730.10	732.9	736.79	755.02	759.89	812.10
719.47	722.70	727.3	730.11	733.00	736.81	755.10	781.93	812.11
719.48	722.71	727.40	730.12	733.01	736.89	755.11	793.7	812.12
719.49	722.72	727.41	730.13	733.02	736.9	755.12	794.17	812.13
719.50	722.73	727.42	730.14	733.03	737.0	755.13	795.6	812.19
719.51	722.80	727.43	730.15	733.09	737.10	755.14	802.8	812.20
719.52	722.81	727.49	730.16	733.10	737.11	755.20	802.9	812.21
719.53	722.82	727.50	730.17	733.11	737.12	755.21	805.00	812.30
719.54	722.83	727.51	730.18	733.12	737.19	755.22	805.01	812.31
719.55	722.90	727.59	730.19	733.13	737.20	755.23	805.02	812.40
719.56	722.91	727.60	730.20	733.14	737.21	755.24	805.03	812.41
719.57	722.92	727.61	730.21	733.15	737.22	755.25	805.04	812.42
719.58	722.93	727.62	730.22	733.16	737.29	755.26	805.05	812.43
719.59	723.0	727.63	730.23	733.19	737.30	755.27	805.06	812.44
719.60	723.1	727.64	730.24	733.20	737.31	755.28	805.07	812.49
719.61	723.5	727.65	730.25	733.21	737.32	755.29	805.08	812.50
719.62	723.7	727.66	730.26	733.22	737.33	755.30	805.10	812.51
719.63	723.8	727.67	730.27	733.29	737.34	755.31	805.11	812.52
719.64	723.9	727.68	730.28	733.3	737.39	755.32	805.12	812.53
719.65	724.00	727.69	730.29	733.40	737.40	755.33	805.13	812.54
719.66	724.01	727.81	730.30	733.41	737.41	755.34	805.14	812.59
719.67	724.02	727.82	730.31	733.42	737.42	755.35	805.15	813.00
719.68	724.03	727.83	730.32	733.43	737.43	755.36	805.16	813.01
719.69	724.09	727.89	730.33	733.44	737.8	755.37	805.17	813.02
719.7	724.1	727.9	730.34	733.45	737.9	755.38	805.18	813.03
719.80	724.2	728.0	730.35	733.49	738.10	755.39	805.2	813.04
719.81	724.3	728.10	730.36	733.5	738.11	755.4	805.3	813.05
719.82	724.4	728.11	730.37	733.7	738.12	755.50	805.4	813.06
719.83	724.5	728.12	730.38	733.81	738.19	755.51	805.5	813.07
719.84	724.6	728.13	730.39	733.82	738.2	755.52	805.6	813.08
719.85	724.70	728.19	730.70	733.90	738.3	755.53	805.7	813.10
719.86	724.71	728.2	730.71	733.91	738.4	755.54	805.8	813.11
719.87	724.79	728.3	730.72	733.92	738.5	755.55	805.9	813.12
719.88	724.8	728.4	730.73	733.93	738.6	755.56	808.0	813.13
719.89	724.9	728.5	730.74	733.94	738.8	755.57	808.1	813.14
719.90	725	728.6	730.75	733.95	738.9	755.58	808.2	813.15
719.91	726.0	728.71	730.76	733.96	739.0	755.59	808.3	813.16
719.92	726.10	728.79	730.77	733.97	739.1	755.60	808.41	813.17
719.93	726.11	728.81	730.78	733.98	739.2	755.61	808.42	813.18
719.94	726.12	728.82	730.79	733.99	739.3	755.62	808.43	813.20
719.95	726.13	728.83	730.80	734	739.4	755.63	808.44	813.21
719.96	726.19	728.84	730.81	735.0	739.5	755.64	808.49	813.22
719.97	726.2	728.85	730.82	735.1	739.6	755.65	808.51	813.23
719.98	726.30	728.86	730.83	735.2	739.7	755.66	808.52	813.30
719.99	726.31	728.87	730.84	735.3	739.8	755.67	808.53	813.31
720.0	726.32	728.88	730.85	735.4	739.9	755.69	808.54	813.32
720.1	726.33	728.89	730.86	735.5	754.0	755.8	808.59	813.33
720.2	726.39	728.9	730.87	735.8	754.1	755.9	808.8	813.40
720.81	726.4	729.0	730.88	735.9	754.2	756.0	808.9	813.41
720.89	726.5	729.1	730.89	736.00	754.30	756.10	809.0	813.42
720.9	726.60	729.4	730.90	736.01	754.31	756.11	809.1	813.43
721.0	726.61	729.5	730.91	736.02	754.32	756.12	810.00	813.44
721.1	726.62	729.6	730.92	736.03	754.33	756.13	810.01	813.45
721.2	726.63	729.71	730.93	736.04	754.35	756.14	810.02	813.46
721.3	726.64	729.72	730.94	736.09	754.40	756.15	810.03	813.47
721.41	726.65	729.73	730.95	736.1	754.41	756.16	810.10	813.50
721.42	726.69	729.79	730.96	736.20	754.42	756.19	810.11	813.51
721.5	726.70	729.81	730.97	736.21	754.43	756.2	810.12	813.52
721.6	726.71	729.82	730.98	736.22	754.44	756.4	810.13	813.53
721.7	726.72	729.89	730.99	736.29	754.50	756.50	811.00	813.54
721.8	726.73	729.90	731.0	736.30	754.51	756.51	811.01	813.80
721.90	726.79	729.91	731.1	736.31	754.52	756.52	811.02	813.81
721.91	726.8	729.92	731.2	736.32	754.53	756.53	811.03	813.82
722.0	726.90	729.99	731.3	736.39	754.59	756.54	811.09	813.83
722.10	726.91	730.00	731.8	736.41	754.60	756.55	811.10	813.90
722.11	727.00	730.01	732.0	736.42	754.61	756.56	811.11	813.91
722.2	727.01	730.02	732.1	736.5	754.62	756.59	811.12	813.92
722.30	727.02	730.03	732.2	736.6	754.69	756.81	811.13	813.93
722.31	727.03	730.04	732.3	736.70	754.70	756.82	811.19	814.00
722.32	727.04	730.05	732.4	736.71	754.71	756.83	812.00	814.01
722.39	727.05	730.06	732.5	736.72	754.79	756.89	812.01	814.02
722.4	727.06	730.07	732.6	736.73	754.89	756.9	812.02	814.03
722.51	727.09	730.08	732.7	736.75	755.00	759.7	812.03	814.04

814.05	820.11	823.82	831.13	836.1	839.12	842.12	881.20	997.69
814.06	820.12	823.90	831.14	836.2	839.13	842.13	881.21	V42.4
814.07	820.13	823.91	831.19	836.3	839.14	842.19	881.22	V43.60
814.08	820.19	823.92	832.00	836.4	839.15	843.0	882.2	V43.61
814.09	820.20	824.0	832.01	836.50	839.16	843.1	883.2	V43.62
814.10	820.21	824.1	832.02	836.51	839.17	843.8	884.2	V43.63
814.11	820.22	824.2	832.03	836.52	839.18	843.9	890.2	V43.64
814.12	820.30	824.3	832.04	836.53	839.20	844.0	891.2	V43.65
814.13	820.31	824.4	832.09	836.54	839.21	844.1	892.2	V43.66
814.14	820.32	824.5	832.10	836.59	839.30	844.2	893.2	V43.69
814.15	820.8	824.6	832.11	836.60	839.31	844.3	894.2	V43.7
814.16	820.9	824.7	832.12	836.61	839.40	844.8	905.1	V52.0
814.17	821.00	824.8	832.13	836.62	839.41	844.9	905.2	V52.1
814.18	821.01	824.9	832.14	836.63	839.42	845.00	905.3	V53.7
814.19	821.10	825.0	832.19	836.64	839.49	845.01	905.4	V54.01
815.00	821.11	825.1	832.2	836.69	839.50	845.02	905.5	V54.02
815.01	821.20	825.20	833.00	837.0	839.51	845.03	905.6	V54.09
815.02	821.21	825.21	833.01	837.1	839.52	845.09	905.7	V54.10
815.03	821.22	825.22	833.02	838.00	839.59	845.10	905.8	V54.11
815.04	821.23	825.23	833.03	838.01	839.69	845.11	905.9	V54.12
815.09	821.29	825.24	833.04	838.02	839.79	845.12	958.6	V54.13
815.10	821.30	825.25	833.05	838.03	839.8	845.13	996.40	V54.14
815.11	821.31	825.29	833.09	838.04	839.9	845.19	996.41	V54.15
815.12	821.32	825.30	833.10	838.05	840.0	846.0	996.42	V54.16
815.13	821.33	825.31	833.11	838.06	840.1	846.1	996.43	V54.17
815.14	821.39	825.32	833.12	838.09	840.2	846.2	996.44	V54.19
815.19	822.0	825.33	833.13	838.10	840.3	846.3	996.45	V54.20
816.00	822.1	825.34	833.14	838.11	840.4	846.8	996.46	V54.21
816.01	823.00	825.35	833.15	838.12	840.5	846.9	996.47	V54.22
816.02	823.01	825.39	833.19	838.13	840.6	847.0	996.49	V54.23
816.03	823.02	826.0	834.00	838.14	840.7	847.1	996.66	V54.24
816.10	823.10	826.1	834.01	838.15	840.8	847.2	996.67	V54.25
816.11	823.11	827.0	834.02	838.16	840.9	847.3	996.77	V54.26
816.12	823.12	827.1	834.10	838.19	841.0	847.4	996.78	V54.27
816.13	823.20	829.0	834.11	839.00	841.1	847.9	996.90	V54.29
817.0	823.21	829.1	834.12	839.01	841.2	848.0	996.91	V54.81
817.1	823.22	831.00	835.00	839.02	841.3	848.2	996.92	V54.82
818.0	823.30	831.01	835.01	839.03	841.8	848.5	996.93	V54.89
818.1	823.31	831.02	835.02	839.04	841.9	848.8	996.94	V54.9
820.00	823.32	831.03	835.03	839.05	842.00	848.9	996.95	V59.2
820.01	823.40	831.04	835.10	839.06	842.01	880.20	996.96	
820.02	823.41	831.09	835.11	839.07	842.02	880.21	996.99	
820.03	823.42	831.10	835.12	839.08	842.09	880.22	997.60	
820.09	823.80	831.11	835.13	839.10	842.10	880.23	997.61	
820.10	823.81	831.12	836.0	839.11	842.11	880.29	997.62	

SURGICAL

DRG 453 Combined Anterior/Posterior Spinal Fusion with MCC
GMLOS 9.7   AMLOS 12.2   RW 11.7453

Operating Room Procedures

81.02	Other cervical fusion of the anterior column, anterior technique
81.04	Dorsal and dorsolumbar fusion of the anterior column, anterior technique
81.06	Lumbar and lumbosacral fusion of the anterior column, anterior technique
81.32	Refusion of other cervical spine, anterior column, anterior technique
81.34	Refusion of dorsal and dorsolumbar spine, anterior column, anterior technique
81.36	Refusion of lumbar and lumbosacral spine, anterior column, anterior technique

AND

Operating Room Procedures

81.03	Other cervical fusion of the posterior column, posterior technique
81.05	Dorsal and dorsolumbar fusion of the posterior column, posterior technique
81.07	Lumbar and lumbosacral fusion of the posterior column, posterior technique
81.08	Lumbar and lumbosacral fusion of the anterior column, posterior technique
81.33	Refusion of other cervical spine, posterior column, posterior technique
81.35	Refusion of dorsal and dorsolumbar spine, posterior column, posterior technique
81.37	Refusion of lumbar and lumbosacral spine, posterior column, posterior technique
81.38	Refusion of lumbar and lumbosacral spine, anterior column, posterior technique

DRG 454 Combined Anterior/Posterior Spinal Fusion with CC
GMLOS 5.1   AMLOS 6.1   RW 8.0200   ☑

Select operating room procedures listed under DRG 453

DRG 455 Combined Anterior/Posterior Spinal Fusion without CC/MCC
GMLOS 3.1   AMLOS 3.6   RW 6.2882   ☑

Select operating room procedures listed under DRG 453

DRG 456 Spinal Fusion Except Cervical with Spinal Curvature/Malignancy/Infection or 9+ Fusions with MCC
GMLOS 10.2   AMLOS 12.5   RW 9.5871   ☑

Principal Diagnosis

015.02	Tuberculosis of vertebral column, bacteriological or histological examination unknown (at present)
015.04	Tuberculosis of vertebral column, tubercle bacilli not found (in sputum) by microscopy, but found by bacterial culture
015.05	Tuberculosis of vertebral column, tubercle bacilli not found by bacteriological examination, but tuberculosis confirmed histologically
170.2	Malignant neoplasm of vertebral column, excluding sacrum and coccyx
198.5	Secondary malignant neoplasm of bone and bone marrow
209.73	Secondary neuroendocrine tumor of bone
213.2	Benign neoplasm of vertebral column, excluding sacrum and coccyx

238.0	Neoplasm of uncertain behavior of bone and articular cartilage
239.2	Neoplasms of unspecified nature of bone, soft tissue, and skin
730.08	Acute osteomyelitis, other specified site
730.18	Chronic osteomyelitis, other specified sites
730.28	Unspecified osteomyelitis, other specified sites
732.0	Juvenile osteochondrosis of spine
733.13	Pathologic fracture of vertebrae
737.0	Adolescent postural kyphosis
737.1*	Kyphosis (acquired)
737.2*	Lordosis (acquired)
737.3*	Kyphoscoliosis and scoliosis
737.8	Other curvatures of spine associated with other conditions
737.9	Unspecified curvature of spine associated with other condition
754.2	Congenital musculoskeletal deformity of spine
756.51	Osteogenesis imperfecta

OR

Secondary Diagnosis

737.4*	Curvature of spine associated with other conditions

AND

Operating Room Procedures

81.00	Spinal fusion, not otherwise specified
81.04	Dorsal and dorsolumbar fusion of the anterior column, anterior technique
81.05	Dorsal and dorsolumbar fusion of the posterior column, posterior technique
81.06	Lumbar and lumbosacral fusion of the anterior column, anterior technique
81.07	Lumbar and lumbosacral fusion of the posterior column, posterior technique
81.08	Lumbar and lumbosacral fusion of the anterior column, posterior technique
81.30	Refusion of spine, not otherwise specified
81.34	Refusion of dorsal and dorsolumbar spine, anterior column, anterior technique
81.35	Refusion of dorsal and dorsolumbar spine, posterior column, posterior technique
81.36	Refusion of lumbar and lumbosacral spine, anterior column, anterior technique
81.37	Refusion of lumbar and lumbosacral spine, posterior column, posterior technique
81.38	Refusion of lumbar and lumbosacral spine, anterior column, posterior technique
81.39	Refusion of spine, not elsewhere classified

OR

Nonoperating Room Procedure

81.64	Fusion or refusion of 9 or more vertebrae

DRG 457 Spinal Fusion Except Cervical with Spinal Curvature/Malignancy/Infection or 9+ Fusions with CC
GMLOS 5.6   AMLOS 6.5   RW 6.8188   ☑

Select principal or secondary diagnosis and operating room procedures listed under DRG 456

OR

Nonoperating room procedure

81.64	Fusion or refusion of 9 or more vertebrae

DRG 458   Spinal Fusion Except Cervical with Spinal Curvature/Malignancy/Infection or 9+ Fusions without CC/MCC

GMLOS 3.3   AMLOS 3.8   RW 5.1378

Select principal or secondary diagnosis and operating room procedures listed under DRG 456

OR

Nonoperating room procedure

81.64   Fusion or refusion of 9 or more vertebrae

DRG 459   Spinal Fusion Except Cervical with MCC

GMLOS 7.1   AMLOS 8.7   RW 6.8163   ☑Ⓣ

Includes any of the following procedure codes, as long as any combination of procedure codes would not otherwise result in assignment to DRG 453

81.00   Spinal fusion, not otherwise specified
81.04   Dorsal and dorsolumbar fusion of the anterior column, anterior technique
81.05   Dorsal and dorsolumbar fusion of the posterior column, posterior technique
81.06   Lumbar and lumbosacral fusion of the anterior column, anterior technique
81.07   Lumbar and lumbosacral fusion of the posterior column, posterior technique
81.08   Lumbar and lumbosacral fusion of the anterior column, posterior technique
81.30   Refusion of spine, not otherwise specified
81.34   Refusion of dorsal and dorsolumbar spine, anterior column, anterior technique
81.35   Refusion of dorsal and dorsolumbar spine, posterior column, posterior technique
81.36   Refusion of lumbar and lumbosacral spine, anterior column, anterior technique
81.37   Refusion of lumbar and lumbosacral spine, posterior column, posterior technique
81.38   Refusion of lumbar and lumbosacral spine, anterior column, posterior technique
81.39   Refusion of spine, not elsewhere classified

DRG 460   Spinal Fusion Except Cervical without MCC

GMLOS 3.1   AMLOS 3.6   RW 4.0221   ☑Ⓣ

Select operating room procedures listed under DRG 459

DRG 461   Bilateral or Multiple Major Joint Procedures of Lower Extremity with MCC

GMLOS 6.1   AMLOS 7.5   RW 5.0254

Any combination of two or more of the following procedures

00.70   Revision of hip replacement, both acetabular and femoral components
00.80   Revision of knee replacement, total (all components)
00.85   Resurfacing hip, total, acetabulum and femoral head
00.86   Resurfacing hip, partial, femoral head
00.87   Resurfacing hip, partial, acetabulum
81.51   Total hip replacement
81.52   Partial hip replacement
81.54   Total knee replacement
81.56   Total ankle replacement

DRG 462   Bilateral or Multiple Major Joint Procedures of Lower Extremity without MCC

GMLOS 3.5   AMLOS 3.8   RW 3.5190   ☑

Select any combination of two or more procedures listed under DRG 461

DRG 463   Wound Debridement and Skin Graft Except Hand, for Musculo-Connective Tissue Disorders with MCC

GMLOS 10.4   AMLOS 14.0   RW 5.1152   Ⓣ

Operating Room Procedures

80.05   Arthrotomy for removal of prosthesis without replacement, hip
80.06   Arthrotomy for removal of prosthesis without replacement, knee
86.22   Excisional debridement of wound, infection, or burn
86.60   Free skin graft, not otherwise specified
86.63   Full-thickness skin graft to other sites
86.65   Heterograft to skin
86.66   Homograft to skin
86.67   Dermal regenerative graft
86.69   Other skin graft to other sites
86.70   Pedicle or flap graft, not otherwise specified
86.71   Cutting and preparation of pedicle grafts or flaps
86.72   Advancement of pedicle graft
86.74   Attachment of pedicle or flap graft to other sites
86.75   Revision of pedicle or flap graft
86.93   Insertion of tissue expander

DRG 464   Wound Debridement and Skin Graft Except Hand, for Musculo-Connective Tissue Disorders with CC

GMLOS 6.2   AMLOS 8.0   RW 3.0243   ☑Ⓣ

Select operating room procedures listed under DRG 463

DRG 465   Wound Debridement and Skin Graft Except Hand, for Musculo-Connective Tissue Disorders without CC/MCC

GMLOS 3.8   AMLOS 4.8   RW 1.9199   ☑Ⓣ

Select operating room procedures listed under DRG 463

DRG 466   Revision of Hip or Knee Replacement with MCC

GMLOS 7.0   AMLOS 8.6   RW 5.2748   Ⓣ

Operating Room Procedures

00.70   Revision of hip replacement, both acetabular and femoral components
00.71   Revision of hip replacement, acetabular component
00.72   Revision of hip replacement, femoral component
00.73   Revision of hip replacement, acetabular liner and/or femoral head only
00.80   Revision of knee replacement, total (all components)
00.81   Revision of knee replacement, tibial component
00.82   Revision of knee replacement, femoral component
81.53   Revision of hip replacement, not otherwise specified
81.55   Revision of knee replacement, not otherwise specified

DRG 467   Revision of Hip or Knee Replacement with CC

GMLOS 3.9   AMLOS 4.5   RW 3.4140   ☑Ⓣ

Select operating room procedures listed under DRG 466

DRG 468   Revision of Hip or Knee Replacement without CC/MCC

GMLOS 3.0   AMLOS 3.2   RW 2.7624   ☑Ⓣ

Select operating room procedures listed under DRG 466

DRG 469   Major Joint Replacement or Reattachment of Lower Extremity with MCC

GMLOS 6.2   AMLOS 7.4   RW 3.4377   ☑Ⓣ

Operating Room Procedures

00.85   Resurfacing hip, total, acetabulum and femoral head
00.86   Resurfacing hip, partial, femoral head
00.87   Resurfacing hip, partial, acetabulum

Ⓣ *Transfer DRG*   Ⓢᴾ *Special Payment*   ☑ *Optimization Potential*   ᵛ *Targeted Potential*   * *Code Range*   ● *New DRG*   ▲ *Revised DRG Title*

81.51   Total hip replacement
81.52   Partial hip replacement
81.54   Total knee replacement
81.56   Total ankle replacement
84.26   Foot reattachment
84.27   Lower leg or ankle reattachment
84.28   Thigh reattachment

DRG 470 Major Joint Replacement or Reattachment of Lower Extremity without MCC

GMLOS 3.1   AMLOS 3.4   RW 2.1463 ☑ T

Select operating room procedures listed under DRG 469

DRG 471 Cervical Spinal Fusion with MCC

GMLOS 6.4   AMLOS 8.9   RW 4.9444 ☑

Operating Room Procedures
81.01   Atlas-axis spinal fusion
81.02   Other cervical fusion of the anterior column, anterior technique
81.03   Other cervical fusion of the posterior column, posterior technique
81.31   Refusion of Atlas-axis spine
81.32   Refusion of other cervical spine, anterior column, anterior technique
81.33   Refusion of other cervical spine, posterior column, posterior technique

DRG 472 Cervical Spinal Fusion with CC

GMLOS 2.5   AMLOS 3.5   RW 2.9288 ☑

Select operating room procedures listed under DRG 471

DRG 473 Cervical Spinal Fusion without CC/MCC

GMLOS 1.5   AMLOS 1.8   RW 2.2458 ☑

Select operating room procedures listed under DRG 471

DRG 474 Amputation for Musculoskeletal System and Connective Tissue Disorders with MCC

GMLOS 8.8   AMLOS 11.2   RW 3.6884 ☑ T

Operating Room Procedures
84.00   Upper limb amputation, not otherwise specified
84.03   Amputation through hand
84.04   Disarticulation of wrist
84.05   Amputation through forearm
84.06   Disarticulation of elbow
84.07   Amputation through humerus
84.08   Disarticulation of shoulder
84.09   Interthoracoscapular amputation
84.10   Lower limb amputation, not otherwise specified
84.12   Amputation through foot
84.13   Disarticulation of ankle
84.14   Amputation of ankle through malleoli of tibia and fibula
84.15   Other amputation below knee
84.16   Disarticulation of knee
84.17   Amputation above knee
84.18   Disarticulation of hip
84.19   Abdominopelvic amputation
84.3   Revision of amputation stump
84.91   Amputation, not otherwise specified

DRG 475 Amputation for Musculoskeletal System and Connective Tissue Disorders with CC

GMLOS 5.7   AMLOS 7.1   RW 2.0488 ☑ T

Select operating room procedures listed under DRG 474

DRG 476 Amputation for Musculoskeletal System and Connective Tissue Disorders without CC/MCC

GMLOS 3.1   AMLOS 3.9   RW 1.0717 ☑ T

Select operating room procedures listed under DRG 474

DRG 477 Biopsies of Musculoskeletal System and Connective Tissue with MCC

GMLOS 8.6   AMLOS 10.8   RW 3.2827 SP

Operating Room Procedures
01.15   Biopsy of skull
01.19   Other diagnostic procedures on skull
76.1*   Diagnostic procedures on facial bones and joints
77.40   Biopsy of bone, unspecified site
77.41   Biopsy of scapula, clavicle, and thorax (ribs and sternum)
77.42   Biopsy of humerus
77.43   Biopsy of radius and ulna
77.45   Biopsy of femur
77.46   Biopsy of patella
77.47   Biopsy of tibia and fibula
77.48   Biopsy of tarsals and metatarsals
77.49   Biopsy of other bone, except facial bones
78.80   Diagnostic procedures on bone, not elsewhere classified, unspecified site
78.81   Diagnostic procedures on scapula, clavicle, and thorax (ribs and sternum) not elsewhere classified
78.82   Diagnostic procedures on humerus, not elsewhere classified
78.83   Diagnostic procedures on radius and ulna, not elsewhere classified
78.85   Diagnostic procedures on femur, not elsewhere classified
78.86   Diagnostic procedures on patella, not elsewhere classified
78.87   Diagnostic procedures on tibia and fibula, not elsewhere classified
78.89   Diagnostic procedures on other bone, except facial bones, not elsewhere classified
81.98   Other diagnostic procedures on joint structures

DRG 478 Biopsies of Musculoskeletal System and Connective Tissue with CC

GMLOS 5.4   AMLOS 6.7   RW 2.2115 ☑ SP

Select operating room procedures listed under DRG 477

DRG 479 Biopsies of Musculoskeletal System and Connective Tissue without CC/MCC

GMLOS 3.3   AMLOS 4.2   RW 1.7340 ☑ SP

Select operating room procedures listed under DRG 477

DRG 480 Hip and Femur Procedures Except Major Joint with MCC

GMLOS 7.1   AMLOS 8.3   RW 3.0694 ☑ SP

Operating Room Procedures
77.05   Sequestrectomy of femur
77.25   Wedge osteotomy of femur
77.35   Other division of femur
77.85   Other partial ostectomy of femur
77.95   Total ostectomy of femur
78.05   Bone graft of femur
78.15   Application of external fixator device, femur
78.25   Limb shortening procedures, femur
78.35   Limb lengthening procedures, femur

MDC 8: Diseases And Disorders Of The Musculoskeletal System And Connective Tissue—SURGICAL

Surgical   Medical   CC Indicator   MCC Indicator   Procedure Proxy

MDC 8: Diseases And Disorders Of The Musculoskeletal System And Connective Tissue—SURGICAL

78.45	Other repair or plastic operations on femur
78.55	Internal fixation of femur without fracture reduction
78.75	Osteoclasis of femur
78.95	Insertion of bone growth stimulator into femur
79.15	Closed reduction of fracture of femur with internal fixation
79.25	Open reduction of fracture of femur without internal fixation
79.35	Open reduction of fracture of femur with internal fixation
79.45	Closed reduction of separated epiphysis of femur
79.55	Open reduction of separated epiphysis of femur
79.65	Debridement of open fracture of femur
79.85	Open reduction of dislocation of hip
79.95	Unspecified operation on bone injury of femur
80.15	Other arthrotomy of hip
80.45	Division of joint capsule, ligament, or cartilage of hip
80.75	Synovectomy of hip
80.95	Other excision of hip joint
81.21	Arthrodesis of hip
81.40	Repair of hip, not elsewhere classified
83.12	Adductor tenotomy of hip

DRG 481 Hip and Femur Procedures Except Major Joint with CC

GMLOS 4.8   AMLOS 5.2   RW 1.9721   ☑ SP

Select operating room procedures listed under DRG 480

DRG 482 Hip and Femur Procedures Except Major Joint without CC/MCC

GMLOS 3.9   AMLOS 4.2   RW 1.6305   ☑ SP

Select operating room procedures listed under DRG 480

DRG 483 Major Joint and Limb Reattachment Procedures of Upper Extremity with CC/MCC

GMLOS 2.8   AMLOS 3.4   RW 2.6488   ☑ T

Operating Room Procedures

81.73	Total wrist replacement
81.80	Other total shoulder replacement
81.81	Partial shoulder replacement
81.84	Total elbow replacement
81.88	Reverse total shoulder replacement
84.23	Forearm, wrist, or hand reattachment
84.24	Upper arm reattachment

DRG 484 Major Joint and Limb Reattachment Procedures of Upper Extremity without CC/MCC

GMLOS 1.8   AMLOS 2.0   RW 2.2298   ☑ T

Select operating room procedures listed under DRG 483

DRG 485 Knee Procedures with Principal Diagnosis of Infection with MCC

GMLOS 8.4   AMLOS 10.3   RW 3.2719   ☑

Principal Diagnosis

711.06	Pyogenic arthritis, lower leg
730.06	Acute osteomyelitis, lower leg
730.16	Chronic osteomyelitis, lower leg
730.26	Unspecified osteomyelitis, lower leg
996.66	Infection and inflammatory reaction due to internal joint prosthesis
996.67	Infection and inflammatory reaction due to other internal orthopedic device, implant, and graft

Operating Room Procedures

00.83	Revision of knee replacement, patellar component
00.84	Revision of total knee replacement, tibial insert (liner)
77.06	Sequestrectomy of patella
77.26	Wedge osteotomy of patella

77.36	Other division of patella
77.86	Other partial ostectomy of patella
77.96	Total ostectomy of patella
78.06	Bone graft of patella
78.16	Application of external fixator device, patella
78.46	Other repair or plastic operations on patella
78.56	Internal fixation of patella without fracture reduction
78.76	Osteoclasis of patella
78.96	Insertion of bone growth stimulator into patella
79.86	Open reduction of dislocation of knee
80.16	Other arthrotomy of knee
80.46	Division of joint capsule, ligament, or cartilage of knee
80.6	Excision of semilunar cartilage of knee
80.76	Synovectomy of knee
80.96	Other excision of knee joint
81.22	Arthrodesis of knee
81.42	Five-in-one repair of knee
81.43	Triad knee repair
81.44	Patellar stabilization
81.45	Other repair of the cruciate ligaments
81.46	Other repair of the collateral ligaments
81.47	Other repair of knee

DRG 486 Knee Procedures with Principal Diagnosis of Infection with CC

GMLOS 5.6   AMLOS 6.5   RW 2.0199   ☑

Select principal diagnosis and operating room procedures listed under DRG 485

DRG 487 Knee Procedures with Principal Diagnosis of Infection without CC/MCC

GMLOS 4.1   AMLOS 4.6   RW 1.5215   ☑

Select principal diagnosis and operating room procedures listed under DRG 485

DRG 488 Knee Procedures without Principal Diagnosis of Infection with CC/MCC

GMLOS 3.5   AMLOS 4.3   RW 1.7379   ☑ T

Select only operating room procedures listed under DRG 485

DRG 489 Knee Procedures without Principal Diagnosis of Infection without CC/MCC

GMLOS 2.5   AMLOS 2.8   RW 1.2799   ☑ T

Select only operating room procedures listed under DRG 485

DRG 490 Back and Neck Procedures Except Spinal Fusion with CC/MCC or Disc Device/Neurostimulator

GMLOS 3.4   AMLOS 4.6   RW 1.8845   ☑

Operating Room Procedures

03.02	Reopening of laminectomy site
03.09	Other exploration and decompression of spinal canal
03.1	Division of intraspinal nerve root
03.32	Biopsy of spinal cord or spinal meninges
03.39	Other diagnostic procedures on spinal cord and spinal canal structures
03.4	Excision or destruction of lesion of spinal cord or spinal meninges
03.53	Repair of vertebral fracture
03.59	Other repair and plastic operations on spinal cord structures
03.6	Lysis of adhesions of spinal cord and nerve roots
03.93	Implantation or replacement of spinal neurostimulator lead(s)
03.94	Removal of spinal neurostimulator lead(s)
03.97	Revision of spinal thecal shunt

T Transfer DRG   SP Special Payment   ☑ Optimization Potential   YES Targeted Potential   * Code Range   ● New DRG   ▲ Revised DRG Title

03.98	Removal of spinal thecal shunt
03.99	Other operations on spinal cord and spinal canal structures
80.50	Excision or destruction of intervertebral disc, unspecified
80.51	Excision of intervertebral disc
80.53	Repair of the anulus fibrosus with graft or prosthesis
80.54	Other and unspecified repair of the anulus fibrosus
80.59	Other destruction of intervertebral disc
84.59	Insertion of other spinal devices
84.6*	Replacement of spinal disc
84.80	Insertion or replacement of interspinous process device(s)
84.82	Insertion or replacement of pedicle-based dynamic stabilization device(s)
84.84	Insertion or replacement of facet replacement device(s)

OR

Any of the following procedure code combinations

03.93	Implantation or replacement of spinal neurostimulator lead(s)
	AND
86.94	Insertion or replacement of single array neurostimulator pulse generator, not specified as rechargeable

OR

03.93	Implantation or replacement of spinal neurostimulator lead(s)
	AND
86.95	Insertion or replacement of multiple array neurostimulator pulse generator, not specified as rechargeable

OR

03.93	Implantation or replacement of spinal neurostimulator lead(s)
	AND
86.97	Insertion or replacement of single array rechargeable neurostimulator pulse generator

OR

03.93	Implantation or replacement of spinal neurostimulator lead(s)
	AND
86.98	Insertion or replacement of multiple array (two or more) rechargeable neurostimulator pulse generator

DRG 491   Back and Neck Procedures Except Spinal Fusion without CC/MCC

GMLOS 1.9   AMLOS 2.3   RW 1.0893   ☑

Operating Room Procedures

03.02	Reopening of laminectomy site
03.09	Other exploration and decompression of spinal canal
03.1	Division of intraspinal nerve root
03.32	Biopsy of spinal cord or spinal meninges
03.39	Other diagnostic procedures on spinal cord and spinal canal structures
03.4	Excision or destruction of lesion of spinal cord or spinal meninges
03.53	Repair of vertebral fracture
03.59	Other repair and plastic operations on spinal cord structures
03.6	Lysis of adhesions of spinal cord and nerve roots
03.93	Implantation or replacement of spinal neurostimulator lead(s)
03.94	Removal of spinal neurostimulator lead(s)
03.97	Revision of spinal thecal shunt
03.98	Removal of spinal thecal shunt
03.99	Other operations on spinal cord and spinal canal structures
80.50	Excision or destruction of intervertebral disc, unspecified
80.51	Excision of intervertebral disc
80.53	Repair of the anulus fibrosus with graft or prosthesis
80.54	Other and unspecified repair of the anulus fibrosus
80.59	Other destruction of intervertebral disc
84.60	Insertion of spinal disc prosthesis, not otherwise specified

84.61	Insertion of partial spinal disc prosthesis, cervical
84.63	Insertion of spinal disc prosthesis, thoracic
84.64	Insertion of partial spinal disc prosthesis, lumbosacral
84.66	Revision or replacement of artificial spinal disc prosthesis, cervical
84.67	Revision or replacement of artificial spinal disc prosthesis, thoracic
84.68	Revision or replacement of artificial spinal disc prosthesis, lumbosacral
84.69	Revision or replacement of artificial spinal disc prosthesis, not otherwise specified

DRG 492   Lower Extremity and Humerus Procedures Except Hip, Foot, Femur with MCC

GMLOS 6.4   AMLOS 8.0   RW 3.1831   ☑ SP

Operating Room Procedures

77.02	Sequestrectomy of humerus
77.07	Sequestrectomy of tibia and fibula
77.22	Wedge osteotomy of humerus
77.27	Wedge osteotomy of tibia and fibula
77.32	Other division of humerus
77.37	Other division of tibia and fibula
77.82	Other partial ostectomy of humerus
77.87	Other partial ostectomy of tibia and fibula
77.92	Total ostectomy of humerus
77.97	Total ostectomy of tibia and fibula
78.02	Bone graft of humerus
78.07	Bone graft of tibia and fibula
78.12	Application of external fixator device, humerus
78.17	Application of external fixator device, tibia and fibula
78.22	Limb shortening procedures, humerus
78.27	Limb shortening procedures, tibia and fibula
78.32	Limb lengthening procedures, humerus
78.37	Limb lengthening procedures, tibia and fibula
78.42	Other repair or plastic operation on humerus
78.47	Other repair or plastic operations on tibia and fibula
78.52	Internal fixation of humerus without fracture reduction
78.57	Internal fixation of tibia and fibula without fracture reduction
78.72	Osteoclasis of humerus
78.77	Osteoclasis of tibia and fibula
78.92	Insertion of bone growth stimulator into humerus
78.97	Insertion of bone growth stimulator into tibia and fibula
79.11	Closed reduction of fracture of humerus with internal fixation
79.16	Closed reduction of fracture of tibia and fibula with internal fixation
79.21	Open reduction of fracture of humerus without internal fixation
79.26	Open reduction of fracture of tibia and fibula without internal fixation
79.31	Open reduction of fracture of humerus with internal fixation
79.36	Open reduction of fracture of tibia and fibula with internal fixation
79.41	Closed reduction of separated epiphysis of humerus
79.46	Closed reduction of separated epiphysis of tibia and fibula
79.51	Open reduction of separated epiphysis of humerus
79.56	Open reduction of separated epiphysis of tibia and fibula
79.61	Debridement of open fracture of humerus
79.66	Debridement of open fracture of tibia and fibula
79.87	Open reduction of dislocation of ankle
79.91	Unspecified operation on bone injury of humerus
79.96	Unspecified operation on bone injury of tibia and fibula
79.97	Unspecified operation on bone injury of tarsals and metatarsals
80.17	Other arthrotomy of ankle
80.47	Division of joint capsule, ligament, or cartilage of ankle
80.77	Synovectomy of ankle
80.87	Other local excision or destruction of lesion of ankle joint

Surgical   **Medical**   **CC Indicator**   **MCC Indicator**   **Procedure Proxy**

80.97	Other excision of ankle joint
80.99	Other excision of joint of other specified site
81.11	Ankle fusion
81.12	Triple arthrodesis
81.49	Other repair of ankle
84.48	Implantation of prosthetic device of leg

DRG 493 Lower Extremity and Humerus Procedures Except Hip, Foot, Femur with CC

| GMLOS 4.0 | AMLOS 4.8 | RW 1.9971 | ☑ SP |

Select operating room procedures listed under DRG 492

DRG 494 Lower Extremity and Humerus Procedures Except Hip, Foot, Femur without CC/MCC

| GMLOS 2.7 | AMLOS 3.2 | RW 1.5073 | ☑ SP |

Select operating room procedures listed under DRG 492

DRG 495 Local Excision and Removal Internal Fixation Devices Except Hip and Femur with MCC

| GMLOS 7.2 | AMLOS 9.6 | RW 2.9110 | ☑ SP |

Operating Room Procedures

01.6	Excision of lesion of skull
34.4	Excision or destruction of lesion of chest wall
76.09	Other incision of facial bone
76.2	Local excision or destruction of lesion of facial bone
76.97	Removal of internal fixation device from facial bone
77.10	Other incision of bone without division, unspecified site
77.11	Other incision of scapula, clavicle, and thorax (ribs and sternum) without division
77.12	Other incision of humerus without division
77.13	Other incision of radius and ulna without division
77.16	Other incision of patella without division
77.17	Other incision of tibia and fibula without division
77.19	Other incision of other bone, except facial bones, without division
77.60	Local excision of lesion or tissue of bone, unspecified site
77.61	Local excision of lesion or tissue of scapula, clavicle, and thorax (ribs and sternum)
77.62	Local excision of lesion or tissue of humerus
77.63	Local excision of lesion or tissue of radius and ulna
77.66	Local excision of lesion or tissue of patella
77.67	Local excision of lesion or tissue of tibia and fibula
77.69	Local excision of lesion or tissue of other bone, except facial bones
77.70	Excision of bone for graft, unspecified site
77.71	Excision of scapula, clavicle, and thorax (ribs and sternum) for graft
77.72	Excision of humerus for graft
77.73	Excision of radius and ulna for graft
77.76	Excision of patella for graft
77.77	Excision of tibia and fibula for graft
77.79	Excision of other bone for graft, except facial bones
78.60	Removal of implanted device, unspecified site
78.61	Removal of implanted device from scapula, clavicle, and thorax (ribs and sternum)
78.62	Removal of implanted device from humerus
78.63	Removal of implanted device from radius and ulna
78.64	Removal of implanted device from carpals and metacarpals
78.66	Removal of implanted device from patella
78.67	Removal of implanted device from tibia and fibula
78.68	Removal of implanted device from tarsal and metatarsals
78.69	Removal of implanted device from other bone
80.00	Arthrotomy for removal of prosthesis without replacement, unspecified site
80.01	Arthrotomy for removal of prosthesis without replacement, shoulder

80.02	Arthrotomy for removal of prosthesis without replacement, elbow
80.03	Arthrotomy for removal of prosthesis without replacement, wrist
80.04	Arthrotomy for removal of prosthesis without replacement, hand and finger
80.07	Arthrotomy for removal of prosthesis without replacement, ankle
80.08	Arthrotomy for removal of prosthesis without replacement, foot and toe
80.09	Arthrotomy for removal of prosthesis without replacement, other specified site
80.80	Other local excision or destruction of lesion of joint, unspecified site
80.81	Other local excision or destruction of lesion of shoulder joint
80.82	Other local excision or destruction of lesion of elbow joint
80.86	Other local excision or destruction of lesion of knee joint
80.89	Other local excision or destruction of lesion of joint of other specified site

DRG 496 Local Excision and Removal Internal Fixation Devices Except Hip and Femur with CC

| GMLOS 4.0 | AMLOS 5.2 | RW 1.7290 | ☑ SP |

Select operating room procedures listed under DRG 495

DRG 497 Local Excision and Removal Internal Fixation Devices Except Hip and Femur without CC/MCC

| GMLOS 2.1 | AMLOS 2.6 | RW 1.1731 | ☑ SP |

Select operating room procedures listed under DRG 495

DRG 498 Local Excision and Removal Internal Fixation Devices of Hip and Femur with CC/MCC

| GMLOS 5.3 | AMLOS 7.2 | RW 2.1924 | ☑ |

Operating Room Procedures

77.15	Other incision of femur without division
77.65	Local excision of lesion or tissue of femur
77.75	Excision of femur for graft
78.65	Removal of implanted device from femur
80.85	Other local excision or destruction of lesion of hip joint

DRG 499 Local Excision and Removal Internal Fixation Devices of Hip and Femur without CC/MCC

| GMLOS 2.1 | AMLOS 2.6 | RW 0.9577 | ☑ |

Select operating room procedures listed under DRG 498

DRG 500 Soft Tissue Procedures with MCC

| GMLOS 7.3 | AMLOS 9.8 | RW 3.0116 | ☑ SP |

Operating Room Procedures

54.3	Excision or destruction of lesion or tissue of abdominal wall or umbilicus
80.70	Synovectomy, unspecified site
80.79	Synovectomy of other specified site
81.95	Suture of capsule or ligament of other lower extremity
83.0*	Incision of muscle, tendon, fascia, and bursa
83.13	Other tenotomy
83.14	Fasciotomy
83.19	Other division of soft tissue
83.2*	Diagnostic procedures on muscle, tendon, fascia, and bursa, including that of hand
83.3*	Excision of lesion of muscle, tendon, fascia, and bursa
83.4*	Other excision of muscle, tendon, and fascia
83.5	Bursectomy
83.61	Suture of tendon sheath
83.62	Delayed suture of tendon

Ⓣ *Transfer DRG*   Ⓢᴾ *Special Payment*   ☑ *Optimization Potential*   ⱽᴱᵍ *Targeted Potential*   * *Code Range*   ● *New DRG*   ▲ *Revised DRG Title*

92   Valid 10/01/2013-09/30/2014   © 2013 OptumInsight, Inc.

MDC 8: Diseases And Disorders Of The Musculoskeletal System And Connective Tissue—SURGICAL

83.64	Other suture of tendon
83.65	Other suture of muscle or fascia
83.7*	Reconstruction of muscle and tendon
83.81	Tendon graft
83.82	Graft of muscle or fascia
83.83	Tendon pulley reconstruction on muscle, tendon, and fascia
83.85	Other change in muscle or tendon length
83.86	Quadricepsplasty
83.87	Other plastic operations on muscle
83.88	Other plastic operations on tendon
83.89	Other plastic operations on fascia
83.91	Lysis of adhesions of muscle, tendon, fascia, and bursa
83.92	Insertion or replacement of skeletal muscle stimulator
83.93	Removal of skeletal muscle stimulator
83.99	Other operations on muscle, tendon, fascia, and bursa
86.4	Radical excision of skin lesion
86.81	Repair for facial weakness

DRG 501   Soft Tissue Procedures with CC
GMLOS 4.4   AMLOS 5.5   RW 1.5804   ☑ SP

Select operating room procedures listed under DRG 500

DRG 502   Soft Tissue Procedures without CC/MCC
GMLOS 2.4   AMLOS 2.9   RW 1.1277   ☑ SP

Select operating room procedures listed under DRG 500

DRG 503   Foot Procedures with MCC
GMLOS 6.3   AMLOS 7.8   RW 2.2584   ☑

Operating Room Procedures

04.44	Release of tarsal tunnel
77.08	Sequestrectomy of tarsals and metatarsals
77.18	Other incision of tarsals and metatarsals without division
77.28	Wedge osteotomy of tarsals and metatarsals
77.38	Other division of tarsals and metatarsals
77.5*	Excision and repair of bunion and other toe deformities
77.68	Local excision of lesion or tissue of tarsals and metatarsals
77.78	Excision of tarsals and metatarsals for graft
77.88	Other partial ostectomy of tarsals and metatarsals
77.98	Total ostectomy of tarsals and metatarsals
78.08	Bone graft of tarsals and metatarsals
78.18	Application of external fixator device, tarsals and metatarsals
78.28	Limb shortening procedures, tarsals and metatarsals
78.38	Limb lengthening procedures, tarsals and metatarsals
78.48	Other repair or plastic operations on tarsals and metatarsals
78.58	Internal fixation of tarsals and metatarsals without fracture reduction
78.78	Osteoclasis of tarsals and metatarsals
78.88	Diagnostic procedures on tarsals and metatarsals, not elsewhere classified
78.98	Insertion of bone growth stimulator into tarsals and metatarsals
79.17	Closed reduction of fracture of tarsals and metatarsals with internal fixation
79.18	Closed reduction of fracture of phalanges of foot with internal fixation
79.27	Open reduction of fracture of tarsals and metatarsals without internal fixation
79.28	Open reduction of fracture of phalanges of foot without internal fixation
79.37	Open reduction of fracture of tarsals and metatarsals with internal fixation
79.38	Open reduction of fracture of phalanges of foot with internal fixation
79.67	Debridement of open fracture of tarsals and metatarsals
79.68	Debridement of open fracture of phalanges of foot
79.88	Open reduction of dislocation of foot and toe

79.98	Unspecified operation on bone injury of phalanges of foot
80.18	Other arthrotomy of foot and toe
80.48	Division of joint capsule, ligament, or cartilage of foot and toe
80.78	Synovectomy of foot and toe
80.88	Other local excision or destruction of lesion of joint of foot and toe
80.98	Other excision of joint of foot and toe
81.13	Subtalar fusion
81.14	Midtarsal fusion
81.15	Tarsometatarsal fusion
81.16	Metatarsophalangeal fusion
81.17	Other fusion of foot
81.57	Replacement of joint of foot and toe
81.94	Suture of capsule or ligament of ankle and foot
83.11	Achillotenotomy
83.84	Release of clubfoot, not elsewhere classified
84.11	Amputation of toe
84.25	Toe reattachment

DRG 504   Foot Procedures with CC
GMLOS 4.9   AMLOS 5.9   RW 1.6133   ☑

Select operating room procedures listed under DRG 503

DRG 505   Foot Procedures without CC/MCC
GMLOS 2.7   AMLOS 3.3   RW 1.2072   ☑

Select operating room procedures listed under DRG 503

DRG 506   Major Thumb or Joint Procedures
GMLOS 2.9   AMLOS 3.8   RW 1.2041   ☑

Operating Room Procedures

80.13	Other arthrotomy of wrist
80.14	Other arthrotomy of hand and finger
81.71	Arthroplasty of metacarpophalangeal and interphalangeal joint with implant
81.72	Arthroplasty of metacarpophalangeal and interphalangeal joint without implant
81.74	Arthroplasty of carpocarpal or carpometacarpal joint with implant
81.75	Arthroplasty of carpocarpal or carpometacarpal joint without implant
81.79	Other repair of hand, fingers, and wrist
82.6*	Reconstruction of thumb

DRG 507   Major Shoulder or Elbow Joint Procedures with CC/MCC
GMLOS 4.1   AMLOS 5.6   RW 1.9667   ☑

Operating Room Procedures

80.11	Other arthrotomy of shoulder
80.12	Other arthrotomy of elbow
81.23	Arthrodesis of shoulder
81.24	Arthrodesis of elbow
81.83	Other repair of shoulder
81.85	Other repair of elbow

DRG 508   Major Shoulder or Elbow Joint Procedures without CC/MCC
GMLOS 2.0   AMLOS 2.4   RW 1.3190   ☑

Select operating room procedures listed under DRG 507

DRG 509   Arthroscopy
GMLOS 2.7   AMLOS 3.5   RW 1.3245   ☑

Operating Room Procedures

80.2*	Arthroscopy

DRG 510 Shoulder, Elbow or Forearm Procedure, Except Major Joint Procedure with MCC

GMLOS 4.8   AMLOS 6.0   RW 2.2717   ☑ⓣ

Operating room procedures

77.03	Sequestrectomy of radius and ulna
77.23	Wedge osteotomy of radius and ulna
77.33	Other division of radius and ulna
77.83	Other partial ostectomy of radius and ulna
77.93	Total ostectomy of radius and ulna
78.03	Bone graft of radius and ulna
78.13	Application of external fixator device, radius and ulna
78.23	Limb shortening procedures, radius and ulna
78.33	Limb lengthening procedures, radius and ulna
78.43	Other repair or plastic operations on radius and ulna
78.53	Internal fixation of radius and ulna without fracture reduction
78.73	Osteoclasis of radius and ulna
78.93	Insertion of bone growth stimulator into radius and ulna
79.12	Closed reduction of fracture of radius and ulna with internal fixation
79.22	Open reduction of fracture of radius and ulna without internal fixation
79.32	Open reduction of fracture of radius and ulna with internal fixation
79.42	Closed reduction of separated epiphysis of radius and ulna
79.52	Open reduction of separated epiphysis of radius and ulna
79.62	Debridement of open fracture of radius and ulna
79.81	Open reduction of dislocation of shoulder
79.82	Open reduction of dislocation of elbow
79.92	Unspecified operation on bone injury of radius and ulna
80.41	Division of joint capsule, ligament, or cartilage of shoulder
80.42	Division of joint capsule, ligament, or cartilage of elbow
80.71	Synovectomy of shoulder
80.72	Synovectomy of elbow
80.91	Other excision of shoulder joint
80.92	Other excision of elbow joint
81.82	Repair of recurrent dislocation of shoulder
81.93	Suture of capsule or ligament of upper extremity
83.63	Rotator cuff repair
84.44	Implantation of prosthetic device of arm

DRG 511 Shoulder, Elbow or Forearm Procedure, Except Major Joint Procedure with CC

GMLOS 3.2   AMLOS 3.8   RW 1.5894   ☑ⓣ

Select operating room procedures listed under DRG 510

DRG 512 Shoulder, Elbow or Forearm Procedure, Except Major Joint Procedure without CC/MCC

GMLOS 2.0   AMLOS 2.3   RW 1.2266   ☑ⓣ

Select operating room procedures listed under DRG 510

DRG 513 Hand or Wrist Procedures, Except Major Thumb or Joint Procedures with CC/MCC

GMLOS 3.7   AMLOS 4.9   RW 1.4122   ☑

Operating Room Procedures

04.43	Release of carpal tunnel
77.04	Sequestrectomy of carpals and metacarpals
77.14	Other incision of carpals and metacarpals without division
77.24	Wedge osteotomy of carpals and metacarpals
77.34	Other division of carpals and metacarpals
77.44	Biopsy of carpals and metacarpals
77.64	Local excision of lesion or tissue of carpals and metacarpals
77.74	Excision of carpals and metacarpals for graft
77.84	Other partial ostectomy of carpals and metacarpals
77.94	Total ostectomy of carpals and metacarpals
78.04	Bone graft of carpals and metacarpals
78.14	Application of external fixator device, carpals and metacarpals
78.24	Limb shortening procedures, carpals and metacarpals
78.34	Limb lengthening procedures, carpals and metacarpals
78.44	Other repair or plastic operations on carpals and metacarpals
78.54	Internal fixation of carpals and metacarpals without fracture reduction
78.74	Osteoclasis of carpals and metacarpals
78.84	Diagnostic procedures on carpals and metacarpals, not elsewhere classified
78.94	Insertion of bone growth stimulator into carpals and metacarpals
79.13	Closed reduction of fracture of carpals and metacarpals with internal fixation
79.14	Closed reduction of fracture of phalanges of hand with internal fixation
79.23	Open reduction of fracture of carpals and metacarpals without internal fixation
79.24	Open reduction of fracture of phalanges of hand without internal fixation
79.33	Open reduction of fracture of carpals and metacarpals with internal fixation
79.34	Open reduction of fracture of phalanges of hand with internal fixation
79.63	Debridement of open fracture of carpals and metacarpals
79.64	Debridement of open fracture of phalanges of hand
79.83	Open reduction of dislocation of wrist
79.84	Open reduction of dislocation of hand and finger
79.93	Unspecified operation on bone injury of carpals and metacarpals
79.94	Unspecified operation on bone injury of phalanges of hand
80.43	Division of joint capsule, ligament, or cartilage of wrist
80.44	Division of joint capsule, ligament, or cartilage of hand and finger
80.73	Synovectomy of wrist
80.74	Synovectomy of hand and finger
80.83	Other local excision or destruction of lesion of wrist joint
80.84	Other local excision or destruction of lesion of joint of hand and finger
80.93	Other excision of wrist joint
80.94	Other excision of joint of hand and finger
81.25	Carporadial fusion
81.26	Metacarpocarpal fusion
81.27	Metacarpophalangeal fusion
81.28	Interphalangeal fusion
82.01	Exploration of tendon sheath of hand
82.02	Myotomy of hand
82.03	Bursotomy of hand
82.09	Other incision of soft tissue of hand
82.1*	Division of muscle, tendon, and fascia of hand
82.2*	Excision of lesion of muscle, tendon, and fascia of hand
82.3*	Other excision of soft tissue of hand
82.4*	Suture of muscle, tendon, and fascia of hand
82.5*	Transplantation of muscle and tendon of hand
82.7*	Plastic operation on hand with graft or implant
82.8*	Other plastic operations on hand
82.91	Lysis of adhesions of hand
82.99	Other operations on muscle, tendon, and fascia of hand
84.01	Amputation and disarticulation of finger
84.02	Amputation and disarticulation of thumb
84.21	Thumb reattachment
84.22	Finger reattachment
86.61	Full-thickness skin graft to hand
86.62	Other skin graft to hand
86.73	Attachment of pedicle or flap graft to hand
86.85	Correction of syndactyly

ⓣ Transfer DRG   ⓢ Special Payment   ☑ Optimization Potential   ⱱ Targeted Potential   * Code Range   ● New DRG   ▲ Revised DRG Title

Valid 10/01/2013–09/30/2014   © 2013 OptumInsight, Inc.

DRG 514   **Hand or Wrist Procedures, Except Major Thumb or Joint Procedures without CC/MCC**
          GMLOS 2.2   AMLOS 2.7   RW 0.8781   ☑

Select operating room procedures listed under DRG 513

DRG 515   **Other Musculoskeletal System and Connective Tissue O.R. Procedure with MCC**
          GMLOS 7.5   AMLOS 9.6   RW 3.3340   SP

Operating Room Procedures

01.25	Other craniectomy
02.0*	Cranioplasty
02.94	Insertion or replacement of skull tongs or halo traction device
02.99	Other operations on skull, brain, and cerebral meninges
04.03	Division or crushing of other cranial and peripheral nerves
04.04	Other incision of cranial and peripheral nerves
04.06	Other cranial or peripheral ganglionectomy
04.07	Other excision or avulsion of cranial and peripheral nerves
04.12	Open biopsy of cranial or peripheral nerve or ganglion
04.19	Other diagnostic procedures on cranial and peripheral nerves and ganglia
04.49	Other peripheral nerve or ganglion decompression or lysis of adhesions
04.92	Implantation or replacement of peripheral neurostimulator lead(s)
04.93	Removal of peripheral neurostimulator lead(s)
04.99	Other operations on cranial and peripheral nerves
06.13	Biopsy of parathyroid gland
06.19	Other diagnostic procedures on thyroid and parathyroid glands
16.51	Exenteration of orbit with removal of adjacent structures
16.59	Other exenteration of orbit
17.56	Atherectomy of other non-coronary vessel(s)
21.72	Open reduction of nasal fracture
21.83	Total nasal reconstruction
21.84	Revision rhinoplasty
21.85	Augmentation rhinoplasty
21.86	Limited rhinoplasty
21.87	Other rhinoplasty
21.88	Other septoplasty
21.89	Other repair and plastic operations on nose
22.62	Excision of lesion of maxillary sinus with other approach
33.20	Thoracoscopic lung biopsy
33.28	Open biopsy of lung
34.74	Repair of pectus deformity
34.79	Other repair of chest wall
34.81	Excision of lesion or tissue of diaphragm
38.21	Biopsy of blood vessel
38.7	Interruption of the vena cava
39.50	Angioplasty of other non-coronary vessel(s)
39.98	Control of hemorrhage, not otherwise specified
40.1*	Diagnostic procedures on lymphatic structures
40.21	Excision of deep cervical lymph node
40.23	Excision of axillary lymph node
40.24	Excision of inguinal lymph node
40.29	Simple excision of other lymphatic structure
40.3	Regional lymph node excision
40.51	Radical excision of axillary lymph nodes
40.52	Radical excision of periaortic lymph nodes
40.53	Radical excision of iliac lymph nodes
40.54	Radical groin dissection
40.59	Radical excision of other lymph nodes
41.43	Partial splenectomy
41.5	Total splenectomy
50.12	Open biopsy of liver
55.24	Open biopsy of kidney
59.00	Retroperitoneal dissection, not otherwise specified
62.41	Removal of both testes at same operative episode

76.01	Sequestrectomy of facial bone
76.31	Partial mandibulectomy
76.39	Partial ostectomy of other facial bone
76.4*	Excision and reconstruction of facial bones
76.5	Temporomandibular arthroplasty
76.6*	Other facial bone repair and orthognathic surgery
76.70	Reduction of facial fracture, not otherwise specified
76.72	Open reduction of malar and zygomatic fracture
76.74	Open reduction of maxillary fracture
76.76	Open reduction of mandibular fracture
76.77	Open reduction of alveolar fracture
76.79	Other open reduction of facial fracture
76.91	Bone graft to facial bone
76.92	Insertion of synthetic implant in facial bone
76.94	Open reduction of temporomandibular dislocation
76.99	Other operations on facial bones and joints
77.00	Sequestrectomy, unspecified site
77.01	Sequestrectomy of scapula, clavicle, and thorax (ribs and sternum)
77.09	Sequestrectomy of other bone, except facial bones
77.20	Wedge osteotomy, unspecified site
77.21	Wedge osteotomy of scapula, clavicle, and thorax (ribs and sternum)
77.29	Wedge osteotomy of other bone, except facial bones
77.30	Other division of bone, unspecified site
77.31	Other division of scapula, clavicle, and thorax (ribs and sternum)
77.39	Other division of other bone, except facial bones
77.80	Other partial ostectomy, unspecified site
77.81	Other partial ostectomy of scapula, clavicle, and thorax (ribs and sternum)
77.89	Other partial ostectomy of other bone, except facial bones
77.90	Total ostectomy, unspecified site
77.91	Total ostectomy of scapula, clavicle, and thorax (ribs and sternum)
77.99	Total ostectomy of other bone, except facial bones
78.00	Bone graft, unspecified site
78.01	Bone graft of scapula, clavicle, and thorax (ribs and sternum)
78.09	Bone graft of other bone, except facial bones
78.10	Application of external fixator device, unspecified site
78.11	Application of external fixator device, scapula, clavicle, and thorax [ribs and sternum]
78.19	Application of external fixator device, other
78.20	Limb shortening procedures, unspecified site
78.29	Limb shortening procedures, other
78.30	Limb lengthening procedures, unspecified site
78.39	Other limb lengthening procedures
78.40	Other repair or plastic operations on bone, unspecified site
78.41	Other repair or plastic operations on scapula, clavicle, and thorax (ribs and sternum)
78.49	Other repair or plastic operations on other bone, except facial bones
78.50	Internal fixation of bone without fracture reduction, unspecified site
78.51	Internal fixation of scapula, clavicle, and thorax (ribs and sternum) without fracture reduction
78.59	Internal fixation of other bone, except facial bones, without fracture reduction
78.70	Osteoclasis, unspecified site
78.71	Osteoclasis of scapula, clavicle, and thorax (ribs and sternum)
78.79	Osteoclasis of other bone, except facial bones
78.90	Insertion of bone growth stimulator, unspecified site
78.91	Insertion of bone growth stimulator into scapula, clavicle and thorax (ribs and sternum)
78.99	Insertion of bone growth stimulator into other bone
79.10	Closed reduction of fracture with internal fixation, unspecified site
79.19	Closed reduction of fracture of other specified bone, except facial bones, with internal fixation

---

Surgical	Medical	CC Indicator	MCC Indicator	Procedure Proxy

MDC 8: Diseases And Disorders Of The Musculoskeletal System And Connective Tissue—MEDICAL

79.20	Open reduction of fracture without internal fixation, unspecified site
79.29	Open reduction of fracture of other specified bone, except facial bones, without internal fixation
79.30	Open reduction of fracture with internal fixation, unspecified site
79.39	Open reduction of fracture of other specified bone, except facial bones, with internal fixation
79.40	Closed reduction of separated epiphysis, unspecified site
79.49	Closed reduction of separated epiphysis of other specified bone
79.50	Open reduction of separated epiphysis, unspecified site
79.59	Open reduction of separated epiphysis of other specified bone
79.60	Debridement of open fracture, unspecified site
79.69	Debridement of open fracture of other specified bone, except facial bones
79.80	Open reduction of dislocation of unspecified site
79.89	Open reduction of dislocation of other specified site, except temporomandibular
79.90	Unspecified operation on bone injury, unspecified site
79.99	Unspecified operation on bone injury of other specified bone
80.10	Other arthrotomy, unspecified site
80.19	Other arthrotomy of other specified site
80.40	Division of joint capsule, ligament, or cartilage, unspecified site
80.49	Division of joint capsule, ligament, or cartilage of other specified site
80.90	Other excision of joint, unspecified site
81.18	Subtalar joint arthroereisis
81.20	Arthrodesis of unspecified joint
81.29	Arthrodesis of other specified joint
81.59	Revision of joint replacement of lower extremity, not elsewhere classified
81.65	Percutaneous vertebroplasty
81.66	Percutaneous vertebral augmentation
81.96	Other repair of joint
81.97	Revision of joint replacement of upper extremity
81.99	Other operations on joint structures
84.29	Other reattachment of extremity
84.40	Implantation or fitting of prosthetic limb device, not otherwise specified
84.81	Revision of interspinous process device(s)
84.83	Revision of pedicle-based dynamic stabilization device(s)
84.85	Revision of facet replacement device(s)
84.92	Separation of equal conjoined twins
84.93	Separation of unequal conjoined twins
84.94	Insertion of sternal fixation device with rigid plates
84.99	Other operations on musculoskeletal system
86.06	Insertion of totally implantable infusion pump

DRG 516   Other Musculoskeletal System and Connective Tissue O.R. Procedure with CC
GMLOS 4.5   AMLOS 5.5   RW 2.0160   ☑ 𝔰ℙ

Select operating room procedures listed under DRG 515

DRG 517   Other Musculoskeletal System and Connective Tissue O.R. Procedure without CC/MCC
GMLOS 2.8   AMLOS 3.4   RW 1.6777   ☑ 𝔰ℙ

Select operating room procedures listed under DRG 515

MEDICAL

DRG 533   Fractures of Femur with MCC
GMLOS 4.3   AMLOS 5.6   RW 1.3759   ☑ 𝚃

Principal Diagnosis
821*   Fracture of other and unspecified parts of femur

DRG 534   Fractures of Femur without MCC
GMLOS 2.9   AMLOS 3.6   RW 0.7364   ☑ 𝚃

Select principal diagnosis listed under DRG 533

DRG 535   Fractures of Hip and Pelvis with MCC
GMLOS 4.2   AMLOS 5.4   RW 1.3085   ☑ 𝚃

Principal Diagnosis
808*   Fracture of pelvis
820*   Fracture of neck of femur

DRG 536   Fractures of Hip and Pelvis without MCC
GMLOS 3.0   AMLOS 3.5   RW 0.7091   ☑ 𝚃

Select principal diagnosis listed under DRG 535

DRG 537   Sprains, Strains, and Dislocations of Hip, Pelvis and Thigh with CC/MCC
GMLOS 3.4   AMLOS 4.0   RW 0.8604   ☑

Principal Diagnosis
835*   Dislocation of hip
843*   Sprains and strains of hip and thigh
848.5   Pelvic sprain and strains

DRG 538   Sprains, Strains, and Dislocations of Hip, Pelvis and Thigh without CC/MCC
GMLOS 2.4   AMLOS 2.8   RW 0.6870   ☑

Select principal diagnosis listed under DRG 537

DRG 539   Osteomyelitis with MCC
GMLOS 6.2   AMLOS 8.1   RW 1.8631   ☑ 𝚃

Principal Diagnosis
003.24   Salmonella osteomyelitis
015.0*   Tuberculosis of vertebral column
015.5*   Tuberculosis of limb bones
015.7*   Tuberculosis of other specified bone
091.61   Early syphilis, secondary syphilitic periostitis
095.5   Syphilis of bone
098.53   Gonococcal spondylitis
730.0*   Acute osteomyelitis
730.1*   Chronic osteomyelitis
730.2*   Unspecified osteomyelitis
730.8*   Other infections involving bone in diseases classified elsewhere
730.9*   Unspecified infection of bone

DRG 540   Osteomyelitis with CC
GMLOS 4.9   AMLOS 6.1   RW 1.3063   ☑ 𝚃

Select principal diagnosis listed under DRG 539

DRG 541   Osteomyelitis without CC/MCC
GMLOS 3.6   AMLOS 4.7   RW 0.9743   ☑ 𝚃

Select principal diagnosis listed under DRG 539

𝚃 *Transfer DRG*   𝔰ℙ *Special Payment*   ☑ *Optimization Potential*   ᵀᴳ *Targeted Potential*   * *Code Range*   ● *New DRG*   ▲ *Revised DRG Title*

DRG 542 Pathological Fractures and Musculoskeletal and Connective Tissue Malignancy with MCC

GMLOS 6.0   AMLOS 7.9   RW 1.9451   ☑ ▽ T

Principal Diagnosis

170*	Malignant neoplasm of bone and articular cartilage
171*	Malignant neoplasm of connective and other soft tissue
198.5	Secondary malignant neoplasm of bone and bone marrow
209.73	Secondary neuroendocrine tumor of bone
238.0	Neoplasm of uncertain behavior of bone and articular cartilage
446.3	Lethal midline granuloma
446.4	Wegener's granulomatosis
733.1*	Pathologic fracture
733.93	Stress fracture of tibia or fibula
733.94	Stress fracture of the metatarsals
733.95	Stress fracture of other bone
733.96	Stress fracture of femoral neck
733.97	Stress fracture of shaft of femur
733.98	Stress fracture of pelvis

DRG 543 Pathological Fractures and Musculoskeletal and Connective Tissue Malignancy with CC

GMLOS 4.2   AMLOS 5.2   RW 1.1267   ☑ ▽ T

Select principal diagnosis listed under DRG 542

DRG 544 Pathological Fractures and Musculoskeletal and Connective Tissue Malignancy without CC/MCC

GMLOS 3.2   AMLOS 3.7   RW 0.7736   ☑ ▽ T

Select principal diagnosis listed under DRG 542

DRG 545 Connective Tissue Disorders with MCC

GMLOS 6.0   AMLOS 8.5   RW 2.4445   T

Principal Diagnosis

099.3	Reiter's disease
136.1	Behcet's syndrome
277.3*	Amyloidosis
279.4*	Autoimmune disease, not elsewhere classified
359.7*	Inflammatory and immune myopathies, NEC
390	Rheumatic fever without mention of heart involvement
443.0	Raynaud's syndrome
446.0	Polyarteritis nodosa
446.1	Acute febrile mucocutaneous lymph node syndrome (MCLS)
446.2*	Hypersensitivity angiitis
446.5	Giant cell arteritis
446.6	Thrombotic microangiopathy
446.7	Takayasu's disease
447.6	Unspecified arteritis
696.0	Psoriatic arthropathy
710*	Diffuse diseases of connective tissue
711.1*	Arthropathy associated with Reiter's disease and nonspecific urethritis
711.2*	Arthropathy in Behcet's syndrome
714.0	Rheumatoid arthritis
714.1	Felty's syndrome
714.2	Other rheumatoid arthritis with visceral or systemic involvement
714.3*	Juvenile chronic polyarthritis
714.89	Other specified inflammatory polyarthropathies
720.0	Ankylosing spondylitis
725	Polymyalgia rheumatica
795.6	False positive serological test for syphilis

DRG 546 Connective Tissue Disorders with CC

GMLOS 4.0   AMLOS 5.0   RW 1.1711   ☑ T

Select principal diagnosis listed under DRG 545

DRG 547 Connective Tissue Disorders without CC/MCC

GMLOS 2.9   AMLOS 3.6   RW 0.8061   ☑ T

Select principal diagnosis listed under DRG 545

DRG 548 Septic Arthritis with MCC

GMLOS 5.9   AMLOS 7.6   RW 1.7811   ☑

Principal Diagnosis

003.23	Salmonella arthritis
015.1*	Tuberculosis of hip
015.2*	Tuberculosis of knee
015.8*	Tuberculosis of other specified joint
015.9*	Tuberculosis of unspecified bones and joints
036.82	Meningococcal arthropathy
098.50	Gonococcal arthritis
098.51	Gonococcal synovitis and tenosynovitis
098.52	Gonococcal bursitis
098.59	Other gonococcal infection of joint
102.6	Bone and joint lesions due to yaws
711.0*	Pyogenic arthritis
711.4*	Arthropathy associated with other bacterial diseases
711.6*	Arthropathy associated with mycoses
711.7*	Arthropathy associated with helminthiasis
711.8*	Arthropathy associated with other infectious and parasitic diseases
711.9*	Unspecified infective arthritis

DRG 549 Septic Arthritis with CC

GMLOS 4.3   AMLOS 5.2   RW 1.1101   ☑

Select principal diagnosis listed under DRG 548

DRG 550 Septic Arthritis without CC/MCC

GMLOS 3.1   AMLOS 3.8   RW 0.8149   ☑

Select principal diagnosis listed under DRG 548

DRG 551 Medical Back Problems with MCC

GMLOS 5.0   AMLOS 6.4   RW 1.6317   ☑ ▽ T

Principal Diagnosis

720.1	Spinal enthesopathy
720.2	Sacroiliitis, not elsewhere classified
720.8*	Other inflammatory spondylopathies
720.9	Unspecified inflammatory spondylopathy
721*	Spondylosis and allied disorders
722*	Intervertebral disc disorders
723.0	Spinal stenosis in cervical region
723.1	Cervicalgia
723.5	Torticollis, unspecified
723.7	Ossification of posterior longitudinal ligament in cervical region
723.8	Other syndromes affecting cervical region
723.9	Unspecified musculoskeletal disorders and symptoms referable to neck
724*	Other and unspecified disorders of back
737*	Curvature of spine
738.4	Acquired spondylolisthesis
738.5	Other acquired deformity of back or spine
739.1	Nonallopathic lesion of cervical region, not elsewhere classified
739.2	Nonallopathic lesion of thoracic region, not elsewhere classified

---

Surgical   Medical   CC Indicator   MCC Indicator   Procedure Proxy

739.3	Nonallopathic lesion of lumbar region, not elsewhere classified
739.4	Nonallopathic lesion of sacral region, not elsewhere classified
756.10	Congenital anomaly of spine, unspecified
756.11	Congenital spondylolysis, lumbosacral region
756.12	Congenital spondylolisthesis
756.13	Congenital absence of vertebra
756.14	Hemivertebra
756.15	Congenital fusion of spine (vertebra)
756.19	Other congenital anomaly of spine
781.93	Ocular torticollis
805*	Fracture of vertebral column without mention of spinal cord injury
839.0*	Closed dislocation, cervical vertebra
839.1*	Open dislocation, cervical vertebra
839.2*	Closed dislocation, thoracic and lumbar vertebra
839.3*	Open dislocation, thoracic and lumbar vertebra
839.4*	Closed dislocation, other vertebra
839.5*	Open dislocation, other vertebra
846*	Sprains and strains of sacroiliac region
847*	Sprains and strains of other and unspecified parts of back
905.1	Late effect of fracture of spine and trunk without mention of spinal cord lesion

DRG 552   Medical Back Problems without MCC
GMLOS 3.2   AMLOS 3.9   RW 0.8467   ☑ ▽ Ⓣ

Select principal diagnosis listed under DRG 551

DRG 553   Bone Diseases and Arthropathies with MCC
GMLOS 4.4   AMLOS 5.6   RW 1.2370   ☑

Principal Diagnosis

056.71	Arthritis due to rubella
268.0	Rickets, active
268.1	Rickets, late effect
268.2	Osteomalacia, unspecified
274.0*	Gouty arthropathy
274.8*	Gout with other specified manifestations
274.9	Gout, unspecified
711.3*	Postdysenteric arthropathy
711.5*	Arthropathy associated with other viral diseases
712*	Crystal arthropathies
713*	Arthropathy associated with other disorders classified elsewhere
714.4	Chronic postrheumatic arthropathy
714.9	Unspecified inflammatory polyarthropathy
715*	Osteoarthrosis and allied disorders
716*	Other and unspecified arthropathies
718.5*	Ankylosis of joint
719.1*	Hemarthrosis
719.2*	Villonodular synovitis
719.3*	Palindromic rheumatism
730.30	Periostitis, without mention of osteomyelitis, unspecified site
730.31	Periostitis, without mention of osteomyelitis, shoulder region
730.32	Periostitis, without mention of osteomyelitis, upper arm
730.33	Periostitis, without mention of osteomyelitis, forearm
730.34	Periostitis, without mention of osteomyelitis, hand
730.35	Periostitis, without mention of osteomyelitis, pelvic region and thigh
730.36	Periostitis, without mention of osteomyelitis, lower leg
731*	Osteitis deformans and osteopathies associated with other disorders classified elsewhere
732*	Osteochondropathies
733.0*	Osteoporosis
733.2*	Cyst of bone
733.4*	Aseptic necrosis of bone

733.5	Osteitis condensans
733.92	Chondromalacia

DRG 554   Bone Diseases and Arthropathies without MCC
GMLOS 2.9   AMLOS 3.6   RW 0.7181   ☑

Select principal diagnosis listed under DRG 553

DRG 555   Signs and Symptoms of Musculoskeletal System and Connective Tissue with MCC
GMLOS 3.7   AMLOS 5.0   RW 1.1974   ☑

Principal Diagnosis

719.4*	Pain in joint
719.5*	Stiffness of joint, not elsewhere classified
719.6*	Other symptoms referable to joint
719.7	Difficulty in walking
719.8*	Other specified disorders of joint
719.9*	Unspecified disorder of joint
728.85	Spasm of muscle
728.87	Muscle weakness (generalized)
729.0	Rheumatism, unspecified and fibrositis
729.1	Unspecified myalgia and myositis
729.5	Pain in soft tissues of limb
729.81	Swelling of limb
729.82	Cramp of limb
729.89	Other musculoskeletal symptoms referable to limbs
729.9*	Other and unspecified disorders of soft tissue
739.0	Nonallopathic lesion of head region, not elsewhere classified
739.5	Nonallopathic lesion of pelvic region, not elsewhere classified
739.6	Nonallopathic lesion of lower extremities, not elsewhere classified
739.7	Nonallopathic lesion of upper extremities, not elsewhere classified
739.8	Nonallopathic lesion of rib cage, not elsewhere classified
739.9	Nonallopathic lesion of abdomen and other sites, not elsewhere classified

DRG 556   Signs and Symptoms of Musculoskeletal System and Connective Tissue without MCC
GMLOS 2.6   AMLOS 3.2   RW 0.7066   ☑

Select principal diagnosis listed under DRG 555

DRG 557   Tendonitis, Myositis and Bursitis with MCC
GMLOS 5.1   AMLOS 6.4   RW 1.4756   ☑ Ⓣ

Principal Diagnosis

040.81	Tropical pyomyositis
095.6	Syphilis of muscle
095.7	Syphilis of synovium, tendon, and bursa
306.0	Musculoskeletal malfunction arising from mental factors
726.0	Adhesive capsulitis of shoulder
726.1*	Rotator cuff syndrome of shoulder and allied disorders
726.2	Other affections of shoulder region, not elsewhere classified
726.3*	Enthesopathy of elbow region
726.4	Enthesopathy of wrist and carpus
726.5	Enthesopathy of hip region
726.6*	Enthesopathy of knee
726.70	Unspecified enthesopathy of ankle and tarsus
726.71	Achilles bursitis or tendinitis
726.72	Tibialis tendinitis
726.79	Other enthesopathy of ankle and tarsus
726.8	Other peripheral enthesopathies
726.9*	Unspecified enthesopathy
727.00	Unspecified synovitis and tenosynovitis
727.01	Synovitis and tenosynovitis in diseases classified elsewhere

---

Ⓣ *Transfer DRG*   ⓢ *Special Payment*   ☑ *Optimization Potential*   ▽ *Targeted Potential*   * *Code Range*   ● *New DRG*   ▲ *Revised DRG Title*

727.03	Trigger finger (acquired)
727.04	Radial styloid tenosynovitis
727.05	Other tenosynovitis of hand and wrist
727.06	Tenosynovitis of foot and ankle
727.09	Other synovitis and tenosynovitis
727.2	Specific bursitides often of occupational origin
727.3	Other bursitis disorders
727.4*	Ganglion and cyst of synovium, tendon, and bursa
727.5*	Rupture of synovium
727.6*	Rupture of tendon, nontraumatic
727.8*	Other disorders of synovium, tendon, and bursa
727.9	Unspecified disorder of synovium, tendon, and bursa
728.0	Infective myositis
728.1*	Muscular calcification and ossification
728.2	Muscular wasting and disuse atrophy, not elsewhere classified
728.3	Other specific muscle disorders
728.4	Laxity of ligament
728.5	Hypermobility syndrome
728.6	Contracture of palmar fascia
728.7*	Other fibromatoses of muscle, ligament, and fascia
728.81	Interstitial myositis
728.82	Foreign body granuloma of muscle
728.83	Rupture of muscle, nontraumatic
728.84	Diastasis of muscle
728.86	Necrotizing fasciitis
728.88	Rhabdomyolysis
728.89	Other disorder of muscle, ligament, and fascia
728.9	Unspecified disorder of muscle, ligament, and fascia
729.4	Unspecified fasciitis
729.7*	Nontraumatic compartment syndrome

DRG 558   Tendonitis, Myositis and Bursitis without MCC
GMLOS 3.4   AMLOS 4.0   RW 0.8337   ☑Ⓣ

Select principal diagnosis listed under DRG 557

DRG 559   Aftercare, Musculoskeletal System and Connective Tissue with MCC
GMLOS 5.0   AMLOS 6.9   RW 1.8639   ☑Ⓣ

Principal Diagnosis

905.2	Late effect of fracture of upper extremities
905.3	Late effect of fracture of neck of femur
905.4	Late effect of fracture of lower extremities
905.5	Late effect of fracture of multiple and unspecified bones
905.8	Late effect of tendon injury
905.9	Late effect of traumatic amputation
996.4*	Mechanical complication of internal orthopedic device, implant, and graft
996.66	Infection and inflammatory reaction due to internal joint prosthesis
996.67	Infection and inflammatory reaction due to other internal orthopedic device, implant, and graft
996.77	Other complications due to internal joint prosthesis
996.78	Other complications due to other internal orthopedic device, implant, and graft
996.9*	Complications of reattached extremity or body part
V52.0	Fitting and adjustment of artificial arm (complete) (partial)
V52.1	Fitting and adjustment of artificial leg (complete) (partial)
V53.7	Fitting and adjustment of orthopedic device
V54.0*	Aftercare involving internal fixation device
V54.1*	Aftercare for healing traumatic fracture
V54.2*	Aftercare for healing pathologic fracture
V54.8*	Other orthopedic aftercare
V54.9	Unspecified orthopedic aftercare

DRG 560   Aftercare, Musculoskeletal System and Connective Tissue with CC
GMLOS 3.4   AMLOS 4.4   RW 1.0260   ☑Ⓣ

Select principal diagnosis listed under DRG 559

DRG 561   Aftercare, Musculoskeletal System and Connective Tissue without CC/MCC
GMLOS 2.0   AMLOS 2.5   RW 0.6408   ☑Ⓣ

Select principal diagnosis listed under DRG 559

DRG 562   Fractures, Sprains, Strains and Dislocations Except Femur, Hip, Pelvis and Thigh with MCC
GMLOS 4.4   AMLOS 5.5   RW 1.3528   ☑Ⓣ

Principal Diagnosis

717.0	Old bucket handle tear of medial meniscus
717.1	Derangement of anterior horn of medial meniscus
717.2	Derangement of posterior horn of medial meniscus
717.3	Other and unspecified derangement of medial meniscus
717.4*	Derangement of lateral meniscus
717.5	Derangement of meniscus, not elsewhere classified
717.7	Chondromalacia of patella
717.8*	Other internal derangement of knee
717.9	Unspecified internal derangement of knee
718.01	Articular cartilage disorder, shoulder region
718.02	Articular cartilage disorder, upper arm
718.03	Articular cartilage disorder, forearm
718.04	Articular cartilage disorder, hand
718.07	Articular cartilage disorder, ankle and foot
718.20	Pathological dislocation of joint, site unspecified
718.21	Pathological dislocation of shoulder joint
718.22	Pathological dislocation of upper arm joint
718.23	Pathological dislocation of forearm joint
718.24	Pathological dislocation of hand joint
718.26	Pathological dislocation of lower leg joint
718.27	Pathological dislocation of ankle and foot joint
718.31	Recurrent dislocation of shoulder joint
718.32	Recurrent dislocation of upper arm joint
718.33	Recurrent dislocation of forearm joint
718.34	Recurrent dislocation of hand joint
718.36	Recurrent dislocation of lower leg joint
718.37	Recurrent dislocation of ankle and foot joint
754.41	Congenital dislocation of knee (with genu recurvatum)
810*	Fracture of clavicle
811.00	Closed fracture of unspecified part of scapula
811.01	Closed fracture of acromial process of scapula
811.02	Closed fracture of coracoid process of scapula
811.03	Closed fracture of glenoid cavity and neck of scapula
811.10	Open fracture of unspecified part of scapula
811.11	Open fracture of acromial process of scapula
811.12	Open fracture of coracoid process
811.13	Open fracture of glenoid cavity and neck of scapula
812*	Fracture of humerus
813*	Fracture of radius and ulna
814*	Fracture of carpal bone(s)
815*	Fracture of metacarpal bone(s)
816*	Fracture of one or more phalanges of hand
817*	Multiple fractures of hand bones
818*	Ill-defined fractures of upper limb
822*	Fracture of patella
823*	Fracture of tibia and fibula
824*	Fracture of ankle
825.0	Closed fracture of calcaneus
825.1	Open fracture of calcaneus
825.2*	Closed fracture of other tarsal and metatarsal bones
825.3*	Open fracture of other tarsal and metatarsal bones
826*	Fracture of one or more phalanges of foot
827*	Other, multiple, and ill-defined fractures of lower limb

---

Surgical	Medical	CC Indicator	MCC Indicator	Procedure Proxy

MDC 8: Diseases And Disorders Of The Musculoskeletal System And Connective Tissue—MEDICAL

829*	Fracture of unspecified bones
831*	Dislocation of shoulder
832*	Dislocation of elbow
833*	Dislocation of wrist
834*	Dislocation of finger
836*	Dislocation of knee
837*	Dislocation of ankle
838*	Dislocation of foot
839.69	Closed dislocation, other location
839.79	Open dislocation, other location
839.8	Closed dislocation, multiple and ill-defined sites
839.9	Open dislocation, multiple and ill-defined sites
840*	Sprains and strains of shoulder and upper arm
841*	Sprains and strains of elbow and forearm
842*	Sprains and strains of wrist and hand
844*	Sprains and strains of knee and leg
845.0*	Ankle sprain and strain
845.1*	Foot sprain and strain
848.8	Other specified sites of sprains and strains
848.9	Unspecified site of sprain and strain
905.6	Late effect of dislocation
905.7	Late effect of sprain and strain without mention of tendon injury

DRG 563   Fractures, Sprains, Strains and Dislocations Except Femur, Hip, Pelvis and Thigh without MCC

GMLOS 3.0   AMLOS 3.5   RW 0.7535   ☑ⓣ

Select principal diagnosis listed under DRG 562

DRG 564   Other Musculoskeletal System and Connective Tissue Diagnoses with MCC

GMLOS 4.5   AMLOS 6.1   RW 1.4855   ☑

Principal Diagnosis

137.3	Late effects of tuberculosis of bones and joints
213.0	Benign neoplasm of bones of skull and face
213.2	Benign neoplasm of vertebral column, excluding sacrum and coccyx
213.4	Benign neoplasm of scapula and long bones of upper limb
213.5	Benign neoplasm of short bones of upper limb
213.6	Benign neoplasm of pelvic bones, sacrum, and coccyx
213.7	Benign neoplasm of long bones of lower limb
213.8	Benign neoplasm of short bones of lower limb
213.9	Benign neoplasm of bone and articular cartilage, site unspecified
215*	Other benign neoplasm of connective and other soft tissue
238.1	Neoplasm of uncertain behavior of connective and other soft tissue
239.2	Neoplasms of unspecified nature of bone, soft tissue, and skin
380.01	Acute perichondritis of pinna
380.02	Chronic perichondritis of pinna
380.03	Chondritis of pinna
717.6	Loose body in knee
718.00	Articular cartilage disorder, site unspecified
718.05	Articular cartilage disorder, pelvic region and thigh
718.08	Articular cartilage disorder, other specified site
718.09	Articular cartilage disorder, multiple sites
718.1*	Loose body in joint
718.25	Pathological dislocation of pelvic region and thigh joint
718.28	Pathological dislocation of joint of other specified site
718.29	Pathological dislocation of joint of multiple sites
718.30	Recurrent dislocation of joint, site unspecified
718.35	Recurrent dislocation of pelvic region and thigh joint
718.38	Recurrent dislocation of joint of other specified site
718.39	Recurrent dislocation of joint of multiple sites
718.4*	Contracture of joint
718.65	Unspecified intrapelvic protrusion acetabulum, pelvic region and thigh

718.7*	Developmental dislocation of joint
718.8*	Other joint derangement, not elsewhere classified
718.9*	Unspecified derangement of joint
719.0*	Effusion of joint
726.73	Calcaneal spur
727.02	Giant cell tumor of tendon sheath
727.1	Bunion
729.6	Residual foreign body in soft tissue
730.37	Periostitis, without mention of osteomyelitis, ankle and foot
730.38	Periostitis, without mention of osteomyelitis, other specified sites
730.39	Periostitis, without mention of osteomyelitis, multiple sites
730.7*	Osteopathy resulting from poliomyelitis
733.3	Hyperostosis of skull
733.7	Algoneurodystrophy
733.8*	Malunion and nonunion of fracture
733.90	Disorder of bone and cartilage, unspecified
733.91	Arrest of bone development or growth
733.99	Other disorders of bone and cartilage
734	Flat foot
735*	Acquired deformities of toe
736.00	Unspecified deformity of forearm, excluding fingers
736.01	Cubitus valgus (acquired)
736.02	Cubitus varus (acquired)
736.03	Valgus deformity of wrist (acquired)
736.04	Varus deformity of wrist (acquired)
736.09	Other acquired deformities of forearm, excluding fingers
736.1	Mallet finger
736.2*	Other acquired deformities of finger
736.3*	Acquired deformities of hip
736.4*	Genu valgum or varum (acquired)
736.5	Genu recurvatum (acquired)
736.6	Other acquired deformities of knee
736.70	Unspecified deformity of ankle and foot, acquired
736.71	Acquired equinovarus deformity
736.72	Equinus deformity of foot, acquired
736.73	Cavus deformity of foot, acquired
736.75	Cavovarus deformity of foot, acquired
736.76	Other acquired calcaneus deformity
736.79	Other acquired deformity of ankle and foot
736.8*	Acquired deformities of other parts of limbs
736.9	Acquired deformity of limb, site unspecified
738.1*	Other acquired deformity of head
738.2	Acquired deformity of neck
738.3	Acquired deformity of chest and rib
738.6	Acquired deformity of pelvis
738.8	Acquired musculoskeletal deformity of other specified site
738.9	Acquired musculoskeletal deformity of unspecified site
754.0	Congenital musculoskeletal deformities of skull, face, and jaw
754.1	Congenital musculoskeletal deformity of sternocleidomastoid muscle
754.2	Congenital musculoskeletal deformity of spine
754.3*	Congenital dislocation of hip
754.40	Congenital genu recurvatum
754.42	Congenital bowing of femur
754.43	Congenital bowing of tibia and fibula
754.44	Congenital bowing of unspecified long bones of leg
754.5*	Congenital varus deformities of feet
754.6*	Congenital valgus deformities of feet
754.7*	Other congenital deformity of feet
754.89	Other specified nonteratogenic anomalies
755*	Other congenital anomalies of limbs
756.0	Congenital anomalies of skull and face bones
756.16	Klippel-Feil syndrome
756.2	Cervical rib
756.4	Chondrodystrophy
756.5*	Congenital osteodystrophies
756.8*	Other specified congenital anomalies of muscle, tendon, fascia, and connective tissue

---

ⓣ *Transfer DRG*   ⓢ *Special Payment*   ☑ *Optimization Potential*   � *Targeted Potential*   * *Code Range*   ● *New DRG*   ▲ *Revised DRG Title*

756.9	Other and unspecified congenital anomaly of musculoskeletal system
759.7	Multiple congenital anomalies, so described
759.81	Prader-Willi syndrome
759.89	Other specified multiple congenital anomalies, so described
793.7	Nonspecific (abnormal) findings on radiological and other examination of musculoskeletal system
794.17	Nonspecific abnormal electromyogram (EMG)
802.8	Other facial bones, closed fracture
802.9	Other facial bones, open fracture
809.0	Fracture of bones of trunk, closed
809.1	Fracture of bones of trunk, open
811.09	Closed fracture of other part of scapula
811.19	Open fracture of other part of scapula
848.0	Sprain and strain of septal cartilage of nose
848.2	Sprain and strain of thyroid region
880.2*	Open wound of shoulder and upper arm, with tendon involvement
881.2*	Open wound of elbow, forearm, and wrist, with tendon involvement
882.2	Open wound of hand except finger(s) alone, with tendon involvement
883.2	Open wound of finger(s), with tendon involvement
884.2	Multiple and unspecified open wound of upper limb, with tendon involvement
890.2	Open wound of hip and thigh, with tendon involvement
891.2	Open wound of knee, leg (except thigh), and ankle, with tendon involvement
892.2	Open wound of foot except toe(s) alone, with tendon involvement
893.2	Open wound of toe(s), with tendon involvement
894.2	Multiple and unspecified open wound of lower limb, with tendon involvement
958.6	Volkmann's ischemic contracture
997.6*	Amputation stump complication
V42.4	Bone replaced by transplant
V43.6*	Joint replaced by other means
V43.7	Limb replaced by other means
V59.2	Bone donor

DRG 565   **Other Musculoskeletal System and Connective Tissue Diagnoses with CC**
   GMLOS 3.6   AMLOS 4.4   RW 0.9281   ☑

Select principal diagnosis listed under DRG 564

DRG 566   **Other Musculoskeletal System and Connective Tissue Diagnoses without CC/MCC**
   GMLOS 2.6   AMLOS 3.3   RW 0.6642   ☑

Select principal diagnosis listed under DRG 564

MDC 8: Diseases And Disorders Of The Musculoskeletal System And Connective Tissue—MEDICAL

MDC 9
Diseases And Disorders Of The Skin, Subcutaneous Tissue And Breast

006.6	132.0	176.0	612.1	693.9	704.09	744.9	906.5	916.4
017.00	132.1	176.1	617.6	694.0	704.1	757.0	906.6	916.5
017.01	132.2	176.8	680.0	694.1	704.2	757.1	906.7	916.6
017.02	132.3	176.9	680.1	694.2	704.3	757.2	906.8	916.7
017.03	132.9	198.2	680.2	694.3	704.41	757.31	906.9	916.8
017.04	133.0	198.81	680.3	694.4	704.42	757.32	910.0	916.9
017.05	133.8	209.31	680.4	694.5	704.8	757.33	910.1	917.0
017.06	133.9	209.32	680.5	694.60	704.9	757.39	910.2	917.1
017.10	134.0	209.33	680.6	694.8	705.0	757.4	910.3	917.2
017.11	134.1	209.34	680.7	694.9	705.1	757.5	910.4	917.3
017.12	134.2	209.35	680.8	695.0	705.21	757.6	910.5	917.4
017.13	134.8	209.36	680.9	695.10	705.22	757.8	910.6	917.5
017.14	134.9	214.0	681.00	695.11	705.81	757.9	910.7	917.6
017.15	172.0	214.1	681.01	695.12	705.82	780.8	910.8	917.7
017.16	172.2	214.8	681.02	695.13	705.83	782.1	910.9	917.8
022.0	172.3	214.9	681.10	695.14	705.89	782.2	911.0	917.9
031.1	172.4	216.0	681.11	695.15	705.9	782.8	911.1	919.0
032.85	172.5	216.2	681.9	695.19	706.0	782.9	911.2	919.2
035	172.6	216.3	682.0	695.2	706.1	784.2	911.3	919.3
039.0	172.7	216.4	682.1	695.3	706.2	793.80	911.4	919.4
039.3	172.8	216.5	682.2	695.4	706.3	793.81	911.5	919.5
039.4	172.9	216.6	682.3	695.50	706.8	793.82	911.6	919.6
051.1	173.00	216.7	682.4	695.51	706.9	793.89	911.7	919.7
051.2	173.01	216.8	682.5	695.52	707.00	873.0	911.8	919.8
053.9	173.02	216.9	682.6	695.53	707.01	873.1	911.9	919.9
054.0	173.09	217	682.7	695.54	707.02	873.40	912.0	920
054.6	173.20	228.01	682.8	695.55	707.03	873.41	912.1	922.0
054.9	173.21	232.0	682.9	695.56	707.04	873.42	912.2	922.1
058.81	173.22	232.2	684	695.57	707.05	873.49	912.3	922.2
058.82	173.29	232.3	685.0	695.58	707.06	873.50	912.4	922.31
058.89	173.30	232.4	685.1	695.59	707.07	873.51	912.5	922.32
078.0	173.31	232.5	686.00	695.81	707.09	873.52	912.6	922.33
078.10	173.32	232.6	686.01	695.89	707.10	873.59	912.7	922.8
078.11	173.39	232.7	686.09	695.9	707.11	873.8	912.8	922.9
078.12	173.40	232.8	686.1	696.1	707.12	873.9	912.9	923.00
078.19	173.41	232.9	686.8	696.2	707.13	874.8	913.0	923.01
085.1	173.42	233.0	686.9	696.3	707.14	874.9	913.1	923.02
085.2	173.49	238.2	690.10	696.4	707.15	875.0	913.2	923.03
085.3	173.50	238.3	690.11	696.5	707.19	876.0	913.3	923.09
085.4	173.51	239.3	690.12	696.8	707.20	876.1	913.4	923.10
085.5	173.52	306.3	690.18	697.0	707.21	877.0	913.5	923.11
091.3	173.59	374.51	690.8	697.1	707.22	877.1	913.6	923.20
091.82	173.60	448.1	691.0	697.8	707.23	879.0	913.7	923.21
102.0	173.61	457.0	691.8	697.9	707.24	879.1	913.8	923.3
102.1	173.62	457.1	692.0	698.0	707.25	879.2	913.9	923.8
102.2	173.69	457.2	692.1	698.2	707.8	879.4	914.0	923.9
102.3	173.70	610.0	692.2	698.3	707.9	879.6	914.1	924.00
102.4	173.71	610.1	692.3	698.4	708.0	879.8	914.2	924.01
103.0	173.72	610.2	692.4	698.8	708.1	880.00	914.3	924.10
103.1	173.79	610.3	692.5	698.9	708.2	880.01	914.4	924.11
103.3	173.80	610.4	692.6	700	708.3	880.02	914.5	924.20
110.0	173.81	610.8	692.70	701.0	708.4	880.03	914.6	924.21
110.1	173.82	610.9	692.71	701.1	708.5	880.09	914.7	924.3
110.2	173.89	611.0	692.72	701.2	708.8	881.00	914.8	924.4
110.3	173.90	611.1	692.73	701.3	708.9	881.01	914.9	924.5
110.4	173.91	611.2	692.74	701.4	709.00	881.02	915.0	924.8
110.5	173.92	611.3	692.75	701.5	709.01	882.0	915.1	924.9
110.6	173.99	611.4	692.76	701.8	709.09	883.0	915.2	996.54
110.8	174.0	611.5	692.77	701.9	709.1	884.0	915.3	V42.3
110.9	174.1	611.6	692.79	702.0	709.2	890.0	915.4	V50.0
111.0	174.2	611.71	692.81	702.11	709.3	891.0	915.5	V50.1
111.1	174.3	611.72	692.82	702.19	709.4	892.0	915.6	V50.41
111.2	174.4	611.79	692.83	702.8	709.8	893.0	915.7	V51.0
111.3	174.5	611.81	692.84	703.0	709.9	894.0	915.8	V51.8
111.8	174.6	611.82	692.89	703.8	723.6	906.0	915.9	V59.1
111.9	174.8	611.83	692.9	703.9	729.30	906.1	916.0	
112.3	174.9	611.89	693.0	704.00	729.31	906.2	916.1	
114.1	175.0	611.9	693.1	704.01	729.39	906.3	916.2	
120.3	175.9	612.0	693.8	704.02	744.5	906.4	916.3	

SURGICAL

DRG 570   Skin Debridement with MCC
GMLOS 7.2   AMLOS 9.4   RW 2.4154   ☑ⓣ

Operating Room Procedure
86.22   Excisional debridement of wound, infection, or burn

DRG 571   Skin Debridement with CC
GMLOS 5.4   AMLOS 6.5   RW 1.4906   ☑ⓣ

Select operating room procedure listed under DRG 570

DRG 572   Skin Debridement without CC/MCC
GMLOS 3.8   AMLOS 4.6   RW 1.0077   ☑ⓣ

Select operating room procedure listed under DRG 570

DRG 573   Skin Graft for Skin Ulcer or Cellulitis with MCC
GMLOS 8.2   AMLOS 12.3   RW 3.4623   ☑ⓣ

Principal Diagnosis
681*   Cellulitis and abscess of finger and toe
682*   Other cellulitis and abscess
707*   Chronic ulcer of skin

Operating Room Procedures
85.82   Split-thickness graft to breast
85.83   Full-thickness graft to breast
85.84   Pedicle graft to breast
85.85   Muscle flap graft to breast
86.4   Radical excision of skin lesion
86.60   Free skin graft, not otherwise specified
86.61   Full-thickness skin graft to hand
86.62   Other skin graft to hand
86.63   Full-thickness skin graft to other sites
86.65   Heterograft to skin
86.66   Homograft to skin
86.67   Dermal regenerative graft
86.69   Other skin graft to other sites
86.7*   Pedicle grafts or flaps
86.91   Excision of skin for graft
86.93   Insertion of tissue expander

DRG 574   Skin Graft for Skin Ulcer or Cellulitis with CC
GMLOS 7.1   AMLOS 9.6   RW 2.6883   ☑ⓣ

Select principal diagnosis and operating room procedures listed under DRG 573

DRG 575   Skin Graft for Skin Ulcer or Cellulitis without CC/MCC
GMLOS 4.2   AMLOS 5.4   RW 1.4376   ☑ⓣ

Select principal diagnosis and operating room procedures listed under DRG 573

DRG 576   Skin Graft Except for Skin Ulcer or Cellulitis with MCC
GMLOS 7.9   AMLOS 12.3   RW 4.2927   ☑

Select only operating room procedures listed under DRG 573

DRG 577   Skin Graft Except for Skin Ulcer or Cellulitis with CC
GMLOS 4.0   AMLOS 5.9   RW 2.0212   ☑

Select only operating room procedures listed under DRG 573

DRG 578   Skin Graft Except for Skin Ulcer or Cellulitis without CC/MCC
GMLOS 2.4   AMLOS 3.3   RW 1.2617   ☑

Select only operating room procedures listed under DRG 573

DRG 579   Other Skin, Subcutaneous Tissue and Breast Procedures with MCC
GMLOS 7.0   AMLOS 9.2   RW 2.6106   ☑ⓣ

Operating Room Procedures
06.09   Other incision of thyroid field
07.22   Unilateral adrenalectomy
07.3   Bilateral adrenalectomy
07.63   Partial excision of pituitary gland, unspecified approach
07.64   Total excision of pituitary gland, transfrontal approach
07.65   Total excision of pituitary gland, transsphenoidal approach
07.68   Total excision of pituitary gland, other specified approach
07.69   Total excision of pituitary gland, unspecified approach
07.72   Incision of pituitary gland
07.79   Other operations on hypophysis
08.20   Removal of lesion of eyelid, not otherwise specified
08.22   Excision of other minor lesion of eyelid
08.23   Excision of major lesion of eyelid, partial-thickness
08.24   Excision of major lesion of eyelid, full-thickness
08.25   Destruction of lesion of eyelid
08.38   Correction of lid retraction
08.44   Repair of entropion or ectropion with lid reconstruction
08.5*   Other adjustment of lid position
08.6*   Reconstruction of eyelid with flaps or grafts
08.7*   Other reconstruction of eyelid
08.99   Other operations on eyelids
09.73   Repair of canaliculus
16.93   Excision of lesion of eye, unspecified structure
17.56   Atherectomy of other non-coronary vessel(s)
18.21   Excision of preauricular sinus
18.3*   Other excision of external ear
18.5   Surgical correction of prominent ear
18.6   Reconstruction of external auditory canal
18.71   Construction of auricle of ear
18.79   Other plastic repair of external ear
18.9   Other operations on external ear
21.4   Resection of nose
21.72   Open reduction of nasal fracture
21.83   Total nasal reconstruction
21.84   Revision rhinoplasty
21.85   Augmentation rhinoplasty
21.86   Limited rhinoplasty
21.87   Other rhinoplasty
21.88   Other septoplasty
21.89   Other repair and plastic operations on nose
21.99   Other operations on nose
27.0   Drainage of face and floor of mouth
27.42   Wide excision of lesion of lip
27.43   Other excision of lesion or tissue of lip
27.54   Repair of cleft lip
27.55   Full-thickness skin graft to lip and mouth
27.56   Other skin graft to lip and mouth
27.57   Attachment of pedicle or flap graft to lip and mouth
27.59   Other plastic repair of mouth
27.63   Revision of cleft palate repair
27.69   Other plastic repair of palate
27.92   Incision of mouth, unspecified structure
29.2   Excision of branchial cleft cyst or vestige
29.52   Closure of branchial cleft fistula
31.72   Closure of external fistula of trachea
31.74   Revision of tracheostomy
34.4   Excision or destruction of lesion of chest wall
34.79   Other repair of chest wall
37.79   Revision or relocation of cardiac device pocket

MDC 9: Diseases And Disorders Of The Skin, Subcutaneous Tissue And Breast—SURGICAL

39.25	Aorta-iliac-femoral bypass
39.29	Other (peripheral) vascular shunt or bypass
39.31	Suture of artery
39.50	Angioplasty of other non-coronary vessel(s)
39.59	Other repair of vessel
39.98	Control of hemorrhage, not otherwise specified
40.0	Incision of lymphatic structures
40.1*	Diagnostic procedures on lymphatic structures
40.2*	Simple excision of lymphatic structure
40.3	Regional lymph node excision
40.4*	Radical excision of cervical lymph nodes
40.5*	Radical excision of other lymph nodes
40.9	Other operations on lymphatic structures
48.35	Local excision of rectal lesion or tissue
48.73	Closure of other rectal fistula
48.8*	Incision or excision of perirectal tissue or lesion
49.01	Incision of perianal abscess
49.02	Other incision of perianal tissue
49.04	Other excision of perianal tissue
49.11	Anal fistulotomy
49.12	Anal fistulectomy
49.39	Other local excision or destruction of lesion or tissue of anus
49.71	Suture of laceration of anus
49.72	Anal cerclage
49.73	Closure of anal fistula
49.75	Implantation or revision of artificial anal sphincter
49.76	Removal of artificial anal sphincter
49.79	Other repair of anal sphincter
50.12	Open biopsy of liver
50.14	Laparoscopic liver biopsy
50.19	Other diagnostic procedures on liver
54.0	Incision of abdominal wall
54.11	Exploratory laparotomy
54.21	Laparoscopy
54.22	Biopsy of abdominal wall or umbilicus
54.3	Excision or destruction of lesion or tissue of abdominal wall or umbilicus
54.63	Other suture of abdominal wall
54.72	Other repair of abdominal wall
59.00	Retroperitoneal dissection, not otherwise specified
64.11	Biopsy of penis
64.2	Local excision or destruction of lesion of penis
64.49	Other repair of penis
65.5*	Bilateral oophorectomy
65.61	Other removal of both ovaries and tubes at same operative episode
65.63	Laparoscopic removal of both ovaries and tubes at same operative episode
67.1*	Diagnostic procedures on cervix
67.39	Other excision or destruction of lesion or tissue of cervix
70.24	Vaginal biopsy
70.33	Excision or destruction of lesion of vagina
70.71	Suture of laceration of vagina
71.09	Other incision of vulva and perineum
71.1*	Diagnostic procedures on vulva
71.24	Excision or other destruction of Bartholin's gland (cyst)
71.3	Other local excision or destruction of vulva and perineum
71.62	Bilateral vulvectomy
71.71	Suture of laceration of vulva or perineum
76.43	Other reconstruction of mandible
77.28	Wedge osteotomy of tarsals and metatarsals
77.4*	Biopsy of bone
80.83	Other local excision or destruction of lesion of wrist joint
82.09	Other incision of soft tissue of hand
82.21	Excision of lesion of tendon sheath of hand
82.29	Excision of other lesion of soft tissue of hand
82.39	Other excision of soft tissue of hand
82.45	Other suture of other tendon of hand
82.72	Plastic operation on hand with graft of muscle or fascia
82.79	Plastic operation on hand with other graft or implant

82.89	Other plastic operations on hand
82.91	Lysis of adhesions of hand
83.02	Myotomy
83.09	Other incision of soft tissue
83.14	Fasciotomy
83.21	Open biopsy of soft tissue
83.32	Excision of lesion of muscle
83.39	Excision of lesion of other soft tissue
83.44	Other fasciectomy
83.45	Other myectomy
83.49	Other excision of soft tissue
83.65	Other suture of muscle or fascia
83.71	Advancement of tendon
83.82	Graft of muscle or fascia
83.87	Other plastic operations on muscle
83.88	Other plastic operations on tendon
83.89	Other plastic operations on fascia
84.0*	Amputation of upper limb
84.1*	Amputation of lower limb
84.3	Revision of amputation stump
84.91	Amputation, not otherwise specified
86.06	Insertion of totally implantable infusion pump
86.21	Excision of pilonidal cyst or sinus
86.25	Dermabrasion
86.8*	Other repair and reconstruction of skin and subcutaneous tissue
86.90	Extraction of fat for graft or banking
92.27	Implantation or insertion of radioactive elements

OR

Nonoperating Room Procedures

86.07	Insertion of totally implantable vascular access device (VAD)
86.09	Other incision of skin and subcutaneous tissue
86.3	Other local excision or destruction of lesion or tissue of skin and subcutaneous tissue

---

DRG 580 **Other Skin, Subcutaneous Tissue and Breast Procedures with CC**

GMLOS 3.8	AMLOS 5.1	RW 1.5398	☑ⓣ

Select operating room procedures or nonoperating room procedures listed under DRG 579

DRG 581 **Other Skin, Subcutaneous Tissue and Breast Procedures without CC/MCC**

GMLOS 2.0	AMLOS 2.6	RW 1.0605	☑ⓣ

Select operating room procedures or nonoperating room procedures listed under DRG 579

DRG 582 **Mastectomy for Malignancy with CC/MCC**

GMLOS 2.0	AMLOS 2.7	RW 1.1913	☑

Principal or Secondary Diagnosis

174*	Malignant neoplasm of female breast
175*	Malignant neoplasm of male breast
198.2	Secondary malignant neoplasm of skin
198.81	Secondary malignant neoplasm of breast
233.0	Carcinoma in situ of breast
238.3	Neoplasm of uncertain behavior of breast

Operating Room Procedures

85.22	Resection of quadrant of breast
85.23	Subtotal mastectomy
85.3*	Reduction mammoplasty and subcutaneous mammectomy
85.4*	Mastectomy
85.7*	Total reconstruction of breast

ⓣ *Transfer DRG*   🅢 *Special Payment*   ☑ *Optimization Potential*   ᵀᴬ *Targeted Potential*   * *Code Range*   ● *New DRG*   ▲ *Revised DRG Title*

Valid 10/01/2013-09/30/2014

DRG 583   Mastectomy for Malignancy without CC/MCC
GMLOS 1.5   AMLOS 1.7   RW 0.9711   ☑

Select principal or secondary diagnosis and operating room procedures listed under DRG 582

DRG 584   Breast Biopsy, Local Excision and Other Breast Procedures with CC/MCC
GMLOS 3.5   AMLOS 4.8   RW 1.6998   ☑

Operating Room Procedures
17.69	Laser interstitial thermal therapy [LITT] of lesion or tissue of other and unspecified site under guidance
85.12	Open biopsy of breast
85.20	Excision or destruction of breast tissue, not otherwise specified
85.21	Local excision of lesion of breast
85.22	Resection of quadrant of breast
85.23	Subtotal mastectomy
85.24	Excision of ectopic breast tissue
85.25	Excision of nipple
85.3*	Reduction mammoplasty and subcutaneous mammectomy
85.4*	Mastectomy
85.50	Augmentation mammoplasty, not otherwise specified
85.53	Unilateral breast implant
85.54	Bilateral breast implant
85.55	Fat graft to breast
85.6	Mastopexy
85.7*	Total reconstruction of breast
85.86	Transposition of nipple
85.87	Other repair or reconstruction of nipple
85.89	Other mammoplasty
85.93	Revision of implant of breast
85.94	Removal of implant of breast
85.95	Insertion of breast tissue expander
85.96	Removal of breast tissue expander (s)
85.99	Other operations on the breast

DRG 585   Breast Biopsy, Local Excision and Other Breast Procedures without CC/MCC
GMLOS 2.0   AMLOS 2.6   RW 1.3162   ☑

Select operating room procedures listed under DRG 584

MEDICAL

DRG 592   Skin Ulcers with MCC
GMLOS 5.1   AMLOS 6.6   RW 1.4131   ☑ Ⓣ

Principal Diagnosis
707*	Chronic ulcer of skin

DRG 593   Skin Ulcers with CC
GMLOS 4.2   AMLOS 5.1   RW 1.0094   ☑ Ⓣ

Select principal diagnosis listed under DRG 592

DRG 594   Skin Ulcers without CC/MCC
GMLOS 3.1   AMLOS 3.9   RW 0.6814   ☑ Ⓣ

Select principal diagnosis listed under DRG 592

DRG 595   Major Skin Disorders with MCC
GMLOS 5.7   AMLOS 7.8   RW 1.9464   ☑

Principal Diagnosis
017.1*	Erythema nodosum with hypersensitivity reaction in tuberculosis
053.9	Herpes zoster without mention of complication
172.0	Malignant melanoma of skin of lip
172.2	Malignant melanoma of skin of ear and external auditory canal
172.3	Malignant melanoma of skin of other and unspecified parts of face
172.4	Malignant melanoma of skin of scalp and neck
172.5	Malignant melanoma of skin of trunk, except scrotum
172.6	Malignant melanoma of skin of upper limb, including shoulder
172.7	Malignant melanoma of skin of lower limb, including hip
172.8	Malignant melanoma of other specified sites of skin
172.9	Melanoma of skin, site unspecified
209.31	Merkel cell carcinoma of the face
209.32	Merkel cell carcinoma of the scalp and neck
209.33	Merkel cell carcinoma of the upper limb
209.34	Merkel cell carcinoma of the lower limb
209.35	Merkel cell carcinoma of the trunk
209.36	Merkel cell carcinoma of other sites
694.4	Pemphigus
694.5	Pemphigoid
694.60	Benign mucous membrane pemphigoid without mention of ocular involvement
694.8	Other specified bullous dermatosis
694.9	Unspecified bullous dermatosis
695.0	Toxic erythema
695.1*	Erythema multiforme
695.2	Erythema nodosum
695.4	Lupus erythematosus
695.81	Ritter's disease
696.1	Other psoriasis
696.2	Parapsoriasis

DRG 596   Major Skin Disorders without MCC
GMLOS 3.6   AMLOS 4.6   RW 0.9284   ☑

Select principal diagnosis listed under DRG 595

DRG 597   Malignant Breast Disorders with MCC
GMLOS 5.2   AMLOS 7.1   RW 1.7064   ☑

Principal Diagnosis
174*	Malignant neoplasm of female breast
175*	Malignant neoplasm of male breast
198.2	Secondary malignant neoplasm of skin
198.81	Secondary malignant neoplasm of breast
233.0	Carcinoma in situ of breast
238.3	Neoplasm of uncertain behavior of breast

DRG 598   Malignant Breast Disorders with CC
GMLOS 3.9   AMLOS 5.1   RW 1.0817   ☑

Select principal diagnosis listed under DRG 597

DRG 599   Malignant Breast Disorders without CC/MCC
GMLOS 2.5   AMLOS 3.1   RW 0.6547   ☑

Select principal diagnosis listed under DRG 597

DRG 600   Nonmalignant Breast Disorders with CC/MCC
GMLOS 3.8   AMLOS 4.7   RW 0.9963   ☑

Principal Diagnosis
239.3	Neoplasm of unspecified nature of breast

Surgical	Medical	CC Indicator	MCC Indicator	Procedure Proxy

457.0	Postmastectomy lymphedema syndrome
610*	Benign mammary dysplasias
611*	Other disorders of breast
612*	Deformity and disproportion of reconstructed breast
757.6	Specified congenital anomalies of breast
793.8*	Nonspecific abnormal findings on radiological and other examinations of body structure, breast
996.54	Mechanical complication due to breast prosthesis
V50.41	Prophylactic breast removal

DRG 601   Nonmalignant Breast Disorders without CC/MCC
GMLOS 2.8   AMLOS 3.4   RW 0.6445   ☑

Select principal diagnosis listed under DRG 600

DRG 602   Cellulitis with MCC
GMLOS 5.0   AMLOS 6.3   RW 1.4607   ☑Ⓣ

Principal Diagnosis

035	Erysipelas
457.2	Lymphangitis
680*	Carbuncle and furuncle
681*	Cellulitis and abscess of finger and toe
682*	Other cellulitis and abscess
684	Impetigo
685*	Pilonidal cyst
686*	Other local infection of skin and subcutaneous tissue
910.1	Face, neck, and scalp except eye, abrasion or friction burn, infected
910.5	Face, neck, and scalp except eye, insect bite, nonvenomous, infected
910.7	Face, neck, and scalp except eye, superficial foreign body (splinter), without major open wound, infected
910.9	Other and unspecified superficial injury of face, neck, and scalp, infected
911.1	Trunk abrasion or friction burn, infected
911.3	Trunk blister, infected
911.5	Trunk, insect bite, nonvenomous, infected
911.7	Trunk, superficial foreign body (splinter), without major open wound, infected
911.9	Other and unspecified superficial injury of trunk, infected
912.1	Shoulder and upper arm, abrasion or friction burn, infected
912.3	Shoulder and upper arm, blister, infected
912.5	Shoulder and upper arm, insect bite, nonvenomous, infected
912.7	Shoulder and upper arm, superficial foreign body (splinter), without major open wound, infected
912.9	Other and unspecified superficial injury of shoulder and upper arm, infected
913.1	Elbow, forearm, and wrist, abrasion or friction burn, infected
913.3	Elbow, forearm, and wrist, blister infected
913.5	Elbow, forearm, and wrist, insect bite, nonvenomous, infected
913.7	Elbow, forearm, and wrist, superficial foreign body (splinter), without major open wound, infected
913.9	Other and unspecified superficial injury of elbow, forearm, and wrist, infected
914.1	Hand(s) except finger(s) alone, abrasion or friction burn, infected
914.3	Hand(s) except finger(s) alone, blister, infected
914.5	Hand(s) except finger(s) alone, insect bite, nonvenomous, infected
914.7	Hand(s) except finger(s) alone, superficial foreign body (splinter) without major open wound, infected
914.9	Other and unspecified superficial injury of hand(s) except finger(s) alone, infected
915.1	Finger, abrasion or friction burn, infected
915.3	Finger, blister, infected
915.5	Finger, insect bite, nonvenomous, infected
915.7	Finger, superficial foreign body (splinter), without major open wound, infected
915.9	Other and unspecified superficial injury of finger, infected
916.1	Hip, thigh, leg, and ankle, abrasion or friction burn, infected
916.3	Hip, thigh, leg, and ankle, blister, infected
916.5	Hip, thigh, leg, and ankle, insect bite, nonvenomous, infected
916.7	Hip, thigh, leg, and ankle, superficial foreign body (splinter), without major open wound, infected
916.9	Other and unspecified superficial injury of hip, thigh, leg, and ankle, infected
917.1	Foot and toe(s), abrasion or friction burn, infected
917.3	Foot and toe(s), blister, infected
917.5	Foot and toe(s), insect bite, nonvenomous, infected
917.7	Foot and toe(s), superficial foreign body (splinter), without major open wound, infected
917.9	Other and unspecified superficial injury of foot and toes, infected
919.1	Other, multiple, and unspecified sites, abrasion or friction burn, infected
919.3	Other, multiple, and unspecified sites, blister, infected
919.5	Other, multiple, and unspecified sites, insect bite, nonvenomous, infected
919.7	Other, multiple, and unspecified sites, superficial foreign body (splinter), without major open wound, infected
919.9	Other and unspecified superficial injury of other, multiple, and unspecified sites, infected

DRG 603   Cellulitis without MCC
GMLOS 3.6   AMLOS 4.2   RW 0.8402   ☑Ⓣ

Select principal diagnosis listed under DRG 602

DRG 604   Trauma to the Skin, Subcutaneous Tissue and Breast with MCC
GMLOS 3.9   AMLOS 5.1   RW 1.3223   ☑

Principal Diagnosis

873.0	Open wound of scalp, without mention of complication
873.1	Open wound of scalp, complicated
873.40	Open wound of face, unspecified site, without mention of complication
873.41	Open wound of cheek, without mention of complication
873.42	Open wound of forehead, without mention of complication
873.49	Open wound of face, other and multiple sites, without mention of complication
873.50	Open wound of face, unspecified site, complicated
873.51	Open wound of cheek, complicated
873.52	Open wound of forehead, complicated
873.59	Open wound of face, other and multiple sites, complicated
873.8	Other and unspecified open wound of head without mention of complication
873.9	Other and unspecified open wound of head, complicated
874.8	Open wound of other and unspecified parts of neck, without mention of complication
874.9	Open wound of other and unspecified parts of neck, complicated
875.0	Open wound of chest (wall), without mention of complication
876*	Open wound of back
877*	Open wound of buttock
879.0	Open wound of breast, without mention of complication
879.1	Open wound of breast, complicated
879.2	Open wound of abdominal wall, anterior, without mention of complication
879.4	Open wound of abdominal wall, lateral, without mention of complication
879.6	Open wound of other and unspecified parts of trunk, without mention of complication

---

Ⓣ *Transfer DRG*   ⑤ᴾ *Special Payment*   ☑ *Optimization Potential*   ᵂᵁ *Targeted Potential*   * *Code Range*   ● *New DRG*   ▲ *Revised DRG Title*

879.8	Open wound(s) (multiple) of unspecified site(s), without mention of complication
880.0*	Open wound of shoulder and upper arm, without mention of complication
881.0*	Open wound of elbow, forearm, and wrist, without mention of complication
882.0	Open wound of hand except finger(s) alone, without mention of complication
883.0	Open wound of finger(s), without mention of complication
884.0	Multiple and unspecified open wound of upper limb, without mention of complication
890.0	Open wound of hip and thigh, without mention of complication
891.0	Open wound of knee, leg (except thigh), and ankle, without mention of complication
892.0	Open wound of foot except toe(s) alone, without mention of complication
893.0	Open wound of toe(s), without mention of complication
894.0	Multiple and unspecified open wound of lower limb, without mention of complication
906*	Late effects of injuries to skin and subcutaneous tissues
910.0	Face, neck, and scalp, except eye, abrasion or friction burn, without mention of infection
910.6	Face, neck, and scalp, except eye, superficial foreign body (splinter), without major open wound or mention of infection
910.8	Other and unspecified superficial injury of face, neck, and scalp, without mention of infection
911.0	Trunk abrasion or friction burn, without mention of infection
911.6	Trunk, superficial foreign body (splinter), without major open wound and without mention of infection
911.8	Other and unspecified superficial injury of trunk, without mention of infection
912.0	Shoulder and upper arm, abrasion or friction burn, without mention of infection
912.2	Shoulder and upper arm, blister, without mention of infection
912.6	Shoulder and upper arm, superficial foreign body (splinter), without major open wound and without mention of infection
912.8	Other and unspecified superficial injury of shoulder and upper arm, without mention of infection
913.0	Elbow, forearm, and wrist, abrasion or friction burn, without mention of infection
913.6	Elbow, forearm, and wrist, superficial foreign body (splinter), without major open wound and without mention of infection
913.8	Other and unspecified superficial injury of elbow, forearm, and wrist, without mention of infection
914.0	Hand(s) except finger(s) alone, abrasion or friction burn, without mention of infection
914.6	Hand(s) except finger(s) alone, superficial foreign body (splinter), without major open wound and without mention of infection
914.8	Other and unspecified superficial injury of hand(s) except finger(s) alone, without mention of infection
915.0	Abrasion or friction burn of finger, without mention of infection
915.6	Finger, superficial foreign body (splinter), without major open wound and without mention of infection
915.8	Other and unspecified superficial injury of finger without mention of infection
916.0	Hip, thigh, leg, and ankle, abrasion or friction burn, without mention of infection
916.6	Hip, thigh, leg, and ankle, superficial foreign body (splinter), without major open wound and without mention of infection
916.8	Other and unspecified superficial injury of hip, thigh, leg, and ankle, without mention of infection
917.0	Abrasion or friction burn of foot and toe(s), without mention of infection
917.6	Foot and toe(s), superficial foreign body (splinter), without major open wound and without mention of infection
917.8	Other and unspecified superficial injury of foot and toes, without mention of infection
919.0	Abrasion or friction burn of other, multiple, and unspecified sites, without mention of infection
919.6	Other, multiple, and unspecified sites, superficial foreign body (splinter), without major open wound and without mention of infection
919.8	Other and unspecified superficial injury of other, multiple, and unspecified sites, without mention of infection
920	Contusion of face, scalp, and neck except eye(s)
922.0	Contusion of breast
922.1	Contusion of chest wall
922.2	Contusion of abdominal wall
922.3*	Contusion of trunk
922.8	Contusion of multiple sites of trunk
922.9	Contusion of unspecified part of trunk
923*	Contusion of upper limb
924*	Contusion of lower limb and of other and unspecified sites

DRG 605   Trauma to the Skin, Subcutaneous Tissue & Breast without MCC

GMLOS 2.6	AMLOS 3.2	RW 0.7372	☑

Select principal diagnosis listed under DRG 604

DRG 606   Minor Skin Disorders with MCC

GMLOS 4.3	AMLOS 6.0	RW 1.3594	☑

Principal Diagnosis

006.6	Amebic skin ulceration
017.0*	Tuberculosis of skin and subcutaneous cellular tissue
022.0	Cutaneous anthrax
031.1	Cutaneous diseases due to other mycobacteria
032.85	Cutaneous diphtheria
039.0	Cutaneous actinomycotic infection
039.3	Cervicofacial actinomycotic infection
039.4	Madura foot
051.1	Pseudocowpox
051.2	Contagious pustular dermatitis
054.0	Eczema herpeticum
054.6	Herpetic whitlow
054.9	Herpes simplex without mention of complication
058.8*	Other human herpesvirus infections
078.0	Molluscum contagiosum
078.1*	Viral warts
085.1	Cutaneous leishmaniasis, urban
085.2	Cutaneous leishmaniasis, Asian desert
085.3	Cutaneous leishmaniasis, Ethiopian
085.4	Cutaneous leishmaniasis, American
085.5	Mucocutaneous leishmaniasis, (American)
091.3	Secondary syphilis of skin or mucous membranes
091.82	Early syphilis, syphilitic alopecia
102.0	Initial lesions of yaws
102.1	Multiple papillomata and wet crab yaws due to yaws
102.2	Other early skin lesions due to yaws
102.3	Hyperkeratosis due to yaws
102.4	Gummata and ulcers due to yaws
103.0	Primary lesions of pinta
103.1	Intermediate lesions of pinta
103.3	Mixed lesions of pinta
110*	Dermatophytosis
111*	Dermatomycosis, other and unspecified
112.3	Candidiasis of skin and nails
114.1	Primary extrapulmonary coccidioidomycosis
120.3	Cutaneous schistosomiasis
132*	Pediculosis and phthirus infestation

Surgical	Medical	CC Indicator	MCC Indicator	Procedure Proxy

MDC 9: Diseases And Disorders Of The Skin, Subcutaneous Tissue And Breast—MEDICAL

133*	Acariasis
134*	Other infestation
173.0*	Other and unspecified malignant neoplasm of skin of lip
173.2*	Other and unspecified malignant neoplasm of skin of ear and external auditory canal
173.3*	Other and unspecified malignant neoplasm of skin of other and unspecified parts of face
173.4*	Other and unspecified malignant neoplasm of scalp and skin of neck
173.5*	Other and unspecified malignant neoplasm of skin of trunk, except scrotum
173.6*	Other and unspecified malignant neoplasm of skin of upper limb, including shoulder
173.7*	Other and unspecified malignant neoplasm of skin of lower limb, including hip
173.8*	Other and unspecified malignant neoplasm of other specified sites of skin
173.9*	Other and unspecified malignant neoplasm of skin, site unspecified
176.0	Kaposi's sarcoma of skin
176.1	Kaposi's sarcoma of soft tissue
176.8	Kaposi's sarcoma of other specified sites
176.9	Kaposi's sarcoma of unspecified site
214.0	Lipoma of skin and subcutaneous tissue of face
214.1	Lipoma of other skin and subcutaneous tissue
214.8	Lipoma of other specified sites
214.9	Lipoma of unspecified site
216.0	Benign neoplasm of skin of lip
216.2	Benign neoplasm of ear and external auditory canal
216.3	Benign neoplasm of skin of other and unspecified parts of face
216.4	Benign neoplasm of scalp and skin of neck
216.5	Benign neoplasm of skin of trunk, except scrotum
216.6	Benign neoplasm of skin of upper limb, including shoulder
216.7	Benign neoplasm of skin of lower limb, including hip
216.8	Benign neoplasm of other specified sites of skin
216.9	Benign neoplasm of skin, site unspecified
217	Benign neoplasm of breast
228.01	Hemangioma of skin and subcutaneous tissue
232.0	Carcinoma in situ of skin of lip
232.2	Carcinoma in situ of skin of ear and external auditory canal
232.3	Carcinoma in situ of skin of other and unspecified parts of face
232.4	Carcinoma in situ of scalp and skin of neck
232.5	Carcinoma in situ of skin of trunk, except scrotum
232.6	Carcinoma in situ of skin of upper limb, including shoulder
232.7	Carcinoma in situ of skin of lower limb, including hip
232.8	Carcinoma in situ of other specified sites of skin
232.9	Carcinoma in situ of skin, site unspecified
238.2	Neoplasm of uncertain behavior of skin
306.3	Skin malfunction arising from mental factors
374.51	Xanthelasma of eyelid
448.1	Nevus, non-neoplastic
457.1	Other noninfectious lymphedema
617.6	Endometriosis in scar of skin
690*	Erythematosquamous dermatosis
691*	Atopic dermatitis and related conditions
692*	Contact dermatitis and other eczema
693*	Dermatitis due to substances taken internally
694.0	Dermatitis herpetiformis
694.1	Subcorneal pustular dermatosis
694.2	Juvenile dermatitis herpetiformis
694.3	Impetigo herpetiformis
695.3	Rosacea
695.5*	Exfoliation due to erythematous conditions according to extent of body surface involved
695.89	Other specified erythematous condition
695.9	Unspecified erythematous condition
696.3	Pityriasis rosea
696.4	Pityriasis rubra pilaris

696.5	Other and unspecified pityriasis
696.8	Psoriasis related disease NEC
697*	Lichen
698.0	Pruritus ani
698.2	Prurigo
698.3	Lichenification and lichen simplex chronicus
698.4	Dermatitis factitia (artefacta)
698.8	Other specified pruritic conditions
698.9	Unspecified pruritic disorder
700	Corns and callosities
701*	Other hypertrophic and atrophic conditions of skin
702*	Other dermatoses
703*	Diseases of nail
704*	Diseases of hair and hair follicles
705*	Disorders of sweat glands
706*	Diseases of sebaceous glands
708*	Urticaria
709*	Other disorders of skin and subcutaneous tissue
723.6	Panniculitis specified as affecting neck
729.3*	Unspecified panniculitis
744.5	Congenital webbing of neck
744.9	Unspecified congenital anomaly of face and neck
757.0	Hereditary edema of legs
757.1	Ichthyosis congenita
757.2	Dermatoglyphic anomalies
757.31	Congenital ectodermal dysplasia
757.32	Congenital vascular hamartomas
757.33	Congenital pigmentary anomaly of skin
757.39	Other specified congenital anomaly of skin
757.4	Specified congenital anomalies of hair
757.5	Specified congenital anomalies of nails
757.8	Other specified congenital anomalies of the integument
757.9	Unspecified congenital anomaly of the integument
780.8	Generalized hyperhidrosis
782.1	Rash and other nonspecific skin eruption
782.2	Localized superficial swelling, mass, or lump
782.8	Changes in skin texture
782.9	Other symptoms involving skin and integumentary tissues
784.2	Swelling, mass, or lump in head and neck
910.2	Face, neck, and scalp except eye, blister, without mention of infection
910.3	Face, neck, and scalp except eye, blister, infected
910.4	Face, neck, and scalp except eye, insect bite, nonvenomous, without mention of infection
911.2	Trunk blister, without mention of infection
911.4	Trunk, insect bite, nonvenomous, without mention of infection
912.4	Shoulder and upper arm, insect bite, nonvenomous, without mention of infection
913.2	Elbow, forearm, and wrist, blister, without mention of infection
913.4	Elbow, forearm, and wrist, insect bite, nonvenomous, without mention of infection
914.2	Hand(s) except finger(s) alone, blister, without mention of infection
914.4	Hand(s) except finger(s) alone, insect bite, nonvenomous, without mention of infection
915.2	Finger, blister, without mention of infection
915.4	Finger, insect bite, nonvenomous, without mention of infection
916.2	Hip, thigh, leg, and ankle, blister, without mention of infection
916.4	Hip, thigh, leg, and ankle, insect bite, nonvenomous, without mention of infection
917.2	Foot and toe(s), blister, without mention of infection
917.4	Foot and toe(s), insect bite, nonvenomous, without mention of infection
919.2	Other, multiple, and unspecified sites, blister, without mention of infection

---

Ⓣ *Transfer DRG*　　Ⓢᴾ *Special Payment*　　☑ *Optimization Potential*　　▽ᵀᴳ *Targeted Potential*　　* *Code Range*　　● *New DRG*　　▲ *Revised DRG Title*

919.4	Other, multiple, and unspecified sites, insect bite, nonvenomous, without mention of infection
V42.3	Skin replaced by transplant
V50.0	Elective hair transplant for purposes other than remedying health states
V50.1	Other plastic surgery for unacceptable cosmetic appearance
V51*	Aftercare involving the use of plastic surgery
V59.1	Skin donor

DRG 607 **Minor Skin Disorders without MCC**

GMLOS 2.8   AMLOS 3.6   RW 0.7043   ☑

Select principal diagnosis listed under DRG 606

MDC 9: Diseases And Disorders Of The Skin, Subcutaneous Tissue And Breast—MEDICAL

Surgical   *Medical*   *CC Indicator*   *MCC Indicator*   *Procedure Proxy*

Endocrine, Nutritional And Metabolic Diseases And Disorders

017.50	240.9	246.2	250.82	255.13	263.0	271.4	276.51	779.34
017.51	241.0	246.3	250.83	255.14	263.1	271.8	276.52	781.7
017.52	241.1	246.8	250.90	255.2	263.2	271.9	276.61	783.0
017.53	241.9	246.9	250.91	255.3	263.8	272.0	276.69	783.1
017.54	242.00	249.00	250.92	255.41	263.9	272.1	276.7	783.21
017.55	242.01	249.01	250.93	255.42	264.8	272.2	276.8	783.22
017.56	242.10	249.10	251.0	255.5	264.9	272.3	276.9	783.3
017.60	242.11	249.11	251.1	255.6	265.0	272.4	277.00	783.40
017.61	242.20	249.20	251.2	255.8	265.1	272.5	277.09	783.41
017.62	242.21	249.21	251.3	255.9	265.2	272.6	277.1	783.42
017.63	242.30	249.30	251.4	257.0	266.0	272.7	277.2	783.43
017.64	242.31	249.31	251.8	257.1	266.1	272.8	277.5	783.5
017.65	242.40	249.80	251.9	257.2	266.2	272.9	277.6	783.6
017.66	242.41	249.81	252.00	257.8	266.9	273.4	277.7	783.7
122.2	242.80	249.90	252.01	257.9	267	275.01	277.81	783.9
193	242.81	249.91	252.02	258.01	268.9	275.02	277.82	790.21
194.0	242.90	250.00	252.08	258.02	269.0	275.03	277.83	790.22
194.1	242.91	250.01	252.1	258.03	269.1	275.09	277.84	790.29
194.3	243	250.02	252.8	258.1	269.2	275.1	277.85	791.5
194.8	244.0	250.03	252.9	258.8	269.3	275.2	277.86	791.6
194.9	244.1	250.10	253.0	258.9	269.8	275.3	277.87	794.5
198.7	244.2	250.11	253.1	259.0	269.9	275.40	277.89	794.6
211.7	244.3	250.12	253.2	259.1	270.0	275.41	277.9	794.7
226	244.8	250.13	253.3	259.2	270.1	275.42	278.00	868.01
227.0	244.9	250.20	253.4	259.3	270.2	275.49	278.01	868.11
227.1	245.0	250.21	253.5	259.4	270.3	275.5	278.02	874.2
227.3	245.1	250.22	253.6	259.50	270.4	275.8	278.1	874.3
227.8	245.2	250.23	253.7	259.51	270.5	275.9	278.2	V85.41
227.9	245.3	250.30	253.8	259.52	270.6	276.0	278.3	V85.42
237.0	245.4	250.31	253.9	259.8	270.7	276.1	278.4	V85.43
237.2	245.8	250.32	255.0	259.9	270.8	276.2	278.8	V85.44
237.4	245.9	250.33	255.10	260	270.9	276.3	306.6	V85.45
239.7	246.0	250.80	255.11	261	271.0	276.4	759.1	
240.0	246.1	250.81	255.12	262	271.1	276.50	759.2	

SURGICAL

DRG 614   Adrenal and Pituitary Procedures with CC/MCC
GMLOS 4.3   AMLOS 5.9   RW 2.5455

Operating Room Procedures
07.0*	Exploration of adrenal field
07.12	Open biopsy of adrenal gland
07.13	Biopsy of pituitary gland, transfrontal approach
07.14	Biopsy of pituitary gland, transsphenoidal approach
07.15	Biopsy of pituitary gland, unspecified approach
07.17	Biopsy of pineal gland
07.19	Other diagnostic procedures on adrenal glands, pituitary gland, pineal gland, and thymus
07.2*	Partial adrenalectomy
07.3	Bilateral adrenalectomy
07.4*	Other operations on adrenal glands, nerves, and vessels
07.5*	Operations on pineal gland
07.6*	Hypophysectomy
07.7*	Other operations on hypophysis

DRG 615   Adrenal and Pituitary Procedures without CC/MCC
GMLOS 2.3   AMLOS 2.7   RW 1.4579   ☑

Select operating room procedures listed under DRG 614

DRG 616   Amputation of Lower Limb for Endocrine, Nutritional, and Metabolic Disorders with MCC
GMLOS 10.9   AMLOS 13.1   RW 4.0773   ☑Ⓣ

Operating Room Procedures
84.10	Lower limb amputation, not otherwise specified
84.11	Amputation of toe
84.12	Amputation through foot
84.13	Disarticulation of ankle
84.14	Amputation of ankle through malleoli of tibia and fibula
84.15	Other amputation below knee
84.16	Disarticulation of knee
84.17	Amputation above knee

DRG 617   Amputation of Lower Limb for Endocrine, Nutritional, and Metabolic Disorders with CC
GMLOS 6.1   AMLOS 7.4   RW 2.0071   ☑Ⓣ

Select operating room procedures listed under DRG 616

DRG 618   Amputation of Lower Limb for Endocrine, Nutritional, and Metabolic Disorders without CC/MCC
GMLOS 4.3   AMLOS 5.2   RW 1.2489   ☑Ⓣ

Select operating room procedures listed under DRG 616

DRG 619   O.R. Procedures for Obesity with MCC
GMLOS 4.8   AMLOS 7.7   RW 3.6200

Operating Room Procedures
43.82	Laparoscopic vertical (sleeve) gastrectomy
43.89	Open and other partial gastrectomy
44.3*	Gastroenterostomy without gastrectomy
44.5	Revision of gastric anastomosis
44.68	Laparoscopic gastroplasty
44.69	Other repair of stomach
44.95	Laparoscopic gastric restrictive procedure
44.96	Laparoscopic revision of gastric restrictive procedure
44.97	Laparoscopic removal of gastric restrictive device(s)
44.98	(Laparoscopic) adjustment of size of adjustable gastric restrictive device
44.99	Other operations on stomach

45.90	Intestinal anastomosis, not otherwise specified
45.91	Small-to-small intestinal anastomosis
85.31	Unilateral reduction mammoplasty
85.32	Bilateral reduction mammoplasty
86.83	Size reduction plastic operation
86.87	Fat graft of skin and subcutaneous tissue
86.89	Other repair and reconstruction of skin and subcutaneous tissue

DRG 620   O.R. Procedures for Obesity with CC
GMLOS 2.7   AMLOS 3.2   RW 1.9399   ☑

Select operating room procedures listed under DRG 619

DRG 621   O.R. Procedures for Obesity without CC/MCC
GMLOS 1.8   AMLOS 2.0   RW 1.5772   ☑

Select operating room procedures listed under DRG 619

DRG 622   Skin Grafts and Wound Debridement for Endocrine, Nutritional and Metabolic Disorders with MCC
GMLOS 9.1   AMLOS 12.2   RW 3.3505   ☑Ⓣ

Operating Room Procedures
84.3	Revision of amputation stump
86.22	Excisional debridement of wound, infection, or burn
86.60	Free skin graft, not otherwise specified
86.63	Full-thickness skin graft to other sites
86.67	Dermal regenerative graft
86.69	Other skin graft to other sites
86.70	Pedicle or flap graft, not otherwise specified
86.71	Cutting and preparation of pedicle grafts or flaps
86.72	Advancement of pedicle graft
86.74	Attachment of pedicle or flap graft to other sites
86.75	Revision of pedicle or flap graft
86.91	Excision of skin for graft
86.93	Insertion of tissue expander

DRG 623   Skin Grafts and Wound Debridement for Endocrine, Nutritional and Metabolic Disorders with CC
GMLOS 5.7   AMLOS 7.1   RW 1.8239   ☑Ⓣ

Select operating room procedures listed under DRG 622

DRG 624   Skin Grafts and Wound Debridement for Endocrine, Nutritional and Metabolic Disorders without CC/MCC
GMLOS 3.5   AMLOS 4.2   RW 0.9635   ☑Ⓣ

Select operating room procedures listed under DRG 622

DRG 625   Thyroid, Parathyroid and Thyroglossal Procedures with MCC
GMLOS 4.4   AMLOS 7.3   RW 2.4009

Operating Room Procedures
06.02	Reopening of wound of thyroid field
06.09	Other incision of thyroid field
06.12	Open biopsy of thyroid gland
06.13	Biopsy of parathyroid gland
06.19	Other diagnostic procedures on thyroid and parathyroid glands
06.2	Unilateral thyroid lobectomy
06.3*	Other partial thyroidectomy
06.4	Complete thyroidectomy
06.5*	Substernal thyroidectomy
06.6	Excision of lingual thyroid
06.7	Excision of thyroglossal duct or tract
06.8*	Parathyroidectomy
06.91	Division of thyroid isthmus

Surgical	Medical	CC Indicator	MCC Indicator	Procedure Proxy

06.92	Ligation of thyroid vessels
06.93	Suture of thyroid gland
06.94	Thyroid tissue reimplantation
06.95	Parathyroid tissue reimplantation
06.98	Other operations on thyroid glands
06.99	Other operations on parathyroid glands
17.62	Laser interstitial thermal therapy [LITT] of lesion or tissue of head and neck under guidance

DRG 626 Thyroid, Parathyroid and Thyroglossal Procedures with CC
GMLOS 2.0   AMLOS 2.8   RW 1.2459   ☑

Select operating room procedures listed under DRG 625

DRG 627 Thyroid, Parathyroid and Thyroglossal Procedures without CC/MCC
GMLOS 1.3   AMLOS 1.4   RW 0.8458   ☑

Select operating room procedures listed under DRG 625

DRG 628 Other Endocrine, Nutritional and Metabolic O.R. Procedures with MCC
GMLOS 6.6   AMLOS 9.6   RW 3.3515   ⊤

Operating Room Procedures

00.70	Revision of hip replacement, both acetabular and femoral components
00.71	Revision of hip replacement, acetabular component
00.72	Revision of hip replacement, femoral component
00.73	Revision of hip replacement, acetabular liner and/or femoral head only
00.86	Resurfacing hip, partial, femoral head
00.87	Resurfacing hip, partial, acetabulum
01.15	Biopsy of skull
07.16	Biopsy of thymus
07.8*	Thymectomy
07.9*	Other operations on thymus
08.20	Removal of lesion of eyelid, not otherwise specified
08.38	Correction of lid retraction
08.70	Reconstruction of eyelid, not otherwise specified
12.64	Trabeculectomy ab externo
12.72	Cyclocryotherapy
12.79	Other glaucoma procedures
13.1*	Intracapsular extraction of lens
13.59	Other extracapsular extraction of lens
14.49	Other scleral buckling
14.54	Repair of retinal detachment with laser photocoagulation
14.6	Removal of surgically implanted material from posterior segment of eye
14.72	Other removal of vitreous
14.74	Other mechanical vitrectomy
16.99	Other operations on eyeball
17.35	Laparoscopic left hemicolectomy
17.56	Atherectomy of other non-coronary vessel(s)
34.26	Open biopsy of mediastinum
34.3	Excision or destruction of lesion or tissue of mediastinum
34.4	Excision or destruction of lesion of chest wall
38.00	Incision of vessel, unspecified site
38.02	Incision of other vessels of head and neck
38.03	Incision of upper limb vessels
38.08	Incision of lower limb arteries
38.12	Endarterectomy of other vessels of head and neck
38.13	Endarterectomy of upper limb vessels
38.18	Endarterectomy of lower limb arteries
38.21	Biopsy of blood vessel
38.29	Other diagnostic procedures on blood vessels
38.30	Resection of vessel with anastomosis, unspecified site
38.33	Resection of upper limb vessels with anastomosis
38.38	Resection of lower limb arteries with anastomosis
38.43	Resection of upper limb vessels with replacement

38.48	Resection of lower limb arteries with replacement
38.55	Ligation and stripping of varicose veins of other thoracic vessel
38.60	Other excision of vessels, unspecified site
38.63	Other excision of upper limb vessels
38.68	Other excision of lower limb arteries
38.7	Interruption of the vena cava
38.83	Other surgical occlusion of upper limb vessels
38.88	Other surgical occlusion of lower limb arteries
39.25	Aorta-iliac-femoral bypass
39.27	Arteriovenostomy for renal dialysis
39.29	Other (peripheral) vascular shunt or bypass
39.31	Suture of artery
39.41	Control of hemorrhage following vascular surgery
39.42	Revision of arteriovenous shunt for renal dialysis
39.49	Other revision of vascular procedure
39.50	Angioplasty of other non-coronary vessel(s)
39.56	Repair of blood vessel with tissue patch graft
39.57	Repair of blood vessel with synthetic patch graft
39.58	Repair of blood vessel with unspecified type of patch graft
39.59	Other repair of vessel
39.91	Freeing of vessel
39.93	Insertion of vessel-to-vessel cannula
39.98	Control of hemorrhage, not otherwise specified
40.1*	Diagnostic procedures on lymphatic structures
40.21	Excision of deep cervical lymph node
40.29	Simple excision of other lymphatic structure
40.3	Regional lymph node excision
40.4*	Radical excision of cervical lymph nodes
40.52	Radical excision of periaortic lymph nodes
40.53	Radical excision of iliac lymph nodes
43.0	Gastrotomy
43.42	Local excision of other lesion or tissue of stomach
43.7	Partial gastrectomy with anastomosis to jejunum
44.92	Intraoperative manipulation of stomach
45.41	Excision of lesion or tissue of large intestine
45.62	Other partial resection of small intestine
45.75	Open and other left hemicolectomy
45.93	Other small-to-large intestinal anastomosis
45.94	Large-to-large intestinal anastomosis
50.12	Open biopsy of liver
52.12	Open biopsy of pancreas
52.19	Other diagnostic procedures on pancreas
52.22	Other excision or destruction of lesion or tissue of pancreas or pancreatic duct
52.5*	Partial pancreatectomy
52.80	Pancreatic transplant, not otherwise specified
52.82	Homotransplant of pancreas
52.83	Heterotransplant of pancreas
54.11	Exploratory laparotomy
54.3	Excision or destruction of lesion or tissue of abdominal wall or umbilicus
54.4	Excision or destruction of peritoneal tissue
54.59	Other lysis of peritoneal adhesions
62.7	Insertion of testicular prosthesis
65.22	Wedge resection of ovary
65.24	Laparoscopic wedge resection of ovary
77.27	Wedge osteotomy of tibia and fibula
77.38	Other division of tarsals and metatarsals
77.4*	Biopsy of bone
77.61	Local excision of lesion or tissue of scapula, clavicle, and thorax (ribs and sternum)
77.68	Local excision of lesion or tissue of tarsals and metatarsals
77.69	Local excision of lesion or tissue of other bone, except facial bones
77.88	Other partial ostectomy of tarsals and metatarsals
77.89	Other partial ostectomy of other bone, except facial bones
78.65	Removal of implanted device from femur
79.35	Open reduction of fracture of femur with internal fixation
80.10	Other arthrotomy, unspecified site

⊤ *Transfer DRG*   ⓢ *Special Payment*   ☑ *Optimization Potential*   ▽ *Targeted Potential*   * *Code Range*   ● *New DRG*   ▲ *Revised DRG Title*

80.12	Other arthrotomy of elbow	
80.16	Other arthrotomy of knee	
80.26	Arthroscopy of knee	
80.6	Excision of semilunar cartilage of knee	
80.82	Other local excision or destruction of lesion of elbow joint	
80.88	Other local excision or destruction of lesion of joint of foot and toe	
80.98	Other excision of joint of foot and toe	
81.11	Ankle fusion	
81.23	Arthrodesis of shoulder	
81.52	Partial hip replacement	
81.53	Revision of hip replacement, not otherwise specified	
82.21	Excision of lesion of tendon sheath of hand	
82.33	Other tenonectomy of hand	
83.13	Other tenotomy	
83.31	Excision of lesion of tendon sheath	
83.39	Excision of lesion of other soft tissue	
83.65	Other suture of muscle or fascia	
83.75	Tendon transfer or transplantation	
83.79	Other muscle transposition	
85.12	Open biopsy of breast	
85.21	Local excision of lesion of breast	
86.06	Insertion of totally implantable infusion pump	
92.27	Implantation or insertion of radioactive elements	

OR

Nonoperating Room Procedures

92.3*   Stereotactic radiosurgery

DRG 629 Other Endocrine, Nutritional and Metabolic O.R. Procedures with CC
GMLOS 6.0   AMLOS 7.2   RW 2.1292   ☑Ⓣ

Select operating or nonoperating room procedures listed under DRG 628

DRG 630 Other Endocrine, Nutritional and Metabolic O.R. Procedures without CC/MCC
GMLOS 3.0   AMLOS 3.8   RW 1.3444   ☑Ⓣ

Select operating or nonoperating room procedures listed under DRG 628

MEDICAL

DRG 637 Diabetes with MCC
GMLOS 4.2   AMLOS 5.5   RW 1.3888   ☑Ⓣ

Principal Diagnosis

249.0*	Secondary diabetes mellitus without mention of complication
249.1*	Secondary diabetes mellitus with ketoacidosis
249.2*	Secondary diabetes mellitus with hyperosmolarity
249.3*	Secondary diabetes mellitus with other coma
249.8*	Secondary diabetes mellitus with other specified manifestations
249.9*	Secondary diabetes mellitus with unspecified complication
250.0*	Diabetes mellitus without mention of complication
250.1*	Diabetes with ketoacidosis
250.2*	Diabetes with hyperosmolarity
250.3*	Diabetes with other coma
250.8*	Diabetes with other specified manifestations
250.9*	Diabetes with unspecified complication
791.5	Glycosuria

DRG 638 Diabetes with CC
GMLOS 3.0   AMLOS 3.7   RW 0.8252   ☑Ⓣ

Select principal diagnosis listed under DRG 637

DRG 639 Diabetes without CC/MCC
GMLOS 2.2   AMLOS 2.6   RW 0.5708   ☑Ⓣ

Select principal diagnosis listed under DRG 637

DRG 640 Miscellaneous Disorders of Nutrition, Metabolism, and Fluids and Electrolytes with MCC
GMLOS 3.3   AMLOS 4.6   RW 1.1111   ☑▽Ⓣ

Principal Diagnosis

251.0	Hypoglycemic coma
251.2	Hypoglycemia, unspecified
251.3	Postsurgical hypoinsulinemia
260	Kwashiorkor
261	Nutritional marasmus
262	Other severe protein-calorie malnutrition
263*	Other and unspecified protein-calorie malnutrition
264.8	Other manifestations of vitamin A deficiency
264.9	Unspecified vitamin A deficiency
265*	Thiamine and niacin deficiency states
266*	Deficiency of B-complex components
267	Ascorbic acid deficiency
268.9	Unspecified vitamin D deficiency
269*	Other nutritional deficiencies
275.2	Disorders of magnesium metabolism
275.4*	Disorders of calcium metabolism
275.5	Hungry bone syndrome
276*	Disorders of fluid, electrolyte, and acid-base balance
277.00	Cystic fibrosis without mention of meconium ileus
277.09	Cystic fibrosis with other manifestations
278.00	Obesity, unspecified
278.01	Morbid obesity
278.02	Overweight
278.1	Localized adiposity
278.2	Hypervitaminosis A
278.3	Hypercarotinemia
278.4	Hypervitaminosis D
278.8	Other hyperalimentation
779.34	Failure to thrive in newborn
781.7	Tetany
783*	Symptoms concerning nutrition, metabolism, and development
790.2*	Abnormal glucose
791.6	Acetonuria
V85.4*	Body Mass Index 40 and over, adult

DRG 641 Miscellaneous Disorders of Nutrition, Metabolism, and Fluids and Electrolytes without MCC
GMLOS 2.8   AMLOS 3.4   RW 0.6992   ☑▽Ⓣ

Select principal diagnosis listed under DRG 640

DRG 642 Inborn and Other Disorders of Metabolism
GMLOS 3.2   AMLOS 4.2   RW 1.0674

Principal Diagnosis

270*	Disorders of amino-acid transport and metabolism
271.0	Glycogenosis
271.1	Galactosemia
271.4	Renal glycosuria
271.8	Other specified disorders of carbohydrate transport and metabolism
271.9	Unspecified disorder of carbohydrate transport and metabolism
272*	Disorders of lipid metabolism

Surgical	Medical	CC Indicator	MCC Indicator	Procedure Proxy

273.4	Alpha-1-antitrypsin deficiency
275.0*	Disorders of iron metabolism
275.1	Disorders of copper metabolism
275.3	Disorders of phosphorus metabolism
275.8	Other specified disorders of mineral metabolism
275.9	Unspecified disorder of mineral metabolism
277.1	Disorders of porphyrin metabolism
277.2	Other disorders of purine and pyrimidine metabolism
277.5	Mucopolysaccharidosis
277.6	Other deficiencies of circulating enzymes
277.7	Dysmetabolic Syndrome X
277.81	Primary carnitine deficiency
277.82	Carnitine deficiency due to inborn errors of metabolism
277.83	Iatrogenic carnitine deficiency
277.84	Other secondary carnitine deficiency
277.85	Disorders of fatty acid oxidation
277.86	Peroxisomal disorders
277.87	Disorders of mitochondrial metabolism
277.89	Other specified disorders of metabolism
277.9	Unspecified disorder of metabolism

DRG 643   Endocrine Disorders with MCC

GMLOS 5.5   **AMLOS 6.9**   **RW 1.6693**   ☑Ⓣ

Principal Diagnosis

017.5*	Tuberculosis of thyroid gland
017.6*	Tuberculosis of adrenal glands
122.2	Echinococcus granulosus infection of thyroid
193	Malignant neoplasm of thyroid gland
194.0	Malignant neoplasm of adrenal gland
194.1	Malignant neoplasm of parathyroid gland
194.3	Malignant neoplasm of pituitary gland and craniopharyngeal duct
194.8	Malignant neoplasm of other endocrine glands and related structures
194.9	Malignant neoplasm of endocrine gland, site unspecified
198.7	Secondary malignant neoplasm of adrenal gland
211.7	Benign neoplasm of islets of Langerhans
226	Benign neoplasm of thyroid glands
227.0	Benign neoplasm of adrenal gland
227.1	Benign neoplasm of parathyroid gland
227.3	Benign neoplasm of pituitary gland and craniopharyngeal duct (pouch)
227.8	Benign neoplasm of other endocrine glands and related structures
227.9	Benign neoplasm of endocrine gland, site unspecified
237.0	Neoplasm of uncertain behavior of pituitary gland and craniopharyngeal duct
237.2	Neoplasm of uncertain behavior of adrenal gland
237.4	Neoplasm of uncertain behavior of other and unspecified endocrine glands
239.7	Neoplasm of unspecified nature of endocrine glands and other parts of nervous system
240*	Simple and unspecified goiter
241*	Nontoxic nodular goiter
242*	Thyrotoxicosis with or without goiter
243	Congenital hypothyroidism
244*	Acquired hypothyroidism
245*	Thyroiditis
246*	Other disorders of thyroid
251.1	Other specified hypoglycemia
251.4	Abnormality of secretion of glucagon
251.8	Other specified disorders of pancreatic internal secretion
251.9	Unspecified disorder of pancreatic internal secretion
252*	Disorders of parathyroid gland
253*	Disorders of the pituitary gland and its hypothalamic control
255*	Disorders of adrenal glands
257*	Testicular dysfunction
258*	Polyglandular dysfunction and related disorders
259*	Other endocrine disorders

306.6	Endocrine malfunction arising from mental factors
759.1	Congenital anomalies of adrenal gland
759.2	Congenital anomalies of other endocrine glands
794.5	Nonspecific abnormal results of thyroid function study
794.6	Nonspecific abnormal results of other endocrine function study
794.7	Nonspecific abnormal results of basal metabolism function study
868.01	Adrenal gland injury without mention of open wound into cavity
868.11	Adrenal gland injury, with open wound into cavity
874.2	Open wound of thyroid gland, without mention of complication
874.3	Open wound of thyroid gland, complicated

DRG 644   Endocrine Disorders with CC

GMLOS 3.9   **AMLOS 4.7**   **RW 1.0194**   ☑Ⓣ

Select principal diagnosis listed under DRG 643

DRG 645   Endocrine Disorders without CC/MCC

GMLOS 2.8   **AMLOS 3.4**   **RW 0.7041**   ☑Ⓣ

Select principal diagnosis listed under DRG 643

Ⓣ *Transfer DRG*   SP *Special Payment*   ☑ *Optimization Potential*   ᵛᵀᴳ *Targeted Potential*   * *Code Range*   ● *New DRG*   ▲ *Revised DRG Title*

114   Valid 10/01/2013-09/30/2014   © 2013 OptumInsight, Inc.

Diseases And Disorders Of The Kidney And Urinary Tract

016.00	098.30	239.4	581.3	589.0	595.3	599.5	788.30	866.13
016.01	098.31	239.5	581.81	589.1	595.4	599.60	788.31	867.0
016.02	099.54	249.40	581.89	589.9	595.81	599.69	788.32	867.1
016.03	120.0	249.41	581.9	590.00	595.82	599.70	788.33	867.2
016.04	137.2	250.40	582.0	590.01	595.89	599.71	788.34	867.3
016.05	188.0	250.41	582.1	590.10	595.9	599.72	788.35	868.04
016.06	188.1	250.42	582.2	590.11	596.0	599.81	788.36	868.14
016.10	188.2	250.43	582.4	590.2	596.1	599.82	788.37	939.0
016.11	188.3	274.10	582.81	590.3	596.2	599.83	788.38	939.9
016.12	188.4	274.11	582.89	590.80	596.3	599.84	788.39	958.5
016.13	188.5	274.19	582.9	590.81	596.4	599.89	788.41	996.30
016.14	188.6	277.88	583.0	590.9	596.51	599.9	788.42	996.31
016.15	188.7	306.50	583.1	591	596.52	753.0	788.43	996.39
016.16	188.8	306.53	583.2	592.0	596.53	753.10	788.5	996.64
016.20	188.9	306.59	583.4	592.1	596.54	753.11	788.61	996.65
016.21	189.0	344.61	583.6	592.9	596.55	753.12	788.62	996.76
016.22	189.1	403.00	583.7	593.0	596.59	753.13	788.63	996.81
016.23	189.2	403.01	583.81	593.1	596.6	753.14	788.64	997.5
016.24	189.3	403.10	583.89	593.2	596.7	753.15	788.65	997.72
016.25	189.4	403.11	583.9	593.3	596.81	753.16	788.69	V42.0
016.26	189.8	403.90	584.5	593.4	596.82	753.17	788.7	V43.5
016.30	189.9	403.91	584.6	593.5	596.83	753.19	788.8	V45.74
016.31	198.0	404.02	584.7	593.6	596.89	753.20	788.91	V53.6
016.32	198.1	404.12	584.8	593.70	596.9	753.21	788.99	V55.5
016.33	209.24	404.92	584.9	593.71	597.0	753.22	791.0	V55.6
016.34	209.64	440.1	585.1	593.72	597.80	753.23	791.1	V56.0
016.35	223.0	442.1	585.2	593.73	597.81	753.29	791.2	V56.1
016.36	223.1	443.23	585.3	593.81	597.89	753.3	791.7	V56.2
016.90	223.2	445.81	585.4	593.82	598.00	753.4	791.9	V56.31
016.91	223.3	447.3	585.5	593.89	598.01	753.5	793.5	V56.32
016.92	223.81	453.3	585.6	593.9	598.1	753.6	794.4	V56.8
016.93	223.89	580.0	585.9	594.0	598.2	753.7	794.9	V59.4
016.94	223.9	580.4	586	594.1	598.8	753.8	866.00	
016.95	233.7	580.81	587	594.2	598.9	753.9	866.01	
016.96	233.9	580.89	588.0	594.8	599.0	788.0	866.02	
032.84	236.7	580.9	588.1	594.9	599.1	788.1	866.03	
078.6	236.90	581.0	588.81	595.0	599.2	788.20	866.10	
095.4	236.91	581.1	588.89	595.1	599.3	788.21	866.11	
098.11	236.99	581.2	588.9	595.2	599.4	788.29	866.12	

SURGICAL

DRG 652   Kidney Transplant
GMLOS 5.8   AMLOS 6.8   RW 3.1530   ☑

Operating Room Procedure
55.69   Other kidney transplantation

DRG 653   Major Bladder Procedures with MCC
GMLOS 12.7   AMLOS 15.4   RW 5.9558   Ⓣ

Operating Room Procedures
57.6   Partial cystectomy
57.7*   Total cystectomy
57.83   Repair of fistula involving bladder and intestine
57.84   Repair of other fistula of bladder
57.85   Cystourethroplasty and plastic repair of bladder neck
57.86   Repair of bladder exstrophy
57.87   Reconstruction of urinary bladder
57.88   Other anastomosis of bladder
57.89   Other repair of bladder
70.53   Repair of cystocele and rectocele with graft or prosthesis

DRG 654   Major Bladder Procedures with CC
GMLOS 7.8   AMLOS 8.9   RW 3.0944   ☑Ⓣ

Select operating room procedures listed under DRG 653

DRG 655   Major Bladder Procedures without CC/MCC
GMLOS 4.7   AMLOS 5.5   RW 2.1671   ☑Ⓣ

Select operating room procedures listed under DRG 653

DRG 656   Kidney and Ureter Procedures for Neoplasm with MCC
GMLOS 7.2   AMLOS 9.3   RW 3.5221   ☑

Principal Diagnosis
188*   Malignant neoplasm of bladder
189*   Malignant neoplasm of kidney and other and unspecified urinary organs
198.0   Secondary malignant neoplasm of kidney
198.1   Secondary malignant neoplasm of other urinary organs
209.24   Malignant carcinoid tumor of the kidney
209.64   Benign carcinoid tumor of the kidney
223*   Benign neoplasm of kidney and other urinary organs
233.7   Carcinoma in situ of bladder
233.9   Carcinoma in situ of other and unspecified urinary organs
236.7   Neoplasm of uncertain behavior of bladder
236.9*   Neoplasm of uncertain behavior of other and unspecified urinary organs
239.4   Neoplasm of unspecified nature of bladder
239.5   Neoplasm of unspecified nature of other genitourinary organs

Operating Room Procedures
39.24   Aorta-renal bypass
39.26   Other intra-abdominal vascular shunt or bypass
39.55   Reimplantation of aberrant renal vessel
40.52   Radical excision of periaortic lymph nodes
40.53   Radical excision of iliac lymph nodes
40.54   Radical groin dissection
40.59   Radical excision of other lymph nodes
55.0*   Nephrotomy and nephrostomy
55.1*   Pyelotomy and pyelostomy
55.24   Open biopsy of kidney
55.29   Other diagnostic procedures on kidney
55.3*   Local excision or destruction of lesion or tissue of kidney
55.4   Partial nephrectomy
55.5*   Complete nephrectomy

55.61   Renal autotransplantation
55.7   Nephropexy
55.8*   Other repair of kidney
55.91   Decapsulation of kidney
55.97   Implantation or replacement of mechanical kidney
55.98   Removal of mechanical kidney
55.99   Other operations on kidney
56.1   Ureteral meatotomy
56.2   Ureterotomy
56.34   Open biopsy of ureter
56.39   Other diagnostic procedures on ureter
56.4*   Ureterectomy
56.5*   Cutaneous uretero-ileostomy
56.6*   Other external urinary diversion
56.7*   Other anastomosis or bypass of ureter
56.8*   Repair of ureter
56.92   Implantation of electronic ureteral stimulator
56.93   Replacement of electronic ureteral stimulator
56.94   Removal of electronic ureteral stimulator
56.95   Ligation of ureter
56.99   Other operations on ureter
59.00   Retroperitoneal dissection, not otherwise specified
59.02   Other lysis of perirenal or periureteral adhesions
59.03   Laparoscopic lysis of perirenal or periureteral adhesions
59.09   Other incision of perirenal or periureteral tissue

DRG 657   Kidney and Ureter Procedures for Neoplasm with CC
GMLOS 4.5   AMLOS 5.4   RW 2.0261   ☑

Select principal diagnosis and operating room procedures listed under DRG 656

DRG 658   Kidney and Ureter Procedures for Neoplasm without CC/MCC
GMLOS 2.8   AMLOS 3.1   RW 1.5074   ☑

Select principal diagnosis and operating room procedures listed under DRG 656

DRG 659   Kidney and Ureter Procedures for Non-neoplasm with MCC
GMLOS 7.6   AMLOS 10.3   RW 3.4051   ☑Ⓣ

Select only operating room procedures listed under DRG 656

DRG 660   Kidney and Ureter Procedures for Non-neoplasm with CC
GMLOS 4.3   AMLOS 5.6   RW 1.8827   ☑Ⓣ

Select only operating room procedures listed under DRG 656

DRG 661   Kidney and Ureter Procedures for Non-neoplasm without CC/MCC
GMLOS 2.3   AMLOS 2.8   RW 1.3435   ☑Ⓣ

Select only operating room procedures listed under DRG 656

DRG 662   Minor Bladder Procedures with MCC
GMLOS 7.7   AMLOS 10.2   RW 2.9801   ☑

Operating Room Procedures
57.12   Lysis of intraluminal adhesions with incision into bladder
57.18   Other suprapubic cystostomy
57.19   Other cystotomy
57.2*   Vesicostomy
57.34   Open biopsy of bladder
57.39   Other diagnostic procedures on bladder
57.5*   Other excision or destruction of bladder tissue
57.81   Suture of laceration of bladder
57.82   Closure of cystostomy
57.91   Sphincterotomy of bladder
57.93   Control of (postoperative) hemorrhage of bladder

Ⓣ *Transfer DRG*   SP *Special Payment*   ☑ *Optimization Potential*   V̄ *Targeted Potential*   * *Code Range*   ● *New DRG*   ▲ *Revised DRG Title*

116   Valid 10/01/2013-09/30/2014   © 2013 OptumInsight, Inc.

MDC 11: Diseases And Disorders Of The Kidney And

57.96	Implantation of electronic bladder stimulator	
57.97	Replacement of electronic bladder stimulator	
57.98	Removal of electronic bladder stimulator	
57.99	Other operations on bladder	
58.93	Implantation of artificial urinary sphincter (AUS)	
59.1*	Incision of perivesical tissue	
59.2*	Diagnostic procedures on perirenal and perivesical tissue	
59.3	Plication of urethrovesical junction	
59.4	Suprapubic sling operation	
59.5	Retropubic urethral suspension	
59.6	Paraurethral suspension	
59.71	Levator muscle operation for urethrovesical suspension	
59.79	Other repair of urinary stress incontinence	
59.91	Excision of perirenal or perivesical tissue	
59.92	Other operations on perirenal or perivesical tissue	
70.50	Repair of cystocele and rectocele	
70.51	Repair of cystocele	
70.54	Repair of cystocele with graft or prosthesis	
70.77	Vaginal suspension and fixation	
70.78	Vaginal suspension and fixation with graft or prosthesis	

DRG 663   Minor Bladder Procedures with CC
GMLOS 3.9   AMLOS 5.3   RW 1.5666   ☑

Select operating room procedures listed under DRG 662

DRG 664   Minor Bladder Procedures without CC/MCC
GMLOS 1.7   AMLOS 2.2   RW 1.2208   ☑

Select operating room procedures listed under DRG 662

DRG 665   Prostatectomy with MCC
GMLOS 9.2   AMLOS 11.7   RW 3.1414   ☑

Operating Room Procedures
60.2*	Transurethral prostatectomy
60.3	Suprapubic prostatectomy
60.4	Retropubic prostatectomy
60.5	Radical prostatectomy
60.62	Perineal prostatectomy
60.69	Other prostatectomy
60.96	Transurethral destruction of prostate tissue by microwave thermotherapy
60.97	Other transurethral destruction of prostate tissue by other thermotherapy

DRG 666   Prostatectomy with CC
GMLOS 4.5   AMLOS 6.2   RW 1.7042   ☑

Select operating room procedures listed under DRG 665

DRG 667   Prostatectomy without CC/MCC
GMLOS 2.0   AMLOS 2.6   RW 0.8949   ☑

Select operating room procedures listed under DRG 665

DRG 668   Transurethral Procedures with MCC
GMLOS 6.6   AMLOS 8.8   RW 2.5573   ☑

Operating Room Procedures
56.0	Transurethral removal of obstruction from ureter and renal pelvis
57.33	Closed (transurethral) biopsy of bladder
57.4*	Transurethral excision or destruction of bladder tissue
60.12	Open biopsy of prostate
60.95	Transurethral balloon dilation of the prostatic urethra

DRG 669   Transurethral Procedures with CC
GMLOS 3.0   AMLOS 4.1   RW 1.2693   ☑

Select operating room procedures listed under DRG 668

DRG 670   Transurethral Procedures without CC/MCC
GMLOS 1.9   AMLOS 2.4   RW 0.8354   ☑

Select operating room procedures listed under DRG 668

DRG 671   Urethral Procedures with CC/MCC
GMLOS 4.3   AMLOS 5.7   RW 1.5887   ☑

Operating Room Procedures
58.0	Urethrotomy
58.1	Urethral meatotomy
58.4*	Repair of urethra
58.5	Release of urethral stricture
58.91	Incision of periurethral tissue
58.92	Excision of periurethral tissue
58.99	Other operations on urethra and periurethral tissue

DRG 672   Urethral Procedures without CC/MCC
GMLOS 1.9   AMLOS 2.3   RW 0.8835   ☑

Select operating room procedures listed under DRG 671

DRG 673   Other Kidney and Urinary Tract Procedures with MCC
GMLOS 6.5   AMLOS 9.7   RW 3.1150

Operating Room Procedures
03.93	Implantation or replacement of spinal neurostimulator lead(s)
03.94	Removal of spinal neurostimulator lead(s)
04.92	Implantation or replacement of peripheral neurostimulator lead(s)
06.8*	Parathyroidectomy
17.56	Atherectomy of other non-coronary vessel(s)
33.20	Thoracoscopic lung biopsy
33.28	Open biopsy of lung
34.02	Exploratory thoracotomy
38.06	Incision of abdominal arteries
38.07	Incision of abdominal veins
38.16	Endarterectomy of abdominal arteries
38.21	Biopsy of blood vessel
38.36	Resection of abdominal arteries with anastomosis
38.37	Resection of abdominal veins with anastomosis
38.46	Resection of abdominal arteries with replacement
38.47	Resection of abdominal veins with replacement
38.66	Other excision of abdominal arteries
38.67	Other excision of abdominal veins
38.7	Interruption of the vena cava
38.86	Other surgical occlusion of abdominal arteries
38.87	Other surgical occlusion of abdominal veins
39.27	Arteriovenostomy for renal dialysis
39.42	Revision of arteriovenous shunt for renal dialysis
39.43	Removal of arteriovenous shunt for renal dialysis
39.49	Other revision of vascular procedure
39.50	Angioplasty of other non-coronary vessel(s)
39.52	Other repair of aneurysm
39.56	Repair of blood vessel with tissue patch graft
39.57	Repair of blood vessel with synthetic patch graft
39.58	Repair of blood vessel with unspecified type of patch graft
39.59	Other repair of vessel
39.71	Endovascular implantation of other graft in abdominal aorta
39.72	Endovascular (total) embolization or occlusion of head and neck vessels
39.73	Endovascular implantation of graft in thoracic aorta
39.75	Endovascular embolization or occlusion of vessel(s) of head or neck using bare coils

Surgical	Medical	CC Indicator	MCC Indicator	Procedure Proxy

MDC 11: Diseases And Disorders Of The Kidney And Urinary Tract—MEDICAL

39.76	Endovascular embolization or occlusion of vessel(s) of head or neck using bioactive coils
39.79	Other endovascular procedures on other vessels
39.93	Insertion of vessel-to-vessel cannula
39.94	Replacement of vessel-to-vessel cannula
39.98	Control of hemorrhage, not otherwise specified
40.11	Biopsy of lymphatic structure
40.19	Other diagnostic procedures on lymphatic structures
40.24	Excision of inguinal lymph node
40.29	Simple excision of other lymphatic structure
40.3	Regional lymph node excision
40.50	Radical excision of lymph nodes, not otherwise specified
40.9	Other operations on lymphatic structures
50.12	Open biopsy of liver
50.14	Laparoscopic liver biopsy
50.19	Other diagnostic procedures on liver
54.0	Incision of abdominal wall
54.1*	Laparotomy
54.21	Laparoscopy
54.5*	Lysis of peritoneal adhesions
54.92	Removal of foreign body from peritoneal cavity
54.93	Creation of cutaneoperitoneal fistula
54.95	Incision of peritoneum
64.95	Insertion or replacement of non-inflatable penile prosthesis
64.96	Removal of internal prosthesis of penis
64.97	Insertion or replacement of inflatable penile prosthesis
77.4*	Biopsy of bone
86.06	Insertion of totally implantable infusion pump
86.22	Excisional debridement of wound, infection, or burn
92.27	Implantation or insertion of radioactive elements

OR

Principal Diagnosis

277.88	Tumor lysis syndrome
403.00	Hypertensive chronic kidney disease, malignant, with chronic kidney disease stage I through stage IV, or unspecified
403.01	Hypertensive chronic kidney disease, malignant, with chronic kidney disease stage V or end stage renal disease
403.10	Hypertensive chronic kidney disease, benign, with chronic kidney disease stage I through stage IV, or unspecified
403.11	Hypertensive chronic kidney disease, benign, with chronic kidney disease stage V or end stage renal disease
403.90	Hypertensive chronic kidney disease, unspecified, with chronic kidney disease stage I through stage IV, or unspecified
403.91	Hypertensive chronic kidney disease, unspecified, with chronic kidney disease stage V or end stage renal disease
404.02	Hypertensive heart and chronic kidney disease, malignant, without heart failure and with chronic kidney disease stage V or end stage renal disease
404.12	Hypertensive heart and chronic kidney disease, benign, without heart failure and with chronic kidney disease stage V or end stage renal disease
404.92	Hypertensive heart and chronic kidney disease, unspecified, without heart failure and with chronic kidney disease stage V or end stage renal disease
584.5	Acute kidney failure with lesion of tubular necrosis
584.6	Acute kidney failure with lesion of renal cortical necrosis
584.7	Acute kidney failure with lesion of medullary [papillary] necrosis
584.8	Acute kidney failure with other specified pathological lesion in kidney
584.9	Acute kidney failure, unspecified
585*	Chronic kidney disease (CKD)
586	Unspecified renal failure
788.5	Oliguria and anuria
958.5	Traumatic anuria

AND

Nonoperating Room Procedure

86.07	Insertion of totally implantable vascular access device (VAD)

OR

Principal Diagnosis

250.41	Diabetes with renal manifestations, type I [juvenile type], not stated as uncontrolled
250.43	Diabetes with renal manifestations, type I [juvenile type], uncontrolled

AND

Nonoperating Room Procedures

52.84	Autotransplantation of cells of islets of Langerhans
52.85	Allotransplantation of cells of islets of Langerhans

DRG 674 **Other Kidney and Urinary Tract Procedures with CC**

GMLOS 5.1	AMLOS 6.9	RW 2.2378	☑

Select principal diagnosis and operating and nonoperating room procedures listed under DRG 673

DRG 675 **Other Kidney and Urinary Tract Procedures without CC/MCC**

GMLOS 1.9	AMLOS 2.7	RW 1.3807	☑

Select principal diagnosis and operating and nonoperating room procedures listed under DRG 673

MEDICAL

DRG 682 **Renal Failure with MCC**

GMLOS 4.7	AMLOS 6.2	RW 1.5401	☑ ⱱ T

Principal Diagnosis

277.88	Tumor lysis syndrome
403.00	Hypertensive chronic kidney disease, malignant, with chronic kidney disease stage I through stage IV, or unspecified
403.01	Hypertensive chronic kidney disease, malignant, with chronic kidney disease stage V or end stage renal disease
403.10	Hypertensive chronic kidney disease, benign, with chronic kidney disease stage I through stage IV, or unspecified
403.11	Hypertensive chronic kidney disease, benign, with chronic kidney disease stage V or end stage renal disease
403.90	Hypertensive chronic kidney disease, unspecified, with chronic kidney disease stage I through stage IV, or unspecified
403.91	Hypertensive chronic kidney disease, unspecified, with chronic kidney disease stage V or end stage renal disease
404.02	Hypertensive heart and chronic kidney disease, malignant, without heart failure and with chronic kidney disease stage V or end stage renal disease
404.12	Hypertensive heart and chronic kidney disease, benign, without heart failure and with chronic kidney disease stage V or end stage renal disease
404.92	Hypertensive heart and chronic kidney disease, unspecified, without heart failure and with chronic kidney disease stage V or end stage renal disease
584.5	Acute kidney failure with lesion of tubular necrosis
584.6	Acute kidney failure with lesion of renal cortical necrosis
584.7	Acute kidney failure with lesion of medullary [papillary] necrosis
584.8	Acute kidney failure with other specified pathological lesion in kidney
584.9	Acute kidney failure, unspecified
585*	Chronic kidney disease (CKD)

T Transfer DRG   SP Special Payment   ☑ Optimization Potential   ⱱ Targeted Potential   * Code Range   ● New DRG   ▲ Revised DRG Title

586	Unspecified renal failure
788.5	Oliguria and anuria
958.5	Traumatic anuria

DRG 683 Renal Failure with CC

GMLOS 3.7   **AMLOS 4.5**   **RW 0.9655**   ☑ ▽ T

Select principal diagnosis listed under DRG 682

DRG 684 Renal Failure without CC/MCC

GMLOS 2.5   **AMLOS 3.0**   **RW 0.6213**   ☑ ▽ T

Select principal diagnosis listed under DRG 682

DRG 685 Admit for Renal Dialysis

GMLOS 2.6   **AMLOS 3.4**   **RW 0.9282**   ☑

Principal Diagnosis
| V56* | Encounter for dialysis and dialysis catheter care |

DRG 686 Kidney and Urinary Tract Neoplasms with MCC

GMLOS 5.4   **AMLOS 7.2**   **RW 1.7237**   ☑

Principal Diagnosis
188*	Malignant neoplasm of bladder
189*	Malignant neoplasm of kidney and other and unspecified urinary organs
198.0	Secondary malignant neoplasm of kidney
198.1	Secondary malignant neoplasm of other urinary organs
209.24	Malignant carcinoid tumor of the kidney
209.64	Benign carcinoid tumor of the kidney
223*	Benign neoplasm of kidney and other urinary organs
233.7	Carcinoma in situ of bladder
233.9	Carcinoma in situ of other and unspecified urinary organs
236.7	Neoplasm of uncertain behavior of bladder
236.9*	Neoplasm of uncertain behavior of other and unspecified urinary organs
239.4	Neoplasm of unspecified nature of bladder
239.5	Neoplasm of unspecified nature of other genitourinary organs

DRG 687 Kidney and Urinary Tract Neoplasms with CC

GMLOS 3.7   **AMLOS 4.8**   **RW 1.0441**   ☑

Select principal diagnosis listed under DRG 686

DRG 688 Kidney and Urinary Tract Neoplasms without CC/MCC

GMLOS 2.2   **AMLOS 2.7**   **RW 0.6867**   ☑

Select principal diagnosis listed under DRG 686

DRG 689 Kidney and Urinary Tract Infections with MCC

GMLOS 4.3   **AMLOS 5.3**   **RW 1.1300**   ☑ ▽ T

Principal Diagnosis
016.0*	Tuberculosis of kidney
016.1*	Tuberculosis of bladder
016.2*	Tuberculosis of ureter
016.3*	Tuberculosis of other urinary organs
016.9*	Genitourinary tuberculosis, unspecified
032.84	Diphtheritic cystitis
078.6	Hemorrhagic nephrosonephritis
095.4	Syphilis of kidney
098.11	Gonococcal cystitis (acute)
098.30	Chronic gonococcal infection of upper genitourinary tract, site unspecified
098.31	Gonococcal cystitis, chronic
099.54	Chlamydia trachomatis infection of other genitourinary sites
120.0	Schistosomiasis due to schistosoma haematobium

137.2	Late effects of genitourinary tuberculosis
590*	Infections of kidney
593.3	Stricture or kinking of ureter
595.0	Acute cystitis
595.1	Chronic interstitial cystitis
595.2	Other chronic cystitis
595.3	Trigonitis
595.4	Cystitis in diseases classified elsewhere
595.81	Cystitis cystica
595.89	Other specified types of cystitis
595.9	Unspecified cystitis
597*	Urethritis, not sexually transmitted, and urethral syndrome
599.0	Urinary tract infection, site not specified

DRG 690 Kidney and Urinary Tract Infections without MCC

GMLOS 3.2   **AMLOS 3.8**   **RW 0.7693**   ☑ ▽ T

Select principal diagnosis listed under DRG 689

DRG 691 Urinary Stones with ESW Lithotripsy with CC/MCC

GMLOS 3.0   **AMLOS 3.8**   **RW 1.5454**   ☑

Principal Diagnosis
274.11	Uric acid nephrolithiasis
591	Hydronephrosis
592*	Calculus of kidney and ureter
593.4	Other ureteric obstruction
593.5	Hydroureter
594.1	Other calculus in bladder
594.2	Calculus in urethra
594.8	Other lower urinary tract calculus
594.9	Unspecified calculus of lower urinary tract
788.0	Renal colic

WITH

Nonoperating Room Procedure
| 98.51 | Extracorporeal shockwave lithotripsy (ESWL) of the kidney, ureter and/or bladder |

DRG 692 Urinary Stones with ESW Lithotripsy without CC/MCC

GMLOS 1.7   **AMLOS 2.0**   **RW 1.0690**   ☑

Select principal diagnosis and nonoperating room procedure listed under DRG 691

DRG 693 Urinary Stones without ESW Lithotripsy with MCC

GMLOS 4.1   **AMLOS 5.3**   **RW 1.4186**   ☑

Select only principal diagnosis listed under DRG 691

DRG 694 Urinary Stones without ESW Lithotripsy without MCC

GMLOS 2.0   **AMLOS 2.4**   **RW 0.6879**   ☑

Select only principal diagnosis listed under DRG 691

DRG 695 Kidney and Urinary Tract Signs and Symptoms with MCC

GMLOS 4.2   **AMLOS 5.5**   **RW 1.2773**   ☑

Principal Diagnosis
599.7*	Hematuria
788.1	Dysuria
788.2*	Retention of urine
788.3*	Urinary incontinence
788.4*	Frequency of urination and polyuria
788.6*	Other abnormality of urination
788.7	Urethral discharge
788.8	Extravasation of urine
788.9*	Other symptoms involving urinary system
791.0	Proteinuria
791.1	Chyluria

Surgical   *Medical*   *CC Indicator*   *MCC Indicator*   *Procedure Proxy*

MDC 11: Diseases And Disorders Of The Kidney And Urinary Tract—MEDICAL

791.2	Hemoglobinuria
791.7	Other cells and casts in urine
791.9	Other nonspecific finding on examination of urine
793.5	Nonspecific (abnormal) findings on radiological and other examination of genitourinary organs
794.4	Nonspecific abnormal results of kidney function study
794.9	Nonspecific abnormal results of other specified function study

DRG 696 Kidney and Urinary Tract Signs and Symptoms without MCC

GMLOS 2.5   **AMLOS 3.1**   **RW 0.6615**   ☑

Select principal diagnosis listed under DRG 695

DRG 697 Urethral Stricture

GMLOS 2.5   **AMLOS 3.2**   **RW 0.8225**   ☑

Principal Diagnosis
598*	Urethral stricture

DRG 698 Other Kidney and Urinary Tract Diagnoses with MCC

GMLOS 5.1   **AMLOS 6.4**   **RW 1.5681**   ☑ ▽ Ⓣ

Principal Diagnosis
249.4*	Secondary diabetes mellitus with renal manifestations
250.4*	Diabetes with renal manifestations
274.10	Gouty nephropathy, unspecified
274.19	Other gouty nephropathy
306.50	Psychogenic genitourinary malfunction, unspecified
306.53	Psychogenic dysuria
306.59	Other genitourinary malfunction arising from mental factors
344.61	Cauda equina syndrome with neurogenic bladder
440.1	Atherosclerosis of renal artery
442.1	Aneurysm of renal artery
443.23	Dissection of renal artery
445.81	Atheroembolism of kidney
447.3	Hyperplasia of renal artery
453.3	Embolism and thrombosis of renal vein
580*	Acute glomerulonephritis
581*	Nephrotic syndrome
582*	Chronic glomerulonephritis
583*	Nephritis and nephropathy, not specified as acute or chronic
587	Unspecified renal sclerosis
588*	Disorders resulting from impaired renal function
589*	Small kidney of unknown cause
593.0	Nephroptosis
593.1	Hypertrophy of kidney
593.2	Acquired cyst of kidney
593.6	Postural proteinuria
593.7*	Vesicoureteral reflux
593.8*	Other specified disorders of kidney and ureter
593.9	Unspecified disorder of kidney and ureter
594.0	Calculus in diverticulum of bladder
595.82	Irradiation cystitis
596*	Other disorders of bladder
599.1	Urethral fistula
599.2	Urethral diverticulum
599.3	Urethral caruncle
599.4	Urethral false passage
599.5	Prolapsed urethral mucosa
599.6*	Urinary obstruction
599.8*	Other specified disorder of urethra and urinary tract
599.9	Unspecified disorder of urethra and urinary tract
753*	Congenital anomalies of urinary system
866*	Injury to kidney
867.0	Bladder and urethra injury without mention of open wound into cavity
867.1	Bladder and urethra injury with open wound into cavity
867.2	Ureter injury without mention of open wound into cavity

867.3	Ureter injury with open wound into cavity
868.04	Retroperitoneum injury without mention of open wound into cavity
868.14	Retroperitoneum injury with open wound into cavity
939.0	Foreign body in bladder and urethra
939.9	Foreign body in unspecified site in genitourinary tract
996.30	Mechanical complication of unspecified genitourinary device, implant, and graft
996.31	Mechanical complication due to urethral (indwelling) catheter
996.39	Mechanical complication of genitourinary device, implant, and graft, other
996.64	Infection and inflammatory reaction due to indwelling urinary catheter
996.65	Infection and inflammatory reaction due to other genitourinary device, implant, and graft
996.76	Other complications due to genitourinary device, implant, and graft
996.81	Complications of transplanted kidney
997.5	Urinary complications
997.72	Vascular complications of renal artery
V42.0	Kidney replaced by transplant
V43.5	Bladder replaced by other means
V45.74	Acquired absence of organ, other parts of urinary tract
V53.6	Fitting and adjustment of urinary device
V55.5	Attention to cystostomy
V55.6	Attention to other artificial opening of urinary tract
V59.4	Kidney donor

DRG 699 Other Kidney and Urinary Tract Diagnoses with CC

GMLOS 3.5   **AMLOS 4.4**   **RW 0.9890**   ☑ ▽ Ⓣ

Select principal diagnosis listed under DRG 698

DRG 700 Other Kidney and Urinary Tract Diagnoses without CC/MCC

GMLOS 2.6   **AMLOS 3.2**   **RW 0.7026**   ☑ ▽ Ⓣ

Select principal diagnosis listed under DRG 698

Ⓣ *Transfer DRG*   🆂🅿 *Special Payment*   ☑ *Optimization Potential*   ▽ *Targeted Potential*   * *Code Range*   ● *New DRG*   ▲ *Revised DRG Title*

MDC 12
Diseases And Disorders Of The Male Reproductive System

016.40	098.10	099.8	198.82	600.11	603.1	607.85	608.9	867.7
016.41	098.12	099.9	214.4	600.20	603.8	607.89	698.1	867.8
016.42	098.13	112.2	222.0	600.21	603.9	607.9	752.51	867.9
016.43	098.14	131.00	222.1	600.3	604.0	608.0	752.52	878.0
016.44	098.19	131.02	222.2	600.90	604.90	608.1	752.61	878.1
016.45	098.2	131.03	222.3	600.91	604.91	608.20	752.62	878.2
016.46	098.32	131.09	222.4	601.0	604.99	608.21	752.63	878.3
016.50	098.33	185	222.8	601.1	605	608.22	752.64	878.8
016.51	098.34	186.0	222.9	601.2	606.0	608.23	752.65	878.9
016.52	098.39	186.9	233.4	601.3	606.1	608.24	752.69	908.2
016.53	099.0	187.1	233.5	601.4	606.8	608.3	752.7	922.4
016.54	099.1	187.2	233.6	601.8	606.9	608.4	752.81	926.0
016.55	099.2	187.3	236.4	601.9	607.0	608.81	752.89	939.3
016.56	099.40	187.4	236.5	602.0	607.1	608.82	752.9	V25.2
054.10	099.41	187.5	236.6	602.1	607.2	608.83	758.6	V26.0
054.13	099.49	187.6	456.4	602.2	607.3	608.84	758.7	V45.77
054.19	099.50	187.7	456.5	602.3	607.81	608.85	758.81	V50.2
072.0	099.53	187.8	600.00	602.8	607.82	608.86	758.89	
091.0	099.55	187.9	600.01	602.9	607.83	608.87	792.2	
098.0	099.59	195.3	600.10	603.0	607.84	608.89	867.6	

SURGICAL

DRG 707 Major Male Pelvic Procedures with CC/MCC
GMLOS 3.0   AMLOS 4.1   RW 1.8265   ☑

Operating Room Procedures

40.52	Radical excision of periaortic lymph nodes
40.53	Radical excision of iliac lymph nodes
40.54	Radical groin dissection
40.59	Radical excision of other lymph nodes
48.69	Other resection of rectum
54.11	Exploratory laparotomy
57.6	Partial cystectomy
57.7*	Total cystectomy
59.00	Retroperitoneal dissection, not otherwise specified
60.3	Suprapubic prostatectomy
60.4	Retropubic prostatectomy
60.5	Radical prostatectomy
60.62	Perineal prostatectomy
60.69	Other prostatectomy

DRG 708 Major Male Pelvic Procedures without CC/MCC
GMLOS 1.4   AMLOS 1.6   RW 1.2928   ☑

Select operating room procedures listed under DRG 707

DRG 709 Penis Procedures with CC/MCC
GMLOS 4.0   AMLOS 6.2   RW 2.1038   ☑

Operating Room Procedures

58.43	Closure of other fistula of urethra
58.45	Repair of hypospadias or epispadias
58.46	Other reconstruction of urethra
58.49	Other repair of urethra
58.5	Release of urethral stricture
64.11	Biopsy of penis
64.2	Local excision or destruction of lesion of penis
64.3	Amputation of penis
64.4*	Repair and plastic operation on penis
64.5	Operations for sex transformation, not elsewhere classified
64.92	Incision of penis
64.93	Division of penile adhesions
64.95	Insertion or replacement of non-inflatable penile prosthesis
64.96	Removal of internal prosthesis of penis
64.97	Insertion or replacement of inflatable penile prosthesis
64.98	Other operations on penis
64.99	Other operations on male genital organs

DRG 710 Penis Procedures without CC/MCC
GMLOS 1.5   AMLOS 1.9   RW 1.3429   ☑

Select operating room procedures listed under DRG 709

DRG 711 Testes Procedures with CC/MCC
GMLOS 5.5   AMLOS 7.6   RW 2.0316

Operating Room Procedures

61.2	Excision of hydrocele (of tunica vaginalis)
61.42	Repair of scrotal fistula
61.49	Other repair of scrotum and tunica vaginalis
61.92	Excision of lesion of tunica vaginalis other than hydrocele
61.99	Other operations on scrotum and tunica vaginalis
62.0	Incision of testis
62.12	Open biopsy of testis
62.19	Other diagnostic procedures on testes
62.2	Excision or destruction of testicular lesion
62.3	Unilateral orchiectomy
62.4*	Bilateral orchiectomy
62.5	Orchiopexy
62.6*	Repair of testes
62.7	Insertion of testicular prosthesis
62.99	Other operations on testes
63.09	Other diagnostic procedures on spermatic cord, epididymis, and vas deferens
63.1	Excision of varicocele and hydrocele of spermatic cord
63.2	Excision of cyst of epididymis
63.3	Excision of other lesion or tissue of spermatic cord and epididymis
63.4	Epididymectomy
63.51	Suture of laceration of spermatic cord and epididymis
63.53	Transplantation of spermatic cord
63.59	Other repair of spermatic cord and epididymis
63.81	Suture of laceration of vas deferens and epididymis
63.82	Reconstruction of surgically divided vas deferens
63.83	Epididymovasostomy
63.85	Removal of valve from vas deferens
63.89	Other repair of vas deferens and epididymis
63.92	Epididymotomy
63.93	Incision of spermatic cord
63.94	Lysis of adhesions of spermatic cord
63.95	Insertion of valve in vas deferens
63.99	Other operations on spermatic card, epididymis, and vas deferens

DRG 712 Testes Procedures without CC/MCC
GMLOS 2.3   AMLOS 3.0   RW 0.9580   ☑

Select operating room procedures listed under DRG 711

DRG 713 Transurethral Prostatectomy with CC/MCC
GMLOS 3.3   AMLOS 4.5   RW 1.3814   ☑

Operating Room Procedures

60.2*	Transurethral prostatectomy
60.96	Transurethral destruction of prostate tissue by microwave thermotherapy
60.97	Other transurethral destruction of prostate tissue by other thermotherapy

DRG 714 Transurethral Prostatectomy without CC/MCC
GMLOS 1.7   AMLOS 2.0   RW 0.7402   ☑

Select operating room procedures listed under DRG 713

DRG 715 Other Male Reproductive System O.R. Procedures for Malignancy with CC/MCC
GMLOS 5.5   AMLOS 7.8   RW 2.2268

Principal Diagnosis

185	Malignant neoplasm of prostate
186*	Malignant neoplasm of testis
187*	Malignant neoplasm of penis and other male genital organs
195.3	Malignant neoplasm of pelvis
198.82	Secondary malignant neoplasm of genital organs
233.4	Carcinoma in situ of prostate
233.5	Carcinoma in situ of penis
233.6	Carcinoma in situ of other and unspecified male genital organs
236.4	Neoplasm of uncertain behavior of testis
236.5	Neoplasm of uncertain behavior of prostate
236.6	Neoplasm of uncertain behavior of other and unspecified male genital organs

Operating Room Procedures

03.93	Implantation or replacement of spinal neurostimulator lead(s)
03.94	Removal of spinal neurostimulator lead(s)

☐ Transfer DRG   ⃝SP Special Payment   ☑ Optimization Potential   ⃝ᵂᴱ Targeted Potential   * Code Range   ● New DRG   ▲ Revised DRG Title

122   Valid 10/01/2013–09/30/2014   © 2013 OptumInsight, Inc.

MDC 12: Diseases And D... Reproductive System—SURGICAL

04.92	Implantation or replacement of peripheral neurostimulator lead(s)
04.93	Removal of peripheral neurostimulator lead(s)
17.69	Laser interstitial thermal therapy [LITT] of lesion or tissue of other and unspecified site under guidance
38.7	Interruption of the vena cava
39.98	Control of hemorrhage, not otherwise specified
40.1*	Diagnostic procedures on lymphatic structures
40.24	Excision of inguinal lymph node
40.29	Simple excision of other lymphatic structure
40.3	Regional lymph node excision
40.50	Radical excision of lymph nodes, not otherwise specified
40.9	Other operations on lymphatic structures
50.12	Open biopsy of liver
56.41	Partial ureterectomy
56.5*	Cutaneous uretero-ileostomy
56.6*	Other external urinary diversion
56.71	Urinary diversion to intestine
56.72	Revision of ureterointestinal anastomosis
56.73	Nephrocystanastomosis, not otherwise specified
56.75	Transureteroureterostomy
56.83	Closure of ureterostomy
56.84	Closure of other fistula of ureter
57.18	Other suprapubic cystostomy
57.2*	Vesicostomy
57.33	Closed (transurethral) biopsy of bladder
57.34	Open biopsy of bladder
57.39	Other diagnostic procedures on bladder
57.49	Other transurethral excision or destruction of lesion or tissue of bladder
57.5*	Other excision or destruction of bladder tissue
57.82	Closure of cystostomy
57.83	Repair of fistula involving bladder and intestine
57.84	Repair of other fistula of bladder
57.88	Other anastomosis of bladder
58.1	Urethral meatotomy
58.47	Urethral meatoplasty
58.99	Other operations on urethra and periurethral tissue
59.02	Other lysis of perirenal or periureteral adhesions
59.03	Laparoscopic lysis of perirenal or periureteral adhesions
59.09	Other incision of perirenal or periureteral tissue
59.1*	Incision of perivesical tissue
59.2*	Diagnostic procedures on perirenal and perivesical tissue
59.91	Excision of perirenal or perivesical tissue
59.92	Other operations on perirenal or perivesical tissue
60.0	Incision of prostate
60.12	Open biopsy of prostate
60.14	Open biopsy of seminal vesicles
60.15	Biopsy of periprostatic tissue
60.18	Other diagnostic procedures on prostate and periprostatic tissue
60.19	Other diagnostic procedures on seminal vesicles
60.61	Local excision of lesion of prostate
60.72	Incision of seminal vesicle
60.73	Excision of seminal vesicle
60.79	Other operations on seminal vesicles
60.8*	Incision or excision of periprostatic tissue
60.93	Repair of prostate
60.94	Control of (postoperative) hemorrhage of prostate
60.95	Transurethral balloon dilation of the prostatic urethra
60.99	Other operations on prostate
77.4*	Biopsy of bone
86.06	Insertion of totally implantable infusion pump
86.22	Excisional debridement of wound, infection, or burn
92.27	Implantation or insertion of radioactive elements

DRG 716 **Other Male Reproductive System O.R. Procedures for Malignancy without CC/MCC**
GMLOS 1.5   AMLOS 1.8   RW 0.9629   ☑

Select principal diagnosis and operating room procedures listed under DRG 715

DRG 717 **Other Male Reproductive System O.R. Procedures Except Malignancy with CC/MCC**
GMLOS 4.9   AMLOS 6.7   RW 1.7495   ☑

Select only operating room procedures listed under DRG 715

DRG 718 **Other Male Reproductive System O.R. Procedures Except Malignancy without CC/MCC**
GMLOS 2.3   AMLOS 2.9   RW 0.8786   ☑

Select only operating room procedures listed under DRG 715

MEDICAL

DRG 722 **Malignancy, Male Reproductive System with MCC**
GMLOS 5.3   AMLOS 7.1   RW 1.6031   ☑

Principal Diagnosis
185	Malignant neoplasm of prostate
186*	Malignant neoplasm of testis
187*	Malignant neoplasm of penis and other male genital organs
195.3	Malignant neoplasm of pelvis
198.82	Secondary malignant neoplasm of genital organs
233.4	Carcinoma in situ of prostate
233.5	Carcinoma in situ of penis
233.6	Carcinoma in situ of other and unspecified male genital organs
236.4	Neoplasm of uncertain behavior of testis
236.5	Neoplasm of uncertain behavior of prostate
236.6	Neoplasm of uncertain behavior of other and unspecified male genital organs

DRG 723 **Malignancy, Male Reproductive System with CC**
GMLOS 3.9   AMLOS 5.0   RW 1.0532   ☑

Select principal diagnosis listed under DRG 722

DRG 724 **Malignancy, Male Reproductive System without CC/MCC**
GMLOS 1.8   AMLOS 2.4   RW 0.5501   ☑

Select principal diagnosis listed under DRG 722

DRG 725 **Benign Prostatic Hypertrophy with MCC**
GMLOS 4.4   AMLOS 5.6   RW 1.2644   ☑

Principal Diagnosis
| 600* | Hyperplasia of prostate |

DRG 726 **Benign Prostatic Hypertrophy without MCC**
GMLOS 2.8   AMLOS 3.4   RW 0.7159   ☑

Select principal diagnosis listed under DRG 725

DRG 727 **Inflammation of the Male Reproductive System with MCC**
GMLOS 4.8   AMLOS 6.2   RW 1.4106

Principal Diagnosis
016.4*	Tuberculosis of epididymis
016.5*	Tuberculosis of other male genital organs
054.10	Unspecified genital herpes

| Surgical | Medical | CC Indicator | MCC Indicator | Procedure Proxy |

054.13	Herpetic infection of penis
054.19	Other genital herpes
072.0	Mumps orchitis
091.0	Genital syphilis (primary)
098.0	Gonococcal infection (acute) of lower genitourinary tract
098.10	Gonococcal infection (acute) of upper genitourinary tract, site unspecified
098.12	Gonococcal prostatitis (acute)
098.13	Gonococcal epididymo-orchitis (acute)
098.14	Gonococcal seminal vesiculitis (acute)
098.19	Other gonococcal infections (acute) of upper genitourinary tract
098.2	Gonococcal infections, chronic, of lower genitourinary tract
098.32	Gonococcal prostatitis, chronic
098.33	Gonococcal epididymo-orchitis, chronic
098.34	Gonococcal seminal vesiculitis, chronic
098.39	Other chronic gonococcal infections of upper genitourinary tract
099.0	Chancroid
099.1	Lymphogranuloma venereum
099.2	Granuloma inguinale
099.4*	Other nongonococcal urethritis (NGU)
099.50	Chlamydia trachomatis infection of unspecified site
099.53	Chlamydia trachomatis infection of lower genitourinary sites
099.55	Chlamydia trachomatis infection of unspecified genitourinary site
099.59	Chlamydia trachomatis infection of other specified site
099.8	Other specified venereal diseases
099.9	Unspecified venereal disease
112.2	Candidiasis of other urogenital sites
131.00	Unspecified urogenital trichomoniasis
131.02	Trichomonal urethritis
131.03	Trichomonal prostatitis
131.09	Other urogenital trichomoniasis
601*	Inflammatory diseases of prostate
603.1	Infected hydrocele
604*	Orchitis and epididymitis
605	Redundant prepuce and phimosis
607.1	Balanoposthitis
607.2	Other inflammatory disorders of penis
607.81	Balanitis xerotica obliterans
608.0	Seminal vesiculitis
608.4	Other inflammatory disorder of male genital organs
V50.2	Routine or ritual circumcision

DRG 728 Inflammation of the Male Reproductive System without MCC

GMLOS 3.2	AMLOS 3.9	RW 0.7821	☑

Select principal diagnosis listed under DRG 727

DRG 729 Other Male Reproductive System Diagnoses with CC/MCC

GMLOS 3.7	AMLOS 5.0	RW 1.1196	☑

Principal Diagnosis

214.4	Lipoma of spermatic cord
222*	Benign neoplasm of male genital organs
456.4	Scrotal varices
456.5	Pelvic varices
602*	Other disorders of prostate
603.0	Encysted hydrocele
603.8	Other specified type of hydrocele
603.9	Unspecified hydrocele
606*	Male infertility
607.0	Leukoplakia of penis
607.3	Priapism
607.82	Vascular disorders of penis
607.83	Edema of penis
607.84	Impotence of organic origin
607.85	Peyronie's disease

607.89	Other specified disorder of penis
607.9	Unspecified disorder of penis
608.1	Spermatocele
608.2*	Torsion of testis
608.3	Atrophy of testis
608.8*	Other specified disorder of male genital organs
608.9	Unspecified disorder of male genital organs
698.1	Pruritus of genital organs
752.5*	Undescended and retractile testicle
752.6*	Hypospadias and epispadias and other penile anomalies
752.7	Indeterminate sex and pseudohermaphroditism
752.8*	Other specified congenital anomalies of genital organs
752.9	Unspecified congenital anomaly of genital organs
758.6	Gonadal dysgenesis
758.7	Klinefelter's syndrome
758.8*	Other conditions due to chromosome anomalies
792.2	Nonspecific abnormal finding in semen
867.6	Injury to other specified pelvic organs without mention of open wound into cavity
867.7	Injury to other specified pelvic organs with open wound into cavity
867.8	Injury to unspecified pelvic organ without mention of open wound into cavity
867.9	Injury to unspecified pelvic organ with open wound into cavity
878.0	Open wound of penis, without mention of complication
878.1	Open wound of penis, complicated
878.2	Open wound of scrotum and testes, without mention of complication
878.3	Open wound of scrotum and testes, complicated
878.8	Open wound of other and unspecified parts of genital organs, without mention of complication
878.9	Open wound of other and unspecified parts of genital organs, complicated
908.2	Late effect of internal injury to other internal organs
922.4	Contusion of genital organs
926.0	Crushing injury of external genitalia
939.3	Foreign body in penis
V25.2	Sterilization
V26.0	Tuboplasty or vasoplasty after previous sterilization
V45.77	Acquired absence of organ, genital organs

DRG 730 Other Male Reproductive System Diagnoses without CC/MCC

GMLOS 2.2	AMLOS 2.8	RW 0.6266	☑

Select principal diagnosis listed under DRG 729

Ⓣ Transfer DRG   ⑤ Special Payment   ☑ Optimization Potential   ⱽ Targeted Potential   * Code Range   ● New DRG   ▲ Revised DRG Title

124   Valid 10/01/2013–09/30/2014   © 2013 OptumInsight, Inc.

MDC 13
Diseases And Disorders Of The Female Reproductive System

016.60	099.59	219.0	614.7	618.82	622.3	625.9	752.10	795.13
016.61	099.8	219.1	614.8	618.83	622.4	626.0	752.11	795.14
016.62	099.9	219.8	614.9	618.84	622.5	626.1	752.19	795.15
016.63	112.1	219.9	615.0	618.89	622.6	626.2	752.2	795.16
016.64	112.2	220	615.1	618.9	622.7	626.3	752.31	795.18
016.65	131.00	221.0	615.9	619.0	622.8	626.4	752.32	795.19
016.66	131.01	221.1	616.0	619.2	622.9	626.5	752.33	867.4
016.70	131.02	221.2	616.10	619.8	623.0	626.6	752.34	867.5
016.71	131.09	221.8	616.11	619.9	623.1	626.7	752.35	867.6
016.72	179	221.9	616.2	620.0	623.2	626.8	752.36	867.7
016.73	180.0	233.1	616.3	620.1	623.3	626.9	752.39	867.8
016.74	180.1	233.2	616.4	620.2	623.4	627.0	752.40	867.9
016.75	180.8	233.30	616.50	620.3	623.5	627.1	752.41	878.4
016.76	180.9	233.31	616.51	620.4	623.6	627.2	752.42	878.5
054.10	181	233.32	616.81	620.5	623.7	627.3	752.43	878.6
054.11	182.0	233.39	616.89	620.6	623.8	627.4	752.44	878.7
054.12	182.1	236.0	616.9	620.7	623.9	627.8	752.45	878.8
054.19	182.8	236.1	617.0	620.8	624.01	627.9	752.46	878.9
091.0	183.0	236.2	617.1	620.9	624.02	628.0	752.47	908.2
098.0	183.2	236.3	617.2	621.0	624.09	628.1	752.49	922.4
098.10	183.3	256.0	617.3	621.1	624.1	628.2	752.7	926.0
098.15	183.4	256.1	617.4	621.2	624.2	628.3	752.89	939.1
098.16	183.5	256.2	617.8	621.30	624.3	628.4	752.9	939.2
098.17	183.8	256.31	617.9	621.31	624.4	628.8	758.6	947.4
098.19	183.9	256.39	618.00	621.32	624.5	628.9	758.81	996.32
098.2	184.0	256.4	618.01	621.33	624.6	629.0	758.89	V25.2
098.35	184.1	256.8	618.02	621.34	624.8	629.1	795.00	V25.3
098.36	184.2	256.9	618.03	621.35	624.9	629.20	795.01	V26.0
098.37	184.3	306.51	618.04	621.4	625.0	629.21	795.02	V45.77
098.39	184.4	306.52	618.05	621.5	625.1	629.22	795.03	V50.42
099.0	184.8	456.5	618.09	621.6	625.2	629.23	795.04	V55.7
099.1	184.9	456.6	618.1	621.7	625.3	629.29	795.05	V61.5
099.2	195.3	614.0	618.2	621.8	625.4	629.31	795.06	V88.01
099.40	198.6	614.1	618.3	621.9	625.5	629.32	795.07	V88.02
099.41	198.82	614.2	618.4	622.0	625.6	629.81	795.08	V88.03
099.49	218.0	614.3	618.5	622.10	625.70	629.89	795.09	
099.50	218.1	614.4	618.6	622.11	625.71	629.9	795.10	
099.53	218.2	614.5	618.7	622.12	625.79	698.1	795.11	
099.55	218.9	614.6	618.81	622.2	625.8	752.0	795.12	

SURGICAL

DRG 734 Pelvic Evisceration, Radical Hysterectomy and Radical Vulvectomy with CC/MCC
GMLOS 4.6   AMLOS 6.7   RW 2.5547   ☑

Operating Room Procedures
40.50	Radical excision of lymph nodes, not otherwise specified
40.52	Radical excision of periaortic lymph nodes
40.53	Radical excision of iliac lymph nodes
40.54	Radical groin dissection
40.59	Radical excision of other lymph nodes
68.61	Laparoscopic radical abdominal hysterectomy
68.69	Other and unspecified radical abdominal hysterectomy
68.71	Laparoscopic radical vaginal hysterectomy [LRVH]
68.79	Other and unspecified radical vaginal hysterectomy
68.8	Pelvic evisceration
71.5	Radical vulvectomy

DRG 735 Pelvic Evisceration, Radical Hysterectomy and Radical Vulvectomy without CC/MCC
GMLOS 1.9   AMLOS 2.3   RW 1.1910   ☑

Select operating room procedures listed under DRG 734

DRG 736 Uterine and Adnexa Procedures for Ovarian or Adnexal Malignancy with MCC
GMLOS 10.1   AMLOS 12.4   RW 4.2211

Principal Diagnosis
183*	Malignant neoplasm of ovary and other uterine adnexa
198.6	Secondary malignant neoplasm of ovary
236.2	Neoplasm of uncertain behavior of ovary

Operating Room Procedures
65*	Operations on ovary
66.0*	Salpingotomy
66.1*	Diagnostic procedures on fallopian tubes
66.4	Total unilateral salpingectomy
66.5*	Total bilateral salpingectomy
66.61	Excision or destruction of lesion of fallopian tube
66.62	Salpingectomy with removal of tubal pregnancy
66.69	Other partial salpingectomy
66.7*	Repair of fallopian tube
66.92	Unilateral destruction or occlusion of fallopian tube
66.93	Implantation or replacement of prosthesis of fallopian tube
66.94	Removal of prosthesis of fallopian tube
66.96	Dilation of fallopian tube
66.97	Burying of fimbriae in uterine wall
66.99	Other operations on fallopian tubes
68.0	Hysterotomy
68.13	Open biopsy of uterus
68.14	Open biopsy of uterine ligaments
68.19	Other diagnostic procedures on uterus and supporting structures
68.23	Endometrial ablation
68.29	Other excision or destruction of lesion of uterus
68.3*	Subtotal abdominal hysterectomy
68.41	Laparoscopic total abdominal hysterectomy
68.49	Other and unspecified total abdominal hysterectomy
68.5*	Vaginal hysterectomy
68.9	Other and unspecified hysterectomy
69.19	Other excision or destruction of uterus and supporting structures
69.3	Paracervical uterine denervation
69.4*	Uterine repair

DRG 737 Uterine and Adnexa Procedures for Ovarian or Adnexal Malignancy with CC
GMLOS 5.3   AMLOS 6.2   RW 2.0310   ☑

Select principal diagnosis and operating room procedures listed under DRG 736

DRG 738 Uterine and Adnexa Procedures for Ovarian or Adnexal Malignancy without CC/MCC
GMLOS 2.9   AMLOS 3.3   RW 1.2602   ☑

Select principal diagnosis and operating room procedures listed under DRG 736

DRG 739 Uterine, Adnexa Procedures for Nonovarian/Adnexal Malignancy with MCC
GMLOS 6.5   AMLOS 8.7   RW 3.1647   ☑

Principal Diagnosis
179	Malignant neoplasm of uterus, part unspecified
180*	Malignant neoplasm of cervix uteri
181	Malignant neoplasm of placenta
182*	Malignant neoplasm of body of uterus
184*	Malignant neoplasm of other and unspecified female genital organs
195.3	Malignant neoplasm of pelvis
198.82	Secondary malignant neoplasm of genital organs
233.1	Carcinoma in situ of cervix uteri
233.2	Carcinoma in situ of other and unspecified parts of uterus
233.3*	Carcinoma in situ, other and unspecified female genital organs
236.0	Neoplasm of uncertain behavior of uterus
236.1	Neoplasm of uncertain behavior of placenta
236.3	Neoplasm of uncertain behavior of other and unspecified female genital organs

Operating Room Procedures
65*	Operations on ovary
66.0*	Salpingotomy
66.1*	Diagnostic procedures on fallopian tubes
66.4	Total unilateral salpingectomy
66.5*	Total bilateral salpingectomy
66.61	Excision or destruction of lesion of fallopian tube
66.62	Salpingectomy with removal of tubal pregnancy
66.69	Other partial salpingectomy
66.7*	Repair of fallopian tube
66.92	Unilateral destruction or occlusion of fallopian tube
66.93	Implantation or replacement of prosthesis of fallopian tube
66.94	Removal of prosthesis of fallopian tube
66.96	Dilation of fallopian tube
66.97	Burying of fimbriae in uterine wall
66.99	Other operations on fallopian tubes
68.0	Hysterotomy
68.13	Open biopsy of uterus
68.14	Open biopsy of uterine ligaments
68.19	Other diagnostic procedures on uterus and supporting structures
68.23	Endometrial ablation
68.29	Other excision or destruction of lesion of uterus
68.3*	Subtotal abdominal hysterectomy
68.41	Laparoscopic total abdominal hysterectomy
68.49	Other and unspecified total abdominal hysterectomy
68.5*	Vaginal hysterectomy
68.9	Other and unspecified hysterectomy
69.19	Other excision or destruction of uterus and supporting structures
69.3	Paracervical uterine denervation
69.4*	Uterine repair

Disorders Of The Female Reproductive System—SURGICAL

Ⓣ *Transfer DRG*   ⒮ᴾ *Special Payment*   ☑ *Optimization Potential*   ▽ᵀᴳᵀ *Targeted Potential*   * *Code Range*   ● *New DRG*   ▲ *Revised DRG Title*

126   Valid 10/01/2013-09/30/2014   © 2013 OptumInsight, Inc.

DRG 740 Uterine, Adnexa Procedures for Nonovarian/Adnexal Malignancy with CC

GMLOS 3.1	AMLOS 4.1	RW 1.5819	☑

Select principal diagnosis and operating room procedures listed under DRG 739

DRG 741 Uterine, Adnexa Procedures for Nonovarian/Adnexal Malignancy without CC/MCC

GMLOS 1.8	AMLOS 2.1	RW 1.1470	☑

Select principal diagnosis and operating room procedures listed under DRG 739

DRG 742 Uterine and Adnexa Procedures for Nonmalignancy with CC/MCC

GMLOS 3.0	AMLOS 4.0	RW 1.4972	☑

Principal Diagnosis

016.6*	Tuberculous oophoritis and salpingitis
016.7*	Tuberculosis of other female genital organs
054.10	Unspecified genital herpes
054.11	Herpetic vulvovaginitis
054.12	Herpetic ulceration of vulva
054.19	Other genital herpes
091.0	Genital syphilis (primary)
098.0	Gonococcal infection (acute) of lower genitourinary tract
098.10	Gonococcal infection (acute) of upper genitourinary tract, site unspecified
098.15	Gonococcal cervicitis (acute)
098.16	Gonococcal endometritis (acute)
098.17	Gonococcal salpingitis, specified as acute
098.19	Other gonococcal infections (acute) of upper genitourinary tract
098.2	Gonococcal infections, chronic, of lower genitourinary tract
098.35	Gonococcal cervicitis, chronic
098.36	Gonococcal endometritis, chronic
098.37	Gonococcal salpingitis (chronic)
098.39	Other chronic gonococcal infections of upper genitourinary tract
099.0	Chancroid
099.1	Lymphogranuloma venereum
099.2	Granuloma inguinale
099.4*	Other nongonococcal urethritis (NGU)
099.50	Chlamydia trachomatis infection of unspecified site
099.53	Chlamydia trachomatis infection of lower genitourinary sites
099.55	Chlamydia trachomatis infection of unspecified genitourinary site
099.59	Chlamydia trachomatis infection of other specified site
099.8	Other specified venereal diseases
099.9	Unspecified venereal disease
112.1	Candidiasis of vulva and vagina
112.2	Candidiasis of other urogenital sites
131.00	Unspecified urogenital trichomoniasis
131.01	Trichomonal vulvovaginitis
131.02	Trichomonal urethritis
131.09	Other urogenital trichomoniasis
218*	Uterine leiomyoma
219*	Other benign neoplasm of uterus
220	Benign neoplasm of ovary
221*	Benign neoplasm of other female genital organs
256*	Ovarian dysfunction
306.51	Psychogenic vaginismus
306.52	Psychogenic dysmenorrhea
456.5	Pelvic varices
456.6	Vulval varices
614*	Inflammatory disease of ovary, fallopian tube, pelvic cellular tissue, and peritoneum
615*	Inflammatory diseases of uterus, except cervix
616.0	Cervicitis and endocervicitis
616.1*	Vaginitis and vulvovaginitis
616.2	Cyst of Bartholin's gland
616.3	Abscess of Bartholin's gland
616.4	Other abscess of vulva
616.5*	Ulceration of vulva
616.8*	Other specified inflammatory diseases of cervix, vagina, and vulva
616.9	Unspecified inflammatory disease of cervix, vagina, and vulva
617.0	Endometriosis of uterus
617.1	Endometriosis of ovary
617.2	Endometriosis of fallopian tube
617.3	Endometriosis of pelvic peritoneum
617.4	Endometriosis of rectovaginal septum and vagina
617.8	Endometriosis of other specified sites
617.9	Endometriosis, site unspecified
618*	Genital prolapse
619.0	Urinary-genital tract fistula, female
619.2	Genital tract-skin fistula, female
619.8	Other specified fistula involving female genital tract
619.9	Unspecified fistula involving female genital tract
620*	Noninflammatory disorders of ovary, fallopian tube, and broad ligament
621*	Disorders of uterus, not elsewhere classified
622*	Noninflammatory disorders of cervix
623*	Noninflammatory disorders of vagina
624*	Noninflammatory disorders of vulva and perineum
625*	Pain and other symptoms associated with female genital organs
626*	Disorders of menstruation and other abnormal bleeding from female genital tract
627*	Menopausal and postmenopausal disorders
628*	Female infertility
629*	Other disorders of female genital organs
698.1	Pruritus of genital organs
752.0	Congenital anomalies of ovaries
752.1*	Congenital anomalies of fallopian tubes and broad ligaments
752.2	Congenital doubling of uterus
752.3*	Other congenital anomaly of uterus
752.4*	Congenital anomalies of cervix, vagina, and external female genitalia
752.7	Indeterminate sex and pseudohermaphroditism
752.89	Other specified anomalies of genital organs
752.9	Unspecified congenital anomaly of genital organs
758.6	Gonadal dysgenesis
758.8*	Other conditions due to chromosome anomalies
795.0*	Abnormal Papanicolaou smear of cervix and cervical HPV
795.1*	Abnormal Papanicolaou smear of vagina and vaginal HPV
867.4	Uterus injury without mention of open wound into cavity
867.5	Uterus injury with open wound into cavity
867.6	Injury to other specified pelvic organs without mention of open wound into cavity
867.7	Injury to other specified pelvic organs with open wound into cavity
867.8	Injury to unspecified pelvic organ without mention of open wound into cavity
867.9	Injury to unspecified pelvic organ with open wound into cavity
878.4	Open wound of vulva, without mention of complication
878.5	Open wound of vulva, complicated
878.6	Open wound of vagina, without mention of complication
878.7	Open wound of vagina, complicated
878.8	Open wound of other and unspecified parts of genital organs, without mention of complication
878.9	Open wound of other and unspecified parts of genital organs, complicated
908.2	Late effect of internal injury to other internal organs
922.4	Contusion of genital organs
926.0	Crushing injury of external genitalia

Surgical	Medical	CC Indicator	MCC Indicator	Procedure Proxy

939.1	Foreign body in uterus, any part
939.2	Foreign body in vulva and vagina
947.4	Burn of vagina and uterus
996.32	Mechanical complication due to intrauterine contraceptive device
V25.2	Sterilization
V25.3	Menstrual extraction
V26.0	Tuboplasty or vasoplasty after previous sterilization
V45.77	Acquired absence of organ, genital organs
V50.42	Prophylactic ovary removal
V55.7	Attention to artificial vagina
V61.5	Multiparity
V88.0*	Acquired absence of cervix and uterus

Operating Room Procedures

65*	Operations on ovary
66.0*	Salpingotomy
66.1*	Diagnostic procedures on fallopian tubes
66.4	Total unilateral salpingectomy
66.5*	Total bilateral salpingectomy
66.61	Excision or destruction of lesion of fallopian tube
66.62	Salpingectomy with removal of tubal pregnancy
66.69	Other partial salpingectomy
66.7*	Repair of fallopian tube
66.92	Unilateral destruction or occlusion of fallopian tube
66.93	Implantation or replacement of prosthesis of fallopian tube
66.94	Removal of prosthesis of fallopian tube
66.96	Dilation of fallopian tube
66.97	Burying of fimbriae in uterine wall
66.99	Other operations on fallopian tubes
68.0	Hysterotomy
68.13	Open biopsy of uterus
68.14	Open biopsy of uterine ligaments
68.19	Other diagnostic procedures on uterus and supporting structures
68.23	Endometrial ablation
68.29	Other excision or destruction of lesion of uterus
68.3*	Subtotal abdominal hysterectomy
68.41	Laparoscopic total abdominal hysterectomy
68.49	Other and unspecified total abdominal hysterectomy
68.5*	Vaginal hysterectomy
68.9	Other and unspecified hysterectomy
69.19	Other excision or destruction of uterus and supporting structures
69.3	Paracervical uterine denervation
69.4*	Uterine repair

DRG 743 **Uterine and Adnexa Procedures for Nonmalignancy without CC/MCC**

GMLOS 1.7   AMLOS 1.9   RW 0.9903   ☑

Select principal diagnosis and operating room procedures listed under DRG 742

DRG 744 **D&C, Conization, Laparoscopy and Tubal Interruption with CC/MCC**

GMLOS 3.9   AMLOS 5.5   RW 1.5084   ☑

Operating Room Procedures

54.21	Laparoscopy
66.2*	Bilateral endoscopic destruction or occlusion of fallopian tubes
66.3*	Other bilateral destruction or occlusion of fallopian tubes
66.63	Bilateral partial salpingectomy, not otherwise specified
67.1*	Diagnostic procedures on cervix
67.2	Conization of cervix
68.15	Closed biopsy of uterine ligaments
68.16	Closed biopsy of uterus
68.21	Division of endometrial synechiae
68.22	Incision or excision of congenital septum of uterus

69.09	Other dilation and curettage of uterus
92.27	Implantation or insertion of radioactive elements

DRG 745 **D&C, Conization, Laparoscopy and Tubal Interruption without CC/MCC**

GMLOS 1.9   AMLOS 2.4   RW 0.8514   ☑

Select operating room procedures listed under DRG 744

DRG 746 **Vagina, Cervix and Vulva Procedures with CC/MCC**

GMLOS 3.0   AMLOS 4.3   RW 1.3694   ☑

Operating Room Procedures

48.73	Closure of other rectal fistula
57.18	Other suprapubic cystostomy
57.21	Vesicostomy
67.3*	Other excision or destruction of lesion or tissue of cervix
67.4	Amputation of cervix
67.51	Transabdominal cerclage of cervix
67.59	Other repair of cervical os
67.6*	Other repair of cervix
69.95	Incision of cervix
69.97	Removal of other penetrating foreign body from cervix
70.13	Lysis of intraluminal adhesions of vagina
70.14	Other vaginotomy
70.23	Biopsy of cul-de-sac
70.24	Vaginal biopsy
70.29	Other diagnostic procedures on vagina and cul-de-sac
70.3*	Local excision or destruction of vagina and cul-de-sac
70.71	Suture of laceration of vagina
70.72	Repair of colovaginal fistula
70.73	Repair of rectovaginal fistula
70.74	Repair of other vaginoenteric fistula
70.75	Repair of other fistula of vagina
70.76	Hymenorrhaphy
70.79	Other repair of vagina
70.91	Other operations on vagina
70.92	Other operations on cul-de-sac
70.93	Other operations on cul-de-sac with graft or prosthesis
71.0*	Incision of vulva and perineum
71.1*	Diagnostic procedures on vulva
71.22	Incision of Bartholin's gland (cyst)
71.23	Marsupialization of Bartholin's gland (cyst)
71.24	Excision or other destruction of Bartholin's gland (cyst)
71.29	Other operations on Bartholin's gland
71.3	Other local excision or destruction of vulva and perineum
71.4	Operations on clitoris
71.6*	Other vulvectomy
71.7*	Repair of vulva and perineum
71.8	Other operations on vulva

DRG 747 **Vagina, Cervix and Vulva Procedures without CC/MCC**

GMLOS 1.6   AMLOS 1.8   RW 0.8814   ☑

Select operating room procedures listed under DRG 746

DRG 748 **Female Reproductive System Reconstructive Procedures**

GMLOS 1.5   AMLOS 1.8   RW 1.0096   ☑

Operating Room Procedures

57.85	Cystourethroplasty and plastic repair of bladder neck
59.4	Suprapubic sling operation
59.5	Retropubic urethral suspension
59.6	Paraurethral suspension
59.71	Levator muscle operation for urethrovesical suspension
59.79	Other repair of urinary stress incontinence
64.5	Operations for sex transformation, not elsewhere classified
69.2*	Repair of uterine supporting structures
69.98	Other operations on supporting structures of uterus
70.4	Obliteration and total excision of vagina

Ⓣ *Transfer DRG*   ⓢ *Special Payment*   ☑ *Optimization Potential*   ⦿ *Targeted Potential*   * *Code Range*   ● *New DRG*   ▲ *Revised DRG Title*

70.5*	Repair of cystocele and rectocele
70.6*	Vaginal construction and reconstruction
70.77	Vaginal suspension and fixation
70.78	Vaginal suspension and fixation with graft or prosthesis
70.8	Obliteration of vaginal vault

DRG 749   **Other Female Reproductive System O.R. Procedures with CC/MCC**

GMLOS 6.1   AMLOS 8.4   RW 2.6239

Operating Room Procedures

03.93	Implantation or replacement of spinal neurostimulator lead(s)
03.94	Removal of spinal neurostimulator lead(s)
04.92	Implantation or replacement of peripheral neurostimulator lead(s)
04.93	Removal of peripheral neurostimulator lead(s)
05.24	Presacral sympathectomy
38.7	Interruption of the vena cava
39.98	Control of hemorrhage, not otherwise specified
40.11	Biopsy of lymphatic structure
40.24	Excision of inguinal lymph node
40.29	Simple excision of other lymphatic structure
40.3	Regional lymph node excision
47.1*	Incidental appendectomy
50.12	Open biopsy of liver
54.1*	Laparotomy
54.23	Biopsy of peritoneum
54.29	Other diagnostic procedures on abdominal region
54.4	Excision or destruction of peritoneal tissue
54.5*	Lysis of peritoneal adhesions
54.61	Reclosure of postoperative disruption of abdominal wall
54.62	Delayed closure of granulating abdominal wound
56.41	Partial ureterectomy
56.5*	Cutaneous uretero-ileostomy
56.6*	Other external urinary diversion
56.71	Urinary diversion to intestine
56.72	Revision of ureterointestinal anastomosis
56.73	Nephrocystanastomosis, not otherwise specified
56.75	Transureteroureterostomy
56.83	Closure of ureterostomy
56.84	Closure of other fistula of ureter
57.22	Revision or closure of vesicostomy
57.33	Closed (transurethral) biopsy of bladder
57.34	Open biopsy of bladder
57.5*	Other excision or destruction of bladder tissue
57.6	Partial cystectomy
57.7*	Total cystectomy
57.82	Closure of cystostomy
57.83	Repair of fistula involving bladder and intestine
57.84	Repair of other fistula of bladder
57.89	Other repair of bladder
58.0	Urethrotomy
58.43	Closure of other fistula of urethra
58.49	Other repair of urethra
58.5	Release of urethral stricture
58.99	Other operations on urethra and periurethral tissue
59.00	Retroperitoneal dissection, not otherwise specified
59.02	Other lysis of perirenal or periureteral adhesions
59.03	Laparoscopic lysis of perirenal or periureteral adhesions
59.09	Other incision of perirenal or periureteral tissue
59.1*	Incision of perivesical tissue
66.95	Insufflation of therapeutic agent into fallopian tubes
68.24	Uterine artery embolization [UAE] with coils
68.25	Uterine artery embolization [UAE] without coils
69.99	Other operations on cervix and uterus
70.12	Culdotomy
71.9	Other operations on female genital organs
86.06	Insertion of totally implantable infusion pump
86.22	Excisional debridement of wound, infection, or burn

DRG 750   **Other Female Reproductive System O.R. Procedures without CC/MCC**

GMLOS 2.2   AMLOS 2.8   RW 1.0854   ☑

Select operating room procedures listed under DRG 749

MEDICAL

DRG 754   **Malignancy, Female Reproductive System with MCC**

GMLOS 5.8   AMLOS 8.4   RW 1.9784   ☑

Principal Diagnosis

179	Malignant neoplasm of uterus, part unspecified
180*	Malignant neoplasm of cervix uteri
181	Malignant neoplasm of placenta
182*	Malignant neoplasm of body of uterus
183*	Malignant neoplasm of ovary and other uterine adnexa
184*	Malignant neoplasm of other and unspecified female genital organs
195.3	Malignant neoplasm of pelvis
198.6	Secondary malignant neoplasm of ovary
198.82	Secondary malignant neoplasm of genital organs
233.1	Carcinoma in situ of cervix uteri
233.2	Carcinoma in situ of other and unspecified parts of uterus
233.3*	Carcinoma in situ, other and unspecified female genital organs
236.0	Neoplasm of uncertain behavior of uterus
236.1	Neoplasm of uncertain behavior of placenta
236.2	Neoplasm of uncertain behavior of ovary
236.3	Neoplasm of uncertain behavior of other and unspecified female genital organs

DRG 755   **Malignancy, Female Reproductive System with CC**

GMLOS 3.7   AMLOS 5.0   RW 1.0880   ☑

Select principal diagnosis listed under DRG 754

DRG 756   **Malignancy, Female Reproductive System without CC/MCC**

GMLOS 2.1   AMLOS 2.6   RW 0.6334   ☑

Select principal diagnosis listed under DRG 754

DRG 757   **Infections, Female Reproductive System with MCC**

GMLOS 5.7   AMLOS 7.2   RW 1.5292   ☑

Principal Diagnosis

016.6*	Tuberculous oophoritis and salpingitis
016.7*	Tuberculosis of other female genital organs
054.10	Unspecified genital herpes
054.11	Herpetic vulvovaginitis
054.12	Herpetic ulceration of vulva
054.19	Other genital herpes
091.0	Genital syphilis (primary)
098.0	Gonococcal infection (acute) of lower genitourinary tract
098.10	Gonococcal infection (acute) of upper genitourinary tract, site unspecified
098.15	Gonococcal cervicitis (acute)
098.16	Gonococcal endometritis (acute)
098.17	Gonococcal salpingitis, specified as acute
098.19	Other gonococcal infections (acute) of upper genitourinary tract
098.2	Gonococcal infections, chronic, of lower genitourinary tract
098.35	Gonococcal cervicitis, chronic
098.36	Gonococcal endometritis, chronic
098.37	Gonococcal salpingitis (chronic)
098.39	Other chronic gonococcal infections of upper genitourinary tract

099.0	Chancroid
099.1	Lymphogranuloma venereum
099.2	Granuloma inguinale
099.4*	Other nongonococcal urethritis (NGU)
099.50	Chlamydia trachomatis infection of unspecified site
099.53	Chlamydia trachomatis infection of lower genitourinary sites
099.55	Chlamydia trachomatis infection of unspecified genitourinary site
099.59	Chlamydia trachomatis infection of other specified site
099.8	Other specified venereal diseases
099.9	Unspecified venereal disease
112.1	Candidiasis of vulva and vagina
112.2	Candidiasis of other urogenital sites
131.00	Unspecified urogenital trichomoniasis
131.01	Trichomonal vulvovaginitis
131.02	Trichomonal urethritis
131.09	Other urogenital trichomoniasis
614.0	Acute salpingitis and oophoritis
614.1	Chronic salpingitis and oophoritis
614.2	Salpingitis and oophoritis not specified as acute, subacute, or chronic
614.3	Acute parametritis and pelvic cellulitis
614.4	Chronic or unspecified parametritis and pelvic cellulitis
614.5	Acute or unspecified pelvic peritonitis, female
614.7	Other chronic pelvic peritonitis, female
614.8	Other specified inflammatory disease of female pelvic organs and tissues
614.9	Unspecified inflammatory disease of female pelvic organs and tissues
615*	Inflammatory diseases of uterus, except cervix
616.0	Cervicitis and endocervicitis
616.1*	Vaginitis and vulvovaginitis
616.3	Abscess of Bartholin's gland
616.4	Other abscess of vulva
616.8*	Other specified inflammatory diseases of cervix, vagina, and vulva
616.9	Unspecified inflammatory disease of cervix, vagina, and vulva
625.71	Vulvar vestibulitis
698.1	Pruritus of genital organs

DRG 758   Infections, Female Reproductive System with CC

GMLOS 4.2   AMLOS 5.2   RW 1.0452   ☑

Select principal diagnosis listed under DRG 757

DRG 759   Infections, Female Reproductive System without CC/MCC

GMLOS 3.2   AMLOS 3.8   RW 0.6995   ☑

Select principal diagnosis listed under DRG 757

DRG 760   Menstrual and Other Female Reproductive System Disorders with CC/MCC

GMLOS 2.8   AMLOS 3.6   RW 0.8063   ☑

Principal Diagnosis

218*	Uterine leiomyoma
219*	Other benign neoplasm of uterus
220	Benign neoplasm of ovary
221*	Benign neoplasm of other female genital organs
256*	Ovarian dysfunction
306.51	Psychogenic vaginismus
306.52	Psychogenic dysmenorrhea
456.5	Pelvic varices
456.6	Vulval varices
614.6	Pelvic peritoneal adhesions, female (postoperative) (postinfection)
616.2	Cyst of Bartholin's gland
616.5*	Ulceration of vulva
617.0	Endometriosis of uterus

617.1	Endometriosis of ovary
617.2	Endometriosis of fallopian tube
617.3	Endometriosis of pelvic peritoneum
617.4	Endometriosis of rectovaginal septum and vagina
617.8	Endometriosis of other specified sites
617.9	Endometriosis, site unspecified
618*	Genital prolapse
619.0	Urinary-genital tract fistula, female
619.2	Genital tract-skin fistula, female
619.8	Other specified fistula involving female genital tract
619.9	Unspecified fistula involving female genital tract
620*	Noninflammatory disorders of ovary, fallopian tube, and broad ligament
621*	Disorders of uterus, not elsewhere classified
622*	Noninflammatory disorders of cervix
623*	Noninflammatory disorders of vagina
624*	Noninflammatory disorders of vulva and perineum
625.0	Dyspareunia
625.1	Vaginismus
625.2	Mittelschmerz
625.3	Dysmenorrhea
625.4	Premenstrual tension syndromes
625.5	Pelvic congestion syndrome
625.6	Female stress incontinence
625.70	Vulvodynia, unspecified
625.79	Other vulvodynia
625.8	Other specified symptom associated with female genital organs
625.9	Unspecified symptom associated with female genital organs
626*	Disorders of menstruation and other abnormal bleeding from female genital tract
627*	Menopausal and postmenopausal disorders
628*	Female infertility
629.0	Hematocele, female, not elsewhere classified
629.1	Hydrocele, canal of Nuck
629.2*	Female genital mutilation status
629.3*	Complication of implanted vaginal mesh and other prosthetic materials
629.8*	Other specified disorders of female genital organs
629.9	Unspecified disorder of female genital organs
752.0	Congenital anomalies of ovaries
752.1*	Congenital anomalies of fallopian tubes and broad ligaments
752.2	Congenital doubling of uterus
752.3*	Other congenital anomaly of uterus
752.4*	Congenital anomalies of cervix, vagina, and external female genitalia
752.7	Indeterminate sex and pseudohermaphroditism
752.89	Other specified anomalies of genital organs
752.9	Unspecified congenital anomaly of genital organs
758.6	Gonadal dysgenesis
758.8*	Other conditions due to chromosome anomalies
795.0*	Abnormal Papanicolaou smear of cervix and cervical HPV
795.1*	Abnormal Papanicolaou smear of vagina and vaginal HPV
867.4	Uterus injury without mention of open wound into cavity
867.5	Uterus injury with open wound into cavity
867.6	Injury to other specified pelvic organs without mention of open wound into cavity
867.7	Injury to other specified pelvic organs with open wound into cavity
867.8	Injury to unspecified pelvic organ without mention of open wound into cavity
867.9	Injury to unspecified pelvic organ with open wound into cavity
878.4	Open wound of vulva, without mention of complication
878.5	Open wound of vulva, complicated
878.6	Open wound of vagina, without mention of complication
878.7	Open wound of vagina, complicated
878.8	Open wound of other and unspecified parts of genital organs, without mention of complication

MDC 13: Diseases And Disorders Of The Female Reproductive System—MEDICAL

Ⓣ *Transfer DRG*   ⓢⓟ *Special Payment*   ☑ *Optimization Potential*   ▽ *Targeted Potential*   * *Code Range*   ● *New DRG*   ▲ *Revised DRG Title*

130   Valid 10/01/2013-09/30/2014   © 2013 OptumInsight, Inc.

878.9	Open wound of other and unspecified parts of genital organs, complicated
908.2	Late effect of internal injury to other internal organs
922.4	Contusion of genital organs
926.0	Crushing injury of external genitalia
939.1	Foreign body in uterus, any part
939.2	Foreign body in vulva and vagina
947.4	Burn of vagina and uterus
996.32	Mechanical complication due to intrauterine contraceptive device
V25.2	Sterilization
V25.3	Menstrual extraction
V26.0	Tuboplasty or vasoplasty after previous sterilization
V45.77	Acquired absence of organ, genital organs
V50.42	Prophylactic ovary removal
V55.7	Attention to artificial vagina
V61.5	Multiparity
V88.0*	Acquired absence of cervix and uterus

DRG 761 **Menstrual and Other Female Reproductive System Disorders without CC/MCC**

GMLOS 1.8   AMLOS 2.2   RW 0.4904   ☑

Select principal diagnosis listed under DRG 760

MDC 13: Diseases And Disorders Of The Female Reproductive System—MEDICAL

630	635.81	638.4	642.52	646.53	648.11	649.50	652.81	654.71
631.0	635.82	638.5	642.53	646.54	648.12	649.51	652.83	654.72
631.8	635.90	638.6	642.54	646.60	648.13	649.53	652.90	654.73
632	635.91	638.7	642.60	646.61	648.14	649.60	652.91	654.74
633.00	635.92	638.8	642.61	646.62	648.20	649.61	652.93	654.80
633.01	636.00	638.9	642.62	646.63	648.21	649.62	653.00	654.81
633.10	636.01	639.0	642.63	646.64	648.22	649.63	653.01	654.82
633.11	636.02	639.1	642.64	646.70	648.23	649.64	653.03	654.83
633.20	636.10	639.2	642.70	646.71	648.24	649.70	653.10	654.84
633.21	636.11	639.3	642.71	646.73	648.30	649.71	653.11	654.90
633.80	636.12	639.4	642.72	646.80	648.31	649.73	653.13	654.91
633.81	636.20	639.5	642.73	646.81	648.32	649.81	653.20	654.92
633.90	636.21	639.6	642.74	646.82	648.33	649.82	653.21	654.93
633.91	636.22	639.8	642.90	646.83	648.34	650	653.23	654.94
634.00	636.30	639.9	642.91	646.84	648.40	651.00	653.30	655.00
634.01	636.31	640.00	642.92	646.90	648.41	651.01	653.31	655.01
634.02	636.32	640.01	642.93	646.91	648.42	651.03	653.33	655.03
634.10	636.40	640.03	642.94	646.93	648.43	651.10	653.40	655.10
634.11	636.41	640.80	643.00	647.00	648.44	651.11	653.41	655.11
634.12	636.42	640.81	643.01	647.01	648.50	651.13	653.43	655.13
634.20	636.50	640.83	643.03	647.02	648.51	651.20	653.50	655.20
634.21	636.51	640.90	643.10	647.03	648.52	651.21	653.51	655.21
634.22	636.52	640.91	643.11	647.04	648.53	651.23	653.53	655.23
634.30	636.60	640.93	643.13	647.10	648.54	651.30	653.60	655.30
634.31	636.61	641.00	643.20	647.11	648.60	651.31	653.61	655.31
634.32	636.62	641.01	643.21	647.12	648.61	651.33	653.63	655.33
634.40	636.70	641.03	643.23	647.13	648.62	651.40	653.70	655.40
634.41	636.71	641.10	643.80	647.14	648.63	651.41	653.71	655.41
634.42	636.72	641.11	643.81	647.20	648.64	651.43	653.73	655.43
634.50	636.80	641.13	643.83	647.21	648.70	651.50	653.80	655.50
634.51	636.81	641.20	643.90	647.22	648.71	651.51	653.81	655.51
634.52	636.82	641.21	643.91	647.23	648.72	651.53	653.83	655.53
634.60	636.90	641.23	643.93	647.24	648.73	651.60	653.90	655.60
634.61	636.91	641.30	644.00	647.30	648.74	651.61	653.91	655.61
634.62	636.92	641.31	644.03	647.31	648.80	651.63	653.93	655.63
634.70	637.00	641.33	644.10	647.32	648.81	651.70	654.00	655.70
634.71	637.01	641.80	644.13	647.33	648.82	651.71	654.01	655.71
634.72	637.02	641.81	644.20	647.34	648.83	651.73	654.02	655.73
634.80	637.10	641.83	644.21	647.40	648.84	651.80	654.03	655.80
634.81	637.11	641.90	645.10	647.41	648.90	651.81	654.04	655.81
634.82	637.12	641.91	645.11	647.42	648.91	651.83	654.10	655.83
634.90	637.20	641.93	645.13	647.43	648.92	651.90	654.11	655.90
634.91	637.21	642.00	645.20	647.44	648.93	651.91	654.12	655.91
634.92	637.22	642.01	645.21	647.50	648.94	651.93	654.13	655.93
635.00	637.30	642.02	645.23	647.51	649.00	652.00	654.14	656.00
635.01	637.31	642.03	646.00	647.52	649.01	652.01	654.20	656.01
635.02	637.32	642.04	646.01	647.53	649.02	652.03	654.21	656.03
635.10	637.40	642.10	646.03	647.54	649.03	652.10	654.23	656.10
635.11	637.41	642.11	646.10	647.60	649.04	652.11	654.30	656.11
635.12	637.42	642.12	646.11	647.61	649.10	652.13	654.31	656.13
635.20	637.50	642.13	646.12	647.62	649.11	652.20	654.32	656.20
635.21	637.51	642.14	646.13	647.63	649.12	652.21	654.33	656.21
635.22	637.52	642.20	646.14	647.64	649.13	652.23	654.34	656.23
635.30	637.60	642.21	646.20	647.80	649.14	652.30	654.40	656.30
635.31	637.61	642.22	646.21	647.81	649.20	652.31	654.41	656.31
635.32	637.62	642.23	646.22	647.82	649.21	652.33	654.42	656.33
635.40	637.70	642.24	646.23	647.83	649.22	652.40	654.43	656.40
635.41	637.71	642.30	646.24	647.84	649.23	652.41	654.44	656.41
635.42	637.72	642.31	646.30	647.90	649.24	652.43	654.50	656.43
635.50	637.80	642.32	646.31	647.91	649.30	652.50	654.51	656.50
635.51	637.81	642.33	646.33	647.92	649.31	652.51	654.52	656.51
635.52	637.82	642.34	646.40	647.93	649.32	652.53	654.53	656.53
635.60	637.90	642.40	646.41	647.94	649.33	652.60	654.54	656.60
635.61	637.91	642.41	646.42	648.00	649.34	652.61	654.60	656.61
635.62	637.92	642.42	646.43	648.01	649.40	652.63	654.61	656.63
635.70	638.0	642.43	646.44	648.02	649.41	652.70	654.62	656.70
635.71	638.1	642.44	646.50	648.03	649.42	652.71	654.63	656.71
635.72	638.2	642.50	646.51	648.04	649.43	652.73	654.64	656.73
635.80	638.3	642.51	646.52	648.10	649.44	652.80	654.70	656.80

656.81	659.91	662.21	664.91	668.03	669.91	672.04	675.03	676.80
656.83	659.93	662.23	664.94	668.04	669.92	673.00	675.04	676.81
656.90	660.00	662.30	665.00	668.10	669.93	673.01	675.10	676.82
656.91	660.01	662.31	665.01	668.11	669.94	673.02	675.11	676.83
656.93	660.03	662.33	665.03	668.12	670.00	673.03	675.12	676.84
657.00	660.10	663.00	665.10	668.13	670.02	673.04	675.13	676.90
657.01	660.11	663.01	665.11	668.14	670.04	673.10	675.14	676.91
657.03	660.13	663.03	665.20	668.20	670.10	673.11	675.20	676.92
658.00	660.20	663.10	665.22	668.21	670.12	673.12	675.21	676.93
658.01	660.21	663.11	665.24	668.22	670.14	673.13	675.22	676.94
658.03	660.23	663.13	665.30	668.23	670.20	673.14	675.23	677
658.10	660.30	663.20	665.31	668.24	670.22	673.20	675.24	678.00
658.11	660.31	663.21	665.34	668.80	670.24	673.21	675.80	678.01
658.13	660.33	663.23	665.40	668.81	670.30	673.22	675.81	678.03
658.20	660.40	663.30	665.41	668.82	670.32	673.23	675.82	678.10
658.21	660.41	663.31	665.44	668.83	670.34	673.24	675.83	678.11
658.23	660.43	663.33	665.50	668.84	670.80	673.30	675.84	678.13
658.30	660.50	663.40	665.51	668.90	670.82	673.31	675.90	679.00
658.31	660.51	663.41	665.54	668.91	670.84	673.32	675.91	679.01
658.33	660.53	663.43	665.60	668.92	671.00	673.33	675.92	679.02
658.40	660.60	663.50	665.61	668.93	671.01	673.34	675.93	679.03
658.41	660.61	663.51	665.64	668.94	671.02	673.80	675.94	679.04
658.43	660.63	663.53	665.70	669.00	671.03	673.81	676.00	679.10
658.80	660.70	663.60	665.71	669.01	671.04	673.82	676.01	679.11
658.81	660.71	663.61	665.72	669.02	671.10	673.83	676.02	679.12
658.83	660.73	663.63	665.74	669.03	671.11	673.84	676.03	679.13
658.90	660.80	663.80	665.80	669.04	671.12	674.00	676.04	679.14
658.91	660.81	663.81	665.81	669.10	671.13	674.01	676.10	792.3
658.93	660.83	663.83	665.82	669.11	671.14	674.02	676.11	796.5
659.00	660.90	663.90	665.83	669.12	671.20	674.03	676.12	V23.0
659.01	660.91	663.91	665.84	669.13	671.21	674.04	676.13	V23.1
659.03	660.93	663.93	665.90	669.14	671.22	674.10	676.14	V23.2
659.10	661.00	664.00	665.91	669.20	671.23	674.12	676.20	V23.3
659.11	661.01	664.01	665.92	669.21	671.24	674.14	676.21	V23.41
659.13	661.03	664.04	665.93	669.22	671.30	674.20	676.22	V23.42
659.20	661.10	664.10	665.94	669.23	671.31	674.22	676.23	V23.49
659.21	661.11	664.11	666.00	669.24	671.33	674.24	676.24	V23.5
659.23	661.13	664.14	666.02	669.30	671.40	674.30	676.30	V23.7
659.30	661.20	664.20	666.04	669.32	671.42	674.32	676.31	V23.81
659.31	661.21	664.21	666.10	669.34	671.44	674.34	676.32	V23.82
659.33	661.23	664.24	666.12	669.40	671.50	674.40	676.33	V23.83
659.40	661.30	664.30	666.14	669.41	671.51	674.42	676.34	V23.84
659.41	661.31	664.31	666.20	669.42	671.52	674.44	676.40	V23.85
659.43	661.33	664.34	666.22	669.43	671.53	674.50	676.41	V23.86
659.50	661.40	664.40	666.24	669.44	671.54	674.51	676.42	V23.87
659.51	661.41	664.41	666.30	669.50	671.80	674.52	676.43	V23.89
659.53	661.43	664.44	666.32	669.51	671.81	674.53	676.44	V23.9
659.60	661.90	664.50	666.34	669.60	671.82	674.54	676.50	V24.0
659.61	661.91	664.51	667.00	669.61	671.83	674.80	676.51	V28.0
659.63	661.93	664.54	667.02	669.70	671.84	674.82	676.52	V28.1
659.70	662.00	664.60	667.04	669.71	671.90	674.84	676.53	V28.2
659.71	662.01	664.61	667.10	669.80	671.91	674.90	676.54	V61.6
659.73	662.03	664.64	667.12	669.81	671.92	674.92	676.60	V61.7
659.80	662.10	664.80	667.14	669.82	671.93	674.94	676.61	
659.81	662.11	664.81	668.00	669.83	671.94	675.00	676.62	
659.83	662.13	664.84	668.01	669.84	672.00	675.01	676.63	
659.90	662.20	664.90	668.02	669.90	672.02	675.02	676.64	

SURGICAL

DRG 765   Cesarean Section with CC/MCC

GMLOS 3.9	AMLOS 4.8	RW 1.1125

Principal Diagnosis

640.01	Threatened abortion, delivered
640.81	Other specified hemorrhage in early pregnancy, delivered
640.91	Unspecified hemorrhage in early pregnancy, delivered
641.01	Placenta previa without hemorrhage, with delivery
641.11	Hemorrhage from placenta previa, with delivery
641.21	Premature separation of placenta, with delivery
641.31	Antepartum hemorrhage associated with coagulation defects, with delivery
641.81	Other antepartum hemorrhage, with delivery
641.91	Unspecified antepartum hemorrhage, with delivery
642.01	Benign essential hypertension with delivery
642.02	Benign essential hypertension, with delivery, with current postpartum complication
642.11	Hypertension secondary to renal disease, with delivery
642.12	Hypertension secondary to renal disease, with delivery, with current postpartum complication
642.21	Other pre-existing hypertension, with delivery
642.22	Other pre-existing hypertension, with delivery, with current postpartum complication
642.31	Transient hypertension of pregnancy, with delivery
642.32	Transient hypertension of pregnancy, with delivery, with current postpartum complication
642.41	Mild or unspecified pre-eclampsia, with delivery
642.42	Mild or unspecified pre-eclampsia, with delivery, with current postpartum complication
642.51	Severe pre-eclampsia, with delivery
642.52	Severe pre-eclampsia, with delivery, with current postpartum complication
642.61	Eclampsia, with delivery
642.62	Eclampsia, with delivery, with current postpartum complication
642.71	Pre-eclampsia or eclampsia superimposed on pre-existing hypertension, with delivery
642.72	Pre-eclampsia or eclampsia superimposed on pre-existing hypertension, with delivery, with current postpartum complication
642.91	Unspecified hypertension, with delivery
642.92	Unspecified hypertension, with delivery, with current postpartum complication
643.01	Mild hyperemesis gravidarum, delivered
643.11	Hyperemesis gravidarum with metabolic disturbance, delivered
643.21	Late vomiting of pregnancy, delivered
643.81	Other vomiting complicating pregnancy, delivered
643.91	Unspecified vomiting of pregnancy, delivered
644.21	Early onset of delivery, delivered, with or without mention of antepartum condition
645.11	Post term pregnancy, delivered, with or without mention of antepartum condition
645.21	Prolonged pregnancy, delivered, with or without mention of antepartum condition
646.00	Papyraceous fetus, unspecified as to episode of care
646.01	Papyraceous fetus, delivered, with or without mention of antepartum condition
646.11	Edema or excessive weight gain in pregnancy, with delivery, with or without mention of antepartum complication
646.12	Edema or excessive weight gain in pregnancy, with delivery, with current postpartum complication
646.21	Unspecified renal disease in pregnancy, with delivery
646.22	Unspecified renal disease in pregnancy, with delivery, with current postpartum complication
646.31	Pregnancy complication, recurrent pregnancy loss, with or without mention of antepartum condition
646.41	Peripheral neuritis in pregnancy, with delivery
646.42	Peripheral neuritis in pregnancy, with delivery, with current postpartum complication
646.51	Asymptomatic bacteriuria in pregnancy, with delivery
646.52	Asymptomatic bacteriuria in pregnancy, with delivery, with current postpartum complication
646.61	Infections of genitourinary tract in pregnancy, with delivery
646.62	Infections of genitourinary tract in pregnancy, with delivery, with current postpartum complication
646.71	Liver and biliary tract disorders in pregnancy, delivered, with or without mention of antepartum condition
646.81	Other specified complication of pregnancy, with delivery
646.82	Other specified complications of pregnancy, with delivery, with current postpartum complication
646.91	Unspecified complication of pregnancy, with delivery
647.01	Maternal syphilis, complicating pregnancy, with delivery
647.02	Maternal syphilis, complicating pregnancy, with delivery, with current postpartum complication
647.11	Maternal gonorrhea with delivery
647.12	Maternal gonorrhea, with delivery, with current postpartum complication
647.21	Other maternal venereal diseases with delivery
647.22	Other maternal venereal diseases with delivery, with current postpartum complication
647.31	Maternal tuberculosis with delivery
647.32	Maternal tuberculosis with delivery, with current postpartum complication
647.41	Maternal malaria with delivery
647.42	Maternal malaria with delivery, with current postpartum complication
647.51	Maternal rubella with delivery
647.52	Maternal rubella with delivery, with current postpartum complication
647.61	Other maternal viral disease with delivery
647.62	Other maternal viral disease with delivery, with current postpartum complication
647.81	Other specified maternal infectious and parasitic disease with delivery
647.82	Other specified maternal infectious and parasitic disease with delivery, with current postpartum complication
647.91	Unspecified maternal infection or infestation with delivery
647.92	Unspecified maternal infection or infestation with delivery, with current postpartum complication
648.01	Maternal diabetes mellitus with delivery
648.02	Maternal diabetes mellitus with delivery, with current postpartum complication
648.11	Maternal thyroid dysfunction with delivery, with or without mention of antepartum condition
648.12	Maternal thyroid dysfunction with delivery, with current postpartum complication
648.21	Maternal anemia, with delivery
648.22	Maternal anemia with delivery, with current postpartum complication
648.31	Maternal drug dependence, with delivery
648.32	Maternal drug dependence, with delivery, with current postpartum complication
648.41	Maternal mental disorders, with delivery
648.42	Maternal mental disorders, with delivery, with current postpartum complication
648.51	Maternal congenital cardiovascular disorders, with delivery
648.52	Maternal congenital cardiovascular disorders, with delivery, with current postpartum complication
648.61	Other maternal cardiovascular diseases, with delivery
648.62	Other maternal cardiovascular diseases, with delivery, with current postpartum complication
648.71	Bone and joint disorders of maternal back, pelvis, and lower limbs, with delivery
648.72	Bone and joint disorders of maternal back, pelvis, and lower limbs, with delivery, with current postpartum complication
648.81	Abnormal maternal glucose tolerance, with delivery

---

1 Transfer DRG   SP Special Payment   ☑ Optimization Potential   ᵀᴾ Targeted Potential   * Code Range   ● New DRG   ▲ Revised DRG Title

648.82	Abnormal maternal glucose tolerance, with delivery, with current postpartum complication
648.91	Other current maternal conditions classifiable elsewhere, with delivery
648.92	Other current maternal conditions classifiable elsewhere, with delivery, with current postpartum complication
649.01	Tobacco use disorder complicating pregnancy, childbirth, or the puerperium, delivered, with or without mention of antepartum condition
649.02	Tobacco use disorder complicating pregnancy, childbirth, or the puerperium, delivered, with mention of postpartum complication
649.11	Obesity complicating pregnancy, childbirth, or the puerperium, delivered, with or without mention of antepartum condition
649.12	Obesity complicating pregnancy, childbirth, or the puerperium, delivered, with mention of postpartum complication
649.21	Bariatric surgery status complicating pregnancy, childbirth, or the puerperium, delivered, with or without mention of antepartum condition
649.22	Bariatric surgery status complicating pregnancy, childbirth, or the puerperium, delivered, with mention of postpartum complication
649.31	Coagulation defects complicating pregnancy, childbirth, or the puerperium, delivered, with or without mention of antepartum condition
649.32	Coagulation defects complicating pregnancy, childbirth, or the puerperium, delivered, with mention of postpartum complication
649.41	Epilepsy complicating pregnancy, childbirth, or the puerperium, delivered, with or without mention of antepartum condition
649.42	Epilepsy complicating pregnancy, childbirth, or the puerperium, delivered, with mention of postpartum complication
649.51	Spotting complicating pregnancy, delivered, with or without mention of antepartum condition
649.61	Uterine size date discrepancy, delivered, with or without mention of antepartum condition
649.62	Uterine size date discrepancy, delivered, with mention of postpartum complication
649.71	Cervical shortening, delivered, with or without mention of antepartum condition
649.8*	Onset (spontaneous) of labor after 37 completed weeks of gestation but before 39 completed weeks gestation, with delivery by (planned) cesarean section
650	Normal delivery
651.01	Twin pregnancy, delivered
651.11	Triplet pregnancy, delivered
651.21	Quadruplet pregnancy, delivered
651.31	Twin pregnancy with fetal loss and retention of one fetus, delivered
651.41	Triplet pregnancy with fetal loss and retention of one or more, delivered
651.51	Quadruplet pregnancy with fetal loss and retention of one or more, delivered
651.61	Other multiple pregnancy with fetal loss and retention of one or more fetus(es), delivered
651.71	Multiple gestation following (elective) fetal reduction, delivered, with or without mention of antepartum condition
651.81	Other specified multiple gestation, delivered
651.91	Unspecified multiple gestation, delivered
652.01	Unstable lie of fetus, delivered
652.11	Breech or other malpresentation successfully converted to cephalic presentation, delivered
652.21	Breech presentation without mention of version, delivered
652.31	Transverse or oblique fetal presentation, delivered
652.41	Fetal face or brow presentation, delivered
652.51	High fetal head at term, delivered

652.61	Multiple gestation with malpresentation of one fetus or more, delivered
652.71	Prolapsed arm of fetus, delivered
652.81	Other specified malposition or malpresentation of fetus, delivered
652.91	Unspecified malposition or malpresentation of fetus, delivered
653.01	Major abnormality of bony pelvis, not further specified, delivered
653.11	Generally contracted pelvis in pregnancy, delivered
653.21	Inlet contraction of pelvis in pregnancy, delivered
653.31	Outlet contraction of pelvis in pregnancy, delivered
653.41	Fetopelvic disproportion, delivered
653.51	Unusually large fetus causing disproportion, delivered
653.61	Hydrocephalic fetus causing disproportion, delivered
653.71	Other fetal abnormality causing disproportion, delivered
653.81	Fetal disproportion of other origin, delivered
653.91	Unspecified fetal disproportion, delivered
654.01	Congenital abnormalities of pregnant uterus, delivered
654.02	Congenital abnormalities of pregnant uterus, delivered, with mention of postpartum complication
654.11	Tumors of body of uterus, delivered
654.12	Tumors of body of uterus, delivered, with mention of postpartum complication
654.21	Previous cesarean delivery, delivered, with or without mention of antepartum condition
654.31	Retroverted and incarcerated gravid uterus, delivered
654.32	Retroverted and incarcerated gravid uterus, delivered, with mention of postpartum complication
654.41	Other abnormalities in shape or position of gravid uterus and of neighboring structures, delivered
654.42	Other abnormalities in shape or position of gravid uterus and of neighboring structures, delivered, with mention of postpartum complication
654.51	Cervical incompetence, delivered
654.52	Cervical incompetence, delivered, with mention of postpartum complication
654.61	Other congenital or acquired abnormality of cervix, with delivery
654.62	Other congenital or acquired abnormality of cervix, delivered, with mention of postpartum complication
654.71	Congenital or acquired abnormality of vagina, with delivery
654.72	Congenital or acquired abnormality of vagina, delivered, with mention of postpartum complication
654.81	Congenital or acquired abnormality of vulva, with delivery
654.82	Congenital or acquired abnormality of vulva, delivered, with mention of postpartum complication
654.91	Other and unspecified abnormality of organs and soft tissues of pelvis, with delivery
654.92	Other and unspecified abnormality of organs and soft tissues of pelvis, delivered, with mention of postpartum complication
655.01	Central nervous system malformation in fetus, with delivery
655.11	Chromosomal abnormality in fetus, affecting management of mother, with delivery
655.21	Hereditary disease in family possibly affecting fetus, affecting management of mother, with delivery
655.31	Suspected damage to fetus from viral disease in mother, affecting management of mother, with delivery
655.41	Suspected damage to fetus from other disease in mother, affecting management of mother, with delivery
655.51	Suspected damage to fetus from drugs, affecting management of mother, delivered
655.61	Suspected damage to fetus from radiation, affecting management of mother, delivered
655.71	Decreased fetal movements, affecting management of mother, delivered
655.81	Other known or suspected fetal abnormality, not elsewhere classified, affecting management of mother, delivery

Surgical	Medical	CC Indicator	MCC Indicator	Procedure Proxy

655.91	Unspecified fetal abnormality affecting management of mother, delivery
656.01	Fetal-maternal hemorrhage, with delivery
656.11	Rhesus isoimmunization affecting management of mother, delivered
656.21	Isoimmunization from other and unspecified blood-group incompatibility, affecting management of mother, delivered
656.30	Fetal distress affecting management of mother, unspecified as to episode of care
656.31	Fetal distress affecting management of mother, delivered
656.40	Intrauterine death affecting management of mother, unspecified as to episode of care
656.41	Intrauterine death affecting management of mother, delivered
656.51	Poor fetal growth, affecting management of mother, delivered
656.61	Excessive fetal growth affecting management of mother, delivered
656.71	Other placental conditions affecting management of mother, delivered
656.81	Other specified fetal and placental problems affecting management of mother, delivered
656.91	Unspecified fetal and placental problem affecting management of mother, delivered
657.01	Polyhydramnios, with delivery
658.01	Oligohydramnios, delivered
658.10	Premature rupture of membranes in pregnancy, unspecified as to episode of care
658.11	Premature rupture of membranes in pregnancy, delivered
658.20	Delayed delivery after spontaneous or unspecified rupture of membranes, unspecified as to episode of care
658.21	Delayed delivery after spontaneous or unspecified rupture of membranes, delivered
658.30	Delayed delivery after artificial rupture of membranes, unspecified as to episode of care
658.31	Delayed delivery after artificial rupture of membranes, delivered
658.40	Infection of amniotic cavity, unspecified as to episode of care
658.41	Infection of amniotic cavity, delivered
658.81	Other problem associated with amniotic cavity and membranes, delivered
658.91	Unspecified problem associated with amniotic cavity and membranes, delivered
659.00	Failed mechanical induction of labor, unspecified as to episode of care
659.01	Failed mechanical induction of labor, delivered
659.10	Failed medical or unspecified induction of labor, unspecified as to episode of care
659.11	Failed medical or unspecified induction of labor, delivered
659.20	Unspecified maternal pyrexia during labor, unspecified as to episode of care
659.21	Unspecified maternal pyrexia during labor, delivered
659.30	Generalized infection during labor, unspecified as to episode of care
659.31	Generalized infection during labor, delivered
659.41	Grand multiparity, delivered, with or without mention of antepartum condition
659.50	Elderly primigravida, unspecified as to episode of care
659.51	Elderly primigravida, delivered
659.60	Elderly multigravida, unspecified as to episode of care or not applicable
659.61	Elderly multigravida, delivered, with mention of antepartum condition
659.70	Abnormality in fetal heart rate or rhythm, unspecified as to episode of care or not applicable
659.71	Abnormality in fetal heart rate or rhythm, delivered, with or without mention of antepartum condition
659.80	Other specified indication for care or intervention related to labor and delivery, unspecified as to episode of care
659.81	Other specified indication for care or intervention related to labor and delivery, delivered
659.90	Unspecified indication for care or intervention related to labor and delivery, unspecified as to episode of care
659.91	Unspecified indication for care or intervention related to labor and delivery, delivered
660.00	Obstruction caused by malposition of fetus at onset of labor, unspecified as to episode of care
660.01	Obstruction caused by malposition of fetus at onset of labor, delivered
660.10	Obstruction by bony pelvis during labor and delivery, unspecified as to episode of care
660.11	Obstruction by bony pelvis during labor and delivery, delivered
660.20	Obstruction by abnormal pelvic soft tissues during labor and delivery, unspecified as to episode of care
660.21	Obstruction by abnormal pelvic soft tissues during labor and delivery, delivered
660.30	Deep transverse arrest and persistent occipitoposterior position during labor and delivery, unspecified as to episode of care
660.31	Deep transverse arrest and persistent occipitoposterior position during labor and deliver, delivered
660.40	Shoulder (girdle) dystocia during labor and delivery, unspecified as to episode of care
660.41	Shoulder (girdle) dystocia during labor and deliver, delivered
660.50	Locked twins during labor and delivery, unspecified as to episode of care in pregnancy
660.51	Locked twins, delivered
660.60	Unspecified failed trial of labor, unspecified as to episode of care
660.61	Unspecified failed trial of labor, delivered
660.70	Unspecified failed forceps or vacuum extractor, unspecified as to episode of care
660.71	Unspecified failed forceps or vacuum extractor, delivered
660.80	Other causes of obstructed labor, unspecified as to episode of care
660.81	Other causes of obstructed labor, delivered
660.90	Unspecified obstructed labor, unspecified as to episode of care
660.91	Unspecified obstructed labor, with delivery
661.00	Primary uterine inertia, unspecified as to episode of care
661.01	Primary uterine inertia, with delivery
661.10	Secondary uterine inertia, unspecified as to episode of care
661.11	Secondary uterine inertia, with delivery
661.20	Other and unspecified uterine inertia, unspecified as to episode of care
661.21	Other and unspecified uterine inertia, with delivery
661.30	Precipitate labor, unspecified as to episode of care
661.31	Precipitate labor, with delivery
661.40	Hypertonic, incoordinate, or prolonged uterine contractions, unspecified as to episode of care
661.41	Hypertonic, incoordinate, or prolonged uterine contractions, with delivery
661.90	Unspecified abnormality of labor, unspecified as to episode of care
661.91	Unspecified abnormality of labor, with delivery
662.00	Prolonged first stage of labor, unspecified as to episode of care
662.01	Prolonged first stage of labor, delivered
662.10	Unspecified prolonged labor, unspecified as to episode of care
662.11	Unspecified prolonged labor, delivered
662.20	Prolonged second stage of labor, unspecified as to episode of care
662.21	Prolonged second stage of labor, delivered
662.30	Delayed delivery of second twin, triplet, etc., unspecified as to episode of care
662.31	Delayed delivery of second twin, triplet, etc., delivered
663.00	Prolapse of cord, complicating labor and delivery, unspecified as to episode of care

T *Transfer DRG*   SP *Special Payment*   ☑ *Optimization Potential*   ▽ *Targeted Potential*   ⌃ *Code Range*   ● *New DRG*   ▲ *Revised DRG Title*

136   Valid 10/01/2013–09/30/2014   © 2013 OptumInsight, Inc.

663.01	Prolapse of cord, complicating labor and delivery, delivered
663.10	Cord around neck, with compression, complicating labor and delivery, unspecified as to episode of care
663.11	Cord around neck, with compression, complicating labor and delivery, delivered
663.20	Other and unspecified cord entanglement, with compression, complicating labor and delivery, unspecified as to episode of care
663.21	Other and unspecified cord entanglement, with compression, complicating labor and delivery, delivered
663.30	Other and unspecified cord entanglement, without mention of compression, complicating labor and delivery, unspecified as to episode of care
663.31	Other and unspecified cord entanglement, without mention of compression, complicating labor and delivery, delivered
663.40	Short cord complicating labor and delivery, unspecified as to episode of care
663.41	Short cord complicating labor and delivery, delivered
663.50	Vasa previa complicating labor and delivery, unspecified as to episode of care
663.51	Vasa previa complicating labor and delivery, delivered
663.60	Vascular lesions of cord complicating labor and delivery, unspecified as to episode of care
663.61	Vascular lesions of cord complicating labor and delivery, delivered
663.80	Other umbilical cord complications during labor and delivery, unspecified as to episode of care
663.81	Other umbilical cord complications during labor and delivery, delivered
663.90	Unspecified umbilical cord complication during labor and delivery, unspecified as to episode of care
663.91	Unspecified umbilical cord complication during labor and delivery, delivered
664.00	First-degree perineal laceration, unspecified as to episode of care in pregnancy
664.01	First-degree perineal laceration, with delivery
664.10	Second-degree perineal laceration, unspecified as to episode of care in pregnancy
664.11	Second-degree perineal laceration, with delivery
664.20	Third-degree perineal laceration, unspecified as to episode of care in pregnancy
664.21	Third-degree perineal laceration, with delivery
664.30	Fourth-degree perineal laceration, unspecified as to episode of care in pregnancy
664.31	Fourth-degree perineal laceration, with delivery
664.40	Unspecified perineal laceration, unspecified as to episode of care in pregnancy
664.41	Unspecified perineal laceration, with delivery
664.50	Vulvar and perineal hematoma, unspecified as to episode of care in pregnancy
664.51	Vulvar and perineal hematoma, with delivery
664.60	Anal sphincter tear complicating delivery, not associated with third-degree perineal laceration, unspecified as to episode of care or not applicable
664.61	Anal sphincter tear complicating delivery, not associated with third-degree perineal laceration, delivered, with or without mention of antepartum condition
664.80	Other specified trauma to perineum and vulva, unspecified as to episode of care in pregnancy
664.81	Other specified trauma to perineum and vulva, with delivery
664.90	Unspecified trauma to perineum and vulva, unspecified as to episode of care in pregnancy
664.91	Unspecified trauma to perineum and vulva, with delivery
665.00	Rupture of uterus before onset of labor, unspecified as to episode of care
665.01	Rupture of uterus before onset of labor, with delivery
665.10	Rupture of uterus during labor, unspecified as to episode
665.11	Rupture of uterus during labor, with delivery
665.20	Inversion of uterus, unspecified as to episode of care in pregnancy
665.22	Inversion of uterus, delivered with postpartum complication
665.30	Laceration of cervix, unspecified as to episode of care in pregnancy
665.31	Laceration of cervix, with delivery
665.40	High vaginal laceration, unspecified as to episode of care in pregnancy
665.41	High vaginal laceration, with delivery
665.50	Other injury to pelvic organs, unspecified as to episode of care in pregnancy
665.51	Other injury to pelvic organs, with delivery
665.60	Damage to pelvic joints and ligaments, unspecified as to episode of care in pregnancy
665.61	Damage to pelvic joints and ligaments, with delivery
665.70	Pelvic hematoma, unspecified as to episode of care
665.71	Pelvic hematoma, with delivery
665.72	Pelvic hematoma, delivered with postpartum complication
665.80	Other specified obstetrical trauma, unspecified as to episode of care
665.81	Other specified obstetrical trauma, with delivery
665.82	Other specified obstetrical trauma, delivered, with postpartum
665.90	Unspecified obstetrical trauma, unspecified as to episode of care
665.91	Unspecified obstetrical trauma, with delivery
665.92	Unspecified obstetrical trauma, delivered, with postpartum complication
666.02	Third-stage postpartum hemorrhage, with delivery
666.12	Other immediate postpartum hemorrhage, with delivery
666.22	Delayed and secondary postpartum hemorrhage, with delivery
666.32	Postpartum coagulation defects, with delivery
667.02	Retained placenta without hemorrhage, with delivery, with mention of postpartum complication
667.12	Retained portions of placenta or membranes, without hemorrhage, delivered, with mention of postpartum complication
668.00	Pulmonary complications of the administration of anesthesia or other sedation in labor and delivery, unspecified as to episode of care
668.01	Pulmonary complications of the administration of anesthesia or other sedation in labor and delivery, delivered
668.02	Pulmonary complications of the administration of anesthesia or other sedation in labor and delivery, delivered, with mention of postpartum complication
668.10	Cardiac complications of the administration of anesthesia or other sedation in labor and delivery, unspecified as to episode of care
668.11	Cardiac complications of the administration of anesthesia or other sedation in labor and delivery, delivered
668.12	Cardiac complications of the administration of anesthesia or other sedation in labor and delivery, delivered, with mention of postpartum complication
668.20	Central nervous system complications of the administration of anesthesia or other sedation in labor and delivery, unspecified as to episode of care
668.21	Central nervous system complications of the administration of anesthesia or other sedation in labor and delivery, delivered
668.22	Central nervous system complications of the administration of anesthesia or other sedation in labor and delivery, delivered, with mention of postpartum complication
668.80	Other complications of the administration of anesthesia or other sedation in labor and delivery, unspecified as to episode of care
668.81	Other complications of the administration of anesthesia or other sedation in labor and delivery, delivered
668.82	Other complications of the administration of anesthesia or other sedation in labor and delivery, delivered, with mention of postpartum complication

MDC 14: Pregnancy, Childbirth And The Puerperium—SURGICAL

Surgical	*Medical*	CC Indicator	MCC Indicator	Procedure Proxy

MDC 14: Pregnancy, Childbirth And The Puerperium—SURGICAL

668.90 Unspecified complication of the administration of anesthesia or other sedation in labor and delivery, unspecified as to episode of care

668.91 Unspecified complication of the administration of anesthesia or other sedation in labor and delivery, delivered

668.92 Unspecified complication of the administration of anesthesia or other sedation in labor and delivery, delivered, with mention of postpartum complication

669.00 Maternal distress complicating labor and delivery, unspecified as to episode of care

669.01 Maternal distress, with delivery, with or without mention of antepartum condition

669.02 Maternal distress, with delivery, with mention of postpartum complication

669.10 Shock during or following labor and delivery, unspecified as to episode of care

669.11 Shock during or following labor and delivery, with delivery, with or without mention of antepartum condition

669.12 Shock during or following labor and delivery, with delivery, with mention of postpartum complication

669.20 Maternal hypotension syndrome complicating labor and delivery, unspecified as to episode of care

669.21 Maternal hypotension syndrome, with delivery, with or without mention of antepartum condition

669.22 Maternal hypotension syndrome, with delivery, with mention of postpartum complication

669.30 Acute kidney failure following labor and delivery, unspecified as to episode of care or not applicable

669.32 Acute kidney failure following labor and delivery, delivered, with mention of postpartum complication

669.40 Other complications of obstetrical surgery and procedures, unspecified as to episode of care

669.41 Other complications of obstetrical surgery and procedures, with delivery, with or without mention of antepartum condition

669.42 Other complications of obstetrical surgery and procedures, with delivery, with mention of postpartum complication

669.50 Forceps or vacuum extractor delivery without mention of indication, unspecified as to episode of care

669.51 Forceps or vacuum extractor delivery without mention of indication, delivered, with or without mention of antepartum condition

669.60 Breech extraction, without mention of indication, unspecified as to episode of care

669.61 Breech extraction, without mention of indication, delivered, with or without mention of antepartum condition

669.70 Cesarean delivery, without mention of indication, unspecified as to episode of care

669.71 Cesarean delivery, without mention of indication, delivered, with or without mention of antepartum condition

669.80 Other complication of labor and delivery, unspecified as to episode of care

669.81 Other complication of labor and delivery, delivered, with or without mention of antepartum condition

669.82 Other complication of labor and delivery, delivered, with mention of postpartum complication

669.90 Unspecified complication of labor and delivery, unspecified as to episode of care

669.91 Unspecified complication of labor and delivery, with delivery, with or without mention of antepartum condition

669.92 Unspecified complication of labor and delivery, with delivery, with mention of postpartum complication

670.02 Major puerperal infection, unspecified, delivered, with mention of postpartum complication

670.12 Puerperal endometritis, delivered, with mention of postpartum complication

670.22 Puerperal sepsis, delivered, with mention of postpartum complication

670.32 Puerperal septic thrombophlebitis, delivered, with mention of postpartum complication

670.82 Other major puerperal infection, delivered, with mention of postpartum complication

671.01 Varicose veins of legs, with delivery, with or without mention of antepartum condition

671.02 Varicose veins of legs, with delivery, with mention of postpartum complication

671.11 Varicose veins of vulva and perineum, with delivery, with or without mention of antepartum condition

671.12 Varicose veins of vulva and perineum, with delivery, with mention of postpartum complication

671.21 Superficial thrombophlebitis with delivery, with or without mention of antepartum condition

671.22 Superficial thrombophlebitis with delivery, with mention of postpartum complication

671.31 Deep phlebothrombosis, antepartum, with delivery

671.42 Deep phlebothrombosis, postpartum, with delivery

671.51 Other phlebitis and thrombosis with delivery, with or without mention of antepartum condition

671.52 Other phlebitis and thrombosis with delivery, with mention of postpartum complication

671.81 Other venous complication, with delivery, with or without mention of antepartum condition

671.82 Other venous complication, with delivery, with mention of postpartum complication

671.91 Unspecified venous complication, with delivery, with or without mention of antepartum condition

671.92 Unspecified venous complication, with delivery, with mention of postpartum complication

672.02 Puerperal pyrexia of unknown origin, delivered, with mention of postpartum complication

673.01 Obstetrical air embolism, with delivery, with or without mention of antepartum condition

673.02 Obstetrical air embolism, with delivery, with mention of postpartum complication

673.11 Amniotic fluid embolism, with delivery, with or without mention of antepartum condition

673.12 Amniotic fluid embolism, with delivery, with mention of postpartum complication

673.21 Obstetrical blood-clot embolism, with delivery, with or without mention of antepartum condition

673.22 Obstetrical blood-clot embolism, with mention of postpartum complication

673.31 Obstetrical pyemic and septic embolism, with delivery, with or without mention of antepartum condition

673.32 Obstetrical pyemic and septic embolism, with delivery, with mention of postpartum complication

673.81 Other obstetrical pulmonary embolism, with delivery, with or without mention of antepartum condition

673.82 Other obstetrical pulmonary embolism, with delivery, with mention of postpartum complication

674.01 Cerebrovascular disorder, with delivery, with or without mention of antepartum condition

674.02 Cerebrovascular disorder, with delivery, with mention of postpartum complication

674.12 Disruption of cesarean wound, with delivery, with mention of postpartum complication

674.22 Disruption of perineal wound, with delivery, with mention of postpartum complication

674.32 Other complication of obstetrical surgical wounds, with delivery, with mention of postpartum complication

674.42 Placental polyp, with delivery, with mention of postpartum complication

674.51 Peripartum cardiomyopathy, delivered, with or without mention of antepartum condition

674.52 Peripartum cardiomyopathy, delivered, with mention of postpartum condition

674.82 Other complication of puerperium, with delivery, with mention of postpartum complication

674.92 Unspecified complications of puerperium, with delivery, with mention of postpartum complication

---

T *Transfer DRG* SP *Special Payment* ☑ *Optimization Potential* ▽ *Targeted Potential* * *Code Range* ● *New DRG* ▲ *Revised DRG Title*

675.01	Infection of nipple associated with childbirth, delivered, with or without mention of antepartum condition
675.02	Infection of nipple associated with childbirth, delivered with mention of postpartum complication
675.11	Abscess of breast associated with childbirth, delivered, with or without mention of antepartum condition
675.12	Abscess of breast associated with childbirth, delivered, with mention of postpartum complication
675.21	Nonpurulent mastitis, delivered, with or without mention of antepartum condition
675.22	Nonpurulent mastitis, delivered, with mention of postpartum complication
675.81	Other specified infection of the breast and nipple associated with childbirth, delivered, with or without mention of antepartum condition
675.82	Other specified infection of the breast and nipple associated with childbirth, delivered, with mention of postpartum complication
675.91	Unspecified infection of the breast and nipple, delivered, with or without mention of antepartum condition
675.92	Unspecified infection of the breast and nipple, delivered, with mention of postpartum complication
676.01	Retracted nipple, delivered, with or without mention of antepartum condition
676.02	Retracted nipple, delivered, with mention of postpartum complication
676.11	Cracked nipple, delivered, with or without mention of antepartum condition
676.12	Cracked nipple, delivered, with mention of postpartum complication
676.21	Engorgement of breasts, delivered, with or without mention of antepartum condition
676.22	Engorgement of breasts, delivered, with mention of postpartum complication
676.31	Other and unspecified disorder of breast associated with childbirth, delivered, with or without mention of antepartum condition
676.32	Other and unspecified disorder of breast associated with childbirth, delivered, with mention of postpartum complication
676.41	Failure of lactation, with delivery, with or without mention of antepartum condition
676.42	Failure of lactation, with delivery, with mention of postpartum complication
676.51	Suppressed lactation, with delivery, with or without mention of antepartum condition
676.52	Suppressed lactation, with delivery, with mention of postpartum complication
676.61	Galactorrhea, with delivery, with or without mention of antepartum condition
676.62	Galactorrhea, with delivery, with mention of postpartum complication
676.81	Other disorder of lactation, with delivery, with or without mention of antepartum condition
676.82	Other disorder of lactation, with delivery, with mention of postpartum complication
676.91	Unspecified disorder of lactation, with delivery, with or without mention of antepartum condition
676.92	Unspecified disorder of lactation, with delivery, with mention of postpartum complication
678.01	Fetal hematologic conditions, delivered, with or without mention of antepartum condition
678.11	Fetal conjoined twins, delivered, with or without mention of antepartum condition
679.00	Maternal complications from in utero procedure, unspecified as to episode of care or not applicable
679.01	Maternal complications from in utero procedure, delivered, with or without mention of antepartum condition
679.02	Maternal complications from in utero procedure, delivered, with mention of postpartum complication

679.11	Fetal complications from in utero procedure, delivered, with or without mention of antepartum condition
679.12	Fetal complications from in utero procedure, delivered, with mention of postpartum complication

Operating Room Procedures

74.0	Classical cesarean section
74.1	Low cervical cesarean section
74.2	Extraperitoneal cesarean section
74.4	Cesarean section of other specified type
74.99	Other cesarean section of unspecified type

DRG 766   Cesarean Section without CC/MCC
GMLOS 2.9   AMLOS 3.1   RW 0.7766   ☑

Select principal diagnosis and operating room procedure listed under DRG 765

DRG 767   Vaginal Delivery with Sterilization and/or D&C
GMLOS 2.7   AMLOS 3.6   RW 0.9235   ☑

Select principal diagnosis listed under DRG 765

Operating Room Procedures

66.2*	Bilateral endoscopic destruction or occlusion of fallopian tubes
66.3*	Other bilateral destruction or occlusion of fallopian tubes
66.4	Total unilateral salpingectomy
66.5*	Total bilateral salpingectomy
66.63	Bilateral partial salpingectomy, not otherwise specified
66.69	Other partial salpingectomy
66.92	Unilateral destruction or occlusion of fallopian tube
66.97	Burying of fimbriae in uterine wall
69.02	Dilation and curettage following delivery or abortion
69.09	Other dilation and curettage of uterus
69.52	Aspiration curettage following delivery or abortion

DRG 768   Vaginal Delivery with O.R. Procedure Except Sterilization and/or D&C
GMLOS 3.1   AMLOS 3.2   RW 1.0976

Select principal diagnosis listed under DRG 765

Operating Room Procedures

38.7	Interruption of the vena cava
39.98	Control of hemorrhage, not otherwise specified
39.99	Other operations on vessels
40.24	Excision of inguinal lymph node
40.3	Regional lymph node excision
48.79	Other repair of rectum
49.46	Excision of hemorrhoids
54.11	Exploratory laparotomy
54.21	Laparoscopy
66.62	Salpingectomy with removal of tubal pregnancy
67.1*	Diagnostic procedures on cervix
67.2	Conization of cervix
67.3*	Other excision or destruction of lesion or tissue of cervix
67.62	Repair of fistula of cervix
68.0	Hysterotomy
68.3*	Subtotal abdominal hysterectomy
68.41	Laparoscopic total abdominal hysterectomy
68.49	Other and unspecified total abdominal hysterectomy
68.5*	Vaginal hysterectomy
68.61	Laparoscopic radical abdominal hysterectomy
68.69	Other and unspecified radical abdominal hysterectomy
68.71	Laparoscopic radical vaginal hysterectomy [LRVH]
68.79	Other and unspecified radical vaginal hysterectomy
68.9	Other and unspecified hysterectomy
69.41	Suture of laceration of uterus
69.49	Other repair of uterus
69.95	Incision of cervix

MDC 14: Pregnancy, Childbirth And The Puerperium—SURGICAL

Surgical	*Medical*	CC Indicator	MCC Indicator	Procedure Proxy

70.12	Culdotomy
70.23	Biopsy of cul-de-sac
70.29	Other diagnostic procedures on vagina and cul-de-sac
70.32	Excision or destruction of lesion of cul-de-sac
71.22	Incision of Bartholin's gland (cyst)
71.23	Marsupialization of Bartholin's gland (cyst)
71.24	Excision or other destruction of Bartholin's gland (cyst)
71.29	Other operations on Bartholin's gland
73.94	Pubiotomy to assist delivery
74.3	Removal of extratubal ectopic pregnancy
75.36	Correction of fetal defect
75.52	Repair of current obstetric laceration of corpus uteri
75.93	Surgical correction of inverted uterus
75.99	Other obstetric operations

DRG 769 Postpartum and Postabortion Diagnoses with O.R. Procedure
GMLOS 4.3   AMLOS 6.4   RW 2.1785

Select principal diagnosis listed under DRG 776 with any operating room procedure

DRG 770 Abortion with D&C, Aspiration Curettage or Hysterotomy
GMLOS 1.6   AMLOS 2.1   RW 0.7070   ☑

Select principal diagnosis listed under DRG 779

Operating Room Procedures

69.0*	Dilation and curettage of uterus
69.51	Aspiration curettage of uterus for termination of pregnancy
69.52	Aspiration curettage following delivery or abortion
74.91	Hysterotomy to terminate pregnancy

MEDICAL

DRG 774 Vaginal Delivery with Complicating Diagnoses
GMLOS 2.5   AMLOS 3.0   RW 0.7137   ☑

Principal Diagnosis

641.01	Placenta previa without hemorrhage, with delivery
641.11	Hemorrhage from placenta previa, with delivery
641.21	Premature separation of placenta, with delivery
641.31	Antepartum hemorrhage associated with coagulation defects, with delivery
641.81	Other antepartum hemorrhage, with delivery
641.91	Unspecified antepartum hemorrhage, with delivery
642.01	Benign essential hypertension with delivery
642.02	Benign essential hypertension, with delivery, with current postpartum complication
642.11	Hypertension secondary to renal disease, with delivery
642.12	Hypertension secondary to renal disease, with delivery, with current postpartum complication
642.21	Other pre-existing hypertension, with delivery
642.22	Other pre-existing hypertension, with delivery, with current postpartum complication
642.41	Mild or unspecified pre-eclampsia, with delivery
642.42	Mild or unspecified pre-eclampsia, with delivery, with current postpartum complication
642.51	Severe pre-eclampsia, with delivery
642.52	Severe pre-eclampsia, with delivery, with current postpartum complication
642.61	Eclampsia, with delivery
642.62	Eclampsia, with delivery, with current postpartum complication
642.71	Pre-eclampsia or eclampsia superimposed on pre-existing hypertension, with delivery

642.72	Pre-eclampsia or eclampsia superimposed on pre-existing hypertension, with delivery, with current postpartum complication
642.91	Unspecified hypertension, with delivery
642.92	Unspecified hypertension, with delivery, with current postpartum complication
647.01	Maternal syphilis, complicating pregnancy, with delivery
647.02	Maternal syphilis, complicating pregnancy, with delivery, with current postpartum complication
647.11	Maternal gonorrhea with delivery
647.12	Maternal gonorrhea, with delivery, with current postpartum complication
647.21	Other maternal venereal diseases with delivery
647.22	Other maternal venereal diseases with delivery, with current postpartum complication
647.31	Maternal tuberculosis with delivery
647.32	Maternal tuberculosis with delivery, with current postpartum complication
647.41	Maternal malaria with delivery
647.42	Maternal malaria with delivery, with current postpartum complication
647.51	Maternal rubella with delivery
647.52	Maternal rubella with delivery, with current postpartum complication
647.61	Other maternal viral disease with delivery
647.62	Other maternal viral disease with delivery, with current postpartum complication
647.81	Other specified maternal infectious and parasitic disease with delivery
647.82	Other specified maternal infectious and parasitic disease with delivery, with current postpartum complication
647.91	Unspecified maternal infection or infestation with delivery
647.92	Unspecified maternal infection or infestation with delivery, with current postpartum complication
648.01	Maternal diabetes mellitus with delivery
648.02	Maternal diabetes mellitus with delivery, with current postpartum complication
648.51	Maternal congenital cardiovascular disorders, with delivery
648.52	Maternal congenital cardiovascular disorders, with delivery, with current postpartum complication
648.61	Other maternal cardiovascular diseases, with delivery
648.62	Other maternal cardiovascular diseases, with delivery, with current postpartum complication
649.8*	Onset (spontaneous) of labor after 37 completed weeks of gestation but before 39 completed weeks gestation, with delivery by (planned) cesarean section
659.21	Unspecified maternal pyrexia during labor, delivered
659.31	Generalized infection during labor, delivered
666.02	Third-stage postpartum hemorrhage, with delivery
666.12	Other immediate postpartum hemorrhage, with delivery
666.22	Delayed and secondary postpartum hemorrhage, with delivery
666.32	Postpartum coagulation defects, with delivery
667.02	Retained placenta without hemorrhage, with delivery, with mention of postpartum complication
667.12	Retained portions of placenta or membranes, without hemorrhage, delivered, with mention of postpartum complication
668.01	Pulmonary complications of the administration of anesthesia or other sedation in labor and delivery, delivered
668.02	Pulmonary complications of the administration of anesthesia or other sedation in labor and delivery, delivered, with mention of postpartum complication
668.11	Cardiac complications of the administration of anesthesia or other sedation in labor and delivery, delivered
668.12	Cardiac complications of the administration of anesthesia or other sedation in labor and delivery, delivered, with mention of postpartum complication

MDC 14: Pregnancy, Childbirth And The Puerperium—MEDICAL

Ⓣ *Transfer DRG*   ⓢ *Special Payment*   ☑ *Optimization Potential*   ⓦ *Targeted Potential*   * *Code Range*   ● *New DRG*   ▲ *Revised DRG Title*

668.21 Central nervous system complications of the administration of anesthesia or other sedation in labor and delivery, delivered

668.22 Central nervous system complications of the administration of anesthesia or other sedation in labor and delivery, delivered, with mention of postpartum complication

668.81 Other complications of the administration of anesthesia or other sedation in labor and delivery, delivered

668.82 Other complications of the administration of anesthesia or other sedation in labor and delivery, delivered, with mention of postpartum complication

668.91 Unspecified complication of the administration of anesthesia or other sedation in labor and delivery, delivered

668.92 Unspecified complication of the administration of anesthesia or other sedation in labor and delivery, delivered, with mention of postpartum complication

669.11 Shock during or following labor and delivery, with delivery, with or without mention of antepartum condition

669.12 Shock during or following labor and delivery, with delivery, with mention of postpartum complication

669.32 Acute kidney failure following labor and delivery, delivered, with mention of postpartum complication

669.41 Other complications of obstetrical surgery and procedures, with delivery, with or without mention of antepartum condition

669.42 Other complications of obstetrical surgery and procedures, with delivery, with mention of postpartum complication

670.02 Major puerperal infection, unspecified, delivered, with mention of postpartum complication

670.12 Puerperal endometritis, delivered, with mention of postpartum complication

670.22 Puerperal sepsis, delivered, with mention of postpartum complication

670.32 Puerperal septic thrombophlebitis, delivered, with mention of postpartum complication

670.82 Other major puerperal infection, delivered, with mention of postpartum complication

671.31 Deep phlebothrombosis, antepartum, with delivery

671.42 Deep phlebothrombosis, postpartum, with delivery

671.51 Other phlebitis and thrombosis with delivery, with or without mention of antepartum condition

671.52 Other phlebitis and thrombosis with delivery, with mention of postpartum complication

672.02 Puerperal pyrexia of unknown origin, delivered, with mention of postpartum complication

673.01 Obstetrical air embolism, with delivery, with or without mention of antepartum condition

673.02 Obstetrical air embolism, with delivery, with mention of postpartum complication

673.11 Amniotic fluid embolism, with delivery, with or without mention of antepartum condition

673.12 Amniotic fluid embolism, with delivery, with mention of postpartum complication

673.21 Obstetrical blood-clot embolism, with delivery, with or without mention of antepartum condition

673.22 Obstetrical blood-clot embolism, with mention of postpartum complication

673.31 Obstetrical pyemic and septic embolism, with delivery, with or without mention of antepartum condition

673.32 Obstetrical pyemic and septic embolism, with delivery, with mention of postpartum complication

673.81 Other obstetrical pulmonary embolism, with delivery, with or without mention of antepartum condition

673.82 Other obstetrical pulmonary embolism, with delivery, with mention of postpartum complication

674.01 Cerebrovascular disorder, with delivery, with or without mention of antepartum condition

674.02 Cerebrovascular disorder, with delivery, with mention of postpartum complication

674.12 Disruption of cesarean wound, with delivery, with mention of postpartum complication

674.22 Disruption of perineal wound, with delivery, with mention of postpartum complication

674.32 Other complication of obstetrical surgical wounds, with delivery, with mention of postpartum complication

674.51 Peripartum cardiomyopathy, delivered, with or without mention of antepartum condition

674.52 Peripartum cardiomyopathy, delivered, with mention of postpartum condition

674.82 Other complication of puerperium, with delivery, with mention of postpartum complication

675.01 Infection of nipple associated with childbirth, delivered, with or without mention of antepartum condition

675.02 Infection of nipple associated with childbirth, delivered with mention of postpartum complication

675.11 Abscess of breast associated with childbirth, delivered, with or without mention of antepartum condition

675.12 Abscess of breast associated with childbirth, delivered, with mention of postpartum complication

675.21 Nonpurulent mastitis, delivered, with or without mention of antepartum condition

675.22 Nonpurulent mastitis, delivered, with mention of postpartum complication

679.01 Maternal complications from in utero procedure, delivered, with or without mention of antepartum condition

679.02 Maternal complications from in utero procedure, delivered, with mention of postpartum complication

OR

Principal Diagnosis

640.01 Threatened abortion, delivered

640.81 Other specified hemorrhage in early pregnancy, delivered

640.91 Unspecified hemorrhage in early pregnancy, delivered

642.31 Transient hypertension of pregnancy, with delivery

642.32 Transient hypertension of pregnancy, with delivery, with current postpartum complication

643.01 Mild hyperemesis gravidarum, delivered

643.11 Hyperemesis gravidarum with metabolic disturbance, delivered

643.21 Late vomiting of pregnancy, delivered

643.81 Other vomiting complicating pregnancy, delivered

643.91 Unspecified vomiting of pregnancy, delivered

644.21 Early onset of delivery, delivered, with or without mention of antepartum condition

645.11 Post term pregnancy, delivered, with or without mention of antepartum condition

645.21 Prolonged pregnancy, delivered, with or without mention of antepartum condition

646.00 Papyraceous fetus, unspecified as to episode of care

646.01 Papyraceous fetus, delivered, with or without mention of antepartum condition

646.11 Edema or excessive weight gain in pregnancy, with delivery, with or without mention of antepartum complication

646.12 Edema or excessive weight gain in pregnancy, with delivery, with current postpartum complication

646.21 Unspecified renal disease in pregnancy, with delivery

646.22 Unspecified renal disease in pregnancy, with delivery, with current postpartum complication

646.31 Pregnancy complication, recurrent pregnancy loss, with or without mention of antepartum condition

646.41 Peripheral neuritis in pregnancy, with delivery

646.42 Peripheral neuritis in pregnancy, with delivery, with current postpartum complication

646.51 Asymptomatic bacteriuria in pregnancy, with delivery

646.52 Asymptomatic bacteriuria in pregnancy, with delivery, with current postpartum complication

646.61 Infections of genitourinary tract in pregnancy, with delivery

646.62 Infections of genitourinary tract in pregnancy, with delivery, with current postpartum complication

Surgical   Medical   CC Indicator   MCC Indicator   Procedure Proxy

646.71	Liver and biliary tract disorders in pregnancy, delivered, with or without mention of antepartum condition
646.81	Other specified complication of pregnancy, with delivery
646.82	Other specified complications of pregnancy, with delivery, with current postpartum complication
646.91	Unspecified complication of pregnancy, with delivery
648.11	Maternal thyroid dysfunction with delivery, with or without mention of antepartum condition
648.12	Maternal thyroid dysfunction with delivery, with current postpartum complication
648.21	Maternal anemia, with delivery
648.22	Maternal anemia with delivery, with current postpartum complication
648.31	Maternal drug dependence, with delivery
648.32	Maternal drug dependence, with delivery, with current postpartum complication
648.41	Maternal mental disorders, with delivery
648.42	Maternal mental disorders, with delivery, with current postpartum complication
648.71	Bone and joint disorders of maternal back, pelvis, and lower limbs, with delivery
648.72	Bone and joint disorders of maternal back, pelvis, and lower limbs, with delivery, with current postpartum complication
648.81	Abnormal maternal glucose tolerance, with delivery
648.82	Abnormal maternal glucose tolerance, with delivery, with current postpartum complication
648.91	Other current maternal conditions classifiable elsewhere, with delivery
648.92	Other current maternal conditions classifiable elsewhere, with delivery, with current postpartum complication
649.01	Tobacco use disorder complicating pregnancy, childbirth, or the puerperium, delivered, with or without mention of antepartum condition
649.02	Tobacco use disorder complicating pregnancy, childbirth, or the puerperium, delivered, with mention of postpartum complication
649.11	Obesity complicating pregnancy, childbirth, or the puerperium, delivered, with or without mention of antepartum condition
649.12	Obesity complicating pregnancy, childbirth, or the puerperium, delivered, with mention of postpartum complication
649.21	Bariatric surgery status complicating pregnancy, childbirth, or the puerperium, delivered, with or without mention of antepartum condition
649.22	Bariatric surgery status complicating pregnancy, childbirth, or the puerperium, delivered, with mention of postpartum complication
649.31	Coagulation defects complicating pregnancy, childbirth, or the puerperium, delivered, with or without mention of antepartum condition
649.32	Coagulation defects complicating pregnancy, childbirth, or the puerperium, delivered, with mention of postpartum complication
649.41	Epilepsy complicating pregnancy, childbirth, or the puerperium, delivered, with or without mention of antepartum condition
649.42	Epilepsy complicating pregnancy, childbirth, or the puerperium, delivered, with mention of postpartum complication
649.51	Spotting complicating pregnancy, delivered, with or without mention of antepartum condition
649.61	Uterine size date discrepancy, delivered, with or without mention of antepartum condition
649.62	Uterine size date discrepancy, delivered, with mention of postpartum complication
649.71	Cervical shortening, delivered, with or without mention of antepartum condition
649.81	Onset (spontaneous) of labor after 37 completed weeks of gestation but before 39 completed weeks gestation, with delivery by (planned) cesarean section, delivered, with or without mention of antepartum condition
649.82	Onset (spontaneous) of labor after 37 completed weeks of gestation but before 39 completed weeks gestation, with delivery by (planned) cesarean section, delivered, with mention of postpartum complication
650	Normal delivery
651.01	Twin pregnancy, delivered
651.11	Triplet pregnancy, delivered
651.21	Quadruplet pregnancy, delivered
651.31	Twin pregnancy with fetal loss and retention of one fetus, delivered
651.41	Triplet pregnancy with fetal loss and retention of one or more, delivered
651.51	Quadruplet pregnancy with fetal loss and retention of one or more, delivered
651.61	Other multiple pregnancy with fetal loss and retention of one or more fetus(es), delivered
651.71	Multiple gestation following (elective) fetal reduction, delivered, with or without mention of antepartum condition
651.81	Other specified multiple gestation, delivered
651.91	Unspecified multiple gestation, delivered
652.01	Unstable lie of fetus, delivered
652.11	Breech or other malpresentation successfully converted to cephalic presentation, delivered
652.21	Breech presentation without mention of version, delivered
652.31	Transverse or oblique fetal presentation, delivered
652.41	Fetal face or brow presentation, delivered
652.51	High fetal head at term, delivered
652.61	Multiple gestation with malpresentation of one fetus or more, delivered
652.71	Prolapsed arm of fetus, delivered
652.81	Other specified malposition or malpresentation of fetus, delivered
652.91	Unspecified malposition or malpresentation of fetus, delivered
653.01	Major abnormality of bony pelvis, not further specified, delivered
653.11	Generally contracted pelvis in pregnancy, delivered
653.21	Inlet contraction of pelvis in pregnancy, delivered
653.31	Outlet contraction of pelvis in pregnancy, delivered
653.41	Fetopelvic disproportion, delivered
653.51	Unusually large fetus causing disproportion, delivered
653.61	Hydrocephalic fetus causing disproportion, delivered
653.71	Other fetal abnormality causing disproportion, delivered
653.81	Fetal disproportion of other origin, delivered
653.91	Unspecified fetal disproportion, delivered
654.01	Congenital abnormalities of pregnant uterus, delivered
654.02	Congenital abnormalities of pregnant uterus, delivered, with mention of postpartum complication
654.11	Tumors of body of uterus, delivered
654.12	Tumors of body of uterus, delivered, with mention of postpartum complication
654.21	Previous cesarean delivery, delivered, with or without mention of antepartum condition
654.31	Retroverted and incarcerated gravid uterus, delivered
654.32	Retroverted and incarcerated gravid uterus, delivered, with mention of postpartum complication
654.41	Other abnormalities in shape or position of gravid uterus and of neighboring structures, delivered
654.42	Other abnormalities in shape or position of gravid uterus and of neighboring structures, delivered, with mention of postpartum complication
654.51	Cervical incompetence, delivered
654.52	Cervical incompetence, delivered, with mention of postpartum complication
654.61	Other congenital or acquired abnormality of cervix, with delivery

---

T *Transfer DRG*　　SP *Special Payment*　　☑ *Optimization Potential*　　TBLS *Targeted Potential*　　* *Code Range*　　● *New DRG*　　▲ *Revised DRG Title*

654.62	Other congenital or acquired abnormality of cervix, delivered, with mention of postpartum complication
654.71	Congenital or acquired abnormality of vagina, with delivery
654.72	Congenital or acquired abnormality of vagina, delivered, with mention of postpartum complication
654.81	Congenital or acquired abnormality of vulva, with delivery
654.82	Congenital or acquired abnormality of vulva, delivered, with mention of postpartum complication
654.91	Other and unspecified abnormality of organs and soft tissues of pelvis, with delivery
654.92	Other and unspecified abnormality of organs and soft tissues of pelvis, delivered, with mention of postpartum complication
655.01	Central nervous system malformation in fetus, with delivery
655.11	Chromosomal abnormality in fetus, affecting management of mother, with delivery
655.21	Hereditary disease in family possibly affecting fetus, affecting management of mother, with delivery
655.31	Suspected damage to fetus from viral disease in mother, affecting management of mother, with delivery
655.41	Suspected damage to fetus from other disease in mother, affecting management of mother, with delivery
655.51	Suspected damage to fetus from drugs, affecting management of mother, delivered
655.61	Suspected damage to fetus from radiation, affecting management of mother, delivered
655.71	Decreased fetal movements, affecting management of mother, delivered
655.81	Other known or suspected fetal abnormality, not elsewhere classified, affecting management of mother, delivery
655.91	Unspecified fetal abnormality affecting management of mother, delivery
656.01	Fetal-maternal hemorrhage, with delivery
656.11	Rhesus isoimmunization affecting management of mother, delivered
656.21	Isoimmunization from other and unspecified blood-group incompatibility, affecting management of mother, delivered
656.30	Fetal distress affecting management of mother, unspecified as to episode of care
656.31	Fetal distress affecting management of mother, delivered
656.40	Intrauterine death affecting management of mother, unspecified as to episode of care
656.41	Intrauterine death affecting management of mother, delivered
656.51	Poor fetal growth, affecting management of mother, delivered
656.61	Excessive fetal growth affecting management of mother, delivered
656.71	Other placental conditions affecting management of mother, delivered
656.81	Other specified fetal and placental problems affecting management of mother, delivered
656.91	Unspecified fetal and placental problem affecting management of mother, delivered
657.01	Polyhydramnios, with delivery
658.01	Oligohydramnios, delivered
658.10	Premature rupture of membranes in pregnancy, unspecified as to episode of care
658.11	Premature rupture of membranes in pregnancy, delivered
658.20	Delayed delivery after spontaneous or unspecified rupture of membranes, unspecified as to episode of care
658.21	Delayed delivery after spontaneous or unspecified rupture of membranes, delivered
658.30	Delayed delivery after artificial rupture of membranes, unspecified as to episode of care
658.31	Delayed delivery after artificial rupture of membranes, delivered
658.40	Infection of amniotic cavity, unspecified as to episode of care
658.41	Infection of amniotic cavity, delivered
658.81	Other problem associated with amniotic cavity and membranes, delivered
658.91	Unspecified problem associated with amniotic cavity and membranes, delivered
659.00	Failed mechanical induction of labor, unspecified as to episode of care
659.01	Failed mechanical induction of labor, delivered
659.10	Failed medical or unspecified induction of labor, unspecified as to episode of care
659.11	Failed medical or unspecified induction of labor, delivered
659.20	Unspecified maternal pyrexia during labor, unspecified as to episode of care
659.30	Generalized infection during labor, unspecified as to episode of care
659.41	Grand multiparity, delivered, with or without mention of antepartum condition
659.50	Elderly primigravida, unspecified as to episode of care
659.51	Elderly primigravida, delivered
659.60	Elderly multigravida, unspecified as to episode of care or not applicable
659.61	Elderly multigravida, delivered, with mention of antepartum condition
659.70	Abnormality in fetal heart rate or rhythm, unspecified as to episode of care or not applicable
659.71	Abnormality in fetal heart rate or rhythm, delivered, with or without mention of antepartum condition
659.80	Other specified indication for care or intervention related to labor and delivery, unspecified as to episode of care
659.81	Other specified indication for care or intervention related to labor and delivery, delivered
659.90	Unspecified indication for care or intervention related to labor and delivery, unspecified as to episode of care
659.91	Unspecified indication for care or intervention related to labor and delivery, delivered
660.00	Obstruction caused by malposition of fetus at onset of labor, unspecified as to episode of care
660.01	Obstruction caused by malposition of fetus at onset of labor, delivered
660.10	Obstruction by bony pelvis during labor and delivery, unspecified as to episode of care
660.11	Obstruction by bony pelvis during labor and delivery, delivered
660.20	Obstruction by abnormal pelvic soft tissues during labor and delivery, unspecified as to episode of care
660.21	Obstruction by abnormal pelvic soft tissues during labor and delivery, delivered
660.30	Deep transverse arrest and persistent occipitoposterior position during labor and delivery, unspecified as to episode of care
660.31	Deep transverse arrest and persistent occipitoposterior position during labor and deliver, delivered
660.40	Shoulder (girdle) dystocia during labor and delivery, unspecified as to episode of care
660.41	Shoulder (girdle) dystocia during labor and deliver, delivered
660.50	Locked twins during labor and delivery, unspecified as to episode of care in pregnancy
660.51	Locked twins, delivered
660.60	Unspecified failed trial of labor, unspecified as to episode
660.61	Unspecified failed trial of labor, delivered
660.70	Unspecified failed forceps or vacuum extractor, unspecified as to episode of care
660.71	Unspecified failed forceps or vacuum extractor, delivered
660.80	Other causes of obstructed labor, unspecified as to episode of care
660.81	Other causes of obstructed labor, delivered
660.90	Unspecified obstructed labor, unspecified as to episode of care
660.91	Unspecified obstructed labor, with delivery
661.00	Primary uterine inertia, unspecified as to episode of care
661.01	Primary uterine inertia, with delivery

MDC 14: Pregnancy, Childbirth And The Puerperium—MEDICAL

Surgical	Medical	CC Indicator	MCC Indicator	Procedure Proxy

661.10	Secondary uterine inertia, unspecified as to episode of care
661.11	Secondary uterine inertia, with delivery
661.20	Other and unspecified uterine inertia, unspecified as to episode of care
661.21	Other and unspecified uterine inertia, with delivery
661.30	Precipitate labor, unspecified as to episode of care
661.31	Precipitate labor, with delivery
661.40	Hypertonic, incoordinate, or prolonged uterine contractions, unspecified as to episode of care
661.41	Hypertonic, incoordinate, or prolonged uterine contractions, with delivery
661.90	Unspecified abnormality of labor, unspecified as to episode of care
661.91	Unspecified abnormality of labor, with delivery
662.00	Prolonged first stage of labor, unspecified as to episode of care
662.01	Prolonged first stage of labor, delivered
662.10	Unspecified prolonged labor, unspecified as to episode of care
662.11	Unspecified prolonged labor, delivered
662.20	Prolonged second stage of labor, unspecified as to episode of care
662.21	Prolonged second stage of labor, delivered
662.30	Delayed delivery of second twin, triplet, etc., unspecified as to episode of care
662.31	Delayed delivery of second twin, triplet, etc., delivered
663.00	Prolapse of cord, complicating labor and delivery, unspecified as to episode of care
663.01	Prolapse of cord, complicating labor and delivery, delivered
663.10	Cord around neck, with compression, complicating labor and delivery, unspecified as to episode of care
663.11	Cord around neck, with compression, complicating labor and delivery, delivered
663.20	Other and unspecified cord entanglement, with compression, complicating labor and delivery, unspecified as to episode of care
663.21	Other and unspecified cord entanglement, with compression, complicating labor and delivery, delivered
663.30	Other and unspecified cord entanglement, without mention of compression, complicating labor and delivery, unspecified as to episode of care
663.31	Other and unspecified cord entanglement, without mention of compression, complicating labor and delivery, delivered
663.40	Short cord complicating labor and delivery, unspecified as to episode of care
663.41	Short cord complicating labor and delivery, delivered
663.50	Vasa previa complicating labor and delivery, unspecified as to episode of care
663.51	Vasa previa complicating labor and delivery, delivered
663.60	Vascular lesions of cord complicating labor and delivery, unspecified as to episode of care
663.61	Vascular lesions of cord complicating labor and delivery, delivered
663.80	Other umbilical cord complications during labor and delivery, unspecified as to episode of care
663.81	Other umbilical cord complications during labor and delivery, delivered
663.90	Unspecified umbilical cord complication during labor and delivery, unspecified as to episode of care
663.91	Unspecified umbilical cord complication during labor and delivery, delivered
664.00	First-degree perineal laceration, unspecified as to episode of care in pregnancy
664.01	First-degree perineal laceration, with delivery
664.10	Second-degree perineal laceration, unspecified as to episode of care in pregnancy
664.11	Second-degree perineal laceration, with delivery
664.20	Third-degree perineal laceration, unspecified as to episode of care in pregnancy
664.21	Third-degree perineal laceration, with delivery
664.30	Fourth-degree perineal laceration, unspecified as to episode of care in pregnancy
664.31	Fourth-degree perineal laceration, with delivery
664.40	Unspecified perineal laceration, unspecified as to episode of care in pregnancy
664.41	Unspecified perineal laceration, with delivery
664.50	Vulvar and perineal hematoma, unspecified as to episode of care in pregnancy
664.51	Vulvar and perineal hematoma, with delivery
664.60	Anal sphincter tear complicating delivery, not associated with third-degree perineal laceration, unspecified as to episode of care or not applicable
664.61	Anal sphincter tear complicating delivery, not associated with third-degree perineal laceration, delivered, with or without mention of antepartum condition
664.80	Other specified trauma to perineum and vulva, unspecified as to episode of care in pregnancy
664.81	Other specified trauma to perineum and vulva, with delivery
664.90	Unspecified trauma to perineum and vulva, unspecified as to episode of care in pregnancy
664.91	Unspecified trauma to perineum and vulva, with delivery
665.00	Rupture of uterus before onset of labor, unspecified as to episode of care
665.01	Rupture of uterus before onset of labor, with delivery
665.10	Rupture of uterus during labor, unspecified as to episode
665.11	Rupture of uterus during labor, with delivery
665.20	Inversion of uterus, unspecified as to episode of care in pregnancy
665.22	Inversion of uterus, delivered with postpartum complication
665.30	Laceration of cervix, unspecified as to episode of care in pregnancy
665.31	Laceration of cervix, with delivery
665.40	High vaginal laceration, unspecified as to episode of care in pregnancy
665.41	High vaginal laceration, with delivery
665.50	Other injury to pelvic organs, unspecified as to episode of care in pregnancy
665.51	Other injury to pelvic organs, with delivery
665.60	Damage to pelvic joints and ligaments, unspecified as to episode of care in pregnancy
665.61	Damage to pelvic joints and ligaments, with delivery
665.70	Pelvic hematoma, unspecified as to episode of care
665.71	Pelvic hematoma, with delivery
665.72	Pelvic hematoma, delivered with postpartum complication
665.80	Other specified obstetrical trauma, unspecified as to episode of care
665.81	Other specified obstetrical trauma, with delivery
665.82	Other specified obstetrical trauma, delivered, with postpartum
665.90	Unspecified obstetrical trauma, unspecified as to episode of care
665.91	Unspecified obstetrical trauma, with delivery
665.92	Unspecified obstetrical trauma, delivered, with postpartum complication
668.00	Pulmonary complications of the administration of anesthesia or other sedation in labor and delivery, unspecified as to episode of care
668.10	Cardiac complications of the administration of anesthesia or other sedation in labor and delivery, unspecified as to episode of care
668.20	Central nervous system complications of the administration of anesthesia or other sedation in labor and delivery, unspecified as to episode of care
668.80	Other complications of the administration of anesthesia or other sedation in labor and delivery, unspecified as to episode of care
668.90	Unspecified complication of the administration of anesthesia or other sedation in labor and delivery, unspecified as to episode of care

---

Ⓣ *Transfer DRG*   ⓢ᷉ *Special Payment*   ☑ *Optimization Potential*   ᵀᴳᵗ *Targeted Potential*   * *Code Range*   ● *New DRG*   ▲ *Revised DRG Title*

669.00	Maternal distress complicating labor and delivery, unspecified as to episode of care
669.01	Maternal distress, with delivery, with or without mention of antepartum condition
669.02	Maternal distress, with delivery, with mention of postpartum complication
669.10	Shock during or following labor and delivery, unspecified as to episode of care
669.20	Maternal hypotension syndrome complicating labor and delivery, unspecified as to episode of care
669.21	Maternal hypotension syndrome, with delivery, with or without mention of antepartum condition
669.22	Maternal hypotension syndrome, with delivery, with mention of postpartum complication
669.30	Acute kidney failure following labor and delivery, unspecified as to episode of care or not applicable
669.40	Other complications of obstetrical surgery and procedures, unspecified as to episode of care
669.50	Forceps or vacuum extractor delivery without mention of indication, unspecified as to episode of care
669.51	Forceps or vacuum extractor delivery without mention of indication, delivered, with or without mention of antepartum condition
669.60	Breech extraction, without mention of indication, unspecified as to episode of care
669.61	Breech extraction, without mention of indication, delivered, with or without mention of antepartum condition
669.70	Cesarean delivery, without mention of indication, unspecified as to episode of care
669.71	Cesarean delivery, without mention of indication, delivered, with or without mention of antepartum condition
669.80	Other complication of labor and delivery, unspecified as to episode of care
669.81	Other complication of labor and delivery, delivered, with or without mention of antepartum condition
669.82	Other complication of labor and delivery, delivered, with mention of postpartum complication
669.90	Unspecified complication of labor and delivery, unspecified as to episode of care
669.91	Unspecified complication of labor and delivery, with delivery, with or without mention of antepartum condition
669.92	Unspecified complication of labor and delivery, with delivery, with mention of postpartum complication
671.01	Varicose veins of legs, with delivery, with or without mention of antepartum condition
671.02	Varicose veins of legs, with delivery, with mention of postpartum complication
671.11	Varicose veins of vulva and perineum, with delivery, with or without mention of antepartum condition
671.12	Varicose veins of vulva and perineum, with delivery, with mention of postpartum complication
671.21	Superficial thrombophlebitis with delivery, with or without mention of antepartum condition
671.22	Superficial thrombophlebitis with delivery, with mention of postpartum complication
671.81	Other venous complication, with delivery, with or without mention of antepartum condition
671.82	Other venous complication, with delivery, with mention of postpartum complication
671.91	Unspecified venous complication, with delivery, with or without mention of antepartum condition
671.92	Unspecified venous complication, with delivery, with mention of postpartum complication
674.42	Placental polyp, with delivery, with mention of postpartum complication
674.92	Unspecified complications of puerperium, with delivery, with mention of postpartum complication
675.81	Other specified infection of the breast and nipple associated with childbirth, delivered, with or without mention of antepartum condition
675.82	Other specified infection of the breast and nipple associated with childbirth, delivered, with mention of postpartum complication
675.91	Unspecified infection of the breast and nipple, delivered, with or without mention of antepartum condition
675.92	Unspecified infection of the breast and nipple, delivered, with mention of postpartum complication
676.01	Retracted nipple, delivered, with or without mention of antepartum condition
676.02	Retracted nipple, delivered, with mention of postpartum complication
676.11	Cracked nipple, delivered, with or without mention of antepartum condition
676.12	Cracked nipple, delivered, with mention of postpartum complication
676.21	Engorgement of breasts, delivered, with or without mention of antepartum condition
676.22	Engorgement of breasts, delivered, with mention of postpartum complication
676.31	Other and unspecified disorder of breast associated with childbirth, delivered, with or without mention of antepartum condition
676.32	Other and unspecified disorder of breast associated with childbirth, delivered, with mention of postpartum complication
676.41	Failure of lactation, with delivery, with or without mention of antepartum condition
676.42	Failure of lactation, with delivery, with mention of postpartum complication
676.51	Suppressed lactation, with delivery, with or without mention of antepartum condition
676.52	Suppressed lactation, with delivery, with mention of postpartum complication
676.61	Galactorrhea, with delivery, with or without mention of antepartum condition
676.62	Galactorrhea, with delivery, with mention of postpartum complication
676.81	Other disorder of lactation, with delivery, with or without mention of antepartum condition
676.82	Other disorder of lactation, with delivery, with mention of postpartum complication
676.91	Unspecified disorder of lactation, with delivery, with or without mention of antepartum condition
676.92	Unspecified disorder of lactation, with delivery, with mention of postpartum complication
678.01	Fetal hematologic conditions, delivered, with or without mention of antepartum condition
678.11	Fetal conjoined twins, delivered, with or without mention of antepartum condition
679.00	Maternal complications from in utero procedure, unspecified as to episode of care or not applicable
679.11	Fetal complications from in utero procedure, delivered, with or without mention of antepartum condition
679.12	Fetal complications from in utero procedure, delivered, with mention of postpartum complication

AND

Secondary Diagnosis

641.01	Placenta previa without hemorrhage, with delivery
641.11	Hemorrhage from placenta previa, with delivery
641.21	Premature separation of placenta, with delivery
641.31	Antepartum hemorrhage associated with coagulation defects, with delivery
641.81	Other antepartum hemorrhage, with delivery
641.91	Unspecified antepartum hemorrhage, with delivery
642.01	Benign essential hypertension with delivery
642.02	Benign essential hypertension, with delivery, with current postpartum complication
642.11	Hypertension secondary to renal disease, with delivery

Surgical	Medical	CC Indicator	MCC Indicator	Procedure Proxy

642.12	Hypertension secondary to renal disease, with delivery, with current postpartum complication		667.12	Retained portions of placenta or membranes, without hemorrhage, delivered, with mention of postpartum complication
642.21	Other pre-existing hypertension, with delivery		668.01	Pulmonary complications of the administration of anesthesia or other sedation in labor and delivery, delivered
642.22	Other pre-existing hypertension, with delivery, with current postpartum complication		668.02	Pulmonary complications of the administration of anesthesia or other sedation in labor and delivery, delivered, with mention of postpartum complication
642.41	Mild or unspecified pre-eclampsia, with delivery		668.11	Cardiac complications of the administration of anesthesia or other sedation in labor and delivery, delivered
642.42	Mild or unspecified pre-eclampsia, with delivery, with current postpartum complication		668.12	Cardiac complications of the administration of anesthesia or other sedation in labor and delivery, delivered, with mention of postpartum complication
642.51	Severe pre-eclampsia, with delivery		668.21	Central nervous system complications of the administration of anesthesia or other sedation in labor and delivery, delivered
642.52	Severe pre-eclampsia, with delivery, with current postpartum complication		668.22	Central nervous system complications of the administration of anesthesia or other sedation in labor and delivery, delivered, with mention of postpartum complication
642.61	Eclampsia, with delivery		668.81	Other complications of the administration of anesthesia or other sedation in labor and delivery, delivered
642.62	Eclampsia, with delivery, with current postpartum complication		668.82	Other complications of the administration of anesthesia or other sedation in labor and delivery, delivered, with mention of postpartum complication
642.71	Pre-eclampsia or eclampsia superimposed on pre-existing hypertension, with delivery		668.91	Unspecified complication of the administration of anesthesia or other sedation in labor and delivery, delivered
642.72	Pre-eclampsia or eclampsia superimposed on pre-existing hypertension, with delivery, with current postpartum complication		668.92	Unspecified complication of the administration of anesthesia or other sedation in labor and delivery, delivered, with mention of postpartum complication
642.91	Unspecified hypertension, with delivery		669.11	Shock during or following labor and delivery, with delivery, with or without mention of antepartum condition
642.92	Unspecified hypertension, with delivery, with current postpartum complication		669.12	Shock during or following labor and delivery, with delivery, with mention of postpartum complication
647.01	Maternal syphilis, complicating pregnancy, with delivery		669.32	Acute kidney failure following labor and delivery, delivered, with mention of postpartum complication
647.02	Maternal syphilis, complicating pregnancy, with delivery, with current postpartum complication		669.41	Other complications of obstetrical surgery and procedures, with delivery, with or without mention of antepartum condition
647.11	Maternal gonorrhea with delivery		669.42	Other complications of obstetrical surgery and procedures, with delivery, with mention of postpartum complication
647.12	Maternal gonorrhea, with delivery, with current postpartum complication		670.02	Major puerperal infection, unspecified, delivered, with mention of postpartum complication
647.21	Other maternal venereal diseases with delivery		670.12	Puerperal endometritis, delivered, with mention of postpartum complication
647.22	Other maternal venereal diseases with delivery, with current postpartum complication		670.22	Puerperal sepsis, delivered, with mention of postpartum complication
647.31	Maternal tuberculosis with delivery		670.32	Puerperal septic thrombophlebitis, delivered, with mention of postpartum complication
647.32	Maternal tuberculosis with delivery, with current postpartum complication		670.82	Other major puerperal infection, delivered, with mention of postpartum complication
647.41	Maternal malaria with delivery		671.31	Deep phlebothrombosis, antepartum, with delivery
647.42	Maternal malaria with delivery, with current postpartum complication		671.42	Deep phlebothrombosis, postpartum, with delivery
647.51	Maternal rubella with delivery		671.51	Other phlebitis and thrombosis with delivery, with or without mention of antepartum condition
647.52	Maternal rubella with delivery, with current postpartum complication		671.52	Other phlebitis and thrombosis with delivery, with mention of postpartum complication
647.61	Other maternal viral disease with delivery		672.02	Puerperal pyrexia of unknown origin, delivered, with mention of postpartum complication
647.62	Other maternal viral disease with delivery, with current postpartum complication		673.01	Obstetrical air embolism, with delivery, with or without mention of antepartum condition
647.81	Other specified maternal infectious and parasitic disease with delivery		673.02	Obstetrical air embolism, with delivery, with mention of postpartum complication
647.82	Other specified maternal infectious and parasitic disease with delivery, with current postpartum complication		673.11	Amniotic fluid embolism, with delivery, with or without mention of antepartum condition
647.91	Unspecified maternal infection or infestation with delivery		673.12	Amniotic fluid embolism, with delivery, with mention of postpartum complication
647.92	Unspecified maternal infection or infestation with delivery, with current postpartum complication		673.21	Obstetrical blood-clot embolism, with delivery, with or without mention of antepartum condition
648.01	Maternal diabetes mellitus with delivery		673.22	Obstetrical blood-clot embolism, with mention of postpartum complication
648.02	Maternal diabetes mellitus with delivery, with current postpartum complication			
648.51	Maternal congenital cardiovascular disorders, with delivery			
648.52	Maternal congenital cardiovascular disorders, with delivery, with current postpartum complication			
648.61	Other maternal cardiovascular diseases, with delivery			
648.62	Other maternal cardiovascular diseases, with delivery, with current postpartum complication			
659.21	Unspecified maternal pyrexia during labor, delivered			
659.31	Generalized infection during labor, delivered			
666.02	Third-stage postpartum hemorrhage, with delivery			
666.12	Other immediate postpartum hemorrhage, with delivery			
666.22	Delayed and secondary postpartum hemorrhage, with delivery			
666.32	Postpartum coagulation defects, with delivery			
667.02	Retained placenta without hemorrhage, with delivery, with mention of postpartum complication			

Ⓣ *Transfer DRG*　　Ⓢ *Special Payment*　　☑ *Optimization Potential*　　▽ *Targeted Potential*　　* *Code Range*　　● *New DRG*　　▲ *Revised DRG Title*

146　　　　　　　　　　　　　　Valid 10/01/2013–09/30/2014　　　　　　　　　　　　© 2013 OptumInsight, Inc.

MDC 14: Pregnancy, Childbirth And The Puerperium—MEDICAL

673.31	Obstetrical pyemic and septic embolism, with delivery, with or without mention of antepartum condition
673.32	Obstetrical pyemic and septic embolism, with delivery, with mention of postpartum complication
673.81	Other obstetrical pulmonary embolism, with delivery, with or without mention of antepartum condition
673.82	Other obstetrical pulmonary embolism, with delivery, with mention of postpartum complication
674.01	Cerebrovascular disorder, with delivery, with or without mention of antepartum condition
674.02	Cerebrovascular disorder, with delivery, with mention of postpartum complication
674.12	Disruption of cesarean wound, with delivery, with mention of postpartum complication
674.22	Disruption of perineal wound, with delivery, with mention of postpartum complication
674.32	Other complication of obstetrical surgical wounds, with delivery, with mention of postpartum complication
674.51	Peripartum cardiomyopathy, delivered, with or without mention of antepartum condition
674.52	Peripartum cardiomyopathy, delivered, with mention of postpartum condition
674.82	Other complication of puerperium, with delivery, with mention of postpartum complication
675.01	Infection of nipple associated with childbirth, delivered, with or without mention of antepartum condition
675.02	Infection of nipple associated with childbirth, delivered with mention of postpartum complication
675.11	Abscess of breast associated with childbirth, delivered, with or without mention of antepartum condition
675.12	Abscess of breast associated with childbirth, delivered, with mention of postpartum complication
675.21	Nonpurulent mastitis, delivered, with or without mention of antepartum condition
675.22	Nonpurulent mastitis, delivered, with mention of postpartum complication
679.01	Maternal complications from in utero procedure, delivered, with or without mention of antepartum condition
679.02	Maternal complications from in utero procedure, delivered, with mention of postpartum complication

AND

Only Operating Room Procedures

48.71	Suture of laceration of rectum
49.59	Other anal sphincterotomy
67.51	Transabdominal cerclage of cervix
67.59	Other repair of cervical os
67.61	Suture of laceration of cervix
67.69	Other repair of cervix
70.13	Lysis of intraluminal adhesions of vagina
70.14	Other vaginotomy
70.24	Vaginal biopsy
70.31	Hymenectomy
70.33	Excision or destruction of lesion of vagina
70.71	Suture of laceration of vagina
70.79	Other repair of vagina
71.0*	Incision of vulva and perineum
71.1*	Diagnostic procedures on vulva
71.3	Other local excision or destruction of vulva and perineum
71.71	Suture of laceration of vulva or perineum
71.79	Other repair of vulva and perineum
73.99	Other operations to assist delivery
75.50	Repair of current obstetric laceration of uterus, not otherwise specified
75.51	Repair of current obstetric laceration of cervix
75.61	Repair of current obstetric laceration of bladder and urethra

OR

No Operating Room Procedures

DRG 775 Vaginal Delivery without Complicating Diagnoses

GMLOS 2.1	AMLOS 2.3	RW 0.5625	☑

Principal Diagnosis

640.01	Threatened abortion, delivered
640.81	Other specified hemorrhage in early pregnancy, delivered
640.91	Unspecified hemorrhage in early pregnancy, delivered
642.31	Transient hypertension of pregnancy, with delivery
642.32	Transient hypertension of pregnancy, with delivery, with current postpartum complication
643.01	Mild hyperemesis gravidarum, delivered
643.11	Hyperemesis gravidarum with metabolic disturbance, delivered
643.21	Late vomiting of pregnancy, delivered
643.81	Other vomiting complicating pregnancy, delivered
643.91	Unspecified vomiting of pregnancy, delivered
644.21	Early onset of delivery, delivered, with or without mention of antepartum condition
645.11	Post term pregnancy, delivered, with or without mention of antepartum condition
645.21	Prolonged pregnancy, delivered, with or without mention of antepartum condition
646.00	Papyraceous fetus, unspecified as to episode of care
646.01	Papyraceous fetus, delivered, with or without mention of antepartum condition
646.11	Edema or excessive weight gain in pregnancy, with delivery, with or without mention of antepartum complication
646.12	Edema or excessive weight gain in pregnancy, with delivery, with current postpartum complication
646.21	Unspecified renal disease in pregnancy, with delivery
646.22	Unspecified renal disease in pregnancy, with delivery, with current postpartum complication
646.31	Pregnancy complication, recurrent pregnancy loss, with or without mention of antepartum condition
646.41	Peripheral neuritis in pregnancy, with delivery
646.42	Peripheral neuritis in pregnancy, with delivery, with current postpartum complication
646.51	Asymptomatic bacteriuria in pregnancy, with delivery
646.52	Asymptomatic bacteriuria in pregnancy, with delivery, with current postpartum complication
646.61	Infections of genitourinary tract in pregnancy, with delivery
646.62	Infections of genitourinary tract in pregnancy, with delivery, with current postpartum complication
646.71	Liver and biliary tract disorders in pregnancy, delivered, with or without mention of antepartum condition
646.81	Other specified complication of pregnancy, with delivery
646.82	Other specified complications of pregnancy, with delivery, with current postpartum complication
646.91	Unspecified complication of pregnancy, with delivery
648.11	Maternal thyroid dysfunction with delivery, with or without mention of antepartum condition
648.12	Maternal thyroid dysfunction with delivery, with current postpartum complication
648.21	Maternal anemia, with delivery
648.22	Maternal anemia with delivery, with current postpartum complication
648.31	Maternal drug dependence, with delivery
648.32	Maternal drug dependence, with delivery, with current postpartum complication
648.41	Maternal mental disorders, with delivery
648.42	Maternal mental disorders, with delivery, with current postpartum complication
648.71	Bone and joint disorders of maternal back, pelvis, and lower limbs, with delivery
648.72	Bone and joint disorders of maternal back, pelvis, and lower limbs, with delivery, with current postpartum complication

MDC 14: Pregnancy, Childbirth And The Puerperium—MEDICAL

648.81	Abnormal maternal glucose tolerance, with delivery
648.82	Abnormal maternal glucose tolerance, with delivery, with current postpartum complication
648.91	Other current maternal conditions classifiable elsewhere, with delivery
648.92	Other current maternal conditions classifiable elsewhere, with delivery, with current postpartum complication
649.01	Tobacco use disorder complicating pregnancy, childbirth, or the puerperium, delivered, with or without mention of antepartum condition
649.02	Tobacco use disorder complicating pregnancy, childbirth, or the puerperium, delivered, with mention of postpartum complication
649.11	Obesity complicating pregnancy, childbirth, or the puerperium, delivered, with or without mention of antepartum condition
649.12	Obesity complicating pregnancy, childbirth, or the puerperium, delivered, with mention of postpartum complication
649.21	Bariatric surgery status complicating pregnancy, childbirth, or the puerperium, delivered, with or without mention of antepartum condition
649.22	Bariatric surgery status complicating pregnancy, childbirth, or the puerperium, delivered, with mention of postpartum complication
649.31	Coagulation defects complicating pregnancy, childbirth, or the puerperium, delivered, with or without mention of antepartum condition
649.32	Coagulation defects complicating pregnancy, childbirth, or the puerperium, delivered, with mention of postpartum complication
649.41	Epilepsy complicating pregnancy, childbirth, or the puerperium, delivered, with or without mention of antepartum condition
649.42	Epilepsy complicating pregnancy, childbirth, or the puerperium, delivered, with mention of postpartum complication
649.51	Spotting complicating pregnancy, delivered, with or without mention of antepartum condition
649.61	Uterine size date discrepancy, delivered, with or without mention of antepartum condition
649.62	Uterine size date discrepancy, delivered, with mention of postpartum complication
649.71	Cervical shortening, delivered, with or without mention of antepartum condition
649.8*	Onset (spontaneous) of labor after 37 completed weeks of gestation but before 39 completed weeks gestation, with delivery by (planned) cesarean section
650	Normal delivery
651.01	Twin pregnancy, delivered
651.11	Triplet pregnancy, delivered
651.21	Quadruplet pregnancy, delivered
651.31	Twin pregnancy with fetal loss and retention of one fetus, delivered
651.41	Triplet pregnancy with fetal loss and retention of one or more, delivered
651.51	Quadruplet pregnancy with fetal loss and retention of one or more, delivered
651.61	Other multiple pregnancy with fetal loss and retention of one or more fetus(es), delivered
651.71	Multiple gestation following (elective) fetal reduction, delivered, with or without mention of antepartum condition
651.81	Other specified multiple gestation, delivered
651.91	Unspecified multiple gestation, delivered
652.01	Unstable lie of fetus, delivered
652.11	Breech or other malpresentation successfully converted to cephalic presentation, delivered
652.21	Breech presentation without mention of version, delivered
652.31	Transverse or oblique fetal presentation, delivered
652.41	Fetal face or brow presentation, delivered

652.51	High fetal head at term, delivered
652.61	Multiple gestation with malpresentation of one fetus or more, delivered
652.71	Prolapsed arm of fetus, delivered
652.81	Other specified malposition or malpresentation of fetus, delivered
652.91	Unspecified malposition or malpresentation of fetus, delivered
653.01	Major abnormality of bony pelvis, not further specified, delivered
653.11	Generally contracted pelvis in pregnancy, delivered
653.21	Inlet contraction of pelvis in pregnancy, delivered
653.31	Outlet contraction of pelvis in pregnancy, delivered
653.41	Fetopelvic disproportion, delivered
653.51	Unusually large fetus causing disproportion, delivered
653.61	Hydrocephalic fetus causing disproportion, delivered
653.71	Other fetal abnormality causing disproportion, delivered
653.81	Fetal disproportion of other origin, delivered
653.91	Unspecified fetal disproportion, delivered
654.01	Congenital abnormalities of pregnant uterus, delivered
654.02	Congenital abnormalities of pregnant uterus, delivered, with mention of postpartum complication
654.11	Tumors of body of uterus, delivered
654.12	Tumors of body of uterus, delivered, with mention of postpartum complication
654.21	Previous cesarean delivery, delivered, with or without mention of antepartum condition
654.31	Retroverted and incarcerated gravid uterus, delivered
654.32	Retroverted and incarcerated gravid uterus, delivered, with mention of postpartum complication
654.41	Other abnormalities in shape or position of gravid uterus and of neighboring structures, delivered
654.42	Other abnormalities in shape or position of gravid uterus and of neighboring structures, delivered, with mention of postpartum complication
654.51	Cervical incompetence, delivered
654.52	Cervical incompetence, delivered, with mention of postpartum complication
654.61	Other congenital or acquired abnormality of cervix, with delivery
654.62	Other congenital or acquired abnormality of cervix, delivered, with mention of postpartum complication
654.71	Congenital or acquired abnormality of vagina, with delivery
654.72	Congenital or acquired abnormality of vagina, delivered, with mention of postpartum complication
654.81	Congenital or acquired abnormality of vulva, with delivery
654.82	Congenital or acquired abnormality of vulva, delivered, with mention of postpartum complication
654.91	Other and unspecified abnormality of organs and soft tissues of pelvis, with delivery
654.92	Other and unspecified abnormality of organs and soft tissues of pelvis, delivered, with mention of postpartum complication
655.01	Central nervous system malformation in fetus, with delivery
655.11	Chromosomal abnormality in fetus, affecting management of mother, with delivery
655.21	Hereditary disease in family possibly affecting fetus, affecting management of mother, with delivery
655.31	Suspected damage to fetus from viral disease in mother, affecting management of mother, with delivery
655.41	Suspected damage to fetus from other disease in mother, affecting management of mother, with delivery
655.51	Suspected damage to fetus from drugs, affecting management of mother, delivered
655.61	Suspected damage to fetus from radiation, affecting management of mother, delivered
655.71	Decreased fetal movements, affecting management of mother, delivered
655.81	Other known or suspected fetal abnormality, not elsewhere classified, affecting management of mother, delivery

Ⓣ Transfer DRG   ⓢ Special Payment   ☑ Optimization Potential   ⓣ Targeted Potential   * Code Range   ● New DRG   ▲ Revised DRG Title

148   Valid 10/01/2013–09/30/2014   © 2013 OptumInsight, Inc.

655.91	Unspecified fetal abnormality affecting management of mother, delivery
656.01	Fetal-maternal hemorrhage, with delivery
656.11	Rhesus isoimmunization affecting management of mother, delivered
656.21	Isoimmunization from other and unspecified blood-group incompatibility, affecting management of mother, delivered
656.30	Fetal distress affecting management of mother, unspecified as to episode of care
656.31	Fetal distress affecting management of mother, delivered
656.40	Intrauterine death affecting management of mother, unspecified as to episode of care
656.41	Intrauterine death affecting management of mother, delivered
656.51	Poor fetal growth, affecting management of mother, delivered
656.61	Excessive fetal growth affecting management of mother, delivered
656.71	Other placental conditions affecting management of mother, delivered
656.81	Other specified fetal and placental problems affecting management of mother, delivered
656.91	Unspecified fetal and placental problem affecting management of mother, delivered
657.01	Polyhydramnios, with delivery
658.01	Oligohydramnios, delivered
658.10	Premature rupture of membranes in pregnancy, unspecified as to episode of care
658.11	Premature rupture of membranes in pregnancy, delivered
658.20	Delayed delivery after spontaneous or unspecified rupture of membranes, unspecified as to episode of care
658.21	Delayed delivery after spontaneous or unspecified rupture of membranes, delivered
658.30	Delayed delivery after artificial rupture of membranes, unspecified as to episode of care
658.31	Delayed delivery after artificial rupture of membranes, delivered
658.40	Infection of amniotic cavity, unspecified as to episode of care
658.41	Infection of amniotic cavity, delivered
658.81	Other problem associated with amniotic cavity and membranes, delivered
658.91	Unspecified problem associated with amniotic cavity and membranes, delivered
659.00	Failed mechanical induction of labor, unspecified as to episode of care
659.01	Failed mechanical induction of labor, delivered
659.10	Failed medical or unspecified induction of labor, unspecified as to episode of care
659.11	Failed medical or unspecified induction of labor, delivered
659.20	Unspecified maternal pyrexia during labor, unspecified as to episode of care
659.30	Generalized infection during labor, unspecified as to episode of care
659.41	Grand multiparity, delivered, with or without mention of antepartum condition
659.50	Elderly primigravida, unspecified as to episode of care
659.51	Elderly primigravida, delivered
659.60	Elderly multigravida, unspecified as to episode of care or not applicable
659.61	Elderly multigravida, delivered, with mention of antepartum condition
659.70	Abnormality in fetal heart rate or rhythm, unspecified as to episode of care or not applicable
659.71	Abnormality in fetal heart rate or rhythm, delivered, with or without mention of antepartum condition
659.80	Other specified indication for care or intervention related to labor and delivery, unspecified as to episode of care
659.81	Other specified indication for care or intervention related to labor and delivery, delivered

659.90	Unspecified indication for care or intervention related to labor and delivery, unspecified as to episode of care
659.91	Unspecified indication for care or intervention related to labor and delivery, delivered
660.00	Obstruction caused by malposition of fetus at onset of labor, unspecified as to episode of care
660.01	Obstruction caused by malposition of fetus at onset of labor, delivered
660.10	Obstruction by bony pelvis during labor and delivery, unspecified as to episode of care
660.11	Obstruction by bony pelvis during labor and delivery, delivered
660.20	Obstruction by abnormal pelvic soft tissues during labor and delivery, unspecified as to episode of care
660.21	Obstruction by abnormal pelvic soft tissues during labor and delivery, delivered
660.30	Deep transverse arrest and persistent occipitoposterior position during labor and delivery, unspecified as to episode of care
660.31	Deep transverse arrest and persistent occipitoposterior position during labor and deliver, delivered
660.40	Shoulder (girdle) dystocia during labor and delivery, unspecified as to episode of care
660.41	Shoulder (girdle) dystocia during labor and deliver, delivered
660.50	Locked twins during labor and delivery, unspecified as to episode of care in pregnancy
660.51	Locked twins, delivered
660.60	Unspecified failed trial of labor, unspecified as to episode
660.61	Unspecified failed trial of labor, delivered
660.70	Unspecified failed forceps or vacuum extractor, unspecified as to episode of care
660.71	Unspecified failed forceps or vacuum extractor, delivered
660.80	Other causes of obstructed labor, unspecified as to episode of care
660.81	Other causes of obstructed labor, delivered
660.90	Unspecified obstructed labor, unspecified as to episode of care
660.91	Unspecified obstructed labor, with delivery
661.00	Primary uterine inertia, unspecified as to episode of care
661.01	Primary uterine inertia, with delivery
661.10	Secondary uterine inertia, unspecified as to episode of care
661.11	Secondary uterine inertia, with delivery
661.20	Other and unspecified uterine inertia, unspecified as to episode of care
661.21	Other and unspecified uterine inertia, with delivery
661.30	Precipitate labor, unspecified as to episode of care
661.31	Precipitate labor, with delivery
661.40	Hypertonic, incoordinate, or prolonged uterine contractions, unspecified as to episode of care
661.41	Hypertonic, incoordinate, or prolonged uterine contractions, with delivery
661.90	Unspecified abnormality of labor, unspecified as to episode of care
661.91	Unspecified abnormality of labor, with delivery
662.00	Prolonged first stage of labor, unspecified as to episode of care
662.01	Prolonged first stage of labor, delivered
662.10	Unspecified prolonged labor, unspecified as to episode of care
662.11	Unspecified prolonged labor, delivered
662.20	Prolonged second stage of labor, unspecified as to episode of care
662.21	Prolonged second stage of labor, delivered
662.30	Delayed delivery of second twin, triplet, etc., unspecified as to episode of care
662.31	Delayed delivery of second twin, triplet, etc., delivered
663.00	Prolapse of cord, complicating labor and delivery, unspecified as to episode of care
663.01	Prolapse of cord, complicating labor and delivery, delivered

MDC 14: Pregnancy, Childbirth And The Puerperium—MEDICAL

Surgical	*Medical*	*CC Indicator*	*MCC Indicator*	*Procedure Proxy*

MDC 14: Pregnancy, Childbirth And The Puerperium—MEDICAL

663.10	Cord around neck, with compression, complicating labor and delivery, unspecified as to episode of care	665.30	Laceration of cervix, unspecified as to episode of care in pregnancy
663.11	Cord around neck, with compression, complicating labor and delivery, delivered	665.31	Laceration of cervix, with delivery
663.20	Other and unspecified cord entanglement, with compression, complicating labor and delivery, unspecified as to episode of care	665.40	High vaginal laceration, unspecified as to episode of care in pregnancy
		665.41	High vaginal laceration, with delivery
663.21	Other and unspecified cord entanglement, with compression, complicating labor and delivery, delivered	665.50	Other injury to pelvic organs, unspecified as to episode of care in pregnancy
663.30	Other and unspecified cord entanglement, without mention of compression, complicating labor and delivery, unspecified as to episode of care	665.51	Other injury to pelvic organs, with delivery
		665.60	Damage to pelvic joints and ligaments, unspecified as to episode of care in pregnancy
663.31	Other and unspecified cord entanglement, without mention of compression, complicating labor and delivery, delivered	665.61	Damage to pelvic joints and ligaments, with delivery
		665.70	Pelvic hematoma, unspecified as to episode of care
663.40	Short cord complicating labor and delivery, unspecified as to episode of care	665.71	Pelvic hematoma, with delivery
		665.72	Pelvic hematoma, delivered with postpartum complication
663.41	Short cord complicating labor and delivery, delivered	665.80	Other specified obstetrical trauma, unspecified as to episode of care
663.50	Vasa previa complicating labor and delivery, unspecified as to episode of care	665.81	Other specified obstetrical trauma, with delivery
663.51	Vasa previa complicating labor and delivery, delivered	665.82	Other specified obstetrical trauma, delivered, with postpartum
663.60	Vascular lesions of cord complicating labor and delivery, unspecified as to episode of care	665.90	Unspecified obstetrical trauma, unspecified as to episode of care
663.61	Vascular lesions of cord complicating labor and delivery, delivered	665.91	Unspecified obstetrical trauma, with delivery
663.80	Other umbilical cord complications during labor and delivery, unspecified as to episode of care	665.92	Unspecified obstetrical trauma, delivered, with postpartum complication
		668.00	Pulmonary complications of the administration of anesthesia or other sedation in labor and delivery, unspecified as to episode of care
663.81	Other umbilical cord complications during labor and delivery, delivered		
663.90	Unspecified umbilical cord complication during labor and delivery, unspecified as to episode of care	668.10	Cardiac complications of the administration of anesthesia or other sedation in labor and delivery, unspecified as to episode of care
663.91	Unspecified umbilical cord complication during labor and delivery, delivered	668.20	Central nervous system complications of the administration of anesthesia or other sedation in labor and delivery, unspecified as to episode of care
664.00	First-degree perineal laceration, unspecified as to episode of care in pregnancy		
664.01	First-degree perineal laceration, with delivery	668.80	Other complications of the administration of anesthesia or other sedation in labor and delivery, unspecified as to episode of care
664.10	Second-degree perineal laceration, unspecified as to episode of care in pregnancy		
664.11	Second-degree perineal laceration, with delivery	668.90	Unspecified complication of the administration of anesthesia or other sedation in labor and delivery, unspecified as to episode of care
664.20	Third-degree perineal laceration, unspecified as to episode of care in pregnancy		
664.21	Third-degree perineal laceration, with delivery	669.00	Maternal distress complicating labor and delivery, unspecified as to episode of care
664.30	Fourth-degree perineal laceration, unspecified as to episode of care in pregnancy	669.01	Maternal distress, with delivery, with or without mention of antepartum condition
664.31	Fourth-degree perineal laceration, with delivery		
664.40	Unspecified perineal laceration, unspecified as to episode of care in pregnancy	669.02	Maternal distress, with delivery, with mention of postpartum complication
		669.10	Shock during or following labor and delivery, unspecified as to episode of care
664.41	Unspecified perineal laceration, with delivery		
664.50	Vulvar and perineal hematoma, unspecified as to episode of care in pregnancy	669.20	Maternal hypotension syndrome complicating labor and delivery, unspecified as to episode of care
664.51	Vulvar and perineal hematoma, with delivery	669.21	Maternal hypotension syndrome, with delivery, with or without mention of antepartum condition
664.60	Anal sphincter tear complicating delivery, not associated with third-degree perineal laceration, unspecified as to episode of care or not applicable		
		669.22	Maternal hypotension syndrome, with delivery, with mention of postpartum complication
664.61	Anal sphincter tear complicating delivery, not associated with third-degree perineal laceration, delivered, with or without mention of antepartum condition	669.30	Acute kidney failure following labor and delivery, unspecified as to episode of care or not applicable
		669.40	Other complications of obstetrical surgery and procedures, unspecified as to episode of care
664.80	Other specified trauma to perineum and vulva, unspecified as to episode of care in pregnancy	669.50	Forceps or vacuum extractor delivery without mention of indication, unspecified as to episode of care
664.81	Other specified trauma to perineum and vulva, with delivery		
664.90	Unspecified trauma to perineum and vulva, unspecified as to episode of care in pregnancy	669.51	Forceps or vacuum extractor delivery without mention of indication, delivered, with or without mention of antepartum condition
664.91	Unspecified trauma to perineum and vulva, with delivery		
665.00	Rupture of uterus before onset of labor, unspecified as to episode of care	669.60	Breech extraction, without mention of indication, unspecified as to episode of care
665.01	Rupture of uterus before onset of labor, with delivery	669.61	Breech extraction, without mention of indication, delivered, with or without mention of antepartum condition
665.10	Rupture of uterus during labor, unspecified as to episode		
665.11	Rupture of uterus during labor, with delivery	669.70	Cesarean delivery, without mention of indication, unspecified as to episode of care
665.20	Inversion of uterus, unspecified as to episode of care in pregnancy		
665.22	Inversion of uterus, delivered with postpartum complication		

Ⓣ *Transfer DRG*   ⓢ *Special Payment*   ☑ *Optimization Potential*   ⱅ *Targeted Potential*   * *Code Range*   ● *New DRG*   ▲ *Revised DRG Title*

Valid 10/01/2013-09/30/2014

669.71	Cesarean delivery, without mention of indication, delivered, with or without mention of antepartum condition
669.80	Other complication of labor and delivery, unspecified as to episode of care
669.81	Other complication of labor and delivery, delivered, with or without mention of antepartum condition
669.82	Other complication of labor and delivery, delivered, with mention of postpartum complication
669.90	Unspecified complication of labor and delivery, unspecified as to episode of care
669.91	Unspecified complication of labor and delivery, with delivery, with or without mention of antepartum condition
669.92	Unspecified complication of labor and delivery, with delivery, with mention of postpartum complication
671.01	Varicose veins of legs, with delivery, with or without mention of antepartum condition
671.02	Varicose veins of legs, with delivery, with mention of postpartum complication
671.11	Varicose veins of vulva and perineum, with delivery, with or without mention of antepartum condition
671.12	Varicose veins of vulva and perineum, with delivery, with mention of postpartum complication
671.21	Superficial thrombophlebitis with delivery, with or without mention of antepartum condition
671.22	Superficial thrombophlebitis with delivery, with mention of postpartum complication
671.81	Other venous complication, with delivery, with or without mention of antepartum condition
671.82	Other venous complication, with delivery, with mention of postpartum complication
671.91	Unspecified venous complication, with delivery, with or without mention of antepartum condition
671.92	Unspecified venous complication, with delivery, with mention of postpartum complication
674.42	Placental polyp, with delivery, with mention of postpartum complication
674.92	Unspecified complications of puerperium, with delivery, with mention of postpartum complication
675.81	Other specified infection of the breast and nipple associated with childbirth, delivered, with or without mention of antepartum condition
675.82	Other specified infection of the breast and nipple associated with childbirth, delivered, with mention of postpartum complication
675.91	Unspecified infection of the breast and nipple, delivered, with or without mention of antepartum condition
675.92	Unspecified infection of the breast and nipple, delivered, with mention of postpartum complication
676.01	Retracted nipple, delivered, with or without mention of antepartum condition
676.02	Retracted nipple, delivered, with mention of postpartum complication
676.11	Cracked nipple, delivered, with or without mention of antepartum condition
676.12	Cracked nipple, delivered, with mention of postpartum complication
676.21	Engorgement of breasts, delivered, with or without mention of antepartum condition
676.22	Engorgement of breasts, delivered, with mention of postpartum complication
676.31	Other and unspecified disorder of breast associated with childbirth, delivered, with or without mention of antepartum condition
676.32	Other and unspecified disorder of breast associated with childbirth, delivered, with mention of postpartum complication
676.41	Failure of lactation, with delivery, with or without mention of antepartum condition
676.42	Failure of lactation, with delivery, with mention of postpartum complication

676.51	Suppressed lactation, with delivery, with or without mention of antepartum condition
676.52	Suppressed lactation, with delivery, with mention of postpartum complication
676.61	Galactorrhea, with delivery, with or without mention of antepartum condition
676.62	Galactorrhea, with delivery, with mention of postpartum complication
676.81	Other disorder of lactation, with delivery, with or without mention of antepartum condition
676.82	Other disorder of lactation, with delivery, with mention of postpartum complication
676.91	Unspecified disorder of lactation, with delivery, with or without mention of antepartum condition
676.92	Unspecified disorder of lactation, with delivery, with mention of postpartum complication
678.01	Fetal hematologic conditions, delivered, with or without mention of antepartum condition
678.11	Fetal conjoined twins, delivered, with or without mention of antepartum condition
679.00	Maternal complications from in utero procedure, unspecified as to episode of care or not applicable
679.11	Fetal complications from in utero procedure, delivered, with or without mention of antepartum condition
679.12	Fetal complications from in utero procedure, delivered, with mention of postpartum complication

AND

Only operating room procedures listed under DRG 774
OR

No operating room procedures

DRG 776 **Postpartum and Postabortion Diagnoses without O.R. Procedure**
          GMLOS 2.5   AMLOS 3.4   RW 0.7075   ☑

Principal Diagnosis

639*	Complications following abortion or ectopic and molar pregnancies
642.04	Benign essential hypertension, complicating pregnancy, childbirth, and the puerperium, postpartum condition or complication
642.14	Hypertension secondary to renal disease, complicating pregnancy, childbirth, and the puerperium, postpartum condition or complication
642.24	Other pre-existing hypertension complicating pregnancy, childbirth, and the puerperium, postpartum condition or complication
642.34	Transient hypertension of pregnancy, postpartum condition or complication
642.44	Mild or unspecified pre-eclampsia, postpartum condition or complication
642.54	Severe pre-eclampsia, postpartum condition or complication
642.64	Eclampsia, postpartum condition or complication
642.74	Pre-eclampsia or eclampsia superimposed on pre-existing hypertension, postpartum condition or complication
642.94	Unspecified hypertension complicating pregnancy, childbirth, or the puerperium, postpartum condition or complication
646.14	Edema or excessive weight gain in pregnancy, without mention of hypertension, postpartum condition or complication
646.24	Unspecified renal disease in pregnancy, without mention of hypertension, postpartum condition or complication
646.44	Peripheral neuritis in pregnancy, postpartum condition or complication
646.54	Asymptomatic bacteriuria in pregnancy, postpartum condition or complication

---

| *Surgical* | *Medical* | *CC Indicator* | *MCC Indicator* | *Procedure Proxy* |

646.64   Infections of genitourinary tract in pregnancy, postpartum condition or complication

646.84   Other specified complications of pregnancy, postpartum condition or complication

647.04   Maternal syphilis complicating pregnancy, childbrith, or the puerperium, postpartum condition or complication

647.14   Maternal gonorrhea complicating pregnancy, childbrith, or the puerperium, postpartum condition or complication

647.24   Other venereal diseases complicating pregnancy, childbrith, or the puerperium, postpartum condition or complication

647.34   Maternal tuberculosis complicating pregnancy, childbirth, or the puerperium, postpartum condition or complication

647.44   Maternal malaria, complicating pregnancy, childbirth, or the puerperium, postpartum condition or complication

647.54   Maternal rubella complicating pregnancy, childbirth, or the puerperium, postpartum condition or complication

647.64   Other maternal viral diseases complicating pregnancy, childbirth, or the puerperium, postpartum condition or complication

647.84   Other specified maternal infectious and parasitic diseases complicating pregnancy, childbirth, or the puerperium, postpartum condition or complication

647.94   Unspecified maternal infection or infestation complicating pregnancy, childbirth, or the puerperium, postpartum condition or complication

648.04   Maternal diabetes mellitus, complicating pregnancy, childbirth, or the puerperium, postpartum condition or complication

648.14   Maternal thyroid dysfunction complicating pregnancy, childbirth, or the puerperium, postpartum condition or complication

648.24   Maternal anemia complicating pregnancy, childbirth, or the puerperium, postpartum condition or complication

648.34   Maternal drug dependence complicating pregnancy, childbirth, or the puerperium, postpartum condition or complication

648.44   Maternal mental disorders complicating pregnancy, childbirth, or the puerperium, postpartum condition or complication

648.54   Maternal congenital cardiovascular disorders complicating pregnancy, childbirth, or the puerperium, postpartum condition or complication

648.64   Other maternal cardiovascular diseases complicating pregnancy, childbirth, or the puerperium, postpartum condition or complication

648.74   Bone and joint disorders of maternal back, pelvis, and lower limbs complicating pregnancy, childbirth, or the puerperium, postpartum condition or complication

648.84   Abnormal maternal glucose tolerance complicating pregnancy, childbirth, or the puerperium, postpartum condition or complication

648.94   Other current maternal conditions classifiable elsewhere complicating pregnancy, childbirth, or the puerperium, postpartum condition or complication

649.04   Tobacco use disorder complicating pregnancy, childbirth, or the puerperium, postpartum condition or complication

649.14   Obesity complicating pregnancy, childbirth, or the puerperium, postpartum condition or complication

649.24   Bariatric surgery status complicating pregnancy, childbirth, or the puerperium, postpartum condition or complication

649.34   Coagulation defects complicating pregnancy, childbirth, or the puerperium, postpartum condition or complication

649.44   Epilepsy complicating pregnancy, childbirth, or the puerperium, postpartum condition or complication

649.64   Uterine size date discrepancy, postpartum condition or complication

654.04   Congenital abnormalities of uterus, postpartum condition or complication

654.14   Tumors of body of uterus, postpartum condition or complication

654.34   Retroverted and incarcerated gravid uterus, postpartum condition or complication

654.44   Other abnormalities in shape or position of gravid uterus and of neighboring structures, postpartum condition or complication

654.54   Cervical incompetence, postpartum condition or complication

654.64   Other congenital or acquired abnormality of cervix, postpartum condition or complication

654.74   Congenital or acquired abnormality of vagina, postpartum condition or complication

654.84   Congenital or acquired abnormality of vulva, postpartum condition or complication

654.94   Other and unspecified abnormality of organs and soft tissues of pelvis, postpartum condition or complication

664.04   First-degree perineal laceration, postpartum condition or complication

664.14   Second-degree perineal laceration, postpartum condition or complication

664.24   Third-degree perineal laceration, postpartum condition or complication

664.34   Fourth-degree perineal laceration, postpartum condition or complication

664.44   Unspecified perineal laceration, postpartum condition or complication

664.54   Vulvar and perineal hematoma, postpartum condition or complication

664.64   Anal sphincter tear complicating delivery, not associated with third-degree perineal laceration, postpartum condition or complication

664.84   Other specified trauma to perineum and vulva, postpartum condition or complication

664.94   Unspecified trauma to perineum and vulva, postpartum condition or complication

665.24   Inversion of uterus, postpartum condition or complication

665.34   Laceration of cervix, postpartum condition or complication

665.44   High vaginal laceration, postpartum condition or complication

665.54   Other injury to pelvic organs, postpartum condition or complication

665.64   Damage to pelvic joints and ligaments, postpartum condition or complication

665.74   Pelvic hematoma, postpartum condition or complication

665.84   Other specified obstetrical trauma, postpartum condition or complication

665.94   Unspecified obstetrical trauma, postpartum condition or complication

666.04   Third-stage postpartum hemorrhage, postpartum condition or complication

666.14   Other immediate postpartum hemorrhage, postpartum condition or complication

666.24   Delayed and secondary postpartum hemorrhage, postpartum condition or complication

666.34   Postpartum coagulation defects, postpartum condition or complication

667.04   Retained placenta without hemorrhage, postpartum condition or complication

667.14   Retained portions of placenta or membranes, without hemorrhage, postpartum condition or complication

668.04   Pulmonary complications of the administration of anesthesia or other sedation in labor and delivery, postpartum condition or complication

668.14   Cardiac complications of the administration of anesthesia or other sedation in labor and delivery, postpartum condition or complication

668.24   Central nervous system complications of the administration of anesthesia or other sedation in labor and delivery, postpartum condition or complication

---

Ⓣ *Transfer DRG*   ⓈⓅ *Special Payment*   ☑ *Optimization Potential*   ▽ *Targeted Potential*   * *Code Range*   ● *New DRG*   ▲ *Revised DRG Title*

    Valid 10/01/2013-09/30/2014

668.84 Other complications of the administration of anesthesia or other sedation in labor and delivery, postpartum condition or complication

668.94 Unspecified complication of the administration of anesthesia or other sedation in labor and delivery, postpartum condition or complication

669.04 Maternal distress complicating labor and delivery, postpartum condition or complication

669.14 Shock during or following labor and delivery, postpartum condition or complication

669.24 Maternal hypotension syndrome, postpartum condition or complication

669.34 Acute kidney failure following labor and delivery, postpartum condition or complication

669.44 Other complications of obstetrical surgery and procedures, postpartum condition or complication

669.84 Other complication of labor and delivery, postpartum condition or complication

669.94 Unspecified complication of labor and delivery, postpartum condition or complication

670.04 Major puerperal infection, unspecified, postpartum condition or complication

670.14 Puerperal endometritis, postpartum condition or complication

670.24 Puerperal sepsis, postpartum condition or complication

670.34 Puerperal septic thrombophlebitis, postpartum condition or complication

670.84 Other major puerperal infection, postpartum condition or complication

671.04 Varicose veins of legs, postpartum condition or complication

671.14 Varicose veins of vulva and perineum, postpartum condition or complication

671.24 Superficial thrombophlebitis, postpartum condition or complication

671.44 Deep phlebothrombosis, postpartum condition or complication

671.54 Other phlebitis and thrombosis, postpartum condition or complication

671.84 Other venous complications, postpartum condition or complication

671.94 Unspecified venous complication, postpartum condition or complication

672.04 Puerperal pyrexia of unknown origin, postpartum condition or complication

673.04 Obstetrical air embolism, postpartum condition or complication

673.14 Amniotic fluid embolism, postpartum condition or complication

673.24 Obstetrical blood-clot embolism, postpartum condition or complication

673.34 Obstetrical pyemic and septic embolism, postpartum condition or complication

673.84 Other obstetrical pulmonary embolism, postpartum condition or complication

674.04 Cerebrovascular disorders in the puerperium, postpartum condition or complication

674.14 Disruption of cesarean wound, postpartum condition or complication

674.24 Disruption of perineal wound, postpartum condition or complication

674.34 Other complications of obstetrical surgical wounds, postpartum condition or complication

674.44 Placental polyp, postpartum condition or complication

674.54 Peripartum cardiomyopathy, postpartum condition or complication

674.84 Other complications of puerperium, postpartum condition or complication

674.94 Unspecified complications of puerperium, postpartum condition or complication

675.04 Infection of nipple, postpartum condition or complication

675.14 Abscess of breast, postpartum condition or complication

675.24 Nonpurulent mastitis, postpartum condition or complication

675.84 Other specified infections of the breast and nipple, postpartum condition or complication

675.94 Unspecified infection of the breast and nipple, postpartum condition or complication

676.04 Retracted nipple, postpartum condition or complication

676.14 Cracked nipple, postpartum condition or complication

676.24 Engorgement of breasts, postpartum condition or complication

676.34 Other and unspecified disorder of breast associated with childbirth, postpartum condition or complication

676.44 Failure of lactation, postpartum condition or complication

676.54 Suppressed lactation, postpartum condition or complication

676.64 Galactorrhea, postpartum condition or complication

676.84 Other disorders of lactation, postpartum condition or complication

676.94 Unspecified disorder of lactation, postpartum condition or complication

679.04 Maternal complications from in utero procedure, postpartum condition or complication

679.14 Fetal complications from in utero procedure, postpartum condition or complication

V24.0 Postpartum care and examination immediately after delivery

DRG 777 Ectopic Pregnancy

| GMLOS 1.6 | AMLOS 2.1 | RW 0.9550 | ☑ |

Principal Diagnosis
633*   Ectopic pregnancy

DRG 778 Threatened Abortion

| GMLOS 1.9 | AMLOS 2.9 | RW 0.5247 | ☑ |

Principal Diagnosis
640.00 Threatened abortion, unspecified as to episode of care
640.03 Threatened abortion, antepartum
640.80 Other specified hemorrhage in early pregnancy, unspecified as to episode of care
640.83 Other specified hemorrhage in early pregnancy, antepartum
640.90 Unspecified hemorrhage in early pregnancy, unspecified as to episode of care
640.93 Unspecified hemorrhage in early pregnancy, antepartum
644.00 Threatened premature labor, unspecified as to episode of care
644.03 Threatened premature labor, antepartum

DRG 779 Abortion without D&C

| GMLOS 1.5 | AMLOS 1.8 | RW 0.4843 | ☑ |

Principal Diagnosis
632   Missed abortion
634*   Spontaneous abortion
635*   Legally induced abortion
636*   Illegally induced abortion
637*   Abortion, unspecified as to legality
638*   Failed attempted abortion
V61.7   Other unwanted pregnancy

DRG 780 False Labor

| GMLOS 1.2 | AMLOS 1.4 | RW 0.2515 | ☑ |

Principal Diagnosis
644.10 Other threatened labor, unspecified as to episode of care
644.13 Other threatened labor, antepartum

| Surgical | Medical | CC Indicator | MCC Indicator | Procedure Proxy |

DRG 781 Other Antepartum Diagnoses with Medical Complications

| GMLOS 2.7 | AMLOS 3.9 | RW 0.7568 | ☑ |

Principal Diagnosis

630	Hydatidiform mole
631*	Other abnormal product of conception
641.03	Placenta previa without hemorrhage, antepartum
641.13	Hemorrhage from placenta previa, antepartum
641.23	Premature separation of placenta, antepartum
641.33	Antepartum hemorrhage associated with coagulation defect, antepartum
641.83	Other antepartum hemorrhage, antepartum
641.93	Unspecified antepartum hemorrhage, antepartum
642.03	Benign essential hypertension antepartum
642.13	Hypertension secondary to renal disease, antepartum
642.23	Other pre-existing hypertension, antepartum
642.33	Transient hypertension of pregnancy, antepartum
642.43	Mild or unspecified pre-eclampsia, antepartum
642.53	Severe pre-eclampsia, antepartum
642.63	Eclampsia, antepartum
642.73	Pre-eclampsia or eclampsia superimposed on pre-existing hypertension, antepartum
642.93	Unspecified hypertension antepartum
643.03	Mild hyperemesis gravidarum, antepartum
643.13	Hyperemesis gravidarum with metabolic disturbance, antepartum
643.23	Late vomiting of pregnancy, antepartum
643.83	Other vomiting complicating pregnancy, antepartum
643.93	Unspecified vomiting of pregnancy, antepartum
644.20	Early onset of delivery, unspecified as to episode of care
645.13	Post term pregnancy, antepartum condition or complication
645.23	Prolonged pregnancy, antepartum condition or complication
646.03	Papyraceous fetus, antepartum
646.13	Edema or excessive weight gain, antepartum
646.23	Unspecified antepartum renal disease
646.33	Pregnancy complication, recurrent pregnancy loss, antepartum condition or complication
646.43	Peripheral neuritis antepartum
646.53	Asymptomatic bacteriuria antepartum
646.63	Infections of genitourinary tract antepartum
646.73	Liver and biliary tract disorders in pregnancy, antepartum condition or complication
646.83	Other specified complication, antepartum
646.93	Unspecified complication of pregnancy, antepartum
647.03	Maternal syphilis, antepartum
647.13	Maternal gonorrhea, antepartum
647.23	Other maternal venereal diseases, antepartum condition or complication
647.33	Maternal tuberculosis, antepartum
647.43	Maternal malaria, antepartum
647.53	Maternal rubella, antepartum
647.63	Other maternal viral disease, antepartum
647.83	Other specified maternal infectious and parasitic disease, antepartum
647.93	Unspecified maternal infection or infestation, antepartum
648.03	Maternal diabetes mellitus, antepartum
648.13	Maternal thyroid dysfunction, antepartum condition or complication
648.23	Maternal anemia, antepartum
648.33	Maternal drug dependence, antepartum
648.43	Maternal mental disorders, antepartum
648.53	Maternal congenital cardiovascular disorders, antepartum
648.63	Other maternal cardiovascular diseases, antepartum
648.73	Bone and joint disorders of maternal back, pelvis, and lower limbs, antepartum
648.83	Abnormal maternal glucose tolerance, antepartum
648.93	Other current maternal conditions classifiable elsewhere, antepartum
649.03	Tobacco use disorder complicating pregnancy, childbirth, or the puerperium, antepartum condition or complication
649.13	Obesity complicating pregnancy, childbirth, or the puerperium, antepartum condition or complication
649.23	Bariatric surgery status complicating pregnancy, childbirth, or the puerperium, antepartum condition or complication
649.33	Coagulation defects complicating pregnancy, childbirth, or the puerperium, antepartum condition or complication
649.43	Epilepsy complicating pregnancy, childbirth, or the puerperium, antepartum condition or complication
649.53	Spotting complicating pregnancy, antepartum condition or complication
649.63	Uterine size date discrepancy, antepartum condition or complication
649.73	Cervical shortening, antepartum condition or complication
651.03	Twin pregnancy, antepartum
651.13	Triplet pregnancy, antepartum
651.23	Quadruplet pregnancy, antepartum
651.33	Twin pregnancy with fetal loss and retention of one fetus, antepartum
651.43	Triplet pregnancy with fetal loss and retention of one or more, antepartum
651.53	Quadruplet pregnancy with fetal loss and retention of one or more, antepartum
651.63	Other multiple pregnancy with fetal loss and retention of one or more fetus(es), antepartum
651.73	Multiple gestation following (elective) fetal reduction, antepartum condition or complication
651.83	Other specified multiple gestation, antepartum
651.93	Unspecified multiple gestation, antepartum
652.03	Unstable lie of fetus, antepartum
652.13	Breech or other malpresentation successfully converted to cephalic presentation, antepartum
652.23	Breech presentation without mention of version, antepartum
652.33	Transverse or oblique fetal presentation, antepartum
652.43	Fetal face or brow presentation, antepartum
652.53	High fetal head at term, antepartum
652.63	Multiple gestation with malpresentation of one fetus or more, antepartum
652.73	Prolapsed arm of fetus, antepartum condition or complication
652.83	Other specified malposition or malpresentation of fetus, antepartum
652.93	Unspecified malposition or malpresentation of fetus, antepartum
653.03	Major abnormality of bony pelvis, not further specified, antepartum
653.13	Generally contracted pelvis in pregnancy, antepartum
653.23	Inlet contraction of pelvis in pregnancy, antepartum
653.33	Outlet contraction of pelvis in pregnancy, antepartum
653.43	Fetopelvic disproportion, antepartum
653.53	Unusually large fetus causing disproportion, antepartum
653.63	Hydrocephalic fetus causing disproportion, antepartum
653.73	Other fetal abnormality causing disproportion, antepartum
653.83	Fetal disproportion of other origin, antepartum
653.93	Unspecified fetal disproportion, antepartum
654.03	Congenital abnormalities of pregnant uterus, antepartum
654.13	Tumors of body of uterus, antepartum condition or complication
654.23	Previous cesarean delivery, antepartum condition or complication
654.33	Retroverted and incarcerated gravid uterus, antepartum
654.43	Other abnormalities in shape or position of gravid uterus and of neighboring structures, antepartum
654.53	Cervical incompetence, antepartum condition or complication
654.63	Other congenital or acquired abnormality of cervix, antepartum condition or complication

T Transfer DRG   SP Special Payment   ☑ Optimization Potential   ᵛᵉᵈ Targeted Potential   * Code Range   ● New DRG   ▲ Revised DRG Title

154   Valid 10/01/2013-09/30/2014   © 2013 OptumInsight, Inc.

654.73	Congenital or acquired abnormality of vagina, antepartum condition or complication
654.83	Congenital or acquired abnormality of vulva, antepartum condition or complication
654.93	Other and unspecified abnormality of organs and soft tissues of pelvis, antepartum condition or complication
655.03	Central nervous system malformation in fetus, antepartum
655.13	Chromosomal abnormality in fetus, affecting management of mother, antepartum
655.23	Hereditary disease in family possibly affecting fetus, affecting management of mother, antepartum condition or complication
655.33	Suspected damage to fetus from viral disease in mother, affecting management of mother, antepartum condition or complication
655.43	Suspected damage to fetus from other disease in mother, affecting management of mother, antepartum condition or complication
655.53	Suspected damage to fetus from drugs, affecting management of mother, antepartum
655.63	Suspected damage to fetus from radiation, affecting management of mother, antepartum condition or complication
655.73	Decreased fetal movements, affecting management of mother, antepartum condition or complication
655.83	Other known or suspected fetal abnormality, not elsewhere classified, affecting management of mother, antepartum condition or complication
655.93	Unspecified fetal abnormality affecting management of mother, antepartum condition or complication
656.03	Fetal-maternal hemorrhage, antepartum condition or complication
656.13	Rhesus isoimmunization affecting management of mother, antepartum condition
656.23	Isoimmunization from other and unspecified blood-group incompatibility, affecting management of mother, antepartum
656.33	Fetal distress affecting management of mother, antepartum
656.43	Intrauterine death affecting management of mother, antepartum
656.53	Poor fetal growth, affecting management of mother, antepartum condition or complication
656.63	Excessive fetal growth affecting management of mother, antepartum
656.73	Other placental conditions affecting management of mother, antepartum
656.83	Other specified fetal and placental problems affecting management of mother, antepartum
656.93	Unspecified fetal and placental problem affecting management of mother, antepartum
657.03	Polyhydramnios, antepartum complication
658.03	Oligohydramnios, antepartum
658.13	Premature rupture of membranes in pregnancy, antepartum
658.23	Delayed delivery after spontaneous or unspecified rupture of membranes, antepartum
658.33	Delayed delivery after artificial rupture of membranes, antepartum
658.43	Infection of amniotic cavity, antepartum
658.83	Other problem associated with amniotic cavity and membranes, antepartum
658.93	Unspecified problem associated with amniotic cavity and membranes, antepartum
659.03	Failed mechanical induction of labor, antepartum
659.13	Failed medical or unspecified induction of labor, antepartum
659.23	Unspecified maternal pyrexia, antepartum
659.33	Generalized infection during labor, antepartum
659.43	Grand multiparity with current pregnancy, antepartum
659.53	Elderly primigravida, antepartum
659.63	Elderly multigravida, with antepartum condition or complication
659.73	Abnormality in fetal heart rate or rhythm, antepartum condition or complication
659.83	Other specified indication for care or intervention related to labor and delivery, antepartum
659.93	Unspecified indication for care or intervention related to labor and delivery, antepartum
660.03	Obstruction caused by malposition of fetus at onset of labor, antepartum
660.13	Obstruction by bony pelvis during labor and delivery, antepartum
660.23	Obstruction by abnormal pelvic soft tissues during labor and delivery, antepartum
660.33	Deep transverse arrest and persistent occipitoposterior position during labor and delivery, antepartum
660.43	Shoulder (girdle) dystocia during labor and delivery, antepartum
660.53	Locked twins, antepartum
660.63	Unspecified failed trial of labor, antepartum
660.73	Failed forceps or vacuum extractor, unspecified, antepartum
660.83	Other causes of obstructed labor, antepartum
660.93	Unspecified obstructed labor, antepartum
661.03	Primary uterine inertia, antepartum
661.13	Secondary uterine inertia, antepartum
661.23	Other and unspecified uterine inertia, antepartum
661.33	Precipitate labor, antepartum
661.43	Hypertonic, incoordinate, or prolonged uterine contractions, antepartum
661.93	Unspecified abnormality of labor, antepartum
662.03	Prolonged first stage of labor, antepartum
662.13	Unspecified prolonged labor, antepartum
662.23	Prolonged second stage of labor, antepartum
662.33	Delayed delivery of second twin, triplet, etc., antepartum
663.03	Prolapse of cord, complicating labor and delivery, antepartum
663.13	Cord around neck, with compression, complicating labor and delivery, antepartum
663.23	Other and unspecified cord entanglement, with compression, complicating labor and delivery, antepartum
663.33	Other and unspecified cord entanglement, without mention of compression, complicating labor and delivery, antepartum
663.43	Short cord complicating labor and delivery, antepartum
663.53	Vasa previa complicating labor and delivery, antepartum
663.63	Vascular lesions of cord complicating labor and delivery, antepartum
663.83	Other umbilical cord complications during labor and delivery, antepartum
663.93	Unspecified umbilical cord complication during labor and delivery, antepartum
665.03	Rupture of uterus before onset of labor, antepartum
665.83	Other specified obstetrical trauma, antepartum
665.93	Unspecified obstetrical trauma, antepartum
668.03	Pulmonary complications of the administration of anesthesia or other sedation in labor and delivery, antepartum
668.13	Cardiac complications of the administration of anesthesia or other sedation in labor and delivery, antepartum
668.23	Central nervous system complications of the administration of anesthesia or other sedation in labor and delivery, antepartum
668.83	Other complications of the administration of anesthesia or other sedation in labor and delivery, antepartum
668.93	Unspecified complication of the administration of anesthesia or other sedation in labor and delivery, antepartum
669.03	Maternal distress complicating labor and delivery, antepartum condition or complication
669.13	Shock during or following labor and delivery, antepartum shock
669.23	Maternal hypotension syndrome, antepartum

Surgical	**Medical**	**CC Indicator**	**MCC Indicator**	**Procedure Proxy**

MDC 14: Pregnancy, Childbirth And The Puerperium—MEDICAL

669.43	Other complications of obstetrical surgery and procedures, antepartum condition or complication
669.83	Other complication of labor and delivery, antepartum condition or complication
669.93	Unspecified complication of labor and delivery, antepartum condition or complication
671.03	Varicose veins of legs, antepartum
671.13	Varicose veins of vulva and perineum, antepartum
671.23	Superficial thrombophlebitis, antepartum
671.33	Deep phlebothrombosis, antepartum
671.53	Other antepartum phlebitis and thrombosis
671.83	Other venous complication, antepartum
671.93	Unspecified venous complication, antepartum
673.03	Obstetrical air embolism, antepartum condition or complication
673.13	Amniotic fluid embolism, antepartum condition or complication
673.23	Obstetrical blood-clot embolism, antepartum
673.33	Obstetrical pyemic and septic embolism, antepartum
673.83	Other obstetrical pulmonary embolism, antepartum
674.03	Cerebrovascular disorder, antepartum
674.53	Peripartum cardiomyopathy, antepartum condition or complication
675.03	Infection of nipple, antepartum
675.13	Abscess of breast, antepartum
675.23	Nonpurulent mastitis, antepartum
675.83	Other specified infection of the breast and nipple, antepartum
675.93	Unspecified infection of the breast and nipple, antepartum
676.03	Retracted nipple, antepartum condition or complication
676.13	Cracked nipple, antepartum condition or complication
676.23	Engorgement of breast, antepartum
676.33	Other and unspecified disorder of breast associated with childbirth, antepartum condition or complication
676.43	Failure of lactation, antepartum condition or complication
676.53	Suppressed lactation, antepartum condition or complication
676.63	Galactorrhea, antepartum condition or complication
676.83	Other disorder of lactation, antepartum condition or complication
676.93	Unspecified disorder of lactation, antepartum condition or complication
678.03	Fetal hematologic conditions, antepartum condition or complication
678.13	Fetal conjoined twins, antepartum condition or complication
679.03	Maternal complications from in utero procedure, antepartum condition or complication
679.13	Fetal complications from in utero procedure, antepartum condition or complication
792.3	Nonspecific abnormal finding in amniotic fluid
796.5	Abnormal finding on antenatal screening
V28.0	Screening for chromosomal anomalies by amniocentesis
V28.1	Screening for raised alpha-fetoprotein levels in amniotic fluid
V28.2	Other antenatal screening based on amniocentesis
V61.6	Illegitimacy or illegitimate pregnancy

AND

Secondary Diagnosis

641.30	Antepartum hemorrhage associated with coagulation defects, unspecified as to episode of care
641.33	Antepartum hemorrhage associated with coagulation defect, antepartum
642.03	Benign essential hypertension antepartum
642.13	Hypertension secondary to renal disease, antepartum
642.23	Other pre-existing hypertension, antepartum
642.43	Mild or unspecified pre-eclampsia, antepartum
642.50	Severe pre-eclampsia, unspecified as to episode of care
642.53	Severe pre-eclampsia, antepartum

642.60	Eclampsia complicating pregnancy, childbirth or the puerperium, unspecified as to episode of care
642.63	Eclampsia, antepartum
642.70	Pre-eclampsia or eclampsia superimposed on pre-existing hypertension, complicating pregnancy, childbirth, or the puerperium, unspecified as to episode of care
642.73	Pre-eclampsia or eclampsia superimposed on pre-existing hypertension, antepartum
642.93	Unspecified hypertension antepartum
643.00	Mild hyperemesis gravidarum, unspecified as to episode of care
643.03	Mild hyperemesis gravidarum, antepartum
643.10	Hyperemesis gravidarum with metabolic disturbance, unspecified as to episode of care
643.13	Hyperemesis gravidarum with metabolic disturbance, antepartum
643.20	Late vomiting of pregnancy, unspecified as to episode of care
643.23	Late vomiting of pregnancy, antepartum
643.80	Other vomiting complicating pregnancy, unspecified as to episode of care
643.83	Other vomiting complicating pregnancy, antepartum
643.90	Unspecified vomiting of pregnancy, unspecified as to episode of care
643.93	Unspecified vomiting of pregnancy, antepartum
646.10	Edema or excessive weight gain in pregnancy, unspecified as to episode of care
646.13	Edema or excessive weight gain, antepartum
646.20	Unspecified renal disease in pregnancy, unspecified as to episode of care
646.23	Unspecified antepartum renal disease
646.43	Peripheral neuritis antepartum
646.60	Infections of genitourinary tract in pregnancy, unspecified as to episode of care
646.63	Infections of genitourinary tract antepartum
646.70	Liver and biliary tract disorders in pregnancy, unspecified as to episode of care or not applicable
646.73	Liver and biliary tract disorders in pregnancy, antepartum condition or complication
646.80	Other specified complication of pregnancy, unspecified as to episode of care
646.83	Other specified complication, antepartum
647.03	Maternal syphilis, antepartum
647.13	Maternal gonorrhea, antepartum
647.23	Other maternal venereal diseases, antepartum condition or complication
647.33	Maternal tuberculosis, antepartum
647.43	Maternal malaria, antepartum
647.53	Maternal rubella, antepartum
647.63	Other maternal viral disease, antepartum
647.83	Other specified maternal infectious and parasitic disease, antepartum
647.93	Unspecified maternal infection or infestation, antepartum
648.03	Maternal diabetes mellitus, antepartum
648.13	Maternal thyroid dysfunction, antepartum condition or complication
648.23	Maternal anemia, antepartum
648.33	Maternal drug dependence, antepartum
648.43	Maternal mental disorders, antepartum
648.53	Maternal congenital cardiovascular disorders, antepartum
648.63	Other maternal cardiovascular diseases, antepartum
648.73	Bone and joint disorders of maternal back, pelvis, and lower limbs, antepartum
648.83	Abnormal maternal glucose tolerance, antepartum
648.93	Other current maternal conditions classifiable elsewhere, antepartum

---

T *Transfer DRG*   SP *Special Payment*   ☑ *Optimization Potential*   ▽ *Targeted Potential*   * *Code Range*   ● *New DRG*   ▲ *Revised DRG Title*

DRG 782   **Other Antepartum Diagnoses without Medical Complications**

GMLOS 1.6   AMLOS 2.3   RW 0.4463   ☑

Principal Diagnosis

630	Hydatidiform mole
631*	Other abnormal product of conception
641.03	Placenta previa without hemorrhage, antepartum
641.13	Hemorrhage from placenta previa, antepartum
641.23	Premature separation of placenta, antepartum
641.83	Other antepartum hemorrhage, antepartum
641.93	Unspecified antepartum hemorrhage, antepartum
642.33	Transient hypertension of pregnancy, antepartum
644.20	Early onset of delivery, unspecified as to episode of care
645.13	Post term pregnancy, antepartum condition or complication
645.23	Prolonged pregnancy, antepartum condition or complication
646.03	Papyraceous fetus, antepartum
646.33	Pregnancy complication, recurrent pregnancy loss, antepartum condition or complication
646.53	Asymptomatic bacteriuria antepartum
646.93	Unspecified complication of pregnancy, antepartum
649.03	Tobacco use disorder complicating pregnancy, childbirth, or the puerperium, antepartum condition or complication
649.13	Obesity complicating pregnancy, childbirth, or the puerperium, antepartum condition or complication
649.23	Bariatric surgery status complicating pregnancy, childbirth, or the puerperium, antepartum condition or complication
649.33	Coagulation defects complicating pregnancy, childbirth, or the puerperium, antepartum condition or complication
649.43	Epilepsy complicating pregnancy, childbirth, or the puerperium, antepartum condition or complication
649.53	Spotting complicating pregnancy, antepartum condition or complication
649.63	Uterine size date discrepancy, antepartum condition or complication
649.73	Cervical shortening, antepartum condition or complication
651.03	Twin pregnancy, antepartum
651.13	Triplet pregnancy, antepartum
651.23	Quadruplet pregnancy, antepartum
651.33	Twin pregnancy with fetal loss and retention of one fetus, antepartum
651.43	Triplet pregnancy with fetal loss and retention of one or more, antepartum
651.53	Quadruplet pregnancy with fetal loss and retention of one or more, antepartum
651.63	Other multiple pregnancy with fetal loss and retention of one or more fetus(es), antepartum
651.73	Multiple gestation following (elective) fetal reduction, antepartum condition or complication
651.83	Other specified multiple gestation, antepartum
651.93	Unspecified multiple gestation, antepartum
652.03	Unstable lie of fetus, antepartum
652.13	Breech or other malpresentation successfully converted to cephalic presentation, antepartum
652.23	Breech presentation without mention of version, antepartum
652.33	Transverse or oblique fetal presentation, antepartum
652.43	Fetal face or brow presentation, antepartum
652.53	High fetal head at term, antepartum
652.63	Multiple gestation with malpresentation of one fetus or more, antepartum
652.73	Prolapsed arm of fetus, antepartum condition or complication
652.83	Other specified malposition or malpresentation of fetus, antepartum
652.93	Unspecified malposition or malpresentation of fetus, antepartum
653.03	Major abnormality of bony pelvis, not further specified, antepartum
653.13	Generally contracted pelvis in pregnancy, antepartum
653.23	Inlet contraction of pelvis in pregnancy, antepartum
653.33	Outlet contraction of pelvis in pregnancy, antepartum
653.43	Fetopelvic disproportion, antepartum
653.53	Unusually large fetus causing disproportion, antepartum
653.63	Hydrocephalic fetus causing disproportion, antepartum
653.73	Other fetal abnormality causing disproportion, antepartum
653.83	Fetal disproportion of other origin, antepartum
653.93	Unspecified fetal disproportion, antepartum
654.03	Congenital abnormalities of pregnant uterus, antepartum
654.13	Tumors of body of uterus, antepartum condition or complication
654.23	Previous cesarean delivery, antepartum condition or complication
654.33	Retroverted and incarcerated gravid uterus, antepartum
654.43	Other abnormalities in shape or position of gravid uterus and of neighboring structures, antepartum
654.53	Cervical incompetence, antepartum condition or complication
654.63	Other congenital or acquired abnormality of cervix, antepartum condition or complication
654.73	Congenital or acquired abnormality of vagina, antepartum condition or complication
654.83	Congenital or acquired abnormality of vulva, antepartum condition or complication
654.93	Other and unspecified abnormality of organs and soft tissues of pelvis, antepartum condition or complication
655.03	Central nervous system malformation in fetus, antepartum
655.13	Chromosomal abnormality in fetus, affecting management of mother, antepartum
655.23	Hereditary disease in family possibly affecting fetus, affecting management of mother, antepartum condition or complication
655.33	Suspected damage to fetus from viral disease in mother, affecting management of mother, antepartum condition or complication
655.43	Suspected damage to fetus from other disease in mother, affecting management of mother, antepartum condition or complication
655.53	Suspected damage to fetus from drugs, affecting management of mother, antepartum
655.63	Suspected damage to fetus from radiation, affecting management of mother, antepartum condition or complication
655.73	Decreased fetal movements, affecting management of mother, antepartum condition or complication
655.83	Other known or suspected fetal abnormality, not elsewhere classified, affecting management of mother, antepartum condition or complication
655.93	Unspecified fetal abnormality affecting management of mother, antepartum condition or complication
656.03	Fetal-maternal hemorrhage, antepartum condition or complication
656.13	Rhesus isoimmunization affecting management of mother, antepartum condition
656.23	Isoimmunization from other and unspecified blood-group incompatibility, affecting management of mother, antepartum
656.33	Fetal distress affecting management of mother, antepartum
656.43	Intrauterine death affecting management of mother, antepartum
656.53	Poor fetal growth, affecting management of mother, antepartum condition or complication
656.63	Excessive fetal growth affecting management of mother, antepartum
656.73	Other placental conditions affecting management of mother, antepartum
656.83	Other specified fetal and placental problems affecting management of mother, antepartum

MDC 14: Pregnancy, Childbirth And The Puerperium—MEDICAL

656.93	Unspecified fetal and placental problem affecting management of mother, antepartum	663.93	Unspecified umbilical cord complication during labor and delivery, antepartum
657.03	Polyhydramnios, antepartum complication	665.03	Rupture of uterus before onset of labor, antepartum
658.03	Oligohydramnios, antepartum	665.83	Other specified obstetrical trauma, antepartum
658.13	Premature rupture of membranes in pregnancy, antepartum	665.93	Unspecified obstetrical trauma, antepartum
658.23	Delayed delivery after spontaneous or unspecified rupture of membranes, antepartum	668.03	Pulmonary complications of the administration of anesthesia or other sedation in labor and delivery, antepartum
658.33	Delayed delivery after artificial rupture of membranes, antepartum	668.13	Cardiac complications of the administration of anesthesia or other sedation in labor and delivery, antepartum
658.43	Infection of amniotic cavity, antepartum	668.23	Central nervous system complications of the administration of anesthesia or other sedation in labor and delivery, antepartum
658.83	Other problem associated with amniotic cavity and membranes, antepartum		
658.93	Unspecified problem associated with amniotic cavity and membranes, antepartum	668.83	Other complications of the administration of anesthesia or other sedation in labor and delivery, antepartum
659.03	Failed mechanical induction of labor, antepartum	668.93	Unspecified complication of the administration of anesthesia or other sedation in labor and delivery, antepartum
659.13	Failed medical or unspecified induction of labor, antepartum		
659.23	Unspecified maternal pyrexia, antepartum	669.03	Maternal distress complicating labor and delivery, antepartum condition or complication
659.33	Generalized infection during labor, antepartum		
659.43	Grand multiparity with current pregnancy, antepartum	669.13	Shock during or following labor and delivery, antepartum shock
659.53	Elderly primigravida, antepartum		
659.63	Elderly multigravida, with antepartum condition or complication	669.23	Maternal hypotension syndrome, antepartum
659.73	Abnormality in fetal heart rate or rhythm, antepartum condition or complication	669.43	Other complications of obstetrical surgery and procedures, antepartum condition or complication
659.83	Other specified indication for care or intervention related to labor and delivery, antepartum	669.83	Other complication of labor and delivery, antepartum condition or complication
659.93	Unspecified indication for care or intervention related to labor and delivery, antepartum	669.93	Unspecified complication of labor and delivery, antepartum condition or complication
660.03	Obstruction caused by malposition of fetus at onset of labor, antepartum	671.03	Varicose veins of legs, antepartum
660.13	Obstruction by bony pelvis during labor and delivery, antepartum	671.13	Varicose veins of vulva and perineum, antepartum
660.23	Obstruction by abnormal pelvic soft tissues during labor and delivery, antepartum	671.23	Superficial thrombophlebitis, antepartum
		671.33	Deep phlebothrombosis, antepartum
660.33	Deep transverse arrest and persistent occipitoposterior position during labor and delivery, antepartum	671.53	Other antepartum phlebitis and thrombosis
		671.83	Other venous complication, antepartum
660.43	Shoulder (girdle) dystocia during labor and delivery, antepartum	671.93	Unspecified venous complication, antepartum
		673.03	Obstetrical air embolism, antepartum condition or complication
660.53	Locked twins, antepartum		
660.63	Unspecified failed trial of labor, antepartum	673.13	Amniotic fluid embolism, antepartum condition or complication
660.73	Failed forceps or vacuum extractor, unspecified, antepartum		
660.83	Other causes of obstructed labor, antepartum	673.23	Obstetrical blood-clot embolism, antepartum
660.93	Unspecified obstructed labor, antepartum	673.33	Obstetrical pyemic and septic embolism, antepartum
661.03	Primary uterine inertia, antepartum	673.83	Other obstetrical pulmonary embolism, antepartum
661.13	Secondary uterine inertia, antepartum	674.03	Cerebrovascular disorder, antepartum
661.23	Other and unspecified uterine inertia, antepartum	674.53	Peripartum cardiomyopathy, antepartum condition or complication
661.33	Precipitate labor, antepartum		
661.43	Hypertonic, incoordinate, or prolonged uterine contractions, antepartum	675.03	Infection of nipple, antepartum
		675.13	Abscess of breast, antepartum
661.93	Unspecified abnormality of labor, antepartum	675.23	Nonpurulent mastitis, antepartum
662.03	Prolonged first stage of labor, antepartum	675.83	Other specified infection of the breast and nipple, antepartum
662.13	Unspecified prolonged labor, antepartum		
662.23	Prolonged second stage of labor, antepartum	675.93	Unspecified infection of the breast and nipple, antepartum
662.33	Delayed delivery of second twin, triplet, etc., antepartum	676.03	Retracted nipple, antepartum condition or complication
663.03	Prolapse of cord, complicating labor and delivery, antepartum	676.13	Cracked nipple, antepartum condition or complication
		676.23	Engorgement of breast, antepartum
663.13	Cord around neck, with compression, complicating labor and delivery, antepartum	676.33	Other and unspecified disorder of breast associated with childbirth, antepartum condition or complication
663.23	Other and unspecified cord entanglement, with compression, complicating labor and delivery, antepartum	676.43	Failure of lactation, antepartum condition or complication
		676.53	Suppressed lactation, antepartum condition or complication
663.33	Other and unspecified cord entanglement, without mention of compression, complicating labor and delivery, antepartum	676.63	Galactorrhea, antepartum condition or complication
		676.83	Other disorder of lactation, antepartum condition or complication
663.43	Short cord complicating labor and delivery, antepartum	676.93	Unspecified disorder of lactation, antepartum condition or complication
663.53	Vasa previa complicating labor and delivery, antepartum		
663.63	Vascular lesions of cord complicating labor and delivery, antepartum	678.03	Fetal hematologic conditions, antepartum condition or complication
		678.13	Fetal conjoined twins, antepartum condition or complication
663.83	Other umbilical cord complications during labor and delivery, antepartum	679.03	Maternal complications from in utero procedure, antepartum condition or complication

---

T Transfer DRG   SP Special Payment   ☑ Optimization Potential   ⱽᴵᴸᴰ Targeted Potential   * Code Range   ● New DRG   ▲ Revised DRG Title

679.13	Fetal complications from in utero procedure, antepartum condition or complication
792.3	Nonspecific abnormal finding in amniotic fluid
796.5	Abnormal finding on antenatal screening
V28.0	Screening for chromosomal anomalies by amniocentesis
V28.1	Screening for raised alpha-fetoprotein levels in amniotic fluid
V28.2	Other antenatal screening based on amniocentesis
V61.6	Illegitimacy or illegitimate pregnancy

DRG 998 Principal Diagnosis Invalid as Discharge Diagnosis
GMLOS 0.0   AMLOS 0.0   RW 0.0000

Note: If there is no value in either the GMLOS or the AMLOS, the volume of cases for this DRG is insufficient to determine a meaningful computation of these statistics.

Principal diagnoses listed for MDC 14 considered invalid as discharge diagnosis

641.00	Placenta previa without hemorrhage, unspecified as to episode of care
641.10	Hemorrhage from placenta previa, unspecified as to episode of care
641.20	Premature separation of placenta, unspecified as to episode of care
641.30	Antepartum hemorrhage associated with coagulation defects, unspecified as to episode of care
641.80	Other antepartum hemorrhage, unspecified as to episode of care
641.90	Unspecified antepartum hemorrhage, unspecified as to episode of care
642.00	Benign essential hypertension complicating pregnancy, childbirth, and the puerperium, unspecified as to episode of care
642.10	Hypertension secondary to renal disease, complicating pregnancy, childbirth, and the puerperium, unspecified as to episode of care
642.20	Other pre-existing hypertension complicating pregnancy, childbirth, and the puerperium, unspecified as to episode of care
642.30	Transient hypertension of pregnancy, unspecified as to episode of care
642.40	Mild or unspecified pre-eclampsia, unspecified as to episode of care
642.50	Severe pre-eclampsia, unspecified as to episode of care
642.60	Eclampsia complicating pregnancy, childbirth or the puerperium, unspecified as to episode of care
642.70	Pre-eclampsia or eclampsia superimposed on pre-existing hypertension, complicating pregnancy, childbirth, or the puerperium, unspecified as to episode of care
642.90	Unspecified hypertension complicating pregnancy, childbirth, or the puerperium, unspecified as to episode of care
643.00	Mild hyperemesis gravidarum, unspecified as to episode of care
643.10	Hyperemesis gravidarum with metabolic disturbance, unspecified as to episode of care
643.20	Late vomiting of pregnancy, unspecified as to episode of care
643.80	Other vomiting complicating pregnancy, unspecified as to episode of care
643.90	Unspecified vomiting of pregnancy, unspecified as to episode of care
645.10	Post term pregnancy, unspecified as to episode of care or not applicable
645.20	Prolonged pregnancy, unspecified as to episode of care or not applicable
646.10	Edema or excessive weight gain in pregnancy, unspecified as to episode of care
646.20	Unspecified renal disease in pregnancy, unspecified as to episode of care
646.30	Pregnancy complication, recurrent pregnancy loss, unspecified as to episode of care
646.40	Peripheral neuritis in pregnancy, unspecified as to episode of care
646.50	Asymptomatic bacteriuria in pregnancy, unspecified as to episode of care
646.60	Infections of genitourinary tract in pregnancy, unspecified as to episode of care
646.70	Liver and biliary tract disorders in pregnancy, unspecified as to episode of care or not applicable
646.80	Other specified complication of pregnancy, unspecified as to episode of care
646.90	Unspecified complication of pregnancy, unspecified as to episode of care
647.00	Maternal syphilis, complicating pregnancy, childbirth, or the puerperium, unspecified as to episode of care
647.10	Maternal gonorrhea complicating pregnancy, childbirth, or the puerperium, unspecified as to episode of care
647.20	Other maternal venereal diseases, complicating pregnancy, childbirth, or the puerperium, unspecified as to episode of care
647.30	Maternal tuberculosis complicating pregnancy, childbirth, or the puerperium, unspecified as to episode of care
647.40	Maternal malaria complicating pregnancy, childbirth or the puerperium, unspecified as to episode of care
647.50	Maternal rubella complicating pregnancy, childbirth, or the puerperium, unspecified as to episode of care
647.60	Other maternal viral disease complicating pregnancy, childbirth, or the puerperium, unspecified as to episode of care
647.80	Other specified maternal infectious and parasitic disease complicating pregnancy, childbirth, or the puerperium, unspecified as to episode of care
647.90	Unspecified maternal infection or infestation complicating pregnancy, childbirth, or the puerperium, unspecified as to episode of care
648.00	Maternal diabetes mellitus, complicating pregnancy, childbirth, or the puerperium, unspecified as to episode of care
648.10	Maternal thyroid dysfunction complicating pregnancy, childbirth, or the puerperium, unspecified as to episode of care or not applicable
648.20	Maternal anemia of mother, complicating pregnancy, childbirth, or the puerperium, unspecified as to episode of care
648.30	Maternal drug dependence complicating pregnancy, childbirth, or the puerperium, unspecified as to episode of care
648.40	Maternal mental disorders, complicating pregnancy, childbirth, or the puerperium, unspecified as to episode of care
648.50	Maternal congenital cardiovascular disorders, complicating pregnancy, childbirth, or the puerperium, unspecified as to episode of care
648.60	Other maternal cardiovascular diseases complicating pregnancy, childbirth, or the puerperium, unspecified as to episode of care
648.70	Bone and joint disorders of maternal back, pelvis, and lower limbs, complicating pregnancy, childbirth, or the puerperium, unspecified as to episode of care
648.80	Abnormal maternal glucose tolerance, complicating pregnancy, childbirth, or the puerperium, unspecified as to episode of care
648.90	Other current maternal conditions classifiable elsewhere, complicating pregnancy, childbirth, or the puerperium, unspecified as to episode of care
649.00	Tobacco use disorder complicating pregnancy, childbirth, or the puerperium, unspecified as to episode of care or not applicable

Surgical		*Medical*		CC Indicator		MCC Indicator		Procedure Proxy

649.10	Obesity complicating pregnancy, childbirth, or the puerperium, unspecified as to episode of care or not applicable	653.90	Unspecified fetal disproportion, unspecified as to episode of care
649.20	Bariatric surgery status complicating pregnancy, childbirth, or the puerperium, unspecified as to episode of care or not applicable	654.00	Congenital abnormalities of pregnant uterus, unspecified as to episode of care
649.30	Coagulation defects complicating pregnancy, childbirth, or the puerperium, unspecified as to episode of care or not applicable	654.10	Tumors of body of pregnant uterus, unspecified as to episode of care in pregnancy
		654.20	Previous cesarean delivery, unspecified as to episode of care or not applicable
649.40	Epilepsy complicating pregnancy, childbirth, or the puerperium, unspecified as to episode of care or not applicable	654.30	Retroverted and incarcerated gravid uterus, unspecified as to episode of care
		654.40	Other abnormalities in shape or position of gravid uterus and of neighboring structures, unspecified as to episode of care
649.50	Spotting complicating pregnancy, unspecified as to episode of care or not applicable		
649.60	Uterine size date discrepancy, unspecified as to episode of care or not applicable	654.50	Cervical incompetence, unspecified as to episode of care in pregnancy
649.70	Cervical shortening, unspecified as to episode of care or not applicable	654.60	Other congenital or acquired abnormality of cervix, unspecified as to episode of care in pregnancy
651.00	Twin pregnancy, unspecified as to episode of care	654.70	Congenital or acquired abnormality of vagina, unspecified as to episode of care in pregnancy
651.10	Triplet pregnancy, unspecified as to episode of care		
651.20	Quadruplet pregnancy, unspecified as to episode of care	654.80	Congenital or acquired abnormality of vulva, unspecified as to episode of care in pregnancy
651.30	Twin pregnancy with fetal loss and retention of one fetus, unspecified as to episode of care or not applicable	654.90	Other and unspecified abnormality of organs and soft tissues of pelvis, unspecified as to episode of care in pregnancy
651.40	Triplet pregnancy with fetal loss and retention of one or more, unspecified as to episode of care or not applicable	655.00	Central nervous system malformation in fetus, unspecified as to episode of care in pregnancy
651.50	Quadruplet pregnancy with fetal loss and retention of one or more, unspecified as to episode of care or not applicable	655.10	Chromosomal abnormality in fetus, affecting management of mother, unspecified as to episode of care in pregnancy
651.60	Other multiple pregnancy with fetal loss and retention of one or more fetus(es), unspecified as to episode of care or not applicable	655.20	Hereditary disease in family possibly affecting fetus, affecting management of mother, unspecified as to episode of care in pregnancy
651.70	Multiple gestation following (elective) fetal reduction, unspecified as to episode of care or not applicable	655.30	Suspected damage to fetus from viral disease in mother, affecting management of mother, unspecified as to episode of care in pregnancy
651.80	Other specified multiple gestation, unspecified as to episode of care		
651.90	Unspecified multiple gestation, unspecified as to episode of care	655.40	Suspected damage to fetus from other disease in mother, affecting management of mother, unspecified as to episode of care in pregnancy
652.00	Unstable lie of fetus, unspecified as to episode of care	655.50	Suspected damage to fetus from drugs, affecting management of mother, unspecified as to episode of care
652.10	Breech or other malpresentation successfully converted to cephalic presentation, unspecified as to episode of care	655.60	Suspected damage to fetus from radiation, affecting management of mother, unspecified as to episode of care
652.20	Breech presentation without mention of version, unspecified as to episode of care	655.70	Decreased fetal movements, unspecified as to episode of care
652.30	Transverse or oblique fetal presentation, unspecified as to episode of care	655.80	Other known or suspected fetal abnormality, not elsewhere classified, affecting management of mother, unspecified as to episode of care
652.40	Fetal face or brow presentation, unspecified as to episode of care		
652.50	High fetal head at term, unspecified as to episode of care	655.90	Unspecified fetal abnormality affecting management of mother, unspecified as to episode of care
652.60	Multiple gestation with malpresentation of one fetus or more, unspecified as to episode of care	656.00	Fetal-maternal hemorrhage, unspecified as to episode of care in pregnancy
652.70	Prolapsed arm of fetus, unspecified as to episode of care	656.10	Rhesus isoimmunization unspecified as to episode of care in pregnancy
652.80	Other specified malposition or malpresentation of fetus, unspecified as to episode of care	656.20	Isoimmunization from other and unspecified blood-group incompatibility, unspecified as to episode of care in pregnancy
652.90	Unspecified malposition or malpresentation of fetus, unspecified as to episode of care		
653.00	Major abnormality of bony pelvis, not further specified in pregnancy, unspecified as to episode of care	656.50	Poor fetal growth, affecting management of mother, unspecified as to episode of care
653.10	Generally contracted pelvis in pregnancy, unspecified as to episode of care in pregnancy	656.60	Excessive fetal growth affecting management of mother, unspecified as to episode of care
653.20	Inlet contraction of pelvis in pregnancy, unspecified as to episode of care in pregnancy	656.70	Other placental conditions affecting management of mother, unspecified as to episode of care
653.30	Outlet contraction of pelvis in pregnancy, unspecified as to episode of care in pregnancy	656.80	Other specified fetal and placental problems affecting management of mother, unspecified as to episode of care
653.40	Fetopelvic disproportion, unspecified as to episode of care	656.90	Unspecified fetal and placental problem affecting management of mother, unspecified as to episode of care
653.50	Unusually large fetus causing disproportion, unspecified as to episode of care	657.00	Polyhydramnios, unspecified as to episode of care
653.60	Hydrocephalic fetus causing disproportion, unspecified as to episode of care	658.00	Oligohydramnios, unspecified as to episode of care
653.70	Other fetal abnormality causing disproportion, unspecified as to episode of care	658.80	Other problem associated with amniotic cavity and membranes, unspecified as to episode of care
653.80	Fetal disproportion of other origin, unspecified as to episode of care		

658.90	Unspecified problem associated with amniotic cavity and membranes, unspecified as to episode of care
659.40	Grand multiparity with current pregnancy, unspecified as to episode of care
666.00	Third-stage postpartum hemorrhage, unspecified as to episode of care
666.10	Other immediate postpartum hemorrhage, unspecified as to episode of care
666.20	Delayed and secondary postpartum hemorrhage, unspecified as to episode of care
666.30	Postpartum coagulation defects, unspecified as to episode of care
667.00	Retained placenta without hemorrhage, unspecified as to episode of care
667.10	Retained portions of placenta or membranes, without hemorrhage, unspecified as to episode of care
670.00	Major puerperal infection, unspecified, unspecified as to episode of care or not applicable
670.10	Puerperal endometritis, unspecified as to episode of care or not applicable
670.20	Puerperal sepsis, unspecified as to episode of care or not applicable
670.30	Puerperal septic thrombophlebitis, unspecified as to episode of care or not applicable
670.80	Other major puerperal infection, unspecified as to episode of care or not applicable
671.00	Varicose veins of legs complicating pregnancy and the puerperium, unspecified as to episode of care
671.10	Varicose veins of vulva and perineum complicating pregnancy and the puerperium, unspecified as to episode of care
671.20	Superficial thrombophlebitis complicating pregnancy and the puerperium, unspecified as to episode of care
671.30	Deep phlebothrombosis, antepartum, unspecified as to episode of care
671.40	Deep phlebothrombosis, postpartum, unspecified as to episode of care
671.50	Other phlebitis and thrombosis complicating pregnancy and the puerperium, unspecified as to episode of care
671.80	Other venous complication of pregnancy and the puerperium, unspecified as to episode of care
671.90	Unspecified venous complication of pregnancy and the puerperium, unspecified as to episode of care
672.00	Puerperal pyrexia of unknown origin, unspecified as to episode of care
673.00	Obstetrical air embolism, unspecified as to episode of care
673.10	Amniotic fluid embolism, unspecified as to episode of care
673.20	Obstetrical blood-clot embolism, unspecified as to episode of care
673.30	Obstetrical pyemic and septic embolism, unspecified as to episode of care
673.80	Other obstetrical pulmonary embolism, unspecified as to episode of care
674.00	Cerebrovascular disorder occurring in pregnancy, childbirth, or the puerperium, unspecified as to episode of care
674.10	Disruption of cesarean wound, unspecified as to episode of care
674.20	Disruption of perineal wound, unspecified as to episode of care in pregnancy
674.30	Other complication of obstetrical surgical wounds, unspecified as to episode of care
674.40	Placental polyp, unspecified as to episode of care
674.50	Peripartum cardiomyopathy, unspecified as to episode of care or not applicable
674.80	Other complication of puerperium, unspecified as to episode of care
674.90	Unspecified complications of puerperium, unspecified as to episode of care
675.00	Infection of nipple associated with childbirth, unspecified as to episode of care
675.10	Abscess of breast associated with childbirth, unspecified as to episode of care
675.20	Nonpurulent mastitis, unspecified as to episode of prenatal or postnatal care
675.80	Other specified infection of the breast and nipple associated with childbirth, unspecified as to episode of care
675.90	Unspecified infection of the breast and nipple, unspecified as to prenatal or postnatal episode of care
676.00	Retracted nipple, unspecified as to prenatal or postnatal episode of care
676.10	Cracked nipple, unspecified as to prenatal or postnatal episode of care
676.20	Engorgement of breasts, unspecified as to prenatal or postnatal episode of care
676.30	Other and unspecified disorder of breast associated with childbirth, unspecified as to episode of care
676.40	Failure of lactation, unspecified as to episode of care
676.50	Suppressed lactation, unspecified as to episode of care
676.60	Galactorrhea associated with childbirth, unspecified as to episode of care
676.80	Other disorder of lactation, unspecified as to episode of care
676.90	Unspecified disorder of lactation, unspecified as to episode of care
677	Late effect of complication of pregnancy, childbirth, and the puerperium
678.00	Fetal hematologic conditions, unspecified as to episode of care or not applicable
678.10	Fetal conjoined twins, unspecified as to episode of care or not applicable
679.10	Fetal complications from in utero procedure, unspecified as to episode of care or not applicable
V23.0	Pregnancy with history of infertility
V23.1	Pregnancy with history of trophoblastic disease
V23.2	Pregnancy with history of abortion
V23.3	Pregnancy with grand multiparity
V23.4*	Pregnancy with other poor obstetric history
V23.5	Pregnancy with other poor reproductive history
V23.7	Insufficient prenatal care
V23.8*	Supervision of other high-risk pregnancy
V23.9	Unspecified high-risk pregnancy

Surgical   **Medical**   **CC Indicator**   **MCC Indicator**   **Procedure Proxy**

277.01	762.2	764.14	765.10	768.1	770.9	774.31	777.8	V32.00
747.83	762.3	764.15	765.11	768.2	771.0	774.39	777.9	V32.01
760.0	762.4	764.16	765.12	768.3	771.1	774.4	778.0	V32.1
760.1	762.5	764.17	765.13	768.4	771.2	774.5	778.1	V32.2
760.2	762.6	764.18	765.14	768.5	771.3	774.6	778.2	V33.00
760.3	762.7	764.19	765.15	768.6	771.4	774.7	778.3	V33.01
760.4	762.8	764.20	765.16	768.70	771.5	775.0	778.4	V33.1
760.5	762.9	764.21	765.17	768.71	771.6	775.1	778.5	V33.2
760.61	763.0	764.22	765.18	768.72	771.7	775.2	778.6	V34.00
760.62	763.1	764.23	765.19	768.73	771.81	775.3	778.7	V34.01
760.63	763.2	764.24	765.20	768.9	771.82	775.4	778.8	V34.1
760.64	763.3	764.25	765.21	769	771.83	775.5	778.9	V34.2
760.70	763.4	764.26	765.22	770.0	771.89	775.6	779.0	V35.00
760.71	763.5	764.27	765.23	770.10	772.0	775.7	779.1	V35.01
760.72	763.6	764.28	765.24	770.11	772.10	775.81	779.2	V35.1
760.73	763.7	764.29	765.25	770.12	772.11	775.89	779.31	V35.2
760.74	763.81	764.90	765.26	770.13	772.12	775.9	779.32	V36.00
760.75	763.82	764.91	765.27	770.14	772.13	776.0	779.33	V36.01
760.76	763.83	764.92	765.28	770.15	772.14	776.1	779.4	V36.1
760.77	763.84	764.93	765.29	770.16	772.2	776.2	779.5	V36.2
760.78	763.89	764.94	766.0	770.17	772.3	776.3	779.6	V37.00
760.79	763.9	764.95	766.1	770.18	772.4	776.4	779.81	V37.01
760.8	764.00	764.96	766.21	770.2	772.5	776.5	779.82	V37.1
760.9	764.01	764.97	766.22	770.3	772.6	776.6	779.83	V37.2
761.0	764.02	764.98	767.0	770.4	772.8	776.7	779.84	V39.00
761.1	764.03	764.99	767.11	770.5	772.9	776.8	779.85	V39.01
761.2	764.04	765.00	767.19	770.6	773.0	776.9	779.89	V39.1
761.3	764.05	765.01	767.2	770.81	773.1	777.1	779.9	V39.2
761.4	764.06	765.02	767.3	770.82	773.2	777.2	V30.00	
761.5	764.07	765.03	767.4	770.83	773.3	777.3	V30.01	
761.6	764.08	765.04	767.5	770.84	773.4	777.4	V30.1	
761.7	764.09	765.05	767.6	770.85	773.5	777.50	V30.2	
761.8	764.10	765.06	767.7	770.86	774.0	777.51	V31.00	
761.9	764.11	765.07	767.8	770.87	774.1	777.52	V31.01	
762.0	764.12	765.08	767.9	770.88	774.2	777.53	V31.1	
762.1	764.13	765.09	768.0	770.89	774.30	777.6	V31.2	

MEDICAL

DRG 789 Neonates, Died or Transferred to Another Acute Care Facility
GMLOS 1.8   **AMLOS 1.8**   **RW 1.5258**

Discharge status of transfer to an acute care facility or expired

DRG 790 Extreme Immaturity or Respiratory Distress Syndrome, Neonate
GMLOS 17.9   **AMLOS 17.9**   **RW 5.0315**

Principal or Secondary Diagnosis
765.01	Extreme fetal immaturity, less than 500 grams
765.02	Extreme fetal immaturity, 500-749 grams
765.03	Extreme fetal immaturity, 750-999 grams
765.04	Extreme fetal immaturity, 1,000-1,249 grams
765.05	Extreme fetal immaturity, 1,250-1,499 grams
765.21	Less than 24 completed weeks of gestation
765.22	24 completed weeks of gestation
765.23	25-26 completed weeks of gestation
769	Respiratory distress syndrome in newborn

DRG 791 Prematurity with Major Problems
GMLOS 13.3   **AMLOS 13.3**   **RW 3.4363**   ☑

Principal or Secondary Diagnosis of Prematurity
765.00	Extreme fetal immaturity, unspecified (weight)
765.06	Extreme fetal immaturity, 1,500-1,749 grams
765.07	Extreme fetal immaturity, 1,750-1,999 grams
765.08	Extreme fetal immaturity, 2,000-2,499 grams
765.1*	Other preterm infants
765.24	27-28 completed weeks of gestation
765.25	29-30 completed weeks of gestation
765.26	31-32 completed weeks of gestation
765.27	33-34 completed weeks of gestation
765.28	35-36 completed weeks of gestation

AND

Principal or Secondary Diagnosis of Major Problem
277.01	Cystic fibrosis with meconium ileus
747.83	Persistent fetal circulation
763.4	Fetus or newborn affected by cesarean delivery
764.11	Light-for-dates with signs of fetal malnutrition, less than 500 grams
764.12	Light-for-dates with signs of fetal malnutrition, 500-749 grams
764.13	Light-for-dates with signs of fetal malnutrition, 750-999 grams
764.14	Light-for-dates with signs of fetal malnutrition, 1,000-1,249 grams
764.15	Light-for-dates with signs of fetal malnutrition, 1,250-1,499 grams
764.16	Light-for-dates with signs of fetal malnutrition, 1,500-1,749 grams
764.17	Light-for-dates with signs of fetal malnutrition, 1,750-1,999 grams
764.18	Light-for-dates with signs of fetal malnutrition, 2,000-2,499 grams
764.21	Fetal malnutrition without mention of "light-for-dates", less than 500 grams
764.22	Fetal malnutrition without mention of "light-for-dates", 500-749 grams
764.23	Fetal malnutrition without mention of "light-for-dates", 750-999 grams
764.24	Fetal malnutrition without mention of "light-for-dates", 1,000-1,249 grams
764.25	Fetal malnutrition without mention of "light-for-dates", 1,250-1,499 grams
764.26	Fetal malnutrition without mention of "light-for-dates", 1,500-1,749 grams
764.27	Fetal malnutrition without mention of "light-for-dates", 1,750-1,999 grams
764.28	Fetal malnutrition without mention of "light-for-dates", 2,000-2,499 grams
767.0	Subdural and cerebral hemorrhage, birth trauma
767.11	Birth trauma, epicranial subaponeurotic hemorrhage (massive)
767.4	Injury to spine and spinal cord, birth trauma
767.7	Other cranial and peripheral nerve injuries, birth trauma
768.5	Severe birth asphyxia
768.72	Moderate hypoxic-ischemic encephalopathy
768.73	Severe hypoxic-ischemic encephalopathy
770.0	Congenital pneumonia
770.1*	Fetal and newborn aspiration
770.2	Interstitial emphysema and related conditions of newborn
770.3	Pulmonary hemorrhage of fetus or newborn
770.4	Primary atelectasis of newborn
770.84	Respiratory failure of newborn
770.85	Aspiration of postnatal stomach contents without respiratory symptoms
770.86	Aspiration of postnatal stomach contents with respiratory symptoms
771.0	Congenital rubella
771.1	Congenital cytomegalovirus infection
771.2	Other congenital infection specific to the perinatal period
771.4	Omphalitis of the newborn
771.5	Neonatal infective mastitis
771.8*	Other infection specific to the perinatal period
772.0	Fetal blood loss affecting newborn
772.1*	Intraventricular hemorrhage
772.2	Fetal and neonatal subarachnoid hemorrhage of newborn
772.4	Fetal and neonatal gastrointestinal hemorrhage
772.5	Fetal and neonatal adrenal hemorrhage
773.2	Hemolytic disease due to other and unspecified isoimmunization of fetus or newborn
773.3	Hydrops fetalis due to isoimmunization
773.4	Kernicterus due to isoimmunization of fetus or newborn
773.5	Late anemia due to isoimmunization of fetus or newborn
774.4	Perinatal jaundice due to hepatocellular damage
774.7	Kernicterus of fetus or newborn not due to isoimmunization
775.1	Neonatal diabetes mellitus
775.2	Neonatal myasthenia gravis
775.3	Neonatal thyrotoxicosis
775.4	Hypocalcemia and hypomagnesemia of newborn
775.5	Other transitory neonatal electrolyte disturbances
775.6	Neonatal hypoglycemia
775.7	Late metabolic acidosis of newborn
776.0	Hemorrhagic disease of newborn
776.1	Transient neonatal thrombocytopenia
776.2	Disseminated intravascular coagulation in newborn
776.3	Other transient neonatal disorders of coagulation
776.6	Anemia of neonatal prematurity
777.1	Fetal and newborn meconium obstruction
777.2	Neonatal intestinal obstruction due to inspissated milk
777.5*	Necrotizing enterocolitis in newborn
777.6	Perinatal intestinal perforation
778.0	Hydrops fetalis not due to isoimmunization
779.0	Convulsions in newborn
779.1	Other and unspecified cerebral irritability in newborn
779.2	Cerebral depression, coma, and other abnormal cerebral signs in fetus or newborn
779.32	Bilious vomiting in newborn
779.4	Drug reactions and intoxications specific to newborn
779.5	Drug withdrawal syndrome in newborn
779.85	Cardiac arrest of newborn

MDC 15: Newborns And Other Neonates With Conditions Originating In The Perinatal Period

OR

Secondary Diagnosis of Major Problem

036.3	Waterhouse-Friderichsen syndrome, meningococcal
036.4*	Meningococcal carditis
036.81	Meningococcal optic neuritis
036.82	Meningococcal arthropathy
037	Tetanus
038*	Septicemia
040.0	Gas gangrene
040.41	Infant botulism
046.2	Subacute sclerosing panencephalitis
052.0	Postvaricella encephalitis
052.1	Varicella (hemorrhagic) pneumonitis
052.7	Chickenpox with other specified complications
052.8	Chickenpox with unspecified complication
052.9	Varicella without mention of complication
053.0	Herpes zoster with meningitis
053.10	Herpes zoster with unspecified nervous system complication
053.11	Geniculate herpes zoster
053.12	Postherpetic trigeminal neuralgia
053.13	Postherpetic polyneuropathy
053.19	Other herpes zoster with nervous system complications
053.20	Herpes zoster dermatitis of eyelid
053.21	Herpes zoster keratoconjunctivitis
053.22	Herpes zoster iridocyclitis
053.29	Other ophthalmic herpes zoster complications
053.71	Otitis externa due to herpes zoster
053.79	Other specified herpes zoster complications
053.8	Unspecified herpes zoster complication
053.9	Herpes zoster without mention of complication
054.0	Eczema herpeticum
054.2	Herpetic gingivostomatitis
054.3	Herpetic meningoencephalitis
054.4*	Herpes simplex with ophthalmic complications
054.5	Herpetic septicemia
054.71	Visceral herpes simplex
054.72	Herpes simplex meningitis
054.73	Herpes simplex otitis externa
054.79	Other specified herpes simplex complications
054.8	Unspecified herpes simplex complication
055.0	Postmeasles encephalitis
055.1	Postmeasles pneumonia
055.2	Postmeasles otitis media
055.7*	Measles, with other specified complications
055.8	Unspecified measles complication
056.0*	Rubella with neurological complications
056.7*	Rubella with other specified complications
056.8	Unspecified rubella complications
058.10	Roseola infantum, unspecified
058.11	Roseola infantum due to human herpesvirus 6
058.12	Roseola infantum due to human herpesvirus 7
058.21	Human herpesvirus 6 encephalitis
058.29	Other human herpesvirus encephalitis
070.2*	Viral hepatitis B with hepatic coma
070.3*	Viral hepatitis B without mention of hepatic coma
070.4*	Other specified viral hepatitis with hepatic coma
070.5*	Other specified viral hepatitis without mention of hepatic coma
070.6	Unspecified viral hepatitis with hepatic coma
070.9	Unspecified viral hepatitis without mention of hepatic coma
072.0	Mumps orchitis
072.1	Mumps meningitis
072.2	Mumps encephalitis
072.3	Mumps pancreatitis
072.7*	Mumps with other specified complications
072.8	Unspecified mumps complication
079.6	Respiratory syncytial virus (RSV)
112.4	Candidiasis of lung
112.5	Disseminated candidiasis
112.81	Candidal endocarditis
112.82	Candidal otitis externa
112.83	Candidal meningitis
112.84	Candidiasis of the esophagus
112.85	Candidiasis of the intestine
114.2	Coccidioidal meningitis
114.3	Other forms of progressive coccidioidomycosis
115.01	Histoplasma capsulatum meningitis
115.02	Histoplasma capsulatum retinitis
115.03	Histoplasma capsulatum pericarditis
115.04	Histoplasma capsulatum endocarditis
115.05	Histoplasma capsulatum pneumonia
115.11	Histoplasma duboisii meningitis
115.12	Histoplasma duboisii retinitis
115.13	Histoplasma duboisii pericarditis
115.14	Histoplasma duboisii endocarditis
115.15	Histoplasma duboisii pneumonia
115.91	Unspecified Histoplasmosis meningitis
115.92	Unspecified Histoplasmosis retinitis
115.93	Unspecified Histoplasmosis pericarditis
115.94	Unspecified Histoplasmosis endocarditis
115.95	Unspecified Histoplasmosis pneumonia
116.0	Blastomycosis
116.1	Paracoccidioidomycosis
117.3	Aspergillosis
117.4	Mycotic mycetomas
117.5	Cryptococcosis
117.6	Allescheriosis (Petriellidiosis)
117.7	Zygomycosis (Phycomycosis or Mucormycosis)
118	Opportunistic mycoses
130.0	Meningoencephalitis due to toxoplasmosis
130.1	Conjunctivitis due to toxoplasmosis
130.2	Chorioretinitis due to toxoplasmosis
130.3	Myocarditis due to toxoplasmosis
130.4	Pneumonitis due to toxoplasmosis
130.5	Hepatitis due to toxoplasmosis
130.7	Toxoplasmosis of other specified sites
130.8	Multisystemic disseminated toxoplasmosis
136.3	Pneumocystosis
251.0	Hypoglycemic coma
252.1	Hypoparathyroidism
253.5	Diabetes insipidus
254.1	Abscess of thymus
261	Nutritional marasmus
262	Other severe protein-calorie malnutrition
263.0	Malnutrition of moderate degree
263.1	Malnutrition of mild degree
263.8	Other protein-calorie malnutrition
263.9	Unspecified protein-calorie malnutrition
276*	Disorders of fluid, electrolyte, and acid-base balance
277.88	Tumor lysis syndrome
282.40	Thalassemia, unspecified
282.41	Sickle-cell thalassemia without crisis
282.42	Sickle-cell thalassemia with crisis
282.43	Alpha thalassemia
282.44	Beta thalassemia
282.45	Delta-beta thalassemia
282.47	Hemoglobin E-beta thalassemia
282.49	Other thalassemia
283.1*	Non-autoimmune hemolytic anemias
283.2	Hemoglobinuria due to hemolysis from external causes
283.9	Acquired hemolytic anemia, unspecified
285.1	Acute posthemorrhagic anemia
286.6	Defibrination syndrome
287.4*	Secondary thrombocytopenia
289.84	Heparin-induced thrombocytopenia [HIT]
292.0	Drug withdrawal
320*	Bacterial meningitis
321*	Meningitis due to other organisms
322.0	Nonpyogenic meningitis

T Transfer DRG   SP Special Payment   ☑ Optimization Potential   ▽ Targeted Potential   * Code Range   ● New DRG   ▲ Revised DRG Title

164   Valid 10/01/2013-09/30/2014   © 2013 OptumInsight, Inc.

322.1	Eosinophilic meningitis
322.9	Unspecified meningitis
324*	Intracranial and intraspinal abscess
348.1	Anoxic brain damage
349.0	Reaction to spinal or lumbar puncture
349.1	Nervous system complications from surgically implanted device
349.3*	Dural tear
349.81	Cerebrospinal fluid rhinorrhea
349.82	Toxic encephalopathy
377.00	Unspecified papilledema
377.01	Papilledema associated with increased intracranial pressure
377.02	Papilledema associated with decreased ocular pressure
383.01	Subperiosteal abscess of mastoid
383.81	Postauricular fistula
398.91	Rheumatic heart failure (congestive)
402.01	Malignant hypertensive heart disease with heart failure
402.11	Benign hypertensive heart disease with heart failure
402.91	Hypertensive heart disease, unspecified, with heart failure
404.01	Hypertensive heart and chronic kidney disease, malignant, with heart failure and with chronic kidney disease stage I through stage IV, or unspecified
404.03	Hypertensive heart and chronic kidney disease, malignant, with heart failure and with chronic kidney disease stage V or end stage renal disease
404.11	Hypertensive heart and chronic kidney disease, benign, with heart failure and with chronic kidney disease stage I through stage IV, or unspecified
404.13	Hypertensive heart and chronic kidney disease, benign, with heart failure and chronic kidney disease stage V or end stage renal disease
404.91	Hypertensive heart and chronic kidney disease, unspecified, with heart failure and with chronic kidney disease stage I through stage IV, or unspecified
404.93	Hypertensive heart and chronic kidney disease, unspecified, with heart failure and chronic kidney disease stage V or end stage renal disease
414.10	Aneurysm of heart
415*	Acute pulmonary heart disease
416.2	Chronic pulmonary embolism
420.0	Acute pericarditis in diseases classified elsewhere
421*	Acute and subacute endocarditis
422.0	Acute myocarditis in diseases classified elsewhere
422.92	Septic myocarditis
423.0	Hemopericardium
424.9*	Endocarditis, valve unspecified
425.8	Cardiomyopathy in other diseases classified elsewhere
426.0	Atrioventricular block, complete
426.53	Other bilateral bundle branch block
426.54	Trifascicular block
426.7	Anomalous atrioventricular excitation
426.89	Other specified conduction disorder
427.1	Paroxysmal ventricular tachycardia
427.3*	Atrial fibrillation and flutter
427.4*	Ventricular fibrillation and flutter
427.5	Cardiac arrest
428.0	Congestive heart failure, unspecified
428.1	Left heart failure
428.2*	Systolic heart failure
428.3*	Diastolic heart failure
428.4*	Combined systolic and diastolic heart failure
428.9	Unspecified heart failure
429.4	Functional disturbances following cardiac surgery
429.81	Other disorders of papillary muscle
429.82	Hyperkinetic heart disease
430	Subarachnoid hemorrhage
431	Intracerebral hemorrhage
432*	Other and unspecified intracranial hemorrhage
433.01	Occlusion and stenosis of basilar artery with cerebral infarction
433.11	Occlusion and stenosis of carotid artery with cerebral infarction
433.21	Occlusion and stenosis of vertebral artery with cerebral infarction
433.31	Occlusion and stenosis of multiple and bilateral precerebral arteries with cerebral infarction
433.81	Occlusion and stenosis of other specified precerebral artery with cerebral infarction
433.91	Occlusion and stenosis of unspecified precerebral artery with cerebral infarction
434*	Occlusion of cerebral arteries
436	Acute, but ill-defined, cerebrovascular disease
440.24	Atherosclerosis of native arteries of the extremities with gangrene
444*	Arterial embolism and thrombosis
449	Septic arterial embolism
451.1*	Phlebitis and thrombophlebitis of deep veins of lower extremities
451.2	Phlebitis and thrombophlebitis of lower extremities, unspecified
451.81	Phlebitis and thrombophlebitis of iliac vein
453.2	Other venous embolism and thrombosis, of inferior vena cava
457.2	Lymphangitis
459.0	Unspecified hemorrhage
478.22	Parapharyngeal abscess
478.24	Retropharyngeal abscess
478.3*	Paralysis of vocal cords or larynx
478.75	Laryngeal spasm
481	Pneumococcal pneumonia (streptococcus pneumoniae pneumonia)
482*	Other bacterial pneumonia
483*	Pneumonia due to other specified organism
485	Bronchopneumonia, organism unspecified
486	Pneumonia, organism unspecified
488.01	Influenza due to identified avian influenza virus with pneumonia
488.02	Influenza due to identified avian influenza virus with other respiratory manifestations
488.11	Influenza due to identified 2009 H1N1 influenza virus with pneumonia
488.12	Influenza due to identified 2009 H1N1 influenza virus with other respiratory manifestations
488.81	Influenza due to identified novel influenza A virus with pneumonia
488.82	Influenza due to identified novel influenza A virus with other respiratory manifestations
493.01	Extrinsic asthma with status asthmaticus
493.11	Intrinsic asthma with status asthmaticus
493.91	Asthma, unspecified with status asthmaticus
507.0	Pneumonitis due to inhalation of food or vomitus
507.8	Pneumonitis due to other solids and liquids
508.0	Acute pulmonary manifestations due to radiation
510*	Empyema
511.1	Pleurisy with effusion, with mention of bacterial cause other than tuberculosis
511.89	Other specified forms of effusion, except tuberculous
511.9	Unspecified pleural effusion
513*	Abscess of lung and mediastinum
516.6*	Interstitial lung diseases of childhood
518.0	Pulmonary collapse
518.1	Interstitial emphysema
518.4	Unspecified acute edema of lung
518.52	Other pulmonary insufficiency, not elsewhere classified, following trauma and surgery
519.2	Mediastinitis
530.4	Perforation of esophagus
530.84	Tracheoesophageal fistula
536.1	Acute dilatation of stomach

Surgical	Medical	CC Indicator	MCC Indicator	Procedure Proxy

MDC 15: Newborns And Other Neonates With Conditions Originating In The Perinatal Period—MEDICAL

550.00	Inguinal hernia with gangrene, unilateral or unspecified, (not specified as recurrent)
550.02	Inguinal hernia with gangrene, bilateral
550.10	Inguinal hernia with obstruction, without mention of gangrene, unilateral or unspecified, (not specified as recurrent)
550.12	Inguinal hernia with obstruction, without mention gangrene, bilateral, (not specified as recurrent)
551.00	Femoral hernia with gangrene, unilateral or unspecified (not specified as recurrent)
551.02	Femoral hernia with gangrene, bilateral, (not specified as recurrent)
551.1	Umbilical hernia with gangrene
551.2*	Ventral hernia with gangrene
551.3	Diaphragmatic hernia with gangrene
551.8	Hernia of other specified sites, with gangrene
551.9	Hernia of unspecified site, with gangrene
552.00	Unilateral or unspecified femoral hernia with obstruction
552.02	Bilateral femoral hernia with obstruction
552.1	Umbilical hernia with obstruction
552.2*	Ventral hernia with obstruction
552.3	Diaphragmatic hernia with obstruction
552.8	Hernia of other specified site, with obstruction
552.9	Hernia of unspecified site, with obstruction
557.0	Acute vascular insufficiency of intestine
558.2	Toxic gastroenteritis and colitis
560.0	Intussusception
560.1	Paralytic ileus
560.2	Volvulus
560.30	Unspecified impaction of intestine
560.32	Fecal impaction
560.39	Impaction of intestine, other
560.89	Other specified intestinal obstruction
560.9	Unspecified intestinal obstruction
566	Abscess of anal and rectal regions
567*	Peritonitis and retroperitoneal infections
568.81	Hemoperitoneum (nontraumatic)
569.3	Hemorrhage of rectum and anus
569.7*	Complications of intestinal pouch
569.83	Perforation of intestine
570	Acute and subacute necrosis of liver
572.0	Abscess of liver
572.1	Portal pyemia
572.2	Hepatic encephalopathy
572.4	Hepatorenal syndrome
573.3	Unspecified hepatitis
573.4	Hepatic infarction
576.1	Cholangitis
577.0	Acute pancreatitis
577.2	Cyst and pseudocyst of pancreas
578*	Gastrointestinal hemorrhage
579.3	Other and unspecified postsurgical nonabsorption
580*	Acute glomerulonephritis
584*	Acute kidney failure
590.1*	Acute pyelonephritis
590.2	Renal and perinephric abscess
590.3	Pyeloureteritis cystica
590.8*	Other pyelonephritis or pyonephrosis, not specified as acute or chronic
590.9	Unspecified infection of kidney
591	Hydronephrosis
593.5	Hydroureter
595.0	Acute cystitis
595.4	Cystitis in diseases classified elsewhere
595.81	Cystitis cystica
595.89	Other specified types of cystitis
595.9	Unspecified cystitis
596.0	Bladder neck obstruction
596.1	Intestinovesical fistula
596.2	Vesical fistula, not elsewhere classified
596.4	Atony of bladder
596.6	Nontraumatic rupture of bladder
596.7	Hemorrhage into bladder wall
597.0	Urethral abscess
599.0	Urinary tract infection, site not specified
599.6*	Urinary obstruction
599.7*	Hematuria
619.1	Digestive-genital tract fistula, female
619.8	Other specified fistula involving female genital tract
620.7	Hematoma of broad ligament
682*	Other cellulitis and abscess
683	Acute lymphadenitis
693.0	Dermatitis due to drugs and medicines taken internally
695.0	Toxic erythema
708.0	Allergic urticaria
733.1*	Pathologic fracture
740*	Anencephalus and similar anomalies
741*	Spina bifida
742*	Other congenital anomalies of nervous system
745.4	Ventricular septal defect
756.72	Omphalocele
756.73	Gastroschisis
759.4	Conjoined twins
779.7	Periventricular leukomalacia
780.01	Coma
780.03	Persistent vegetative state
780.31	Febrile convulsions (simple), unspecified
780.39	Other convulsions
781.7	Tetany
785.0	Unspecified tachycardia
785.4	Gangrene
785.50	Unspecified shock
788.2*	Retention of urine
790.7	Bacteremia
791.1	Chyluria
799.1	Respiratory arrest
820*	Fracture of neck of femur
821.0*	Closed fracture of shaft or unspecified part of femur
821.1*	Open fracture of shaft or unspecified part of femur
860*	Traumatic pneumothorax and hemothorax
865*	Injury to spleen
900.0*	Injury to carotid artery
900.1	Internal jugular vein injury
900.81	External jugular vein injury
901.0	Thoracic aorta injury
901.1	Innominate and subclavian artery injury
901.2	Superior vena cava injury
901.3	Innominate and subclavian vein injury
901.41	Pulmonary artery injury
901.42	Pulmonary vein injury
902.0	Abdominal aorta injury
902.10	Unspecified inferior vena cava injury
953.4	Injury to brachial plexus
958.0	Air embolism as an early complication of trauma
958.1	Fat embolism as an early complication of trauma
958.2	Secondary and recurrent hemorrhage as an early complication of trauma
958.3	Posttraumatic wound infection not elsewhere classified
958.4	Traumatic shock
958.5	Traumatic anuria
958.7	Traumatic subcutaneous emphysema
995.20	Unspecified adverse effect of unspecified drug, medicinal and biological substance
995.21	Arthus phenomenon
995.22	Unspecified adverse effect of anesthesia
995.23	Unspecified adverse effect of insulin
995.27	Other drug allergy
995.29	Unspecified adverse effect of other drug, medicinal and biological substance
995.4	Shock due to anesthesia not elsewhere classified

Ⓣ *Transfer DRG*　　ⓈⓅ *Special Payment*　　☑ *Optimization Potential*　　▽ *Targeted Potential*　　* *Code Range*　　● *New DRG*　　▲ *Revised DRG Title*

997.0*	Nervous system complications
997.1	Cardiac complications
997.2	Peripheral vascular complications
997.3*	Respiratory complications
997.4*	Digestive system complications, not elsewhere classified
997.5	Urinary complications
997.71	Vascular complications of mesenteric artery
997.72	Vascular complications of renal artery
997.79	Vascular complications of other vessels
998.0*	Postoperative shock
998.11	Hemorrhage complicating a procedure
998.12	Hematoma complicating a procedure
998.13	Seroma complicating a procedure
998.2	Accidental puncture or laceration during procedure
998.4	Foreign body accidentally left during procedure, not elsewhere classified
998.51	Infected postoperative seroma
998.59	Other postoperative infection
998.6	Persistent postoperative fistula, not elsewhere classified
998.7	Acute reaction to foreign substance accidentally left during procedure, not elsewhere classified
998.9	Unspecified complication of procedure, not elsewhere classified
999.1	Air embolism as complication of medical care, not elsewhere classified
999.2	Other vascular complications of medical care, not elsewhere classified
999.34	Acute infection following transfusion, infusion, or injection of blood and blood products
999.39	Complications of medical care, NEC, infection following other infusion, injection, transfusion, or vaccination
999.4*	Anaphylactic reaction due to serum
999.5*	Other serum reaction, not elsewhere classified
999.6*	ABO incompatibility reaction due to transfusion of blood or blood products
999.7*	Rh and other non-ABO incompatibility reaction due to transfusion of blood or blood products
999.8*	Other and unspecified infusion and transfusion reaction

DRG 792   Prematurity without Major Problems
GMLOS 8.6   AMLOS 8.6   RW 2.0734   ☑

Principal or Secondary Diagnosis of Prematurity

765.00	Extreme fetal immaturity, unspecified (weight)
765.06	Extreme fetal immaturity, 1,500-1,749 grams
765.07	Extreme fetal immaturity, 1,750-1,999 grams
765.08	Extreme fetal immaturity, 2,000-2,499 grams
765.1*	Other preterm infants
765.24	27-28 completed weeks of gestation
765.25	29-30 completed weeks of gestation
765.26	31-32 completed weeks of gestation
765.27	33-34 completed weeks of gestation
765.28	35-36 completed weeks of gestation

DRG 793   Full Term Neonate with Major Problems
GMLOS 4.7   AMLOS 4.7   RW 3.5299   ☑

Principal or Secondary Diagnosis of Major Problem

277.01	Cystic fibrosis with meconium ileus
747.83	Persistent fetal circulation
763.4	Fetus or newborn affected by cesarean delivery
764.11	Light-for-dates with signs of fetal malnutrition, less than 500 grams
764.12	Light-for-dates with signs of fetal malnutrition, 500-749 grams
764.13	Light-for-dates with signs of fetal malnutrition, 750-999 grams
764.14	Light-for-dates with signs of fetal malnutrition, 1,000-1,249 grams

764.15	Light-for-dates with signs of fetal malnutrition, 1,250-1,499 grams
764.16	Light-for-dates with signs of fetal malnutrition, 1,500-1,749 grams
764.17	Light-for-dates with signs of fetal malnutrition, 1,750-1,999 grams
764.18	Light-for-dates with signs of fetal malnutrition, 2,000-2,499 grams
764.21	Fetal malnutrition without mention of "light-for-dates", less than 500 grams
764.22	Fetal malnutrition without mention of "light-for-dates", 500-749 grams
764.23	Fetal malnutrition without mention of "light-for-dates", 750-999 grams
764.24	Fetal malnutrition without mention of "light-for-dates", 1,000-1,249 grams
764.25	Fetal malnutrition without mention of "light-for-dates", 1,250-1,499 grams
764.26	Fetal malnutrition without mention of "light-for-dates", 1,500-1,749 grams
764.27	Fetal malnutrition without mention of "light-for-dates", 1,750-1,999 grams
764.28	Fetal malnutrition without mention of "light-for-dates", 2,000-2,499 grams
767.0	Subdural and cerebral hemorrhage, birth trauma
767.11	Birth trauma, epicranial subaponeurotic hemorrhage (massive)
767.4	Injury to spine and spinal cord, birth trauma
767.7	Other cranial and peripheral nerve injuries, birth trauma
768.5	Severe birth asphyxia
768.72	Moderate hypoxic-ischemic encephalopathy
768.73	Severe hypoxic-ischemic encephalopathy
770.0	Congenital pneumonia
770.1*	Fetal and newborn aspiration
770.2	Interstitial emphysema and related conditions of newborn
770.3	Pulmonary hemorrhage of fetus or newborn
770.4	Primary atelectasis of newborn
770.84	Respiratory failure of newborn
770.85	Aspiration of postnatal stomach contents without respiratory symptoms
770.86	Aspiration of postnatal stomach contents with respiratory symptoms
771.0	Congenital rubella
771.1	Congenital cytomegalovirus infection
771.2	Other congenital infection specific to the perinatal period
771.4	Omphalitis of the newborn
771.5	Neonatal infective mastitis
771.8*	Other infection specific to the perinatal period
772.0	Fetal blood loss affecting newborn
772.1*	Intraventricular hemorrhage
772.2	Fetal and neonatal subarachnoid hemorrhage of newborn
772.4	Fetal and neonatal gastrointestinal hemorrhage
772.5	Fetal and neonatal adrenal hemorrhage
773.2	Hemolytic disease due to other and unspecified isoimmunization of fetus or newborn
773.3	Hydrops fetalis due to isoimmunization
773.4	Kernicterus due to isoimmunization of fetus or newborn
773.5	Late anemia due to isoimmunization of fetus or newborn
774.4	Perinatal jaundice due to hepatocellular damage
774.7	Kernicterus of fetus or newborn not due to isoimmunization
775.1	Neonatal diabetes mellitus
775.2	Neonatal myasthenia gravis
775.3	Neonatal thyrotoxicosis
775.4	Hypocalcemia and hypomagnesemia of newborn
775.5	Other transitory neonatal electrolyte disturbances
775.6	Neonatal hypoglycemia
775.7	Late metabolic acidosis of newborn
776.0	Hemorrhagic disease of newborn
776.1	Transient neonatal thrombocytopenia
776.2	Disseminated intravascular coagulation in newborn

Surgical	Medical	CC Indicator	MCC Indicator	Procedure Proxy

776.3	Other transient neonatal disorders of coagulation
776.6	Anemia of neonatal prematurity
777.1	Fetal and newborn meconium obstruction
777.2	Neonatal intestinal obstruction due to inspissated milk
777.5*	Necrotizing enterocolitis in newborn
777.6	Perinatal intestinal perforation
778.0	Hydrops fetalis not due to isoimmunization
779.0	Convulsions in newborn
779.1	Other and unspecified cerebral irritability in newborn
779.2	Cerebral depression, coma, and other abnormal cerebral signs in fetus or newborn
779.32	Bilious vomiting in newborn
779.4	Drug reactions and intoxications specific to newborn
779.5	Drug withdrawal syndrome in newborn
779.85	Cardiac arrest of newborn

OR

Secondary Diagnosis of Major Problem

036.3	Waterhouse-Friderichsen syndrome, meningococcal
036.4*	Meningococcal carditis
036.81	Meningococcal optic neuritis
036.82	Meningococcal arthropathy
037	Tetanus
038*	Septicemia
040.0	Gas gangrene
040.41	Infant botulism
046.2	Subacute sclerosing panencephalitis
052.0	Postvaricella encephalitis
052.1	Varicella (hemorrhagic) pneumonitis
052.7	Chickenpox with other specified complications
052.8	Chickenpox with unspecified complication
052.9	Varicella without mention of complication
053.0	Herpes zoster with meningitis
053.10	Herpes zoster with unspecified nervous system complication
053.11	Geniculate herpes zoster
053.12	Postherpetic trigeminal neuralgia
053.13	Postherpetic polyneuropathy
053.19	Other herpes zoster with nervous system complications
053.20	Herpes zoster dermatitis of eyelid
053.21	Herpes zoster keratoconjunctivitis
053.22	Herpes zoster iridocyclitis
053.29	Other ophthalmic herpes zoster complications
053.71	Otitis externa due to herpes zoster
053.79	Other specified herpes zoster complications
053.8	Unspecified herpes zoster complication
053.9	Herpes zoster without mention of complication
054.0	Eczema herpeticum
054.2	Herpetic gingivostomatitis
054.3	Herpetic meningoencephalitis
054.4*	Herpes simplex with ophthalmic complications
054.5	Herpetic septicemia
054.71	Visceral herpes simplex
054.72	Herpes simplex meningitis
054.73	Herpes simplex otitis externa
054.79	Other specified herpes simplex complications
054.8	Unspecified herpes simplex complication
055.0	Postmeasles encephalitis
055.1	Postmeasles pneumonia
055.2	Postmeasles otitis media
055.7*	Measles, with other specified complications
055.8	Unspecified measles complication
056.0*	Rubella with neurological complications
056.7*	Rubella with other specified complications
056.8	Unspecified rubella complications
058.10	Roseola infantum, unspecified
058.11	Roseola infantum due to human herpesvirus 6
058.12	Roseola infantum due to human herpesvirus 7
058.21	Human herpesvirus 6 encephalitis
058.29	Other human herpesvirus encephalitis

070.2*	Viral hepatitis B with hepatic coma
070.3*	Viral hepatitis B without mention of hepatic coma
070.4*	Other specified viral hepatitis with hepatic coma
070.5*	Other specified viral hepatitis without mention of hepatic coma
070.6	Unspecified viral hepatitis with hepatic coma
070.9	Unspecified viral hepatitis without mention of hepatic coma
072.0	Mumps orchitis
072.1	Mumps meningitis
072.2	Mumps encephalitis
072.3	Mumps pancreatitis
072.7*	Mumps with other specified complications
072.8	Unspecified mumps complication
079.6	Respiratory syncytial virus (RSV)
112.4	Candidiasis of lung
112.5	Disseminated candidiasis
112.81	Candidal endocarditis
112.82	Candidal otitis externa
112.83	Candidal meningitis
112.84	Candidiasis of the esophagus
112.85	Candidiasis of the intestine
114.2	Coccidioidal meningitis
114.3	Other forms of progressive coccidioidomycosis
115.01	Histoplasma capsulatum meningitis
115.02	Histoplasma capsulatum retinitis
115.03	Histoplasma capsulatum pericarditis
115.04	Histoplasma capsulatum endocarditis
115.05	Histoplasma capsulatum pneumonia
115.11	Histoplasma duboisii meningitis
115.12	Histoplasma duboisii retinitis
115.13	Histoplasma duboisii pericarditis
115.14	Histoplasma duboisii endocarditis
115.15	Histoplasma duboisii pneumonia
115.91	Unspecified Histoplasmosis meningitis
115.92	Unspecified Histoplasmosis retinitis
115.93	Unspecified Histoplasmosis pericarditis
115.94	Unspecified Histoplasmosis endocarditis
115.95	Unspecified Histoplasmosis pneumonia
116.0	Blastomycosis
116.1	Paracoccidioidomycosis
117.3	Aspergillosis
117.4	Mycotic mycetomas
117.5	Cryptococcosis
117.6	Allescheriosis (Petriellidiosis)
117.7	Zygomycosis (Phycomycosis or Mucormycosis)
118	Opportunistic mycoses
130.0	Meningoencephalitis due to toxoplasmosis
130.1	Conjunctivitis due to toxoplasmosis
130.2	Chorioretinitis due to toxoplasmosis
130.3	Myocarditis due to toxoplasmosis
130.4	Pneumonitis due to toxoplasmosis
130.5	Hepatitis due to toxoplasmosis
130.7	Toxoplasmosis of other specified sites
130.8	Multisystemic disseminated toxoplasmosis
136.3	Pneumocystosis
251.0	Hypoglycemic coma
252.1	Hypoparathyroidism
253.5	Diabetes insipidus
254.1	Abscess of thymus
261	Nutritional marasmus
262	Other severe protein-calorie malnutrition
263.0	Malnutrition of moderate degree
263.1	Malnutrition of mild degree
263.8	Other protein-calorie malnutrition
263.9	Unspecified protein-calorie malnutrition
276*	Disorders of fluid, electrolyte, and acid-base balance
277.88	Tumor lysis syndrome
282.40	Thalassemia, unspecified
282.41	Sickle-cell thalassemia without crisis
282.42	Sickle-cell thalassemia with crisis

T Transfer DRG   SP Special Payment   ☑ Optimization Potential   ▽ Targeted Potential   * Code Range   ● New DRG   ▲ Revised DRG Title

168   Valid 10/01/2013-09/30/2014   © 2013 OptumInsight, Inc.

282.43	Alpha thalassemia
282.44	Beta thalassemia
282.45	Delta-beta thalassemia
282.47	Hemoglobin E-beta thalassemia
282.49	Other thalassemia
283.1*	Non-autoimmune hemolytic anemias
283.2	Hemoglobinuria due to hemolysis from external causes
283.9	Acquired hemolytic anemia, unspecified
285.1	Acute posthemorrhagic anemia
286.6	Defibrination syndrome
287.4*	Secondary thrombocytopenia
289.84	Heparin-induced thrombocytopenia [HIT]
292.0	Drug withdrawal
320*	Bacterial meningitis
321*	Meningitis due to other organisms
322.0	Nonpyogenic meningitis
322.1	Eosinophilic meningitis
322.9	Unspecified meningitis
324*	Intracranial and intraspinal abscess
348.1	Anoxic brain damage
349.0	Reaction to spinal or lumbar puncture
349.1	Nervous system complications from surgically implanted device
349.3*	Dural tear
349.81	Cerebrospinal fluid rhinorrhea
349.82	Toxic encephalopathy
377.00	Unspecified papilledema
377.01	Papilledema associated with increased intracranial pressure
377.02	Papilledema associated with decreased ocular pressure
383.01	Subperiosteal abscess of mastoid
383.81	Postauricular fistula
398.91	Rheumatic heart failure (congestive)
402.01	Malignant hypertensive heart disease with heart failure
402.11	Benign hypertensive heart disease with heart failure
402.91	Hypertensive heart disease, unspecified, with heart failure
404.01	Hypertensive heart and chronic kidney disease, malignant, with heart failure and with chronic kidney disease stage I through stage IV, or unspecified
404.03	Hypertensive heart and chronic kidney disease, malignant, with heart failure and with chronic kidney disease stage V or end stage renal disease
404.11	Hypertensive heart and chronic kidney disease, benign, with heart failure and with chronic kidney disease stage I through stage IV, or unspecified
404.13	Hypertensive heart and chronic kidney disease, benign, with heart failure and chronic kidney disease stage V or end stage renal disease
404.91	Hypertensive heart and chronic kidney disease, unspecified, with heart failure and with chronic kidney disease stage I through stage IV, or unspecified
404.93	Hypertensive heart and chronic kidney disease, unspecified, with heart failure and with chronic kidney disease stage V or end stage renal disease
414.10	Aneurysm of heart
415*	Acute pulmonary heart disease
416.2	Chronic pulmonary embolism
420.0	Acute pericarditis in diseases classified elsewhere
421*	Acute and subacute endocarditis
422.0	Acute myocarditis in diseases classified elsewhere
422.92	Septic myocarditis
423.0	Hemopericardium
424.9*	Endocarditis, valve unspecified
425.8	Cardiomyopathy in other diseases classified elsewhere
426.0	Atrioventricular block, complete
426.53	Other bilateral bundle branch block
426.54	Trifascicular block
426.7	Anomalous atrioventricular excitation
426.89	Other specified conduction disorder
427.1	Paroxysmal ventricular tachycardia
427.3*	Atrial fibrillation and flutter
427.4*	Ventricular fibrillation and flutter
427.5	Cardiac arrest
428.0	Congestive heart failure, unspecified
428.1	Left heart failure
428.2*	Systolic heart failure
428.3*	Diastolic heart failure
428.4*	Combined systolic and diastolic heart failure
428.9	Unspecified heart failure
429.4	Functional disturbances following cardiac surgery
429.81	Other disorders of papillary muscle
429.82	Hyperkinetic heart disease
430	Subarachnoid hemorrhage
431	Intracerebral hemorrhage
432*	Other and unspecified intracranial hemorrhage
433.01	Occlusion and stenosis of basilar artery with cerebral infarction
433.11	Occlusion and stenosis of carotid artery with cerebral infarction
433.21	Occlusion and stenosis of vertebral artery with cerebral infarction
433.31	Occlusion and stenosis of multiple and bilateral precerebral arteries with cerebral infarction
433.81	Occlusion and stenosis of other specified precerebral artery with cerebral infarction
433.91	Occlusion and stenosis of unspecified precerebral artery with cerebral infarction
434*	Occlusion of cerebral arteries
436	Acute, but ill-defined, cerebrovascular disease
440.24	Atherosclerosis of native arteries of the extremities with gangrene
444*	Arterial embolism and thrombosis
449	Septic arterial embolism
451.1*	Phlebitis and thrombophlebitis of deep veins of lower extremities
451.2	Phlebitis and thrombophlebitis of lower extremities, unspecified
451.81	Phlebitis and thrombophlebitis of iliac vein
453.2	Other venous embolism and thrombosis, of inferior vena cava
457.2	Lymphangitis
459.0	Unspecified hemorrhage
478.22	Parapharyngeal abscess
478.24	Retropharyngeal abscess
478.3*	Paralysis of vocal cords or larynx
478.75	Laryngeal spasm
481	Pneumococcal pneumonia (streptococcus pneumoniae pneumonia)
482*	Other bacterial pneumonia
483*	Pneumonia due to other specified organism
485	Bronchopneumonia, organism unspecified
486	Pneumonia, organism unspecified
488.01	Influenza due to identified avian influenza virus with pneumonia
488.02	Influenza due to identified avian influenza virus with other respiratory manifestations
488.11	Influenza due to identified 2009 H1N1 influenza virus with pneumonia
488.12	Influenza due to identified 2009 H1N1 influenza virus with other respiratory manifestations
488.81	Influenza due to identified novel influenza A virus with pneumonia
488.82	Influenza due to identified novel influenza A virus with other respiratory manifestations
493.01	Extrinsic asthma with status asthmaticus
493.11	Intrinsic asthma with status asthmaticus
493.91	Asthma, unspecified with status asthmaticus
507.0	Pneumonitis due to inhalation of food or vomitus
507.8	Pneumonitis due to other solids and liquids
508.0	Acute pulmonary manifestations due to radiation
510*	Empyema

Surgical	*Medical*	CC Indicator	MCC Indicator	*Procedure Proxy*

511.1	Pleurisy with effusion, with mention of bacterial cause other than tuberculosis
511.89	Other specified forms of effusion, except tuberculous
511.9	Unspecified pleural effusion
513*	Abscess of lung and mediastinum
516.6*	Interstitial lung diseases of childhood
518.0	Pulmonary collapse
518.1	Interstitial emphysema
518.4	Unspecified acute edema of lung
518.52	Other pulmonary insufficiency, not elsewhere classified, following trauma and surgery
519.2	Mediastinitis
530.4	Perforation of esophagus
530.84	Tracheoesophageal fistula
536.1	Acute dilatation of stomach
550.00	Inguinal hernia with gangrene, unilateral or unspecified, (not specified as recurrent)
550.02	Inguinal hernia with gangrene, bilateral
550.10	Inguinal hernia with obstruction, without mention of gangrene, unilateral or unspecified, (not specified as recurrent)
550.12	Inguinal hernia with obstruction, without mention gangrene, bilateral, (not specified as recurrent)
551.00	Femoral hernia with gangrene, unilateral or unspecified (not specified as recurrent)
551.02	Femoral hernia with gangrene, bilateral, (not specified as recurrent)
551.1	Umbilical hernia with gangrene
551.2*	Ventral hernia with gangrene
551.3	Diaphragmatic hernia with gangrene
551.8	Hernia of other specified sites, with gangrene
551.9	Hernia of unspecified site, with gangrene
552.00	Unilateral or unspecified femoral hernia with obstruction
552.02	Bilateral femoral hernia with obstruction
552.1	Umbilical hernia with obstruction
552.2*	Ventral hernia with obstruction
552.3	Diaphragmatic hernia with obstruction
552.8	Hernia of other specified site, with obstruction
552.9	Hernia of unspecified site, with obstruction
557.0	Acute vascular insufficiency of intestine
558.2	Toxic gastroenteritis and colitis
560.0	Intussusception
560.1	Paralytic ileus
560.2	Volvulus
560.30	Unspecified impaction of intestine
560.32	Fecal impaction
560.39	Impaction of intestine, other
560.89	Other specified intestinal obstruction
560.9	Unspecified intestinal obstruction
566	Abscess of anal and rectal regions
567*	Peritonitis and retroperitoneal infections
568.81	Hemoperitoneum (nontraumatic)
569.3	Hemorrhage of rectum and anus
569.7*	Complications of intestinal pouch
569.83	Perforation of intestine
570	Acute and subacute necrosis of liver
572.0	Abscess of liver
572.1	Portal pyemia
572.2	Hepatic encephalopathy
572.4	Hepatorenal syndrome
573.3	Unspecified hepatitis
573.4	Hepatic infarction
576.1	Cholangitis
577.0	Acute pancreatitis
577.2	Cyst and pseudocyst of pancreas
578*	Gastrointestinal hemorrhage
579.3	Other and unspecified postsurgical nonabsorption
580*	Acute glomerulonephritis
584*	Acute kidney failure
590.1*	Acute pyelonephritis
590.2	Renal and perinephric abscess
590.3	Pyeloureteritis cystica
590.8*	Other pyelonephritis or pyonephrosis, not specified as acute or chronic
590.9	Unspecified infection of kidney
591	Hydronephrosis
593.5	Hydroureter
595.0	Acute cystitis
595.4	Cystitis in diseases classified elsewhere
595.81	Cystitis cystica
595.89	Other specified types of cystitis
595.9	Unspecified cystitis
596.0	Bladder neck obstruction
596.1	Intestinovesical fistula
596.2	Vesical fistula, not elsewhere classified
596.4	Atony of bladder
596.6	Nontraumatic rupture of bladder
596.7	Hemorrhage into bladder wall
597.0	Urethral abscess
599.0	Urinary tract infection, site not specified
599.6*	Urinary obstruction
599.7*	Hematuria
619.1	Digestive-genital tract fistula, female
619.8	Other specified fistula involving female genital tract
620.7	Hematoma of broad ligament
682*	Other cellulitis and abscess
683	Acute lymphadenitis
693.0	Dermatitis due to drugs and medicines taken internally
695.0	Toxic erythema
708.0	Allergic urticaria
733.1*	Pathologic fracture
740*	Anencephalus and similar anomalies
741*	Spina bifida
742*	Other congenital anomalies of nervous system
745.4	Ventricular septal defect
756.72	Omphalocele
756.73	Gastroschisis
759.4	Conjoined twins
779.7	Periventricular leukomalacia
780.01	Coma
780.03	Persistent vegetative state
780.31	Febrile convulsions (simple), unspecified
780.39	Other convulsions
781.7	Tetany
785.0	Unspecified tachycardia
785.4	Gangrene
785.50	Unspecified shock
788.2*	Retention of urine
790.7	Bacteremia
791.1	Chyluria
799.1	Respiratory arrest
820*	Fracture of neck of femur
821.0*	Closed fracture of shaft or unspecified part of femur
821.1*	Open fracture of shaft or unspecified part of femur
860*	Traumatic pneumothorax and hemothorax
865*	Injury to spleen
900.0*	Injury to carotid artery
900.1	Internal jugular vein injury
900.81	External jugular vein injury
901.0	Thoracic aorta injury
901.1	Innominate and subclavian artery injury
901.2	Superior vena cava injury
901.3	Innominate and subclavian vein injury
901.41	Pulmonary artery injury
901.42	Pulmonary vein injury
902.0	Abdominal aorta injury
902.10	Unspecified inferior vena cava injury
953.4	Injury to brachial plexus
958.0	Air embolism as an early complication of trauma
958.1	Fat embolism as an early complication of trauma

Ⓣ *Transfer DRG*   ⓈⓅ *Special Payment*   ☑ *Optimization Potential*   ⱽᴱˢ *Targeted Potential*   * *Code Range*   ● *New DRG*   ▲ *Revised DRG Title*

Valid 10/01/2013-09/30/2014   © 2013 OptumInsight, Inc.

958.2	Secondary and recurrent hemorrhage as an early complication of trauma
958.3	Posttraumatic wound infection not elsewhere classified
958.4	Traumatic shock
958.5	Traumatic anuria
958.7	Traumatic subcutaneous emphysema
995.20	Unspecified adverse effect of unspecified drug, medicinal and biological substance
995.21	Arthus phenomenon
995.22	Unspecified adverse effect of anesthesia
995.23	Unspecified adverse effect of insulin
995.27	Other drug allergy
995.29	Unspecified adverse effect of other drug, medicinal and biological substance
995.4	Shock due to anesthesia not elsewhere classified
997.0*	Nervous system complications
997.1	Cardiac complications
997.2	Peripheral vascular complications
997.3*	Respiratory complications
997.4*	Digestive system complications, not elsewhere classified
997.5	Urinary complications
997.71	Vascular complications of mesenteric artery
997.72	Vascular complications of renal artery
997.79	Vascular complications of other vessels
998.0*	Postoperative shock
998.11	Hemorrhage complicating a procedure
998.12	Hematoma complicating a procedure
998.13	Seroma complicating a procedure
998.2	Accidental puncture or laceration during procedure
998.4	Foreign body accidentally left during procedure, not elsewhere classified
998.51	Infected postoperative seroma
998.59	Other postoperative infection
998.6	Persistent postoperative fistula, not elsewhere classified
998.7	Acute reaction to foreign substance accidentally left during procedure, not elsewhere classified
998.9	Unspecified complication of procedure, not elsewhere classified
999.1	Air embolism as complication of medical care, not elsewhere classified
999.2	Other vascular complications of medical care, not elsewhere classified
999.34	Acute infection following transfusion, infusion, or injection of blood and blood products
999.39	Complications of medical care, NEC, infection following other infusion, injection, transfusion, or vaccination
999.4*	Anaphylactic reaction due to serum
999.5*	Other serum reaction, not elsewhere classified
999.6*	ABO incompatibility reaction due to transfusion of blood or blood products
999.7*	Rh and other non-ABO incompatibility reaction due to transfusion of blood or blood products
999.8*	Other and unspecified infusion and transfusion reaction

DRG 794 Neonate with Other Significant Problems

GMLOS 3.4	**AMLOS 3.4**	**RW 1.2494**	☑

Principal or secondary diagnosis of newborn or neonate with other significant problems, not assigned to DRGs 789-793, 795 or 998

DRG 795 Normal Newborn

GMLOS 3.1	**AMLOS 3.1**	**RW 0.1692**	☑

Principal Diagnosis

762.4	Fetus or newborn affected by prolapsed cord
762.5	Fetus or newborn affected by other compression of umbilical cord
762.6	Fetus or newborn affected by other and unspecified conditions of umbilical cord
763.0	Fetus or newborn affected by breech delivery and extraction

763.1	Fetus or newborn affected by other malpresentation, malposition, and disproportion during labor and delivery
763.2	Fetus or newborn affected by forceps delivery
763.3	Fetus or newborn affected by delivery by vacuum extractor
763.6	Fetus or newborn affected by precipitate delivery
763.9	Unspecified complication of labor and delivery affecting fetus or newborn
764.08	Light-for-dates without mention of fetal malnutrition, 2,000-2,499 grams
764.09	Light-for-dates without mention of fetal malnutrition, 2,500 or more grams
764.98	Unspecified fetal growth retardation, 2,000-2,499 grams
764.99	Unspecified fetal growth retardation, 2,500 or more grams
765.20	Unspecified weeks of gestation
765.29	37 or more completed weeks of gestation
766.0	Exceptionally large baby relating to long gestation
766.1	Other "heavy-for-dates" infants not related to gestation period
766.2*	Late infant, not "heavy-for-dates"
767.19	Birth trauma, other injuries to scalp
768.6	Mild or moderate birth asphyxia
772.6	Fetal and neonatal cutaneous hemorrhage
774.3*	Neonatal jaundice due to delayed conjugation from other causes
774.5	Perinatal jaundice from other causes
774.6	Unspecified fetal and neonatal jaundice
778.8	Other specified condition involving the integument of fetus and newborn
779.31	Feeding problems in newborn
779.33	Other vomiting in newborn
779.83	Delayed separation of umbilical cord
V30.00	Single liveborn, born in hospital, delivered without mention of cesarean delivery
V30.01	Single liveborn, born in hospital, delivered by cesarean delivery
V30.1	Single liveborn, born before admission to hospital
V31.00	Twin, mate liveborn, born in hospital, delivered without mention of cesarean delivery
V31.01	Twin, mate liveborn, born in hospital, delivered by cesarean delivery
V31.1	Twin birth, mate liveborn, born before admission to hospital
V32.00	Twin, mate stillborn, born in hospital, delivered without mention of cesarean delivery
V32.01	Twin, mate stillborn, born in hospital, delivered by cesarean delivery
V32.1	Twin birth, mate stillborn, born before admission to hospital
V33.00	Twin, unspecified whether mate stillborn or liveborn, born in hospital, delivered without mention of cesarean delivery
V33.01	Twin, unspecified whether mate stillborn or liveborn, born in hospital, delivered by cesarean delivery
V33.1	Twin birth, unspecified whether mate liveborn or stillborn, born before admission to hospital
V34.00	Other multiple, mates all liveborn, born in hospital, delivered without mention of cesarean delivery
V34.01	Other multiple, mates all liveborn, born in hospital, delivered by cesarean delivery
V34.1	Other multiple birth (three or more), mates all liveborn, born before admission to hospital
V35.00	Other multiple, mates all stillborn, born in hospital, delivered without mention of cesarean delivery
V35.01	Other multiple, mates all stillborn, born in hospital, delivered by cesarean delivery
V35.1	Other multiple birth (three or more), mates all stillborn, born before admission to hospital
V36.00	Other multiple, mates liveborn and stillborn, born in hospital, delivered without mention of cesarean delivery
V36.01	Other multiple, mates liveborn and stillborn, born in hospital, delivered by cesarean delivery
V36.1	Other multiple birth (three or more), mates liveborn and stillborn, born before admission to hospital

Surgical	Medical	CC Indicator	MCC Indicator	Procedure Proxy

MDC 15: Newborns And Other Neonates With Conditions Originating In The Perinatal Period—MEDICAL

V37.00 Other multiple, unspecified whether mates stillborn or liveborn, born in hospital, delivered without mention of cesarean delivery
V37.01 Other multiple, unspecified whether mates stillborn or liveborn, born in hospital, delivered by cesarean delivery
V37.1   Other multiple birth (three or more), unspecified whether mates liveborn or stillborn, born before admission to hospital
V39.00 Liveborn infant, unspecified whether single, twin, or multiple, born in hospital, delivered without mention of cesarean delivery
V39.01 Liveborn infant, unspecified whether single, twin, or multiple, born in hospital, delivered by cesarean
V39.1   Liveborn, unspecified whether single, twin or multiple, born before admission to hospital

AND

No Secondary Diagnosis

OR

Only Secondary Diagnosis
478.11 Nasal mucositis (ulcerative)
478.19 Other diseases of nasal cavity and sinuses
520.6   Disturbances in tooth eruption
605   Redundant prepuce and phimosis
623.8   Other specified noninflammatory disorder of vagina
686.9   Unspecified local infection of skin and subcutaneous tissue
691.0   Diaper or napkin rash
709.00 Dyschromia, unspecified
709.01 Vitiligo
709.09 Other dyschromia
744.1   Congenital anomalies of accessory auricle
752.5* Undescended and retractile testicle
754.61 Congenital pes planus
757.33 Congenital pigmentary anomaly of skin
757.39 Other specified congenital anomaly of skin
762.4   Fetus or newborn affected by prolapsed cord
762.5   Fetus or newborn affected by other compression of umbilical cord
762.6   Fetus or newborn affected by other and unspecified conditions of umbilical cord
763.0   Fetus or newborn affected by breech delivery and extraction
763.1   Fetus or newborn affected by other malpresentation, malposition, and disproportion during labor and delivery
763.2   Fetus or newborn affected by forceps delivery
763.3   Fetus or newborn affected by delivery by vacuum extractor
763.6   Fetus or newborn affected by precipitate delivery
763.9   Unspecified complication of labor and delivery affecting fetus or newborn
764.08 Light-for-dates without mention of fetal malnutrition, 2,000-2,499 grams
764.09 Light-for-dates without mention of fetal malnutrition, 2,500 or more grams
764.98 Unspecified fetal growth retardation, 2,000-2,499 grams
764.99 Unspecified fetal growth retardation, 2,500 or more grams
765.20 Unspecified weeks of gestation
765.29 37 or more completed weeks of gestation
766.0   Exceptionally large baby relating to long gestation
766.1   Other "heavy-for-dates" infants not related to gestation period
766.2* Late infant, not "heavy-for-dates"
767.19 Birth trauma, other injuries to scalp
768.6   Mild or moderate birth asphyxia
772.6   Fetal and neonatal cutaneous hemorrhage
774.3* Neonatal jaundice due to delayed conjugation from other causes
774.5   Perinatal jaundice from other causes
774.6   Unspecified fetal and neonatal jaundice
778.8   Other specified condition involving the integument of fetus and newborn
794.15 Nonspecific abnormal auditory function studies

795.4   Other nonspecific abnormal histological findings
796.4   Other abnormal clinical finding
V01.81 Contact with or exposure to anthrax
V01.89 Contact or exposure to other communicable diseases
V05.3   Need for prophylactic vaccination and inoculation against viral hepatitis
V05.4   Need for prophylactic vaccination and inoculation against varicella
V05.8   Need for prophylactic vaccination and inoculation against other specified disease
V20.1   Health supervision of other healthy infant or child receiving care
V20.2   Routine infant or child health check
V20.3* Newborn health supervision
V29*   Observation and evaluation of newborns and infants for suspected condition not found
V30.00 Single liveborn, born in hospital, delivered without mention of cesarean delivery
V30.01 Single liveborn, born in hospital, delivered by cesarean delivery
V30.1   Single liveborn, born before admission to hospital
V31.00 Twin, mate liveborn, born in hospital, delivered without mention of cesarean delivery
V31.01 Twin, mate liveborn, born in hospital, delivered by cesarean delivery
V31.1   Twin birth, mate liveborn, born before admission to hospital
V32.00 Twin, mate stillborn, born in hospital, delivered without mention of cesarean delivery
V32.01 Twin, mate stillborn, born in hospital, delivered by cesarean delivery
V32.1   Twin birth, mate stillborn, born before admission to hospital
V33.00 Twin, unspecified whether mate stillborn or liveborn, born in hospital, delivered without mention of cesarean delivery
V33.01 Twin, unspecified whether mate stillborn or liveborn, born in hospital, delivered by cesarean delivery
V33.1   Twin birth, unspecified whether mate liveborn or stillborn, born before admission to hospital
V34.00 Other multiple, mates all liveborn, born in hospital, delivered without mention of cesarean delivery
V34.01 Other multiple, mates all liveborn, born in hospital, delivered by cesarean delivery
V34.1   Other multiple birth (three or more), mates all liveborn, born before admission to hospital
V35.00 Other multiple, mates all stillborn, born in hospital, delivered without mention of cesarean delivery
V35.01 Other multiple, mates all stillborn, born in hospital, delivered by cesarean delivery
V35.1   Other multiple birth (three or more), mates all stillborn, born before admission to hospital
V36.00 Other multiple, mates liveborn and stillborn, born in hospital, delivered without mention of cesarean delivery
V36.01 Other multiple, mates liveborn and stillborn, born in hospital, delivered by cesarean delivery
V36.1   Other multiple birth (three or more), mates liveborn and stillborn, born before admission to hospital
V37.00 Other multiple, unspecified whether mates stillborn or liveborn, born in hospital, delivered without mention of cesarean delivery
V37.01 Other multiple, unspecified whether mates stillborn or liveborn, born in hospital, delivered by cesarean delivery
V37.1   Other multiple birth (three or more), unspecified whether mates liveborn or stillborn, born before admission to hospital
V39.00 Liveborn infant, unspecified whether single, twin, or multiple, born in hospital, delivered without mention of cesarean delivery
V39.01 Liveborn infant, unspecified whether single, twin, or multiple, born in hospital, delivered by cesarean
V39.1   Liveborn, unspecified whether single, twin or multiple, born before admission to hospital

---

Ⓣ *Transfer DRG*   Ⓢ *Special Payment*   ☑ *Optimization Potential*   Ⓦ *Targeted Potential*   * *Code Range*   ● *New DRG*   ▲ *Revised DRG Title*

V50.2   Routine or ritual circumcision
V64.0*   Vaccination not carried out
V64.1   Surgical or other procedure not carried out because of
         contraindication
V64.2   Surgical or other procedure not carried out because of
         patient's decision
V64.3   Procedure not carried out for other reasons
V70.3   Other general medical exami for administrative purposes
V72.1*   Examination of ears and hearing
V77.3   Screening for phenylketonuria (PKU)

DRG 998   Principal Diagnosis Invalid as Discharge Diagnosis
            GMLOS 0.0   AMLOS 0.0   RW 0.0000

Note: If there is no value in either the GMLOS or the AMLOS, the volume
of cases is insufficient to determine a meaningful computation of these
statistics.

Principal diagnoses listed for MDC 15 considered invalid as discharge
diagnosis
V30.2   Single liveborn, born outside hospital and not hospitalized
V31.2   Twin birth, mate liveborn, born outside hospital and not
         hospitalized
V32.2   Twin birth, mate stillborn, born outside hospital and not
         hospitalized
V33.2   Twin birth, unspecified whether mate liveborn or stillborn,
         born outside hospital and not hospitalized
V34.2   Other multiple birth (three or more), mates all liveborn, born
         outside hospital and not hospitalized
V35.2   Other multiple birth (three or more), mates all stillborn, born
         outside of hospital and not hospitalized
V36.2   Other multiple birth (three or more), mates liveborn and
         stillborn, born outside hospital and not hospitalized
V37.2   Other multiple birth (three or more), unspecified whether
         mates liveborn or stillborn, born outside of hospital
V39.2   Liveborn, unspecified whether single, twin or multiple, born
         outside hospital and not hospitalized

Surgical	Medical	CC Indicator	MCC Indicator	Procedure Proxy

MDC 16
Diseases And Disorders Of The Blood And Blood-Forming Organs And Immunological Disorders

017.20	254.0	279.8	282.49	284.9	287.32	288.64	759.0	999.69
017.21	254.1	279.9	282.5	285.0	287.33	288.65	782.7	999.70
017.22	254.8	280.0	282.60	285.1	287.39	288.66	785.6	999.71
017.23	254.9	280.1	282.61	285.21	287.41	288.69	789.2	999.72
017.24	273.0	280.8	282.62	285.22	287.49	288.8	790.01	999.73
017.25	273.1	280.9	282.63	285.29	287.5	288.9	790.09	999.74
017.26	279.00	281.0	282.64	285.3	287.8	289.0	795.71	999.75
017.70	279.01	281.1	282.68	285.8	287.9	289.1	795.79	999.76
017.71	279.02	281.2	282.69	285.9	288.00	289.3	865.00	999.77
017.72	279.03	281.3	282.7	286.0	288.01	289.4	865.01	999.78
017.73	279.04	281.4	282.8	286.1	288.02	289.50	865.02	999.79
017.74	279.05	281.8	282.9	286.2	288.03	289.51	865.03	999.80
017.75	279.06	281.9	283.0	286.3	288.04	289.52	865.04	999.83
017.76	279.09	282.0	283.10	286.4	288.09	289.53	865.09	999.84
078.3	279.10	282.1	283.11	286.52	288.1	289.59	865.10	999.85
091.4	279.11	282.2	283.19	286.53	288.2	289.6	865.11	999.89
209.62	279.12	282.3	283.2	286.59	288.3	289.7	865.12	V42.81
212.6	279.13	282.40	283.9	286.6	288.4	289.81	865.13	V42.82
228.1	279.19	282.41	284.01	286.7	288.50	289.82	865.14	
229.0	279.2	282.42	284.09	286.9	288.51	289.84	865.19	
238.71	279.3	282.43	284.11	287.0	288.59	289.89	996.85	
238.72	279.50	282.44	284.12	287.1	288.60	289.9	999.60	
238.73	279.51	282.45	284.19	287.2	288.61	457.8	999.61	
238.74	279.52	282.46	284.81	287.30	288.62	457.9	999.62	
238.75	279.53	282.47	284.89	287.31	288.63	683	999.63	

SURGICAL

DRG 799   Splenectomy with MCC
GMLOS 9.9   AMLOS 12.9   RW 5.0639   ☑

Operating Room Procedures
41.2	Splenotomy
41.33	Open biopsy of spleen
41.4*	Excision or destruction of lesion or tissue of spleen
41.5	Total splenectomy
41.93	Excision of accessory spleen
41.94	Transplantation of spleen
41.95	Repair and plastic operations on spleen
41.99	Other operations on spleen

DRG 800   Splenectomy with CC
GMLOS 5.2   AMLOS 6.8   RW 2.5234   ☑

Select operating room procedures listed under DRG 799

DRG 801   Splenectomy without CC/MCC
GMLOS 2.8   AMLOS 3.5   RW 1.5980   ☑

Select operating room procedures listed under DRG 799

DRG 802   Other O.R. Procedures of the Blood and Blood-Forming Organs with MCC
GMLOS 7.7   AMLOS 10.4   RW 3.1642   ☑

Operating Room Procedures
07.16	Biopsy of thymus
07.8*	Thymectomy
07.9*	Other operations on thymus
26.30	Sialoadenectomy, not otherwise specified
34.22	Mediastinoscopy
34.26	Open biopsy of mediastinum
38.7	Interruption of the vena cava
40.0	Incision of lymphatic structures
40.1*	Diagnostic procedures on lymphatic structures
40.2*	Simple excision of lymphatic structure
40.3	Regional lymph node excision
40.4*	Radical excision of cervical lymph nodes
40.5*	Radical excision of other lymph nodes
40.9	Other operations on lymphatic structures
50.12	Open biopsy of liver
50.14	Laparoscopic liver biopsy
50.19	Other diagnostic procedures on liver
54.11	Exploratory laparotomy
54.19	Other laparotomy
54.21	Laparoscopy
54.23	Biopsy of peritoneum
54.29	Other diagnostic procedures on abdominal region
55.24	Open biopsy of kidney
55.29	Other diagnostic procedures on kidney
77.49	Biopsy of other bone, except facial bones
83.21	Open biopsy of soft tissue
86.06	Insertion of totally implantable infusion pump
86.22	Excisional debridement of wound, infection, or burn

DRG 803   Other O.R. Procedures of the Blood and Blood-Forming Organs with CC
GMLOS 4.7   AMLOS 6.3   RW 1.8831   ☑

Select operating room procedures listed under DRG 802

DRG 804   Other O.R. Procedures of the Blood and Blood-Forming Organs without CC/MCC
GMLOS 2.3   AMLOS 3.0   RW 1.1558   ☑

Select operating room procedures listed under DRG 802

MEDICAL

DRG 808   Major Hematologic/Immunologic Diagnoses Except Sickle Cell Crisis and Coagulation with MCC
GMLOS 6.1   AMLOS 8.1   RW 2.2217

Principal Diagnosis
279.11	DiGeorge's syndrome
279.12	Wiskott-Aldrich syndrome
279.13	Nezelof's syndrome
279.19	Other deficiency of cell-mediated immunity
279.2	Combined immunity deficiency
279.5*	Graft-versus-host disease
283.0	Autoimmune hemolytic anemias
283.10	Unspecified non-autoimmune hemolytic anemia
283.19	Other non-autoimmune hemolytic anemias
283.2	Hemoglobinuria due to hemolysis from external causes
283.9	Acquired hemolytic anemia, unspecified
284.0*	Constitutional aplastic anemia
284.1*	Pancytopenia
284.8*	Other specified aplastic anemias
284.9	Unspecified aplastic anemia
288.0*	Neutropenia
288.1	Functional disorders of polymorphonuclear neutrophils
288.2	Genetic anomalies of leukocytes
996.85	Complications of bone marrow transplant

DRG 809   Major Hematologic/Immunologic Diagnoses Except Sickle Cell Crisis and Coagulation with CC
GMLOS 3.8   AMLOS 4.8   RW 1.1901   ☑

Select principal diagnosis listed under DRG 808

DRG 810   Major Hematologic/Immunologic Diagnoses Except Sickle Cell Crisis and Coagulation without CC/MCC
GMLOS 2.7   AMLOS 3.3   RW 0.8226   ☑

Select principal diagnosis listed under DRG 808

DRG 811   Red Blood Cell Disorders with MCC
GMLOS 3.6   AMLOS 4.8   RW 1.2488   ☑

Principal Diagnosis
238.72	Low grade myelodysplastic syndrome lesions
238.73	High grade myelodysplastic syndrome lesions
238.74	Myelodysplastic syndrome with 5q deletion
238.75	Myelodysplastic syndrome, unspecified
280*	Iron deficiency anemias
281*	Other deficiency anemias
282*	Hereditary hemolytic anemias
283.11	Hemolytic-uremic syndrome
285*	Other and unspecified anemias
289.7	Methemoglobinemia
790.0*	Abnormality of red blood cells

Surgical	Medical	CC Indicator	MCC Indicator	Procedure Proxy

999.6*	ABO incompatibility reaction due to transfusion of blood or blood products
999.7*	Rh and other non-ABO incompatibility reaction due to transfusion of blood or blood products
999.80	Transfusion reaction, unspecified
999.83	Hemolytic transfusion reaction, incompatibility unspecified
999.84	Acute hemolytic transfusion reaction, incompatibility unspecified
999.85	Delayed hemolytic transfusion reaction, incompatibility unspecified
999.89	Other transfusion reaction

DRG 812   Red Blood Cell Disorders without MCC

| GMLOS 2.6 | AMLOS 3.4 | RW 0.7985 | ☑ |

Select principal diagnosis listed under DRG 811

DRG 813   Coagulation Disorders

| GMLOS 3.6 | AMLOS 5.0 | RW 1.6433 | ☑ |

Principal Diagnosis

286.0	Congenital factor VIII disorder
286.1	Congenital factor IX disorder
286.2	Congenital factor XI deficiency
286.3	Congenital deficiency of other clotting factors
286.4	Von Willebrand's disease
286.52	Acquired hemophilia
286.59	Other hemorrhagic disorder due to intrinsic circulating anticoagulants, antibodies, or inhibitors
286.6	Defibrination syndrome
286.7	Acquired coagulation factor deficiency
286.9	Other and unspecified coagulation defects
287*	Purpura and other hemorrhagic conditions
289.84	Heparin-induced thrombocytopenia [HIT]
782.7	Spontaneous ecchymoses

DRG 814   Reticuloendothelial and Immunity Disorders with MCC

| GMLOS 4.9 | AMLOS 6.8 | RW 1.6910 | ☑ |

Principal Diagnosis

017.2*	Tuberculosis of peripheral lymph nodes
017.7*	Tuberculosis of spleen
078.3	Cat-scratch disease
091.4	Adenopathy due to secondary syphilis
209.62	Benign carcinoid tumor of the thymus
212.6	Benign neoplasm of thymus
228.1	Lymphangioma, any site
229.0	Benign neoplasm of lymph nodes
238.71	Essential thrombocythemia
254*	Diseases of thymus gland
273.0	Polyclonal hypergammaglobulinemia
273.1	Monoclonal paraproteinemia
279.0*	Deficiency of humoral immunity
279.10	Unspecified immunodeficiency with predominant T-cell defect
279.3	Unspecified immunity deficiency
279.8	Other specified disorders involving the immune mechanism
279.9	Unspecified disorder of immune mechanism
286.53	Antiphospholipid antibody with hemorrhagic disorder
288.3	Eosinophilia
288.4	Hemophagocytic syndromes
288.5*	Decreased white blood cell count
288.6*	Elevated white blood cell count
288.8	Other specified disease of white blood cells
288.9	Unspecified disease of white blood cells
289.0	Polycythemia, secondary
289.1	Chronic lymphadenitis
289.3	Lymphadenitis, unspecified, except mesenteric
289.4	Hypersplenism
289.5*	Other diseases of spleen

289.6	Familial polycythemia
289.81	Primary hypercoagulable state
289.82	Secondary hypercoagulable state
289.89	Other specified diseases of blood and blood-forming organs
289.9	Unspecified diseases of blood and blood-forming organs
457.8	Other noninfectious disorders of lymphatic channels
457.9	Unspecified noninfectious disorder of lymphatic channels
683	Acute lymphadenitis
759.0	Congenital anomalies of spleen
785.6	Enlargement of lymph nodes
789.2	Splenomegaly
795.7*	Other nonspecific immunological findings
865*	Injury to spleen
V42.81	Bone marrow replaced by transplant
V42.82	Peripheral stem cells replaced by transplant

DRG 815   Reticuloendothelial and Immunity Disorders with CC

| GMLOS 3.3 | AMLOS 4.2 | RW 0.9844 | ☑ |

Select principal diagnosis listed under DRG 814

DRG 816   Reticuloendothelial and Immunity Disorders without CC/MCC

| GMLOS 2.4 | AMLOS 2.9 | RW 0.6655 | ☑ |

Select principal diagnosis listed under DRG 814

[T] *Transfer DRG*   [SP] *Special Payment*   ☑ *Optimization Potential*   [YES] *Targeted Potential*   * *Code Range*   ● *New DRG*   ▲ *Revised DRG Title*

MDC 17
Myeloproliferative Diseases And Disorders And Poorly Differentiated Neoplasms

158.0	200.33	200.87	201.62	202.26	202.81	205.22	208.90	V10.3
159.1	200.34	200.88	201.63	202.27	202.82	205.30	208.91	V10.40
164.0	200.35	201.00	201.64	202.28	202.83	205.31	208.92	V10.41
176.5	200.36	201.01	201.65	202.30	202.84	205.32	209.20	V10.42
195.4	200.37	201.02	201.66	202.31	202.85	205.80	209.22	V10.43
195.5	200.38	201.03	201.67	202.32	202.86	205.81	209.29	V10.44
195.8	200.40	201.04	201.68	202.33	202.87	205.82	209.30	V10.45
196.0	200.41	201.05	201.70	202.34	202.88	205.90	209.60	V10.46
196.1	200.42	201.06	201.71	202.35	202.90	205.91	209.69	V10.47
196.2	200.43	201.07	201.72	202.36	202.91	205.92	209.70	V10.48
196.3	200.44	201.08	201.73	202.37	202.92	206.00	209.71	V10.49
196.5	200.45	201.10	201.74	202.38	202.93	206.01	209.75	V10.50
196.6	200.46	201.11	201.75	202.40	202.94	206.02	209.79	V10.51
196.8	200.47	201.12	201.76	202.41	202.95	206.10	229.8	V10.52
196.9	200.48	201.13	201.77	202.42	202.96	206.11	229.9	V10.53
198.89	200.50	201.14	201.78	202.43	202.97	206.12	234.8	V10.59
199.0	200.51	201.15	201.90	202.44	202.98	206.20	234.9	V10.60
199.1	200.52	201.16	201.91	202.45	203.00	206.21	238.4	V10.61
199.2	200.53	201.17	201.92	202.46	203.01	206.22	238.5	V10.62
200.00	200.54	201.18	201.93	202.47	203.02	206.80	238.6	V10.63
200.01	200.55	201.20	201.94	202.48	203.10	206.81	238.76	V10.69
200.02	200.56	201.21	201.95	202.50	203.11	206.82	238.79	V10.71
200.03	200.57	201.22	201.96	202.51	203.12	206.90	238.8	V10.72
200.04	200.58	201.23	201.97	202.52	203.80	206.91	238.9	V10.79
200.05	200.60	201.24	201.98	202.53	203.81	206.92	239.81	V10.81
200.06	200.61	201.25	202.00	202.54	203.82	207.00	239.89	V10.82
200.07	200.62	201.26	202.01	202.55	204.00	207.01	239.9	V10.83
200.08	200.63	201.27	202.02	202.56	204.01	207.02	273.2	V10.84
200.10	200.64	201.28	202.03	202.57	204.02	207.10	273.3	V10.85
200.11	200.65	201.40	202.04	202.58	204.10	207.11	273.8	V10.86
200.12	200.66	201.41	202.05	202.60	204.11	207.12	273.9	V10.87
200.13	200.67	201.42	202.06	202.61	204.12	207.20	284.2	V10.88
200.14	200.68	201.43	202.07	202.62	204.20	207.21	289.83	V10.89
200.15	200.70	201.44	202.08	202.63	204.21	207.22	759.6	V10.90
200.16	200.71	201.45	202.10	202.64	204.22	207.80	V10.00	V10.91
200.17	200.72	201.46	202.11	202.65	204.80	207.81	V10.01	V13.22
200.18	200.73	201.47	202.12	202.66	204.81	207.82	V10.02	V58.0
200.20	200.74	201.48	202.13	202.67	204.82	208.00	V10.03	V58.11
200.21	200.75	201.50	202.14	202.68	204.90	208.01	V10.04	V58.12
200.22	200.76	201.51	202.15	202.70	204.91	208.02	V10.05	V67.1
200.23	200.77	201.52	202.16	202.71	204.92	208.10	V10.06	V67.2
200.24	200.78	201.53	202.17	202.72	205.00	208.11	V10.07	V71.1
200.25	200.80	201.54	202.18	202.73	205.01	208.12	V10.09	
200.26	200.81	201.55	202.20	202.74	205.02	208.20	V10.11	
200.27	200.82	201.56	202.21	202.75	205.10	208.21	V10.12	
200.28	200.83	201.57	202.22	202.76	205.11	208.22	V10.20	
200.30	200.84	201.58	202.23	202.77	205.12	208.80	V10.21	
200.31	200.85	201.60	202.24	202.78	205.20	208.81	V10.22	
200.32	200.86	201.61	202.25	202.80	205.21	208.82	V10.29	

SURGICAL

DRG 820	Lymphoma and Leukemia with Major O.R. Procedure with MCC

GMLOS 13.0   **AMLOS 17.1**   **RW 5.8779**   ☑

Principal Diagnosis
159.1	Malignant neoplasm of spleen, not elsewhere classified
176.5	Kaposi's sarcoma of lymph nodes
196*	Secondary and unspecified malignant neoplasm of lymph nodes
200*	Lymphosarcoma and reticulosarcoma and other specified malignant tumors of lymphatic tissue
201*	Hodgkin's disease
202.0*	Nodular lymphoma
202.1*	Mycosis fungoides
202.2*	Sezary's disease
202.3*	Malignant histiocytosis
202.4*	Leukemic reticuloendotheliosis
202.6*	Malignant mast cell tumors
202.7*	Peripheral T-cell lymphoma
202.8*	Other malignant lymphomas
202.9*	Other and unspecified malignant neoplasms of lymphoid and histiocytic tissue
203*	Multiple myeloma and immunoproliferative neoplasms
204*	Lymphoid leukemia
205*	Myeloid leukemia
206*	Monocytic leukemia
207*	Other specified leukemia
208*	Leukemia of unspecified cell type
209.71	Secondary neuroendocrine tumor of distant lymph nodes
238.4	Neoplasm of uncertain behavior of polycythemia vera
238.5	Neoplasm of uncertain behavior of histiocytic and mast cells
238.6	Neoplasm of uncertain behavior of plasma cells
238.76	Myelofibrosis with myeloid metaplasia
238.79	Other lymphatic and hematopoietic tissues
273.2	Other paraproteinemias
273.3	Macroglobulinemia
284.2	Myelophthisis
289.83	Myelofibrosis

Operating Room Procedures
01.12	Open biopsy of cerebral meninges
01.14	Open biopsy of brain
01.18	Other diagnostic procedures on brain and cerebral meninges
01.22	Removal of intracranial neurostimulator lead(s)
01.23	Reopening of craniotomy site
01.24	Other craniotomy
01.25	Other craniectomy
01.28	Placement of intracerebral catheter(s) via burr hole(s)
01.31	Incision of cerebral meninges
01.32	Lobotomy and tractotomy
01.39	Other incision of brain
01.4*	Operations on thalamus and globus pallidus
01.5*	Other excision or destruction of brain and meninges
01.6	Excision of lesion of skull
02.2*	Ventriculostomy
02.3*	Extracranial ventricular shunt
02.42	Replacement of ventricular shunt
02.91	Lysis of cortical adhesions
02.93	Implantation or replacement of intracranial neurostimulator lead(s)
02.99	Other operations on skull, brain, and cerebral meninges
03.02	Reopening of laminectomy site
03.09	Other exploration and decompression of spinal canal
03.1	Division of intraspinal nerve root
03.2*	Chordotomy
03.32	Biopsy of spinal cord or spinal meninges
03.39	Other diagnostic procedures on spinal cord and spinal canal structures
03.4	Excision or destruction of lesion of spinal cord or spinal meninges
03.53	Repair of vertebral fracture
03.59	Other repair and plastic operations on spinal cord structures
03.6	Lysis of adhesions of spinal cord and nerve roots
03.7*	Shunt of spinal theca
03.93	Implantation or replacement of spinal neurostimulator lead(s)
03.97	Revision of spinal thecal shunt
03.99	Other operations on spinal cord and spinal canal structures
07.16	Biopsy of thymus
07.8*	Thymectomy
07.9*	Other operations on thymus
17.31	Laparoscopic multiple segmental resection of large intestine
17.33	Laparoscopic right hemicolectomy
17.34	Laparoscopic resection of transverse colon
17.35	Laparoscopic left hemicolectomy
17.36	Laparoscopic sigmoidectomy
17.39	Other laparoscopic partial excision of large intestine
17.62	Laser interstitial thermal therapy [LITT] of lesion or tissue of head and neck under guidance
17.69	Laser interstitial thermal therapy [LITT] of lesion or tissue of other and unspecified site under guidance
32.20	Thoracoscopic excision of lesion or tissue of lung
32.23	Open ablation of lung lesion or tissue
32.25	Thoracoscopic ablation of lung lesion or tissue
32.29	Other local excision or destruction of lesion or tissue of lung
32.3*	Segmental resection of lung
33.28	Open biopsy of lung
34.02	Exploratory thoracotomy
34.22	Mediastinoscopy
34.26	Open biopsy of mediastinum
34.3	Excision or destruction of lesion or tissue of mediastinum
34.4	Excision or destruction of lesion of chest wall
34.51	Decortication of lung
34.52	Thoracoscopic decortication of lung
34.6	Scarification of pleura
37.12	Pericardiotomy
37.24	Biopsy of pericardium
37.31	Pericardiectomy
37.91	Open chest cardiac massage
38.08	Incision of lower limb arteries
39.98	Control of hemorrhage, not otherwise specified
39.99	Other operations on vessels
40.3	Regional lymph node excision
40.4*	Radical excision of cervical lymph nodes
40.5*	Radical excision of other lymph nodes
40.9	Other operations on lymphatic structures
41.2	Splenotomy
41.33	Open biopsy of spleen
41.4*	Excision or destruction of lesion or tissue of spleen
41.5	Total splenectomy
41.93	Excision of accessory spleen
41.94	Transplantation of spleen
41.95	Repair and plastic operations on spleen
41.99	Other operations on spleen
42.1*	Esophagostomy
42.21	Operative esophagoscopy by incision
42.25	Open biopsy of esophagus
42.32	Local excision of other lesion or tissue of esophagus
42.39	Other destruction of lesion or tissue of esophagus
42.4*	Excision of esophagus
42.5*	Intrathoracic anastomosis of esophagus
42.6*	Antesternal anastomosis of esophagus
42.7	Esophagomyotomy
42.82	Suture of laceration of esophagus
42.83	Closure of esophagostomy
42.84	Repair of esophageal fistula, not elsewhere classified

⊤ Transfer DRG   ⑤ Special Payment   ☑ Optimization Potential   ▽ Targeted Potential   * Code Range   ● New DRG   ▲ Revised DRG Title

178   Valid 10/01/2013-09/30/2014   © 2013 OptumInsight, Inc.

MDC 17: Myeloproliferative Diseases   y Differentiated Neoplasms—SURGICAL

42.85	Repair of esophageal stricture
42.86	Production of subcutaneous tunnel without esophageal anastomosis
42.87	Other graft of esophagus
42.89	Other repair of esophagus
43.0	Gastrotomy
43.5	Partial gastrectomy with anastomosis to esophagus
43.6	Partial gastrectomy with anastomosis to duodenum
43.7	Partial gastrectomy with anastomosis to jejunum
43.8*	Other partial gastrectomy
43.9*	Total gastrectomy
44.11	Transabdominal gastroscopy
44.3*	Gastroenterostomy without gastrectomy
44.63	Closure of other gastric fistula
45.02	Other incision of small intestine
45.03	Incision of large intestine
45.11	Transabdominal endoscopy of small intestine
45.31	Other local excision of lesion of duodenum
45.32	Other destruction of lesion of duodenum
45.33	Local excision of lesion or tissue of small intestine, except duodenum
45.34	Other destruction of lesion of small intestine, except duodenum
45.41	Excision of lesion or tissue of large intestine
45.49	Other destruction of lesion of large intestine
45.50	Isolation of intestinal segment, not otherwise specified
45.61	Multiple segmental resection of small intestine
45.62	Other partial resection of small intestine
45.63	Total removal of small intestine
45.71	Open and other multiple segmental resection of large intestine
45.73	Open and other right hemicolectomy
45.74	Open and other resection of transverse colon
45.75	Open and other left hemicolectomy
45.76	Open and other sigmoidectomy
45.79	Other and unspecified partial excision of large intestine
45.8*	Total intra-abdominal colectomy
45.90	Intestinal anastomosis, not otherwise specified
45.91	Small-to-small intestinal anastomosis
45.92	Anastomosis of small intestine to rectal stump
45.93	Other small-to-large intestinal anastomosis
45.94	Large-to-large intestinal anastomosis
45.95	Anastomosis to anus
46.0*	Exteriorization of intestine
46.10	Colostomy, not otherwise specified
46.11	Temporary colostomy
46.13	Permanent colostomy
46.20	Ileostomy, not otherwise specified
46.21	Temporary ileostomy
46.22	Continent ileostomy
46.23	Other permanent ileostomy
46.40	Revision of intestinal stoma, not otherwise specified
46.41	Revision of stoma of small intestine
46.80	Intra-abdominal manipulation of intestine, not otherwise specified
46.81	Intra-abdominal manipulation of small intestine
46.82	Intra-abdominal manipulation of large intestine
46.99	Other operations on intestines
48.4*	Pull-through resection of rectum
48.5*	Abdominoperineal resection of rectum
48.6*	Other resection of rectum
50.12	Open biopsy of liver
50.14	Laparoscopic liver biopsy
50.19	Other diagnostic procedures on liver
51.2*	Cholecystectomy
51.3*	Anastomosis of gallbladder or bile duct
51.42	Common duct exploration for relief of other obstruction
51.43	Insertion of choledochohepatic tube for decompression
51.49	Incision of other bile ducts for relief of obstruction
51.59	Incision of other bile duct

51.93	Closure of other biliary fistula
51.94	Revision of anastomosis of biliary tract
51.95	Removal of prosthetic device from bile duct
51.99	Other operations on biliary tract
52.12	Open biopsy of pancreas
52.19	Other diagnostic procedures on pancreas
52.92	Cannulation of pancreatic duct
54.0	Incision of abdominal wall
54.11	Exploratory laparotomy
54.12	Reopening of recent laparotomy site
54.19	Other laparotomy
54.22	Biopsy of abdominal wall or umbilicus
54.29	Other diagnostic procedures on abdominal region
54.3	Excision or destruction of lesion or tissue of abdominal wall or umbilicus
54.4	Excision or destruction of peritoneal tissue
54.63	Other suture of abdominal wall
54.64	Suture of peritoneum
54.72	Other repair of abdominal wall
54.73	Other repair of peritoneum
54.74	Other repair of omentum
54.75	Other repair of mesentery
54.93	Creation of cutaneoperitoneal fistula
54.94	Creation of peritoneovascular shunt
54.95	Incision of peritoneum
55.24	Open biopsy of kidney
55.29	Other diagnostic procedures on kidney
56.5*	Cutaneous uretero-ileostomy
56.6*	Other external urinary diversion
56.71	Urinary diversion to intestine
56.72	Revision of ureterointestinal anastomosis
56.73	Nephrocystanastomosis, not otherwise specified
56.75	Transureteroureterostomy
56.83	Closure of ureterostomy
56.84	Closure of other fistula of ureter
57.18	Other suprapubic cystostomy
57.21	Vesicostomy
57.22	Revision or closure of vesicostomy
57.34	Open biopsy of bladder
57.39	Other diagnostic procedures on bladder
57.59	Open excision or destruction of other lesion or tissue of bladder
57.6	Partial cystectomy
57.7*	Total cystectomy
57.82	Closure of cystostomy
57.83	Repair of fistula involving bladder and intestine
57.84	Repair of other fistula of bladder
57.88	Other anastomosis of bladder
58.43	Closure of other fistula of urethra
59.00	Retroperitoneal dissection, not otherwise specified
59.02	Other lysis of perirenal or periureteral adhesions
59.03	Laparoscopic lysis of perirenal or periureteral adhesions
59.09	Other incision of perirenal or periureteral tissue
59.1*	Incision of perivesical tissue
59.2*	Diagnostic procedures on perirenal and perivesical tissue
59.91	Excision of perirenal or perivesical tissue
59.92	Other operations on perirenal or perivesical tissue
70.72	Repair of colovaginal fistula
70.73	Repair of rectovaginal fistula
70.74	Repair of other vaginoenteric fistula
70.75	Repair of other fistula of vagina
80.53	Repair of the anulus fibrosus with graft or prosthesis
80.54	Other and unspecified repair of the anulus fibrosus

DRG 821   Lymphoma and Leukemia with Major O.R. Procedure with CC

GMLOS 4.8	AMLOS 6.9	RW 2.4025	☑

Select principal diagnosis and operating room procedures listed under **DRG 820**

Surgical	Medical	CC Indicator	MCC Indicator	Procedure Proxy

DRG 822 **Lymphoma and Leukemia with Major O.R. Procedure without CC/MCC**
      GMLOS 2.2   AMLOS 2.8   RW 1.2336   ☑

Select principal diagnosis and operating room procedures listed under DRG 820

DRG 823 **Lymphoma and Nonacute Leukemia with Other O.R. Procedure with MCC**
      GMLOS 11.3   AMLOS 14.7   RW 4.4850   ☑

Select principal diagnosis listed under DRG 820
AND

Select any other operating room procedures not listed under DRG 820
OR

Nonoperating Room Procedures
92.3*   Stereotactic radiosurgery

DRG 824 **Lymphoma and Nonacute Leukemia with Other O.R. Procedure with CC**
      GMLOS 5.9   AMLOS 7.7   RW 2.1684   ☑

Select principal diagnosis listed under DRG 820

Select any other operating room procedures not listed under DRG 820
OR

Nonoperating Room Procedures
92.3*   Stereotactic radiosurgery

DRG 825 **Lymphoma and Nonacute Leukemia with Other O.R. Procedure without CC/MCC**
      GMLOS 2.9   AMLOS 4.0   RW 1.2935   ☑

Select principal diagnosis listed under DRG 820

Select any other operating room procedures not listed under DRG 820
OR

Nonoperating Room Procedures
92.3*   Stereotactic radiosurgery

DRG 826 **Myeloproliferative Disorders or Poorly Differentiated Neoplasms with Major O.R. Procedure with MCC**
      GMLOS 10.8   AMLOS 14.0   RW 4.9280

Principal Diagnosis
158.0   Malignant neoplasm of retroperitoneum
164.0   Malignant neoplasm of thymus
195.4   Malignant neoplasm of upper limb
195.5   Malignant neoplasm of lower limb
195.8   Malignant neoplasm of other specified sites
198.89   Secondary malignant neoplasm of other specified sites
199.0   Disseminated malignant neoplasm
199.1   Other malignant neoplasm of unspecified site
199.2   Malignant neoplasm associated with transplanted organ
202.5*   Letterer-Siwe disease
209.20   Malignant carcinoid tumor of unknown primary site
209.22   Malignant carcinoid tumor of the thymus
209.29   Malignant carcinoid tumor of other sites
209.30   Malignant poorly differentiated neuroendocrine carcinoma, any site
209.60   Benign carcinoid tumor of unknown primary site
209.69   Benign carcinoid tumor of other sites
209.70   Secondary neuroendocrine tumor, unspecified site
209.75   Secondary Merkel cell carcinoma
209.79   Secondary neuroendocrine tumor of other sites
229.8   Benign neoplasm of other specified sites
229.9   Benign neoplasm of unspecified site
234.8   Carcinoma in situ of other specified sites
234.9   Carcinoma in situ, site unspecified
238.8   Neoplasm of uncertain behavior of other specified sites
238.9   Neoplasm of uncertain behavior, site unspecified
239.8*   Neoplasm of unspecified nature of other specified sites
239.9   Neoplasm of unspecified nature, site unspecified
273.8   Other disorders of plasma protein metabolism
273.9   Unspecified disorder of plasma protein metabolism
759.6   Other congenital hamartoses, not elsewhere classified
V10*   Personal history of malignant neoplasm
V13.22   Personal history of cervical dysplasia
V58.0   Radiotherapy
V58.1*   Encounter for antineoplastic chemotherapy and immunotherapy
V67.1   Radiotherapy follow-up examination
V67.2   Chemotherapy follow-up examination
V71.1   Observation for suspected malignant neoplasm

Select operating room procedures listed under DRG 820

DRG 827 **Myeloproliferative Disorders or Poorly Differentiated Neoplasms with Major O.R. Procedure with CC**
      GMLOS 5.3   AMLOS 6.8   RW 2.2746   ☑

Select principal diagnosis listed under DRG 826 with operating room procedures listed under DRG 820

DRG 828 **Myeloproliferative Disorders or Poorly Differentiated Neoplasms with Major O.R. Procedure without CC/MCC**
      GMLOS 2.7   AMLOS 3.3   RW 1.3642   ☑

Select principal diagnosis listed under DRG 826 with operating room procedures listed under DRG 820

DRG 829 **Myeloproliferative Disorders or Poorly Differentiated Neoplasms with Other O.R. Procedure with CC/MCC**
      GMLOS 6.7   AMLOS 10.2   RW 3.1769   ☑

Select principal diagnosis listed under DRG 826

Select any other operating room procedures not listed under DRG 820
OR

Nonoperating Room Procedures
92.3*   Stereotactic radiosurgery

DRG 830 **Myeloproliferative Disorders or Poorly Differentiated Neoplasms with Other O.R. Procedure without CC/MCC**
      GMLOS 2.4   AMLOS 3.1   RW 1.2781   ☑

Select principal diagnosis listed under DRG 826

Select any other operating room procedures not listed under DRG 820
OR

Nonoperating Room Procedures
92.3*   Stereotactic radiosurgery

MEDICAL

DRG 834 **Acute Leukemia without Major O.R. Procedure with MCC**
      GMLOS 10.3   AMLOS 16.8   RW 5.3828   ☑

Principal Diagnosis
204.0*   Acute lymphoid leukemia
205.0*   Acute myeloid leukemia
206.0*   Acute monocytic leukemia
207.0*   Acute erythremia and erythroleukemia
208.0*   Acute leukemia of unspecified cell type

Ⓣ *Transfer DRG*   ⓈⓅ *Special Payment*   ☑ *Optimization Potential*   ⚁ *Targeted Potential*   * *Code Range*   ● *New DRG*   ▲ *Revised DRG Title*

DRG 835 Acute Leukemia without Major O.R. Procedure with CC
GMLOS 4.6   AMLOS 7.5   RW 2.1606   ☑

Select principal diagnosis listed under DRG 834

DRG 836 Acute Leukemia without Major O.R. Procedure without CC/MCC
GMLOS 2.9   AMLOS 4.3   RW 1.2240   ☑

Select principal diagnosis listed under DRG 834

DRG 837 Chemotherapy with Acute Leukemia as Secondary Diagnosis or with High Dose Chemotherapy Agent with MCC
GMLOS 15.6   AMLOS 21.2   RW 6.0485

Principal Diagnosis
V58.1*   Encounter for antineoplastic chemotherapy and immunotherapy
V67.2   Chemotherapy follow-up examination
AND

Secondary Diagnosis
204.0*   Acute lymphoid leukemia
205.0*   Acute myeloid leukemia
206.0*   Acute monocytic leukemia
207.0*   Acute erythremia and erythroleukemia
208.0*   Acute leukemia of unspecified cell type
OR

Nonoperating Room Procedure
00.15   High-dose infusion interleukin-2 [IL-2]

DRG 838 Chemotherapy with Acute Leukemia as Secondary Diagnosis with CC or High Dose Chemotherapy Agent
GMLOS 6.7   AMLOS 9.7   RW 2.8181   ☑

Select principal and secondary diagnosis or nonoperating procedure listed under DRG 837

DRG 839 Chemotherapy with Acute Leukemia as Secondary Diagnosis without CC/MCC
GMLOS 4.8   AMLOS 5.5   RW 1.3175   ☑

Principal Diagnosis
V58.1*   Encounter for antineoplastic chemotherapy and immunotherapy
V67.2   Chemotherapy follow-up examination
AND

Secondary Diagnosis
204.0*   Acute lymphoid leukemia
205.0*   Acute myeloid leukemia
206.0*   Acute monocytic leukemia
207.0*   Acute erythremia and erythroleukemia
208.0*   Acute leukemia of unspecified cell type

DRG 840 Lymphoma and Nonacute Leukemia with MCC
GMLOS 7.5   AMLOS 10.5   RW 3.0843   ☑Ⓣ

Principal Diagnosis
159.1   Malignant neoplasm of spleen, not elsewhere classified
176.5   Kaposi's sarcoma of lymph nodes
196*   Secondary and unspecified malignant neoplasm of lymph nodes
200*   Lymphosarcoma and reticulosarcoma and other specified malignant tumors of lymphatic tissue
201*   Hodgkin's disease
202.0*   Nodular lymphoma
202.1*   Mycosis fungoides

202.2*   Sezary's disease
202.3*   Malignant histiocytosis
202.4*   Leukemic reticuloendotheliosis
202.6*   Malignant mast cell tumors
202.7*   Peripheral T-cell lymphoma
202.8*   Other malignant lymphomas
202.9*   Other and unspecified malignant neoplasms of lymphoid and histiocytic tissue
203*   Multiple myeloma and immunoproliferative neoplasms
204.1*   Chronic lymphoid leukemia
204.2*   Subacute lymphoid leukemia
204.8*   Other lymphoid leukemia
204.9*   Unspecified lymphoid leukemia
205.1*   Chronic myeloid leukemia
205.2*   Subacute myeloid leukemia
205.3*   Myeloid sarcoma
205.8*   Other myeloid leukemia
205.9*   Unspecified myeloid leukemia
206.1*   Chronic monocytic leukemia
206.2*   Subacute monocytic leukemia
206.8*   Other monocytic leukemia
206.9*   Unspecified monocytic leukemia
207.1*   Chronic erythremia
207.2*   Megakaryocytic leukemia
207.8*   Other specified leukemia
208.1*   Chronic leukemia of unspecified cell type
208.2*   Subacute leukemia of unspecified cell type
208.8*   Other leukemia of unspecified cell type
208.9*   Unspecified leukemia
209.71   Secondary neuroendocrine tumor of distant lymph nodes
238.4   Neoplasm of uncertain behavior of polycythemia vera
238.5   Neoplasm of uncertain behavior of histiocytic and mast cells
238.6   Neoplasm of uncertain behavior of plasma cells
238.76   Myelofibrosis with myeloid metaplasia
238.79   Other lymphatic and hematopoietic tissues
273.2   Other paraproteinemias
273.3   Macroglobulinemia
284.2   Myelophthisis
289.83   Myelofibrosis

DRG 841 Lymphoma and Nonacute Leukemia with CC
GMLOS 4.8   AMLOS 6.3   RW 1.6167   ☑Ⓣ

Select principal diagnosis listed under DRG 840

DRG 842 Lymphoma and Nonacute Leukemia without CC/MCC
GMLOS 3.1   AMLOS 4.1   RW 1.0830   ☑Ⓣ

Select principal diagnosis listed under DRG 840

DRG 843 Other Myeloproliferative Disorders or Poorly Differentiated Neoplasm Diagnoses with MCC
GMLOS 5.3   AMLOS 7.2   RW 1.7768   ☑

Principal Diagnosis
158.0   Malignant neoplasm of retroperitoneum
164.0   Malignant neoplasm of thymus
195.4   Malignant neoplasm of upper limb
195.5   Malignant neoplasm of lower limb
195.8   Malignant neoplasm of other specified sites
198.89   Secondary malignant neoplasm of other specified sites
199*   Malignant neoplasm without specification of site
202.5*   Letterer-Siwe disease
209.20   Malignant carcinoid tumor of unknown primary site
209.22   Malignant carcinoid tumor of the thymus
209.29   Malignant carcinoid tumor of other sites
209.30   Malignant poorly differentiated neuroendocrine carcinoma, any site
209.60   Benign carcinoid tumor of unknown primary site
209.69   Benign carcinoid tumor of other sites

| Surgical | Medical | CC Indicator | MCC Indicator | Procedure Proxy |

209.70	Secondary neuroendocrine tumor, unspecified site
209.75	Secondary Merkel cell carcinoma
209.79	Secondary neuroendocrine tumor of other sites
229.8	Benign neoplasm of other specified sites
229.9	Benign neoplasm of unspecified site
234.8	Carcinoma in situ of other specified sites
234.9	Carcinoma in situ, site unspecified
238.8	Neoplasm of uncertain behavior of other specified sites
238.9	Neoplasm of uncertain behavior, site unspecified
239.8*	Neoplasm of unspecified nature of other specified sites
239.9	Neoplasm of unspecified nature, site unspecified
273.8	Other disorders of plasma protein metabolism
273.9	Unspecified disorder of plasma protein metabolism
759.6	Other congenital hamartoses, not elsewhere classified
V10*	Personal history of malignant neoplasm
V13.22	Personal history of cervical dysplasia
V71.1	Observation for suspected malignant neoplasm

DRG 844 Other Myeloproliferative Disorders or Poorly Differentiated Neoplasm Diagnoses with CC

GMLOS 4.1   AMLOS 5.3   RW 1.1701   ☑

Select principal diagnosis listed under DRG 843

DRG 845 Other Myeloproliferative Disorders or Poorly Differentiated Neoplasm Diagnoses without CC/MCC

GMLOS 2.8   AMLOS 3.7   RW 0.7830   ☑

Select principal diagnosis listed under DRG 843

DRG 846 Chemotherapy without Acute Leukemia as Secondary Diagnosis with MCC

GMLOS 5.7   AMLOS 8.2   RW 2.4337   ☑

Principal Diagnosis

| V58.1* | Encounter for antineoplastic chemotherapy and immunotherapy |
| V67.2 | Chemotherapy follow-up examination |

DRG 847 Chemotherapy without Acute Leukemia as Secondary Diagnosis with CC

GMLOS 3.0   AMLOS 3.6   RW 1.1062   ☑

Select principal diagnosis listed under DRG 846

DRG 848 Chemotherapy without Acute Leukemia as Secondary Diagnosis without CC/MCC

GMLOS 2.5   AMLOS 3.0   RW 0.8635   ☑

Select principal diagnosis listed under DRG 846

DRG 849 Radiotherapy

GMLOS 4.6   AMLOS 6.0   RW 1.4239   ☑

Principal Diagnosis

| V58.0 | Radiotherapy |
| V67.1 | Radiotherapy follow-up examination |

Infectious And Parasitic Diseases

002.0	021.3	038.41	045.23	065.3	081.0	090.5	117.6	488.09
002.1	021.8	038.42	050.0	065.4	081.1	090.6	117.7	488.19
002.2	021.9	038.43	050.1	065.8	081.2	090.7	117.8	488.89
002.3	022.3	038.44	050.2	065.9	081.9	090.9	117.9	780.60
002.9	022.8	038.49	050.9	066.0	082.0	091.2	118	780.61
003.1	022.9	038.8	051.01	066.1	082.1	091.7	120.2	780.62
003.20	023.0	038.9	051.02	066.3	082.2	091.89	120.8	780.63
003.29	023.1	039.8	051.9	066.40	082.3	091.9	120.9	780.66
003.8	023.2	039.9	052.7	066.41	082.40	092.0	121.5	785.52
003.9	023.3	040.0	052.8	066.42	082.41	092.9	121.6	785.59
005.1	023.8	040.1	052.9	066.49	082.49	095.8	121.8	790.7
006.8	023.9	040.3	053.79	066.8	082.8	095.9	121.9	790.8
006.9	024	040.41	053.8	066.9	082.9	096	122.3	795.31
017.90	025	040.42	054.5	072.79	083.0	097.0	122.4	795.39
017.91	026.0	040.82	054.79	072.8	083.1	097.1	122.6	958.3
017.92	026.1	040.89	054.8	072.9	083.2	097.9	122.7	995.90
017.93	026.9	041.00	055.79	073.7	083.8	098.89	122.9	995.91
017.94	027.0	041.01	055.8	073.8	083.9	100.0	124	995.92
017.95	027.1	041.02	055.9	073.9	084.0	100.9	125.0	995.93
017.96	027.2	041.03	056.79	074.3	084.1	102.7	125.1	995.94
018.00	027.8	041.04	056.8	074.8	084.2	102.8	125.2	998.51
018.01	027.9	041.05	056.9	075	084.3	102.9	125.3	998.59
018.02	030.0	041.09	057.0	078.2	084.4	103.2	125.4	999.0
018.03	030.1	041.10	057.8	078.4	084.5	103.9	125.5	999.34
018.04	030.2	041.11	057.9	078.5	084.6	104.0	125.6	999.39
018.05	030.3	041.12	058.10	078.7	084.7	104.8	125.7	V08
018.06	030.8	041.19	058.11	078.88	084.8	104.9	125.9	V09.0
018.80	030.9	041.2	058.12	078.89	084.9	112.5	127.8	V09.1
018.81	031.2	041.3	059.00	079.0	085.0	112.89	128.0	V09.2
018.82	031.8	041.41	059.01	079.1	085.9	112.9	128.1	V09.3
018.83	031.9	041.42	059.09	079.2	086.1	114.3	128.8	V09.4
018.84	032.89	041.43	059.10	079.3	086.2	114.9	128.9	V09.50
018.85	032.9	041.49	059.11	079.4	086.3	115.00	130.7	V09.51
018.86	034.1	041.5	059.12	079.50	086.4	115.09	130.8	V09.6
018.90	036.2	041.6	059.19	079.51	086.5	115.10	130.9	V09.70
018.91	036.3	041.7	059.20	079.52	086.9	115.19	131.8	V09.71
018.92	036.89	041.81	059.21	079.53	087.0	115.90	131.9	V09.80
018.93	036.9	041.82	059.22	079.59	087.1	115.99	136.0	V09.81
018.94	037	041.83	059.8	079.6	087.9	116.0	136.21	V09.90
018.95	038.0	041.84	059.9	079.81	088.0	116.1	136.29	V09.91
018.96	038.10	041.85	060.0	079.82	088.81	116.2	136.4	
020.0	038.11	041.86	060.1	079.83	088.82	117.0	136.5	
020.1	038.12	041.89	060.9	079.88	088.89	117.1	136.8	
020.2	038.19	041.9	061	079.89	088.9	117.2	136.9	
020.8	038.2	045.20	065.0	079.98	090.0	117.3	137.4	
020.9	038.3	045.21	065.1	079.99	090.1	117.4	139.8	
021.0	038.40	045.22	065.2	080	090.2	117.5	487.8	

SURGICAL

DRG 853   Infectious and Parasitic Diseases with O.R. Procedure with MCC

| GMLOS 11.1 | AMLOS 14.3 | RW 5.3491 | ☑T |

Select any principal diagnosis from MDC 18 excluding

958.3	Posttraumatic wound infection not elsewhere classified
998.51	Infected postoperative seroma
998.59	Other postoperative infection
999.39	Complications of medical care, NEC, infection following other infusion, injection, transfusion, or vaccination

AND

Select any operating room procedure

DRG 854   Infectious and Parasitic Diseases with O.R. Procedure with CC

| GMLOS 7.0 | AMLOS 8.5 | RW 2.4891 | ☑T |

Select principal diagnosis and operating room procedure listed under DRG 853

DRG 855   Infectious and Parasitic Diseases with O.R. Procedure without CC/MCC

| GMLOS 3.6 | AMLOS 4.9 | RW 1.5849 | ☑T |

Select principal diagnosis and operating room procedure listed under DRG 853

DRG 856   Postoperative or Posttraumatic Infections with O.R. Procedure with MCC

| GMLOS 10.1 | AMLOS 13.4 | RW 4.7874 | ☑T |

Principal Diagnosis

958.3	Posttraumatic wound infection not elsewhere classified
998.51	Infected postoperative seroma
998.59	Other postoperative infection
999.34	Acute infection following transfusion, infusion, or injection of blood and blood products
999.39	Complications of medical care, NEC, infection following other infusion, injection, transfusion, or vaccination

AND

Select any operating room procedure

DRG 857   Postoperative or Posttraumatic Infections with O.R. Procedure with CC

| GMLOS 5.7 | AMLOS 7.1 | RW 2.0412 | ☑T |

Select principal diagnosis and operating room procedure listed under DRG 856

DRG 858   Postoperative or Posttraumatic Infections with O.R. Procedure without CC/MCC

| GMLOS 3.9 | AMLOS 4.8 | RW 1.3115 | ☑T |

Select principal diagnosis and operating room procedure listed under DRG 856

MEDICAL

DRG 862   Postoperative and Posttraumatic Infections with MCC

| GMLOS 5.6 | AMLOS 7.4 | RW 1.8903 | ☑T |

Principal Diagnosis

958.3	Posttraumatic wound infection not elsewhere classified
998.5*	Postoperative infection, not elsewhere classified

DRG 863   Postoperative and Posttraumatic Infections without MCC

| GMLOS 3.8 | AMLOS 4.6 | RW 0.9845 | ☑T |

Select principal diagnosis listed under DRG 862

DRG 864   Fever

| GMLOS 2.9 | AMLOS 3.6 | RW 0.8441 | ☑ |

Principal Diagnosis

780.60	Fever, unspecified
780.61	Fever presenting with conditions classified elsewhere
780.62	Postprocedural fever
780.63	Postvaccination fever
780.66	Febrile nonhemolytic transfusion reaction

DRG 865   Viral Illness with MCC

| GMLOS 4.9 | AMLOS 6.8 | RW 1.7351 | ☑ |

Principal Diagnosis

045.2*	Acute nonparalytic poliomyelitis
050*	Smallpox
051.0*	Cowpox and vaccinia not from vaccination
051.9	Unspecified paravaccinia
052.7	Chickenpox with other specified complications
052.8	Chickenpox with unspecified complication
052.9	Varicella without mention of complication
053.79	Other specified herpes zoster complications
053.8	Unspecified herpes zoster complication
054.79	Other specified herpes simplex complications
054.8	Unspecified herpes simplex complication
055.79	Other specified measles complications
055.8	Unspecified measles complication
055.9	Measles without mention of complication
056.79	Rubella with other specified complications
056.8	Unspecified rubella complications
056.9	Rubella without mention of complication
057*	Other viral exanthemata
058.10	Roseola infantum, unspecified
058.11	Roseola infantum due to human herpesvirus 6
058.12	Roseola infantum due to human herpesvirus 7
059*	Other poxvirus infections
060*	Yellow fever
061	Dengue
065*	Arthropod-borne hemorrhagic fever
066.0	Phlebotomus fever
066.1	Tick-borne fever
066.3	Other mosquito-borne fever
066.4*	West Nile fever
066.8	Other specified arthropod-borne viral diseases
066.9	Unspecified arthropod-borne viral disease
072.79	Mumps with other specified complications
072.8	Unspecified mumps complication
072.9	Mumps without mention of complication
073.7	Ornithosis with other specified complications
073.8	Ornithosis with unspecified complication
073.9	Unspecified ornithosis
074.3	Hand, foot, and mouth disease
074.8	Other specified diseases due to Coxsackievirus
075	Infectious mononucleosis

T Transfer DRG   SP Special Payment   ☑ Optimization Potential   ᵀᴾ Targeted Potential   * Code Range   ● New DRG   ▲ Revised DRG Title

078.2	Sweating fever
078.4	Foot and mouth disease
078.5	Cytomegaloviral disease
078.7	Arenaviral hemorrhagic fever
078.88	Other specified diseases due to Chlamydiae
078.89	Other specified diseases due to viruses
079*	Viral and chlamydial infection in conditions classified elsewhere and of unspecified site
487.8	Influenza with other manifestations
488.09	Influenza due to identified avian influenza virus with other manifestations
488.19	Influenza due to identified 2009 H1N1 influenza virus with other manifestations
488.89	Influenza due to identified novel influenza A virus with other manifestations
790.8	Unspecified viremia
999.0	Generalized vaccinia as complication of medical care, not elsewhere classified
V08	Asymptomatic human immunodeficiency virus (HIV) infection status

DRG 866 Viral Illness without MCC

GMLOS 2.9   **AMLOS 3.5**   **RW 0.7855**   ☑

Select principal diagnosis listed under DRG 865

DRG 867 Other Infectious and Parasitic Diseases Diagnoses with MCC

GMLOS 6.8   **AMLOS 9.2**   **RW 2.6139**   ☑ⓣ

Principal Diagnosis

002*	Typhoid and paratyphoid fevers
003.20	Unspecified localized salmonella infection
003.29	Other localized salmonella infections
003.8	Other specified salmonella infections
003.9	Unspecified salmonella infection
005.1	Botulism food poisoning
006.8	Amebic infection of other sites
006.9	Unspecified amebiasis
017.9*	Tuberculosis of other specified organs
018.0*	Acute miliary tuberculosis
018.8*	Other specified miliary tuberculosis
018.9*	Unspecified miliary tuberculosis
020.0	Bubonic plague
020.1	Cellulocutaneous plague
020.8	Other specified types of plague
020.9	Unspecified plague
021.0	Ulceroglandular tularemia
021.3	Oculoglandular tularemia
021.8	Other specified tularemia
021.9	Unspecified tularemia
022.8	Other specified manifestations of anthrax
022.9	Unspecified anthrax
023*	Brucellosis
024	Glanders
025	Melioidosis
026*	Rat-bite fever
027*	Other zoonotic bacterial diseases
030*	Leprosy
031.2	Disseminated diseases due to other mycobacteria
031.8	Other specified diseases due to other mycobacteria
031.9	Unspecified diseases due to mycobacteria
032.89	Other specified diphtheria
032.9	Unspecified diphtheria
034.1	Scarlet fever
037	Tetanus
039.8	Actinomycotic infection of other specified sites
039.9	Actinomycotic infection of unspecified site
040.0	Gas gangrene
040.1	Rhinoscleroma
040.3	Necrobacillosis
040.41	Infant botulism
040.42	Wound botulism
040.82	Toxic shock syndrome
040.89	Other specified bacterial diseases
041*	Bacterial infection in conditions classified elsewhere and of unspecified site
080	Louse-borne (epidemic) typhus
081*	Other typhus
082*	Tick-borne rickettsioses
083*	Other rickettsioses
084*	Malaria
085.0	Visceral leishmaniasis (kala-azar)
085.9	Unspecified leishmaniasis
086.1	Chagas' disease with other organ involvement
086.2	Chagas' disease without mention of organ involvement
086.3	Gambian trypanosomiasis
086.4	Rhodesian trypanosomiasis
086.5	African trypanosomiasis, unspecified
086.9	Unspecified trypanosomiasis
087*	Relapsing fever
088*	Other arthropod-borne diseases
090.0	Early congenital syphilis, symptomatic
090.1	Early congenital syphilis, latent
090.2	Unspecified early congenital syphilis
090.5	Other late congenital syphilis, symptomatic
090.6	Late congenital syphilis, latent
090.7	Late congenital syphilis, unspecified
090.9	Congenital syphilis, unspecified
091.2	Other primary syphilis
091.7	Early syphilis, secondary syphilis, relapse
091.89	Early syphilis, other forms of secondary syphilis
091.9	Early syphilis, unspecified secondary syphilis
092*	Early syphilis, latent
095.8	Other specified forms of late symptomatic syphilis
095.9	Unspecified late symptomatic syphilis
096	Late syphilis, latent
097*	Other and unspecified syphilis
098.89	Gonococcal infection of other specified sites
100.0	Leptospirosis icterohemorrhagica
100.9	Unspecified leptospirosis
102.7	Other manifestations due to yaws
102.8	Latent yaws
102.9	Unspecified yaws
103.2	Late lesions of pinta
103.9	Unspecified pinta
104*	Other spirochetal infection
112.5	Disseminated candidiasis
112.89	Other candidiasis of other specified sites
112.9	Candidiasis of unspecified site
114.3	Other forms of progressive coccidioidomycosis
114.9	Unspecified coccidioidomycosis
115.00	Histoplasma capsulatum, without mention of manifestation
115.09	Histoplasma capsulatum, with mention of other manifestation
115.10	Histoplasma duboisii, without mention of manifestation
115.19	Histoplasma duboisii with mention of other manifestation
115.90	Unspecified Histoplasmosis without mention of manifestation
115.99	Unspecified Histoplasmosis with mention of other manifestation
116*	Blastomycotic infection
117*	Other mycoses
118	Opportunistic mycoses
120.2	Schistosomiasis due to schistosoma japonicum
120.8	Other specified schistosomiasis
120.9	Unspecified schistosomiasis
121.5	Metagonimiasis
121.6	Heterophyiasis
121.8	Other specified trematode infections

Surgical	Medical	CC Indicator	MCC Indicator	Procedure Proxy

121.9	Unspecified trematode infection
122.3	Other echinococcus granulosus infection
122.4	Unspecified echinococcus granulosus infection
122.6	Other echinococcus multilocularis infection
122.7	Unspecified echinococcus multilocularis infection
122.9	Other and unspecified echinococcosis
124	Trichinosis
125*	Filarial infection and dracontiasis
127.8	Mixed intestinal helminthiasis
128*	Other and unspecified helminthiases
130.7	Toxoplasmosis of other specified sites
130.8	Multisystemic disseminated toxoplasmosis
130.9	Unspecified toxoplasmosis
131.8	Trichomoniasis of other specified sites
131.9	Unspecified trichomoniasis
136.0	Ainhum
136.2*	Specific infections by free-living amebae
136.4	Psorospermiasis
136.5	Sarcosporidiosis
136.8	Other specified infectious and parasitic diseases
136.9	Unspecified infectious and parasitic diseases
137.4	Late effects of tuberculosis of other specified organs
139.8	Late effects of other and unspecified infectious and parasitic diseases
795.3*	Nonspecific positive culture findings
999.34	Acute infection following transfusion, infusion, or injection of blood and blood products
999.39	Complications of medical care, NEC, infection following other infusion, injection, transfusion, or vaccination
V09*	Infection with drug-resistant microorganisms

DRG 868 Other Infectious and Parasitic Diseases Diagnoses with CC
GMLOS 4.0   AMLOS 5.0   RW 1.0775 ☑Ⓣ

Select principal diagnosis listed under DRG 867

DRG 869 Other Infectious and Parasitic Diseases Diagnoses without CC/MCC
GMLOS 2.9   AMLOS 3.5   RW 0.7406 ☑Ⓣ

Select principal diagnosis listed under DRG 867

DRG 870 Septicemia or Severe Sepsis with Mechanical Ventilation 96+ Hours
GMLOS 12.5   AMLOS 14.6   RW 5.9187 ▽Ⓣ

Principal Diagnosis

003.1	Salmonella septicemia
020.2	Septicemic plague
022.3	Anthrax septicemia
036.2	Meningococcemia
036.3	Waterhouse-Friderichsen syndrome, meningococcal
036.89	Other specified meningococcal infections
036.9	Unspecified meningococcal infection
038*	Septicemia
054.5	Herpetic septicemia
785.52	Septic shock
785.59	Other shock without mention of trauma
790.7	Bacteremia
995.9*	Systemic inflammatory response syndrome (SIRS)

AND

Nonoperating Room Procedure

96.72	Continuous invasive mechanical ventilation for 96 consecutive hours or more

DRG 871 Septicemia or Severe Sepsis without Mechanical Ventilation 96+ Hours with MCC
GMLOS 5.1   AMLOS 6.7   RW 1.8527 ☑▽Ⓣ

Principal Diagnosis

003.1	Salmonella septicemia
020.2	Septicemic plague
022.3	Anthrax septicemia
036.2	Meningococcemia
036.3	Waterhouse-Friderichsen syndrome, meningococcal
036.89	Other specified meningococcal infections
036.9	Unspecified meningococcal infection
038*	Septicemia
054.5	Herpetic septicemia
785.52	Septic shock
785.59	Other shock without mention of trauma
790.7	Bacteremia
995.9*	Systemic inflammatory response syndrome (SIRS)

DRG 872 Septicemia or Severe Sepsis without Mechanical Ventilation 96+ Hours without MCC
GMLOS 4.1   AMLOS 4.9   RW 1.0687 ☑▽Ⓣ

Select principal diagnosis listed under DRG 871

Mental Diseases And Disorders

290.0	295.24	296.01	296.64	300.22	302.72	308.9	313.1	327.15
290.10	295.25	296.02	296.65	300.23	302.73	309.0	313.21	327.19
290.11	295.30	296.03	296.66	300.29	302.74	309.1	313.22	388.45
290.12	295.31	296.04	296.7	300.3	302.75	309.21	313.23	758.0
290.13	295.32	296.05	296.80	300.4	302.76	309.22	313.3	758.1
290.20	295.33	296.06	296.81	300.5	302.79	309.23	313.81	758.2
290.21	295.34	296.10	296.82	300.6	302.81	309.24	313.82	758.31
290.3	295.35	296.11	296.89	300.7	302.82	309.28	313.83	758.32
290.40	295.40	296.12	296.90	300.81	302.83	309.29	313.89	758.33
290.41	295.41	296.13	296.99	300.82	302.84	309.3	313.9	758.39
290.42	295.42	296.14	297.0	300.89	302.85	309.4	314.00	759.83
290.43	295.43	296.15	297.1	300.9	302.89	309.81	314.01	780.02
290.8	295.44	296.16	297.2	301.0	302.9	309.82	314.1	780.1
290.9	295.45	296.20	297.3	301.10	306.7	309.83	314.2	780.50
293.0	295.50	296.21	297.8	301.11	306.8	309.89	314.8	780.52
293.1	295.51	296.22	297.9	301.12	306.9	309.9	314.9	780.54
293.81	295.52	296.23	298.0	301.13	307.0	310.0	315.00	780.55
293.82	295.53	296.24	298.1	301.20	307.1	310.1	315.01	780.56
293.83	295.54	296.25	298.2	301.21	307.3	310.9	315.02	780.58
293.84	295.55	296.26	298.3	301.22	307.40	311	315.09	780.59
293.89	295.60	296.30	298.4	301.3	307.41	312.00	315.1	784.60
293.9	295.61	296.31	298.8	301.4	307.42	312.01	315.2	784.61
294.0	295.62	296.32	298.9	301.50	307.43	312.02	315.31	784.69
294.10	295.63	296.33	299.00	301.51	307.44	312.03	315.32	797
294.11	295.64	296.34	299.01	301.59	307.45	312.10	315.34	799.21
294.20	295.65	296.35	299.10	301.6	307.46	312.11	315.39	799.22
294.21	295.70	296.36	299.11	301.7	307.47	312.12	315.4	799.23
294.8	295.71	296.40	299.80	301.81	307.48	312.13	315.5	799.24
294.9	295.72	296.41	299.81	301.82	307.49	312.20	315.8	799.25
295.00	295.73	296.42	299.90	301.83	307.50	312.21	315.9	799.29
295.01	295.74	296.43	299.91	301.84	307.51	312.22	316	799.51
295.02	295.75	296.44	300.00	301.89	307.52	312.23	317	799.52
295.03	295.80	296.45	300.01	301.9	307.53	312.30	318.0	799.54
295.04	295.81	296.46	300.02	302.0	307.54	312.31	318.1	799.55
295.05	295.82	296.50	300.09	302.1	307.59	312.32	318.2	799.59
295.10	295.83	296.51	300.10	302.2	307.6	312.33	319	V62.84
295.11	295.84	296.52	300.11	302.3	307.7	312.34	327.00	V71.01
295.12	295.85	296.53	300.12	302.4	307.80	312.35	327.01	V71.02
295.13	295.90	296.54	300.13	302.50	307.89	312.39	327.02	V71.09
295.14	295.91	296.55	300.14	302.51	307.9	312.4	327.09	
295.15	295.92	296.56	300.15	302.52	308.0	312.81	327.10	
295.20	295.93	296.60	300.16	302.53	308.1	312.82	327.11	
295.21	295.94	296.61	300.19	302.6	308.2	312.89	327.12	
295.22	295.95	296.62	300.20	302.70	308.3	312.9	327.13	
295.23	296.00	296.63	300.21	302.71	308.4	313.0	327.14	

MDC 19: Mental Diseases And Disorders—SURGICAL

SURGICAL

DRG 876   O.R. Procedure with Principal Diagnoses of Mental Illness
GMLOS 7.5   AMLOS 12.3   RW 2.8172

Select any operating room procedure

MEDICAL

DRG 880   Acute Adjustment Reaction and Psychosocial Dysfunction
GMLOS 2.2   AMLOS 2.9   RW 0.6388   ☑ ▽

Principal Diagnosis

293.0	Delirium due to conditions classified elsewhere
293.1	Subacute delirium
293.9	Unspecified transient mental disorder in conditions classified elsewhere
300.0*	Anxiety states
300.10	Hysteria, unspecified
300.11	Conversion disorder
300.12	Dissociative amnesia
300.13	Dissociative fugue
300.15	Dissociative disorder or reaction, unspecified
300.16	Factitious disorder with predominantly psychological signs and symptoms
300.19	Other and unspecified factitious illness
300.9	Unspecified nonpsychotic mental disorder
308*	Acute reaction to stress
780.1	Hallucinations
799.21	Nervousness
799.22	Irritability
799.25	Demoralization and apathy
799.29	Other signs and symptoms involving emotional state
V62.84	Suicidal ideation
V71.01	Observation of adult antisocial behavior
V71.02	Observation of childhood or adolescent antisocial behavior

DRG 881   Depressive Neuroses
GMLOS 3.2   AMLOS 4.4   RW 0.6541   ☑

Principal Diagnosis

300.4	Dysthymic disorder
301.12	Chronic depressive personality disorder
309.0	Adjustment disorder with depressed mood
309.1	Prolonged depressive reaction as adjustment reaction
311	Depressive disorder, not elsewhere classified

DRG 882   Neuroses Except Depressive
GMLOS 3.2   AMLOS 4.4   RW 0.6953   ☑

Principal Diagnosis

300.2*	Phobic disorders
300.3	Obsessive-compulsive disorders
300.5	Neurasthenia
300.6	Depersonalization disorder
300.7	Hypochondriasis
300.8*	Somatoform disorders
306.7	Malfunction of organs of special sense arising from mental factors
306.9	Unspecified psychophysiological malfunction
307.53	Rumination disorder
307.54	Psychogenic vomiting
307.80	Psychogenic pain, site unspecified
307.89	Other pain disorder related to psychological factors
309.2*	Predominant disturbance of other emotions as adjustment reaction

309.3	Adjustment disorder with disturbance of conduct
309.4	Adjustment disorder with mixed disturbance of emotions and conduct
309.8*	Other specified adjustment reactions
309.9	Unspecified adjustment reaction
313.0	Overanxious disorder specific to childhood and adolescence
313.1	Misery and unhappiness disorder specific to childhood and adolescence
799.23	Impulsiveness

DRG 883   Disorders of Personality and Impulse Control
GMLOS 4.7   AMLOS 7.7   RW 1.2682

Principal Diagnosis

300.14	Dissociative identity disorder
301.0	Paranoid personality disorder
301.10	Affective personality disorder, unspecified
301.11	Chronic hypomanic personality disorder
301.13	Cyclothymic disorder
301.2*	Schizoid personality disorder
301.3	Explosive personality disorder
301.4	Obsessive-compulsive personality disorder
301.5*	Histrionic personality disorder
301.6	Dependent personality disorder
301.7	Antisocial personality disorder
301.8*	Other personality disorders
301.9	Unspecified personality disorder
307.1	Anorexia nervosa
312.31	Pathological gambling
312.32	Kleptomania
312.34	Intermittent explosive disorder
312.35	Isolated explosive disorder
312.39	Other disorder of impulse control
799.24	Emotional lability

DRG 884   Organic Disturbances and Mental Retardation
GMLOS 4.0   AMLOS 5.7   RW 1.0060   ☑ Ⓣ

Principal Diagnosis

290*	Dementias
293.8*	Other specified transient mental disorders due to conditions classified elsewhere
294*	Persistent mental disorders due to conditions classified elsewhere
299.0*	Autistic disorder
299.1*	Childhood disintegrative disorder
307.9	Other and unspecified special symptom or syndrome, not elsewhere classified
310.0	Frontal lobe syndrome
310.1	Personality change due to conditions classified elsewhere
310.9	Unspecified nonpsychotic mental disorder following organic brain damage
316	Psychic factors associated with diseases classified elsewhere
317	Mild intellectual disabilities
318*	Other specified intellectual disabilities
319	Unspecified intellectual disabilities
758.0	Down's syndrome
758.1	Patau's syndrome
758.2	Edwards' syndrome
758.3*	Autosomal deletion syndromes
759.83	Fragile X syndrome
780.02	Transient alteration of awareness
797	Senility without mention of psychosis
799.52	Cognitive communication deficit
799.54	Psychomotor deficit
799.55	Frontal lobe and executive function deficit
799.59	Other signs and symptoms involving cognition

Ⓣ *Transfer DRG*   ⑤ *Special Payment*   ☑ *Optimization Potential*   ▽ *Targeted Potential*   * *Code Range*   ● *New DRG*   ▲ *Revised DRG Title*

188   Valid 10/01/2013–09/30/2014   © 2013 OptumInsight, Inc.

DRG 885 **Psychoses**

GMLOS 5.4   AMLOS 7.3   RW 1.0048   ▽

Principal Diagnosis

295*	Schizophrenic disorders
296*	Episodic mood disorders
297*	Delusional disorders
298.0	Depressive type psychosis
298.1	Excitative type psychosis
298.3	Acute paranoid reaction
298.4	Psychogenic paranoid psychosis
298.8	Other and unspecified reactive psychosis
298.9	Unspecified psychosis
299.8*	Other specified pervasive developmental disorders
299.9*	Unspecified pervasive developmental disorder

DRG 886 **Behavioral and Developmental Disorders**

GMLOS 4.2   AMLOS 7.1   RW 0.9173

Principal Diagnosis

307.52	Pica
307.6	Enuresis
307.7	Encopresis
312.0*	Undersocialized conduct disorder, aggressive type
312.1*	Undersocialized conduct disorder, unaggressive type
312.2*	Socialized conduct disorder
312.30	Impulse control disorder, unspecified
312.33	Pyromania
312.4	Mixed disturbance of conduct and emotions
312.8*	Other specified disturbances of conduct, not elsewhere classified
312.9	Unspecified disturbance of conduct
313.2*	Sensitivity, shyness, and social withdrawal disorder specific to childhood and adolescence
313.3	Relationship problems specific to childhood and adolescence
313.8*	Other or mixed emotional disturbances of childhood or adolescence
313.9	Unspecified emotional disturbance of childhood or adolescence
314*	Hyperkinetic syndrome of childhood
315.00	Developmental reading disorder, unspecified
315.01	Alexia
315.02	Developmental dyslexia
315.09	Other specific developmental reading disorder
315.1	Mathematics disorder
315.2	Other specific developmental learning difficulties
315.31	Expressive language disorder
315.32	Mixed receptive-expressive language disorder
315.34	Speech and language developmental delay due to hearing loss
315.39	Other developmental speech or language disorder
315.4	Developmental coordination disorder
315.5	Mixed development disorder
315.8	Other specified delay in development
315.9	Unspecified delay in development
388.45	Acquired auditory processing disorder
784.61	Alexia and dyslexia
784.69	Other symbolic dysfunction
799.51	Attention or concentration deficit

DRG 887 **Other Mental Disorder Diagnoses**

GMLOS 2.9   AMLOS 4.5   RW 0.9795   ☑

Principal Diagnosis

298.2	Reactive confusion
302*	Sexual and gender identity disorders
306.8	Other specified psychophysiological malfunction
307.0	Adult onset fluency disorder
307.3	Stereotypic movement disorder

307.4*	Specific disorders of sleep of nonorganic origin
307.50	Eating disorder, unspecified
307.51	Bulimia nervosa
307.59	Other disorder of eating
327.0*	Organic disorders of initiating and maintaining sleep [Organic insomnia]
327.1*	Organic disorders of excessive somnolence [Organic hypersomnia]
780.50	Unspecified sleep disturbance
780.52	Insomnia, unspecified
780.54	Hypersomnia, unspecified
780.55	Disruption of 24 hour sleep wake cycle, unspecified
780.56	Dysfunctions associated with sleep stages or arousal from sleep
780.58	Sleep related movement disorder, unspecified
780.59	Other sleep disturbances
784.60	Symbolic dysfunction, unspecified
V71.09	Observation of other suspected mental condition

Surgical	Medical	CC Indicator	MCC Indicator	Procedure Proxy

Valid 10/01/2013–09/30/2014

291.0	292.12	303.03	304.13	304.43	304.73	305.03	305.43	305.73
291.1	292.2	303.90	304.20	304.50	304.80	305.20	305.50	305.80
291.2	292.81	303.91	304.21	304.51	304.81	305.21	305.51	305.81
291.3	292.82	303.92	304.22	304.52	304.82	305.22	305.52	305.82
291.4	292.83	303.93	304.23	304.53	304.83	305.23	305.53	305.83
291.5	292.84	304.00	304.30	304.60	304.90	305.30	305.60	305.90
291.81	292.85	304.01	304.31	304.61	304.91	305.31	305.61	305.91
291.82	292.89	304.02	304.32	304.62	304.92	305.32	305.62	305.92
291.89	292.9	304.03	304.33	304.63	304.93	305.33	305.63	305.93
291.9	303.00	304.10	304.40	304.70	305.00	305.40	305.70	790.3
292.0	303.01	304.11	304.41	304.71	305.01	305.41	305.71	
292.11	303.02	304.12	304.42	304.72	305.02	305.42	305.72	

MEDICAL

DRG 894   Alcohol/Drug Abuse or Dependence, Left Against Medical Advice

GMLOS 2.1   AMLOS 2.9   RW 0.4509   ☑

Select principal diagnosis in MDC 20
AND

Discharge status of against medical advice (AMA)

DRG 895   Alcohol/Drug Abuse or Dependence with Rehabilitation Therapy

GMLOS 9.1   AMLOS 11.7   RW 1.1939   ☑

Principal Diagnosis

291*	Alcohol-induced mental disorders
292*	Drug-induced mental disorders
303.0*	Acute alcoholic intoxication
303.9*	Other and unspecified alcohol dependence
304*	Drug dependence
305.0*	Nondependent alcohol abuse
305.2*	Nondependent cannabis abuse
305.3*	Nondependent hallucinogen abuse
305.4*	Nondependent sedative, hypnotic or anxiolytic abuse
305.5*	Nondependent opioid abuse
305.6*	Nondependent cocaine abuse
305.7*	Nondependent amphetamine or related acting sympathomimetic abuse
305.8*	Nondependent antidepressant type abuse
305.9*	Other, mixed, or unspecified nondependent drug abuse
790.3	Excessive blood level of alcohol

AND

Nonoperating Room Procedures

94.61	Alcohol rehabilitation
94.63	Alcohol rehabilitation and detoxification
94.64	Drug rehabilitation
94.66	Drug rehabilitation and detoxification
94.67	Combined alcohol and drug rehabilitation
94.69	Combined alcohol and drug rehabilitation and detoxification

DRG 896   Alcohol/Drug Abuse or Dependence without Rehabilitation Therapy with MCC

GMLOS 4.7   AMLOS 6.5   RW 1.5146   ☑Ⓣ

Select only principal diagnosis listed under DRG 895

DRG 897   Alcohol/Drug Abuse or Dependence without Rehabilitation Therapy without MCC

GMLOS 3.2   AMLOS 4.0   RW 0.6824   ☑Ⓣ

Select only principal diagnosis listed under DRG 895

Surgical	Medical	CC Indicator	MCC Indicator	Procedure Proxy

238.77	900.02	903.9	958.93	964.8	971.1	978.8	989.6	995.63
349.31	900.03	904.0	958.99	964.9	971.2	978.9	989.7	995.64
349.39	900.1	904.1	959.01	965.00	971.3	979.0	989.81	995.65
796.0	900.81	904.2	959.09	965.01	971.9	979.1	989.82	995.66
819.0	900.82	904.3	959.11	965.02	972.0	979.2	989.83	995.67
819.1	900.89	904.40	959.12	965.09	972.1	979.3	989.84	995.68
828.0	900.9	904.41	959.13	965.1	972.2	979.4	989.89	995.69
828.1	901.0	904.42	959.14	965.4	972.3	979.5	989.9	995.7
862.8	901.1	904.50	959.19	965.5	972.4	979.6	990	995.80
862.9	901.2	904.51	959.2	965.61	972.5	979.7	991.0	995.81
868.09	901.3	904.52	959.3	965.69	972.6	979.9	991.1	995.82
868.19	901.40	904.53	959.4	965.7	972.7	980.0	991.2	995.83
869.0	901.41	904.54	959.5	965.8	972.8	980.1	991.3	995.84
869.1	901.42	904.6	959.6	965.9	972.9	980.2	991.4	995.85
875.1	901.81	904.7	959.7	966.0	973.0	980.3	991.5	995.86
879.3	901.82	904.8	959.8	966.1	973.1	980.8	991.6	995.89
879.5	901.83	904.9	959.9	966.2	973.2	980.9	991.8	996.52
879.7	901.89	908.5	960.0	966.3	973.3	981	991.9	996.55
879.9	901.9	908.6	960.1	966.4	973.4	982.0	992.0	996.56
880.10	902.0	908.9	960.2	967.0	973.5	982.1	992.1	996.57
880.11	902.10	909.0	960.3	967.1	973.6	982.2	992.2	996.59
880.12	902.11	909.1	960.4	967.2	973.8	982.3	992.3	996.60
880.13	902.19	909.2	960.5	967.3	973.9	982.4	992.4	996.68
880.19	902.20	909.3	960.6	967.4	974.0	982.8	992.5	996.69
881.10	902.21	909.4	960.7	967.5	974.1	983.0	992.6	996.70
881.11	902.22	909.5	960.8	967.6	974.2	983.1	992.7	996.79
881.12	902.23	909.9	960.9	967.8	974.3	983.2	992.8	996.80
882.1	902.24	925.1	961.0	967.9	974.4	983.9	992.9	996.87
883.1	902.25	925.2	961.1	968.0	974.5	984.0	993.2	996.88
884.1	902.26	926.11	961.2	968.1	974.6	984.1	993.3	996.89
885.0	902.27	926.12	961.3	968.2	974.7	984.8	993.4	997.91
885.1	902.29	926.19	961.4	968.3	975.0	984.9	993.8	997.99
886.0	902.31	926.8	961.5	968.4	975.1	985.0	993.9	998.00
886.1	902.32	926.9	961.6	968.5	975.2	985.1	994.0	998.01
887.0	902.33	927.00	961.7	968.6	975.3	985.2	994.1	998.02
887.1	902.34	927.01	961.8	968.7	975.4	985.3	994.2	998.09
887.2	902.39	927.02	961.9	968.9	975.5	985.4	994.3	998.11
887.3	902.40	927.03	962.0	969.00	975.6	985.5	994.4	998.12
887.4	902.41	927.09	962.1	969.01	975.7	985.6	994.5	998.13
887.5	902.42	927.10	962.2	969.02	975.8	985.8	994.7	998.2
887.6	902.49	927.11	962.3	969.03	976.0	985.9	994.8	998.30
887.7	902.50	927.20	962.4	969.04	976.1	986	994.9	998.31
890.1	902.51	927.21	962.5	969.05	976.2	987.0	995.0	998.32
891.1	902.52	927.3	962.6	969.09	976.3	987.1	995.1	998.33
892.1	902.53	927.8	962.7	969.1	976.4	987.2	995.20	998.4
893.1	902.54	927.9	962.8	969.2	976.6	987.3	995.21	998.6
894.1	902.55	928.00	962.9	969.3	976.7	987.4	995.22	998.7
895.0	902.56	928.01	963.0	969.4	976.8	987.5	995.23	998.81
895.1	902.59	928.10	963.1	969.5	976.9	987.6	995.24	998.83
896.0	902.81	928.11	963.2	969.6	977.0	987.7	995.27	998.89
896.1	902.82	928.20	963.3	969.70	977.1	987.8	995.29	998.9
896.2	902.87	928.21	963.4	969.71	977.2	987.9	995.3	999.41
896.3	902.89	928.3	963.5	969.72	977.3	988.0	995.4	999.42
897.0	902.9	928.8	963.8	969.73	977.4	988.1	995.50	999.49
897.1	903.00	928.9	963.9	969.79	977.8	988.2	995.51	999.51
897.2	903.01	929.0	964.0	969.8	977.9	988.8	995.52	999.52
897.3	903.02	929.9	964.1	969.9	978.0	988.9	995.53	999.59
897.4	903.1	958.2	964.2	970.0	978.1	989.0	995.54	999.9
897.5	903.2	958.4	964.3	970.1	978.2	989.1	995.55	V71.3
897.6	903.3	958.8	964.4	970.81	978.3	989.2	995.59	V71.4
897.7	903.4	958.90	964.5	970.89	978.4	989.3	995.60	V71.6
900.00	903.5	958.91	964.6	970.9	978.5	989.4	995.61	
900.01	903.8	958.92	964.7	971.0	978.6	989.5	995.62	

SURGICAL

DRG 901   Wound Debridements for Injuries with MCC
GMLOS 9.3   AMLOS 13.9   RW 4.0316   ☑

Operating Room Procedure
86.22   Excisional debridement of wound, infection, or burn

DRG 902   Wound Debridements for Injuries with CC
GMLOS 4.9   AMLOS 6.6   RW 1.7077   ☑

Select operating room procedure listed under DRG 901

DRG 903   Wound Debridements for Injuries without CC/MCC
GMLOS 3.1   AMLOS 4.2   RW 1.0527   ☑

Select operating room procedure listed under DRG 901

DRG 904   Skin Grafts for Injuries with CC/MCC
GMLOS 7.2   AMLOS 10.7   RW 3.1738   ☑

Operating Room Procedures
85.82   Split-thickness graft to breast
85.83   Full-thickness graft to breast
85.84   Pedicle graft to breast
86.60   Free skin graft, not otherwise specified
86.63   Full-thickness skin graft to other sites
86.65   Heterograft to skin
86.66   Homograft to skin
86.67   Dermal regenerative graft
86.69   Other skin graft to other sites
86.70   Pedicle or flap graft, not otherwise specified
86.71   Cutting and preparation of pedicle grafts or flaps
86.72   Advancement of pedicle graft
86.74   Attachment of pedicle or flap graft to other sites
86.75   Revision of pedicle or flap graft
86.93   Insertion of tissue expander

DRG 905   Skin Grafts for Injuries without CC/MCC
GMLOS 3.2   AMLOS 4.3   RW 1.2475   ☑

Select operating room procedures listed under DRG 904

DRG 906   Hand Procedures for Injuries
GMLOS 2.4   AMLOS 3.5   RW 1.2228   ☑

Operating Room Procedures
04.43   Release of carpal tunnel
77.04   Sequestrectomy of carpals and metacarpals
77.14   Other incision of carpals and metacarpals without division
77.24   Wedge osteotomy of carpals and metacarpals
77.34   Other division of carpals and metacarpals
77.44   Biopsy of carpals and metacarpals
77.64   Local excision of lesion or tissue of carpals and metacarpals
77.74   Excision of carpals and metacarpals for graft
77.84   Other partial ostectomy of carpals and metacarpals
77.94   Total ostectomy of carpals and metacarpals
78.04   Bone graft of carpals and metacarpals
78.14   Application of external fixator device, carpals and metacarpals
78.24   Limb shortening procedures, carpals and metacarpals
78.34   Limb lengthening procedures, carpals and metacarpals
78.44   Other repair or plastic operations on carpals and metacarpals
78.54   Internal fixation of carpals and metacarpals without fracture reduction
78.64   Removal of implanted device from carpals and metacarpals
78.74   Osteoclasis of carpals and metacarpals

78.84   Diagnostic procedures on carpals and metacarpals, not elsewhere classified
78.94   Insertion of bone growth stimulator into carpals and metacarpals
79.13   Closed reduction of fracture of carpals and metacarpals with internal fixation
79.14   Closed reduction of fracture of phalanges of hand with internal fixation
79.23   Open reduction of fracture of carpals and metacarpals without internal fixation
79.24   Open reduction of fracture of phalanges of hand without internal fixation
79.33   Open reduction of fracture of carpals and metacarpals with internal fixation
79.34   Open reduction of fracture of phalanges of hand with internal fixation
79.63   Debridement of open fracture of carpals and metacarpals
79.64   Debridement of open fracture of phalanges of hand
79.83   Open reduction of dislocation of wrist
79.84   Open reduction of dislocation of hand and finger
79.93   Unspecified operation on bone injury of carpals and metacarpals
79.94   Unspecified operation on bone injury of phalanges of hand
80.03   Arthrotomy for removal of prosthesis without replacement, wrist
80.04   Arthrotomy for removal of prosthesis without replacement, hand and finger
80.13   Other arthrotomy of wrist
80.14   Other arthrotomy of hand and finger
80.43   Division of joint capsule, ligament, or cartilage of wrist
80.44   Division of joint capsule, ligament, or cartilage of hand and finger
80.73   Synovectomy of wrist
80.74   Synovectomy of hand and finger
80.83   Other local excision or destruction of lesion of wrist joint
80.84   Other local excision or destruction of lesion of joint of hand and finger
80.93   Other excision of wrist joint
80.94   Other excision of joint of hand and finger
81.25   Carporadial fusion
81.26   Metacarpocarpal fusion
81.27   Metacarpophalangeal fusion
81.28   Interphalangeal fusion
81.71   Arthroplasty of metacarpophalangeal and interphalangeal joint with implant
81.72   Arthroplasty of metacarpophalangeal and interphalangeal joint without implant
81.74   Arthroplasty of carpocarpal or carpometacarpal joint with implant
81.75   Arthroplasty of carpocarpal or carpometacarpal joint without implant
81.79   Other repair of hand, fingers, and wrist
82.01   Exploration of tendon sheath of hand
82.02   Myotomy of hand
82.03   Bursotomy of hand
82.09   Other incision of soft tissue of hand
82.1*   Division of muscle, tendon, and fascia of hand
82.2*   Excision of lesion of muscle, tendon, and fascia of hand
82.3*   Other excision of soft tissue of hand
82.4*   Suture of muscle, tendon, and fascia of hand
82.5*   Transplantation of muscle and tendon of hand
82.6*   Reconstruction of thumb
82.7*   Plastic operation on hand with graft or implant
82.8*   Other plastic operations on hand
82.91   Lysis of adhesions of hand
82.99   Other operations on muscle, tendon, and fascia of hand
84.01   Amputation and disarticulation of finger
84.02   Amputation and disarticulation of thumb
84.21   Thumb reattachment
84.22   Finger reattachment

Surgical   *Medical*   *CC Indicator*   *MCC Indicator*   *Procedure Proxy*

86.61	Full-thickness skin graft to hand
86.62	Other skin graft to hand
86.73	Attachment of pedicle or flap graft to hand
86.85	Correction of syndactyly

DRG 907 Other O.R. Procedures for Injuries with MCC

GMLOS 7.7   **AMLOS 10.7**   **RW 3.9235**   ☑Ⓣ

Operating Room Procedures

00.61	Percutaneous angioplasty of extracranial vessel(s)
00.62	Percutaneous angioplasty of intracranial vessel(s)
00.70	Revision of hip replacement, both acetabular and femoral components
00.71	Revision of hip replacement, acetabular component
00.72	Revision of hip replacement, femoral component
00.73	Revision of hip replacement, acetabular liner and/or femoral head only
00.8*	Other knee and hip procedures
01.18	Other diagnostic procedures on brain and cerebral meninges
01.19	Other diagnostic procedures on skull
01.23	Reopening of craniotomy site
01.24	Other craniotomy
01.25	Other craniectomy
01.28	Placement of intracerebral catheter(s) via burr hole(s)
01.3*	Incision of brain and cerebral meninges
01.41	Operations on thalamus
01.52	Hemispherectomy
01.53	Lobectomy of brain
01.59	Other excision or destruction of lesion or tissue of brain
02.0*	Cranioplasty
02.11	Simple suture of dura mater of brain
02.12	Other repair of cerebral meninges
02.13	Ligation of meningeal vessel
02.2*	Ventriculostomy
02.3*	Extracranial ventricular shunt
02.42	Replacement of ventricular shunt
02.43	Removal of ventricular shunt
02.91	Lysis of cortical adhesions
02.92	Repair of brain
02.93	Implantation or replacement of intracranial neurostimulator lead(s)
02.94	Insertion or replacement of skull tongs or halo traction device
02.99	Other operations on skull, brain, and cerebral meninges
03.0*	Exploration and decompression of spinal canal structures
03.1	Division of intraspinal nerve root
03.2*	Chordotomy
03.53	Repair of vertebral fracture
03.59	Other repair and plastic operations on spinal cord structures
03.6	Lysis of adhesions of spinal cord and nerve roots
03.93	Implantation or replacement of spinal neurostimulator lead(s)
03.94	Removal of spinal neurostimulator lead(s)
03.97	Revision of spinal thecal shunt
03.98	Removal of spinal thecal shunt
03.99	Other operations on spinal cord and spinal canal structures
04.02	Division of trigeminal nerve
04.03	Division or crushing of other cranial and peripheral nerves
04.04	Other incision of cranial and peripheral nerves
04.05	Gasserian ganglionectomy
04.06	Other cranial or peripheral ganglionectomy
04.07	Other excision or avulsion of cranial and peripheral nerves
04.12	Open biopsy of cranial or peripheral nerve or ganglion
04.19	Other diagnostic procedures on cranial and peripheral nerves and ganglia
04.3	Suture of cranial and peripheral nerves
04.41	Decompression of trigeminal nerve root
04.42	Other cranial nerve decompression
04.44	Release of tarsal tunnel
04.49	Other peripheral nerve or ganglion decompression or lysis of adhesions
04.5	Cranial or peripheral nerve graft
04.6	Transposition of cranial and peripheral nerves
04.7*	Other cranial or peripheral neuroplasty
04.9*	Other operations on cranial and peripheral nerves
05.9	Other operations on nervous system
06.02	Reopening of wound of thyroid field
06.09	Other incision of thyroid field
06.92	Ligation of thyroid vessels
06.93	Suture of thyroid gland
07.43	Ligation of adrenal vessels
07.44	Repair of adrenal gland
07.45	Reimplantation of adrenal tissue
07.49	Other operations on adrenal glands, nerves, and vessels
07.8*	Thymectomy
07.91	Exploration of thymus field
07.92	Other incision of thymus
07.93	Repair of thymus
07.95	Thoracoscopic incision of thymus
07.98	Other and unspecified thoracoscopic operations on thymus
08.11	Biopsy of eyelid
08.2*	Excision or destruction of lesion or tissue of eyelid
08.3*	Repair of blepharoptosis and lid retraction
08.4*	Repair of entropion or ectropion
08.5*	Other adjustment of lid position
08.6*	Reconstruction of eyelid with flaps or grafts
08.7*	Other reconstruction of eyelid
08.9*	Other operations on eyelids
09.11	Biopsy of lacrimal gland
09.19	Other diagnostic procedures on lacrimal system
09.21	Excision of lesion of lacrimal gland
09.22	Other partial dacryoadenectomy
09.23	Total dacryoadenectomy
09.3	Other operations on lacrimal gland
09.44	Intubation of nasolacrimal duct
09.52	Incision of lacrimal canaliculi
09.6	Excision of lacrimal sac and passage
09.7*	Repair of canaliculus and punctum
09.8*	Fistulization of lacrimal tract to nasal cavity
09.9*	Other operations on lacrimal system
10.0	Removal of embedded foreign body from conjunctiva by incision
10.3*	Excision or destruction of lesion or tissue of conjunctiva
10.4*	Conjunctivoplasty
10.6	Repair of laceration of conjunctiva
11.0	Magnetic removal of embedded foreign body from cornea
11.1	Incision of cornea
11.22	Biopsy of cornea
11.32	Excision of pterygium with corneal graft
11.42	Thermocauterization of corneal lesion
11.43	Cryotherapy of corneal lesion
11.49	Other removal or destruction of corneal lesion
11.5*	Repair of cornea
11.6*	Corneal transplant
11.7*	Other reconstructive and refractive surgery on cornea
11.9*	Other operations on cornea
12.0*	Removal of intraocular foreign body from anterior segment of eye
12.1*	Iridotomy and simple iridectomy
12.2*	Diagnostic procedures on iris, ciliary body, sclera, and anterior chamber
12.3*	Iridoplasty and coreoplasty
12.4*	Excision or destruction of lesion of iris and ciliary body
12.5*	Facilitation of intraocular circulation
12.6*	Scleral fistulization
12.8*	Operations on sclera
12.91	Therapeutic evacuation of anterior chamber
12.92	Injection into anterior chamber
12.97	Other operations on iris

12.98	Other operations on ciliary body
12.99	Other operations on anterior chamber
13.0*	Removal of foreign body from lens
13.72	Secondary insertion of intraocular lens prosthesis
13.8	Removal of implanted lens
13.9*	Other operations on lens
14.0*	Removal of foreign body from posterior segment of eye
14.31	Repair of retinal tear by diathermy
14.4*	Repair of retinal detachment with scleral buckling and implant
14.5*	Other repair of retinal detachment
14.6	Removal of surgically implanted material from posterior segment of eye
14.7*	Operations on vitreous
14.8*	Implantation of epiretinal visual prosthesis
14.9	Other operations on retina, choroid, and posterior chamber
15.7	Repair of injury of extraocular muscle
15.9	Other operations on extraocular muscles and tendons
16.0*	Orbitotomy
16.1	Removal of penetrating foreign body from eye, not otherwise specified
16.3*	Evisceration of eyeball
16.4*	Enucleation of eyeball
16.5*	Exenteration of orbital contents
16.6*	Secondary procedures after removal of eyeball
16.7*	Removal of ocular or orbital implant
16.8*	Repair of injury of eyeball and orbit
16.92	Excision of lesion of orbit
16.93	Excision of lesion of eye, unspecified structure
16.98	Other operations on orbit
16.99	Other operations on eyeball
17.3*	Laparoscopic partial excision of large intestine
17.53	Percutaneous atherectomy of extracranial vessel(s)
17.54	Percutaneous atherectomy of intracranial vessel(s)
17.56	Atherectomy of other non-coronary vessel(s)
18.39	Other excision of external ear
18.6	Reconstruction of external auditory canal
18.7*	Other plastic repair of external ear
18.9	Other operations on external ear
21.04	Control of epistaxis by ligation of ethmoidal arteries
21.05	Control of epistaxis by (transantral) ligation of the maxillary artery
21.06	Control of epistaxis by ligation of the external carotid artery
21.07	Control of epistaxis by excision of nasal mucosa and skin grafting of septum and lateral nasal wall
21.09	Control of epistaxis by other means
21.4	Resection of nose
21.5	Submucous resection of nasal septum
21.62	Fracture of the turbinates
21.69	Other turbinectomy
21.72	Open reduction of nasal fracture
21.83	Total nasal reconstruction
21.84	Revision rhinoplasty
21.85	Augmentation rhinoplasty
21.86	Limited rhinoplasty
21.87	Other rhinoplasty
21.88	Other septoplasty
21.89	Other repair and plastic operations on nose
21.99	Other operations on nose
24.2	Gingivoplasty
24.5	Alveoloplasty
25.59	Other repair and plastic operations on tongue
26.4*	Repair of salivary gland or duct
27.0	Drainage of face and floor of mouth
27.49	Other excision of mouth
27.53	Closure of fistula of mouth
27.54	Repair of cleft lip
27.55	Full-thickness skin graft to lip and mouth
27.56	Other skin graft to lip and mouth
27.57	Attachment of pedicle or flap graft to lip and mouth

27.59	Other plastic repair of mouth
27.61	Suture of laceration of palate
27.92	Incision of mouth, unspecified structure
27.99	Other operations on oral cavity
28.7	Control of hemorrhage after tonsillectomy and adenoidectomy
28.91	Removal of foreign body from tonsil and adenoid by incision
29.0	Pharyngotomy
29.4	Plastic operation on pharynx
29.51	Suture of laceration of pharynx
29.53	Closure of other fistula of pharynx
29.59	Other repair of pharynx
29.99	Other operations on pharynx
30.1	Hemilaryngectomy
30.2*	Other partial laryngectomy
31.61	Suture of laceration of larynx
31.64	Repair of laryngeal fracture
31.69	Other repair of larynx
31.7*	Repair and plastic operations on trachea
31.92	Lysis of adhesions of trachea or larynx
31.99	Other operations on trachea
32.1	Other excision of bronchus
32.20	Thoracoscopic excision of lesion or tissue of lung
32.3*	Segmental resection of lung
32.4*	Lobectomy of lung
32.5*	Pneumonectomy
32.9	Other excision of lung
33.0	Incision of bronchus
33.1	Incision of lung
33.4*	Repair and plastic operation on lung and bronchus
33.92	Ligation of bronchus
33.98	Other operations on bronchus
33.99	Other operations on lung
34.02	Exploratory thoracotomy
34.03	Reopening of recent thoracotomy site
34.1	Incision of mediastinum
34.21	Transpleural thoracoscopy
34.5*	Pleurectomy
34.6	Scarification of pleura
34.73	Closure of other fistula of thorax
34.79	Other repair of chest wall
34.82	Suture of laceration of diaphragm
34.83	Closure of fistula of diaphragm
34.84	Other repair of diaphragm
34.85	Implantation of diaphragmatic pacemaker
34.89	Other operations on diaphragm
34.93	Repair of pleura
34.99	Other operations on thorax
37.11	Cardiotomy
37.12	Pericardiotomy
37.31	Pericardiectomy
37.49	Other repair of heart and pericardium
37.74	Insertion or replacement of epicardial lead (electrode) into epicardium
37.75	Revision of lead (electrode)
37.76	Replacement of transvenous atrial and/or ventricular lead(s) (electrode(s))
37.77	Removal of lead(s) (electrodes) without replacement
37.79	Revision or relocation of cardiac device pocket
37.80	Insertion of permanent pacemaker, initial or replacement, type of device not specified
37.85	Replacement of any type of pacemaker device with single-chamber device, not specified as rate responsive
37.86	Replacement of any type of pacemaker device with single-chamber device, rate responsive
37.87	Replacement of any type of pacemaker device with dual-chamber device
37.89	Revision or removal of pacemaker device
37.91	Open chest cardiac massage
38.0*	Incision of vessel

MDC 21: Injuries, Poisonings And Toxic Effects Of Drugs—SURGICAL

MDC 21: Injuries, Poisonings And Toxic Effects Of Drugs—SURGICAL

38.10	Endarterectomy, unspecified site
38.12	Endarterectomy of other vessels of head and neck
38.13	Endarterectomy of upper limb vessels
38.14	Endarterectomy of aorta
38.15	Endarterectomy of other thoracic vessels
38.16	Endarterectomy of abdominal arteries
38.18	Endarterectomy of lower limb arteries
38.3*	Resection of vessel with anastomosis
38.4*	Resection of vessel with replacement
38.6*	Other excision of vessels
38.7	Interruption of the vena cava
38.8*	Other surgical occlusion of vessels
39.22	Aorta-subclavian-carotid bypass
39.23	Other intrathoracic vascular shunt or bypass
39.24	Aorta-renal bypass
39.25	Aorta-iliac-femoral bypass
39.26	Other intra-abdominal vascular shunt or bypass
39.27	Arteriovenostomy for renal dialysis
39.28	Extracranial-intracranial (EC-IC) vascular bypass
39.29	Other (peripheral) vascular shunt or bypass
39.3*	Suture of vessel
39.4*	Revision of vascular procedure
39.50	Angioplasty of other non-coronary vessel(s)
39.52	Other repair of aneurysm
39.56	Repair of blood vessel with tissue patch graft
39.57	Repair of blood vessel with synthetic patch graft
39.58	Repair of blood vessel with unspecified type of patch graft
39.59	Other repair of vessel
39.71	Endovascular implantation of other graft in abdominal aorta
39.72	Endovascular (total) embolization or occlusion of head and neck vessels
39.73	Endovascular implantation of graft in thoracic aorta
39.74	Endovascular removal of obstruction from head and neck vessel(s)
39.75	Endovascular embolization or occlusion of vessel(s) of head or neck using bare coils
39.76	Endovascular embolization or occlusion of vessel(s) of head or neck using bioactive coils
39.77	Temporary (partial) therapeutic endovascular occlusion of vessel
39.79	Other endovascular procedures on other vessels
39.91	Freeing of vessel
39.93	Insertion of vessel-to-vessel cannula
39.98	Control of hemorrhage, not otherwise specified
39.99	Other operations on vessels
40.29	Simple excision of other lymphatic structure
40.6*	Operations on thoracic duct
40.9	Other operations on lymphatic structures
41.2	Splenotomy
41.42	Excision of lesion or tissue of spleen
41.43	Partial splenectomy
41.5	Total splenectomy
41.93	Excision of accessory spleen
41.95	Repair and plastic operations on spleen
41.99	Other operations on spleen
42.09	Other incision of esophagus
42.1*	Esophagostomy
42.21	Operative esophagoscopy by incision
42.4*	Excision of esophagus
42.5*	Intrathoracic anastomosis of esophagus
42.6*	Antesternal anastomosis of esophagus
42.7	Esophagomyotomy
42.82	Suture of laceration of esophagus
42.83	Closure of esophagostomy
42.84	Repair of esophageal fistula, not elsewhere classified
42.85	Repair of esophageal stricture
42.86	Production of subcutaneous tunnel without esophageal anastomosis
42.87	Other graft of esophagus
42.89	Other repair of esophagus
43.0	Gastrotomy
43.5	Partial gastrectomy with anastomosis to esophagus
43.6	Partial gastrectomy with anastomosis to duodenum
43.7	Partial gastrectomy with anastomosis to jejunum
43.8*	Other partial gastrectomy
43.9*	Total gastrectomy
44.11	Transabdominal gastroscopy
44.5	Revision of gastric anastomosis
44.61	Suture of laceration of stomach
44.63	Closure of other gastric fistula
44.64	Gastropexy
44.65	Esophagogastroplasty
44.66	Other procedures for creation of esophagogastric sphincteric competence
44.67	Laparoscopic procedures for creation of esophagogastric sphincteric competence
44.68	Laparoscopic gastroplasty
44.69	Other repair of stomach
44.92	Intraoperative manipulation of stomach
44.99	Other operations on stomach
45.0*	Enterotomy
45.11	Transabdominal endoscopy of small intestine
45.21	Transabdominal endoscopy of large intestine
45.6*	Other excision of small intestine
45.7*	Open and other partial excision of large intestine
45.8*	Total intra-abdominal colectomy
45.9*	Intestinal anastomosis
46.0*	Exteriorization of intestine
46.10	Colostomy, not otherwise specified
46.11	Temporary colostomy
46.13	Permanent colostomy
46.20	Ileostomy, not otherwise specified
46.21	Temporary ileostomy
46.22	Continent ileostomy
46.23	Other permanent ileostomy
46.4*	Revision of intestinal stoma
46.5*	Closure of intestinal stoma
46.7*	Other repair of intestine
46.80	Intra-abdominal manipulation of intestine, not otherwise specified
46.81	Intra-abdominal manipulation of small intestine
46.82	Intra-abdominal manipulation of large intestine
46.93	Revision of anastomosis of small intestine
46.94	Revision of anastomosis of large intestine
46.99	Other operations on intestines
47.1*	Incidental appendectomy
47.92	Closure of appendiceal fistula
48.0	Proctotomy
48.1	Proctostomy
48.21	Transabdominal proctosigmoidoscopy
48.40	Pull-through resection of rectum, not otherwise specified
48.42	Laparoscopic pull-through resection of rectum
48.43	Open pull-through resection of rectum
48.49	Other pull-through resection of rectum
48.5*	Abdominoperineal resection of rectum
48.6*	Other resection of rectum
48.7*	Repair of rectum
48.8*	Incision or excision of perirectal tissue or lesion
48.91	Incision of rectal stricture
49.1*	Incision or excision of anal fistula
49.71	Suture of laceration of anus
49.73	Closure of anal fistula
49.75	Implantation or revision of artificial anal sphincter
49.76	Removal of artificial anal sphincter
49.79	Other repair of anal sphincter
49.95	Control of (postoperative) hemorrhage of anus
49.99	Other operations on anus
50.0	Hepatotomy
50.12	Open biopsy of liver
50.14	Laparoscopic liver biopsy

T Transfer DRG   SP Special Payment   ☑ Optimization Potential   ▽ Targeted Potential   * Code Range   ● New DRG   ▲ Revised DRG Title

50.19	Other diagnostic procedures on liver
50.22	Partial hepatectomy
50.3	Lobectomy of liver
50.4	Total hepatectomy
50.6*	Repair of liver
51.2*	Cholecystectomy
51.3*	Anastomosis of gallbladder or bile duct
51.42	Common duct exploration for relief of other obstruction
51.43	Insertion of choledochohepatic tube for decompression
51.59	Incision of other bile duct
51.61	Excision of cystic duct remnant
51.7*	Repair of bile ducts
51.81	Dilation of sphincter of Oddi
51.82	Pancreatic sphincterotomy
51.83	Pancreatic sphincteroplasty
51.89	Other operations on sphincter of Oddi
51.91	Repair of laceration of gallbladder
51.92	Closure of cholecystostomy
51.93	Closure of other biliary fistula
51.94	Revision of anastomosis of biliary tract
51.95	Removal of prosthetic device from bile duct
51.99	Other operations on biliary tract
52.12	Open biopsy of pancreas
52.19	Other diagnostic procedures on pancreas
52.5*	Partial pancreatectomy
52.6	Total pancreatectomy
52.7	Radical pancreaticoduodenectomy
52.92	Cannulation of pancreatic duct
52.95	Other repair of pancreas
52.96	Anastomosis of pancreas
52.99	Other operations on pancreas
53.43	Other laparoscopic umbilical herniorrhaphy
53.49	Other open umbilical herniorrhaphy
53.61	Other open incisional hernia repair with graft or prosthesis
53.62	Laparoscopic incisional hernia repair with graft or prosthesis
53.7*	Repair of diaphragmatic hernia, abdominal approach
53.8*	Repair of diaphragmatic hernia, thoracic approach
54.0	Incision of abdominal wall
54.1*	Laparotomy
54.21	Laparoscopy
54.22	Biopsy of abdominal wall or umbilicus
54.29	Other diagnostic procedures on abdominal region
54.5*	Lysis of peritoneal adhesions
54.6*	Suture of abdominal wall and peritoneum
54.7*	Other repair of abdominal wall and peritoneum
54.92	Removal of foreign body from peritoneal cavity
54.93	Creation of cutaneoperitoneal fistula
54.95	Incision of peritoneum
55.0*	Nephrotomy and nephrostomy
55.1*	Pyelotomy and pyelostomy
55.24	Open biopsy of kidney
55.29	Other diagnostic procedures on kidney
55.31	Marsupialization of kidney lesion
55.4	Partial nephrectomy
55.5*	Complete nephrectomy
55.61	Renal autotransplantation
55.81	Suture of laceration of kidney
55.82	Closure of nephrostomy and pyelostomy
55.83	Closure of other fistula of kidney
55.84	Reduction of torsion of renal pedicle
55.86	Anastomosis of kidney
55.87	Correction of ureteropelvic junction
55.89	Other repair of kidney
55.97	Implantation or replacement of mechanical kidney
55.98	Removal of mechanical kidney
55.99	Other operations on kidney
56.0	Transurethral removal of obstruction from ureter and renal pelvis
56.1	Ureteral meatotomy
56.2	Ureterotomy
56.4*	Ureterectomy
56.5*	Cutaneous uretero-ileostomy
56.6*	Other external urinary diversion
56.7*	Other anastomosis or bypass of ureter
56.81	Lysis of intraluminal adhesions of ureter
56.82	Suture of laceration of ureter
56.83	Closure of ureterostomy
56.84	Closure of other fistula of ureter
56.86	Removal of ligature from ureter
56.89	Other repair of ureter
56.95	Ligation of ureter
56.99	Other operations on ureter
57.12	Lysis of intraluminal adhesions with incision into bladder
57.18	Other suprapubic cystostomy
57.19	Other cystotomy
57.2*	Vesicostomy
57.39	Other diagnostic procedures on bladder
57.6	Partial cystectomy
57.79	Other total cystectomy
57.81	Suture of laceration of bladder
57.82	Closure of cystostomy
57.83	Repair of fistula involving bladder and intestine
57.84	Repair of other fistula of bladder
57.87	Reconstruction of urinary bladder
57.89	Other repair of bladder
57.93	Control of (postoperative) hemorrhage of bladder
57.99	Other operations on bladder
58.0	Urethrotomy
58.1	Urethral meatotomy
58.41	Suture of laceration of urethra
58.42	Closure of urethrostomy
58.43	Closure of other fistula of urethra
58.44	Reanastomosis of urethra
58.46	Other reconstruction of urethra
58.49	Other repair of urethra
58.5	Release of urethral stricture
58.93	Implantation of artificial urinary sphincter (AUS)
59.02	Other lysis of perirenal or periureteral adhesions
59.03	Laparoscopic lysis of perirenal or periureteral adhesions
59.09	Other incision of perirenal or periureteral tissue
59.1*	Incision of perivesical tissue
59.2*	Diagnostic procedures on perirenal and perivesical tissue
60.93	Repair of prostate
60.94	Control of (postoperative) hemorrhage of prostate
61.42	Repair of scrotal fistula
61.49	Other repair of scrotum and tunica vaginalis
61.99	Other operations on scrotum and tunica vaginalis
62.0	Incision of testis
62.3	Unilateral orchiectomy
62.4*	Bilateral orchiectomy
62.6*	Repair of testes
62.99	Other operations on testes
63.51	Suture of laceration of spermatic cord and epididymis
63.53	Transplantation of spermatic cord
63.59	Other repair of spermatic cord and epididymis
63.81	Suture of laceration of vas deferens and epididymis
63.82	Reconstruction of surgically divided vas deferens
63.89	Other repair of vas deferens and epididymis
63.94	Lysis of adhesions of spermatic cord
63.99	Other operations on spermatic cord, epididymis, and vas deferens
64.41	Suture of laceration of penis
64.43	Construction of penis
64.44	Reconstruction of penis
64.45	Replantation of penis
64.49	Other repair of penis
65.7*	Repair of ovary
65.8*	Lysis of adhesions of ovary and fallopian tube
66.71	Simple suture of fallopian tube
66.79	Other repair of fallopian tube

MDC 21: Injuries, Poisonings And Toxic Effects Of Drugs—SURGICAL

67.5*	Repair of internal cervical os	77.32	Other division of humerus
67.6*	Other repair of cervix	77.33	Other division of radius and ulna
68.0	Hysterotomy	77.35	Other division of femur
69.23	Vaginal repair of chronic inversion of uterus	77.36	Other division of patella
69.29	Other repair of uterus and supporting structures	77.37	Other division of tibia and fibula
69.4*	Uterine repair	77.38	Other division of tarsals and metatarsals
69.97	Removal of other penetrating foreign body from cervix	77.39	Other division of other bone, except facial bones
70.13	Lysis of intraluminal adhesions of vagina	77.58	Other excision, fusion, and repair of toes
70.62	Vaginal reconstruction	77.60	Local excision of lesion or tissue of bone, unspecified site
70.64	Vaginal reconstruction with graft or prosthesis	77.61	Local excision of lesion or tissue of scapula, clavicle, and thorax (ribs and sternum)
70.71	Suture of laceration of vagina		
70.72	Repair of colovaginal fistula	77.62	Local excision of lesion or tissue of humerus
70.73	Repair of rectovaginal fistula	77.63	Local excision of lesion or tissue of radius and ulna
70.74	Repair of other vaginoenteric fistula	77.65	Local excision of lesion or tissue of femur
70.75	Repair of other fistula of vagina	77.66	Local excision of lesion or tissue of patella
70.79	Other repair of vagina	77.67	Local excision of lesion or tissue of tibia and fibula
71.01	Lysis of vulvar adhesions	77.68	Local excision of lesion or tissue of tarsals and metatarsals
71.7*	Repair of vulva and perineum	77.69	Local excision of lesion or tissue of other bone, except facial bones
76.0*	Incision of facial bone without division		
76.1*	Diagnostic procedures on facial bones and joints	77.70	Excision of bone for graft, unspecified site
76.2	Local excision or destruction of lesion of facial bone	77.71	Excision of scapula, clavicle, and thorax (ribs and sternum) for graft
76.3*	Partial ostectomy of facial bone		
76.4*	Excision and reconstruction of facial bones	77.72	Excision of humerus for graft
76.5	Temporomandibular arthroplasty	77.73	Excision of radius and ulna for graft
76.6*	Other facial bone repair and orthognathic surgery	77.75	Excision of femur for graft
76.70	Reduction of facial fracture, not otherwise specified	77.76	Excision of patella for graft
76.72	Open reduction of malar and zygomatic fracture	77.77	Excision of tibia and fibula for graft
76.74	Open reduction of maxillary fracture	77.78	Excision of tarsals and metatarsals for graft
76.76	Open reduction of mandibular fracture	77.79	Excision of other bone for graft, except facial bones
76.77	Open reduction of alveolar fracture	77.80	Other partial ostectomy, unspecified site
76.79	Other open reduction of facial fracture	77.81	Other partial ostectomy of scapula, clavicle, and thorax (ribs and sternum)
76.91	Bone graft to facial bone		
76.92	Insertion of synthetic implant in facial bone	77.82	Other partial ostectomy of humerus
76.94	Open reduction of temporomandibular dislocation	77.83	Other partial ostectomy of radius and ulna
76.97	Removal of internal fixation device from facial bone	77.85	Other partial ostectomy of femur
76.99	Other operations on facial bones and joints	77.86	Other partial ostectomy of patella
77.00	Sequestrectomy, unspecified site	77.87	Other partial ostectomy of tibia and fibula
77.01	Sequestrectomy of scapula, clavicle, and thorax (ribs and sternum)	77.88	Other partial ostectomy of tarsals and metatarsals
		77.89	Other partial ostectomy of other bone, except facial bones
77.02	Sequestrectomy of humerus	77.90	Total ostectomy, unspecified site
77.03	Sequestrectomy of radius and ulna	77.91	Total ostectomy of scapula, clavicle, and thorax (ribs and sternum)
77.05	Sequestrectomy of femur		
77.06	Sequestrectomy of patella	77.92	Total ostectomy of humerus
77.07	Sequestrectomy of tibia and fibula	77.93	Total ostectomy of radius and ulna
77.08	Sequestrectomy of tarsals and metatarsals	77.95	Total ostectomy of femur
77.09	Sequestrectomy of other bone, except facial bones	77.96	Total ostectomy of patella
77.10	Other incision of bone without division, unspecified site	77.97	Total ostectomy of tibia and fibula
77.11	Other incision of scapula, clavicle, and thorax (ribs and sternum) without division	77.98	Total ostectomy of tarsals and metatarsals
		77.99	Total ostectomy of other bone, except facial bones
77.12	Other incision of humerus without division	78.00	Bone graft, unspecified site
77.13	Other incision of radius and ulna without division	78.01	Bone graft of scapula, clavicle, and thorax (ribs and sternum)
77.15	Other incision of femur without division	78.02	Bone graft of humerus
77.16	Other incision of patella without division	78.03	Bone graft of radius and ulna
77.17	Other incision of tibia and fibula without division	78.05	Bone graft of femur
77.18	Other incision of tarsals and metatarsals without division	78.06	Bone graft of patella
77.19	Other incision of other bone, except facial bones, without division	78.07	Bone graft of tibia and fibula
		78.08	Bone graft of tarsals and metatarsals
77.20	Wedge osteotomy, unspecified site	78.09	Bone graft of other bone, except facial bones
77.21	Wedge osteotomy of scapula, clavicle, and thorax (ribs and sternum)	78.10	Application of external fixator device, unspecified site
		78.11	Application of external fixator device, scapula, clavicle, and thorax [ribs and sternum]
77.22	Wedge osteotomy of humerus		
77.23	Wedge osteotomy of radius and ulna	78.12	Application of external fixator device, humerus
77.25	Wedge osteotomy of femur	78.13	Application of external fixator device, radius and ulna
77.26	Wedge osteotomy of patella	78.15	Application of external fixator device, femur
77.27	Wedge osteotomy of tibia and fibula	78.16	Application of external fixator device, patella
77.28	Wedge osteotomy of tarsals and metatarsals	78.17	Application of external fixator device, tibia and fibula
77.29	Wedge osteotomy of other bone, except facial bones	78.18	Application of external fixator device, tarsals and metatarsals
77.30	Other division of bone, unspecified site		
77.31	Other division of scapula, clavicle, and thorax (ribs and sternum)	78.19	Application of external fixator device, other
		78.20	Limb shortening procedures, unspecified site

MDC 21: Injuries, Poisonings And Toxic Effects Of Drugs—SURGICAL

T *Transfer DRG*   SP *Special Payment*   ☑ *Optimization Potential*   ▽ *Targeted Potential*   * *Code Range*   ● *New DRG*   ▲ *Revised DRG Title*

Valid 10/01/2013-09/30/2014   © 2013 OptumInsight, Inc.

78.22	Limb shortening procedures, humerus
78.23	Limb shortening procedures, radius and ulna
78.25	Limb shortening procedures, femur
78.27	Limb shortening procedures, tibia and fibula
78.28	Limb shortening procedures, tarsals and metatarsals
78.29	Limb shortening procedures, other
78.30	Limb lengthening procedures, unspecified site
78.32	Limb lengthening procedures, humerus
78.33	Limb lengthening procedures, radius and ulna
78.35	Limb lengthening procedures, femur
78.37	Limb lengthening procedures, tibia and fibula
78.38	Limb lengthening procedures, tarsals and metatarsals
78.39	Other limb lengthening procedures
78.40	Other repair or plastic operations on bone, unspecified site
78.41	Other repair or plastic operations on scapula, clavicle, and thorax (ribs and sternum)
78.42	Other repair or plastic operation on humerus
78.43	Other repair or plastic operations on radius and ulna
78.45	Other repair or plastic operations on femur
78.46	Other repair or plastic operations on patella
78.47	Other repair or plastic operations on tibia and fibula
78.48	Other repair or plastic operations on tarsals and metatarsals
78.49	Other repair or plastic operations on other bone, except facial bones
78.50	Internal fixation of bone without fracture reduction, unspecified site
78.51	Internal fixation of scapula, clavicle, and thorax (ribs and sternum) without fracture reduction
78.52	Internal fixation of humerus without fracture reduction
78.53	Internal fixation of radius and ulna without fracture reduction
78.55	Internal fixation of femur without fracture reduction
78.56	Internal fixation of patella without fracture reduction
78.57	Internal fixation of tibia and fibula without fracture reduction
78.58	Internal fixation of tarsals and metatarsals without fracture reduction
78.59	Internal fixation of other bone, except facial bones, without fracture reduction
78.60	Removal of implanted device, unspecified site
78.61	Removal of implanted device from scapula, clavicle, and thorax (ribs and sternum)
78.62	Removal of implanted device from humerus
78.63	Removal of implanted device from radius and ulna
78.65	Removal of implanted device from femur
78.66	Removal of implanted device from patella
78.67	Removal of implanted device from tibia and fibula
78.68	Removal of implanted device from tarsal and metatarsals
78.69	Removal of implanted device from other bone
78.70	Osteoclasis, unspecified site
78.71	Osteoclasis of scapula, clavicle, and thorax (ribs and sternum)
78.72	Osteoclasis of humerus
78.73	Osteoclasis of radius and ulna
78.75	Osteoclasis of femur
78.76	Osteoclasis of patella
78.77	Osteoclasis of tibia and fibula
78.78	Osteoclasis of tarsals and metatarsals
78.79	Osteoclasis of other bone, except facial bones
78.90	Insertion of bone growth stimulator, unspecified site
78.91	Insertion of bone growth stimulator into scapula, clavicle and thorax (ribs and sternum)
78.92	Insertion of bone growth stimulator into humerus
78.93	Insertion of bone growth stimulator into radius and ulna
78.95	Insertion of bone growth stimulator into femur
78.96	Insertion of bone growth stimulator into patella
78.97	Insertion of bone growth stimulator into tibia and fibula
78.98	Insertion of bone growth stimulator into tarsals and metatarsals
78.99	Insertion of bone growth stimulator into other bone
79.10	Closed reduction of fracture with internal fixation, unspecified site
79.11	Closed reduction of fracture of humerus with internal fixation
79.12	Closed reduction of fracture of radius and ulna with internal fixation
79.15	Closed reduction of fracture of femur with internal fixation
79.16	Closed reduction of fracture of tibia and fibula with internal fixation
79.17	Closed reduction of fracture of tarsals and metatarsals with internal fixation
79.18	Closed reduction of fracture of phalanges of foot with internal fixation
79.19	Closed reduction of fracture of other specified bone, except facial bones, with internal fixation
79.20	Open reduction of fracture without internal fixation, unspecified site
79.21	Open reduction of fracture of humerus without internal fixation
79.22	Open reduction of fracture of radius and ulna without internal fixation
79.25	Open reduction of fracture of femur without internal fixation
79.26	Open reduction of fracture of tibia and fibula without internal fixation
79.27	Open reduction of fracture of tarsals and metatarsals without internal fixation
79.28	Open reduction of fracture of phalanges of foot without internal fixation
79.29	Open reduction of fracture of other specified bone, except facial bones, without internal fixation
79.30	Open reduction of fracture with internal fixation, unspecified site
79.31	Open reduction of fracture of humerus with internal fixation
79.32	Open reduction of fracture of radius and ulna with internal fixation
79.35	Open reduction of fracture of femur with internal fixation
79.36	Open reduction of fracture of tibia and fibula with internal fixation
79.37	Open reduction of fracture of tarsals and metatarsals with internal fixation
79.38	Open reduction of fracture of phalanges of foot with internal fixation
79.39	Open reduction of fracture of other specified bone, except facial bones, with internal fixation
79.40	Closed reduction of separated epiphysis, unspecified site
79.41	Closed reduction of separated epiphysis of humerus
79.42	Closed reduction of separated epiphysis of radius and ulna
79.45	Closed reduction of separated epiphysis of femur
79.46	Closed reduction of separated epiphysis of tibia and fibula
79.49	Closed reduction of separated epiphysis of other specified bone
79.50	Open reduction of separated epiphysis, unspecified site
79.51	Open reduction of separated epiphysis of humerus
79.52	Open reduction of separated epiphysis of radius and ulna
79.55	Open reduction of separated epiphysis of femur
79.56	Open reduction of separated epiphysis of tibia and fibula
79.59	Open reduction of separated epiphysis of other specified bone
79.60	Debridement of open fracture, unspecified site
79.61	Debridement of open fracture of humerus
79.62	Debridement of open fracture of radius and ulna
79.65	Debridement of open fracture of femur
79.66	Debridement of open fracture of tibia and fibula
79.67	Debridement of open fracture of tarsals and metatarsals
79.68	Debridement of open fracture of phalanges of foot
79.69	Debridement of open fracture of other specified bone, except facial bones
79.80	Open reduction of dislocation of unspecified site
79.81	Open reduction of dislocation of shoulder
79.82	Open reduction of dislocation of elbow

Surgical	Medical	CC Indicator	MCC Indicator	Procedure Proxy

79.85	Open reduction of dislocation of hip	80.85	Other local excision or destruction of lesion of hip joint
79.86	Open reduction of dislocation of knee	80.86	Other local excision or destruction of lesion of knee joint
79.87	Open reduction of dislocation of ankle	80.87	Other local excision or destruction of lesion of ankle joint
79.88	Open reduction of dislocation of foot and toe	80.88	Other local excision or destruction of lesion of joint of foot and toe
79.89	Open reduction of dislocation of other specified site, except temporomandibular	80.89	Other local excision or destruction of lesion of joint of other specified site
79.90	Unspecified operation on bone injury, unspecified site	80.90	Other excision of joint, unspecified site
79.91	Unspecified operation on bone injury of humerus	80.91	Other excision of shoulder joint
79.92	Unspecified operation on bone injury of radius and ulna	80.92	Other excision of elbow joint
79.95	Unspecified operation on bone injury of femur	80.95	Other excision of hip joint
79.96	Unspecified operation on bone injury of tibia and fibula	80.96	Other excision of knee joint
79.97	Unspecified operation on bone injury of tarsals and metatarsals	80.97	Other excision of ankle joint
79.98	Unspecified operation on bone injury of phalanges of foot	80.98	Other excision of joint of foot and toe
79.99	Unspecified operation on bone injury of other specified bone	80.99	Other excision of joint of other specified site
80.00	Arthrotomy for removal of prosthesis without replacement, unspecified site	81.00	Spinal fusion, not otherwise specified
		81.01	Atlas-axis spinal fusion
80.01	Arthrotomy for removal of prosthesis without replacement, shoulder	81.02	Other cervical fusion of the anterior column, anterior technique
80.02	Arthrotomy for removal of prosthesis without replacement, elbow	81.03	Other cervical fusion of the posterior column, posterior technique
80.05	Arthrotomy for removal of prosthesis without replacement, hip	81.04	Dorsal and dorsolumbar fusion of the anterior column, anterior technique
80.06	Arthrotomy for removal of prosthesis without replacement, knee	81.05	Dorsal and dorsolumbar fusion of the posterior column, posterior technique
80.07	Arthrotomy for removal of prosthesis without replacement, ankle	81.06	Lumbar and lumbosacral fusion of the anterior column, anterior technique
80.08	Arthrotomy for removal of prosthesis without replacement, foot and toe	81.07	Lumbar and lumbosacral fusion of the posterior column, posterior technique
80.09	Arthrotomy for removal of prosthesis without replacement, other specified site	81.08	Lumbar and lumbosacral fusion of the anterior column, posterior technique
80.10	Other arthrotomy, unspecified site	81.1*	Arthrodesis and arthroereisis of foot and ankle
80.11	Other arthrotomy of shoulder	81.20	Arthrodesis of unspecified joint
80.12	Other arthrotomy of elbow	81.21	Arthrodesis of hip
80.15	Other arthrotomy of hip	81.22	Arthrodesis of knee
80.16	Other arthrotomy of knee	81.23	Arthrodesis of shoulder
80.17	Other arthrotomy of ankle	81.24	Arthrodesis of elbow
80.18	Other arthrotomy of foot and toe	81.29	Arthrodesis of other specified joint
80.19	Other arthrotomy of other specified site	81.3*	Refusion of spine
80.2*	Arthroscopy	81.4*	Other repair of joint of lower extremity
80.40	Division of joint capsule, ligament, or cartilage, unspecified site	81.5*	Joint replacement of lower extremity
		81.65	Percutaneous vertebroplasty
80.41	Division of joint capsule, ligament, or cartilage of shoulder	81.66	Percutaneous vertebral augmentation
80.42	Division of joint capsule, ligament, or cartilage of elbow	81.73	Total wrist replacement
80.45	Division of joint capsule, ligament, or cartilage of hip	81.8*	Arthroplasty and repair of shoulder and elbow
80.46	Division of joint capsule, ligament, or cartilage of knee	81.93	Suture of capsule or ligament of upper extremity
80.47	Division of joint capsule, ligament, or cartilage of ankle	81.94	Suture of capsule or ligament of ankle and foot
80.48	Division of joint capsule, ligament, or cartilage of foot and toe	81.95	Suture of capsule or ligament of other lower extremity
		81.96	Other repair of joint
80.49	Division of joint capsule, ligament, or cartilage of other specified site	81.97	Revision of joint replacement of upper extremity
		81.98	Other diagnostic procedures on joint structures
80.50	Excision or destruction of intervertebral disc, unspecified	81.99	Other operations on joint structures
80.51	Excision of intervertebral disc	83.0*	Incision of muscle, tendon, fascia, and bursa
80.53	Repair of the anulus fibrosus with graft or prosthesis	83.1*	Division of muscle, tendon, and fascia
80.54	Other and unspecified repair of the anulus fibrosus	83.29	Other diagnostic procedures on muscle, tendon, fascia, and bursa, including that of hand
80.59	Other destruction of intervertebral disc		
80.6	Excision of semilunar cartilage of knee	83.3*	Excision of lesion of muscle, tendon, fascia, and bursa
80.70	Synovectomy, unspecified site	83.4*	Other excision of muscle, tendon, and fascia
80.71	Synovectomy of shoulder	83.5	Bursectomy
80.72	Synovectomy of elbow	83.6*	Suture of muscle, tendon, and fascia
80.75	Synovectomy of hip	83.7*	Reconstruction of muscle and tendon
80.76	Synovectomy of knee	83.8*	Other plastic operations on muscle, tendon, and fascia
80.77	Synovectomy of ankle	83.91	Lysis of adhesions of muscle, tendon, fascia, and bursa
80.78	Synovectomy of foot and toe	83.92	Insertion or replacement of skeletal muscle stimulator
80.79	Synovectomy of other specified site	83.93	Removal of skeletal muscle stimulator
80.80	Other local excision or destruction of lesion of joint, unspecified site	83.99	Other operations on muscle, tendon, fascia, and bursa
		84.00	Upper limb amputation, not otherwise specified
		84.03	Amputation through hand
80.81	Other local excision or destruction of lesion of shoulder joint	84.04	Disarticulation of wrist
80.82	Other local excision or destruction of lesion of elbow joint	84.05	Amputation through forearm

---

Ⓣ *Transfer DRG*   ⓢⓟ *Special Payment*   ☑ *Optimization Potential*   ▽ *Targeted Potential*   * *Code Range*   ● *New DRG*   ▲ *Revised DRG Title*

84.06	Disarticulation of elbow
84.07	Amputation through humerus
84.08	Disarticulation of shoulder
84.09	Interthoracoscapular amputation
84.1*	Amputation of lower limb
84.23	Forearm, wrist, or hand reattachment
84.24	Upper arm reattachment
84.25	Toe reattachment
84.26	Foot reattachment
84.27	Lower leg or ankle reattachment
84.28	Thigh reattachment
84.29	Other reattachment of extremity
84.3	Revision of amputation stump
84.40	Implantation or fitting of prosthetic limb device, not otherwise specified
84.44	Implantation of prosthetic device of arm
84.48	Implantation of prosthetic device of leg
84.59	Insertion of other spinal devices
84.6*	Replacement of spinal disc
84.8*	Insertion, replacement and revision of posterior spinal motion preservation device(s)
84.91	Amputation, not otherwise specified
84.94	Insertion of sternal fixation device with rigid plates
84.99	Other operations on musculoskeletal system
85.12	Open biopsy of breast
85.2*	Excision or destruction of breast tissue
85.3*	Reduction mammoplasty and subcutaneous mammectomy
85.4*	Mastectomy
85.50	Augmentation mammoplasty, not otherwise specified
85.53	Unilateral breast implant
85.54	Bilateral breast implant
85.6	Mastopexy
85.7*	Total reconstruction of breast
85.85	Muscle flap graft to breast
85.86	Transposition of nipple
85.87	Other repair or reconstruction of nipple
85.89	Other mammoplasty
85.93	Revision of implant of breast
85.94	Removal of implant of breast
85.95	Insertion of breast tissue expander
85.96	Removal of breast tissue expander (s)
85.99	Other operations on the breast
86.06	Insertion of totally implantable infusion pump
86.21	Excision of pilonidal cyst or sinus
86.4	Radical excision of skin lesion
86.81	Repair for facial weakness
86.82	Facial rhytidectomy
86.83	Size reduction plastic operation
86.84	Relaxation of scar or web contracture of skin
86.86	Onychoplasty
86.87	Fat graft of skin and subcutaneous tissue
86.89	Other repair and reconstruction of skin and subcutaneous tissue
86.91	Excision of skin for graft
92.27	Implantation or insertion of radioactive elements

OR

Any of the following procedure combinations

37.70	Initial insertion of lead (electrode), not otherwise specified
	AND
37.80	Insertion of permanent pacemaker, initial or replacement, type of device not specified

OR

37.70	Initial insertion of lead (electrode), not otherwise specified
	AND
37.81	Initial insertion of single-chamber device, not specified as rate responsive

OR

37.70	Initial insertion of lead (electrode), not otherwise specified

	AND
37.82	Initial insertion of single-chamber device, rate responsive

OR

37.70	Initial insertion of lead (electrode), not otherwise specified
	AND
37.85	Replacement of any type of pacemaker device with single-chamber device, not specified as rate responsive

OR

37.70	Initial insertion of lead (electrode), not otherwise specified
	AND
37.86	Replacement of any type of pacemaker device with single-chamber device, rate responsive

OR

37.70	Initial insertion of lead (electrode), not otherwise specified
	AND
37.87	Replacement of any type of pacemaker device with dual-chamber device

OR

37.71	Initial insertion of transvenous lead (electrode) into ventricle
	AND
37.80	Insertion of permanent pacemaker, initial or replacement, type of device not specified

OR

37.71	Initial insertion of transvenous lead (electrode) into ventricle
	AND
37.81	Initial insertion of single-chamber device, not specified as rate responsive

OR

37.71	Initial insertion of transvenous lead (electrode) into ventricle
	AND
37.82	Initial insertion of single-chamber device, rate responsive

OR

37.71	Initial insertion of transvenous lead (electrode) into ventricle
	AND
37.85	Replacement of any type of pacemaker device with single-chamber device, not specified as rate responsive

OR

37.71	Initial insertion of transvenous lead (electrode) into ventricle
	AND
37.86	Replacement of any type of pacemaker device with single-chamber device, rate responsive

OR

37.71	Initial insertion of transvenous lead (electrode) into ventricle
	AND
37.87	Replacement of any type of pacemaker device with dual-chamber device

OR

37.72	Initial insertion of transvenous leads (electrodes) into atrium and ventricle
	AND
37.80	Insertion of permanent pacemaker, initial or replacement, type of device not specified

OR

37.72	Initial insertion of transvenous leads (electrodes) into atrium and ventricle
	AND
37.83	Initial insertion of dual-chamber device

OR

37.73	Initial insertion of transvenous lead (electrode) into atrium
	AND
37.80	Insertion of permanent pacemaker, initial or replacement, type of device not specified

---

Surgical   *Medical*   CC Indicator   *MCC Indicator*   **Procedure Proxy**

MDC 21: Injuries, Poisonings And Toxic Effects Of Drugs—SURGICAL

OR

37.73 Initial insertion of transvenous lead (electrode) into atrium
AND
37.81 Initial insertion of single-chamber device, not specified as rate responsive

OR

37.73 Initial insertion of transvenous lead (electrode) into atrium
AND
37.82 Initial insertion of single-chamber device, rate responsive

OR

37.73 Initial insertion of transvenous lead (electrode) into atrium
AND
37.85 Replacement of any type of pacemaker device with single-chamber device, not specified as rate responsive

OR

37.73 Initial insertion of transvenous lead (electrode) into atrium
AND
37.86 Replacement of any type of pacemaker device with single-chamber device, rate responsive

OR

37.73 Initial insertion of transvenous lead (electrode) into atrium
AND
37.87 Replacement of any type of pacemaker device with dual-chamber device

OR

37.74 Insertion or replacement of epicardial lead (electrode) into epicardium
AND
37.80 Insertion of permanent pacemaker, initial or replacement, type of device not specified

OR

37.74 Insertion or replacement of epicardial lead (electrode) into epicardium
AND
37.81 Initial insertion of single-chamber device, not specified as rate responsive

OR

37.74 Insertion or replacement of epicardial lead (electrode) into epicardium
AND
37.82 Initial insertion of single-chamber device, rate responsive

OR

37.74 Insertion or replacement of epicardial lead (electrode) into epicardium
AND
37.83 Initial insertion of dual-chamber device

OR

37.74 Insertion or replacement of epicardial lead (electrode) into epicardium
AND
37.85 Replacement of any type of pacemaker device with single-chamber device, not specified as rate responsive

OR

37.74 Insertion or replacement of epicardial lead (electrode) into epicardium
AND
37.86 Replacement of any type of pacemaker device with single-chamber device, rate responsive

OR

37.74 Insertion or replacement of epicardial lead (electrode) into epicardium
AND
37.87 Replacement of any type of pacemaker device with dual-chamber device

OR

37.76 Replacement of transvenous atrial and/or ventricular lead(s) (electrode(s))
AND
37.80 Insertion of permanent pacemaker, initial or replacement, type of device not specified

OR

37.76 Replacement of transvenous atrial and/or ventricular lead(s) (electrode(s))
AND
37.85 Replacement of any type of pacemaker device with single-chamber device, not specified as rate responsive

OR

37.76 Replacement of transvenous atrial and/or ventricular lead(s) (electrode(s))
AND
37.86 Replacement of any type of pacemaker device with single-chamber device, rate responsive

OR

37.76 Replacement of transvenous atrial and/or ventricular lead(s) (electrode(s))
AND
37.87 Replacement of any type of pacemaker device with dual-chamber device

DRG 908 Other O.R. Procedures for Injuries with CC
GMLOS 4.4   AMLOS 5.8   RW 1.9485   ☑Ⓣ

Select operating room procedure and combination procedures listed under DRG 907

DRG 909 Other O.R. Procedures for Injuries without CC/MCC
GMLOS 2.5   AMLOS 3.2   RW 1.2150   ☑Ⓣ

Select operating room procedure and combination procedures listed under DRG 907

MEDICAL

DRG 913 Traumatic Injury with MCC
GMLOS 3.7   AMLOS 5.0   RW 1.1683   ☑

Principal Diagnosis
819* Multiple fractures involving both upper limbs, and upper limb with rib(s) and sternum
828* Multiple fractures involving both lower limbs, lower with upper limb, and lower limb(s) with rib(s) and sternum
862.8 Injury to multiple and unspecified intrathoracic organs without mention of open wound into cavity
862.9 Injury to multiple and unspecified intrathoracic organs with open wound into cavity
868.09 Injury to other and multiple intra-abdominal organs without mention of open wound into cavity
868.19 Injury to other and multiple intra-abdominal organs, with open wound into cavity
869* Internal injury to unspecified or ill-defined organs
875.1 Open wound of chest (wall), complicated
879.3 Open wound of abdominal wall, anterior, complicated
879.5 Open wound of abdominal wall, lateral, complicated
879.7 Open wound of other and unspecified parts of trunk, complicated
879.9 Open wound(s) (multiple) of unspecified site(s), complicated
880.1* Open wound of shoulder and upper arm, complicated
881.1* Open wound of elbow, forearm, and wrist, complicated
882.1 Open wound of hand except finger(s) alone, complicated
883.1 Open wound of finger(s), complicated

884.1	Multiple and unspecified open wound of upper limb, complicated
885*	Traumatic amputation of thumb (complete) (partial)
886*	Traumatic amputation of other finger(s) (complete) (partial)
887*	Traumatic amputation of arm and hand (complete) (partial)
890.1	Open wound of hip and thigh, complicated
891.1	Open wound of knee, leg (except thigh), and ankle, complicated
892.1	Open wound of foot except toe(s) alone, complicated
893.1	Open wound of toe(s), complicated
894.1	Multiple and unspecified open wound of lower limb, complicated
895*	Traumatic amputation of toe(s) (complete) (partial)
896*	Traumatic amputation of foot (complete) (partial)
897*	Traumatic amputation of leg(s) (complete) (partial)
900*	Injury to blood vessels of head and neck
901*	Injury to blood vessels of thorax
902*	Injury to blood vessels of abdomen and pelvis
903*	Injury to blood vessels of upper extremity
904*	Injury to blood vessels of lower extremity and unspecified sites
908.5	Late effect of foreign body in orifice
908.6	Late effect of certain complications of trauma
908.9	Late effect of unspecified injury
925*	Crushing injury of face, scalp, and neck
926.1*	Crushing injury of other specified sites of trunk
926.8	Crushing injury of multiple sites of trunk
926.9	Crushing injury of unspecified site of trunk
927*	Crushing injury of upper limb
928*	Crushing injury of lower limb
929*	Crushing injury of multiple and unspecified sites
959*	Injury, other and unspecified

DRG 914 Traumatic Injury without MCC

GMLOS 2.5	AMLOS 3.1	RW 0.7110	☑

Select principal diagnosis listed under DRG 913

DRG 915 Allergic Reactions with MCC

GMLOS 3.6	AMLOS 4.9	RW 1.4721	☑

Principal Diagnosis

995.0	Other anaphylactic reaction
995.1	Angioneurotic edema not elsewhere classified
995.3	Allergy, unspecified not elsewhere classified
995.6*	Anaphylactic reaction due to food
999.4*	Anaphylactic reaction due to serum
999.5*	Other serum reaction, not elsewhere classified

DRG 916 Allergic Reactions without MCC

GMLOS 1.7	AMLOS 2.1	RW 0.5139	☑

Select principal diagnosis listed under DRG 915

DRG 917 Poisoning and Toxic Effects of Drugs with MCC

GMLOS 3.5	AMLOS 4.8	RW 1.4093	☑ⓣ

Principal Diagnosis

960*	Poisoning by antibiotics
961*	Poisoning by other anti-infectives
962*	Poisoning by hormones and synthetic substitutes
963*	Poisoning by primarily systemic agents
964*	Poisoning by agents primarily affecting blood constituents
965*	Poisoning by analgesics, antipyretics, and antirheumatics
966*	Poisoning by anticonvulsants and anti-Parkinsonism drugs
967*	Poisoning by sedatives and hypnotics
968*	Poisoning by other central nervous system depressants and anesthetics
969*	Poisoning by psychotropic agents
970*	Poisoning by central nervous system stimulants
971*	Poisoning by drugs primarily affecting the autonomic nervous system
972*	Poisoning by agents primarily affecting the cardiovascular system
973*	Poisoning by agents primarily affecting the gastrointestinal system
974*	Poisoning by water, mineral, and uric acid metabolism drugs
975*	Poisoning by agents primarily acting on the smooth and skeletal muscles and respiratory system
976.0	Poisoning by local anti-infectives and anti-inflammatory drugs
976.1	Poisoning by antipruritics
976.2	Poisoning by local astringents and local detergents
976.3	Poisoning by emollients, demulcents, and protectants
976.4	Poisoning by keratolytics, keratoplastics, other hair treatment drugs and preparations
976.6	Poisoning by anti-infectives and other drugs and preparations for ear, nose, and throat
976.7	Poisoning by dental drugs topically applied
976.8	Poisoning by other agents primarily affecting skin and mucous membrane
976.9	Poisoning by unspecified agent primarily affecting skin and mucous membrane
977*	Poisoning by other and unspecified drugs and medicinal substances
978*	Poisoning by bacterial vaccines
979*	Poisoning by other vaccines and biological substances
980*	Toxic effect of alcohol
981	Toxic effect of petroleum products
982*	Toxic effect of solvents other than petroleum-based
983*	Toxic effect of corrosive aromatics, acids, and caustic alkalis
984*	Toxic effect of lead and its compounds (including fumes)
985*	Toxic effect of other metals
986	Toxic effect of carbon monoxide
987*	Toxic effect of other gases, fumes, or vapors
988*	Toxic effect of noxious substances eaten as food
989*	Toxic effect of other substances, chiefly nonmedicinal as to source
995.2*	Other and unspecified adverse effect of drug, medicinal and biological substance

DRG 918 Poisoning and Toxic Effects of Drugs without MCC

GMLOS 2.1	AMLOS 2.7	RW 0.6346	☑ⓣ

Select principal diagnosis listed under DRG 917

DRG 919 Complications of Treatment with MCC

GMLOS 4.4	AMLOS 6.1	RW 1.7206	☑

Principal Diagnosis

238.77	Post-transplant lymphoproliferative disorder [PTLD]
349.3*	Dural tear
996.52	Mechanical complication due to other tissue graft, not elsewhere classified
996.55	Mechanical complications due to artificial skin graft and decellularized allodermis
996.56	Mechanical complications due to peritoneal dialysis catheter
996.57	Mechanical complication due to insulin pump
996.59	Mechanical complication due to other implant and internal device, not elsewhere classified
996.60	Infection and inflammatory reaction due to unspecified device, implant, and graft
996.68	Infection and inflammatory reaction due to peritoneal dialysis catheter
996.69	Infection and inflammatory reaction due to other internal prosthetic device, implant, and graft
996.70	Other complications due to unspecified device, implant, and graft
996.79	Other complications due to other internal prosthetic device, implant, and graft

Surgical	Medical	CC Indicator	MCC Indicator	Procedure Proxy

Code	Description
996.80	Complications of transplanted organ, unspecified site
996.87	Complications of transplanted organ, intestine
996.88	Complications of transplanted organ, stem cell
996.89	Complications of other transplanted organ
997.9*	Complications affecting other specified body systems, not elsewhere classified
998.0*	Postoperative shock
998.1*	Hemorrhage or hematoma or seroma complicating procedure, not elsewhere classified
998.2	Accidental puncture or laceration during procedure
998.3*	Disruption of wound
998.4	Foreign body accidentally left during procedure, not elsewhere classified
998.6	Persistent postoperative fistula, not elsewhere classified
998.7	Acute reaction to foreign substance accidentally left during procedure, not elsewhere classified
998.81	Emphysema (subcutaneous) (surgical) resulting from a procedure
998.83	Non-healing surgical wound
998.89	Other specified complications
998.9	Unspecified complication of procedure, not elsewhere classified
999.9	Other and unspecified complications of medical care, not elsewhere classified

DRG 920   Complications of Treatment with CC
GMLOS 3.1   AMLOS 4.0   RW 0.9779   ☑

Select principal diagnosis listed under DRG 919

DRG 921   Complications of Treatment without CC/MCC
GMLOS 2.2   AMLOS 2.8   RW 0.6522   ☑

Select principal diagnosis listed under DRG 919

DRG 922   Other Injury, Poisoning and Toxic Effect Diagnoses with MCC
GMLOS 4.0   AMLOS 5.6   RW 1.5088   ☑

Principal Diagnosis

Code	Description
796.0	Nonspecific abnormal toxicological findings
909*	Late effects of other and unspecified external causes
958.2	Secondary and recurrent hemorrhage as an early complication of trauma
958.4	Traumatic shock
958.8	Other early complications of trauma
958.9*	Traumatic compartment syndrome
990	Effects of radiation, unspecified
991*	Effects of reduced temperature
992*	Effects of heat and light
993.2	Other and unspecified effects of high altitude
993.3	Caisson disease
993.4	Effects of air pressure caused by explosion
993.8	Other specified effects of air pressure
993.9	Unspecified effect of air pressure
994.0	Effects of lightning
994.1	Drowning and nonfatal submersion
994.2	Effects of hunger
994.3	Effects of thirst
994.4	Exhaustion due to exposure
994.5	Exhaustion due to excessive exertion
994.7	Asphyxiation and strangulation
994.8	Electrocution and nonfatal effects of electric current
994.9	Other effects of external causes
995.4	Shock due to anesthesia not elsewhere classified
995.5*	Child maltreatment syndrome
995.7	Other adverse food reactions, not elsewhere classified
995.8*	Other specified adverse effects, not elsewhere classified
V71.3	Observation following accident at work
V71.4	Observation following other accident

Code	Description
V71.6	Observation following other inflicted injury

DRG 923   Other Injury, Poisoning and Toxic Effect Diagnoses without MCC
GMLOS 2.2   AMLOS 2.9   RW 0.6620   ☑

Select principal diagnosis listed under DRG 922

Ⓣ Transfer DRG   🆂🅿 Special Payment   ☑ Optimization Potential   ▽ Targeted Potential   * Code Range   ● New DRG   ▲ Revised DRG Title

204   Valid 10/01/2013-09/30/2014   © 2013 OptumInsight, Inc.

MDC 21: Injuries, Poisonings And Toxic Effects Of Drugs—MEDICAL

Burns

941.00	941.40	942.24	943.14	944.00	944.40	945.22	947.8	948.76
941.01	941.41	942.25	943.15	944.01	944.41	945.23	947.9	948.77
941.03	941.43	942.29	943.16	944.02	944.42	945.24	948.00	948.80
941.04	941.44	942.30	943.19	944.03	944.43	945.25	948.10	948.81
941.05	941.45	942.31	943.20	944.04	944.44	945.26	948.11	948.82
941.06	941.46	942.32	943.21	944.05	944.45	945.29	948.20	948.83
941.07	941.47	942.33	943.22	944.06	944.46	945.30	948.21	948.84
941.08	941.48	942.34	943.23	944.07	944.47	945.31	948.22	948.85
941.09	941.49	942.35	943.24	944.08	944.48	945.32	948.30	948.86
941.10	941.50	942.39	943.25	944.10	944.50	945.33	948.31	948.87
941.11	941.51	942.40	943.26	944.11	944.51	945.34	948.32	948.88
941.13	941.53	942.41	943.29	944.12	944.52	945.35	948.33	948.90
941.14	941.54	942.42	943.30	944.13	944.53	945.36	948.40	948.91
941.15	941.55	942.43	943.31	944.14	944.54	945.39	948.41	948.92
941.16	941.56	942.44	943.32	944.15	944.55	945.40	948.42	948.93
941.17	941.57	942.45	943.33	944.16	944.56	945.41	948.43	948.94
941.18	941.58	942.49	943.34	944.17	944.57	945.42	948.44	948.95
941.19	941.59	942.50	943.35	944.18	944.58	945.43	948.50	948.96
941.20	942.00	942.51	943.36	944.20	945.00	945.44	948.51	948.97
941.21	942.01	942.52	943.39	944.21	945.01	945.45	948.52	948.98
941.23	942.02	942.53	943.40	944.22	945.02	945.46	948.53	948.99
941.24	942.03	942.54	943.41	944.23	945.03	945.49	948.54	949.0
941.25	942.04	942.55	943.42	944.24	945.04	945.50	948.55	949.1
941.26	942.05	942.59	943.43	944.25	945.05	945.51	948.60	949.2
941.27	942.09	943.00	943.44	944.26	945.06	945.52	948.61	949.3
941.28	942.10	943.01	943.45	944.27	945.09	945.53	948.62	949.4
941.29	942.11	943.02	943.46	944.28	945.10	945.54	948.63	949.5
941.30	942.12	943.03	943.49	944.30	945.11	945.55	948.64	
941.31	942.13	943.04	943.50	944.31	945.12	945.56	948.65	
941.33	942.14	943.05	943.51	944.32	945.13	945.59	948.66	
941.34	942.15	943.06	943.52	944.33	945.14	946.0	948.70	
941.35	942.19	943.09	943.53	944.34	945.15	946.1	948.71	
941.36	942.20	943.10	943.54	944.35	945.16	946.2	948.72	
941.37	942.21	943.11	943.55	944.36	945.19	946.3	948.73	
941.38	942.22	943.12	943.56	944.37	945.20	946.4	948.74	
941.39	942.23	943.13	943.59	944.38	945.21	946.5	948.75	

SURGICAL

DRG 927 **Extensive Burns or Full Thickness Burns with Mechanical Ventilation 96+ Hours with Skin Graft**
GMLOS 22.3   AMLOS 30.7   RW 16.4534

Principal or Secondary Diagnosis

941.3* Full-thickness skin loss due to burn (third degree NOS) of face, head, and neck
941.4* Deep necrosis of underlying tissues due to burn (deep third degree) of face, head, and neck without mention of loss of a body part
941.5* Deep necrosis of underlying tissues due to burn (deep third degree) of face, head, and neck with loss of a body part
942.3* Full-thickness skin loss due to burn (third degree NOS) of trunk
942.4* Deep necrosis of underlying tissues due to burn (deep third degree) of trunk without mention of loss of a body part
942.5* Deep necrosis of underlying tissues due to burn (deep third degree) of trunk with loss of a body part
943.3* Full-thickness skin loss due to burn (third degree NOS) of upper limb, except wrist and hand
943.4* Deep necrosis of underlying tissues due to burn (deep third degree) of upper limb, except wrist and hand, without mention of loss of a body part
943.5* Deep necrosis of underlying tissues due to burn (deep third degree) of upper limb, except wrist and hand, with loss of a body part
944.3* Full-thickness skin loss due to burn (third degree NOS) of wrist(s) and hand(s)
944.4* Deep necrosis of underlying tissues due to burn (deep third degree) of wrist(s) and hand(s), without mention of loss of a body part
944.5* Deep necrosis of underlying tissues due to burn (deep third degree) of wrist(s) and hand(s), with loss of a body part
945.3* Full-thickness skin loss due to burn (third degree NOS) of lower limb(s)
945.4* Deep necrosis of underlying tissues due to burn (deep third degree) of lower limb(s) without mention of loss of a body part
945.5* Deep necrosis of underlying tissues due to burn (deep third degree) of lower limb(s) with loss of a body part
946.3 Full-thickness skin loss due to burn (third degree NOS) of multiple specified sites
946.4 Deep necrosis of underlying tissues due to burn (deep third degree) of multiple specified sites, without mention of loss of a body part
946.5 Deep necrosis of underlying tissues due to burn (deep third degree) of multiple specified sites, with loss of a body part
948.11 Burn (any degree) involving 10-19% of body surface with third degree burn of 10-19%
949.3 Full-thickness skin loss due to burn (third degree NOS), unspecified site
949.4 Deep necrosis of underlying tissue due to burn (deep third degree), unspecified site without mention of loss of body part
949.5 Deep necrosis of underlying tissues due to burn (deep third degree, unspecified site with loss of body part

AND

Nonoperating Room Procedure

96.72 Continuous invasive mechanical ventilation for 96 consecutive hours or more

AND

Operating Room Procedures

85.82 Split-thickness graft to breast
85.83 Full-thickness graft to breast
85.84 Pedicle graft to breast

86.60 Free skin graft, not otherwise specified
86.61 Full-thickness skin graft to hand
86.62 Other skin graft to hand
86.63 Full-thickness skin graft to other sites
86.65 Heterograft to skin
86.66 Homograft to skin
86.67 Dermal regenerative graft
86.69 Other skin graft to other sites
86.7* Pedicle grafts or flaps
86.93 Insertion of tissue expander

OR

Principal or Secondary Diagnosis

948.21 Burn (any degree) involving 20-29% of body surface with third degree burn of 10-19%
948.22 Burn (any degree) involving 20-29% of body surface with third degree burn of 20-29%
948.31 Burn (any degree) involving 30-39% of body surface with third degree burn of 10-19%
948.32 Burn (any degree) involving 30-39% of body surface with third degree burn of 20-29%
948.33 Burn (any degree) involving 30-39% of body surface with third degree burn of 30-39%
948.41 Burn (any degree) involving 40-49% of body surface with third degree burn of 10-19%
948.42 Burn (any degree) involving 40-49% of body surface with third degree burn of 20-29%
948.43 Burn (any degree) involving 40-49% of body surface with third degree burn of 30-39%
948.44 Burn (any degree) involving 40-49% of body surface with third degree burn of 40-49%
948.51 Burn (any degree) involving 50-59% of body surface with third degree burn of 10-19%
948.52 Burn (any degree) involving 50-59% of body surface with third degree burn of 20-29%
948.53 Burn (any degree) involving 50-59% of body surface with third degree burn of 30-39%
948.54 Burn (any degree) involving 50-59% of body surface with third degree burn of 40-49%
948.55 Burn (any degree) involving 50-59% of body surface with third degree burn of 50-59%
948.61 Burn (any degree) involving 60-69% of body surface with third degree burn of 10-19%
948.62 Burn (any degree) involving 60-69% of body surface with third degree burn of 20-29%
948.63 Burn (any degree) involving 60-69% of body surface with third degree burn of 30-39%
948.64 Burn (any degree) involving 60-69% of body surface with third degree burn of 40-49%
948.65 Burn (any degree) involving 60-69% of body surface with third degree burn of 50-59%
948.66 Burn (any degree) involving 60-69% of body surface with third degree burn of 60-69%
948.71 Burn (any degree) involving 70-79% of body surface with third degree burn of 10-19%
948.72 Burn (any degree) involving 70-79% of body surface with third degree burn of 20-29%
948.73 Burn (any degree) involving 70-79% of body surface with third degree burn of 30-39%
948.74 Burn (any degree) involving 70-79% of body surface with third degree burn of 40-49%
948.75 Burn (any degree) involving 70-79% of body surface with third degree burn of 50-59%
948.76 Burn (any degree) involving 70-79% of body surface with third degree burn of 60-69%
948.77 Burn (any degree) involving 70-79% of body surface with third degree burn of 70-79%
948.81 Burn (any degree) involving 80-89% of body surface with third degree burn of 10-19%

T Transfer DRG   SP Special Payment   ☑ Optimization Potential   Targeted Potential   * Code Range   ● New DRG   ▲ Revised DRG Title

206   Valid 10/01/2013-09/30/2014   © 2013 OptumInsight, Inc.

948.82	Burn (any degree) involving 80-89% of body surface with third degree burn of 20-29%
948.83	Burn (any degree) involving 80-89% of body surface with third degree burn of 30-39%
948.84	Burn (any degree) involving 80-89% of body surface with third degree burn of 40-49%
948.85	Burn (any degree) involving 80-89% of body surface with third degree burn of 50-59%
948.86	Burn (any degree) involving 80-89% of body surface with third degree burn of 60-69%
948.87	Burn (any degree) involving 80-89% of body surface with third degree burn of 70-79%
948.88	Burn (any degree) involving 80-89% of body surface with third degree burn of 80-89%
948.91	Burn (any degree) involving 90% or more of body surface with third degree burn of 10-19%
948.92	Burn (any degree) involving 90% or more of body surface with third degree burn of 20-29%
948.93	Burn (any degree) involving 90% or more of body surface with third degree burn of 30-39%
948.94	Burn (any degree) involving 90% or more of body surface with third degree burn of 40-49%
948.95	Burn (any degree) involving 90% or more of body surface with third degree burn of 50-59%
948.96	Burn (any degree) involving 90% or more of body surface with third degree burn of 60-69%
948.97	Burn (any degree) involving 90% or more of body surface with third degree burn of 70-79%
948.98	Burn (any degree) involving 90% or more of body surface with third degree burn of 80-89%
948.99	Burn (any degree) involving 90% or more of body surface with third degree burn of 90% or more of body surface

AND

Operating Room Procedures

85.82	Split-thickness graft to breast
85.83	Full-thickness graft to breast
85.84	Pedicle graft to breast
86.60	Free skin graft, not otherwise specified
86.61	Full-thickness skin graft to hand
86.62	Other skin graft to hand
86.63	Full-thickness skin graft to other sites
86.65	Heterograft to skin
86.66	Homograft to skin
86.67	Dermal regenerative graft
86.69	Other skin graft to other sites
86.7*	Pedicle grafts or flaps
86.93	Insertion of tissue expander

DRG 928   Full Thickness Burn with Skin Graft or Inhalation Injury with CC/MCC

| GMLOS 11.9 | AMLOS 16.1 | RW 5.7744 | ☑ |

Principal or Secondary Diagnosis

941.3*	Full-thickness skin loss due to burn (third degree NOS) of face, head, and neck
941.4*	Deep necrosis of underlying tissues due to burn (deep third degree) of face, head, and neck without mention of loss of a body part
941.5*	Deep necrosis of underlying tissues due to burn (deep third degree) of face, head, and neck with loss of a body part
942.3*	Full-thickness skin loss due to burn (third degree NOS) of trunk
942.4*	Deep necrosis of underlying tissues due to burn (deep third degree) of trunk without mention of loss of a body part
942.5*	Deep necrosis of underlying tissues due to burn (deep third degree) of trunk with loss of a body part
943.3*	Full-thickness skin loss due to burn (third degree NOS) of upper limb, except wrist and hand

943.4*	Deep necrosis of underlying tissues due to burn (deep third degree) of upper limb, except wrist and hand, without mention of loss of a body part
943.5*	Deep necrosis of underlying tissues due to burn (deep third degree) of upper limb, except wrist and hand, with loss of a body part
944.3*	Full-thickness skin loss due to burn (third degree NOS) of wrist(s) and hand(s)
944.4*	Deep necrosis of underlying tissues due to burn (deep third degree) of wrist(s) and hand(s), without mention of loss of a body part
944.5*	Deep necrosis of underlying tissues due to burn (deep third degree) of wrist(s) and hand(s), with loss of a body part
945.3*	Full-thickness skin loss due to burn (third degree NOS) of lower limb(s)
945.4*	Deep necrosis of underlying tissues due to burn (deep third degree) of lower limb(s) without mention of loss of a body part
945.5*	Deep necrosis of underlying tissues due to burn (deep third degree) of lower limb(s) with loss of a body part
946.3	Full-thickness skin loss due to burn (third degree NOS) of multiple specified sites
946.4	Deep necrosis of underlying tissues due to burn (deep third degree) of multiple specified sites, without mention of loss of a body part
946.5	Deep necrosis of underlying tissues due to burn (deep third degree) of multiple specified sites, with loss of a body part
948.11	Burn (any degree) involving 10-19% of body surface with third degree burn of 10-19%
949.3	Full-thickness skin loss due to burn (third degree NOS), unspecified site
949.4	Deep necrosis of underlying tissue due to burn (deep third degree), unspecified site without mention of loss of body part
949.5	Deep necrosis of underlying tissues due to burn (deep third degree, unspecified site with loss of body part

AND

Operating Room Procedures

85.82	Split-thickness graft to breast
85.83	Full-thickness graft to breast
85.84	Pedicle graft to breast
86.60	Free skin graft, not otherwise specified
86.61	Full-thickness skin graft to hand
86.62	Other skin graft to hand
86.63	Full-thickness skin graft to other sites
86.65	Heterograft to skin
86.66	Homograft to skin
86.67	Dermal regenerative graft
86.69	Other skin graft to other sites
86.7*	Pedicle grafts or flaps
86.93	Insertion of tissue expander

OR

Secondary Diagnosis

508.2	Respiratory conditions due to smoke inhalation
518.5*	Pulmonary insufficiency following trauma and surgery
518.81	Acute respiratory failure
518.84	Acute and chronic respiratory failure
947.1	Burn of larynx, trachea, and lung
987.9	Toxic effect of unspecified gas, fume, or vapor

| Surgical | Medical | CC Indicator | MCC Indicator | Procedure Proxy |

DRG 929　Full Thickness Burn with Skin Graft or Inhalation Injury without CC/MCC

GMLOS 5.1　　　　AMLOS 7.2　　　　RW 2.2090　　　☑

Select principal or secondary diagnosis and operating room procedure or secondary diagnosis listed under DRG 928

Select principal or secondary diagnosis in combination with secondary diagnosis of inhalation injury and operating room procedures listed under DRG 928

MEDICAL

DRG 933　Extensive Burns or Full Thickness Burns with Mechanical Ventilation 96+ Hours without Skin Graft

GMLOS 2.6　　　　AMLOS 8.2　　　　RW 3.2785　　　☑

Principal or Secondary Diagnosis

941.3*　Full-thickness skin loss due to burn (third degree NOS) of face, head, and neck

941.4*　Deep necrosis of underlying tissues due to burn (deep third degree) of face, head, and neck without mention of loss of a body part

941.5*　Deep necrosis of underlying tissues due to burn (deep third degree) of face, head, and neck with loss of a body part

942.3*　Full-thickness skin loss due to burn (third degree NOS) of trunk

942.4*　Deep necrosis of underlying tissues due to burn (deep third degree) of trunk without mention of loss of a body part

942.5*　Deep necrosis of underlying tissues due to burn (deep third degree) of trunk with loss of a body part

943.3*　Full-thickness skin loss due to burn (third degree NOS) of upper limb, except wrist and hand

943.4*　Deep necrosis of underlying tissues due to burn (deep third degree) of upper limb, except wrist and hand, without mention of loss of a body part

943.5*　Deep necrosis of underlying tissues due to burn (deep third degree) of upper limb, except wrist and hand, with loss of a body part

944.3*　Full-thickness skin loss due to burn (third degree NOS) of wrist(s) and hand(s)

944.4*　Deep necrosis of underlying tissues due to burn (deep third degree) of wrist(s) and hand(s), without mention of loss of a body part

944.5*　Deep necrosis of underlying tissues due to burn (deep third degree) of wrist(s) and hand(s), with loss of a body part

945.3*　Full-thickness skin loss due to burn (third degree NOS) of lower limb(s)

945.4*　Deep necrosis of underlying tissues due to burn (deep third degree) of lower limb(s) without mention of loss of a body part

945.5*　Deep necrosis of underlying tissues due to burn (deep third degree) of lower limb(s) with loss of a body part

946.3　Full-thickness skin loss due to burn (third degree NOS) of multiple specified sites

946.4　Deep necrosis of underlying tissues due to burn (deep third degree) of multiple specified sites, without mention of loss of a body part

946.5　Deep necrosis of underlying tissues due to burn (deep third degree) of multiple specified sites, with loss of a body part

948.11　Burn (any degree) involving 10-19% of body surface with third degree burn of 10-19%

949.3　Full-thickness skin loss due to burn (third degree NOS), unspecified site

949.4　Deep necrosis of underlying tissue due to burn (deep third degree), unspecified site without mention of loss of body part

949.5　Deep necrosis of underlying tissues due to burn (deep third degree, unspecified site with loss of body part

AND

Nonoperating Room Procedure

96.72　Continuous invasive mechanical ventilation for 96 consecutive hours or more

OR

Principal or Secondary Diagnosis

948.21　Burn (any degree) involving 20-29% of body surface with third degree burn of 10-19%

948.22　Burn (any degree) involving 20-29% of body surface with third degree burn of 20-29%

948.31　Burn (any degree) involving 30-39% of body surface with third degree burn of 10-19%

948.32　Burn (any degree) involving 30-39% of body surface with third degree burn of 20-29%

948.33　Burn (any degree) involving 30-39% of body surface with third degree burn of 30-39%

948.41　Burn (any degree) involving 40-49% of body surface with third degree burn of 10-19%

948.42　Burn (any degree) involving 40-49% of body surface with third degree burn of 20-29%

948.43　Burn (any degree) involving 40-49% of body surface with third degree burn of 30-39%

948.44　Burn (any degree) involving 40-49% of body surface with third degree burn of 40-49%

948.51　Burn (any degree) involving 50-59% of body surface with third degree burn of 10-19%

948.52　Burn (any degree) involving 50-59% of body surface with third degree burn of 20-29%

948.53　Burn (any degree) involving 50-59% of body surface with third degree burn of 30-39%

948.54　Burn (any degree) involving 50-59% of body surface with third degree burn of 40-49%

948.55　Burn (any degree) involving 50-59% of body surface with third degree burn of 50-59%

948.61　Burn (any degree) involving 60-69% of body surface with third degree burn of 10-19%

948.62　Burn (any degree) involving 60-69% of body surface with third degree burn of 20-29%

948.63　Burn (any degree) involving 60-69% of body surface with third degree burn of 30-39%

948.64　Burn (any degree) involving 60-69% of body surface with third degree burn of 40-49%

948.65　Burn (any degree) involving 60-69% of body surface with third degree burn of 50-59%

948.66　Burn (any degree) involving 60-69% of body surface with third degree burn of 60-69%

948.71　Burn (any degree) involving 70-79% of body surface with third degree burn of 10-19%

948.72　Burn (any degree) involving 70-79% of body surface with third degree burn of 20-29%

948.73　Burn (any degree) involving 70-79% of body surface with third degree burn of 30-39%

948.74　Burn (any degree) involving 70-79% of body surface with third degree burn of 40-49%

948.75　Burn (any degree) involving 70-79% of body surface with third degree burn of 50-59%

948.76　Burn (any degree) involving 70-79% of body surface with third degree burn of 60-69%

948.77　Burn (any degree) involving 70-79% of body surface with third degree burn of 70-79%

948.81　Burn (any degree) involving 80-89% of body surface with third degree burn of 10-19%

948.82　Burn (any degree) involving 80-89% of body surface with third degree burn of 20-29%

948.83　Burn (any degree) involving 80-89% of body surface with third degree burn of 30-39%

Ⓣ *Transfer DRG*　　Ⓢ *Special Payment*　　☑ *Optimization Potential*　　▽ *Targeted Potential*　　＊ *Code Range*　　● *New DRG*　　▲ *Revised DRG Title*

948.84 Burn (any degree) involving 80-89% of body surface with third degree burn of 40-49%

948.85 Burn (any degree) involving 80-89% of body surface with third degree burn of 50-59%

948.86 Burn (any degree) involving 80-89% of body surface with third degree burn of 60-69%

948.87 Burn (any degree) involving 80-89% of body surface with third degree burn of 70-79%

948.88 Burn (any degree) involving 80-89% of body surface with third degree burn of 80-89%

948.91 Burn (any degree) involving 90% or more of body surface with third degree burn of 10-19%

948.92 Burn (any degree) involving 90% or more of body surface with third degree burn of 20-29%

948.93 Burn (any degree) involving 90% or more of body surface with third degree burn of 30-39%

948.94 Burn (any degree) involving 90% or more of body surface with third degree burn of 40-49%

948.95 Burn (any degree) involving 90% or more of body surface with third degree burn of 50-59%

948.96 Burn (any degree) involving 90% or more of body surface with third degree burn of 60-69%

948.97 Burn (any degree) involving 90% or more of body surface with third degree burn of 70-79%

948.98 Burn (any degree) involving 90% or more of body surface with third degree burn of 80-89%

948.99 Burn (any degree) involving 90% or more of body surface with third degree burn of 90% or more of body surface

DRG 934 Full Thickness Burn without Skin Graft or Inhalation Injury

| GMLOS 4.2 | AMLOS 6.1 | RW 1.6045 | ☑ |

Principal Diagnosis

941.3* Full-thickness skin loss due to burn (third degree NOS) of face, head, and neck

941.4* Deep necrosis of underlying tissues due to burn (deep third degree) of face, head, and neck without mention of loss of a body part

941.5* Deep necrosis of underlying tissues due to burn (deep third degree) of face, head, and neck with loss of a body part

942.3* Full-thickness skin loss due to burn (third degree NOS) of trunk

942.4* Deep necrosis of underlying tissues due to burn (deep third degree) of trunk without mention of loss of a body part

942.5* Deep necrosis of underlying tissues due to burn (deep third degree) of trunk with loss of a body part

943.3* Full-thickness skin loss due to burn (third degree NOS) of upper limb, except wrist and hand

943.4* Deep necrosis of underlying tissues due to burn (deep third degree) of upper limb, except wrist and hand, without mention of loss of a body part

943.5* Deep necrosis of underlying tissues due to burn (deep third degree) of upper limb, except wrist and hand, with loss of a body part

944.3* Full-thickness skin loss due to burn (third degree NOS) of wrist(s) and hand(s)

944.4* Deep necrosis of underlying tissues due to burn (deep third degree) of wrist(s) and hand(s), without mention of loss of a body part

944.5* Deep necrosis of underlying tissues due to burn (deep third degree) of wrist(s) and hand(s), with loss of a body part

945.3* Full-thickness skin loss due to burn (third degree NOS) of lower limb(s)

945.4* Deep necrosis of underlying tissues due to burn (deep third degree) of lower limb(s) without mention of loss of a body part

945.5* Deep necrosis of underlying tissues due to burn (deep third degree) of lower limb(s) with loss of a body part

946.3 Full-thickness skin loss due to burn (third degree NOS) of multiple specified sites

946.4 Deep necrosis of underlying tissues due to burn (deep third degree) of multiple specified sites, without mention of loss of a body part

946.5 Deep necrosis of underlying tissues due to burn (deep third degree) of multiple specified sites, with loss of a body part

948.11 Burn (any degree) involving 10-19% of body surface with third degree burn of 10-19%

949.3 Full-thickness skin loss due to burn (third degree NOS), unspecified site

949.4 Deep necrosis of underlying tissue due to burn (deep third degree), unspecified site without mention of loss of body part

949.5 Deep necrosis of underlying tissues due to burn (deep third degree, unspecified site with loss of body part

DRG 935 Nonextensive Burns

| GMLOS 3.2 | AMLOS 4.8 | RW 1.3909 | ☑ |

Principal Diagnosis

941.00 Burn of unspecified degree of unspecified site of face and head

941.01 Burn of unspecified degree of ear (any part)

941.03 Burn of unspecified degree of lip(s)

941.04 Burn of unspecified degree of chin

941.05 Burn of unspecified degree of nose (septum)

941.06 Burn of unspecified degree of scalp (any part)

941.07 Burn of unspecified degree of forehead and cheek

941.08 Burn of unspecified degree of neck

941.09 Burn of unspecified degree of multiple sites (except with eye) of face, head, and neck

941.10 Erythema due to burn (first degree) of unspecified site of face and head

941.11 Erythema due to burn (first degree) of ear (any part)

941.13 Erythema due to burn (first degree) of lip(s)

941.14 Erythema due to burn (first degree) of chin

941.15 Erythema due to burn (first degree) of nose (septum)

941.16 Erythema due to burn (first degree) of scalp (any part)

941.17 Erythema due to burn (first degree) of forehead and cheek

941.18 Erythema due to burn (first degree) of neck

941.19 Erythema due to burn (first degree) of multiple sites (except with eye) of face, head, and neck

941.20 Blisters, with epidermal loss due to burn (second degree) of face and head, unspecified site

941.21 Blisters, with epidermal loss due to burn (second degree) of ear (any part)

941.23 Blisters, with epidermal loss due to burn (second degree) of lip(s)

941.24 Blisters, with epidermal loss due to burn (second degree) of chin

941.25 Blisters, with epidermal loss due to burn (second degree) of nose (septum)

941.26 Blisters, with epidermal loss due to burn (second degree) of scalp (any part)

941.27 Blisters, with epidermal loss due to burn (second degree) of forehead and cheek

941.28 Blisters, with epidermal loss due to burn (second degree) of neck

941.29 Blisters, with epidermal loss due to burn (second degree) of multiple sites (except with eye) of face, head, and neck

942.0* Burn of trunk, unspecified degree

942.1* Erythema due to burn (first degree) of trunk

942.2* Blisters with epidermal loss due to burn (second degree) of trunk

943.0* Burn of upper limb, except wrist and hand, unspecified degree

943.1* Erythema due to burn (first degree) of upper limb, except wrist and hand

943.2*	Blisters with epidermal loss due to burn (second degree) of upper limb, except wrist and hand
944.0*	Burn of wrist(s) and hand(s), unspecified degree
944.1*	Erythema due to burn (first degree) of wrist(s) and hand(s)
944.2*	Blisters with epidermal loss due to burn (second degree) of wrist(s) and hand(s)
945.0*	Burn of lower limb(s), unspecified degree
945.1*	Erythema due to burn (first degree) of lower limb(s)
945.2*	Blisters with epidermal loss due to burn (second degree) of lower limb(s)
946.0	Burns of multiple specified sites, unspecified degree
946.1	Erythema due to burn (first degree) of multiple specified sites
946.2	Blisters with epidermal loss due to burn (second degree) of multiple specified sites
947.8	Burn of other specified sites of internal organs
947.9	Burn of internal organs, unspecified site
948.00	Burn (any degree) involving less than 10% of body surface with third degree burn of less than 10% or unspecified amount
948.10	Burn (any degree) involving 10-19% of body surface with third degree burn of less than 10% or unspecified amount
948.20	Burn (any degree) involving 20-29% of body surface with third degree burn of less than 10% or unspecified amount
948.30	Burn (any degree) involving 30-39% of body surface with third degree burn of less than 10% or unspecified amount
948.40	Burn (any degree) involving 40-49% of body surface with third degree burn of less than 10% or unspecified amount
948.50	Burn (any degree) involving 50-59% of body surface with third degree burn of less than 10% or unspecified amount
948.60	Burn (any degree) involving 60-69% of body surface with third degree burn of less than 10% or unspecified amount
948.70	Burn (any degree) involving 70-79% of body surface with third degree burn of less than 10% or unspecified amount
948.80	Burn (any degree) involving 80-89% of body surface with third degree burn of less than 10% or unspecified amount
948.90	Burn (any degree) involving 90% or more of body surface with third degree burn of less than 10% or unspecified amount
949.0	Burn of unspecified site, unspecified degree
949.1	Erythema due to burn (first degree), unspecified site
949.2	Blisters with epidermal loss due to burn (second degree), unspecified site

---

Ⓣ *Transfer DRG*   ⓢ *Special Payment*   ☑ *Optimization Potential*   ▽ *Targeted Potential*   * *Code Range*   ● *New DRG*   ▲ *Revised DRG Title*

MDC 23
Factors Influencing Health Status And Other Contacts With Health Services

305.1	V01.81	V07.8	V14.2	V17.81	V26.32	V44.52	V49.61	V58.67
338.11	V01.82	V07.9	V14.3	V17.89	V26.33	V44.59	V49.62	V58.68
338.12	V01.83	V11.0	V14.4	V18.0	V26.34	V44.6	V49.63	V58.69
338.18	V01.84	V11.1	V14.5	V18.11	V26.35	V44.7	V49.64	V58.71
338.19	V01.89	V11.2	V14.6	V18.19	V26.39	V44.8	V49.65	V58.72
338.3	V01.9	V11.3	V14.7	V18.2	V26.41	V44.9	V49.66	V58.73
758.4	V02.0	V11.4	V14.8	V18.3	V26.42	V45.00	V49.67	V58.74
758.5	V02.1	V11.8	V14.9	V18.4	V26.49	V45.01	V49.70	V58.75
758.9	V02.2	V11.9	V15.01	V18.51	V26.51	V45.02	V49.71	V58.76
759.9	V02.3	V12.00	V15.02	V18.59	V26.52	V45.09	V49.72	V58.77
780.64	V02.4	V12.01	V15.03	V18.61	V26.81	V45.11	V49.73	V58.78
780.65	V02.51	V12.02	V15.04	V18.69	V26.82	V45.12	V49.74	V58.81
780.71	V02.52	V12.03	V15.05	V18.7	V26.89	V45.2	V49.75	V58.82
780.79	V02.53	V12.04	V15.06	V18.8	V26.9	V45.3	V49.76	V58.83
780.91	V02.54	V12.09	V15.07	V18.9	V27.0	V45.4	V49.77	V58.89
780.92	V02.59	V12.1	V15.08	V19.0	V27.1	V45.51	V49.81	V58.9
780.93	V02.7	V12.21	V15.09	V19.11	V27.2	V45.52	V49.82	V59.01
780.94	V02.8	V12.29	V15.1	V19.19	V27.3	V45.59	V49.83	V59.02
780.95	V02.9	V12.3	V15.21	V19.2	V27.4	V45.61	V49.84	V59.09
780.96	V03.0	V12.40	V15.22	V19.3	V27.5	V45.69	V49.85	V59.3
780.97	V03.1	V12.41	V15.29	V19.4	V27.6	V45.71	V49.86	V59.5
780.99	V03.2	V12.42	V15.3	V19.5	V27.7	V45.72	V49.87	V59.70
782.3	V03.3	V12.49	V15.41	V19.6	V27.9	V45.73	V49.89	V59.71
782.5	V03.4	V12.50	V15.42	V19.7	V28.3	V45.75	V49.9	V59.72
782.61	V03.5	V12.51	V15.49	V19.8	V28.4	V45.79	V50.3	V59.73
782.62	V03.6	V12.52	V15.51	V20.0	V28.5	V45.81	V50.49	V59.74
789.51	V03.7	V12.53	V15.52	V20.1	V28.6	V45.82	V50.8	V59.8
789.59	V03.81	V12.54	V15.53	V20.2	V28.81	V45.83	V50.9	V59.9
790.1	V03.82	V12.55	V15.59	V20.31	V28.82	V45.84	V52.2	V60.0
790.4	V03.89	V12.59	V15.6	V20.32	V28.89	V45.85	V52.3	V60.1
790.5	V03.9	V12.60	V15.7	V21.0	V28.9	V45.86	V52.4	V60.2
790.6	V04.0	V12.61	V15.80	V21.1	V29.0	V45.87	V52.8	V60.3
790.91	V04.1	V12.69	V15.81	V21.2	V29.1	V45.88	V52.9	V60.4
790.92	V04.2	V12.70	V15.82	V21.30	V29.2	V45.89	V53.1	V60.5
790.93	V04.3	V12.71	V15.83	V21.31	V29.3	V46.0	V53.2	V60.6
790.94	V04.4	V12.72	V15.84	V21.32	V29.8	V46.11	V53.4	V60.81
790.95	V04.5	V12.79	V15.85	V21.33	V29.9	V46.12	V53.8	V60.89
790.99	V04.6	V13.00	V15.86	V21.34	V40.0	V46.13	V53.90	V60.9
791.3	V04.7	V13.01	V15.87	V21.35	V40.1	V46.14	V53.91	V61.01
792.5	V04.81	V13.02	V15.88	V21.8	V40.2	V46.2	V53.99	V61.02
792.9	V04.82	V13.03	V15.89	V21.9	V40.31	V46.3	V55.8	V61.03
793.91	V04.89	V13.09	V15.9	V22.0	V40.39	V46.8	V55.9	V61.04
793.99	V05.0	V13.1	V16.0	V22.1	V40.9	V46.9	V57.0	V61.05
795.2	V05.1	V13.21	V16.1	V22.2	V41.0	V47.0	V57.1	V61.06
795.4	V05.2	V13.23	V16.2	V24.1	V41.1	V47.1	V57.21	V61.07
795.81	V05.3	V13.24	V16.3	V24.2	V41.2	V47.2	V57.22	V61.08
795.82	V05.4	V13.29	V16.40	V25.01	V41.3	V47.3	V57.3	V61.09
795.89	V05.8	V13.3	V16.41	V25.02	V41.4	V47.4	V57.4	V61.10
796.4	V05.9	V13.4	V16.42	V25.03	V41.5	V47.5	V57.81	V61.11
796.6	V06.0	V13.51	V16.43	V25.04	V41.6	V47.9	V57.89	V61.12
796.9	V06.1	V13.52	V16.49	V25.09	V41.7	V48.0	V57.9	V61.20
798.9	V06.2	V13.59	V16.51	V25.11	V41.8	V48.1	V58.2	V61.21
799.3	V06.3	V13.61	V16.52	V25.12	V41.9	V48.2	V58.30	V61.22
799.4	V06.4	V13.62	V16.59	V25.13	V42.84	V48.3	V58.31	V61.23
799.81	V06.5	V13.63	V16.6	V25.40	V42.89	V48.4	V58.32	V61.24
799.82	V06.6	V13.64	V16.7	V25.41	V42.9	V48.5	V58.41	V61.25
799.89	V06.8	V13.65	V16.8	V25.42	V43.81	V48.6	V58.42	V61.29
799.9	V06.9	V13.66	V16.9	V25.43	V43.82	V48.7	V58.43	V61.3
V01.0	V07.0	V13.67	V17.0	V25.49	V43.83	V48.8	V58.44	V61.41
V01.1	V07.1	V13.68	V17.1	V25.5	V43.89	V48.9	V58.49	V61.42
V01.2	V07.2	V13.69	V17.2	V25.8	V44.0	V49.0	V58.5	V61.49
V01.3	V07.31	V13.7	V17.3	V25.9	V44.1	V49.1	V58.61	V61.8
V01.4	V07.39	V13.81	V17.41	V26.1	V44.2	V49.2	V58.62	V61.9
V01.5	V07.4	V13.89	V17.49	V26.21	V44.3	V49.3	V58.63	V62.0
V01.6	V07.51	V13.9	V17.5	V26.22	V44.4	V49.4	V58.64	V62.1
V01.71	V07.52	V14.0	V17.6	V26.29	V44.50	V49.5	V58.65	V62.21
V01.79	V07.59	V14.1	V17.7	V26.31	V44.51	V49.60	V58.66	V62.22

V62.29	V65.2	V68.81	V72.41	V74.8	V77.2	V82.2	V85.37	V89.05
V62.3	V65.3	V68.89	V72.42	V74.9	V77.3	V82.3	V85.38	V89.09
V62.4	V65.40	V68.9	V72.5	V75.0	V77.4	V82.4	V85.39	V90.01
V62.5	V65.41	V69.0	V72.60	V75.1	V77.5	V82.5	V85.51	V90.09
V62.6	V65.42	V69.1	V72.61	V75.2	V77.6	V82.6	V85.52	V90.10
V62.81	V65.43	V69.2	V72.62	V75.3	V77.7	V82.71	V85.53	V90.11
V62.82	V65.44	V69.3	V72.63	V75.4	V77.8	V82.79	V85.54	V90.12
V62.83	V65.45	V69.4	V72.69	V75.5	V77.91	V82.81	V86.0	V90.2
V62.85	V65.46	V69.5	V72.7	V75.6	V77.99	V82.89	V86.1	V90.31
V62.89	V65.49	V69.8	V72.81	V75.7	V78.0	V82.9	V87.01	V90.32
V62.9	V65.5	V69.9	V72.82	V75.8	V78.1	V83.01	V87.02	V90.33
V63.0	V65.8	V70.0	V72.83	V75.9	V78.2	V83.02	V87.09	V90.39
V63.1	V65.9	V70.1	V72.84	V76.0	V78.3	V83.81	V87.11	V90.81
V63.2	V66.0	V70.2	V72.85	V76.10	V78.8	V83.89	V87.12	V90.83
V63.8	V66.1	V70.3	V72.86	V76.11	V78.9	V84.01	V87.19	V90.89
V63.9	V66.2	V70.4	V72.9	V76.12	V79.0	V84.02	V87.2	V90.9
V64.00	V66.3	V70.5	V73.0	V76.19	V79.1	V84.03	V87.31	V91.00
V64.01	V66.4	V70.6	V73.1	V76.2	V79.2	V84.04	V87.32	V91.01
V64.02	V66.5	V70.7	V73.2	V76.3	V79.3	V84.09	V87.39	V91.02
V64.03	V66.6	V70.8	V73.3	V76.41	V79.8	V84.81	V87.41	V91.03
V64.04	V66.7	V70.9	V73.4	V76.42	V79.9	V84.89	V87.42	V91.09
V64.05	V66.9	V71.5	V73.5	V76.43	V80.01	V85.0	V87.43	V91.10
V64.06	V67.00	V71.81	V73.6	V76.44	V80.09	V85.1	V87.44	V91.11
V64.07	V67.01	V71.82	V73.81	V76.45	V80.1	V85.21	V87.45	V91.12
V64.08	V67.09	V71.83	V73.88	V76.46	V80.2	V85.22	V87.46	V91.19
V64.09	V67.3	V71.89	V73.89	V76.47	V80.3	V85.23	V87.49	V91.20
V64.1	V67.4	V71.9	V73.98	V76.49	V81.0	V85.24	V88.11	V91.21
V64.2	V67.51	V72.0	V73.99	V76.50	V81.1	V85.25	V88.12	V91.22
V64.3	V67.59	V72.11	V74.0	V76.51	V81.2	V85.30	V88.21	V91.29
V64.41	V67.6	V72.12	V74.1	V76.52	V81.3	V85.31	V88.22	V91.90
V64.42	V67.9	V72.19	V74.2	V76.81	V81.4	V85.32	V88.29	V91.91
V64.43	V68.01	V72.2	V74.3	V76.89	V81.5	V85.33	V89.01	V91.92
V65.0	V68.09	V72.31	V74.4	V76.9	V81.6	V85.34	V89.02	V91.99
V65.11	V68.1	V72.32	V74.5	V77.0	V82.0	V85.35	V89.03	
V65.19	V68.2	V72.40	V74.6	V77.1	V82.1	V85.36	V89.04	

MDC 23: Factors Influencing Health Status And Other Contacts With Health Services—SURGICAL

SURGICAL

DRG 939 O.R. Procedure with Diagnoses of Other Contact with Health Services with MCC
GMLOS 6.6   AMLOS 9.8   RW 3.1182

Select any operating room procedure

DRG 940 O.R. Procedure with Diagnoses of Other Contact with Health Services with CC
GMLOS 3.7   AMLOS 5.3   RW 1.7675   ☑

Select any operating room procedure

DRG 941 O.R. Procedure with Diagnoses of Other Contact with Health Services without CC/MCC
GMLOS 2.2   AMLOS 2.8   RW 1.3403   ☑

Select any operating room procedure

MEDICAL

DRG 945 Rehabilitation with CC/MCC
GMLOS 8.3   AMLOS 10.1   RW 1.3804   ☑Ⓣ

Principal Diagnosis
V52.8   Fitting and adjustment of other specified prosthetic device
V52.9   Fitting and adjustment of unspecified prosthetic device
V57.1   Other physical therapy
V57.2*   Occupational therapy and vocational rehabilitation
V57.3   Care involving use of rehabilitation speech-language therapy
V57.89   Other specified rehabilitation procedure
V57.9   Unspecified rehabilitation procedure

DRG 946 Rehabilitation without CC/MCC
GMLOS 6.5   AMLOS 7.4   RW 1.2037   ☑Ⓣ

Select principal diagnosis listed under DRG 945

DRG 947 Signs and Symptoms with MCC
GMLOS 3.6   AMLOS 4.8   RW 1.1324   ☑Ⓣ

Principal Diagnosis
338.1*   Acute pain
338.3   Neoplasm related pain (acute) (chronic)
780.64   Chills (without fever)
780.65   Hypothermia not associated with low environmental temperature
780.71   Chronic fatigue syndrome
780.79   Other malaise and fatigue
780.9*   Other general symptoms
782.3   Edema
782.5   Cyanosis
782.6*   Pallor and flushing
789.5*   Ascites
790.1   Elevated sedimentation rate
790.4   Nonspecific elevation of levels of transaminase or lactic acid dehydrogenase (LDH)
790.5   Other nonspecific abnormal serum enzyme levels
790.6   Other abnormal blood chemistry
790.9*   Other nonspecific findings on examination of blood
791.3   Myoglobinuria
792.5   Cloudy (hemodialysis) (peritoneal) dialysis affluent
792.9   Other nonspecific abnormal finding in body substances

793.9*   Other nonspecific abnormal findings on radiological and other examinations of body structure
795.4   Other nonspecific abnormal histological findings
795.8*   Abnormal tumor markers
796.4   Other abnormal clinical finding
796.6   Nonspecific abnormal findings on neonatal screening
796.9   Other nonspecific abnormal finding
799.3   Unspecified debility
799.4   Cachexia

DRG 948 Signs and Symptoms without MCC
GMLOS 2.6   AMLOS 3.3   RW 0.6897   ☑Ⓣ

Select principal diagnosis listed under DRG 947

DRG 949 Aftercare with CC/MCC
GMLOS 2.8   AMLOS 4.1   RW 1.0038   ☑

Principal Diagnosis
V58.4*   Other aftercare following surgery
V58.5   Orthodontics aftercare
V58.6*   Long-term (current) drug use
V58.7*   Aftercare following surgery to specified body systems, not elsewhere classified
V58.8*   Other specified aftercare
V58.9   Unspecified aftercare
V67.0*   Surgery follow-up examination
V67.4   Treatment of healed fracture follow-up examination
V87.4*   Personal history of drug therapy

DRG 950 Aftercare without CC/MCC
GMLOS 2.3   AMLOS 3.5   RW 0.6005   ☑

Select principal diagnosis listed under DRG 949

DRG 951 Other Factors Influencing Health Status
GMLOS 2.4   AMLOS 5.5   RW 0.8578   ☑

Principal Diagnosis
305.1   Nondependent tobacco use disorder
758.4   Balanced autosomal translocation in normal individual
758.5   Other conditions due to autosomal anomalies
758.9   Conditions due to anomaly of unspecified chromosome
759.9   Unspecified congenital anomaly
795.2   Nonspecific abnormal findings on chromosomal analysis
798.9   Unattended death
799.8*   Other ill-defined conditions
799.9   Other unknown and unspecified cause of morbidity or mortality
V01*   Contact with or exposure to communicable diseases
V02.0   Carrier or suspected carrier of cholera
V02.1   Carrier or suspected carrier of typhoid
V02.2   Carrier or suspected carrier of amebiasis
V02.3   Carrier or suspected carrier of other gastrointestinal pathogens
V02.4   Carrier or suspected carrier of diphtheria
V02.5*   Carrier or suspected carrier of other specified bacterial diseases
V02.7   Carrier or suspected carrier of gonorrhea
V02.8   Carrier or suspected carrier of other venereal diseases
V02.9   Carrier or suspected carrier of other specified infectious organism
V03*   Need for prophylactic vaccination and inoculation against bacterial diseases
V04*   Need for prophylactic vaccination and inoculation against certain viral diseases
V05*   Need for other prophylactic vaccination and inoculation against single diseases
V06*   Need for prophylactic vaccination and inoculation against combinations of diseases

---

Surgical	Medical	CC Indicator	MCC Indicator	Procedure Proxy

MDC 23: Factors Influencing Health Status And Other Contacts With Health Services—MEDICAL

V07*	Need for isolation and other prophylactic or treatment measures
V11*	Personal history of mental disorder
V12*	Personal history of certain other diseases
V13.0*	Personal history of disorders of urinary system
V13.1	Personal history of trophoblastic disease
V13.21	Personal history of pre-term labor
V13.23	Personal history of vaginal dysplasia
V13.24	Personal history of vulvar dysplasia
V13.29	Personal history of other genital system and obstetric disorders
V13.3	Personal history of diseases of skin and subcutaneous tissue
V13.4	Personal history of arthritis
V13.5*	Personal history of other musculoskeletal disorders
V13.6*	Personal history of congenital (corrected) malformations
V13.7	Personal history of perinatal problems
V13.8*	Personal history of other specified diseases
V13.9	Personal history of unspecified disease
V14*	Personal history of allergy to medicinal agents
V15*	Other personal history presenting hazards to health
V16*	Family history of malignant neoplasm
V17*	Family history of certain chronic disabling diseases
V18*	Family history of certain other specific conditions
V19*	Family history of other conditions
V20*	Health supervision of infant or child
V21*	Constitutional states in development
V22*	Normal pregnancy
V24.1	Postpartum care and examination of lactating mother
V24.2	Routine postpartum follow-up
V25.0*	General counseling and advice for contraceptive management
V25.1*	Encounter for insertion or removal of intrauterine contraceptive device
V25.4*	Surveillance of previously prescribed contraceptive methods
V25.5	Insertion of implantable subdermal contraceptive
V25.8	Other specified contraceptive management
V25.9	Unspecified contraceptive management
V26.1	Artificial insemination
V26.2*	Investigation and testing for procreation management
V26.3*	Genetic counseling and testing
V26.4*	Procreative management, general counseling and advice
V26.5*	Sterilization status
V26.8*	Other specified procreative management
V26.9	Unspecified procreative management
V27*	Outcome of delivery
V28.3	Encounter for routine screening for malformation using ultrasonics
V28.4	Antenatal screening for fetal growth retardation using ultrasonics
V28.5	Antenatal screening for isoimmunization
V28.6	Screening of Streptococcus B
V28.8*	Encounter for other specified antenatal screening
V28.9	Unspecified antenatal screening
V29*	Observation and evaluation of newborns and infants for suspected condition not found
V40*	Mental and behavioral problems
V41*	Problems with special senses and other special functions
V42.84	Organ or tissue replaced by transplant, intestines
V42.89	Other organ or tissue replaced by transplant
V42.9	Unspecified organ or tissue replaced by transplant
V43.8*	Other organ or tissue replaced by other means
V44*	Artificial opening status
V45.0*	Postsurgical cardiac pacemaker in situ
V45.1*	Renal dialysis status
V45.2	Presence of cerebrospinal fluid drainage device
V45.3	Intestinal bypass or anastomosis status
V45.4	Arthrodesis status
V45.5*	Presence of contraceptive device
V45.61	Cataract extraction status
V45.69	Other states following surgery of eye and adnexa

V45.71	Acquired absence of breast and nipple
V45.72	Acquired absence of intestine (large) (small)
V45.73	Acquired absence of kidney
V45.75	Acquired absence of organ, stomach
V45.79	Other acquired absence of organ
V45.8*	Other postprocedural status
V46*	Other dependence on machines and devices
V47*	Other problems with internal organs
V48*	Problems with head, neck, and trunk
V49*	Problems with limbs and other problems
V50.3	Ear piercing
V50.49	Other prophylactic organ removal
V50.8	Other elective surgery for purposes other than remedying health states
V50.9	Unspecified elective surgery for purposes other than remedying health states
V52.2	Fitting and adjustment of artificial eye
V52.3	Fitting and adjustment of dental prosthetic device
V52.4	Fitting and adjustment of breast prosthesis and implant
V53.1	Fitting and adjustment of spectacles and contact lenses
V53.2	Fitting and adjustment of hearing aid
V53.4	Fitting and adjustment of orthodontic devices
V53.8	Fitting and adjustment of wheelchair
V53.9*	Fitting and adjustment of other and unspecified device
V55.8	Attention to other specified artificial opening
V55.9	Attention to unspecified artificial opening
V57.0	Care involving breathing exercises
V57.4	Orthoptic training
V57.81	Orthotic training
V58.2	Blood transfusion, without reported diagnosis
V58.3*	Attention to dressings and sutures
V59.0*	Blood donor
V59.3	Bone marrow donor
V59.5	Cornea donor
V59.7*	Egg (oocyte) (ovum) Donor
V59.8	Donor of other specified organ or tissue
V59.9	Donor of unspecified organ or tissue
V60*	Housing, household, and economic circumstances
V61.0*	Family disruption
V61.10	Counseling for marital and partner problems, unspecified
V61.11	Counseling for victim of spousal and partner abuse
V61.12	Counseling for perpetrator of spousal and partner abuse
V61.2*	Parent-child problems
V61.3	Problems with aged parents or in-laws
V61.4*	Health problems within family
V61.8	Other specified family circumstance
V61.9	Unspecified family circumstance
V62.0	Unemployment
V62.1	Adverse effects of work environment
V62.2*	Other occupational circumstances or maladjustment
V62.3	Educational circumstance
V62.4	Social maladjustment
V62.5	Legal circumstance
V62.6	Refusal of treatment for reasons of religion or conscience
V62.81	Interpersonal problem, not elsewhere classified
V62.82	Bereavement, uncomplicated
V62.83	Counseling for perpetrator of physical/sexual abuse
V62.85	Homicidal ideation
V62.89	Other psychological or physical stress, not elsewhere classified
V62.9	Unspecified psychosocial circumstance
V63*	Unavailability of other medical facilities for care
V64*	Persons encountering health services for specific procedures, not carried out
V65*	Other persons seeking consultation
V66*	Convalescence and palliative care
V67.3	Psychotherapy and other treatment for mental disorder follow-up examination
V67.5*	Other follow-up examination
V67.6	Combined treatment follow-up examination

T *Transfer DRG*   SP *Special Payment*   ☑ *Optimization Potential*   ▽ *Targeted Potential*   * *Code Range*   ● *New DRG*   ▲ *Revised DRG Title*

V67.9	Unspecified follow-up examination
V68*	Encounters for administrative purposes
V69*	Problems related to lifestyle
V70*	General medical examination
V71.5	Observation following alleged rape or seduction
V71.8*	Observation and evaluation for other specified suspected conditions
V71.9	Observation for unspecified suspected condition
V72*	Special investigations and examinations
V73*	Special screening examination for viral and chlamydial diseases
V74*	Special screening examination for bacterial and spirochetal diseases
V75*	Special screening examination for other infectious diseases
V76*	Special screening for malignant neoplasms
V77*	Special screening for endocrine, nutritional, metabolic, and immunity disorders
V78*	Special screening for disorders of blood and blood-forming organs
V79*	Special screening for mental disorders and developmental handicaps
V80*	Special screening for neurological, eye, and ear diseases
V81*	Special screening for cardiovascular, respiratory, and genitourinary diseases
V82*	Special screening for other condition
V83.01	Asymptomatic hemophilia A carrier
V83.02	Symptomatic hemophilia A carrier
V83.8*	Other genetic carrier status
V84.0*	Genetic susceptibility to malignant neoplasm
V84.8*	Genetic susceptibility to other disease
V85.0	Body Mass Index less than 19, adult
V85.1	Body Mass Index between 19-24, adult
V85.2*	Body Mass Index between 25-29, adult
V85.3*	Body Mass Index between 30-39, adult
V85.5*	Body Mass Index, pediatric
V86*	Estrogen receptor status
V87.0*	Contact with and (suspected) exposure to hazardous metals
V87.1*	Contact with and (suspected) exposure to hazardous aromatic compounds
V87.2	Contact with and (suspected) exposure to other potentially hazardous chemicals
V87.3*	Contact with and (suspected) exposure to other potentially hazardous substances
V88.1*	Acquired absence of pancreas
V88.2*	Acquired absence of joint
V89.0*	Suspected maternal and fetal conditions not found
V90.0*	Retained radioactive fragment
V90.1*	Retained metal fragments
V90.2	Retained plastic fragments
V90.3*	Retained organic fragments
V90.8*	Other specified retained foreign body
V90.9	Retained foreign body, unspecified material
V91.0*	Twin gestation placenta status
V91.1*	Triplet gestation placenta status
V91.2*	Quadruplet gestation placenta status
V91.9*	Other specified multiple gestation placenta status

MDC 23: Factors Influencing Health Status And Other Contacts With Health Services—MEDICAL

Surgical	Medical	CC Indicator	MCC Indicator	Procedure Proxy

800.00	800.85	801.72	803.23	804.10	804.95	806.4	811.11	813.80
800.01	800.86	801.73	803.24	804.11	804.96	806.5	811.12	813.81
800.02	800.89	801.74	803.25	804.12	804.99	806.60	811.13	813.82
800.03	800.90	801.75	803.26	804.13	805.00	806.61	811.19	813.83
800.04	800.91	801.76	803.29	804.14	805.01	806.62	812.00	813.90
800.05	800.92	801.79	803.30	804.15	805.02	806.69	812.01	813.91
800.06	800.93	801.80	803.31	804.16	805.03	806.70	812.02	813.92
800.09	800.94	801.81	803.32	804.19	805.04	806.71	812.03	813.93
800.10	800.95	801.82	803.33	804.20	805.05	806.72	812.09	814.00
800.11	800.96	801.83	803.34	804.21	805.06	806.79	812.10	814.01
800.12	800.99	801.84	803.35	804.22	805.07	806.8	812.11	814.02
800.13	801.00	801.85	803.36	804.23	805.08	806.9	812.12	814.03
800.14	801.01	801.86	803.39	804.24	805.10	807.00	812.13	814.04
800.15	801.02	801.89	803.40	804.25	805.11	807.01	812.19	814.05
800.16	801.03	801.90	803.41	804.26	805.12	807.02	812.20	814.06
800.19	801.04	801.91	803.42	804.29	805.13	807.03	812.21	814.07
800.20	801.05	801.92	803.43	804.30	805.14	807.04	812.30	814.08
800.21	801.06	801.93	803.44	804.31	805.15	807.05	812.31	814.09
800.22	801.09	801.94	803.45	804.32	805.16	807.06	812.40	814.10
800.23	801.10	801.95	803.46	804.33	805.17	807.07	812.41	814.11
800.24	801.11	801.96	803.49	804.34	805.18	807.08	812.42	814.12
800.25	801.12	801.99	803.50	804.35	805.2	807.09	812.43	814.13
800.26	801.13	802.0	803.51	804.36	805.3	807.10	812.44	814.14
800.29	801.14	802.1	803.52	804.39	805.4	807.11	812.49	814.15
800.30	801.15	802.20	803.53	804.40	805.5	807.12	812.50	814.16
800.31	801.16	802.21	803.54	804.41	805.6	807.13	812.51	814.17
800.32	801.19	802.22	803.55	804.42	805.7	807.14	812.52	814.18
800.33	801.20	802.23	803.56	804.43	805.8	807.15	812.53	814.19
800.34	801.21	802.24	803.59	804.44	805.9	807.16	812.54	815.00
800.35	801.22	802.25	803.60	804.45	806.00	807.17	812.59	815.01
800.36	801.23	802.26	803.61	804.46	806.01	807.18	813.00	815.02
800.39	801.24	802.27	803.62	804.49	806.02	807.19	813.01	815.03
800.40	801.25	802.28	803.63	804.50	806.03	807.2	813.02	815.04
800.41	801.26	802.29	803.64	804.51	806.04	807.3	813.03	815.09
800.42	801.29	802.30	803.65	804.52	806.05	807.4	813.04	815.10
800.43	801.30	802.31	803.66	804.53	806.06	807.5	813.05	815.11
800.44	801.31	802.32	803.69	804.54	806.07	807.6	813.06	815.12
800.45	801.32	802.33	803.70	804.55	806.08	808.0	813.07	815.13
800.46	801.33	802.34	803.71	804.56	806.09	808.1	813.08	815.14
800.49	801.34	802.35	803.72	804.59	806.10	808.2	813.10	815.19
800.50	801.35	802.36	803.73	804.60	806.11	808.3	813.11	816.00
800.51	801.36	802.37	803.74	804.61	806.12	808.41	813.12	816.01
800.52	801.39	802.38	803.75	804.62	806.13	808.42	813.13	816.02
800.53	801.40	802.39	803.76	804.63	806.14	808.43	813.14	816.03
800.54	801.41	802.4	803.79	804.64	806.15	808.44	813.15	816.10
800.55	801.42	802.5	803.80	804.65	806.16	808.49	813.16	816.11
800.56	801.43	802.6	803.81	804.66	806.17	808.51	813.17	816.12
800.59	801.44	802.7	803.82	804.69	806.18	808.52	813.18	816.13
800.60	801.45	802.8	803.83	804.70	806.19	808.53	813.20	817.0
800.61	801.46	802.9	803.84	804.71	806.20	808.54	813.21	817.1
800.62	801.49	803.00	803.85	804.72	806.21	808.59	813.22	818.0
800.63	801.50	803.01	803.86	804.73	806.22	808.8	813.23	818.1
800.64	801.51	803.02	803.89	804.74	806.23	808.9	813.30	819.0
800.65	801.52	803.03	803.90	804.75	806.24	809.0	813.31	819.1
800.66	801.53	803.04	803.91	804.76	806.25	809.1	813.32	820.00
800.69	801.54	803.05	803.92	804.79	806.26	810.00	813.33	820.01
800.70	801.55	803.06	803.93	804.80	806.27	810.01	813.40	820.02
800.71	801.56	803.09	803.94	804.81	806.28	810.02	813.41	820.03
800.72	801.59	803.10	803.95	804.82	806.29	810.03	813.42	820.09
800.73	801.60	803.11	803.96	804.83	806.30	810.10	813.43	820.10
800.74	801.61	803.12	803.99	804.84	806.31	810.11	813.44	820.11
800.75	801.62	803.13	804.00	804.85	806.32	810.12	813.45	820.12
800.76	801.63	803.14	804.01	804.86	806.33	810.13	813.46	820.13
800.79	801.64	803.15	804.02	804.89	806.34	811.00	813.47	820.19
800.80	801.65	803.16	804.03	804.90	806.35	811.01	813.50	820.20
800.81	801.66	803.19	804.04	804.91	806.36	811.02	813.51	820.21
800.82	801.69	803.20	804.05	804.92	806.37	811.03	813.52	820.22
800.83	801.70	803.21	804.06	804.93	806.38	811.09	813.53	820.30
800.84	801.71	803.22	804.09	804.94	806.39	811.10	813.54	820.31

820.32	830.0	838.00	842.12	851.24	852.16	861.02	865.00	872.74
820.8	830.1	838.01	842.13	851.25	852.19	861.03	865.01	872.79
820.9	831.00	838.02	842.19	851.26	852.20	861.10	865.02	872.8
821.00	831.01	838.03	843.0	851.29	852.21	861.11	865.03	872.9
821.01	831.02	838.04	843.1	851.30	852.22	861.12	865.04	873.0
821.10	831.03	838.05	843.8	851.31	852.23	861.13	865.09	873.1
821.11	831.04	838.06	843.9	851.32	852.24	861.20	865.10	873.20
821.20	831.09	838.09	844.0	851.33	852.25	861.21	865.11	873.21
821.21	831.10	838.10	844.1	851.34	852.26	861.22	865.12	873.22
821.22	831.11	838.11	844.2	851.35	852.29	861.30	865.13	873.23
821.23	831.12	838.12	844.3	851.36	852.30	861.31	865.14	873.29
821.29	831.13	838.13	844.8	851.39	852.31	861.32	865.19	873.30
821.30	831.14	838.14	844.9	851.40	852.32	862.0	866.00	873.31
821.31	831.19	838.15	845.00	851.41	852.33	862.1	866.01	873.32
821.32	832.00	838.16	845.01	851.42	852.34	862.21	866.02	873.33
821.33	832.01	838.19	845.02	851.43	852.35	862.22	866.03	873.39
821.39	832.02	839.00	845.03	851.44	852.36	862.29	866.10	873.40
822.0	832.03	839.01	845.09	851.45	852.39	862.31	866.11	873.41
822.1	832.04	839.02	845.10	851.46	852.40	862.32	866.12	873.42
823.00	832.09	839.03	845.11	851.49	852.41	862.39	866.13	873.43
823.01	832.10	839.04	845.12	851.50	852.42	862.8	867.0	873.44
823.02	832.11	839.05	845.13	851.51	852.43	862.9	867.1	873.49
823.10	832.12	839.06	845.19	851.52	852.44	863.0	867.2	873.50
823.11	832.13	839.07	846.0	851.53	852.45	863.1	867.3	873.51
823.12	832.14	839.08	846.1	851.54	852.46	863.20	867.4	873.52
823.20	832.19	839.10	846.2	851.55	852.49	863.21	867.5	873.53
823.21	832.2	839.11	846.3	851.56	852.50	863.29	867.6	873.54
823.22	833.00	839.12	846.8	851.59	852.51	863.30	867.7	873.59
823.30	833.01	839.13	846.9	851.60	852.52	863.31	867.8	873.60
823.31	833.02	839.14	847.0	851.61	852.53	863.39	867.9	873.61
823.32	833.03	839.15	847.1	851.62	852.54	863.40	868.00	873.62
823.40	833.04	839.16	847.2	851.63	852.55	863.41	868.01	873.63
823.41	833.05	839.17	847.3	851.64	852.56	863.42	868.02	873.64
823.42	833.09	839.18	847.4	851.65	852.59	863.43	868.03	873.65
823.80	833.10	839.20	847.9	851.66	853.00	863.44	868.04	873.69
823.81	833.11	839.21	848.0	851.69	853.01	863.45	868.09	873.70
823.82	833.12	839.30	848.1	851.70	853.02	863.46	868.10	873.71
823.90	833.13	839.31	848.2	851.71	853.03	863.49	868.11	873.72
823.91	833.14	839.40	848.3	851.72	853.04	863.50	868.12	873.73
823.92	833.15	839.41	848.40	851.73	853.05	863.51	868.13	873.74
824.0	833.19	839.42	848.41	851.74	853.06	863.52	868.14	873.75
824.1	834.00	839.49	848.42	851.75	853.09	863.53	868.19	873.79
824.2	834.01	839.50	848.49	851.76	853.10	863.54	869.0	873.8
824.3	834.02	839.51	848.5	851.79	853.11	863.55	869.1	873.9
824.4	834.10	839.52	848.8	851.80	853.12	863.56	870.0	874.00
824.5	834.11	839.59	848.9	851.81	853.13	863.59	870.1	874.01
824.6	834.12	839.61	850.0	851.82	853.14	863.80	870.2	874.02
824.7	835.00	839.69	850.11	851.83	853.15	863.81	870.3	874.10
824.8	835.01	839.71	850.12	851.84	853.16	863.82	870.4	874.11
824.9	835.02	839.79	850.2	851.85	853.19	863.83	870.8	874.12
825.0	835.03	839.8	850.3	851.86	854.00	863.84	870.9	874.2
825.1	835.10	839.9	850.4	851.89	854.01	863.85	871.0	874.3
825.20	835.11	840.0	850.5	851.90	854.02	863.89	871.1	874.4
825.21	835.12	840.1	850.9	851.91	854.03	863.90	871.2	874.5
825.22	835.13	840.2	851.00	851.92	854.04	863.91	871.3	874.8
825.23	836.0	840.3	851.01	851.93	854.05	863.92	871.4	874.9
825.24	836.1	840.4	851.02	851.94	854.06	863.93	871.5	875.0
825.25	836.2	840.5	851.03	851.95	854.09	863.94	871.6	875.1
825.29	836.3	840.6	851.04	851.96	854.10	863.95	871.7	876.0
825.30	836.4	840.7	851.05	851.99	854.11	863.99	871.9	876.1
825.31	836.50	840.8	851.06	852.00	854.12	864.00	872.00	877.0
825.32	836.51	840.9	851.09	852.01	854.13	864.01	872.01	877.1
825.33	836.52	841.0	851.10	852.02	854.14	864.02	872.02	878.0
825.34	836.53	841.1	851.11	852.03	854.15	864.03	872.10	878.1
825.35	836.54	841.2	851.12	852.04	854.16	864.04	872.11	878.2
825.39	836.59	841.3	851.13	852.05	854.19	864.05	872.12	878.3
826.0	836.60	841.8	851.14	852.06	860.0	864.09	872.61	878.4
826.1	836.61	841.9	851.15	852.09	860.1	864.10	872.62	878.5
827.0	836.62	842.00	851.16	852.10	860.2	864.11	872.63	878.6
827.1	836.63	842.01	851.19	852.11	860.3	864.12	872.64	878.7
828.0	836.64	842.02	851.20	852.12	860.4	864.13	872.69	878.8
828.1	836.69	842.09	851.21	852.13	860.5	864.14	872.71	878.9
829.0	837.0	842.10	851.22	852.14	861.00	864.15	872.72	879.0
829.1	837.1	842.11	851.23	852.15	861.01	864.19	872.73	879.1

MDC 24: Multiple Significant Trauma

879.2	887.3	901.41	903.4	912.8	917.6	924.11	951.4	955.5
879.3	887.4	901.42	903.5	912.9	917.7	924.20	951.5	955.6
879.4	887.5	901.81	903.8	913.0	917.8	924.21	951.6	955.7
879.5	887.6	901.82	903.9	913.1	917.9	924.3	951.7	955.8
879.6	887.7	901.83	904.0	913.2	918.0	924.4	951.8	955.9
879.7	890.0	901.89	904.1	913.3	918.1	924.5	951.9	956.0
879.8	890.1	901.9	904.2	913.4	918.2	924.8	952.00	956.1
879.9	890.2	902.0	904.3	913.5	918.9	924.9	952.01	956.2
880.00	891.0	902.10	904.40	913.6	919.0	925.1	952.02	956.3
880.01	891.1	902.11	904.41	913.7	919.1	925.2	952.03	956.4
880.02	891.2	902.19	904.42	913.8	919.2	926.0	952.04	956.5
880.03	892.0	902.20	904.50	913.9	919.3	926.12	952.05	956.8
880.09	892.1	902.21	904.51	914.0	919.4	926.19	952.06	956.9
880.10	892.2	902.22	904.52	914.1	919.5	926.8	952.07	957.0
880.11	893.0	902.23	904.53	914.2	919.6	926.9	952.08	957.1
880.12	893.1	902.24	904.54	914.3	919.7	927.00	952.09	957.8
880.13	893.2	902.25	904.6	914.4	919.8	927.01	952.10	957.9
880.19	894.0	902.26	904.7	914.5	919.9	927.02	952.11	958.0
880.20	894.1	902.27	904.8	914.6	920	927.02	952.12	958.1
880.21	894.2	902.29	904.9	914.7	921.0	927.03	952.13	958.2
880.22	895.0	902.31	910.0	914.8	921.1	927.09	952.14	958.3
880.23	895.1	902.32	910.1	914.9	921.2	927.10	952.15	958.4
880.29	896.0	902.33	910.2	915.0	921.3	927.11	952.16	958.5
881.00	896.1	902.34	910.3	915.1	921.9	927.20	952.17	958.6
881.01	896.2	902.39	910.4	915.2	922.0	927.21	952.18	958.7
881.02	896.3	902.40	910.5	915.3	922.1	927.3	952.19	958.8
881.10	897.0	902.41	910.6	915.4	922.2	927.8	952.2	958.90
881.11	897.1	902.42	910.7	915.5	922.31	927.9	952.3	958.91
881.12	897.2	902.49	910.8	915.6	922.32	928.00	952.4	958.92
881.20	897.3	902.50	910.9	915.7	922.33	928.01	952.8	958.93
881.21	897.4	902.51	911.0	915.8	922.4	928.10	952.9	958.99
881.22	897.5	902.52	911.1	915.9	922.8	928.11	953.0	959.01
882.0	897.6	902.53	911.2	916.0	922.9	928.20	953.1	959.09
882.1	897.7	902.54	911.3	916.1	923.00	928.21	953.2	959.11
882.2	900.00	902.55	911.4	916.2	923.01	928.3	953.3	959.12
883.0	900.01	902.56	911.5	916.3	923.02	928.8	953.4	959.13
883.1	900.02	902.59	911.6	916.4	923.03	928.9	953.5	959.14
883.2	900.03	902.81	911.7	916.5	923.09	929.0	953.8	959.19
884.0	900.1	902.82	911.8	916.6	923.10	929.9	953.9	959.2
884.1	900.81	902.87	911.9	916.7	923.11	950.0	954.0	959.3
884.2	900.82	902.89	912.0	916.8	923.20	950.1	954.1	959.4
885.0	900.89	902.9	912.1	916.9	923.21	950.2	954.8	959.5
885.1	900.9	903.00	912.2	917.0	923.3	950.3	954.9	959.6
886.0	901.0	903.01	912.3	917.1	923.8	950.9	955.0	959.7
886.1	901.1	903.02	912.4	917.2	923.9	951.0	955.1	959.8
887.0	901.2	903.1	912.5	917.3	924.00	951.1	955.2	959.9
887.1	901.3	903.2	912.6	917.4	924.01	951.2	955.3	
887.2	901.40	903.3	912.7	917.5	924.10	951.3	955.4	

SURGICAL

DRG 955 **Craniotomy for Multiple Significant Trauma**
       GMLOS 7.2   AMLOS 10.6   RW 5.4056

Select the principal diagnosis from the Trauma Diagnosis List located in DRG 963
AND

At least two different diagnoses from two different Significant Trauma Body Site Categories located in DRG 963
AND

Operating Room Procedures
01.21   Incision and drainage of cranial sinus
01.23   Reopening of craniotomy site
01.24   Other craniotomy
01.25   Other craniectomy
01.28   Placement of intracerebral catheter(s) via burr hole(s)
01.31   Incision of cerebral meninges
01.32   Lobotomy and tractotomy
01.39   Other incision of brain
01.41   Operations on thalamus
01.42   Operations on globus pallidus
01.51   Excision of lesion or tissue of cerebral meninges
01.52   Hemispherectomy
01.53   Lobectomy of brain
01.59   Other excision or destruction of lesion or tissue of brain
01.6   Excision of lesion of skull
02.01   Opening of cranial suture
02.02   Elevation of skull fracture fragments
02.03   Formation of cranial bone flap
02.04   Bone graft to skull
02.05   Insertion of skull plate
02.06   Other cranial osteoplasty
02.11   Simple suture of dura mater of brain
02.12   Other repair of cerebral meninges
02.13   Ligation of meningeal vessel
02.14   Choroid plexectomy
02.2*   Ventriculostomy
02.92   Repair of brain
02.94   Insertion or replacement of skull tongs or halo traction device
02.99   Other operations on skull, brain, and cerebral meninges
04.41   Decompression of trigeminal nerve root
38.81   Other surgical occlusion of intracranial vessels
OR

Select a principal diagnosis from one Significant Trauma Body Site Category located in DRG 963
AND

Two or more significant trauma diagnoses from different Significant Trauma Body Site Categories located in DRG 963
AND

Any operating room procedure listed above

DRG 956 **Limb Reattachment, Hip and Femur Procedures for Multiple Significant Trauma**
       GMLOS 6.8   AMLOS 8.3   RW 3.8321   ☑ⓣ

Select principal diagnosis from Trauma Diagnosis List located in DRG 963
AND

At least two different diagnoses from two different Significant Trauma Body Site Categories located in DRG 963
AND

Operating Room Procedures
00.70   Revision of hip replacement, both acetabular and femoral components
00.71   Revision of hip replacement, acetabular component
00.72   Revision of hip replacement, femoral component
00.73   Revision of hip replacement, acetabular liner and/or femoral head only
00.85   Resurfacing hip, total, acetabulum and femoral head
00.86   Resurfacing hip, partial, femoral head
00.87   Resurfacing hip, partial, acetabulum
77.05   Sequestrectomy of femur
77.25   Wedge osteotomy of femur
77.35   Other division of femur
77.85   Other partial ostectomy of femur
77.95   Total ostectomy of femur
78.05   Bone graft of femur
78.15   Application of external fixator device, femur
78.25   Limb shortening procedures, femur
78.35   Limb lengthening procedures, femur
78.45   Other repair or plastic operations on femur
78.55   Internal fixation of femur without fracture reduction
78.75   Osteoclasis of femur
78.95   Insertion of bone growth stimulator into femur
79.15   Closed reduction of fracture of femur with internal fixation
79.25   Open reduction of fracture of femur without internal fixation
79.35   Open reduction of fracture of femur with internal fixation
79.45   Closed reduction of separated epiphysis of femur
79.55   Open reduction of separated epiphysis of femur
79.65   Debridement of open fracture of femur
79.85   Open reduction of dislocation of hip
79.95   Unspecified operation on bone injury of femur
80.05   Arthrotomy for removal of prosthesis without replacement, hip
80.15   Other arthrotomy of hip
80.45   Division of joint capsule, ligament, or cartilage of hip
80.95   Other excision of hip joint
81.21   Arthrodesis of hip
81.40   Repair of hip, not elsewhere classified
81.51   Total hip replacement
81.52   Partial hip replacement
81.53   Revision of hip replacement, not otherwise specified
83.12   Adductor tenotomy of hip
84.23   Forearm, wrist, or hand reattachment
84.24   Upper arm reattachment
84.26   Foot reattachment
84.27   Lower leg or ankle reattachment
84.28   Thigh reattachment
OR

Select a principal diagnosis from one Significant Trauma Body Site Category located in DRG 963
AND

Two or more significant trauma diagnoses from different Significant Trauma Body Site Categories located in DRG 963
AND

Operating room procedure listed above

DRG 957 **Other O.R. Procedures for Multiple Significant Trauma with MCC**
       GMLOS 9.7   AMLOS 13.9   RW 6.7306

Select principal diagnosis from Trauma Diagnosis List located in DRG 963
AND

At least two different diagnoses from two different Significant Trauma Body Site Categories located in DRG 963
AND

| Surgical | Medical | CC Indicator | MCC Indicator | Procedure Proxy |

Any operating room procedure from MDC 21

EXCLUDING

Pacemaker leads and devices and any procedure listed under DRGs 955 and 956

OR

Select a principal diagnosis from one Significant Trauma Body Site Category located in DRG 963

AND

Two or more significant trauma diagnoses from different Significant Trauma Body Site Categories located in DRG 963

AND

Any operating room procedure from MDC 21

EXCLUDING

Pacemaker leads and devices

All procedures listed under DRGs 955 and 956

DRG 958   Other O.R. Procedures for Multiple Significant Trauma with CC
GMLOS 7.3   AMLOS 8.9   RW 3.8734   ☑

Select principal diagnosis from Trauma Diagnosis List located in DRG 963

AND

At least two different diagnoses from two different Significant Trauma Body Site Categories located in DRG 963

AND

Any operating room procedure from MDC 21

EXCLUDING

Pacemaker leads and devices and any procedure listed under DRGs 955 and 956

OR

Select a principal diagnosis from one Significant Trauma Body Site Category located in DRG 963

AND

Two or more significant trauma diagnoses from different Significant Trauma Body Site Categories located in DRG 963

AND

Any operating room procedure from MDC 21

EXCLUDING

Pacemaker leads and devices

All procedures listed under DRGs 955 and 956

DRG 959   Other O.R. Procedures for Multiple Significant Trauma without CC/MCC
GMLOS 4.3   AMLOS 5.4   RW 2.5391   ☑

Select principal diagnosis from Trauma Diagnosis List located in DRG 963

AND

At least two different diagnoses from two different Significant Trauma Body Site Categories located in DRG 963

AND

Any operating room procedure from MDC 21

EXCLUDING

Pacemaker leads and devices and any procedure listed under DRGs 955 and 956

OR

Select a principal diagnosis from one Significant Trauma Body Site Category located in DRG 963

AND

Two or more significant trauma diagnoses from different Significant Trauma Body Site Categories located in DRG 963

AND

Any operating room procedure from MDC 21

EXCLUDING

Pacemaker leads and devices

All procedures listed under DRGs 955 and 956

MEDICAL

DRG 963   Other Multiple Significant Trauma with MCC
GMLOS 5.5   AMLOS 8.1   RW 2.6733   ☑

Select principal diagnosis from list of the Trauma Diagnosis List located below

WITH

At least two different diagnoses from two different Significant Trauma Body Site Categories located in DRG 963

OR

Select a principal diagnosis from one Significant Trauma Body Site Category

AND

Two or more significant trauma diagnoses from different Significant Trauma Body Site Categories located in DRG 963

Trauma Diagnosis

800.0*	Closed fracture of vault of skull without mention of intracranial injury
800.1*	Closed fracture of vault of skull with cerebral laceration and contusion
800.2*	Closed fracture of vault of skull with subarachnoid, subdural, and extradural hemorrhage
800.3*	Closed fracture of vault of skull with other and unspecified intracranial hemorrhage
800.4*	Closed fracture of vault of skull with intercranial injury of other and unspecified nature
800.5*	Open fracture of vault of skull without mention of intracranial injury
800.6*	Open fracture of vault of skull with cerebral laceration and contusion
800.7*	Open fracture of vault of skull with subarachnoid, subdural, and extradural hemorrhage
800.8*	Open fracture of vault of skull with other and unspecified intracranial hemorrhage
800.9*	Open fracture of vault of skull with intracranial injury of other and unspecified nature
801.0*	Closed fracture of base of skull without mention of intracranial injury
801.1*	Closed fracture of base of skull with cerebral laceration and contusion
801.2*	Closed fracture of base of skull with subarachnoid, subdural, and extradural hemorrhage
801.3*	Closed fracture of base of skull with other and unspecified intracranial hemorrhage
801.4*	Closed fracture of base of skull with intracranial injury of other and unspecified nature
801.5*	Open fracture of base of skull without mention of intracranial injury

Ⓣ *Transfer DRG*   ⓈⓅ *Special Payment*   ☑ *Optimization Potential*   ☝ *Targeted Potential*   * *Code Range*   ● *New DRG*   ▲ *Revised DRG Title*

220   Valid 10/01/2013–09/30/2014   © 2013 OptumInsight, Inc.

801.6*	Open fracture of base of skull with cerebral laceration and contusion
801.7*	Open fracture of base of skull with subarachnoid, subdural, and extradural hemorrhage
801.8*	Open fracture of base of skull with other and unspecified intracranial hemorrhage
801.9*	Open fracture of base of skull with intracranial injury of other and unspecified nature
802.0	Nasal bones, closed fracture
802.1	Nasal bones, open fracture
802.2*	Mandible, closed fracture
802.3*	Mandible, open fracture
802.4	Malar and maxillary bones, closed fracture
802.5	Malar and maxillary bones, open fracture
802.6	Orbital floor (blow-out), closed fracture
802.7	Orbital floor (blow-out), open fracture
802.8	Other facial bones, closed fracture
802.9	Other facial bones, open fracture
803.0*	Other closed skull fracture without mention of intracranial injury
803.1*	Other closed skull fracture with cerebral laceration and contusion
803.2*	Other closed skull fracture with subarachnoid, subdural, and extradural hemorrhage
803.3*	Closed skull fracture with other and unspecified intracranial hemorrhage
803.4*	Other closed skull fracture with intracranial injury of other and unspecified nature
803.5*	Other open skull fracture without mention of intracranial injury
803.6*	Other open skull fracture with cerebral laceration and contusion
803.7*	Other open skull fracture with subarachnoid, subdural, and extradural hemorrhage
803.8*	Other open skull fracture with other and unspecified intracranial hemorrhage
803.9*	Other open skull fracture with intracranial injury of other and unspecified nature
804.0*	Closed fractures involving skull or face with other bones, without mention of intracranial injury
804.1*	Closed fractures involving skull or face with other bones, with cerebral laceration and contusion
804.2*	Closed fractures involving skull or face with other bones with subarachnoid, subdural, and extradural hemorrhage
804.3*	Closed fractures involving skull or face with other bones, with other and unspecified intracranial hemorrhage
804.4*	Closed fractures involving skull or face with other bones, with intracranial injury of other and unspecified nature
804.5*	Open fractures involving skull or face with other bones, without mention of intracranial injury
804.6*	Open fractures involving skull or face with other bones, with cerebral laceration and contusion
804.7*	Open fractures involving skull or face with other bones with subarachnoid, subdural, and extradural hemorrhage
804.8*	Open fractures involving skull or face with other bones, with other and unspecified intracranial hemorrhage
804.9*	Open fractures involving skull or face with other bones, with intracranial injury of other and unspecified nature
805.0*	Closed fracture of cervical vertebra without mention of spinal cord injury
805.1*	Open fracture of cervical vertebra without mention of spinal cord injury
805.2	Closed fracture of dorsal (thoracic) vertebra without mention of spinal cord injury
805.3	Open fracture of dorsal (thoracic) vertebra without mention of spinal cord injury
805.4	Closed fracture of lumbar vertebra without mention of spinal cord injury
805.5	Open fracture of lumbar vertebra without mention of spinal cord injury
805.6	Closed fracture of sacrum and coccyx without mention of spinal cord injury
805.7	Open fracture of sacrum and coccyx without mention of spinal cord injury
805.8	Closed fracture of unspecified part of vertebral column without mention of spinal cord injury
805.9	Open fracture of unspecified part of vertebral column without mention of spinal cord injury
806.0*	Closed fracture of cervical vertebra with spinal cord injury
806.1*	Open fracture of cervical vertebra with spinal cord injury
806.2*	Closed fracture of dorsal (thoracic) vertebra with spinal cord injury
806.3*	Open fracture of dorsal vertebra with spinal cord injury
806.4	Closed fracture of lumbar spine with spinal cord injury
806.5	Open fracture of lumbar spine with spinal cord injury
806.6*	Closed fracture of sacrum and coccyx with spinal cord injury
806.7*	Open fracture of sacrum and coccyx with spinal cord injury
806.8	Closed fracture of unspecified vertebra with spinal cord injury
806.9	Open fracture of unspecified vertebra with spinal cord injury
807.0*	Closed fracture of rib(s)
807.1*	Open fracture of rib(s)
807.2	Closed fracture of sternum
807.3	Open fracture of sternum
807.4	Flail chest
807.5	Closed fracture of larynx and trachea
807.6	Open fracture of larynx and trachea
808.0	Closed fracture of acetabulum
808.1	Open fracture of acetabulum
808.2	Closed fracture of pubis
808.3	Open fracture of pubis
808.4*	Closed fracture of other specified part of pelvis
808.5*	Open fracture of other specified part of pelvis
808.8	Unspecified closed fracture of pelvis
808.9	Unspecified open fracture of pelvis
809.0	Fracture of bones of trunk, closed
809.1	Fracture of bones of trunk, open
810.0*	Closed fracture of clavicle
810.1*	Open fracture of clavicle
811.0*	Closed fracture of scapula
811.1*	Open fracture of scapula
812.0*	Closed fracture of upper end of humerus
812.1*	Open fracture of upper end of humerus
812.2*	Closed fracture of shaft or unspecified part of humerus
812.3*	Open fracture of shaft or unspecified part of humerus
812.4*	Closed fracture of lower end of humerus
812.5*	Open fracture of lower end of humerus
813.0*	Closed fracture of upper end of radius and ulna
813.1*	Open fracture of upper end of radius and ulna
813.2*	Closed fracture of shaft of radius and ulna
813.3*	Open fracture of shaft of radius and ulna
813.4*	Closed fracture of lower end of radius and ulna
813.5*	Open fracture of lower end of radius and ulna
813.8*	Closed fracture of unspecified part of radius with ulna
813.9*	Open fracture of unspecified part of radius with ulna
814.0*	Closed fractures of carpal bones
814.1*	Open fractures of carpal bones
815.0*	Closed fracture of metacarpal bones
815.1*	Open fracture of metacarpal bones
816.0*	Closed fracture of one or more phalanges of hand
816.1*	Open fracture of one or more phalanges of hand
817.0	Multiple closed fractures of hand bones
817.1	Multiple open fractures of hand bones
818.0	Ill-defined closed fractures of upper limb
818.1	Ill-defined open fractures of upper limb
819.0	Multiple closed fractures involving both upper limbs, and upper limb with rib(s) and sternum
819.1	Multiple open fractures involving both upper limbs, and upper limb with rib(s) and sternum
820.0*	Closed transcervical fracture

| Surgical | Medical | CC Indicator | MCC Indicator | Procedure Proxy |

820.1*	Open transcervical fracture
820.2*	Closed pertrochanteric fracture of femur
820.3*	Open pertrochanteric fracture of femur
820.8	Closed fracture of unspecified part of neck of femur
820.9	Open fracture of unspecified part of neck of femur
821.0*	Closed fracture of shaft or unspecified part of femur
821.1*	Open fracture of shaft or unspecified part of femur
821.2*	Closed fracture of lower end of femur
821.3*	Open fracture of lower end of femur
822.0	Closed fracture of patella
822.1	Open fracture of patella
823.0*	Closed fracture of upper end of tibia and fibula
823.1*	Open fracture of upper end of tibia and fibula
823.2*	Closed fracture of shaft of tibia and fibula
823.3*	Open fracture of shaft of tibia and fibula
823.4*	Torus fracture of tibia and fibula
823.8*	Closed fracture of unspecified part of tibia and fibula
823.9*	Open fracture of unspecified part of tibia and fibula
824.0	Closed fracture of medial malleolus
824.1	Open fracture of medial malleolus
824.2	Closed fracture of lateral malleolus
824.3	Open fracture of lateral malleolus
824.4	Closed bimalleolar fracture
824.5	Open bimalleolar fracture
824.6	Closed trimalleolar fracture
824.7	Open trimalleolar fracture
824.8	Unspecified closed fracture of ankle
824.9	Unspecified open fracture of ankle
825.0	Closed fracture of calcaneus
825.1	Open fracture of calcaneus
825.2*	Closed fracture of other tarsal and metatarsal bones
825.3*	Open fracture of other tarsal and metatarsal bones
826.0	Closed fracture of one or more phalanges of foot
826.1	Open fracture of one or more phalanges of foot
827.0	Other, multiple and ill-defined closed fractures of lower limb
827.1	Other, multiple and ill-defined open fractures of lower limb
828.0	Multiple closed fractures involving both lower limbs, lower with upper limb, and lower limb(s) with rib(s) and sternum
828.1	Multiple fractures involving both lower limbs, lower with upper limb, and lower limb(s) with rib(s) and sternum, open
829.0	Closed fracture of unspecified bone
829.1	Open fracture of unspecified bone
830.0	Closed dislocation of jaw
830.1	Open dislocation of jaw
831.0*	Closed dislocation of shoulder, unspecified
831.1*	Open dislocation of shoulder
832.0*	Closed dislocation of elbow
832.1*	Open dislocation of elbow
832.2	Nursemaid's elbow
833.0*	Closed dislocation of wrist
833.1*	Open dislocation of wrist
834.0*	Closed dislocation of finger
834.1*	Open dislocation of finger
835.0*	Closed dislocation of hip
835.1*	Open dislocation of hip
836.0	Tear of medial cartilage or meniscus of knee, current
836.1	Tear of lateral cartilage or meniscus of knee, current
836.2	Other tear of cartilage or meniscus of knee, current
836.3	Closed dislocation of patella
836.4	Open dislocation of patella
836.5*	Other closed dislocation of knee
836.6*	Other open dislocation of knee
837.0	Closed dislocation of ankle
837.1	Open dislocation of ankle
838.0*	Closed dislocation of foot
838.1*	Open dislocation of foot
839.0*	Closed dislocation, cervical vertebra
839.1*	Open dislocation, cervical vertebra
839.2*	Closed dislocation, thoracic and lumbar vertebra
839.3*	Open dislocation, thoracic and lumbar vertebra
839.4*	Closed dislocation, other vertebra
839.5*	Open dislocation, other vertebra
839.6*	Closed dislocation, other location
839.71	Open dislocation, sternum
839.79	Open dislocation, other location
839.8	Closed dislocation, multiple and ill-defined sites
839.9	Open dislocation, multiple and ill-defined sites
840.0	Acromioclavicular (joint) (ligament) sprain and strain
840.1	Coracoclavicular (ligament) sprain and strain
840.2	Coracohumeral (ligament) sprain and strain
840.3	Infraspinatus (muscle) (tendon) sprain and strain
840.4	Rotator cuff (capsule) sprain and strain
840.5	Subscapularis (muscle) sprain and strain
840.6	Supraspinatus (muscle) (tendon) sprain and strain
840.7	Superior glenoid labrum lesions (SLAP)
840.8	Sprain and strain of other specified sites of shoulder and upper arm
840.9	Sprain and strain of unspecified site of shoulder and upper arm
841*	Sprains and strains of elbow and forearm
842*	Sprains and strains of wrist and hand
843*	Sprains and strains of hip and thigh
844*	Sprains and strains of knee and leg
845*	Sprains and strains of ankle and foot
846*	Sprains and strains of sacroiliac region
847*	Sprains and strains of other and unspecified parts of back
848*	Other and ill-defined sprains and strains
850.0	Concussion with no loss of consciousness
850.1*	Concussion with brief (less than one hour) loss of consciousness
850.2	Concussion with moderate (1-24 hours) loss of consciousness
850.3	Concussion with prolonged (more than 24 hours) loss of consciousness and return to pre-existing conscious level
850.4	Concussion with prolonged (more than 24 hours) loss of consciousness, without return to pre-existing conscious level
850.5	Concussion with loss of consciousness of unspecified duration
850.9	Unspecified concussion
851.0*	Cortex (cerebral) contusion without mention of open intracranial wound
851.1*	Cortex (cerebral) contusion with open intracranial wound
851.2*	Cortex (cerebral) laceration without mention of open intracranial wound
851.3*	Cortex (cerebral) laceration with open intracranial wound
851.4*	Cerebellar or brain stem contusion without mention of open intracranial wound
851.5*	Cerebellar or brain stem contusion with open intracranial wound
851.6*	Cerebellar or brain stem laceration without mention of open intracranial wound
851.7*	Cerebellar or brain stem laceration with open intracranial wound
851.8*	Other and unspecified cerebral laceration and contusion, without mention of open intracranial wound
851.9*	Other and unspecified cerebral laceration and contusion, with open intracranial wound
852*	Subarachnoid, subdural, and extradural hemorrhage, following injury
853*	Other and unspecified intracranial hemorrhage following injury
854*	Intracranial injury of other and unspecified nature
860*	Traumatic pneumothorax and hemothorax
861*	Injury to heart and lung
862*	Injury to other and unspecified intrathoracic organs
863.0	Stomach injury without mention of open wound into cavity
863.1	Stomach injury with open wound into cavity
863.2*	Small intestine injury without mention of open wound into cavity

---

T Transfer DRG   SP Special Payment   ☑ Optimization Potential   ▽ Targeted Potential   * Code Range   ● New DRG   ▲ Revised DRG Title

863.3*	Small intestine injury with open wound into cavity
863.4*	Colon or rectal injury without mention of open wound into cavity
863.5*	Injury to colon or rectum with open wound into cavity
863.8*	Injury to other and unspecified gastrointestinal sites without mention of open wound into cavity
863.9*	Injury to other and unspecified gastrointestinal sites, with open wound into cavity
864.0*	Liver injury without mention of open wound into cavity
864.1*	Liver injury with open wound into cavity
865*	Injury to spleen
866*	Injury to kidney
867*	Injury to pelvic organs
868.0*	Injury to other intra-abdominal organs without mention of open wound into cavity
868.1*	Injury to other intra-abdominal organs with open wound into cavity
869*	Internal injury to unspecified or ill-defined organs
870*	Open wound of ocular adnexa
871*	Open wound of eyeball
872*	Open wound of ear
873*	Other open wound of head
874.0*	Open wound of larynx and trachea, without mention of complication
874.1*	Open wound of larynx and trachea, complicated
874.2	Open wound of thyroid gland, without mention of complication
874.3	Open wound of thyroid gland, complicated
874.4	Open wound of pharynx, without mention of complication
874.5	Open wound of pharynx, complicated
874.8	Open wound of other and unspecified parts of neck, without mention of complication
874.9	Open wound of other and unspecified parts of neck, complicated
875*	Open wound of chest (wall)
876*	Open wound of back
877*	Open wound of buttock
878*	Open wound of genital organs (external), including traumatic amputation
879*	Open wound of other and unspecified sites, except limbs
880*	Open wound of shoulder and upper arm
881*	Open wound of elbow, forearm, and wrist
882*	Open wound of hand except finger(s) alone
883*	Open wound of finger(s)
884*	Multiple and unspecified open wound of upper limb
885*	Traumatic amputation of thumb (complete) (partial)
886*	Traumatic amputation of other finger(s) (complete) (partial)
887*	Traumatic amputation of arm and hand (complete) (partial)
890*	Open wound of hip and thigh
891*	Open wound of knee, leg (except thigh), and ankle
892*	Open wound of foot except toe(s) alone
893*	Open wound of toe(s)
894*	Multiple and unspecified open wound of lower limb
895*	Traumatic amputation of toe(s) (complete) (partial)
896*	Traumatic amputation of foot (complete) (partial)
897*	Traumatic amputation of leg(s) (complete) (partial)
900.0*	Injury to carotid artery
900.1	Internal jugular vein injury
900.8*	Injury to other specified blood vessels of head and neck
900.9	Injury to unspecified blood vessel of head and neck
901.0	Thoracic aorta injury
901.1	Innominate and subclavian artery injury
901.2	Superior vena cava injury
901.3	Innominate and subclavian vein injury
901.4*	Pulmonary blood vessel injury
901.8*	Injury to other specified blood vessels of thorax
901.9	Injury to unspecified blood vessel of thorax
902*	Injury to blood vessels of abdomen and pelvis
903*	Injury to blood vessels of upper extremity
904.0	Common femoral artery injury
904.1	Superficial femoral artery injury
904.2	Femoral vein injury
904.3	Saphenous vein injury
904.4*	Popliteal blood vessel vein
904.5*	Tibial blood vessel(s) injury
904.6	Deep plantar blood vessels injury
904.7	Injury to specified blood vessels of lower extremity, other
904.8	Injury to unspecified blood vessel of lower extremity
904.9	Injury to blood vessels, unspecified site
910*	Superficial injury of face, neck, and scalp, except eye
911*	Superficial injury of trunk
912*	Superficial injury of shoulder and upper arm
913*	Superficial injury of elbow, forearm, and wrist
914*	Superficial injury of hand(s) except finger(s) alone
915*	Superficial injury of finger(s)
916*	Superficial injury of hip, thigh, leg, and ankle
917*	Superficial injury of foot and toe(s)
918*	Superficial injury of eye and adnexa
919*	Superficial injury of other, multiple, and unspecified sites
920	Contusion of face, scalp, and neck except eye(s)
921*	Contusion of eye and adnexa
922*	Contusion of trunk
923*	Contusion of upper limb
924*	Contusion of lower limb and of other and unspecified sites
925*	Crushing injury of face, scalp, and neck
926.0	Crushing injury of external genitalia
926.1*	Crushing injury of other specified sites of trunk
926.8	Crushing injury of multiple sites of trunk
926.9	Crushing injury of unspecified site of trunk
927.0*	Crushing injury of shoulder and upper arm
927.1*	Crushing injury of elbow and forearm
927.2*	Crushing injury of wrist and hand(s), except finger(s) alone
927.3	Crushing injury of finger(s)
927.8	Crushing injury of multiple sites of upper limb
927.9	Crushing injury of unspecified site of upper limb
928.0*	Crushing injury of hip and thigh
928.1*	Crushing injury of knee and lower leg
928.2*	Crushing injury of ankle and foot, excluding toe(s) alone
928.3	Crushing injury of toe(s)
928.8	Crushing injury of multiple sites of lower limb
928.9	Crushing injury of unspecified site of lower limb
929*	Crushing injury of multiple and unspecified sites
950*	Injury to optic nerve and pathways
951*	Injury to other cranial nerve(s)
952*	Spinal cord injury without evidence of spinal bone injury
953*	Injury to nerve roots and spinal plexus
953.1	Injury to dorsal nerve root
953.2	Injury to lumbar nerve root
953.3	Injury to sacral nerve root
953.4	Injury to brachial plexus
953.5	Injury to lumbosacral plexus
953.8	Injury to multiple sites of nerve roots and spinal plexus
953.9	Injury to unspecified site of nerve roots and spinal plexus
954.0	Injury to cervical sympathetic nerve, excluding shoulder and pelvic girdles
954.1	Injury to other sympathetic nerve, excluding shoulder and pelvic girdles
954.8	Injury to other specified nerve(s) of trunk, excluding shoulder and pelvic girdles
954.9	Injury to unspecified nerve of trunk, excluding shoulder and pelvic girdles
955.0	Injury to axillary nerve
955.1	Injury to median nerve
955.2	Injury to ulnar nerve
955.3	Injury to radial nerve
955.4	Injury to musculocutaneous nerve
955.5	Injury to cutaneous sensory nerve, upper limb
955.6	Injury to digital nerve, upper limb
955.7	Injury to other specified nerve(s) of shoulder girdle and upper limb

Surgical   Medical   CC Indicator   MCC Indicator   Procedure Proxy

MDC 24: Multiple Significant Trauma—MEDICAL

955.8	Injury to multiple nerves of shoulder girdle and upper limb
955.9	Injury to unspecified nerve of shoulder girdle and upper limb
956.0	Injury to sciatic nerve
956.1	Injury to femoral nerve
956.2	Injury to posterior tibial nerve
956.3	Injury to peroneal nerve
956.4	Injury to cutaneous sensory nerve, lower limb
956.5	Injury to other specified nerve(s) of pelvic girdle and lower limb
956.8	Injury to multiple nerves of pelvic girdle and lower limb
956.9	Injury to unspecified nerve of pelvic girdle and lower limb
957*	Injury to other and unspecified nerves
958.0	Air embolism as an early complication of trauma
958.1	Fat embolism as an early complication of trauma
958.2	Secondary and recurrent hemorrhage as an early complication of trauma
958.3	Posttraumatic wound infection not elsewhere classified
958.4	Traumatic shock
958.5	Traumatic anuria
958.6	Volkmann's ischemic contracture
958.7	Traumatic subcutaneous emphysema
958.8	Other early complications of trauma
958.90	Compartment syndrome, unspecified
958.91	Traumatic compartment syndrome of upper extremity
958.92	Traumatic compartment syndrome of lower extremity
958.93	Traumatic compartment syndrome of abdomen
958.99	Traumatic compartment syndrome of other sites
959.0*	Injury, other and unspecified, head, face, and neck
959.1*	Injury, other and unspecified, trunk
959.2	Injury, other and unspecified, shoulder and upper arm
959.3	Injury, other and unspecified, elbow, forearm, and wrist
959.4	Injury, other and unspecified, hand, except finger
959.5	Injury, other and unspecified, finger
959.6	Injury, other and unspecified, hip and thigh
959.7	Injury, other and unspecified, knee, leg, ankle, and foot
959.8	Injury, other and unspecified, other specified sites, including multiple
959.9	Injury, other and unspecified, unspecified site

Significant Trauma Body Site Category 1—Head

800.02	Closed fracture of vault of skull without mention of intracranial injury, brief (less than one hour) loss of consciousness
800.03	Closed fracture of vault of skull without mention of intracranial injury, moderate (1-24 hours) loss of consciousness
800.04	Closed fracture of vault of skull without mention of intracranial injury, prolonged (more than 24 hours) loss of consciousness and return to pre-existing conscious level
800.05	Closed fracture of vault of skull without mention of intracranial injury, prolonged (more than 24 hours) loss of consciousness, without return to pre-existing conscious level
800.10	Closed fracture of vault of skull with cerebral laceration and contusion, unspecified state of consciousness
800.12	Closed fracture of vault of skull with cerebral laceration and contusion, brief (less than one hour) loss of consciousness
800.13	Closed fracture of vault of skull with cerebral laceration and contusion, moderate (1-24 hours) loss of consciousness
800.14	Closed fracture of vault of skull with cerebral laceration and contusion, prolonged (more than 24 hours) loss of consciousness and return to pre-existing conscious level
800.15	Closed fracture of vault of skull with cerebral laceration and contusion, prolonged (more than 24 hours) loss of consciousness, without return to pre-existing conscious level
800.16	Closed fracture of vault of skull with cerebral laceration and contusion, loss of consciousness of unspecified duration
800.19	Closed fracture of vault of skull with cerebral laceration and contusion, unspecified concussion

800.20	Closed fracture of vault of skull with subarachnoid, subdural, and extradural hemorrhage, unspecified state of consciousness
800.22	Closed fracture of vault of skull with subarachnoid, subdural, and extradural hemorrhage, brief (less than one hour) loss of consciousness
800.23	Closed fracture of vault of skull with subarachnoid, subdural, and extradural hemorrhage, moderate (1-24 hours) loss of consciousness
800.24	Closed fracture of vault of skull with subarachnoid, subdural, and extradural hemorrhage, prolonged (more than 24 hours) loss of consciousness and return to pre-existing conscious level
800.25	Closed fracture of vault of skull with subarachnoid, subdural, and extradural hemorrhage, prolonged (more than 24 hours) loss of consciousness, without return to pre-existing conscious level
800.26	Closed fracture of vault of skull with subarachnoid, subdural, and extradural hemorrhage, loss of consciousness of unspecified duration
800.29	Closed fracture of vault of skull with subarachnoid, subdural, and extradural hemorrhage, unspecified concussion
800.30	Closed fracture of vault of skull with other and unspecified intracranial hemorrhage, unspecified state of consciousness
800.32	Closed fracture of vault of skull with other and unspecified intracranial hemorrhage, brief (less than one hour) loss of consciousness
800.33	Closed fracture of vault of skull with other and unspecified intracranial hemorrhage, moderate (1-24 hours) loss of consciousness
800.34	Closed fracture of vault of skull with other and unspecified intracranial hemorrhage, prolonged (more than 24 hours) loss of consciousness and return to pre-existing conscious level
800.35	Closed fracture of vault of skull with other and unspecified intracranial hemorrhage, prolonged (more than 24 hours) loss of consciousness, without return to pre-existing conscious level
800.36	Closed fracture of vault of skull with other and unspecified intracranial hemorrhage, loss of consciousness of unspecified duration
800.39	Closed fracture of vault of skull with other and unspecified intracranial hemorrhage, unspecified concussion
800.40	Closed fracture of vault of skull with intracranial injury of other and unspecified nature, unspecified state of consciousness
800.42	Closed fracture of vault of skull with intracranial injury of other and unspecified nature, brief (less than one hour) loss of consciousness
800.43	Closed fracture of vault of skull with intracranial injury of other and unspecified nature, moderate (1-24 hours) loss of consciousness
800.44	Closed fracture of vault of skull with intracranial injury of other and unspecified nature, prolonged (more than 24 hours) loss of consciousness and return to pre-existing conscious level
800.45	Closed fracture of vault of skull with intracranial injury of other and unspecified nature, prolonged (more than 24 hours) loss of consciousness, without return to pre-existing conscious level
800.46	Closed fracture of vault of skull with intracranial injury of other and unspecified nature, loss of consciousness of unspecified duration
800.49	Closed fracture of vault of skull with intracranial injury of other and unspecified nature, unspecified concussion
800.52	Open fracture of vault of skull without mention of intracranial injury, brief (less than one hour) loss of consciousness

T Transfer DRG   SP Special Payment   ☑ Optimization Potential   TP Targeted Potential   * Code Range   ● New DRG   ▲ Revised DRG Title

224   Valid 10/01/2013-09/30/2014   © 2013 OptumInsight, Inc.

MDC 24: Multiple Significant Trauma—MEDICAL

800.53   Open fracture of vault of skull without mention of intracranial injury, moderate (1-24 hours) loss of consciousness

800.54   Open fracture of vault of skull without mention of intracranial injury, prolonged (more than 24 hours) loss of consciousness and return to pre-existing conscious level

800.55   Open fracture of vault of skull without mention of intracranial injury, prolonged (more than 24 hours) loss of consciousness, without return to pre-existing conscious level

800.6*   Open fracture of vault of skull with cerebral laceration and contusion

800.7*   Open fracture of vault of skull with subarachnoid, subdural, and extradural hemorrhage

800.8*   Open fracture of vault of skull with other and unspecified intracranial hemorrhage

800.9*   Open fracture of vault of skull with intracranial injury of other and unspecified nature

801.02   Closed fracture of base of skull without mention of intracranial injury, brief (less than one hour) loss of consciousness

801.03   Closed fracture of base of skull without mention of intracranial injury, moderate (1-24 hours) loss of consciousness

801.04   Closed fracture of base of skull without mention of intracranial injury, prolonged (more than 24 hours) loss of consciousness and return to pre-existing conscious level

801.05   Closed fracture of base of skull without mention of intracranial injury, prolonged (more than 24 hours) loss of consciousness, without return to pre-existing conscious level

801.1*   Closed fracture of base of skull with cerebral laceration and contusion

801.2*   Closed fracture of base of skull with subarachnoid, subdural, and extradural hemorrhage

801.3*   Closed fracture of base of skull with other and unspecified intracranial hemorrhage

801.4*   Closed fracture of base of skull with intracranial injury of other and unspecified nature

801.52   Open fracture of base of skull without mention of intracranial injury, brief (less than one hour) loss of consciousness

801.53   Open fracture of base of skull without mention of intracranial injury, moderate (1-24 hours) loss of consciousness

801.54   Open fracture of base of skull without mention of intracranial injury, prolonged (more than 24 hours) loss of consciousness and return to pre-existing conscious level

801.55   Open fracture of base of skull without mention of intracranial injury, prolonged (more than 24 hours) loss of consciousness, without return to pre-existing conscious level

801.6*   Open fracture of base of skull with cerebral laceration and contusion

801.7*   Open fracture of base of skull with subarachnoid, subdural, and extradural hemorrhage

801.8*   Open fracture of base of skull with other and unspecified intracranial hemorrhage

801.9*   Open fracture of base of skull with intracranial injury of other and unspecified nature

803.02   Other closed skull fracture without mention of intracranial injury, brief (less than one hour) loss of consciousness

803.03   Other closed skull fracture without mention of intracranial injury, moderate (1-24 hours) loss of consciousness

803.04   Other closed skull fracture without mention of intracranial injury, prolonged (more than 24 hours) loss of consciousness and return to pre-existing conscious level

803.05   Other closed skull fracture without mention of intracranial injury, prolonged (more than 24 hours) loss of consciousness, without return to pre-existing conscious level

803.1*   Other closed skull fracture with cerebral laceration and contusion

803.2*   Other closed skull fracture with subarachnoid, subdural, and extradural hemorrhage

803.3*   Closed skull fracture with other and unspecified intracranial hemorrhage

803.4*   Other closed skull fracture with intracranial injury of other and unspecified nature

803.52   Other open skull fracture without mention of intracranial injury, brief (less than one hour) loss of consciousness

803.53   Other open skull fracture without mention of intracranial injury, moderate (1-24 hours) loss of consciousness

803.54   Other open skull fracture without mention of intracranial injury, prolonged (more than 24 hours) loss of consciousness and return to pre-existing conscious level

803.55   Other open skull fracture without mention of intracranial injury, prolonged (more than 24 hours) loss of consciousness, without return to pre-existing conscious level

803.6*   Other open skull fracture with cerebral laceration and contusion

803.7*   Other open skull fracture with subarachnoid, subdural, and extradural hemorrhage

803.8*   Other open skull fracture with other and unspecified intracranial hemorrhage

803.9*   Other open skull fracture with intracranial injury of other and unspecified nature

804.02   Closed fractures involving skull or face with other bones, without mention of intracranial injury, brief (less than one hour) loss of consciousness

804.03   Closed fractures involving skull or face with other bones, without mention of intracranial injury, moderate (1-24 hours) loss of consciousness

804.04   Closed fractures involving skull or face with other bones, without mention or intracranial injury, prolonged (more than 24 hours) loss of consciousness and return to pre-existing conscious level

804.05   Closed fractures involving skull of face with other bones, without mention of intracranial injury, prolonged (more than 24 hours) loss of consciousness, without return to pre-existing conscious level

804.06   Closed fractures involving skull of face with other bones, without mention of intracranial injury, loss of consciousness of unspecified duration

804.1*   Closed fractures involving skull or face with other bones, with cerebral laceration and contusion

804.2*   Closed fractures involving skull of face with other bones with subarachnoid, subdural, and extradural hemorrhage

804.3*   Closed fractures involving skull or face with other bones, with other and unspecified intracranial hemorrhage

804.40   Closed fractures involving skull or face with other bones, with intracranial injury of other and unspecified nature, unspecified state of consciousness

804.41   Closed fractures involving skull or face with other bones, with intracranial injury of other and unspecified nature, no loss of consciousness

804.42   Closed fractures involving skull or face with other bones, with intracranial injury of other and unspecified nature, brief (less than one hour) loss of consciousness

804.43   Closed fractures involving skull or face with other bones, with intracranial injury of other and unspecified nature, moderate (1-24 hours) loss of consciousness

804.44   Closed fractures involving skull or face with other bones, with intracranial injury of other and unspecified nature, prolonged (more than 24 hours) loss of consciousness and return to pre-existing conscious level

Surgical	Medical	CC Indicator	MCC Indicator	Procedure Proxy

804.45 Closed fractures involving skull or face with other bones, with intracranial injury of other and unspecified nature, prolonged (more than 24 hours) loss of consciousness, without return to pre-existing conscious level

804.46 Closed fractures involving skull or face with other bones, with intracranial injury of other and unspecified nature, loss of consciousness of unspecified duration

804.52 Open fractures involving skull or face with other bones, without mention of intracranial injury, brief (less than one hour) loss of consciousness

804.53 Open fractures involving skull or face with other bones, without mention of intracranial injury, moderate (1-24 hours) loss of consciousness

804.54 Open fractures involving skull or face with other bones, without mention of intracranial injury, prolonged (more than 24 hours) loss of consciousness and return to pre-existing conscious level

804.55 Open fractures involving skull or face with other bones, without mention of intracranial injury, prolonged (more than 24 hours) loss of consciousness, without return to pre-existing conscious level

804.60 Open fractures involving skull or face with other bones, with cerebral laceration and contusion, unspecified state of consciousness

804.61 Open fractures involving skull or face with other bones, with cerebral laceration and contusion, no loss of consciousness

804.62 Open fractures involving skull or face with other bones, with cerebral laceration and contusion, brief (less than one hour) loss of consciousness

804.63 Open fractures involving skull or face with other bones, with cerebral laceration and contusion, moderate (1-24 hours) loss of consciousness

804.64 Open fractures involving skull or face with other bones, with cerebral laceration and contusion, prolonged (more than 24 hours) loss of consciousness and return to pre-existing conscious level

804.65 Open fractures involving skull or face with other bones, with cerebral laceration and contusion, prolonged (more than 24 hours) loss of consciousness, without return to pre-existing conscious level

804.66 Open fractures involving skull or face with other bones, with cerebral laceration and contusion, loss of consciousness of unspecified duration

804.7* Open fractures involving skull or face with other bones with subarachnoid, subdural, and extradural hemorrhage

804.8* Open fractures involving skull or face with other bones, with other and unspecified intracranial hemorrhage

804.9* Open fractures involving skull or face with other bones, with intracranial injury of other and unspecified nature

850.2 Concussion with moderate (1-24 hours) loss of consciousness

850.3 Concussion with prolonged (more than 24 hours) loss of consciousness and return to pre-existing conscious level

850.4 Concussion with prolonged (more than 24 hours) loss of consciousness, without return to pre-existing conscious level

851.00 Cortex (cerebral) contusion without mention of open intracranial wound, state of consciousness unspecified

851.01 Cortex (cerebral) contusion without mention of open intracranial wound, no loss of consciousness

851.02 Cortex (cerebral) contusion without mention of open intracranial wound, brief (less than 1 hour) loss of consciousness

851.03 Cortex (cerebral) contusion without mention of open intracranial wound, moderate (1-24 hours) loss of consciousness

851.04 Cortex (cerebral) contusion without mention of open intracranial wound, prolonged (more than 24 hours) loss of consciousness and return to pre-existing conscious level

851.05 Cortex (cerebral) contusion without mention of open intracranial wound, prolonged (more than 24 hours) loss of consciousness, without return to pre-existing conscious level

851.06 Cortex (cerebral) contusion without mention of open intracranial wound, loss of consciousness of unspecified duration

851.09 Cortex (cerebral) contusion without mention of open intracranial wound, unspecified concussion

851.1* Cortex (cerebral) contusion with open intracranial wound

851.2* Cortex (cerebral) laceration without mention of open intracranial wound

851.3* Cortex (cerebral) laceration with open intracranial wound

851.4* Cerebellar or brain stem contusion without mention of open intracranial wound

851.5* Cerebellar or brain stem contusion with open intracranial wound

851.6* Cerebellar or brain stem laceration without mention of open intracranial wound

851.7* Cerebellar or brain stem laceration with open intracranial wound

851.8* Other and unspecified cerebral laceration and contusion, without mention of open intracranial wound

851.9* Other and unspecified cerebral laceration and contusion, with open intracranial wound

852* Subarachnoid, subdural, and extradural hemorrhage, following injury

853* Other and unspecified intracranial hemorrhage following injury

854* Intracranial injury of other and unspecified nature

900.01 Common carotid artery injury

900.02 External carotid artery injury

900.03 Internal carotid artery injury

900.1 Internal jugular vein injury

900.81 External jugular vein injury

900.82 Injury to multiple blood vessels of head and neck

925.1 Crushing injury of face and scalp

925.2 Crushing injury of neck

Significant Trauma Body Site Category 2—Chest

807.07 Closed fracture of seven ribs

807.08 Closed fracture of eight or more ribs

807.14 Open fracture of four ribs

807.15 Open fracture of five ribs

807.16 Open fracture of six ribs

807.17 Open fracture of seven ribs

807.18 Open fracture of eight or more ribs

807.19 Open fracture of multiple ribs, unspecified

807.3 Open fracture of sternum

807.4 Flail chest

807.5 Closed fracture of larynx and trachea

807.6 Open fracture of larynx and trachea

819.1 Multiple open fractures involving both upper limbs, and upper limb with rib(s) and sternum

839.71 Open dislocation, sternum

860* Traumatic pneumothorax and hemothorax

861* Injury to heart and lung

862* Injury to other and unspecified intrathoracic organs

874.10 Open wound of larynx with trachea, complicated

874.11 Open wound of larynx, complicated

874.12 Open wound of trachea, complicated

901.0 Thoracic aorta injury

901.1 Innominate and subclavian artery injury

901.2 Superior vena cava injury

901.3 Innominate and subclavian vein injury

901.4* Pulmonary blood vessel injury

901.83 Injury to multiple blood vessels of thorax

901.89 Injury to specified blood vessels of thorax, other

901.9 Injury to unspecified blood vessel of thorax

927.01 Crushing injury of scapular region

958.0 Air embolism as an early complication of trauma

 Valid 10/01/2013-09/30/2014

MDC 24: Multiple Significant Trauma—MEDICAL

958.1   Fat embolism as an early complication of trauma

Significant Trauma Body Site Category 3—Abdomen

863.0   Stomach injury without mention of open wound into cavity
863.1   Stomach injury with open wound into cavity
863.2*   Small intestine injury without mention of open wound into cavity
863.3*   Small intestine injury with open wound into cavity
863.4*   Colon or rectal injury without mention of open wound into cavity
863.5*   Injury to colon or rectum with open wound into cavity
863.81   Pancreas head injury without mention of open wound into cavity
863.82   Pancreas body injury without mention of open wound into cavity
863.83   Pancreas tail injury without mention of open wound into cavity
863.84   Pancreas injury, multiple and unspecified sites, without mention of open wound into cavity
863.85   Appendix injury without mention of open wound into cavity
863.89   Injury to other and unspecified gastrointestinal sites without mention of open wound into cavity
863.9*   Injury to other and unspecified gastrointestinal sites, with open wound into cavity
864*   Injury to liver
865*   Injury to spleen
868.02   Bile duct and gallbladder injury without mention of open wound into cavity
868.09   Injury to other and multiple intra-abdominal organs without mention of open wound into cavity
868.12   Bile duct and gallbladder injury, with open wound into cavity
868.13   Peritoneum injury with open wound into cavity
868.14   Retroperitoneum injury with open wound into cavity
868.19   Injury to other and multiple intra-abdominal organs, with open wound into cavity
902*   Injury to blood vessels of abdomen and pelvis
958.93   Traumatic compartment syndrome of abdomen

Significant Trauma Body Site Category 4—Kidney

866*   Injury to kidney
868.01   Adrenal gland injury without mention of open wound into cavity
868.11   Adrenal gland injury, with open wound into cavity

Significant Trauma Body Site Category 5—Urinary

867*   Injury to pelvic organs

Significant Trauma Body Site Category 6—Pelvis and Spine

805.6   Closed fracture of sacrum and coccyx without mention of spinal cord injury
805.7   Open fracture of sacrum and coccyx without mention of spinal cord injury
806.0*   Closed fracture of cervical vertebra with spinal cord injury
806.1*   Open fracture of cervical vertebra with spinal cord injury
806.2*   Closed fracture of dorsal (thoracic) vertebra with spinal cord injury
806.3*   Open fracture of dorsal vertebra with spinal cord injury
806.4   Closed fracture of lumbar spine with spinal cord injury
806.5   Open fracture of lumbar spine with spinal cord injury
806.60   Closed fracture of sacrum and coccyx with unspecified spinal cord injury
806.7*   Open fracture of sacrum and coccyx with spinal cord injury
806.8   Closed fracture of unspecified vertebra with spinal cord injury
806.9   Open fracture of unspecified vertebra with spinal cord injury
808*   Fracture of pelvis
809.1   Fracture of bones of trunk, open
839.0*   Closed dislocation, cervical vertebra
839.1*   Open dislocation, cervical vertebra
839.52   Open dislocation, sacrum

839.59   Open dislocation, other vertebra
868.03   Peritoneum injury without mention of open wound into cavity
868.04   Retroperitoneum injury without mention of open wound into cavity
926.11   Crushing injury of back
926.19   Crushing injury of other specified sites of trunk
926.8   Crushing injury of multiple sites of trunk
926.9   Crushing injury of unspecified site of trunk
952*   Spinal cord injury without evidence of spinal bone injury
953.5   Injury to lumbosacral plexus
953.8   Injury to multiple sites of nerve roots and spinal plexus
954.8   Injury to other specified nerve(s) of trunk, excluding shoulder and pelvic girdles
954.9   Injury to unspecified nerve of trunk, excluding shoulder and pelvic girdles

Significant Trauma Body Site Category 7—Upper Limb

812.1*   Open fracture of upper end of humerus
812.30   Open fracture of unspecified part of humerus
812.31   Open fracture of shaft of humerus
812.5*   Open fracture of lower end of humerus
813.1*   Open fracture of upper end of radius and ulna
813.3*   Open fracture of shaft of radius and ulna
813.5*   Open fracture of lower end of radius and ulna
813.9*   Open fracture of unspecified part of radius with ulna
818.1   Ill-defined open fractures of upper limb
831.1*   Open dislocation of shoulder
832.1*   Open dislocation of elbow
887*   Traumatic amputation of arm and hand (complete) (partial)
903*   Injury to blood vessels of upper extremity
927.0*   Crushing injury of shoulder and upper arm
927.1*   Crushing injury of elbow and forearm
927.8   Crushing injury of multiple sites of upper limb
927.9   Crushing injury of unspecified site of upper limb
953.4   Injury to brachial plexus
955.0   Injury to axillary nerve
955.1   Injury to median nerve
955.2   Injury to ulnar nerve
955.3   Injury to radial nerve
955.8   Injury to multiple nerves of shoulder girdle and upper limb
958.6   Volkmann's ischemic contracture
958.91   Traumatic compartment syndrome of upper extremity

Significant Trauma Body Site Category 8—Lower Limb

820*   Fracture of neck of femur
821*   Fracture of other and unspecified parts of femur
823.1*   Open fracture of upper end of tibia and fibula
823.3*   Open fracture of shaft of tibia and fibula
823.4*   Torus fracture of tibia and fibula
823.9*   Open fracture of unspecified part of tibia and fibula
828*   Multiple fractures involving both lower limbs, lower with upper limb, and lower limb(s) with rib(s) and sternum
835.1*   Open dislocation of hip
836.6*   Other open dislocation of knee
837.1   Open dislocation of ankle
896*   Traumatic amputation of foot (complete) (partial)
897*   Traumatic amputation of leg(s) (complete) (partial)
904.0   Common femoral artery injury
904.1   Superficial femoral artery injury
904.2   Femoral vein injury
904.4*   Popliteal blood vessel vein
904.5*   Tibial blood vessel(s) injury
904.7   Injury to specified blood vessels of lower extremity, other
926.12   Crushing injury of buttock
928.0*   Crushing injury of hip and thigh
928.1*   Crushing injury of knee and lower leg
928.8   Crushing injury of multiple sites of lower limb
928.9   Crushing injury of unspecified site of lower limb
956.0   Injury to sciatic nerve
956.1   Injury to femoral nerve

Surgical	Medical	CC Indicator	MCC Indicator	Procedure Proxy

956.2	Injury to posterior tibial nerve
956.3	Injury to peroneal nerve
956.8	Injury to multiple nerves of pelvic girdle and lower limb
956.9	Injury to unspecified nerve of pelvic girdle and lower limb
958.92	Traumatic compartment syndrome of lower extremity

DRG 964   Other Multiple Significant Trauma with CC

  GMLOS 4.1 **AMLOS 5.0** **RW 1.3904** ☑

Select principal diagnosis from list of the Trauma Diagnosis List under DRG 963
WITH

At least two different diagnoses from two different Significant Trauma Body Site Categories located in DRG 963
OR

Select a principal diagnosis from one Significant Trauma Body Site Category
AND

Two or more significant trauma diagnoses from different Significant Trauma Body Site Categories listed under DRG 963

DRG 965   Other Multiple Significant Trauma without CC/MCC

  GMLOS 3.0 **AMLOS 3.6** **RW 0.9824** ☑

Select principal diagnosis from list of the Trauma Diagnosis List under DRG 963
WITH

At least two different diagnoses from two different Significant Trauma Body Site Categories located in DRG 963
OR

Select a principal diagnosis from one Significant Trauma Body Site Category
AND

Two or more significant trauma diagnoses from different Significant Trauma Body Site Categories listed under DRG 963

MDC 24: Multiple Significant Trauma—MEDICAL

Ⓣ *Transfer DRG* ⓈⓅ *Special Payment* ☑ *Optimization Potential* ▽ *Targeted Potential* * *Code Range* ● *New DRG* ▲ *Revised DRG Title*

228   Valid 10/01/2013-09/30/2014   © 2013 OptumInsight, Inc.

Note: MDC 25 contains diagnosis code 042 only.

SURGICAL

DRG 969 HIV with Extensive O.R. Procedure with MCC
GMLOS 12.0   AMLOS 16.7   RW 5.4896

Principal Diagnosis
042   Human immunodeficiency virus [HIV]
AND

Any operating room procedures excluding nonextensive operating room procedures (those procedures assigned to DRGs 987 - 989)
OR

Secondary Diagnosis
042   Human immunodeficiency virus [HIV]
WITH

Principal Diagnosis

Any major or significant HIV-related condition listed in DRG 974 or DRG 977
AND

Any operating room procedures excluding nonextensive operating room procedures (those procedures assigned to DRGs 987 - 989)

DRG 970 HIV with Extensive O.R. Procedure without MCC
GMLOS 4.9   AMLOS 7.1   RW 2.2785   ☑

Principal Diagnosis
042   Human immunodeficiency virus [HIV]
AND

Any operating room procedures excluding nonextensive operating room procedures (those procedures assigned to DRGs 987 - 989)
OR

Secondary Diagnosis
042   Human immunodeficiency virus [HIV]
WITH

Principal Diagnosis

Any major or significant HIV-related condition listed in DRG 974 or DRG 977
AND

Any operating room procedures excluding nonextensive operating room procedures (those procedures assigned to DRGs 987 - 989)

MEDICAL

DRG 974 HIV with Major Related Condition with MCC
GMLOS 6.7   AMLOS 9.3   RW 2.6335   ☑

Principal or Secondary Diagnosis
042   Human immunodeficiency virus [HIV]
AND

Major HIV-related Diagnosis
003.1   Salmonella septicemia
003.2*   Localized salmonella infections

003.8   Other specified salmonella infections
003.9   Unspecified salmonella infection
007.2   Coccidiosis
010*   Primary tuberculous infection
011*   Pulmonary tuberculosis
012*   Other respiratory tuberculosis
013*   Tuberculosis of meninges and central nervous system
014*   Tuberculosis of intestines, peritoneum, and mesenteric glands
015*   Tuberculosis of bones and joints
016*   Tuberculosis of genitourinary system
017*   Tuberculosis of other organs
018*   Miliary tuberculosis
031.2   Disseminated diseases due to other mycobacteria
031.8   Other specified diseases due to other mycobacteria
031.9   Unspecified diseases due to mycobacteria
038*   Septicemia
039*   Actinomycotic infections
046.3   Progressive multifocal leukoencephalopathy
046.7*   Other specified prion diseases of central nervous system
046.8   Other specified slow virus infection of central nervous system
046.9   Unspecified slow virus infection of central nervous system
049.8   Other specified non-arthropod-borne viral diseases of central nervous system
049.9   Unspecified non-arthropod-borne viral disease of central nervous system
053.0   Herpes zoster with meningitis
053.10   Herpes zoster with unspecified nervous system complication
053.11   Geniculate herpes zoster
053.12   Postherpetic trigeminal neuralgia
053.13   Postherpetic polyneuropathy
053.19   Other herpes zoster with nervous system complications
053.20   Herpes zoster dermatitis of eyelid
053.21   Herpes zoster keratoconjunctivitis
053.22   Herpes zoster iridocyclitis
053.29   Other ophthalmic herpes zoster complications
053.71   Otitis externa due to herpes zoster
053.79   Other specified herpes zoster complications
053.8   Unspecified herpes zoster complication
053.9   Herpes zoster without mention of complication
054.0   Eczema herpeticum
054.10   Unspecified genital herpes
054.11   Herpetic vulvovaginitis
054.12   Herpetic ulceration of vulva
054.13   Herpetic infection of penis
054.19   Other genital herpes
054.2   Herpetic gingivostomatitis
054.3   Herpetic meningoencephalitis
054.40   Unspecified ophthalmic complication herpes simplex
054.41   Herpes simplex dermatitis of eyelid
054.42   Dendritic keratitis
054.43   Herpes simplex disciform keratitis
054.44   Herpes simplex iridocyclitis
054.49   Herpes simplex with other ophthalmic complications
054.5   Herpetic septicemia
054.6   Herpetic whitlow
054.71   Visceral herpes simplex
054.72   Herpes simplex meningitis
054.73   Herpes simplex otitis externa
054.79   Other specified herpes simplex complications
054.8   Unspecified herpes simplex complication
054.9   Herpes simplex without mention of complication
058.21   Human herpesvirus 6 encephalitis
058.29   Other human herpesvirus encephalitis

Surgical	Medical	CC Indicator	MCC Indicator	Procedure Proxy

078.5	Cytomegaloviral disease
112.0	Candidiasis of mouth
112.3	Candidiasis of skin and nails
112.4	Candidiasis of lung
112.5	Disseminated candidiasis
112.8*	Candidiasis of other specified sites
112.9	Candidiasis of unspecified site
114*	Coccidioidomycosis
115*	Histoplasmosis
117.5	Cryptococcosis
118	Opportunistic mycoses
127.2	Strongyloidiasis
130*	Toxoplasmosis
136.3	Pneumocystosis
136.8	Other specified infectious and parasitic diseases
176*	Kaposi's sarcoma
200.0*	Reticulosarcoma
200.2*	Burkitt's tumor or lymphoma
200.3*	Marginal zone lymphoma
200.4*	Mantle cell lymphoma
200.5*	Primary central nervous system lymphoma
200.6*	Anaplastic large cell lymphoma
200.7*	Large cell lymphoma
200.8*	Other named variants of lymphosarcoma and reticulosarcoma
202.7*	Peripheral T-cell lymphoma
202.8*	Other malignant lymphomas
290.1*	Presenile dementia
294.9	Unspecified persistent mental disorders due to conditions classified elsewhere
298.9	Unspecified psychosis
310.9	Unspecified nonpsychotic mental disorder following organic brain damage
323.81	Other causes of encephalitis and encephalomyelitis
323.82	Other causes of myelitis
323.9	Unspecified causes of encephalitis, myelitis, and encephalomyelitis
336.9	Unspecified disease of spinal cord
341.9	Unspecified demyelinating disease of central nervous system
348.3*	Encephalopathy, not elsewhere classified
348.9	Unspecified condition of brain
349.9	Unspecified disorders of nervous system
421.0	Acute and subacute bacterial endocarditis
421.9	Unspecified acute endocarditis
422.9*	Other and unspecified acute myocarditis
480.3	Pneumonia due to SARS-associated coronavirus
480.8	Pneumonia due to other virus not elsewhere classified
480.9	Unspecified viral pneumonia
481	Pneumococcal pneumonia (streptococcus pneumoniae pneumonia)
482*	Other bacterial pneumonia
486	Pneumonia, organism unspecified
488.01	Influenza due to identified avian influenza virus with pneumonia
488.11	Influenza due to identified 2009 H1N1 influenza virus with pneumonia
488.81	Influenza due to identified novel influenza A virus with pneumonia

DRG 975   HIV with Major Related Condition with CC
GMLOS 4.7   AMLOS 6.1   RW 1.3383   ☑

Select principal and secondary diagnoses listed under DRG 974

DRG 976   HIV with Major Related Condition without CC/MCC
GMLOS 3.3   AMLOS 4.2   RW 0.8627   ☑

Select principal and secondary diagnoses listed under DRG 974

DRG 977   HIV with or without Other Related Condition
GMLOS 3.6   AMLOS 4.8   RW 1.1194   ☑

Principal Diagnosis

042	Human immunodeficiency virus [HIV]

OR

Secondary Diagnosis of HIV Infection

042	Human immunodeficiency virus [HIV]

AND

Principal Diagnosis of Significant HIV-Related Condition

009*	Ill-defined intestinal infections
047.9	Unspecified viral meningitis
079.9*	Unspecified viral and chlamydial infections, in conditions classified elsewhere and of unspecified site
110*	Dermatophytosis
111*	Dermatomycosis, other and unspecified
260	Kwashiorkor
261	Nutritional marasmus
262	Other severe protein-calorie malnutrition
263*	Other and unspecified protein-calorie malnutrition
264*	Vitamin A deficiency
265*	Thiamine and niacin deficiency states
266*	Deficiency of B-complex components
267	Ascorbic acid deficiency
268*	Vitamin D deficiency
269*	Other nutritional deficiencies
276.5*	Volume depletion
279*	Disorders involving the immune mechanism
280*	Iron deficiency anemias
281*	Other deficiency anemias
283*	Acquired hemolytic anemias
284.8*	Other specified aplastic anemias
284.9	Unspecified aplastic anemia
285.9	Unspecified anemia
287.4*	Secondary thrombocytopenia
287.5	Unspecified thrombocytopenia
288.0*	Neutropenia
289.4	Hypersplenism
289.84	Heparin-induced thrombocytopenia [HIT]
289.9	Unspecified diseases of blood and blood-forming organs
357.0	Acute infective polyneuritis
357.9	Unspecified inflammatory and toxic neuropathy
362.1*	Other background retinopathy and retinal vascular changes
369*	Blindness and low vision
425.9	Unspecified secondary cardiomyopathy
516.30	Idiopathic interstitial pneumonia, not otherwise specified
516.35	Idiopathic lymphoid interstitial pneumonia
516.36	Cryptogenic organizing pneumonia
516.37	Desquamative interstitial pneumonia
516.8	Other specified alveolar and parietoalveolar pneumonopathies
527.9	Unspecified disease of the salivary glands
528.6	Leukoplakia of oral mucosa, including tongue
558.1	Gastroenteritis and colitis due to radiation
558.2	Toxic gastroenteritis and colitis
558.4*	Eosinophilic gastroenteritis and colitis
558.9	Other and unspecified noninfectious gastroenteritis and colitis
579.9	Unspecified intestinal malabsorption
580*	Acute glomerulonephritis
581*	Nephrotic syndrome
582*	Chronic glomerulonephritis
583*	Nephritis and nephropathy, not specified as acute or chronic
683	Acute lymphadenitis
709.9	Unspecified disorder of skin and subcutaneous tissue
711.0*	Pyogenic arthritis
711.9*	Unspecified infective arthritis
716.9*	Unspecified arthropathy
729.2	Unspecified neuralgia, neuritis, and radiculitis

Ⓣ *Transfer DRG*   ⓈⓅ *Special Payment*   ☑ *Optimization Potential*   ⱳ *Targeted Potential*   * *Code Range*   ● *New DRG*   ▲ *Revised DRG Title*

779.34	Failure to thrive in newborn
780.60	Fever, unspecified
780.61	Fever presenting with conditions classified elsewhere
780.62	Postprocedural fever
780.63	Postvaccination fever
780.66	Febrile nonhemolytic transfusion reaction
780.7*	Malaise and fatigue
780.8	Generalized hyperhidrosis
782.1	Rash and other nonspecific skin eruption
783.2*	Abnormal loss of weight
783.4*	Lack of expected normal physiological development
785.6	Enlargement of lymph nodes
786.0*	Dyspnea and respiratory abnormalities
789.1	Hepatomegaly
789.2	Splenomegaly
799.4	Cachexia

Surgical   Medical   CC Indicator   MCC Indicator   Procedure Proxy

DRGs Associated with All MDCs

SURGICAL

DRG 981   **Extensive O.R. Procedure Unrelated to Principal Diagnosis with MCC**

       GMLOS 10.1   AMLOS 13.1   RW 4.9319   [T]

Discharges with all operating room procedures not listed for DRG 984 and DRG 987 that are unrelated to principal diagnosis

DRG 982   **Extensive O.R. Procedure Unrelated to Principal Diagnosis with CC**

       GMLOS 5.9   AMLOS 7.6   RW 2.8504   ☑[T]

Discharges with all operating room procedures not listed for DRG 984 and DRG 987 that are unrelated to principal diagnosis

DRG 983   **Extensive O.R. Procedure Unrelated to Principal Diagnosis without CC/MCC**

       GMLOS 2.8   AMLOS 3.8   RW 1.7462   ☑[T]

Discharges with all operating room procedures not listed for DRG 984 and DRG 987 that are unrelated to principal diagnosis

DRG 984   **Prostatic O.R. Procedure Unrelated to Principal Diagnosis with MCC**

       GMLOS 9.3   AMLOS 12.5   RW 3.4143

Operating Room Procedures
60.0	Incision of prostate
60.12	Open biopsy of prostate
60.15	Biopsy of periprostatic tissue
60.18	Other diagnostic procedures on prostate and periprostatic tissue
60.2*	Transurethral prostatectomy
60.61	Local excision of lesion of prostate
60.69	Other prostatectomy
60.8*	Incision or excision of periprostatic tissue
60.93	Repair of prostate
60.94	Control of (postoperative) hemorrhage of prostate
60.95	Transurethral balloon dilation of the prostatic urethra
60.96	Transurethral destruction of prostate tissue by microwave thermotherapy
60.97	Other transurethral destruction of prostate tissue by other thermotherapy
60.99	Other operations on prostate

With or without operating room procedures listed under DRG 987

DRG 985   **Prostatic O.R. Procedure Unrelated to Principal Diagnosis with CC**

       GMLOS 5.1   AMLOS 7.2   RW 1.8859   ☑

Select operating room procedures listed under DRG 984 with or without operating room procedures listed under DRG 987

DRG 986   **Prostatic O.R. Procedure Unrelated to Principal Diagnosis without CC/MCC**

       GMLOS 2.1   AMLOS 3.0   RW 1.0389   ☑

Select operating room procedures listed under DRG 984 with or without operating room procedures listed under DRG 987

DRG 987   **Nonextensive O.R. Procedure Unrelated to Principal Diagnosis with MCC**

       GMLOS 8.4   AMLOS 11.2   RW 3.3422   ☑[T]

Operating Room Procedures
04.07	Other excision or avulsion of cranial and peripheral nerves
04.4*	Lysis of adhesions and decompression of cranial and peripheral nerves
04.99	Other operations on cranial and peripheral nerves
05.23	Lumbar sympathectomy
06.02	Reopening of wound of thyroid field
08.11	Biopsy of eyelid
08.2*	Excision or destruction of lesion or tissue of eyelid
08.3*	Repair of blepharoptosis and lid retraction
08.4*	Repair of entropion or ectropion
08.5*	Other adjustment of lid position
08.6*	Reconstruction of eyelid with flaps or grafts
08.7*	Other reconstruction of eyelid
08.9*	Other operations on eyelids
09.0	Incision of lacrimal gland
09.1*	Diagnostic procedures on lacrimal system
09.2*	Excision of lesion or tissue of lacrimal gland
09.3	Other operations on lacrimal gland
09.4*	Manipulation of lacrimal passage
09.5*	Incision of lacrimal sac and passages
09.6	Excision of lacrimal sac and passage
09.7*	Repair of canaliculus and punctum
09.8*	Fistulization of lacrimal tract to nasal cavity
09.9*	Other operations on lacrimal system
10.0	Removal of embedded foreign body from conjunctiva by incision
10.1	Other incision of conjunctiva
10.2*	Diagnostic procedures on conjunctiva
10.3*	Excision or destruction of lesion or tissue of conjunctiva
10.4*	Conjunctivoplasty
10.5	Lysis of adhesions of conjunctiva and eyelid
10.6	Repair of laceration of conjunctiva
10.9*	Other operations on conjunctiva
11.0	Magnetic removal of embedded foreign body from cornea
11.1	Incision of cornea
11.2*	Diagnostic procedures on cornea
11.3*	Excision of pterygium
11.4*	Excision or destruction of tissue or other lesion of cornea
11.5*	Repair of cornea
11.6*	Corneal transplant
11.7*	Other reconstructive and refractive surgery on cornea
11.9*	Other operations on cornea
12.0*	Removal of intraocular foreign body from anterior segment of eye
12.1*	Iridotomy and simple iridectomy
12.2*	Diagnostic procedures on iris, ciliary body, sclera, and anterior chamber
12.3*	Iridoplasty and coreoplasty
12.4*	Excision or destruction of lesion of iris and ciliary body
12.5*	Facilitation of intraocular circulation
12.61	Trephination of sclera with iridectomy
12.62	Thermocauterization of sclera with iridectomy
12.63	Iridencleisis and iridotasis
12.64	Trabeculectomy ab externo
12.65	Other scleral fistulization with iridectomy
12.66	Postoperative revision of scleral fistulization procedure
12.69	Other scleral fistulizing procedure
12.7*	Other procedures for relief of elevated intraocular pressure
12.8*	Operations on sclera
12.9*	Other operations on iris, ciliary body, and anterior chamber

---

[T] Transfer DRG   SP Special Payment   ☑ Optimization Potential   ▽ Targeted Potential   * Code Range   ● New DRG   ▲ Revised DRG Title

13.0*	Removal of foreign body from lens
13.1*	Intracapsular extraction of lens
13.2	Extracapsular extraction of lens by linear extraction technique
13.3	Extracapsular extraction of lens by simple aspiration (and irrigation) technique
13.4*	Extracapsular extraction of lens by fragmentation and aspiration technique
13.5*	Other extracapsular extraction of lens
13.6*	Other cataract extraction
13.70	Insertion of pseudophakos, not otherwise specified
13.71	Insertion of intraocular lens prosthesis at time of cataract extraction, one-stage
13.72	Secondary insertion of intraocular lens prosthesis
13.8	Removal of implanted lens
13.9*	Other operations on lens
14.0*	Removal of foreign body from posterior segment of eye
14.1*	Diagnostic procedures on retina, choroid, vitreous, and posterior chamber
14.21	Destruction of chorioretinal lesion by diathermy
14.22	Destruction of chorioretinal lesion by cryotherapy
14.26	Destruction of chorioretinal lesion by radiation therapy
14.27	Destruction of chorioretinal lesion by implantation of radiation source
14.29	Other destruction of chorioretinal lesion
14.31	Repair of retinal tear by diathermy
14.32	Repair of retinal tear by cryotherapy
14.39	Other repair of retinal tear
14.4*	Repair of retinal detachment with scleral buckling and implant
14.5*	Other repair of retinal detachment
14.6	Removal of surgically implanted material from posterior segment of eye
14.7*	Operations on vitreous
14.9	Other operations on retina, choroid, and posterior chamber
15.0*	Diagnostic procedures on extraocular muscles or tendons
15.1*	Operations on one extraocular muscle involving temporary detachment from globe
15.2*	Other operations on one extraocular muscle
15.3	Operations on two or more extraocular muscles involving temporary detachment from globe, one or both eyes
15.4	Other operations on two or more extraocular muscles, one or both eyes
15.5	Transposition of extraocular muscles
15.6	Revision of extraocular muscle surgery
15.7	Repair of injury of extraocular muscle
15.9	Other operations on extraocular muscles and tendons
16.0*	Orbitotomy
16.1	Removal of penetrating foreign body from eye, not otherwise specified
16.22	Diagnostic aspiration of orbit
16.23	Biopsy of eyeball and orbit
16.29	Other diagnostic procedures on orbit and eyeball
16.3*	Evisceration of eyeball
16.4*	Enucleation of eyeball
16.5*	Exenteration of orbital contents
16.6*	Secondary procedures after removal of eyeball
16.7*	Removal of ocular or orbital implant
16.8*	Repair of injury of eyeball and orbit
16.92	Excision of lesion of orbit
16.93	Excision of lesion of eye, unspecified structure
16.98	Other operations on orbit
16.99	Other operations on eyeball
18.21	Excision of preauricular sinus
18.31	Radical excision of lesion of external ear
18.39	Other excision of external ear
18.5	Surgical correction of prominent ear
18.6	Reconstruction of external auditory canal
18.71	Construction of auricle of ear
18.72	Reattachment of amputated ear
18.79	Other plastic repair of external ear
18.9	Other operations on external ear
19.1*	Stapedectomy
19.4	Myringoplasty
19.9	Other repair of middle ear
20.01	Myringotomy with insertion of tube
20.2*	Incision of mastoid and middle ear
20.32	Biopsy of middle and inner ear
20.39	Other diagnostic procedures on middle and inner ear
20.51	Excision of lesion of middle ear
21.09	Control of epistaxis by other means
21.5	Submucous resection of nasal septum
21.62	Fracture of the turbinates
21.69	Other turbinectomy
21.72	Open reduction of nasal fracture
21.82	Closure of nasal fistula
21.83	Total nasal reconstruction
21.84	Revision rhinoplasty
21.85	Augmentation rhinoplasty
21.86	Limited rhinoplasty
21.87	Other rhinoplasty
21.88	Other septoplasty
21.89	Other repair and plastic operations on nose
21.99	Other operations on nose
22.63	Ethmoidectomy
24.4	Excision of dental lesion of jaw
24.5	Alveoloplasty
25.1	Excision or destruction of lesion or tissue of tongue
26.12	Open biopsy of salivary gland or duct
26.2*	Excision of lesion of salivary gland
26.3*	Sialoadenectomy
27.21	Biopsy of bony palate
27.22	Biopsy of uvula and soft palate
27.3*	Excision of lesion or tissue of bony palate
27.42	Wide excision of lesion of lip
27.43	Other excision of lesion or tissue of lip
27.49	Other excision of mouth
27.53	Closure of fistula of mouth
27.54	Repair of cleft lip
27.55	Full-thickness skin graft to lip and mouth
27.56	Other skin graft to lip and mouth
27.57	Attachment of pedicle or flap graft to lip and mouth
27.59	Other plastic repair of mouth
27.7*	Operations on uvula
27.92	Incision of mouth, unspecified structure
27.99	Other operations on oral cavity
28.11	Biopsy of tonsils and adenoids
28.2	Tonsillectomy without adenoidectomy
29.4	Plastic operation on pharynx
30.09	Other excision or destruction of lesion or tissue of larynx
31.98	Other operations on larynx
33.27	Closed endoscopic biopsy of lung
34.3	Excision or destruction of lesion or tissue of mediastinum
34.4	Excision or destruction of lesion of chest wall
37.89	Revision or removal of pacemaker device
38.00	Incision of vessel, unspecified site
38.09	Incision of lower limb veins
38.21	Biopsy of blood vessel
38.59	Ligation and stripping of lower limb varicose veins
38.86	Other surgical occlusion of abdominal arteries
39.94	Replacement of vessel-to-vessel cannula
40.0	Incision of lymphatic structures
40.1*	Diagnostic procedures on lymphatic structures
40.21	Excision of deep cervical lymph node
40.23	Excision of axillary lymph node
40.24	Excision of inguinal lymph node
40.29	Simple excision of other lymphatic structure
40.3	Regional lymph node excision
43.49	Other destruction of lesion or tissue of stomach
44.15	Open biopsy of stomach

Surgical	*Medical*	*CC Indicator*	*MCC Indicator*	*Procedure Proxy*

44.67	Laparoscopic procedures for creation of esophagogastric sphincteric competence
44.68	Laparoscopic gastroplasty
44.95	Laparoscopic gastric restrictive procedure
44.96	Laparoscopic revision of gastric restrictive procedure
44.97	Laparoscopic removal of gastric restrictive device(s)
44.98	(Laparoscopic) adjustment of size of adjustable gastric restrictive device
45.11	Transabdominal endoscopy of small intestine
45.21	Transabdominal endoscopy of large intestine
45.26	Open biopsy of large intestine
45.31	Other local excision of lesion of duodenum
45.32	Other destruction of lesion of duodenum
45.33	Local excision of lesion or tissue of small intestine, except duodenum
45.34	Other destruction of lesion of small intestine, except duodenum
45.41	Excision of lesion or tissue of large intestine
45.49	Other destruction of lesion of large intestine
46.41	Revision of stoma of small intestine
46.43	Other revision of stoma of large intestine
46.52	Closure of stoma of large intestine
48.25	Open biopsy of rectum
48.35	Local excision of rectal lesion or tissue
48.8*	Incision or excision of perirectal tissue or lesion
49.1*	Incision or excision of anal fistula
49.39	Other local excision or destruction of lesion or tissue of anus
49.44	Destruction of hemorrhoids by cryotherapy
49.45	Ligation of hemorrhoids
49.46	Excision of hemorrhoids
49.49	Other procedures on hemorrhoids
49.5*	Division of anal sphincter
49.6	Excision of anus
49.79	Other repair of anal sphincter
51.23	Laparoscopic cholecystectomy
51.99	Other operations on biliary tract
53.0*	Other unilateral repair of inguinal hernia
53.1*	Other bilateral repair of inguinal hernia
53.2*	Unilateral repair of femoral hernia
53.3*	Bilateral repair of femoral hernia
53.41	Other and open repair of umbilical hernia with graft or prosthesis
53.49	Other open umbilical herniorrhaphy
53.51	Incisional hernia repair
53.61	Other open incisional hernia repair with graft or prosthesis
53.69	Other and open repair of other hernia of anterior abdominal wall with graft or prosthesis
54.21	Laparoscopy
54.22	Biopsy of abdominal wall or umbilicus
54.29	Other diagnostic procedures on abdominal region
54.3	Excision or destruction of lesion or tissue of abdominal wall or umbilicus
54.4	Excision or destruction of peritoneal tissue
54.64	Suture of peritoneum
55.12	Pyelostomy
56.0	Transurethral removal of obstruction from ureter and renal pelvis
56.1	Ureteral meatotomy
56.2	Ureterotomy
56.39	Other diagnostic procedures on ureter
56.52	Revision of cutaneous uretero-ileostomy
57.22	Revision or closure of vesicostomy
57.33	Closed (transurethral) biopsy of bladder
57.39	Other diagnostic procedures on bladder
57.49	Other transurethral excision or destruction of lesion or tissue of bladder
57.59	Open excision or destruction of other lesion or tissue of bladder
57.82	Closure of cystostomy
57.91	Sphincterotomy of bladder
57.97	Replacement of electronic bladder stimulator
57.98	Removal of electronic bladder stimulator
58.0	Urethrotomy
58.1	Urethral meatotomy
58.5	Release of urethral stricture
58.99	Other operations on urethra and periurethral tissue
59.79	Other repair of urinary stress incontinence
61.2	Excision of hydrocele (of tunica vaginalis)
63.09	Other diagnostic procedures on spermatic cord, epididymis, and vas deferens
63.1	Excision of varicocele and hydrocele of spermatic cord
63.2	Excision of cyst of epididymis
63.3	Excision of other lesion or tissue of spermatic cord and epididymis
64.11	Biopsy of penis
64.2	Local excision or destruction of lesion of penis
64.49	Other repair of penis
64.92	Incision of penis
64.93	Division of penile adhesions
64.95	Insertion or replacement of non-inflatable penile prosthesis
64.96	Removal of internal prosthesis of penis
64.97	Insertion or replacement of inflatable penile prosthesis
64.98	Other operations on penis
64.99	Other operations on male genital organs
65.61	Other removal of both ovaries and tubes at same operative episode
66.2*	Bilateral endoscopic destruction or occlusion of fallopian tubes
66.3*	Other bilateral destruction or occlusion of fallopian tubes
66.92	Unilateral destruction or occlusion of fallopian tube
67.1*	Diagnostic procedures on cervix
67.2	Conization of cervix
67.3*	Other excision or destruction of lesion or tissue of cervix
68.15	Closed biopsy of uterine ligaments
68.16	Closed biopsy of uterus
68.29	Other excision or destruction of lesion of uterus
68.5*	Vaginal hysterectomy
69.01	Dilation and curettage for termination of pregnancy
69.09	Other dilation and curettage of uterus
69.51	Aspiration curettage of uterus for termination of pregnancy
69.52	Aspiration curettage following delivery or abortion
69.95	Incision of cervix
70.14	Other vaginotomy
70.23	Biopsy of cul-de-sac
70.24	Vaginal biopsy
70.29	Other diagnostic procedures on vagina and cul-de-sac
70.3*	Local excision or destruction of vagina and cul-de-sac
70.76	Hymenorrhaphy
71.09	Other incision of vulva and perineum
71.1*	Diagnostic procedures on vulva
71.22	Incision of Bartholin's gland (cyst)
71.23	Marsupialization of Bartholin's gland (cyst)
71.24	Excision or other destruction of Bartholin's gland (cyst)
71.29	Other operations on Bartholin's gland
71.3	Other local excision or destruction of vulva and perineum
71.4	Operations on clitoris
71.71	Suture of laceration of vulva or perineum
71.79	Other repair of vulva and perineum
76.11	Biopsy of facial bone
76.2	Local excision or destruction of lesion of facial bone
77.38	Other division of tarsals and metatarsals
77.4*	Biopsy of bone
77.5*	Excision and repair of bunion and other toe deformities
77.6*	Local excision of lesion or tissue of bone
77.88	Other partial ostectomy of tarsals and metatarsals
77.98	Total ostectomy of tarsals and metatarsals
78.03	Bone graft of radius and ulna
78.6*	Removal of implanted device from bone
79.12	Closed reduction of fracture of radius and ulna with internal fixation

---

Ⓣ *Transfer DRG*   Ⓢ *Special Payment*   ☑ *Optimization Potential*   ▽ *Targeted Potential*   * *Code Range*   ● *New DRG*   ▲ *Revised DRG Title*

Valid 10/01/2013-09/30/2014

© 2013 OptumInsight, Inc.

80.16	Other arthrotomy of knee
80.18	Other arthrotomy of foot and toe
80.26	Arthroscopy of knee
80.46	Division of joint capsule, ligament, or cartilage of knee
80.6	Excision of semilunar cartilage of knee
80.7*	Synovectomy
80.86	Other local excision or destruction of lesion of knee joint
80.88	Other local excision or destruction of lesion of joint of foot and toe
80.98	Other excision of joint of foot and toe
81.57	Replacement of joint of foot and toe
81.83	Other repair of shoulder
82.01	Exploration of tendon sheath of hand
82.09	Other incision of soft tissue of hand
82.11	Tenotomy of hand
82.21	Excision of lesion of tendon sheath of hand
82.29	Excision of other lesion of soft tissue of hand
82.41	Suture of tendon sheath of hand
82.45	Other suture of other tendon of hand
82.46	Suture of muscle or fascia of hand
83.0*	Incision of muscle, tendon, fascia, and bursa
83.13	Other tenotomy
83.19	Other division of soft tissue
83.21	Open biopsy of soft tissue
83.32	Excision of lesion of muscle
83.39	Excision of lesion of other soft tissue
83.5	Bursectomy
83.6*	Suture of muscle, tendon, and fascia
84.01	Amputation and disarticulation of finger
85.12	Open biopsy of breast
85.20	Excision or destruction of breast tissue, not otherwise specified
85.21	Local excision of lesion of breast
85.23	Subtotal mastectomy
85.50	Augmentation mammoplasty, not otherwise specified
85.53	Unilateral breast implant
85.54	Bilateral breast implant
85.93	Revision of implant of breast
85.94	Removal of implant of breast
85.95	Insertion of breast tissue expander
85.96	Removal of breast tissue expander (s)
85.99	Other operations on the breast
86.21	Excision of pilonidal cyst or sinus
86.25	Dermabrasion
86.4	Radical excision of skin lesion
86.60	Free skin graft, not otherwise specified
86.62	Other skin graft to hand
86.65	Heterograft to skin
86.82	Facial rhytidectomy
86.83	Size reduction plastic operation
86.84	Relaxation of scar or web contracture of skin
86.89	Other repair and reconstruction of skin and subcutaneous tissue
87.53	Intraoperative cholangiogram
92.27	Implantation or insertion of radioactive elements
95.04	Eye examination under anesthesia

DRG 988   **Nonextensive O.R. Procedure Unrelated to Principal Diagnosis with CC**

     GMLOS 4.8   AMLOS 6.4   RW 1.7554   ☑ⓣ

Select operating room procedures listed under DRG 987

DRG 989   **Nonextensive O.R. Procedure Unrelated to Principal Diagnosis without CC/MCC**

     GMLOS 2.3   AMLOS 3.0   RW 1.0430   ☑ⓣ

Select operating room procedures listed under DRG 987

DRG 999   **Ungroupable**

     GMLOS 0.0   AMLOS 0.0   RW 0.0000

Discharges with invalid ICD-9-CM principal diagnosis, sex or discharge status field(s) missing or invalid and necessary for DRG assignment

---

Surgical   *Medical*   *CC Indicator*   *MCC Indicator*   *Procedure Proxy*

Alphabetic Index to Diseases

765.22	24 completed weeks of gestation **163**	
765.23	25-26 completed weeks of gestation **163**	
765.24	27-28 completed weeks of gestation **163, 167**	
765.25	29-30 completed weeks of gestation **163, 167**	
765.26	31-32 completed weeks of gestation **163, 167**	
765.27	33-34 completed weeks of gestation **163, 167**	
765.28	35-36 completed weeks of gestation **163, 167**	
765.29	37 or more completed weeks of gestation **171, 172**	
039.2	Abdominal actinomycotic infection **75**	
441.4	Abdominal aneurysm without mention of rupture **66**	
441.3	Abdominal aneurysm, ruptured **66**	
902.0	Abdominal aorta injury **166, 170**	
789.3*	Abdominal or pelvic swelling, mass, or lump **78**	
789.0*	Abdominal pain **78**	
789.4*	Abdominal rigidity **79**	
789.6*	Abdominal tenderness **78**	
786.7	Abnormal chest sounds **54**	
796.7*	Abnormal cytologic smear of anus and anal HPV **79**	
796.5	Abnormal finding on antenatal screening **156, 159**	
790.2*	Abnormal glucose **113**	
374.43	Abnormal innervation syndrome of eyelid **39**	
781.0	Abnormal involuntary movements **33**	
783.2*	Abnormal loss of weight **231**	
648.84	Abnormal maternal glucose tolerance complicating pregnancy, childbirth, or the puerperium, postpartum condition or complication **152**	
648.83	Abnormal maternal glucose tolerance, antepartum **154, 156**	
648.80	Abnormal maternal glucose tolerance, complicating pregnancy, childbirth, or the puerperium, unspecified as to episode of care **159**	
648.81	Abnormal maternal glucose tolerance, with delivery **134, 142, 148**	
648.82	Abnormal maternal glucose tolerance, with delivery, with current postpartum complication **135, 142, 148**	
795.0*	Abnormal Papanicolaou smear of cervix and cervical HPV **127, 130**	
795.1*	Abnormal Papanicolaou smear of vagina and vaginal HPV **127, 130**	
781.92	Abnormal posture **33**	
796.1	Abnormal reflex **33**	
786.4	Abnormal sputum **54**	
795.8*	Abnormal tumor markers **213**	
659.73	Abnormality in fetal heart rate or rhythm, antepartum condition or complication **155, 158**	
659.71	Abnormality in fetal heart rate or rhythm, delivered, with or without mention of antepartum condition **136, 143, 149**	
659.70	Abnormality in fetal heart rate or rhythm, unspecified as to episode of care or not applicable **136, 143, 149**	
781.2	Abnormality of gait **33**	
790.0*	Abnormality of red blood cells **175**	
251.5	Abnormality of secretion of gastrin **77**	
251.4	Abnormality of secretion of glucagon **114**	
999.6*	ABO incompatibility reaction due to transfusion of blood or blood products **167, 171, 176**	
637*	Abortion, unspecified as to legality **153**	
915.0	Abrasion or friction burn of finger, without mention of infection **107**	

917.0	Abrasion or friction burn of foot and toe(s), without mention of infection **107**
919.0	Abrasion or friction burn of other, multiple, and unspecified sites, without mention of infection **107**
566	Abscess of anal and rectal regions **79, 166, 170**
616.3	Abscess of Bartholin's gland **127, 130**
675.12	Abscess of breast associated with childbirth, delivered, with mention of postpartum complication **139, 141, 147**
675.11	Abscess of breast associated with childbirth, delivered, with or without mention of antepartum condition **139, 141, 147**
675.10	Abscess of breast associated with childbirth, unspecified as to episode of care **161**
675.13	Abscess of breast, antepartum **156, 158**
675.14	Abscess of breast, postpartum condition or complication **153**
569.5	Abscess of intestine **76**
572.0	Abscess of liver **166, 170**
513*	Abscess of lung and mediastinum **51, 165, 170**
254.1	Abscess of thymus **164, 168**
133*	Acariasis **108**
998.2	Accidental puncture or laceration during procedure **167, 171, 204**
791.6	Acetonuria **113**
530.0	Achalasia and cardiospasm **78**
726.71	Achilles bursitis or tendinitis **98**
536.0	Achlorhydria **78**
368.54	Achromatopsia **39**
V45.71	Acquired absence of breast and nipple **214**
V88.0*	Acquired absence of cervix and uterus **128, 131**
V45.72	Acquired absence of intestine (large) (small) **214**
V88.2*	Acquired absence of joint **215**
V45.73	Acquired absence of kidney **214**
V45.78	Acquired absence of organ, eye **40**
V45.77	Acquired absence of organ, genital organs **124, 128, 131**
V45.76	Acquired absence of organ, lung **54**
V45.74	Acquired absence of organ, other parts of urinary tract **120**
V45.75	Acquired absence of organ, stomach **214**
V88.1*	Acquired absence of pancreas **215**
388.45	Acquired auditory processing disorder **189**
429.71	Acquired cardiac septal defect **69**
286.7	Acquired coagulation factor deficiency **176**
368.55	Acquired color vision deficiencies **38**
593.2	Acquired cyst of kidney **120**
736.3*	Acquired deformities of hip **100**
736.8*	Acquired deformities of other parts of limbs **100**
735*	Acquired deformities of toe **100**
738.3	Acquired deformity of chest and rib **100**
736.9	Acquired deformity of limb, site unspecified **100**
738.2	Acquired deformity of neck **100**
738.0	Acquired deformity of nose **47**
738.6	Acquired deformity of pelvis **100**
736.71	Acquired equinovarus deformity **100**
283.9	Acquired hemolytic anemia, unspecified **164, 169, 175**
283*	Acquired hemolytic anemias **230**
286.52	Acquired hemophilia **176**
537.0	Acquired hypertrophic pyloric stenosis **77**
244*	Acquired hypothyroidism **114**

738.8	Acquired musculoskeletal deformity of other specified site **100**
738.9	Acquired musculoskeletal deformity of unspecified site **100**
738.4	Acquired spondylolisthesis **97**
380.5*	Acquired stenosis of external ear canal **47**
840.0	Acromioclavicular (joint) (ligament) sprain and strain **222**
039.8	Actinomycotic infection of other specified sites **185**
039.9	Actinomycotic infection of unspecified site **185**
039*	Actinomycotic infections **229**
341.2*	Acute (transverse) myelitis **9**, **34**
341.21	Acute (transverse) myelitis in conditions classified elsewhere **10**
341.20	Acute (transverse) myelitis NOS **10**
571.1	Acute alcoholic hepatitis **82**
303.0*	Acute alcoholic intoxication **191**
006.0	Acute amebic dysentery without mention of abscess **75**
518.84	Acute and chronic respiratory failure **52**, **207**
421.0	Acute and subacute bacterial endocarditis **65**, **230**
421*	Acute and subacute endocarditis **165**, **169**
421.1	Acute and subacute infective endocarditis in diseases classified elsewhere **65**
364.0*	Acute and subacute iridocyclitis **39**
570	Acute and subacute necrosis of liver **83**, **166**, **170**
540.0	Acute appendicitis with generalized peritonitis **73**, **76**
540.1	Acute appendicitis with peritoneal abscess **73**, **76**
540.9	Acute appendicitis without mention of peritonitis **78**
466*	Acute bronchitis and bronchiolitis **53**
519.11	Acute bronchospasm **3**
375.31	Acute canaliculitis, lacrimal **38**
517.3	Acute chest syndrome **53**
415.0	Acute cor pulmonale **69**
411.81	Acute coronary occlusion without myocardial infarction **68**
595.0	Acute cystitis **119**, **166**, **170**
375.01	Acute dacryoadenitis **38**
375.32	Acute dacryocystitis **38**
536.1	Acute dilatation of stomach **78**, **165**, **170**
532.0*	Acute duodenal ulcer with hemorrhage **76**
532.2*	Acute duodenal ulcer with hemorrhage and perforation **76**
532.1*	Acute duodenal ulcer with perforation **77**
532.31	Acute duodenal ulcer without mention of hemorrhage or perforation, with obstruction **77**
532.30	Acute duodenal ulcer without mention of hemorrhage, perforation, or obstruction **77**
333.72	Acute dystonia due to drugs **32**
360.01	Acute endophthalmitis **38**
464.3*	Acute epiglottitis **3**, **46**
207.0*	Acute erythremia and erythroleukemia **180**, **181**
446.1	Acute febrile mucocutaneous lymph node syndrome (MCLS) **97**
531.0*	Acute gastric ulcer with hemorrhage **76**
531.2*	Acute gastric ulcer with hemorrhage and perforation **76**
531.1*	Acute gastric ulcer with perforation **77**
531.31	Acute gastric ulcer without mention of hemorrhage or perforation, with obstruction **77**
531.30	Acute gastric ulcer without mention of hemorrhage, perforation, or obstruction **77**
535.01	Acute gastritis with hemorrhage **76**
535.00	Acute gastritis without mention of hemorrhage **78**
534.0*	Acute gastrojejunal ulcer with hemorrhage **76**
534.2*	Acute gastrojejunal ulcer with hemorrhage and perforation **76**
534.1*	Acute gastrojejunal ulcer with perforation **77**
534.3*	Acute gastrojejunal ulcer without mention of hemorrhage or perforation **77**

580*	Acute glomerulonephritis **120**, **166**, **170**, **230**
999.84	Acute hemolytic transfusion reaction, incompatibility unspecified **176**
999.34	Acute infection following transfusion, infusion, or injection of blood and blood products **167**, **171**, **184**, **186**
357.0	Acute infective polyneuritis **33**, **230**
584*	Acute kidney failure **166**, **170**
669.32	Acute kidney failure following labor and delivery, delivered, with mention of postpartum complication **138**, **141**, **146**
669.34	Acute kidney failure following labor and delivery, postpartum condition or complication **153**
669.30	Acute kidney failure following labor and delivery, unspecified as to episode of care or not applicable **138**, **145**, **150**
584.7	Acute kidney failure with lesion of medullary [papillary] necrosis **118**
584.6	Acute kidney failure with lesion of renal cortical necrosis **118**
584.5	Acute kidney failure with lesion of tubular necrosis **118**
584.8	Acute kidney failure with other specified pathological lesion in kidney **118**
584.9	Acute kidney failure, unspecified **118**
464.01	Acute laryngitis, with obstruction **3**, **46**
464.00	Acute laryngitis, without mention of obstruction **3**, **46**
464.2*	Acute laryngotracheitis **3**, **46**
208.0*	Acute leukemia of unspecified cell type **180**, **181**
683	Acute lymphadenitis **166**, **170**, **176**, **230**
204.0*	Acute lymphoid leukemia **180**, **181**
383.0*	Acute mastoiditis **46**
018.0*	Acute miliary tuberculosis **185**
206.0*	Acute monocytic leukemia **180**, **181**
205.0*	Acute myeloid leukemia **180**, **181**
410.00	Acute myocardial infarction of anterolateral wall, episode of care unspecified **68**
410.01	Acute myocardial infarction of anterolateral wall, initial episode of care **56**, **65**
410.02	Acute myocardial infarction of anterolateral wall, subsequent episode of care **68**
410.20	Acute myocardial infarction of inferolateral wall, episode of care unspecified **69**
410.21	Acute myocardial infarction of inferolateral wall, initial episode of care **56**, **65**
410.22	Acute myocardial infarction of inferolateral wall, subsequent episode of care **69**
410.30	Acute myocardial infarction of inferoposterior wall, episode of care unspecified **69**
410.31	Acute myocardial infarction of inferoposterior wall, initial episode of care **56**, **65**
410.32	Acute myocardial infarction of inferoposterior wall, subsequent episode of care **69**
410.10	Acute myocardial infarction of other anterior wall, episode of care unspecified **68**
410.11	Acute myocardial infarction of other anterior wall, initial episode of care **56**, **65**
410.12	Acute myocardial infarction of other anterior wall, subsequent episode of care **68**
410.40	Acute myocardial infarction of other inferior wall, episode of care unspecified **69**
410.41	Acute myocardial infarction of other inferior wall, initial episode of care **56**, **65**
410.42	Acute myocardial infarction of other inferior wall, subsequent episode of care **69**
410.50	Acute myocardial infarction of other lateral wall, episode of care unspecified **69**
410.51	Acute myocardial infarction of other lateral wall, initial episode of care **56**, **65**

410.52	Acute myocardial infarction of other lateral wall, subsequent episode of care **69**
410.80	Acute myocardial infarction of other specified sites, episode of care unspecified **69**
410.81	Acute myocardial infarction of other specified sites, initial episode of care **57, 65**
410.82	Acute myocardial infarction of other specified sites, subsequent episode of care **69**
410.70	Acute myocardial infarction, subendocardial infarction, episode of care unspecified **69**
410.71	Acute myocardial infarction, subendocardial infarction, initial episode of care **57, 65**
410.72	Acute myocardial infarction, subendocardial infarction, subsequent episode of care **69**
410.60	Acute myocardial infarction, true posterior wall infarction, episode of care unspecified **69**
410.61	Acute myocardial infarction, true posterior wall infarction, initial episode of care **57, 65**
410.62	Acute myocardial infarction, true posterior wall infarction, subsequent episode of care **69**
410.90	Acute myocardial infarction, unspecified site, episode of care unspecified **69**
410.91	Acute myocardial infarction, unspecified site, initial episode of care **57, 65**
410.92	Acute myocardial infarction, unspecified site, subsequent episode of care **69**
422*	Acute myocarditis **69**
422.0	Acute myocarditis in diseases classified elsewhere **165, 169**
384.0*	Acute myringitis without mention of otitis media **46**
460	Acute nasopharyngitis (common cold) **3, 46**
045.2*	Acute nonparalytic poliomyelitis **184**
381.0*	Acute nonsuppurative otitis media **46**
614.5	Acute or unspecified pelvic peritonitis, female **130**
730.0*	Acute osteomyelitis **96**
730.06	Acute osteomyelitis, lower leg **90**
730.08	Acute osteomyelitis, other specified site **87**
338.1*	Acute pain **213**
577.0	Acute pancreatitis **166, 170**
045.0*	Acute paralytic poliomyelitis specified as bulbar **8, 10, 33**
614.3	Acute parametritis and pelvic cellulitis **130**
298.3	Acute paranoid reaction **189**
533.0*	Acute peptic ulcer, unspecified site, with hemorrhage **76**
533.2*	Acute peptic ulcer, unspecified site, with hemorrhage and perforation **76**
533.1*	Acute peptic ulcer, unspecified site, with perforation **77**
533.31	Acute peptic ulcer, unspecified site, without mention of hemorrhage and perforation, with obstruction **77**
533.30	Acute peptic ulcer, unspecified site, without mention of hemorrhage, perforation, or obstruction **77**
420*	Acute pericarditis **69**
420.0	Acute pericarditis in diseases classified elsewhere **165, 169**
380.01	Acute perichondritis of pinna **100**
462	Acute pharyngitis **3, 46**
045.1*	Acute poliomyelitis with other paralysis **8, 10, 33**
285.1	Acute posthemorrhagic anemia **164, 169**
506.1	Acute pulmonary edema due to fumes and vapors **52**
415*	Acute pulmonary heart disease **165, 169**
508.0	Acute pulmonary manifestations due to radiation **54, 165, 169**
590.1*	Acute pyelonephritis **166, 170**
998.7	Acute reaction to foreign substance accidentally left during procedure, not elsewhere classified **167, 171, 204**
308*	Acute reaction to stress **188**
518.81	Acute respiratory failure **52, 207**
391.1	Acute rheumatic endocarditis **67**
391.2	Acute rheumatic myocarditis **68**
391.0	Acute rheumatic pericarditis **68**
614.0	Acute salpingitis and oophoritis **130**
461*	Acute sinusitis **46**
463	Acute tonsillitis **3, 46**
464.1*	Acute tracheitis **53**
045.9*	Acute unspecified poliomyelitis **8, 10, 33**
465*	Acute upper respiratory infections of multiple or unspecified sites **3, 46**
557.0	Acute vascular insufficiency of intestine **166, 170**
453.4*	Acute venous embolism and thrombosis of deep vessels of lower extremity **67**
453.8*	Acute venous embolism and thrombosis of other specified veins **67**
436	Acute, but ill-defined, cerebrovascular disease **20, 165, 169**
474.2	Adenoid vegetations **47**
091.4	Adenopathy due to secondary syphilis **176**
364.7*	Adhesions and disruptions of iris and ciliary body **39**
726.0	Adhesive capsulitis of shoulder **98**
309.0	Adjustment disorder with depressed mood **188**
309.3	Adjustment disorder with disturbance of conduct **188**
309.4	Adjustment disorder with mixed disturbance of emotions and conduct **188**
737.0	Adolescent postural kyphosis **87**
868.01	Adrenal gland injury without mention of open wound into cavity **114, 227**
868.11	Adrenal gland injury, with open wound into cavity **114, 227**
307.0	Adult onset fluency disorder **189**
V62.1	Adverse effects of work environment **214**
301.10	Affective personality disorder, unspecified **188**
086.5	African trypanosomiasis, unspecified **185**
V58.7*	Aftercare following surgery to specified body systems, not elsewhere classified **213**
V54.2*	Aftercare for healing pathologic fracture **99**
V54.1*	Aftercare for healing traumatic fracture **99**
V54.0*	Aftercare involving internal fixation device **99**
V51*	Aftercare involving the use of plastic surgery **109**
136.0	Ainhum **186**
958.0	Air embolism as an early complication of trauma **51, 166, 170, 224, 226**
999.1	Air embolism as complication of medical care, not elsewhere classified **51, 167, 171**
291*	Alcohol-induced mental disorders **191**
571.2	Alcoholic cirrhosis of liver **82**
571.0	Alcoholic fatty liver **83**
535.31	Alcoholic gastritis with hemorrhage **76**
535.30	Alcoholic gastritis without mention of hemorrhage **78**
357.5	Alcoholic polyneuropathy **21**
315.01	Alexia **189**
784.61	Alexia and dyslexia **189**
733.7	Algoneurodystrophy **100**
518.6	Allergic bronchopulmonary aspergillosis **53**
477*	Allergic rhinitis **46**
708.0	Allergic urticaria **166, 170**
995.3	Allergy, unspecified not elsewhere classified **203**
117.6	Allescheriosis (Petriellidiosis) **164, 168**
282.43	Alpha thalassemia **164, 169**
273.4	Alpha-1-antitrypsin deficiency **114**

331.0   Alzheimer's disease **19**

368.0*   Amblyopia ex anopsia **39**

006.5   Amebic brain abscess **8, 10, 33**

006.8   Amebic infection of other sites **185**

006.3   Amebic liver abscess **83**

006.4   Amebic lung abscess **51**

006.2   Amebic nondysenteric colitis **75**

006.6   Amebic skin ulceration **107**

673.13   Amniotic fluid embolism, antepartum condition or complication **156, 158**

673.14   Amniotic fluid embolism, postpartum condition or complication **153**

673.10   Amniotic fluid embolism, unspecified as to episode of care **161**

673.12   Amniotic fluid embolism, with delivery, with mention of postpartum complication **138, 141, 146**

673.11   Amniotic fluid embolism, with delivery, with or without mention of antepartum condition **138, 141, 146**

997.6*   Amputation stump complication **101**

277.3*   Amyloidosis **97**

569.0   Anal and rectal polyp **79**

565*   Anal fissure and fistula **79**

564.6   Anal spasm **78**

664.61   Anal sphincter tear complicating delivery, not associated with third-degree perineal laceration, delivered, with or without mention of antepartum condition **137, 144, 150**

664.64   Anal sphincter tear complicating delivery, not associated with third-degree perineal laceration, postpartum condition or complication **152**

664.60   Anal sphincter tear complicating delivery, not associated with third-degree perineal laceration, unspecified as to episode of care or not applicable **137, 144, 150**

995.6*   Anaphylactic reaction due to food **203**

999.4*   Anaphylactic reaction due to serum **167, 171, 203**

200.6*   Anaplastic large cell lymphoma **230**

126*   Ancylostomiasis and necatoriasis **76**

776.6   Anemia of neonatal prematurity **163, 168**

740*   Anencephalus and similar anomalies **33, 166, 170**

414.1*   Aneurysm and dissection of heart **69**

093.0   Aneurysm of aorta, specified as syphilitic **67**

442.3   Aneurysm of artery of lower extremity **66**

442.0   Aneurysm of artery of upper extremity **66**

414.10   Aneurysm of heart **165, 169**

442.2   Aneurysm of iliac artery **66**

442.8*   Aneurysm of other specified artery **66**

442.1   Aneurysm of renal artery **120**

413.0   Angina decubitus **68**

569.84   Angiodysplasia of intestine (without mention of hemorrhage) **79**

569.85   Angiodysplasia of intestine with hemorrhage **76**

537.82   Angiodysplasia of stomach and duodenum (without mention of hemorrhage) **78**

537.83   Angiodysplasia of stomach and duodenum with hemorrhage **76**

995.1   Angioneurotic edema not elsewhere classified **203**

127.1   Anisakiasis **77**

379.41   Anisocoria **38**

367.3*   Anisometropia and aniseikonia **39**

845.0*   Ankle sprain and strain **100**

720.0   Ankylosing spondylitis **97**

718.5*   Ankylosis of joint **98**

378.85   Anomalies of divergence in binocular eye movement **40**

747.3*   Anomalies of pulmonary artery **68**

426.7   Anomalous atrioventricular excitation **165, 169**

307.1   Anorexia nervosa **188**

348.1   Anoxic brain damage **32, 165, 169**

V28.4   Antenatal screening for fetal growth retardation using ultrasonics **214**

V28.5   Antenatal screening for isoimmunization **214**

641.33   Antepartum hemorrhage associated with coagulation defect, antepartum **154, 156**

641.30   Antepartum hemorrhage associated with coagulation defects, unspecified as to episode of care **156, 159**

641.31   Antepartum hemorrhage associated with coagulation defects, with delivery **134, 140, 145**

335*   Anterior horn cell disease **19**

032.2   Anterior nasal diphtheria **2, 47**

022.3   Anthrax septicemia **186**

286.53   Antiphospholipid antibody with hemorrhagic disorder **176**

301.7   Antisocial personality disorder **188**

300.0*   Anxiety states **188**

441.9   Aortic aneurysm of unspecified site without mention of rupture **66**

441.5   Aortic aneurysm of unspecified site, ruptured **66**

447.7*   Aortic ectasia **66**

379.3*   Aphakia and other disorders of lens **40**

784.3   Aphasia **33**

541   Appendicitis, unqualified **78**

863.95   Appendix injury with open wound into cavity **79**

863.85   Appendix injury without mention of open wound into cavity **79, 227**

078.7   Arenaviral hemorrhagic fever **185**

379.45   Argyll Robertson pupil, atypical **19**

733.91   Arrest of bone development or growth **100**

444*   Arterial embolism and thrombosis **165, 169**

444.0*   Arterial embolism and thrombosis of abdominal aorta **66**

447.0   Arteriovenous fistula, acquired **66**

056.71   Arthritis due to rubella **98**

V45.4   Arthrodesis status **214**

711.7*   Arthropathy associated with helminthiasis **97**

711.6*   Arthropathy associated with mycoses **97**

711.4*   Arthropathy associated with other bacterial diseases **97**

713*   Arthropathy associated with other disorders classified elsewhere **98**

711.8*   Arthropathy associated with other infectious and parasitic diseases **97**

711.5*   Arthropathy associated with other viral diseases **98**

711.1*   Arthropathy associated with Reiter's disease and nonspecific urethritis **97**

711.2*   Arthropathy in Behcet's syndrome **97**

065*   Arthropod-borne hemorrhagic fever **184**

995.21   Arthus phenomenon **166, 171**

718.07   Articular cartilage disorder, ankle and foot **99**

718.03   Articular cartilage disorder, forearm **99**

718.04   Articular cartilage disorder, hand **99**

718.09   Articular cartilage disorder, multiple sites **100**

718.08   Articular cartilage disorder, other specified site **100**

718.05   Articular cartilage disorder, pelvic region and thigh **100**

718.01   Articular cartilage disorder, shoulder region **99**

718.00   Articular cartilage disorder, site unspecified **100**

718.02   Articular cartilage disorder, upper arm **99**

V26.1   Artificial insemination **214**

V44*   Artificial opening status **214**

501   Asbestosis **53**

127.0   Ascariasis **77**

789.5*	Ascites **213**
267	Ascorbic acid deficiency **113, 230**
733.4*	Aseptic necrosis of bone **98**
117.3	Aspergillosis **164, 168**
799.0*	Asphyxia and hypoxemia **54**
994.7	Asphyxiation and strangulation **204**
770.86	Aspiration of postnatal stomach contents with respiratory symptoms **163, 167**
770.85	Aspiration of postnatal stomach contents without respiratory symptoms **163, 167**
493.91	Asthma, unspecified with status asthmaticus **165, 169**
367.2*	Astigmatism **39**
646.53	Asymptomatic bacteriuria antepartum **154, 157**
646.54	Asymptomatic bacteriuria in pregnancy, postpartum condition or complication **151**
646.50	Asymptomatic bacteriuria in pregnancy, unspecified as to episode of care **159**
646.51	Asymptomatic bacteriuria in pregnancy, with delivery **134, 141, 147**
646.52	Asymptomatic bacteriuria in pregnancy, with delivery, with current postpartum complication **134, 141, 147**
V83.01	Asymptomatic hemophilia A carrier **215**
V08	Asymptomatic human immunodeficiency virus (HIV) infection status **185**
094.3	Asymptomatic neurosyphilis **34**
454.9	Asymptomatic varicose veins **67**
445.0*	Atheroembolism of extremities **66**
445.81	Atheroembolism of kidney **120**
445.89	Atheroembolism of other site **66**
440.0	Atherosclerosis of aorta **66**
440.3*	Atherosclerosis of bypass graft of extremities **66**
440.2*	Atherosclerosis of native arteries of the extremities **66**
440.24	Atherosclerosis of native arteries of the extremities with gangrene **165, 169**
440.8	Atherosclerosis of other specified arteries **66**
440.1	Atherosclerosis of renal artery **120**
333.71	Athetoid cerebral palsy **19**
596.4	Atony of bladder **166, 170**
691*	Atopic dermatitis and related conditions **108**
427.3*	Atrial fibrillation and flutter **68, 165, 169**
426.0	Atrioventricular block, complete **165, 169**
535.11	Atrophic gastritis with hemorrhage **76**
535.10	Atrophic gastritis without mention of hemorrhage **78**
608.3	Atrophy of testis **124**
799.51	Attention or concentration deficit **189**
V55.7	Attention to artificial vagina **128, 131**
V55.3	Attention to colostomy **79**
V55.5	Attention to cystostomy **120**
V58.3*	Attention to dressings and sutures **214**
V55.1	Attention to gastrostomy **79**
V55.2	Attention to ileostomy **79**
V55.4	Attention to other artificial opening of digestive tract **79**
V55.6	Attention to other artificial opening of urinary tract **120**
V55.8	Attention to other specified artificial opening **214**
V55.0	Attention to tracheostomy **54**
V55.9	Attention to unspecified artificial opening **214**
299.0*	Autistic disorder **188**
279.4*	Autoimmune disease, not elsewhere classified **97**
283.0	Autoimmune hemolytic anemias **175**
758.3*	Autosomal deletion syndromes **188**

790.7	Bacteremia **166, 170, 186**
041*	Bacterial infection in conditions classified elsewhere and of unspecified site **185**
320*	Bacterial meningitis **9, 10, 33, 164, 169**
758.4	Balanced autosomal translocation in normal individual **213**
607.81	Balanitis xerotica obliterans **124**
607.1	Balanoposthitis **124**
649.23	Bariatric surgery status complicating pregnancy, childbirth, or the puerperium, antepartum condition or complication **154, 157**
649.22	Bariatric surgery status complicating pregnancy, childbirth, or the puerperium, delivered, with mention of postpartum complication **135, 142, 148**
649.21	Bariatric surgery status complicating pregnancy, childbirth, or the puerperium, delivered, with or without mention of antepartum condition **135, 142, 148**
649.24	Bariatric surgery status complicating pregnancy, childbirth, or the puerperium, postpartum condition or complication **152**
649.20	Bariatric surgery status complicating pregnancy, childbirth, or the puerperium, unspecified as to episode of care or not applicable **160**
993.0	Barotrauma, otitic **46**
993.1	Barotrauma, sinus **46**
530.85	Barrett's esophagus **77**
136.1	Behcet's syndrome **97**
209.65	Benign carcinoid tumor of foregut, not otherwise specified **78**
209.67	Benign carcinoid tumor of hindgut, not otherwise specified **78**
209.66	Benign carcinoid tumor of midgut, not otherwise specified **78**
209.69	Benign carcinoid tumor of other sites **180, 181**
209.61	Benign carcinoid tumor of the bronchus and lung **52**
209.64	Benign carcinoid tumor of the kidney **116, 119**
209.63	Benign carcinoid tumor of the stomach **78**
209.62	Benign carcinoid tumor of the thymus **176**
209.60	Benign carcinoid tumor of unknown primary site **180, 181**
209.5*	Benign carcinoid tumors of the appendix, large intestine, and rectum **78**
209.4*	Benign carcinoid tumors of the small intestine **78**
642.03	Benign essential hypertension antepartum **154, 156**
642.00	Benign essential hypertension complicating pregnancy, childbirth, and the puerperium, unspecified as to episode of care **159**
642.01	Benign essential hypertension with delivery **134, 140, 145**
642.04	Benign essential hypertension, complicating pregnancy, childbirth, and the puerperium, postpartum condition or complication **151**
642.02	Benign essential hypertension, with delivery, with current postpartum complication **134, 140, 145**
402.11	Benign hypertensive heart disease with heart failure **56, 66, 165, 169**
402.10	Benign hypertensive heart disease without heart failure **67**
348.2	Benign intracranial hypertension **34**
610*	Benign mammary dysplasias **106**
694.61	Benign mucous membrane pemphigoid with ocular involvement **40**
694.60	Benign mucous membrane pemphigoid without mention of ocular involvement **105**
227.0	Benign neoplasm of adrenal gland **114**
227.6	Benign neoplasm of aortic body and other paraganglia **19**
213.9	Benign neoplasm of bone and articular cartilage, site unspecified **100**
213.0	Benign neoplasm of bones of skull and face **3, 100**
225*	Benign neoplasm of brain and other parts of nervous system **19**
217	Benign neoplasm of breast **108**
212.3	Benign neoplasm of bronchus and lung **52**

*Code Range

227.5	Benign neoplasm of carotid body **19**
211.3	Benign neoplasm of colon **78**
211.2	Benign neoplasm of duodenum, jejunum, and ileum **78**
216.2	Benign neoplasm of ear and external auditory canal **108**
227.9	Benign neoplasm of endocrine gland, site unspecified **114**
211.0	Benign neoplasm of esophagus **78**
224*	Benign neoplasm of eye **38**
216.1	Benign neoplasm of eyelid, including canthus **38**
210.3	Benign neoplasm of floor of mouth **48**
212.7	Benign neoplasm of heart **68**
210.8	Benign neoplasm of hypopharynx **47**
211.7	Benign neoplasm of islets of Langerhans **114**
223*	Benign neoplasm of kidney and other urinary organs **116**, **119**
212.1	Benign neoplasm of larynx **3**, **47**
210.0	Benign neoplasm of lip **48**
210*	Benign neoplasm of lip, oral cavity, and pharynx **3**
211.5	Benign neoplasm of liver and biliary passages **83**
213.7	Benign neoplasm of long bones of lower limb **100**
213.1	Benign neoplasm of lower jaw bone **3**, **48**
229.0	Benign neoplasm of lymph nodes **176**
210.2	Benign neoplasm of major salivary glands **47**
222*	Benign neoplasm of male genital organs **124**
212.5	Benign neoplasm of mediastinum **52**
212.0	Benign neoplasm of nasal cavities, middle ear, and accessory sinuses **3**, **47**
210.7	Benign neoplasm of nasopharynx **47**
210.4	Benign neoplasm of other and unspecified parts of mouth **48**
211.9	Benign neoplasm of other and unspecified site of the digestive system **78**
227.8	Benign neoplasm of other endocrine glands and related structures **114**
221*	Benign neoplasm of other female genital organs **127**, **130**
210.6	Benign neoplasm of other parts of oropharynx **47**
229.8	Benign neoplasm of other specified sites **180**, **182**
212.8	Benign neoplasm of other specified sites of respiratory and intrathoracic organs **52**
216.8	Benign neoplasm of other specified sites of skin **108**
220	Benign neoplasm of ovary **127**, **130**
211.6	Benign neoplasm of pancreas, except islets of Langerhans **83**
227.1	Benign neoplasm of parathyroid gland **114**
213.6	Benign neoplasm of pelvic bones, sacrum, and coccyx **100**
210.9	Benign neoplasm of pharynx, unspecified **47**
227.4	Benign neoplasm of pineal gland **19**
227.3	Benign neoplasm of pituitary gland and craniopharyngeal duct (pouch) **114**
212.4	Benign neoplasm of pleura **52**
211.4	Benign neoplasm of rectum and anal canal **78**
212.9	Benign neoplasm of respiratory and intrathoracic organs, site unspecified **52**
211.8	Benign neoplasm of retroperitoneum and peritoneum **78**
213.3	Benign neoplasm of ribs, sternum, and clavicle **52**
216.4	Benign neoplasm of scalp and skin of neck **108**
213.4	Benign neoplasm of scapula and long bones of upper limb **100**
213.8	Benign neoplasm of short bones of lower limb **100**
213.5	Benign neoplasm of short bones of upper limb **100**
216.0	Benign neoplasm of skin of lip **108**
216.7	Benign neoplasm of skin of lower limb, including hip **108**
216.3	Benign neoplasm of skin of other and unspecified parts of face **108**
216.5	Benign neoplasm of skin of trunk, except scrotum **108**

216.6	Benign neoplasm of skin of upper limb, including shoulder **108**
216.9	Benign neoplasm of skin, site unspecified **108**
211.1	Benign neoplasm of stomach **78**
212.6	Benign neoplasm of thymus **176**
226	Benign neoplasm of thyroid glands **3**, **114**
210.1	Benign neoplasm of tongue **48**
210.5	Benign neoplasm of tonsil **47**
212.2	Benign neoplasm of trachea **52**
229.9	Benign neoplasm of unspecified site **180**, **182**
213.2	Benign neoplasm of vertebral column, excluding sacrum and coccyx **87**, **100**
333.93	Benign shuddering attacks **32**
V62.82	Bereavement, uncomplicated **214**
282.44	Beta thalassemia **164**, **169**
552.02	Bilateral femoral hernia with obstruction **166**, **170**
868.02	Bile duct and gallbladder injury without mention of open wound into cavity **83**, **227**
868.12	Bile duct and gallbladder injury, with open wound into cavity **83**, **227**
571.6	Biliary cirrhosis **82**
779.32	Bilious vomiting in newborn **163**, **168**
791.4	Biliuria **83**
767.11	Birth trauma, epicranial subaponeurotic hemorrhage (massive) **163**, **167**
767.19	Birth trauma, other injuries to scalp **171**, **172**
921.0	Black eye, not otherwise specified **40**
867.1	Bladder and urethra injury with open wound into cavity **120**
867.0	Bladder and urethra injury without mention of open wound into cavity **120**
596.0	Bladder neck obstruction **166**, **170**
V43.5	Bladder replaced by other means **120**
116.0	Blastomycosis **164**, **168**
116*	Blastomycotic infection **185**
374.34	Blepharochalasis **39**
374.46	Blepharophimosis **39**
333.81	Blepharospasm **39**
369*	Blindness and low vision **39**, **230**
945.2*	Blisters with epidermal loss due to burn (second degree) of lower limb(s) **210**
946.2	Blisters with epidermal loss due to burn (second degree) of multiple specified sites **210**
942.2*	Blisters with epidermal loss due to burn (second degree) of trunk **209**
943.2*	Blisters with epidermal loss due to burn (second degree) of upper limb, except wrist and hand **210**
944.2*	Blisters with epidermal loss due to burn (second degree) of wrist(s) and hand(s) **210**
949.2	Blisters with epidermal loss due to burn (second degree), unspecified site **210**
941.24	Blisters, with epidermal loss due to burn (second degree) of chin **209**
941.21	Blisters, with epidermal loss due to burn (second degree) of ear (any part) **209**
941.22	Blisters, with epidermal loss due to burn (second degree) of eye (with other parts of face, head, and neck) **40**
941.20	Blisters, with epidermal loss due to burn (second degree) of face and head, unspecified site **209**
941.27	Blisters, with epidermal loss due to burn (second degree) of forehead and cheek **209**
941.23	Blisters, with epidermal loss due to burn (second degree) of lip(s) **209**
941.29	Blisters, with epidermal loss due to burn (second degree) of multiple sites (except with eye) of face, head, and neck **209**

*Code Range

941.28	Blisters, with epidermal loss due to burn (second degree) of neck **209**
941.25	Blisters, with epidermal loss due to burn (second degree) of nose (septum) **209**
941.26	Blisters, with epidermal loss due to burn (second degree) of scalp (any part) **209**
V59.0*	Blood donor **214**
V58.2	Blood transfusion, without reported diagnosis **214**
V43.4	Blood vessel replaced by other means **69**
999.32	Bloodstream infection due to central venous catheter **69**
V85.4*	Body Mass Index 40 and over, adult **113**
V85.1	Body Mass Index between 19-24, adult **215**
V85.2*	Body Mass Index between 25-29, adult **215**
V85.3*	Body Mass Index between 30-39, adult **215**
V85.0	Body Mass Index less than 19, adult **215**
V85.5*	Body Mass Index, pediatric **215**
648.74	Bone and joint disorders of maternal back, pelvis, and lower limbs complicating pregnancy, childbirth, or the puerperium, postpartum condition or complication **152**
648.73	Bone and joint disorders of maternal back, pelvis, and lower limbs, antepartum **154**, **156**
648.70	Bone and joint disorders of maternal back, pelvis, and lower limbs, complicating pregnancy, childbirth, or the puerperium, unspecified as to episode of care **159**
648.71	Bone and joint disorders of maternal back, pelvis, and lower limbs, with delivery **134**, **142**, **147**
648.72	Bone and joint disorders of maternal back, pelvis, and lower limbs, with delivery, with current postpartum complication **134**, **142**, **147**
102.6	Bone and joint lesions due to yaws **97**
V59.2	Bone donor **101**
V59.3	Bone marrow donor **214**
V42.81	Bone marrow replaced by transplant **176**
V42.4	Bone replaced by transplant **101**
365.0*	Borderline glaucoma (glaucoma suspect) **39**
005.1	Botulism food poisoning **185**
723.4	Brachial neuritis or radiculitis NOS **21**
348.82	Brain death **21**
669.61	Breech extraction, without mention of indication, delivered, with or without mention of antepartum condition **138**, **145**, **150**
669.60	Breech extraction, without mention of indication, unspecified as to episode of care **138**, **145**, **150**
652.13	Breech or other malpresentation successfully converted to cephalic presentation, antepartum **154**, **157**
652.11	Breech or other malpresentation successfully converted to cephalic presentation, delivered **135**, **142**, **148**
652.10	Breech or other malpresentation successfully converted to cephalic presentation, unspecified as to episode of care **160**
652.23	Breech presentation without mention of version, antepartum **154**, **157**
652.21	Breech presentation without mention of version, delivered **135**, **142**, **148**
652.20	Breech presentation without mention of version, unspecified as to episode of care **160**
494*	Bronchiectasis **53**
506.0	Bronchitis and pneumonitis due to fumes and vapors **54**
490	Bronchitis, not specified as acute or chronic **53**
485	Bronchopneumonia, organism unspecified **53**, **165**, **169**
862.31	Bronchus injury with open wound into cavity **52**
862.21	Bronchus injury without mention of open wound into cavity **52**
023*	Brucellosis **185**
020.0	Bubonic plague **185**
453.0	Budd-Chiari syndrome **83**

745.0	Bulbus cordis anomalies and anomalies of cardiac septal closure, common truncus **67**
745.3	Bulbus cordis anomalies and anomalies of cardiac septal closure, common ventricle **67**
307.51	Bulimia nervosa **189**
727.1	Bunion **100**
200.2*	Burkitt's tumor or lymphoma **230**
200.21	Burkitt's tumor or lymphoma of lymph nodes of head, face, and neck **2**
948.11	Burn (any degree) involving 10-19% of body surface with third degree burn of 10-19% **206**, **207**, **208**, **209**
948.10	Burn (any degree) involving 10-19% of body surface with third degree burn of less than 10% or unspecified amount **210**
948.21	Burn (any degree) involving 20-29% of body surface with third degree burn of 10-19% **206**, **208**
948.22	Burn (any degree) involving 20-29% of body surface with third degree burn of 20-29% **206**, **208**
948.20	Burn (any degree) involving 20-29% of body surface with third degree burn of less than 10% or unspecified amount **210**
948.31	Burn (any degree) involving 30-39% of body surface with third degree burn of 10-19% **206**, **208**
948.32	Burn (any degree) involving 30-39% of body surface with third degree burn of 20-29% **206**, **208**
948.33	Burn (any degree) involving 30-39% of body surface with third degree burn of 30-39% **206**, **208**
948.30	Burn (any degree) involving 30-39% of body surface with third degree burn of less than 10% or unspecified amount **210**
948.41	Burn (any degree) involving 40-49% of body surface with third degree burn of 10-19% **206**, **208**
948.42	Burn (any degree) involving 40-49% of body surface with third degree burn of 20-29% **206**, **208**
948.43	Burn (any degree) involving 40-49% of body surface with third degree burn of 30-39% **206**, **208**
948.44	Burn (any degree) involving 40-49% of body surface with third degree burn of 40-49% **206**, **208**
948.40	Burn (any degree) involving 40-49% of body surface with third degree burn of less than 10% or unspecified amount **210**
948.51	Burn (any degree) involving 50-59% of body surface with third degree burn of 10-19% **206**, **208**
948.52	Burn (any degree) involving 50-59% of body surface with third degree burn of 20-29% **206**, **208**
948.53	Burn (any degree) involving 50-59% of body surface with third degree burn of 30-39% **206**, **208**
948.54	Burn (any degree) involving 50-59% of body surface with third degree burn of 40-49% **206**, **208**
948.55	Burn (any degree) involving 50-59% of body surface with third degree burn of 50-59% **206**, **208**
948.50	Burn (any degree) involving 50-59% of body surface with third degree burn of less than 10% or unspecified amount **210**
948.61	Burn (any degree) involving 60-69% of body surface with third degree burn of 10-19% **206**, **208**
948.62	Burn (any degree) involving 60-69% of body surface with third degree burn of 20-29% **206**, **208**
948.63	Burn (any degree) involving 60-69% of body surface with third degree burn of 30-39% **206**, **208**
948.64	Burn (any degree) involving 60-69% of body surface with third degree burn of 40-49% **206**, **208**
948.65	Burn (any degree) involving 60-69% of body surface with third degree burn of 50-59% **206**, **208**
948.66	Burn (any degree) involving 60-69% of body surface with third degree burn of 60-69% **206**, **208**
948.60	Burn (any degree) involving 60-69% of body surface with third degree burn of less than 10% or unspecified amount **210**
948.71	Burn (any degree) involving 70-79% of body surface with third degree burn of 10-19% **206**, **208**

948.72	Burn (any degree) involving 70-79% of body surface with third degree burn of 20-29% **206, 208**
948.73	Burn (any degree) involving 70-79% of body surface with third degree burn of 30-39% **206, 208**
948.74	Burn (any degree) involving 70-79% of body surface with third degree burn of 40-49% **206, 208**
948.75	Burn (any degree) involving 70-79% of body surface with third degree burn of 50-59% **206, 208**
948.76	Burn (any degree) involving 70-79% of body surface with third degree burn of 60-69% **206, 208**
948.77	Burn (any degree) involving 70-79% of body surface with third degree burn of 70-79% **206, 208**
948.70	Burn (any degree) involving 70-79% of body surface with third degree burn of less than 10% or unspecified amount **210**
948.81	Burn (any degree) involving 80-89% of body surface with third degree burn of 10-19% **206, 208**
948.82	Burn (any degree) involving 80-89% of body surface with third degree burn of 20-29% **207, 208**
948.83	Burn (any degree) involving 80-89% of body surface with third degree burn of 30-39% **207, 208**
948.84	Burn (any degree) involving 80-89% of body surface with third degree burn of 40-49% **207, 209**
948.85	Burn (any degree) involving 80-89% of body surface with third degree burn of 50-59% **207, 209**
948.86	Burn (any degree) involving 80-89% of body surface with third degree burn of 60-69% **207, 209**
948.87	Burn (any degree) involving 80-89% of body surface with third degree burn of 70-79% **207, 209**
948.88	Burn (any degree) involving 80-89% of body surface with third degree burn of 80-89% **207, 209**
948.80	Burn (any degree) involving 80-89% of body surface with third degree burn of less than 10% or unspecified amount **210**
948.91	Burn (any degree) involving 90% or more of body surface with third degree burn of 10-19% **207, 209**
948.92	Burn (any degree) involving 90% or more of body surface with third degree burn of 20-29% **207, 209**
948.93	Burn (any degree) involving 90% or more of body surface with third degree burn of 30-39% **207, 209**
948.94	Burn (any degree) involving 90% or more of body surface with third degree burn of 40-49% **207, 209**
948.95	Burn (any degree) involving 90% or more of body surface with third degree burn of 50-59% **207, 209**
948.96	Burn (any degree) involving 90% or more of body surface with third degree burn of 60-69% **207, 209**
948.97	Burn (any degree) involving 90% or more of body surface with third degree burn of 70-79% **207, 209**
948.98	Burn (any degree) involving 90% or more of body surface with third degree burn of 80-89% **207, 209**
948.99	Burn (any degree) involving 90% or more of body surface with third degree burn of 90% or more of body surface **207, 209**
948.90	Burn (any degree) involving 90% or more of body surface with third degree burn of less than 10% or unspecified amount **210**
948.00	Burn (any degree) involving less than 10% of body surface with third degree burn of less than 10% or unspecified amount **210**
940*	Burn confined to eye and adnexa **40**
947.2	Burn of esophagus **75**
947.3	Burn of gastrointestinal tract **79**
947.9	Burn of internal organs, unspecified site **210**
947.1	Burn of larynx, trachea, and lung **54, 207**
945.0*	Burn of lower limb(s), unspecified degree **210**
947.0	Burn of mouth and pharynx **4, 48**
947.8	Burn of other specified sites of internal organs **210**
942.0*	Burn of trunk, unspecified degree **209**
941.04	Burn of unspecified degree of chin **209**
941.01	Burn of unspecified degree of ear (any part) **209**
941.02	Burn of unspecified degree of eye (with other parts of face, head, and neck) **40**
941.07	Burn of unspecified degree of forehead and cheek **209**
941.03	Burn of unspecified degree of lip(s) **209**
941.09	Burn of unspecified degree of multiple sites (except with eye) of face, head, and neck **209**
941.08	Burn of unspecified degree of neck **209**
941.05	Burn of unspecified degree of nose (septum) **209**
941.06	Burn of unspecified degree of scalp (any part) **209**
941.00	Burn of unspecified degree of unspecified site of face and head **209**
949.0	Burn of unspecified site, unspecified degree **210**
943.0*	Burn of upper limb, except wrist and hand, unspecified degree **209**
947.4	Burn of vagina and uterus **128, 131**
944.0*	Burn of wrist(s) and hand(s), unspecified degree **210**
946.0	Burns of multiple specified sites, unspecified degree **210**
799.4	Cachexia **213, 231**
993.3	Caisson disease **204**
726.73	Calcaneal spur **100**
594.0	Calculus in diverticulum of bladder **120**
594.2	Calculus in urethra **119**
592*	Calculus of kidney and ureter **119**
112.81	Candidal endocarditis **65, 164, 168**
112.83	Candidal meningitis **9, 10, 34, 164, 168**
112.82	Candidal otitis externa **47, 164, 168**
112.4	Candidiasis of lung **51, 164, 168, 230**
112.0	Candidiasis of mouth **2, 48, 230**
112.8*	Candidiasis of other specified sites **230**
112.2	Candidiasis of other urogenital sites **124, 127, 130**
112.3	Candidiasis of skin and nails **107, 230**
112.84	Candidiasis of the esophagus **75, 164, 168**
112.85	Candidiasis of the intestine **77, 164, 168**
112.9	Candidiasis of unspecified site **185, 230**
112.1	Candidiasis of vulva and vagina **127, 130**
127.5	Capillariasis **78**
680*	Carbuncle and furuncle **106**
230.5	Carcinoma in situ of anal canal **76**
230.6	Carcinoma in situ of anus, unspecified **76**
233.7	Carcinoma in situ of bladder **116, 119**
233.0	Carcinoma in situ of breast **104, 105**
231.2	Carcinoma in situ of bronchus and lung **52**
233.1	Carcinoma in situ of cervix uteri **126, 129**
230.3	Carcinoma in situ of colon **76**
230.1	Carcinoma in situ of esophagus **76**
234.0	Carcinoma in situ of eye **38**
232.1	Carcinoma in situ of eyelid, including canthus **38**
231.0	Carcinoma in situ of larynx **3, 46**
230.0	Carcinoma in situ of lip, oral cavity, and pharynx **3, 46**
230.8	Carcinoma in situ of liver and biliary system **83**
230.9	Carcinoma in situ of other and unspecified digestive organs **76**
233.6	Carcinoma in situ of other and unspecified male genital organs **122, 123**
230.7	Carcinoma in situ of other and unspecified parts of intestine **76**
233.2	Carcinoma in situ of other and unspecified parts of uterus **126, 129**
233.9	Carcinoma in situ of other and unspecified urinary organs **116, 119**
231.8	Carcinoma in situ of other specified parts of respiratory system **52**
234.8	Carcinoma in situ of other specified sites **180, 182**

232.8	Carcinoma in situ of other specified sites of skin **108**
233.5	Carcinoma in situ of penis **122, 123**
233.4	Carcinoma in situ of prostate **122, 123**
230.4	Carcinoma in situ of rectum **76**
231.9	Carcinoma in situ of respiratory system, part unspecified **52**
232.4	Carcinoma in situ of scalp and skin of neck **108**
232.2	Carcinoma in situ of skin of ear and external auditory canal **108**
232.0	Carcinoma in situ of skin of lip **108**
232.7	Carcinoma in situ of skin of lower limb, including hip **108**
232.3	Carcinoma in situ of skin of other and unspecified parts of face **108**
232.5	Carcinoma in situ of skin of trunk, except scrotum **108**
232.6	Carcinoma in situ of skin of upper limb, including shoulder **108**
232.9	Carcinoma in situ of skin, site unspecified **108**
230.2	Carcinoma in situ of stomach **76**
231.1	Carcinoma in situ of trachea **52**
233.3*	Carcinoma in situ, other and unspecified female genital organs **126, 129**
234.9	Carcinoma in situ, site unspecified **180, 182**
427.5	Cardiac arrest **66, 165, 169**
779.85	Cardiac arrest of newborn **163, 168**
997.1	Cardiac complications **69, 167, 171**
668.13	Cardiac complications of the administration of anesthesia or other sedation in labor and delivery, antepartum **155, 158**
668.11	Cardiac complications of the administration of anesthesia or other sedation in labor and delivery, delivered **137, 140, 146**
668.12	Cardiac complications of the administration of anesthesia or other sedation in labor and delivery, delivered, with mention of postpartum complication **137, 140, 146**
668.14	Cardiac complications of the administration of anesthesia or other sedation in labor and delivery, postpartum condition or complication **152**
668.10	Cardiac complications of the administration of anesthesia or other sedation in labor and delivery, unspecified as to episode of care **137, 144, 150**
785.51	Cardiogenic shock **57, 66**
429.3	Cardiomegaly **67**
425*	Cardiomyopathy **69**
425.8	Cardiomyopathy in other diseases classified elsewhere **165, 169**
306.2	Cardiovascular malfunction arising from mental factors **68**
V57.0	Care involving breathing exercises **214**
V57.3	Care involving use of rehabilitation speech-language therapy **213**
277.82	Carnitine deficiency due to inborn errors of metabolism **114**
V02.2	Carrier or suspected carrier of amebiasis **213**
V02.0	Carrier or suspected carrier of cholera **213**
V02.4	Carrier or suspected carrier of diphtheria **213**
V02.7	Carrier or suspected carrier of gonorrhea **213**
V02.3	Carrier or suspected carrier of other gastrointestinal pathogens **213**
V02.5*	Carrier or suspected carrier of other specified bacterial diseases **213**
V02.9	Carrier or suspected carrier of other specified infectious organism **213**
V02.8	Carrier or suspected carrier of other venereal diseases **213**
V02.1	Carrier or suspected carrier of typhoid **213**
V02.6*	Carrier or suspected carrier of viral hepatitis **83**
078.3	Cat-scratch disease **176**
347*	Cataplexy and narcolepsy **32**
366*	Cataract **39**
V45.61	Cataract extraction status **214**
998.82	Cataract fragments in eye following surgery **40**
344.61	Cauda equina syndrome with neurogenic bladder **120**

344.60	Cauda equina syndrome without mention of neurogenic bladder **21**
738.7	Cauliflower ear **47**
736.75	Cavovarus deformity of foot, acquired **100**
736.73	Cavus deformity of foot, acquired **100**
447.4	Celiac artery compression syndrome **78**
682.0	Cellulitis and abscess of face **3**
681*	Cellulitis and abscess of finger and toe **103, 106**
682.1	Cellulitis and abscess of neck **3**
478.71	Cellulitis and perichondritis of larynx **46**
478.21	Cellulitis of pharynx or nasopharynx **46**
020.1	Cellulocutaneous plague **185**
370.03	Central corneal ulcer **38**
668.23	Central nervous system complications of the administration of anesthesia or other sedation in labor and delivery, antepartum **155, 158**
668.21	Central nervous system complications of the administration of anesthesia or other sedation in labor and delivery, delivered **137, 141, 146**
668.22	Central nervous system complications of the administration of anesthesia or other sedation in labor and delivery, delivered, with mention of postpartum complication **137, 141, 146**
668.24	Central nervous system complications of the administration of anesthesia or other sedation in labor and delivery, postpartum condition or complication **152**
668.20	Central nervous system complications of the administration of anesthesia or other sedation in labor and delivery, unspecified as to episode of care **137, 144, 150**
655.03	Central nervous system malformation in fetus, antepartum **155, 157**
655.00	Central nervous system malformation in fetus, unspecified as to episode of care in pregnancy **160**
655.01	Central nervous system malformation in fetus, with delivery **135, 143, 148**
338.0	Central pain syndrome **32**
327.27	Central sleep apnea in conditions classified elsewhere **32**
851.5*	Cerebellar or brain stem contusion with open intracranial wound **9, 11, 222, 226**
851.52	Cerebellar or brain stem contusion with open intracranial wound, brief (less than 1 hour) loss of consciousness **30**
851.56	Cerebellar or brain stem contusion with open intracranial wound, loss of consciousness of unspecified duration **26**
851.53	Cerebellar or brain stem contusion with open intracranial wound, moderate (1-24 hours) loss of consciousness **26**
851.51	Cerebellar or brain stem contusion with open intracranial wound, no loss of consciousness **30**
851.54	Cerebellar or brain stem contusion with open intracranial wound, prolonged (more than 24 hours) loss of consciousness and return to pre-existing conscious level **26**
851.55	Cerebellar or brain stem contusion with open intracranial wound, prolonged (more than 24 hours) loss of consciousness, without return to pre-existing conscious level **26**
851.59	Cerebellar or brain stem contusion with open intracranial wound, unspecified concussion **30**
851.50	Cerebellar or brain stem contusion with open intracranial wound, unspecified state of consciousness **30**
851.4*	Cerebellar or brain stem contusion without mention of open intracranial wound **222, 226**
851.42	Cerebellar or brain stem contusion without mention of open intracranial wound, brief (less than 1 hour) loss of consciousness **30**
851.46	Cerebellar or brain stem contusion without mention of open intracranial wound, loss of consciousness of unspecified duration **26**

851.43 Cerebellar or brain stem contusion without mention of open intracranial wound, moderate (1-24 hours) loss of consciousness **26**

851.41 Cerebellar or brain stem contusion without mention of open intracranial wound, no loss of consciousness **30**

851.44 Cerebellar or brain stem contusion without mention of open intracranial wound, prolonged (more than 24 hours) loss consciousness and return to pre-existing conscious level **26**

851.45 Cerebellar or brain stem contusion without mention of open intracranial wound, prolonged (more than 24 hours) loss of consciousness, without return to pre-existing conscious level **26**

851.49 Cerebellar or brain stem contusion without mention of open intracranial wound, unspecified concussion **30**

851.40 Cerebellar or brain stem contusion without mention of open intracranial wound, unspecified state of consciousness **30**

851.7* Cerebellar or brain stem laceration with open intracranial wound **9, 11, 222, 226**

851.72 Cerebellar or brain stem laceration with open intracranial wound, brief (less than one hour) loss of consciousness **31**

851.76 Cerebellar or brain stem laceration with open intracranial wound, loss of consciousness of unspecified duration **26**

851.73 Cerebellar or brain stem laceration with open intracranial wound, moderate (1-24 hours) loss of consciousness **26**

851.71 Cerebellar or brain stem laceration with open intracranial wound, no loss of consciousness **31**

851.74 Cerebellar or brain stem laceration with open intracranial wound, prolonged (more than 24 hours) loss of consciousness and return to pre-existing conscious level **26**

851.75 Cerebellar or brain stem laceration with open intracranial wound, prolonged (more than 24 hours) loss of consciousness, without return to pre-existing conscious level **26**

851.70 Cerebellar or brain stem laceration with open intracranial wound, state of consciousness unspecified **31**

851.79 Cerebellar or brain stem laceration with open intracranial wound, unspecified concussion **31**

851.6* Cerebellar or brain stem laceration without mention of open intracranial wound **9, 11, 222, 226**

851.62 Cerebellar or brain stem laceration without mention of open intracranial wound, brief (less than 1 hour) loss of consciousness **31**

851.66 Cerebellar or brain stem laceration without mention of open intracranial wound, loss of consciousness of unspecified duration **26**

851.63 Cerebellar or brain stem laceration without mention of open intracranial wound, moderate (1-24 hours) loss of consciousness **26**

851.61 Cerebellar or brain stem laceration without mention of open intracranial wound, no loss of consciousness **30**

851.64 Cerebellar or brain stem laceration without mention of open intracranial wound, prolonged (more than 24 hours) loss of consciousness and return to pre-existing conscious level **26**

851.65 Cerebellar or brain stem laceration without mention of open intracranial wound, prolonged (more than 24 hours) loss of consciousness, without return to pre-existing conscious level **26**

851.69 Cerebellar or brain stem laceration without mention of open intracranial wound, unspecified concussion **31**

851.60 Cerebellar or brain stem laceration without mention of open intracranial wound, unspecified state of consciousness **30**

437.3 Cerebral aneurysm, nonruptured **33**

437.4 Cerebral arteritis **34**

437.0 Cerebral atherosclerosis **20**

348.0 Cerebral cysts **32**

331.7 Cerebral degeneration in diseases classified elsewhere **19**

330* Cerebral degenerations usually manifest in childhood **19**

779.2 Cerebral depression, coma, and other abnormal cerebral signs in fetus or newborn **163, 168**

348.5 Cerebral edema **21**

434.11 Cerebral embolism with cerebral infarction **9, 10, 20**

434.10 Cerebral embolism without mention of cerebral infarction **20**

434.01 Cerebral thrombosis with cerebral infarction **9, 10, 20**

434.00 Cerebral thrombosis without mention of cerebral infarction **20**

388.61 Cerebrospinal fluid otorrhea **33**

349.81 Cerebrospinal fluid rhinorrhea **32, 165, 169**

674.00 Cerebrovascular disorder occurring in pregnancy, childbirth, or the puerperium, unspecified as to episode of care **161**

674.03 Cerebrovascular disorder, antepartum **156, 158**

674.02 Cerebrovascular disorder, with delivery, with mention of postpartum complication **138, 141, 147**

674.01 Cerebrovascular disorder, with delivery, with or without mention of antepartum condition **138, 141, 147**

674.04 Cerebrovascular disorders in the puerperium, postpartum condition or complication **153**

364.2* Certain types of iridocyclitis **39**

370.3* Certain types of keratoconjunctivitis **39**

654.53 Cervical incompetence, antepartum condition or complication **154, 157**

654.51 Cervical incompetence, delivered **135, 142, 148**

654.52 Cervical incompetence, delivered, with mention of postpartum complication **135, 142, 148**

654.54 Cervical incompetence, postpartum condition or complication **152**

654.50 Cervical incompetence, unspecified as to episode of care in pregnancy **160**

756.2 Cervical rib **100**

649.73 Cervical shortening, antepartum condition or complication **154, 157**

649.71 Cervical shortening, delivered, with or without mention of antepartum condition **135, 142, 148**

649.70 Cervical shortening, unspecified as to episode of care or not applicable **160**

723.1 Cervicalgia **97**

616.0 Cervicitis and endocervicitis **127, 130**

723.3 Cervicobrachial syndrome (diffuse) **21**

723.2 Cervicocranial syndrome **21**

039.3 Cervicofacial actinomycotic infection **107**

669.71 Cesarean delivery, without mention of indication, delivered, with or without mention of antepartum condition **138, 145, 151**

669.70 Cesarean delivery, without mention of indication, unspecified as to episode of care **138, 145, 150**

086.0 Chagas' disease with heart involvement **68**

086.1 Chagas' disease with other organ involvement **185**

086.2 Chagas' disease without mention of organ involvement **185**

099.0 Chancroid **124, 127, 130**

782.8 Changes in skin texture **108**

V67.2 Chemotherapy follow-up examination **180, 181, 182**

786.59 Chest pain, other **68**

786.50 Chest pain, unspecified **68**

052.7 Chickenpox with other specified complications **164, 168, 184**

052.8 Chickenpox with unspecified complication **164, 168, 184**

995.5* Child maltreatment syndrome **204**

299.1* Childhood disintegrative disorder **188**

315.35 Childhood onset fluency disorder **32**

780.64 Chills (without fever) **213**

099.52 Chlamydia trachomatis infection of anus and rectum **78**

099.53 Chlamydia trachomatis infection of lower genitourinary sites **124, 127, 130**

099.54 Chlamydia trachomatis infection of other genitourinary sites **119**

*Code Range

© 2013 OptumInsight, Inc.

099.59	Chlamydia trachomatis infection of other specified site **124, 127, 130**	
099.56	Chlamydia trachomatis infection of peritoneum **78**	
099.51	Chlamydia trachomatis infection of pharynx **2, 46**	
099.55	Chlamydia trachomatis infection of unspecified genitourinary site **124, 127, 130**	
099.50	Chlamydia trachomatis infection of unspecified site **124, 127, 130**	
576.1	Cholangitis **166, 170**	
574*	Cholelithiasis **83**	
567.81	Choleperitonitis **79**	
001*	Cholera **75**	
380.03	Chondritis of pinna **100**	
756.4	Chondrodystrophy **100**	
733.92	Chondromalacia **98**	
717.7	Chondromalacia of patella **99**	
363*	Chorioretinal inflammations, scars, and other disorders of choroid **39**	
130.2	Chorioretinitis due to toxoplasmosis **38, 164, 168**	
655.13	Chromosomal abnormality in fetus, affecting management of mother, antepartum **155, 157**	
655.10	Chromosomal abnormality in fetus, affecting management of mother, unspecified as to episode of care in pregnancy **160**	
655.11	Chromosomal abnormality in fetus, affecting management of mother, with delivery **135, 143, 148**	
474.01	Chronic adenoiditis **46**	
496	Chronic airway obstruction, not elsewhere classified **53**	
508.1	Chronic and other pulmonary manifestations due to radiation **53**	
375.02	Chronic dacryoadenitis **39**	
301.12	Chronic depressive personality disorder **188**	
474*	Chronic disease of tonsils and adenoids **3**	
537.2	Chronic duodenal ileus **78**	
532.71	Chronic duodenal ulcer without mention of hemorrhage or perforation, with obstruction **77**	
532.70	Chronic duodenal ulcer without mention of hemorrhage, perforation, or obstruction **77**	
360.03	Chronic endophthalmitis **39**	
375.03	Chronic enlargement of lacrimal gland **39**	
207.1*	Chronic erythremia **181**	
780.71	Chronic fatigue syndrome **213**	
531.71	Chronic gastric ulcer without mention of hemorrhage or perforation, with obstruction **77**	
531.70	Chronic gastric ulcer without mention of hemorrhage, perforation, without mention of obstruction **77**	
534.7*	Chronic gastrojejunal ulcer without mention of hemorrhage or perforation **77**	
582*	Chronic glomerulonephritis **120, 230**	
098.30	Chronic gonococcal infection of upper genitourinary tract, site unspecified **119**	
571.4*	Chronic hepatitis **83**	
301.11	Chronic hypomanic personality disorder **188**	
458.1	Chronic hypotension **69**	
375.4*	Chronic inflammation of lacrimal passages **39**	
376.1*	Chronic inflammatory disorders of orbit **39**	
595.1	Chronic interstitial cystitis **119**	
006.1	Chronic intestinal amebiasis without mention of abscess **75**	
364.1*	Chronic iridocyclitis **39**	
585*	Chronic kidney disease (CKD) **2, 118**	
476.0	Chronic laryngitis **3**	
476*	Chronic laryngitis and laryngotracheitis **46**	
476.1	Chronic laryngotracheitis **3**	
208.1*	Chronic leukemia of unspecified cell type **181**	

289.1	Chronic lymphadenitis **176**
204.1*	Chronic lymphoid leukemia **181**
383.1	Chronic mastoiditis **46**
206.1*	Chronic monocytic leukemia **181**
381.2*	Chronic mucoid otitis media **46**
205.1*	Chronic myeloid leukemia **181**
384.1	Chronic myringitis without mention of otitis media **46**
472.2	Chronic nasopharyngitis **3**
493.21	Chronic obstructive asthma with status asthmaticus **53**
493.20	Chronic obstructive asthma, unspecified **53**
493.22	Chronic obstructive asthma, with (acute) exacerbation **53**
532.4*	Chronic or unspecified duodenal ulcer with hemorrhage **76**
532.6*	Chronic or unspecified duodenal ulcer with hemorrhage and perforation **76**
532.5*	Chronic or unspecified duodenal ulcer with perforation **77**
531.4*	Chronic or unspecified gastric ulcer with hemorrhage **76**
531.6*	Chronic or unspecified gastric ulcer with hemorrhage and perforation **76**
531.5*	Chronic or unspecified gastric ulcer with perforation **77**
534.4*	Chronic or unspecified gastrojejunal ulcer with hemorrhage **76**
534.6*	Chronic or unspecified gastrojejunal ulcer with hemorrhage and perforation **76**
534.5*	Chronic or unspecified gastrojejunal ulcer with perforation **77**
614.4	Chronic or unspecified parametritis and pelvic cellulitis **130**
533.4*	Chronic or unspecified peptic ulcer, unspecified site, with hemorrhage **76**
533.6*	Chronic or unspecified peptic ulcer, unspecified site, with hemorrhage and perforation **76**
533.5*	Chronic or unspecified peptic ulcer, unspecified site, with perforation **77**
730.1*	Chronic osteomyelitis **96**
730.16	Chronic osteomyelitis, lower leg **90**
730.18	Chronic osteomyelitis, other specified sites **87**
338.2*	Chronic pain **32**
338.4	Chronic pain syndrome **32**
573.0	Chronic passive congestion of liver **83**
533.71	Chronic peptic ulcer of unspecified site without mention of hemorrhage or perforation, with obstruction **77**
533.70	Chronic peptic ulcer, unspecified site, without mention of hemorrhage, perforation, or obstruction **77**
380.02	Chronic perichondritis of pinna **100**
472.1	Chronic pharyngitis **3**
472*	Chronic pharyngitis and nasopharyngitis **46**
714.4	Chronic postrheumatic arthropathy **98**
114.4	Chronic pulmonary coccidioidomycosis **51**
416.2	Chronic pulmonary embolism **51, 165, 169**
506.4	Chronic respiratory conditions due to fumes and vapors **53**
770.7	Chronic respiratory disease arising in the perinatal period **53**
518.83	Chronic respiratory failure **52**
393	Chronic rheumatic pericarditis **68**
614.1	Chronic salpingitis and oophoritis **130**
381.1*	Chronic serous otitis media **46**
473*	Chronic sinusitis **46**
474.00	Chronic tonsillitis **46**
474.02	Chronic tonsillitis and adenoiditis **46**
440.4	Chronic total occlusion of artery of the extremities **66**
414.2	Chronic total occlusion of coronary artery **67**
707*	Chronic ulcer of skin **103, 105**
453.5*	Chronic venous embolism and thrombosis of deep vessels of lower extremity **67**

453.7*	Chronic venous embolism and thrombosis of other specified vessels **67**	
459.3*	Chronic venous hypertension **67**	
791.1	Chyluria **119**, **166**, **170**	
327.3*	Circadian rhythm sleep disorder **3**, **32**	
571.5	Cirrhosis of liver without mention of alcohol **82**	
736.74	Claw foot, acquired **21**	
736.06	Claw hand (acquired) **21**	
749.1*	Cleft lip **3**	
749.0*	Cleft palate **3**	
749*	Cleft palate and cleft lip **48**	
749.2*	Cleft palate with cleft lip **3**	
121.1	Clonorchiasis **83**	
824.4	Closed bimalleolar fracture **222**	
837.0	Closed dislocation of ankle **222**	
832.0*	Closed dislocation of elbow **222**	
834.0*	Closed dislocation of finger **222**	
838.0*	Closed dislocation of foot **222**	
835.0*	Closed dislocation of hip **222**	
830.0	Closed dislocation of jaw **222**	
836.3	Closed dislocation of patella **222**	
831.0*	Closed dislocation of shoulder, unspecified **222**	
833.0*	Closed dislocation of wrist **222**	
839.0*	Closed dislocation, cervical vertebra **98**, **222**, **227**	
839.8	Closed dislocation, multiple and ill-defined sites **100**, **222**	
839.69	Closed dislocation, other location **100**	
839.6*	Closed dislocation, other location **222**	
839.4*	Closed dislocation, other vertebra **98**, **222**	
839.61	Closed dislocation, sternum **52**	
839.2*	Closed dislocation, thoracic and lumbar vertebra **98**, **222**	
808.0	Closed fracture of acetabulum **221**	
811.01	Closed fracture of acromial process of scapula **99**	
801.1*	Closed fracture of base of skull with cerebral laceration and contusion **220**, **225**	
801.12	Closed fracture of base of skull with cerebral laceration and contusion, brief (less than one hour) loss of consciousness **28**	
801.16	Closed fracture of base of skull with cerebral laceration and contusion, loss of consciousness of unspecified duration **23**	
801.13	Closed fracture of base of skull with cerebral laceration and contusion, moderate (1-24 hours) loss of consciousness **23**	
801.11	Closed fracture of base of skull with cerebral laceration and contusion, no loss of consciousness **28**	
801.14	Closed fracture of base of skull with cerebral laceration and contusion, prolonged (more than 24 hours) loss of consciousness and return to pre-existing conscious level **23**	
801.15	Closed fracture of base of skull with cerebral laceration and contusion, prolonged (more than 24 hours) loss of consciousness, without return to pre-existing conscious level **23**	
801.19	Closed fracture of base of skull with cerebral laceration and contusion, unspecified concussion **28**	
801.10	Closed fracture of base of skull with cerebral laceration and contusion, unspecified state of consciousness **28**	
801.4*	Closed fracture of base of skull with intracranial injury of other and unspecified nature **220**, **225**	
801.42	Closed fracture of base of skull with intracranial injury of other and unspecified nature, brief (less than one hour) loss of consciousness **28**	
801.46	Closed fracture of base of skull with intracranial injury of other and unspecified nature, loss of consciousness of unspecified duration **23**	
801.43	Closed fracture of base of skull with intracranial injury of other and unspecified nature, moderate (1-24 hours) loss of consciousness **23**	

801.41	Closed fracture of base of skull with intracranial injury of other and unspecified nature, no loss of consciousness **28**
801.44	Closed fracture of base of skull with intracranial injury of other and unspecified nature, prolonged (more than 24 hours) loss of consciousness and return to pre-existing conscious level **23**
801.45	Closed fracture of base of skull with intracranial injury of other and unspecified nature, prolonged (more than 24 hours) loss of consciousness, without return to pre-existing conscious level **23**
801.49	Closed fracture of base of skull with intracranial injury of other and unspecified nature, unspecified concussion **28**
801.40	Closed fracture of base of skull with intracranial injury of other and unspecified nature, unspecified state of consciousness **28**
801.3*	Closed fracture of base of skull with other and unspecified intracranial hemorrhage **220**, **225**
801.32	Closed fracture of base of skull with other and unspecified intracranial hemorrhage, brief (less than one hour) loss of consciousness **28**
801.36	Closed fracture of base of skull with other and unspecified intracranial hemorrhage, loss of consciousness of unspecified duration **23**
801.33	Closed fracture of base of skull with other and unspecified intracranial hemorrhage, moderate (1-24 hours) loss of consciousness **23**
801.31	Closed fracture of base of skull with other and unspecified intracranial hemorrhage, no loss of consciousness **28**
801.34	Closed fracture of base of skull with other and unspecified intracranial hemorrhage, prolonged (more than 24 hours) loss of consciousness and return to pre-existing conscious level **23**
801.35	Closed fracture of base of skull with other and unspecified intracranial hemorrhage, prolonged (more than 24 hours) loss of consciousness, without return to pre-existing conscious level **23**
801.39	Closed fracture of base of skull with other and unspecified intracranial hemorrhage, unspecified concussion **28**
801.30	Closed fracture of base of skull with other and unspecified intracranial hemorrhage, unspecified state of consciousness **28**
801.2*	Closed fracture of base of skull with subarachnoid, subdural, and extradural hemorrhage **220**, **225**
801.22	Closed fracture of base of skull with subarachnoid, subdural, and extradural hemorrhage, brief (less than one hour) loss of consciousness **28**
801.26	Closed fracture of base of skull with subarachnoid, subdural, and extradural hemorrhage, loss of consciousness of unspecified duration **23**
801.23	Closed fracture of base of skull with subarachnoid, subdural, and extradural hemorrhage, moderate (1-24 hours) loss of consciousness **23**
801.21	Closed fracture of base of skull with subarachnoid, subdural, and extradural hemorrhage, no loss of consciousness **28**
801.24	Closed fracture of base of skull with subarachnoid, subdural, and extradural hemorrhage, prolonged (more than 24 hours) loss of consciousness and return to pre-existing conscious level **23**
801.25	Closed fracture of base of skull with subarachnoid, subdural, and extradural hemorrhage, prolonged (more than 24 hours) loss of consciousness, without return to pre-existing conscious level **23**
801.29	Closed fracture of base of skull with subarachnoid, subdural, and extradural hemorrhage, unspecified concussion **28**
801.20	Closed fracture of base of skull with subarachnoid, subdural, and extradural hemorrhage, unspecified state of consciousness **28**
801.0*	Closed fracture of base of skull without mention of intracranial injury **220**
801.02	Closed fracture of base of skull without mention of intracranial injury, brief (less than one hour) loss of consciousness **28**, **225**
801.06	Closed fracture of base of skull without mention of intracranial injury, loss of consciousness of unspecified duration **23**
801.03	Closed fracture of base of skull without mention of intracranial injury, moderate (1-24 hours) loss of consciousness **23**, **225**

801.01	Closed fracture of base of skull without mention of intracranial injury, no loss of consciousness **28**	807.03	Closed fracture of three ribs **52**
		807.02	Closed fracture of two ribs **54**
801.04	Closed fracture of base of skull without mention of intracranial injury, prolonged (more than 24 hours) loss of consciousness and return to pre-existing conscious level **23, 225**	829.0	Closed fracture of unspecified bone **222**
		820.8	Closed fracture of unspecified part of neck of femur **222**
		813.8*	Closed fracture of unspecified part of radius with ulna **221**
801.05	Closed fracture of base of skull without mention of intracranial injury, prolonged (more than 24 hours) loss of consciousness, without return to pre-existing conscious level **23, 225**	811.00	Closed fracture of unspecified part of scapula **99**
		823.8*	Closed fracture of unspecified part of tibia and fibula **222**
		805.8	Closed fracture of unspecified part of vertebral column without mention of spinal cord injury **221**
801.09	Closed fracture of base of skull without mention of intracranial injury, unspecified concussion **28**	806.8	Closed fracture of unspecified vertebra with spinal cord injury **221, 227**
801.00	Closed fracture of base of skull without mention of intracranial injury, unspecified state of consciousness **28**	812.0*	Closed fracture of upper end of humerus **221**
825.0	Closed fracture of calcaneus **99, 222**	813.0*	Closed fracture of upper end of radius and ulna **221**
806.0*	Closed fracture of cervical vertebra with spinal cord injury **221, 227**	823.0*	Closed fracture of upper end of tibia and fibula **222**
		800.1*	Closed fracture of vault of skull with cerebral laceration and contusion **220**
805.0*	Closed fracture of cervical vertebra without mention of spinal cord injury **221**	800.12	Closed fracture of vault of skull with cerebral laceration and contusion, brief (less than one hour) loss of consciousness **27, 224**
810.0*	Closed fracture of clavicle **221**		
811.02	Closed fracture of coracoid process of scapula **99**	800.16	Closed fracture of vault of skull with cerebral laceration and contusion, loss of consciousness of unspecified duration **22, 224**
806.2*	Closed fracture of dorsal (thoracic) vertebra with spinal cord injury **221, 227**	800.13	Closed fracture of vault of skull with cerebral laceration and contusion, moderate (1-24 hours) loss of consciousness **22, 224**
805.2	Closed fracture of dorsal (thoracic) vertebra without mention of spinal cord injury **221**	800.11	Closed fracture of vault of skull with cerebral laceration and contusion, no loss of consciousness **27**
807.08	Closed fracture of eight or more ribs **52, 226**	800.14	Closed fracture of vault of skull with cerebral laceration and contusion, prolonged (more than 24 hours) loss of consciousness and return to pre-existing conscious level **22, 224**
807.05	Closed fracture of five ribs **52**		
807.04	Closed fracture of four ribs **52**		
811.03	Closed fracture of glenoid cavity and neck of scapula **99**	800.15	Closed fracture of vault of skull with cerebral laceration and contusion, prolonged (more than 24 hours) loss of consciousness, without return to pre-existing conscious level **22, 224**
807.5	Closed fracture of larynx and trachea **3, 47, 221, 226**		
824.2	Closed fracture of lateral malleolus **222**	800.19	Closed fracture of vault of skull with cerebral laceration and contusion, unspecified concussion **27, 224**
821.2*	Closed fracture of lower end of femur **222**		
812.4*	Closed fracture of lower end of humerus **221**	800.10	Closed fracture of vault of skull with cerebral laceration and contusion, unspecified state of consciousness **27, 224**
813.4*	Closed fracture of lower end of radius and ulna **221**		
806.4	Closed fracture of lumbar spine with spinal cord injury **221, 227**	800.4*	Closed fracture of vault of skull with intercranial injury of other and unspecified nature **220**
805.4	Closed fracture of lumbar vertebra without mention of spinal cord injury **221**	800.42	Closed fracture of vault of skull with intracranial injury of other and unspecified nature, brief (less than one hour) loss of consciousness **28, 224**
824.0	Closed fracture of medial malleolus **222**		
815.0*	Closed fracture of metacarpal bones **221**	800.46	Closed fracture of vault of skull with intracranial injury of other and unspecified nature, loss of consciousness of unspecified duration **22, 224**
807.09	Closed fracture of multiple ribs, unspecified **52**		
826.0	Closed fracture of one or more phalanges of foot **222**	800.43	Closed fracture of vault of skull with intracranial injury of other and unspecified nature, moderate (1-24 hours) loss of consciousness **22, 224**
816.0*	Closed fracture of one or more phalanges of hand **221**		
807.01	Closed fracture of one rib **54**	800.41	Closed fracture of vault of skull with intracranial injury of other and unspecified nature, no loss of consciousness **28**
811.09	Closed fracture of other part of scapula **101**		
808.4*	Closed fracture of other specified part of pelvis **221**	800.44	Closed fracture of vault of skull with intracranial injury of other and unspecified nature, prolonged (more than 24 hours) loss of consciousness and return to pre-existing conscious level **22, 224**
825.2*	Closed fracture of other tarsal and metatarsal bones **99, 222**		
822.0	Closed fracture of patella **222**	800.45	Closed fracture of vault of skull with intracranial injury of other and unspecified nature, prolonged (more than 24 hours) loss of consciousness, without return to pre-existing conscious level **22, 224**
808.2	Closed fracture of pubis **221**		
807.0*	Closed fracture of rib(s) **221**		
807.00	Closed fracture of rib(s), unspecified **54**		
806.6*	Closed fracture of sacrum and coccyx with spinal cord injury **221**	800.49	Closed fracture of vault of skull with intracranial injury of other and unspecified nature, unspecified concussion **28, 224**
806.60	Closed fracture of sacrum and coccyx with unspecified spinal cord injury **227**	800.40	Closed fracture of vault of skull with intracranial injury of other and unspecified nature, unspecified state of consciousness **28, 224**
805.6	Closed fracture of sacrum and coccyx without mention of spinal cord injury **221, 227**		
		800.3*	Closed fracture of vault of skull with other and unspecified intracranial hemorrhage **220**
811.0*	Closed fracture of scapula **221**		
807.07	Closed fracture of seven ribs **52, 226**	800.32	Closed fracture of vault of skull with other and unspecified intracranial hemorrhage, brief (less than one hour) loss of consciousness **28, 224**
813.2*	Closed fracture of shaft of radius and ulna **221**		
823.2*	Closed fracture of shaft of tibia and fibula **222**		
821.0*	Closed fracture of shaft or unspecified part of femur **166, 170, 222**		
812.2*	Closed fracture of shaft or unspecified part of humerus **221**		
807.06	Closed fracture of six ribs **52**		
807.2	Closed fracture of sternum **52, 221**		

Alphabetic Index to Diseases

800.36	Closed fracture of vault of skull with other and unspecified intracranial hemorrhage, loss of consciousness of unspecified duration **22, 224**
800.33	Closed fracture of vault of skull with other and unspecified intracranial hemorrhage, moderate (1-24 hours) loss of consciousness **22, 224**
800.31	Closed fracture of vault of skull with other and unspecified intracranial hemorrhage, no loss of consciousness **28**
800.34	Closed fracture of vault of skull with other and unspecified intracranial hemorrhage, prolonged (more than 24 hours) loss of consciousness and return to pre-existing conscious level **22, 224**
800.35	Closed fracture of vault of skull with other and unspecified intracranial hemorrhage, prolonged (more than 24 hours) loss of consciousness, without return to pre-existing conscious level **22, 224**
800.39	Closed fracture of vault of skull with other and unspecified intracranial hemorrhage, unspecified concussion **28, 224**
800.30	Closed fracture of vault of skull with other and unspecified intracranial hemorrhage, unspecified state of consciousness **28, 224**
800.2*	Closed fracture of vault of skull with subarachnoid, subdural, and extradural hemorrhage **220**
800.22	Closed fracture of vault of skull with subarachnoid, subdural, and extradural hemorrhage, brief (less than one hour) loss of consciousness **27, 224**
800.26	Closed fracture of vault of skull with subarachnoid, subdural, and extradural hemorrhage, loss of consciousness of unspecified duration **22, 224**
800.23	Closed fracture of vault of skull with subarachnoid, subdural, and extradural hemorrhage, moderate (1-24 hours) loss of consciousness **22, 224**
800.21	Closed fracture of vault of skull with subarachnoid, subdural, and extradural hemorrhage, no loss of consciousness **27**
800.24	Closed fracture of vault of skull with subarachnoid, subdural, and extradural hemorrhage, prolonged (more than 24 hours) loss of consciousness and return to pre-existing conscious level **22, 224**
800.25	Closed fracture of vault of skull with subarachnoid, subdural, and extradural hemorrhage, prolonged (more than 24 hours) loss of consciousness, without return to pre-existing conscious level **22, 224**
800.29	Closed fracture of vault of skull with subarachnoid, subdural, and extradural hemorrhage, unspecified concussion **27, 224**
800.20	Closed fracture of vault of skull with subarachnoid, subdural, and extradural hemorrhage, unspecified state of consciousness **27, 224**
800.0*	Closed fracture of vault of skull without mention of intracranial injury **220**
800.02	Closed fracture of vault of skull without mention of intracranial injury, brief (less than one hour) loss of consciousness **27, 224**
800.06	Closed fracture of vault of skull without mention of intracranial injury, loss of consciousness of unspecified duration **22**
800.03	Closed fracture of vault of skull without mention of intracranial injury, moderate (1-24 hours) loss of consciousness **22, 224**
800.01	Closed fracture of vault of skull without mention of intracranial injury, no loss of consciousness **27**
800.04	Closed fracture of vault of skull without mention of intracranial injury, prolonged (more than 24 hours) loss of consciousness and return to pre-existing conscious level **22, 224**
800.05	Closed fracture of vault of skull without mention of intracranial injury, prolonged (more than 24 hours) loss of consciousness, without return to pre-existing conscious level **22, 224**
800.09	Closed fracture of vault of skull without mention of intracranial injury, unspecified concussion **27**
800.00	Closed fracture of vault of skull without mention of intracranial injury, unspecified state of consciousness **27**
804.06	Closed fractures involving skull of face with other bones, without mention of intracranial injury, loss of consciousness of unspecified duration **24, 225**
804.05	Closed fractures involving skull of face with other bones, without mention of intracranial injury, prolonged (more than 24 hours) loss of consciousness, without return to pre-existing conscious level **24, 225**
804.09	Closed fractures involving skull of face with other bones, without mention of intracranial injury, unspecified concussion **29**
804.2*	Closed fractures involving skull or face with other bones with subarachnoid, subdural, and extradural hemorrhage **221, 225**
804.22	Closed fractures involving skull or face with other bones with subarachnoid, subdural, and extradural hemorrhage, brief (less than one hour) loss of consciousness **29**
804.26	Closed fractures involving skull or face with other bones with subarachnoid, subdural, and extradural hemorrhage, loss of consciousness of unspecified duration **25**
804.23	Closed fractures involving skull or face with other bones with subarachnoid, subdural, and extradural hemorrhage, moderate (1-24 hours) loss of consciousness **25**
804.21	Closed fractures involving skull or face with other bones with subarachnoid, subdural, and extradural hemorrhage, no loss of consciousness **29**
804.24	Closed fractures involving skull or face with other bones with subarachnoid, subdural, and extradural hemorrhage, prolonged (more than 24 hours) loss of consciousness and return to pre-existing conscious level **25**
804.25	Closed fractures involving skull or face with other bones with subarachnoid, subdural, and extradural hemorrhage, prolonged (more than 24 hours) loss of consciousness, without return to pre-existing conscious level **25**
804.29	Closed fractures involving skull or face with other bones with subarachnoid, subdural, and extradural hemorrhage, unspecified concussion **30**
804.20	Closed fractures involving skull or face with other bones with subarachnoid, subdural, and extradural hemorrhage, unspecified state of consciousness **29**
804.1*	Closed fractures involving skull or face with other bones, with cerebral laceration and contusion **221, 225**
804.12	Closed fractures involving skull or face with other bones, with cerebral laceration and contusion, brief (less than one hour) loss of consciousness **29**
804.16	Closed fractures involving skull or face with other bones, with cerebral laceration and contusion, loss of consciousness of unspecified duration **25**
804.13	Closed fractures involving skull or face with other bones, with cerebral laceration and contusion, moderate (1-24 hours) loss of consciousness **25**
804.11	Closed fractures involving skull or face with other bones, with cerebral laceration and contusion, no loss of consciousness **29**
804.14	Closed fractures involving skull or face with other bones, with cerebral laceration and contusion, prolonged (more than 24 hours) loss of consciousness and return to pre-existing conscious level **25**
804.15	Closed fractures involving skull or face with other bones, with cerebral laceration and contusion, prolonged (more than 24 hours) loss of consciousness, without return to pre-existing conscious level **25**
804.19	Closed fractures involving skull or face with other bones, with cerebral laceration and contusion, unspecified concussion **29**
804.10	Closed fractures involving skull or face with other bones, with cerebral laceration and contusion, unspecified state of consciousness **29**
804.4*	Closed fractures involving skull or face with other bones, with intracranial injury of other and unspecified nature **221**
804.42	Closed fractures involving skull or face with other bones, with intracranial injury of other and unspecified nature, brief (less than one hour) loss of consciousness **30, 225**
804.46	Closed fractures involving skull or face with other bones, with intracranial injury of other and unspecified nature, loss of consciousness of unspecified duration **25, 226**

804.43   Closed fractures involving skull or face with other bones, with intracranial injury of other and unspecified nature, moderate (1-24 hours) loss of consciousness **25, 225**

804.41   Closed fractures involving skull or face with other bones, with intracranial injury of other and unspecified nature, no loss of consciousness **30, 225**

804.44   Closed fractures involving skull or face with other bones, with intracranial injury of other and unspecified nature, prolonged (more than 24 hours) loss of consciousness and return to pre-existing conscious level **25, 225**

804.45   Closed fractures involving skull or face with other bones, with intracranial injury of other and unspecified nature, prolonged (more than 24 hours) loss of consciousness, without return to pre-existing conscious level **25, 226**

804.49   Closed fractures involving skull or face with other bones, with intracranial injury of other and unspecified nature, unspecified concussion **30**

804.40   Closed fractures involving skull or face with other bones, with intracranial injury of other and unspecified nature, unspecified state of consciousness **30, 225**

804.3*   Closed fractures involving skull or face with other bones, with other and unspecified intracranial hemorrhage **221, 225**

804.32   Closed fractures involving skull or face with other bones, with other and unspecified intracranial hemorrhage, brief (less than one hour) loss of consciousness **30**

804.36   Closed fractures involving skull or face with other bones, with other and unspecified intracranial hemorrhage, loss of consciousness of unspecified duration **25**

804.33   Closed fractures involving skull or face with other bones, with other and unspecified intracranial hemorrhage, moderate (1-24 hours) loss of consciousness **25**

804.31   Closed fractures involving skull or face with other bones, with other and unspecified intracranial hemorrhage, no loss of consciousness **30**

804.34   Closed fractures involving skull or face with other bones, with other and unspecified intracranial hemorrhage, prolonged (more than 24 hours) loss of consciousness and return to preexisting conscious level **25**

804.35   Closed fractures involving skull or face with other bones, with other and unspecified intracranial hemorrhage, prolonged (more than 24 hours) loss of consciousness, without return to pre-existing conscious level **25**

804.39   Closed fractures involving skull or face with other bones, with other and unspecified intracranial hemorrhage, unspecified concussion **30**

804.30   Closed fractures involving skull or face with other bones, with other and unspecified intracranial hemorrhage, unspecified state of consciousness **30**

804.0*   Closed fractures involving skull or face with other bones, without mention of intracranial injury **221**

804.02   Closed fractures involving skull or face with other bones, without mention of intracranial injury, brief (less than one hour) loss of consciousness **29, 225**

804.03   Closed fractures involving skull or face with other bones, without mention of intracranial injury, moderate (1-24 hours) loss of consciousness **24, 225**

804.01   Closed fractures involving skull or face with other bones, without mention of intracranial injury, no loss of consciousness **29**

804.00   Closed fractures involving skull or face with other bones, without mention of intracranial injury, unspecified state of consciousness **29**

804.04   Closed fractures involving skull or face with other bones, without mention or intracranial injury, prolonged (more than 24 hours) loss of consciousness and return to pre-existing conscious level **24, 225**

814.0*   Closed fractures of carpal bones **221**

820.2*   Closed pertrochanteric fracture of femur **222**

803.3*   Closed skull fracture with other and unspecified intracranial hemorrhage **221, 225**

820.0*   Closed transcervical fracture **221**

824.6   Closed trimalleolar fracture **222**

792.5   Cloudy (hemodialysis) (peritoneal) dialysis affluent **213**

736.07   Club hand, acquired **21**

781.5   Clubbing of fingers **54**

649.33   Coagulation defects complicating pregnancy, childbirth, or the puerperium, antepartum condition or complication **154, 157**

649.32   Coagulation defects complicating pregnancy, childbirth, or the puerperium, delivered, with mention of postpartum complication **135, 142, 148**

649.31   Coagulation defects complicating pregnancy, childbirth, or the puerperium, delivered, with or without mention of antepartum condition **135, 142, 148**

649.34   Coagulation defects complicating pregnancy, childbirth, or the puerperium, postpartum condition or complication **152**

649.30   Coagulation defects complicating pregnancy, childbirth, or the puerperium, unspecified as to episode of care or not applicable **160**

500   Coal workers' pneumoconiosis **53**

747.1*   Coarctation of aorta **68**

114.2   Coccidioidal meningitis **9, 10, 34, 164, 168**

114*   Coccidioidomycosis **230**

007.2   Coccidiosis **229**

799.52   Cognitive communication deficit **188**

789.7   Colic **78**

377.23   Coloboma of optic disc **40**

863.4*   Colon or rectal injury without mention of open wound into cavity **79, 223, 227**

569.6*   Colostomy and enterostomy complications **79**

780.01   Coma **21, 166, 170**

279.2   Combined immunity deficiency **175**

428.4*   Combined systolic and diastolic heart failure **57, 165, 169**

V67.6   Combined treatment follow-up examination **214**

900.01   Common carotid artery injury **226**

904.0   Common femoral artery injury **223, 227**

331.3   Communicating hydrocephalus **19**

958.90   Compartment syndrome, unspecified **224**

518.2   Compensatory emphysema **54**

629.3*   Complication of implanted vaginal mesh and other prosthetic materials **130**

997.9*   Complications affecting other specified body systems, not elsewhere classified **204**

639*   Complications following abortion or ectopic and molar pregnancies **151**

383.3*   Complications following mastoidectomy **47**

539*   Complications of bariatric procedures **78**

996.85   Complications of bone marrow transplant **175**

569.7*   Complications of intestinal pouch **79, 166, 170**

999.39   Complications of medical care, NEC, infection following other infusion, injection, transfusion, or vaccination **167, 171, 184, 186**

996.89   Complications of other transplanted organ **204**

996.9*   Complications of reattached extremity or body part **99**

996.83   Complications of transplanted heart **69**

996.81   Complications of transplanted kidney **120**

996.82   Complications of transplanted liver **83**

996.84   Complications of transplanted lung **54**

996.87   Complications of transplanted organ, intestine **204**

996.88   Complications of transplanted organ, stem cell **204**

996.80   Complications of transplanted organ, unspecified site **204**

996.86	Complications of transplanted pancreas **83**	754.43	Congenital bowing of tibia and fibula **100**
348.4	Compression of brain **21**	754.44	Congenital bowing of unspecified long bones of leg **100**
459.2	Compression of vein **67**	744.4*	Congenital branchial cleft cyst or fistula; preauricular sinus **47**
850*	Concussion **32**	748.61	Congenital bronchiectasis **53**
850.1*	Concussion with brief (less than one hour) loss of consciousness **222**	327.25	Congenital central alveolar hypoventilation syndrome **32**
850.5	Concussion with loss of consciousness of unspecified duration **222**	748.0	Congenital choanal atresia **47**
850.2	Concussion with moderate (1-24 hours) loss of consciousness **222, 226**	746.85	Congenital coronary artery anomaly **68**
		751.62	Congenital cystic disease of liver **83**
850.0	Concussion with no loss of consciousness **222**	748.4	Congenital cystic lung **54**
850.3	Concussion with prolonged (more than 24 hours) loss of consciousness and return to pre-existing conscious level **222, 226**	771.1	Congenital cytomegalovirus infection **163, 167**
		286.3	Congenital deficiency of other clotting factors **176**
		754.3*	Congenital dislocation of hip **100**
850.4	Concussion with prolonged (more than 24 hours) loss of consciousness, without return to pre-existing conscious level **222, 226**	754.41	Congenital dislocation of knee (with genu recurvatum) **99**
		750.27	Congenital diverticulum of pharynx **3, 47**
758.9	Conditions due to anomaly of unspecified chromosome **213**	752.2	Congenital doubling of uterus **127, 130**
426*	Conduction disorders **68**	757.31	Congenital ectodermal dysplasia **108**
327.41	Confusional arousals **32**	286.1	Congenital factor IX disorder **176**
654.03	Congenital abnormalities of pregnant uterus, antepartum **154, 157**	286.0	Congenital factor VIII disorder **176**
		286.2	Congenital factor XI deficiency **176**
654.01	Congenital abnormalities of pregnant uterus, delivered **135, 142, 148**	750.25	Congenital fistula of lip **3, 48**
		750.24	Congenital fistula of salivary gland **3, 47**
654.02	Congenital abnormalities of pregnant uterus, delivered, with mention of postpartum complication **135, 142, 148**	756.15	Congenital fusion of spine (vertebra) **98**
		754.40	Congenital genu recurvatum **100**
654.00	Congenital abnormalities of pregnant uterus, unspecified as to episode of care **160**	746.86	Congenital heart block **68**
		359.0	Congenital hereditary muscular dystrophy **32**
654.04	Congenital abnormalities of uterus, postpartum condition or complication **152**	750.6	Congenital hiatus hernia **79**
		750.5	Congenital hypertrophic pyloric stenosis **79**
750.21	Congenital absence of salivary gland **3, 47**	243	Congenital hypothyroidism **114**
756.13	Congenital absence of vertebra **98**	746.83	Congenital infundibular pulmonic stenosis **68**
747.5	Congenital absence or hypoplasia of umbilical artery **67**	746.4	Congenital insufficiency of aortic valve **68**
750.22	Congenital accessory salivary gland **3, 47**	746.87	Congenital malposition of heart and cardiac apex **68**
748.5	Congenital agenesis, hypoplasia, and dysplasia of lung **54**	746.6	Congenital mitral insufficiency **68**
744.1	Congenital anomalies of accessory auricle **47, 172**	746.5	Congenital mitral stenosis **68**
759.1	Congenital anomalies of adrenal gland **114**	754.0	Congenital musculoskeletal deformities of skull, face, and jaw **100**
752.4*	Congenital anomalies of cervix, vagina, and external female genitalia **127, 130**	754.2	Congenital musculoskeletal deformity of spine **87, 100**
744.0*	Congenital anomalies of ear causing impairment of hearing **47**	754.1	Congenital musculoskeletal deformity of sternocleidomastoid muscle **100**
743*	Congenital anomalies of eye **40**	379.51	Congenital nystagmus **40**
752.1*	Congenital anomalies of fallopian tubes and broad ligaments **127, 130**	746.84	Congenital obstructive anomalies of heart, not elsewhere classified **68**
747.4*	Congenital anomalies of great veins **68**	654.73	Congenital or acquired abnormality of vagina, antepartum condition or complication **155, 157**
751.4	Congenital anomalies of intestinal fixation **79**		
759.2	Congenital anomalies of other endocrine glands **114**	654.72	Congenital or acquired abnormality of vagina, delivered, with mention of postpartum complication **135, 143, 148**
752.0	Congenital anomalies of ovaries **127, 130**		
751.7	Congenital anomalies of pancreas **83**	654.74	Congenital or acquired abnormality of vagina, postpartum condition or complication **152**
746.0*	Congenital anomalies of pulmonary valve **68**		
756.0	Congenital anomalies of skull and face bones **100**	654.70	Congenital or acquired abnormality of vagina, unspecified as to episode of care in pregnancy **160**
759.0	Congenital anomalies of spleen **176**		
753*	Congenital anomalies of urinary system **120**	654.71	Congenital or acquired abnormality of vagina, with delivery **135, 143, 148**
756.7*	Congenital anomaly of abdominal wall **79**		
747.81	Congenital anomaly of cerebrovascular system **33**	654.83	Congenital or acquired abnormality of vulva, antepartum condition or complication **155, 157**
756.6	Congenital anomaly of diaphragm **54**		
756.10	Congenital anomaly of spine, unspecified **98**	654.82	Congenital or acquired abnormality of vulva, delivered, with mention of postpartum complication **135, 143, 148**
751.2	Congenital atresia and stenosis of large intestine, rectum, and anal canal **79**		
		654.84	Congenital or acquired abnormality of vulva, postpartum condition or complication **152**
751.1	Congenital atresia and stenosis of small intestine **79**		
750.23	Congenital atresia, salivary duct **3, 47**	654.80	Congenital or acquired abnormality of vulva, unspecified as to episode of care in pregnancy **160**
751.61	Congenital biliary atresia **83**		
754.42	Congenital bowing of femur **100**	654.81	Congenital or acquired abnormality of vulva, with delivery **135, 143, 148**
		756.5*	Congenital osteodystrophies **100**

*Code Range

754.61	Congenital pes planus **172**
757.33	Congenital pigmentary anomaly of skin **108**, **172**
770.0	Congenital pneumonia **163**, **167**
771.0	Congenital rubella **163**, **167**
747.82	Congenital spinal vessel anomaly **33**
756.12	Congenital spondylolisthesis **98**
756.11	Congenital spondylolysis, lumbosacral region **98**
746.3	Congenital stenosis of aortic valve **68**
746.81	Congenital subaortic stenosis **68**
090.9	Congenital syphilis, unspecified **185**
750.3	Congenital tracheoesophageal fistula, esophageal atresia and stenosis **75**
746.1	Congenital tricuspid atresia and stenosis **68**
754.6*	Congenital valgus deformities of feet **100**
754.5*	Congenital varus deformities of feet **100**
757.32	Congenital vascular hamartomas **108**
748.2	Congenital web of larynx **3**, **47**
744.5	Congenital webbing of neck **108**
428.0	Congestive heart failure, unspecified **57**, **165**, **169**
759.4	Conjoined twins **79**, **166**, **170**
032.81	Conjunctival diphtheria **38**
130.1	Conjunctivitis due to toxoplasmosis **38**, **164**, **168**
376.31	Constant exophthalmos **39**
564.0*	Constipation **78**
284.0*	Constitutional aplastic anemia **175**
V21*	Constitutional states in development **214**
692*	Contact dermatitis and other eczema **108**
V01.89	Contact or exposure to other communicable diseases **172**
V87.1*	Contact with and (suspected) exposure to hazardous aromatic compounds **215**
V87.0*	Contact with and (suspected) exposure to hazardous metals **215**
V87.2	Contact with and (suspected) exposure to other potentially hazardous chemicals **215**
V87.3*	Contact with and (suspected) exposure to other potentially hazardous substances **215**
V01.81	Contact with or exposure to anthrax **172**
V01*	Contact with or exposure to communicable diseases **213**
051.2	Contagious pustular dermatitis **107**
718.4*	Contracture of joint **100**
728.6	Contracture of palmar fascia **99**
922.2	Contusion of abdominal wall **107**
922.0	Contusion of breast **107**
922.1	Contusion of chest wall **107**
921*	Contusion of eye and adnexa **223**
921.3	Contusion of eyeball **40**
921.1	Contusion of eyelids and periocular area **40**
920	Contusion of face, scalp, and neck except eye(s) **107**, **223**
922.4	Contusion of genital organs **124**, **127**, **131**
924*	Contusion of lower limb and of other and unspecified sites **107**, **223**
922.8	Contusion of multiple sites of trunk **107**
921.2	Contusion of orbital tissues **40**
922.3*	Contusion of trunk **107**
922*	Contusion of trunk **223**
922.9	Contusion of unspecified part of trunk **107**
923*	Contusion of upper limb **107**, **223**
V66*	Convalescence and palliative care **214**
378.84	Convergence excess or spasm in binocular eye movement **40**
378.83	Convergence insufficiency or palsy in binocular eye movement **40**
300.11	Conversion disorder **188**

780.3*	Convulsions **34**
779.0	Convulsions in newborn **163**, **168**
745.7	Cor biloculare **68**
746.82	Cor triatriatum **68**
840.1	Coracoclavicular (ligament) sprain and strain **222**
840.2	Coracohumeral (ligament) sprain and strain **222**
663.13	Cord around neck, with compression, complicating labor and delivery, antepartum **155**, **158**
663.11	Cord around neck, with compression, complicating labor and delivery, delivered **137**, **144**, **150**
663.10	Cord around neck, with compression, complicating labor and delivery, unspecified as to episode of care **137**, **144**, **150**
V59.5	Cornea donor **214**
V42.5	Cornea replaced by transplant **40**
370.55	Corneal abscess **38**
370.6*	Corneal neovascularization **39**
371*	Corneal opacity and other disorders of cornea **39**
700	Corns and callosities **108**
414.0*	Coronary atherosclerosis **67**
414.4	Coronary atherosclerosis due to calcified coronary lesion **67**
414.3	Coronary atherosclerosis due to lipid rich plaque **67**
851.1*	Cortex (cerebral) contusion with open intracranial wound **9**, **11**, **222**, **226**
851.12	Cortex (cerebral) contusion with open intracranial wound, brief (less than 1 hour) loss of consciousness **30**
851.16	Cortex (cerebral) contusion with open intracranial wound, loss of consciousness of unspecified duration **26**
851.13	Cortex (cerebral) contusion with open intracranial wound, moderate (1-24 hours) loss of consciousness **26**
851.11	Cortex (cerebral) contusion with open intracranial wound, no loss of consciousness **30**
851.14	Cortex (cerebral) contusion with open intracranial wound, prolonged (more than 24 hours) loss of consciousness and return to pre-existing conscious level **26**
851.15	Cortex (cerebral) contusion with open intracranial wound, prolonged (more than 24 hours) loss of consciousness, without return to pre-existing conscious level **26**
851.19	Cortex (cerebral) contusion with open intracranial wound, unspecified concussion **30**
851.10	Cortex (cerebral) contusion with open intracranial wound, unspecified state of consciousness **30**
851.0*	Cortex (cerebral) contusion without mention of open intracranial wound **222**
851.02	Cortex (cerebral) contusion without mention of open intracranial wound, brief (less than 1 hour) loss of consciousness **30**, **226**
851.06	Cortex (cerebral) contusion without mention of open intracranial wound, loss of consciousness of unspecified duration **25**, **226**
851.03	Cortex (cerebral) contusion without mention of open intracranial wound, moderate (1-24 hours) loss of consciousness **25**, **226**
851.01	Cortex (cerebral) contusion without mention of open intracranial wound, no loss of consciousness **30**, **226**
851.04	Cortex (cerebral) contusion without mention of open intracranial wound, prolonged (more than 24 hours) loss of consciousness and return to pre-existing conscious level **25**, **226**
851.05	Cortex (cerebral) contusion without mention of open intracranial wound, prolonged (more than 24 hours) loss of consciousness, without return to pre-existing conscious level **25**, **226**
851.00	Cortex (cerebral) contusion without mention of open intracranial wound, state of consciousness unspecified **30**, **226**
851.09	Cortex (cerebral) contusion without mention of open intracranial wound, unspecified concussion **30**, **226**
851.3*	Cortex (cerebral) laceration with open intracranial wound **9**, **11**, **222**, **226**
851.32	Cortex (cerebral) laceration with open intracranial wound, brief (less than 1 hour) loss of consciousness **30**

*Code Range

851.36	Cortex (cerebral) laceration with open intracranial wound, loss of consciousness of unspecified duration **26**
851.33	Cortex (cerebral) laceration with open intracranial wound, moderate (1-24 hours) loss of consciousness **26**
851.31	Cortex (cerebral) laceration with open intracranial wound, no loss of consciousness **30**
851.34	Cortex (cerebral) laceration with open intracranial wound, prolonged (more than 24 hours) loss of consciousness and return to pre-existing conscious level **26**
851.35	Cortex (cerebral) laceration with open intracranial wound, prolonged (more than 24 hours) loss of consciousness, without return to pre-existing conscious level **26**
851.39	Cortex (cerebral) laceration with open intracranial wound, unspecified concussion **30**
851.30	Cortex (cerebral) laceration with open intracranial wound, unspecified state of consciousness **30**
851.2*	Cortex (cerebral) laceration without mention of open intracranial wound **9, 11, 222, 226**
851.22	Cortex (cerebral) laceration without mention of open intracranial wound, brief (less than 1 hour) loss of consciousness **30**
851.26	Cortex (cerebral) laceration without mention of open intracranial wound, loss of consciousness of unspecified duration **26**
851.23	Cortex (cerebral) laceration without mention of open intracranial wound, moderate (1-24 hours) loss of consciousness **26**
851.21	Cortex (cerebral) laceration without mention of open intracranial wound, no loss of consciousness **30**
851.24	Cortex (cerebral) laceration without mention of open intracranial wound, prolonged (more than 24 hours) loss of consciousness and return to pre-existing conscious level **26**
851.25	Cortex (cerebral) laceration without mention of open intracranial wound, prolonged (more than 24 hours) loss of consciousness, without return to pre-existing conscious level **26**
851.29	Cortex (cerebral) laceration without mention of open intracranial wound, unspecified concussion **30**
851.20	Cortex (cerebral) laceration without mention of open intracranial wound, unspecified state of consciousness **30**
331.6	Corticobasal degeneration **19**
365.3*	Corticosteroid-induced glaucoma **39**
786.2	Cough **54**
V61.10	Counseling for marital and partner problems, unspecified **214**
V62.83	Counseling for perpetrator of physical/sexual abuse **214**
V61.12	Counseling for perpetrator of spousal and partner abuse **214**
V61.11	Counseling for victim of spousal and partner abuse **214**
051.0*	Cowpox and vaccinia not from vaccination **184**
074.20	Coxsackie carditis, unspecified **68**
074.22	Coxsackie endocarditis **67**
074.23	Coxsackie myocarditis **68**
074.21	Coxsackie pericarditis **68**
676.13	Cracked nipple, antepartum condition or complication **156, 158**
676.12	Cracked nipple, delivered, with mention of postpartum complication **139, 145, 151**
676.11	Cracked nipple, delivered, with or without mention of antepartum condition **139, 145, 151**
676.14	Cracked nipple, postpartum condition or complication **153**
676.10	Cracked nipple, unspecified as to prenatal or postnatal episode of care **161**
729.82	Cramp of limb **98**
377.22	Crater-like holes of optic disc **40**
359.81	Critical illness myopathy **33**
464.4	Croup **3, 46**
928.2*	Crushing injury of ankle and foot, excluding toe(s) alone **223**
926.11	Crushing injury of back **227**
926.12	Crushing injury of buttock **227**
927.1*	Crushing injury of elbow and forearm **223, 227**

926.0	Crushing injury of external genitalia **124, 127, 131, 223**
925.1	Crushing injury of face and scalp **226**
925*	Crushing injury of face, scalp, and neck **4, 203, 223**
927.3	Crushing injury of finger(s) **223**
928.0*	Crushing injury of hip and thigh **223, 227**
928.1*	Crushing injury of knee and lower leg **223, 227**
928*	Crushing injury of lower limb **203**
929*	Crushing injury of multiple and unspecified sites **203, 223**
928.8	Crushing injury of multiple sites of lower limb **223, 227**
926.8	Crushing injury of multiple sites of trunk **203, 223, 227**
927.8	Crushing injury of multiple sites of upper limb **223, 227**
925.2	Crushing injury of neck **226**
926.1*	Crushing injury of other specified sites of trunk **203, 223**
926.19	Crushing injury of other specified sites of trunk **227**
927.01	Crushing injury of scapular region **226**
927.0*	Crushing injury of shoulder and upper arm **223, 227**
928.3	Crushing injury of toe(s) **223**
928.9	Crushing injury of unspecified site of lower limb **223, 227**
926.9	Crushing injury of unspecified site of trunk **203, 223, 227**
927.9	Crushing injury of unspecified site of upper limb **223, 227**
927*	Crushing injury of upper limb **203**
927.2*	Crushing injury of wrist and hand(s), except finger(s) alone **223**
321.0	Cryptococcal meningitis **9, 10**
117.5	Cryptococcosis **164, 168, 230**
516.36	Cryptogenic organizing pneumonia **230**
712*	Crystal arthropathies **98**
736.01	Cubitus valgus (acquired) **100**
736.02	Cubitus varus (acquired) **100**
737*	Curvature of spine **97**
737.4*	Curvature of spine associated with other conditions **87**
039.0	Cutaneous actinomycotic infection **107**
022.0	Cutaneous anthrax **107**
032.85	Cutaneous diphtheria **107**
031.1	Cutaneous diseases due to other mycobacteria **107**
085.4	Cutaneous leishmaniasis, American **107**
085.2	Cutaneous leishmaniasis, Asian desert **107**
085.3	Cutaneous leishmaniasis, Ethiopian **107**
085.1	Cutaneous leishmaniasis, urban **107**
120.3	Cutaneous schistosomiasis **107**
782.5	Cyanosis **213**
301.13	Cyclothymic disorder **188**
577.2	Cyst and pseudocyst of pancreas **166, 170**
616.2	Cyst of Bartholin's gland **127, 130**
733.2*	Cyst of bone **98**
478.26	Cyst of pharynx or nasopharynx **47**
246.2	Cyst of thyroid **3**
277.03	Cystic fibrosis with gastrointestinal manifestations **78**
277.01	Cystic fibrosis with meconium ileus **163, 167**
277.09	Cystic fibrosis with other manifestations **113**
277.02	Cystic fibrosis with pulmonary manifestations **51**
277.00	Cystic fibrosis without mention of meconium ileus **113**
123.1	Cysticercosis **75**
595.81	Cystitis cystica **119, 166, 170**
595.4	Cystitis in diseases classified elsewhere **119, 166, 170**
364.6*	Cysts of iris, ciliary body, and anterior chamber **39**
078.5	Cytomegaloviral disease **185, 230**
665.64	Damage to pelvic joints and ligaments, postpartum condition or complication **152**

665.60	Damage to pelvic joints and ligaments, unspecified as to episode of care in pregnancy **137, 144, 150**
665.61	Damage to pelvic joints and ligaments, with delivery **137, 144, 150**
798.2	Death occurring in less than 24 hours from onset of symptoms, not otherwise explained **66**
655.73	Decreased fetal movements, affecting management of mother, antepartum condition or complication **155, 157**
655.71	Decreased fetal movements, affecting management of mother, delivered **135, 143, 148**
655.70	Decreased fetal movements, unspecified as to episode of care **160**
288.5*	Decreased white blood cell count **176**
949.4	Deep necrosis of underlying tissue due to burn (deep third degree), unspecified site without mention of loss of body part **206, 207, 208, 209**
949.5	Deep necrosis of underlying tissues due to burn (deep third degree, unspecified site with loss of body part **206, 207, 208, 209**
941.52	Deep necrosis of underlying tissues due to burn (deep third degree) of eye (with other parts of face, head, and neck), with loss of a body part **40**
941.42	Deep necrosis of underlying tissues due to burn (deep third degree) of eye (with other parts of face, head, and neck), without mention of loss of a body part **40**
941.5*	Deep necrosis of underlying tissues due to burn (deep third degree) of face, head, and neck with loss of a body part **206, 207, 208, 209**
941.4*	Deep necrosis of underlying tissues due to burn (deep third degree) of face, head, and neck without mention of loss of a body part **206, 207, 208, 209**
945.5*	Deep necrosis of underlying tissues due to burn (deep third degree) of lower limb(s) with loss of a body part **206, 207, 208, 209**
945.4*	Deep necrosis of underlying tissues due to burn (deep third degree) of lower limb(s) without mention of loss of a body part **206, 207, 208, 209**
946.5	Deep necrosis of underlying tissues due to burn (deep third degree) of multiple specified sites, with loss of a body part **206, 207, 208, 209**
946.4	Deep necrosis of underlying tissues due to burn (deep third degree) of multiple specified sites, without mention of loss of a body part **206, 207, 208, 209**
942.5*	Deep necrosis of underlying tissues due to burn (deep third degree) of trunk with loss of a body part **206, 207, 208, 209**
942.4*	Deep necrosis of underlying tissues due to burn (deep third degree) of trunk without mention of loss of a body part **206, 207, 208, 209**
943.5*	Deep necrosis of underlying tissues due to burn (deep third degree) of upper limb, except wrist and hand, with loss of a body part **206, 207, 208, 209**
943.4*	Deep necrosis of underlying tissues due to burn (deep third degree) of upper limb, except wrist and hand, without mention of loss of a body part **206, 207, 208, 209**
944.5*	Deep necrosis of underlying tissues due to burn (deep third degree) of wrist(s) and hand(s), with loss of a body part **206, 207, 208, 209**
944.4*	Deep necrosis of underlying tissues due to burn (deep third degree) of wrist(s) and hand(s), without mention of loss of a body part **206, 207, 208, 209**
671.33	Deep phlebothrombosis, antepartum **156, 158**
671.30	Deep phlebothrombosis, antepartum, unspecified as to episode of care **161**
671.31	Deep phlebothrombosis, antepartum, with delivery **138, 141, 146**
671.44	Deep phlebothrombosis, postpartum condition or complication **153**
671.40	Deep phlebothrombosis, postpartum, unspecified as to episode of care **161**
671.42	Deep phlebothrombosis, postpartum, with delivery **138, 141, 146**
904.6	Deep plantar blood vessels injury **223**
660.31	Deep transverse arrest and persistent occipitoposterior position during labor and deliver, delivered **136, 143, 149**
660.33	Deep transverse arrest and persistent occipitoposterior position during labor and delivery, antepartum **155, 158**
660.30	Deep transverse arrest and persistent occipitoposterior position during labor and delivery, unspecified as to episode of care **136, 143, 149**
286.6	Defibrination syndrome **164, 169, 176**
266*	Deficiency of B-complex components **113, 230**
279.0*	Deficiency of humoral immunity **176**
612*	Deformity and disproportion of reconstructed breast **106**
376.4*	Deformity of orbit **39**
360.4*	Degenerated conditions of globe **39**
362.5*	Degeneration of macula and posterior pole of retina **39**
364.5*	Degenerations of iris and ciliary body **39**
388.0*	Degenerative and vascular disorders of ear **47**
360.2*	Degenerative disorders of globe **39**
666.24	Delayed and secondary postpartum hemorrhage, postpartum condition or complication **152**
666.20	Delayed and secondary postpartum hemorrhage, unspecified as to episode of care **161**
666.22	Delayed and secondary postpartum hemorrhage, with delivery **137, 140, 146**
658.33	Delayed delivery after artificial rupture of membranes, antepartum **155, 158**
658.31	Delayed delivery after artificial rupture of membranes, delivered **136, 143, 149**
658.30	Delayed delivery after artificial rupture of membranes, unspecified as to episode of care **136, 143, 149**
658.23	Delayed delivery after spontaneous or unspecified rupture of membranes, antepartum **155, 158**
658.21	Delayed delivery after spontaneous or unspecified rupture of membranes, delivered **136, 143, 149**
658.20	Delayed delivery after spontaneous or unspecified rupture of membranes, unspecified as to episode of care **136, 143, 149**
662.33	Delayed delivery of second twin, triplet, etc., antepartum **155, 158**
662.31	Delayed delivery of second twin, triplet, etc., delivered **136, 144, 149**
662.30	Delayed delivery of second twin, triplet, etc., unspecified as to episode of care **136, 144, 149**
999.85	Delayed hemolytic transfusion reaction, incompatibility unspecified **176**
779.83	Delayed separation of umbilical cord **171**
293.0	Delirium due to conditions classified elsewhere **188**
282.45	Delta-beta thalassemia **164, 169**
297*	Delusional disorders **189**
331.82	Dementia with Lewy bodies **19**
290*	Dementias **188**
799.25	Demoralization and apathy **188**
054.42	Dendritic keratitis **229**
061	Dengue **184**
524*	Dentofacial anomalies, including malocclusion **3, 48**
301.6	Dependent personality disorder **188**
300.6	Depersonalization disorder **188**
311	Depressive disorder, not elsewhere classified **188**
298.0	Depressive type psychosis **189**
717.1	Derangement of anterior horn of medial meniscus **99**

*Code Range

© 2013 OptumInsight, Inc.

674.14	Disruption of cesarean wound, postpartum condition or complication **153**
674.10	Disruption of cesarean wound, unspecified as to episode of care **161**
674.12	Disruption of cesarean wound, with delivery, with mention of postpartum complication **138, 141, 147**
674.24	Disruption of perineal wound, postpartum condition or complication **153**
674.20	Disruption of perineal wound, unspecified as to episode of care in pregnancy **161**
674.22	Disruption of perineal wound, with delivery, with mention of postpartum complication **138, 141, 147**
998.3*	Disruption of wound **204**
441.0*	Dissection of aorta **66**
443.21	Dissection of carotid artery **66**
443.22	Dissection of iliac artery **66**
443.29	Dissection of other artery **66**
443.23	Dissection of renal artery **120**
443.24	Dissection of vertebral artery **66**
112.5	Disseminated candidiasis **164, 168, 185, 230**
031.2	Disseminated diseases due to other mycobacteria **185, 229**
776.2	Disseminated intravascular coagulation in newborn **163, 167**
199.0	Disseminated malignant neoplasm **180**
379.55	Dissociated nystagmus **38**
300.12	Dissociative amnesia **188**
300.15	Dissociative disorder or reaction, unspecified **188**
300.13	Dissociative fugue **188**
300.14	Dissociative identity disorder **188**
782.0	Disturbance of skin sensation **33**
520.6	Disturbances in tooth eruption **172**
781.1	Disturbances of sensation of smell and taste **33**
562.11	Diverticulitis of colon (without mention of hemorrhage) **78**
562.13	Diverticulitis of colon with hemorrhage **76**
562.01	Diverticulitis of small intestine (without mention of hemorrhage) **78**
562.03	Diverticulitis of small intestine with hemorrhage **76**
562.10	Diverticulosis of colon (without mention of hemorrhage) **78**
562.12	Diverticulosis of colon with hemorrhage **76**
562.00	Diverticulosis of small intestine (without mention of hemorrhage) **78**
562.02	Diverticulosis of small intestine with hemorrhage **76**
530.6	Diverticulum of esophagus, acquired **78**
780.4	Dizziness and giddiness **46**
V59.8	Donor of other specified organ or tissue **214**
V59.9	Donor of unspecified organ or tissue **214**
758.0	Down's syndrome **188**
994.1	Drowning and nonfatal submersion **204**
304*	Drug dependence **191**
779.4	Drug reactions and intoxications specific to newborn **163, 168**
292.0	Drug withdrawal **164, 169**
779.5	Drug withdrawal syndrome in newborn **163, 168**
292*	Drug-induced mental disorders **191**
359.24	Drug-induced myotonia **32**
377.21	Drusen of optic disc **38**
378.71	Duane's syndrome **40**
532.90	Duodenal ulcer, unspecified as acute or chronic, without hemorrhage, perforation, or obstruction **77**
532.91	Duodenal ulcer, unspecified as acute or chronic, without mention of hemorrhage or perforation, with obstruction **77**
535.61	Duodenitis with hemorrhage **76**
535.60	Duodenitis without mention of hemorrhage **78**
349.3*	Dural tear **165, 169, 203**
709.00	Dyschromia, unspecified **172**
780.56	Dysfunctions associated with sleep stages or arousal from sleep **189**
530.5	Dyskinesia of esophagus **78**
625.3	Dysmenorrhea **130**
277.7	Dysmetabolic Syndrome X **114**
625.0	Dyspareunia **130**
536.8	Dyspepsia and other specified disorders of function of stomach **78**
786.0*	Dyspnea and respiratory abnormalities **54, 231**
300.4	Dysthymic disorder **188**
788.1	Dysuria **119**
V50.3	Ear piercing **214**
090.1	Early congenital syphilis, latent **185**
090.0	Early congenital syphilis, symptomatic **185**
644.21	Early onset of delivery, delivered, with or without mention of antepartum condition **134, 141, 147**
644.20	Early onset of delivery, unspecified as to episode of care **154, 157**
091.81	Early syphilis, acute syphilitic meningitis (secondary) **9, 10, 34**
092*	Early syphilis, latent **185**
091.89	Early syphilis, other forms of secondary syphilis **185**
091.69	Early syphilis, secondary syphilis of other viscera **78**
091.7	Early syphilis, secondary syphilis, relapse **185**
091.62	Early syphilis, secondary syphilitic hepatitis **83**
091.61	Early syphilis, secondary syphilitic periostitis **96**
091.82	Early syphilis, syphilitic alopecia **107**
091.9	Early syphilis, unspecified secondary syphilis **185**
091.5*	Early syphilis, uveitis due to secondary syphilis **38**
307.50	Eating disorder, unspecified **189**
746.2	Ebstein's anomaly **68**
122.0	Echinococcus granulosus infection of liver **83**
122.1	Echinococcus granulosus infection of lung **51**
122.2	Echinococcus granulosus infection of thyroid **114**
122.5	Echinococcus multilocularis infection of liver **83**
642.60	Eclampsia complicating pregnancy, childbirth or the puerperium, unspecified as to episode of care **156, 159**
642.63	Eclampsia, antepartum **154, 156**
642.64	Eclampsia, postpartum condition or complication **151**
642.61	Eclampsia, with delivery **134, 140, 146**
642.62	Eclampsia, with delivery, with current postpartum complication **134, 140, 146**
633*	Ectopic pregnancy **153**
374.1*	Ectropion **39**
054.0	Eczema herpeticum **107, 164, 168, 229**
782.3	Edema **213**
478.6	Edema of larynx **3, 47**
607.83	Edema of penis **124**
478.25	Edema of pharynx or nasopharynx **47**
646.10	Edema or excessive weight gain in pregnancy, unspecified as to episode of care **156, 159**
646.12	Edema or excessive weight gain in pregnancy, with delivery, with current postpartum complication **134, 141, 147**
646.11	Edema or excessive weight gain in pregnancy, with delivery, with or without mention of antepartum complication **134, 141, 147**
646.14	Edema or excessive weight gain in pregnancy, without mention of hypertension, postpartum condition or complication **151**
646.13	Edema or excessive weight gain, antepartum **154, 156**
V62.3	Educational circumstance **214**
758.2	Edwards' syndrome **188**
993.4	Effects of air pressure caused by explosion **204**

Alphabetic Index to Diseases

992*	Effects of heat and light **204**
994.2	Effects of hunger **204**
994.0	Effects of lightning **204**
990	Effects of radiation, unspecified **204**
991*	Effects of reduced temperature **204**
994.3	Effects of thirst **204**
719.0*	Effusion of joint **100**
V59.7*	Egg (oocyte) (ovum) Donor **214**
913.1	Elbow, forearm, and wrist, abrasion or friction burn, infected **106**
913.0	Elbow, forearm, and wrist, abrasion or friction burn, without mention of infection **107**
913.3	Elbow, forearm, and wrist, blister infected **106**
913.2	Elbow, forearm, and wrist, blister, without mention of infection **108**
913.5	Elbow, forearm, and wrist, insect bite, nonvenomous, infected **106**
913.4	Elbow, forearm, and wrist, insect bite, nonvenomous, without mention of infection **108**
913.6	Elbow, forearm, and wrist, superficial foreign body (splinter), without major open wound and without mention of infection **107**
913.7	Elbow, forearm, and wrist, superficial foreign body (splinter), without major open wound, infected **106**
659.61	Elderly multigravida, delivered, with mention of antepartum condition **136, 143, 149**
659.60	Elderly multigravida, unspecified as to episode of care or not applicable **136, 143, 149**
659.63	Elderly multigravida, with antepartum condition or complication **155, 158**
659.53	Elderly primigravida, antepartum **155, 158**
659.51	Elderly primigravida, delivered **136, 143, 149**
659.50	Elderly primigravida, unspecified as to episode of care **136, 143, 149**
V50.0	Elective hair transplant for purposes other than remedying health states **109**
994.8	Electrocution and nonfatal effects of electric current **204**
796.2	Elevated blood pressure reading without diagnosis of hypertension **69**
790.1	Elevated sedimentation rate **213**
288.6*	Elevated white blood cell count **176**
444.2*	Embolism and thrombosis of arteries of the extremities **66**
444.8*	Embolism and thrombosis of other specified artery **66**
453.3	Embolism and thrombosis of renal vein **120**
444.1	Embolism and thrombosis of thoracic aorta **66**
444.9	Embolism and thrombosis of unspecified artery **66**
453.9	Embolism and thrombosis of unspecified site **67**
799.24	Emotional lability **188**
998.81	Emphysema (subcutaneous) (surgical) resulting from a procedure **204**
492.0	Emphysematous bleb **53**
510*	Empyema **51, 165, 169**
323.51	Encephalitis and encephalomyelitis following immunization procedures **10**
323.01	Encephalitis and encephalomyelitis in viral diseases classified elsewhere **10**
323.5*	Encephalitis, myelitis, and encephalomyelitis following immunization procedures **9, 34**
323.2	Encephalitis, myelitis, and encephalomyelitis in protozoal diseases classified elsewhere **9, 10, 34**
323.1	Encephalitis, myelitis, and encephalomyelitis in rickettsial diseases classified elsewhere **9, 10, 34**
323.0*	Encephalitis, myelitis, and encephalomyelitis in viral diseases classified elsewhere **9, 34**
056.01	Encephalomyelitis due to rubella **33**
348.3*	Encephalopathy, not elsewhere classified **20, 230**
307.7	Encopresis **189**
V58.1*	Encounter for antineoplastic chemotherapy and immunotherapy **180, 181, 182**
V56*	Encounter for dialysis and dialysis catheter care **119**
V25.1*	Encounter for insertion or removal of intrauterine contraceptive device **214**
V28.8*	Encounter for other specified antenatal screening **214**
V28.3	Encounter for routine screening for malformation using ultrasonics **214**
V68*	Encounters for administrative purposes **215**
603.0	Encysted hydrocele **124**
424.9*	Endocarditis, valve unspecified **165, 169**
376.2*	Endocrine exophthalmos **39**
306.6	Endocrine malfunction arising from mental factors **114**
617.6	Endometriosis in scar of skin **108**
617.2	Endometriosis of fallopian tube **127, 130**
617.5	Endometriosis of intestine **78**
617.8	Endometriosis of other specified sites **127, 130**
617.1	Endometriosis of ovary **127, 130**
617.3	Endometriosis of pelvic peritoneum **127, 130**
617.4	Endometriosis of rectovaginal septum and vagina **127, 130**
617.0	Endometriosis of uterus **127, 130**
617.9	Endometriosis, site unspecified **127, 130**
676.23	Engorgement of breast, antepartum **156, 158**
676.22	Engorgement of breasts, delivered, with mention of postpartum complication **139, 145, 151**
676.21	Engorgement of breasts, delivered, with or without mention of antepartum condition **139, 145, 151**
676.24	Engorgement of breasts, postpartum condition or complication **153**
676.20	Engorgement of breasts, unspecified as to prenatal or postnatal episode of care **161**
785.6	Enlargement of lymph nodes **176, 231**
376.5*	Enophthalmos **40**
021.1	Enteric tularemia **75**
127.4	Enterobiasis **78**
726.3*	Enthesopathy of elbow region **98**
726.5	Enthesopathy of hip region **98**
726.6*	Enthesopathy of knee **98**
726.4	Enthesopathy of wrist and carpus **98**
374.0*	Entropion and trichiasis of eyelid **39**
307.6	Enuresis **189**
288.3	Eosinophilia **176**
535.71	Eosinophilic gastritis with hemorrhage **76**
535.70	Eosinophilic gastritis without mention of hemorrhage **78**
558.4*	Eosinophilic gastroenteritis and colitis **78, 230**
322.1	Eosinophilic meningitis **165, 169**
074.1	Epidemic pleurodynia **53**
078.81	Epidemic vertigo **32**
078.82	Epidemic vomiting syndrome **77**
345*	Epilepsy and recurrent seizures **34**
649.43	Epilepsy complicating pregnancy, childbirth, or the puerperium, antepartum condition or complication **154, 157**
649.42	Epilepsy complicating pregnancy, childbirth, or the puerperium, delivered, with mention of postpartum complication **135, 142, 148**
649.41	Epilepsy complicating pregnancy, childbirth, or the puerperium, delivered, with or without mention of antepartum condition **135, 142, 148**

*Code Range

649.44	Epilepsy complicating pregnancy, childbirth, or the puerperium, postpartum condition or complication **152**	
649.40	Epilepsy complicating pregnancy, childbirth, or the puerperium, unspecified as to episode of care or not applicable **160**	
375.2*	Epiphora **39**	
296*	Episodic mood disorders **189**	
784.7	Epistaxis **46**	
736.72	Equinus deformity of foot, acquired **100**	
035	Erysipelas **106**	
941.14	Erythema due to burn (first degree) of chin **209**	
941.11	Erythema due to burn (first degree) of ear (any part) **209**	
941.12	Erythema due to burn (first degree) of eye (with other parts face, head, and neck) **40**	
941.17	Erythema due to burn (first degree) of forehead and cheek **209**	
941.13	Erythema due to burn (first degree) of lip(s) **209**	
945.1*	Erythema due to burn (first degree) of lower limb(s) **210**	
941.19	Erythema due to burn (first degree) of multiple sites (except with eye) of face, head, and neck **209**	
946.1	Erythema due to burn (first degree) of multiple specified sites **210**	
941.18	Erythema due to burn (first degree) of neck **209**	
941.15	Erythema due to burn (first degree) of nose (septum) **209**	
941.16	Erythema due to burn (first degree) of scalp (any part) **209**	
942.1*	Erythema due to burn (first degree) of trunk **209**	
941.10	Erythema due to burn (first degree) of unspecified site of face and head **209**	
943.1*	Erythema due to burn (first degree) of upper limb, except wrist and hand **209**	
944.1*	Erythema due to burn (first degree) of wrist(s) and hand(s) **210**	
949.1	Erythema due to burn (first degree), unspecified site **210**	
695.1*	Erythema multiforme **105**	
695.2	Erythema nodosum **105**	
017.1*	Erythema nodosum with hypersensitivity reaction in tuberculosis **105**	
690*	Erythematosquamous dermatosis **108**	
530.82	Esophageal hemorrhage **75**	
530.83	Esophageal leukoplakia **78**	
530.81	Esophageal reflux **78**	
456.0	Esophageal varices with bleeding **75**	
456.20	Esophageal varices with bleeding in diseases classified elsewhere **75**	
456.1	Esophageal varices without mention of bleeding **75**	
456.21	Esophageal varices without mention of bleeding in diseases classified elsewhere **78**	
530.1*	Esophagitis **78**	
862.32	Esophagus injury with open wound into cavity **79**	
862.22	Esophagus injury without mention of open wound into cavity **75**	
378.0*	Esotropia **40**	
333.1	Essential and other specified forms of tremor **32**	
401.1	Essential hypertension, benign **67**	
401.0	Essential hypertension, malignant **67**	
238.71	Essential thrombocythemia **176**	
V86*	Estrogen receptor status **215**	
381.5*	Eustachian salpingitis **46**	
V72.1*	Examination of ears and hearing **173**	
766.0	Exceptionally large baby relating to long gestation **171**, **172**	
790.3	Excessive blood level of alcohol **191**	
656.63	Excessive fetal growth affecting management of mother, antepartum **155**, **157**	
656.61	Excessive fetal growth affecting management of mother, delivered **136**, **143**, **149**	

656.60	Excessive fetal growth affecting management of mother, unspecified as to episode of care **160**
298.1	Excitative type psychosis **189**
695.5*	Exfoliation due to erythematous conditions according to extent of body surface involved **108**
994.5	Exhaustion due to excessive exertion **204**
994.4	Exhaustion due to exposure **204**
378.1*	Exotropia **40**
301.3	Explosive personality disorder **188**
315.31	Expressive language disorder **189**
900.02	External carotid artery injury **226**
900.81	External jugular vein injury **166**, **170**, **226**
852.52	Extradural hemorrhage following injury, with open intracranial wound, brief (less than 1 hour) loss of consciousness **31**
852.56	Extradural hemorrhage following injury, with open intracranial wound, loss of consciousness of unspecified duration **27**
852.53	Extradural hemorrhage following injury, with open intracranial wound, moderate (1-24 hours) loss of consciousness **27**
852.51	Extradural hemorrhage following injury, with open intracranial wound, no loss of consciousness **31**
852.54	Extradural hemorrhage following injury, with open intracranial wound, prolonged (more than 24 hours) loss of consciousness and return to pre-existing conscious level **27**
852.55	Extradural hemorrhage following injury, with open intracranial wound, prolonged (more than 24 hours) loss of consciousness, without return to pre-existing conscious level **27**
852.50	Extradural hemorrhage following injury, with open intracranial wound, state of consciousness unspecified **31**
852.59	Extradural hemorrhage following injury, with open intracranial wound, unspecified concussion **31**
852.42	Extradural hemorrhage following injury, without mention of open intracranial wound, brief (less than 1 hour) loss of consciousness **31**
852.46	Extradural hemorrhage following injury, without mention of open intracranial wound, loss of consciousness of unspecified duration **27**
852.43	Extradural hemorrhage following injury, without mention of open intracranial wound, moderate (1-24 hours) loss of consciousness **27**
852.41	Extradural hemorrhage following injury, without mention of open intracranial wound, no loss of consciousness **31**
852.44	Extradural hemorrhage following injury, without mention of open intracranial wound, prolonged (more than 24 hours) loss of consciousness and return to pre-existing conscious level **27**
852.45	Extradural hemorrhage following injury, without mention of open intracranial wound, prolonged (more than 24 hours) loss of consciousness, without return to pre-existing conscious level **27**
852.49	Extradural hemorrhage following injury, without mention of open intracranial wound, unspecified concussion **31**
852.40	Extradural hemorrhage following injury, without mention of open intracranial wound, unspecified state of consciousness **31**
999.82	Extravasation of other vesicant agent **69**
788.8	Extravasation of urine **119**
999.81	Extravasation of vesicant chemotherapy **69**
765.04	Extreme fetal immaturity, 1,000-1,249 grams **163**
765.05	Extreme fetal immaturity, 1,250-1,499 grams **163**
765.06	Extreme fetal immaturity, 1,500-1,749 grams **163**, **167**
765.07	Extreme fetal immaturity, 1,750-1,999 grams **163**, **167**
765.08	Extreme fetal immaturity, 2,000-2,499 grams **163**, **167**
765.02	Extreme fetal immaturity, 500-749 grams **163**
765.03	Extreme fetal immaturity, 750-999 grams **163**
765.01	Extreme fetal immaturity, less than 500 grams **163**
765.00	Extreme fetal immaturity, unspecified (weight) **163**, **167**
495*	Extrinsic allergic alveolitis **53**

*Code Range

Alphabetic Index to Diseases

493.0*	Extrinsic asthma **53**	
493.01	Extrinsic asthma with status asthmaticus **165, 169**	
V43.0	Eye globe replaced by other means **40**	
374.41	Eyelid retraction or lag **39**	
910.1	Face, neck, and scalp except eye, abrasion or friction burn, infected **106**	
910.3	Face, neck, and scalp except eye, blister, infected **108**	
910.2	Face, neck, and scalp except eye, blister, without mention of infection **108**	
910.5	Face, neck, and scalp except eye, insect bite, nonvenomous, infected **106**	
910.4	Face, neck, and scalp except eye, insect bite, nonvenomous, without mention of infection **108**	
910.7	Face, neck, and scalp except eye, superficial foreign body (splinter), without major open wound, infected **106**	
910.0	Face, neck, and scalp, except eye, abrasion or friction burn, without mention of infection **107**	
910.6	Face, neck, and scalp, except eye, superficial foreign body (splinter), without major open wound or mention of infection **107**	
351*	Facial nerve disorders **21**	
781.94	Facial weakness **33**	
300.16	Factitious disorder with predominantly psychological signs and symptoms **188**	
638*	Failed attempted abortion **153**	
660.73	Failed forceps or vacuum extractor, unspecified, antepartum **155, 158**	
659.03	Failed mechanical induction of labor, antepartum **155, 158**	
659.01	Failed mechanical induction of labor, delivered **136, 143, 149**	
659.00	Failed mechanical induction of labor, unspecified as to episode of care **136, 143, 149**	
659.13	Failed medical or unspecified induction of labor, antepartum **155, 158**	
659.11	Failed medical or unspecified induction of labor, delivered **136, 143, 149**	
659.10	Failed medical or unspecified induction of labor, unspecified as to episode of care **136, 143, 149**	
676.43	Failure of lactation, antepartum condition or complication **156, 158**	
676.44	Failure of lactation, postpartum condition or complication **153**	
676.40	Failure of lactation, unspecified as to episode of care **161**	
676.42	Failure of lactation, with delivery, with mention of postpartum complication **139, 145, 151**	
676.41	Failure of lactation, with delivery, with or without mention of antepartum condition **139, 145, 151**	
779.34	Failure to thrive in newborn **113, 231**	
795.6	False positive serological test for syphilis **97**	
289.6	Familial polycythemia **176**	
V61.0*	Family disruption **214**	
V17*	Family history of certain chronic disabling diseases **214**	
V18*	Family history of certain other specific conditions **214**	
V16*	Family history of malignant neoplasm **214**	
V19*	Family history of other conditions **214**	
121.3	Fascioliasis **83**	
121.4	Fasciolopsiasis **83**	
958.1	Fat embolism as an early complication of trauma **51, 166, 170, 224, 227**	
032.0	Faucial diphtheria **2, 47**	
780.31	Febrile convulsions (simple), unspecified **166, 170**	
780.66	Febrile nonhemolytic transfusion reaction **184, 231**	
560.32	Fecal impaction **166, 170**	
779.31	Feeding problems in newborn **171**	
714.1	Felty's syndrome **97**	

629.2*	Female genital mutilation status **130**	
628*	Female infertility **127, 130**	
625.6	Female stress incontinence **130**	
551.02	Femoral hernia with gangrene, bilateral, (not specified as recurrent) **166, 170**	
551.00	Femoral hernia with gangrene, unilateral or unspecified (not specified as recurrent) **166, 170**	
552.0*	Femoral hernia with obstruction **78**	
553.0*	Femoral hernia without mention of obstruction or gangrene **79**	
904.2	Femoral vein injury **223, 227**	
772.5	Fetal and neonatal adrenal hemorrhage **163, 167**	
772.6	Fetal and neonatal cutaneous hemorrhage **171, 172**	
772.4	Fetal and neonatal gastrointestinal hemorrhage **163, 167**	
772.2	Fetal and neonatal subarachnoid hemorrhage of newborn **163, 167**	
770.1*	Fetal and newborn aspiration **163, 167**	
777.1	Fetal and newborn meconium obstruction **163, 168**	
772.0	Fetal blood loss affecting newborn **163, 167**	
679.13	Fetal complications from in utero procedure, antepartum condition or complication **156, 159**	
679.12	Fetal complications from in utero procedure, delivered, with mention of postpartum complication **139, 145, 151**	
679.11	Fetal complications from in utero procedure, delivered, with or without mention of antepartum condition **139, 145, 151**	
679.14	Fetal complications from in utero procedure, postpartum condition or complication **153**	
679.10	Fetal complications from in utero procedure, unspecified as to episode of care or not applicable **161**	
678.13	Fetal conjoined twins, antepartum condition or complication **156, 158**	
678.11	Fetal conjoined twins, delivered, with or without mention of antepartum condition **139, 145, 151**	
678.10	Fetal conjoined twins, unspecified as to episode of care or not applicable **161**	
653.83	Fetal disproportion of other origin, antepartum **154, 157**	
653.81	Fetal disproportion of other origin, delivered **135, 142, 148**	
653.80	Fetal disproportion of other origin, unspecified as to episode of care **160**	
656.33	Fetal distress affecting management of mother, antepartum **155, 157**	
656.31	Fetal distress affecting management of mother, delivered **136, 143, 149**	
656.30	Fetal distress affecting management of mother, unspecified as to episode of care **136, 143, 149**	
652.43	Fetal face or brow presentation, antepartum **154, 157**	
652.41	Fetal face or brow presentation, delivered **135, 142, 148**	
652.40	Fetal face or brow presentation, unspecified as to episode of care **160**	
678.03	Fetal hematologic conditions, antepartum condition or complication **156, 158**	
678.01	Fetal hematologic conditions, delivered, with or without mention of antepartum condition **139, 145, 151**	
678.00	Fetal hematologic conditions, unspecified as to episode of care or not applicable **161**	
764.24	Fetal malnutrition without mention of "light-for-dates", 1,000-1,249 grams **163, 167**	
764.25	Fetal malnutrition without mention of "light-for-dates", 1,250-1,499 grams **163, 167**	
764.26	Fetal malnutrition without mention of "light-for-dates", 1,500-1,749 grams **163, 167**	
764.27	Fetal malnutrition without mention of "light-for-dates", 1,750-1,999 grams **163, 167**	
764.28	Fetal malnutrition without mention of "light-for-dates", 2,000-2,499 grams **163, 167**	

*Code Range

764.22	Fetal malnutrition without mention of "light-for-dates", 500-749 grams **163, 167**	
764.23	Fetal malnutrition without mention of "light-for-dates", 750-999 grams **163, 167**	
764.21	Fetal malnutrition without mention of "light-for-dates", less than 500 grams **163, 167**	
656.03	Fetal-maternal hemorrhage, antepartum condition or complication **155, 157**	
656.00	Fetal-maternal hemorrhage, unspecified as to episode of care in pregnancy **160**	
656.01	Fetal-maternal hemorrhage, with delivery **136, 143, 149**	
653.43	Fetopelvic disproportion, antepartum **154, 157**	
653.41	Fetopelvic disproportion, delivered **135, 142, 148**	
653.40	Fetopelvic disproportion, unspecified as to episode of care **160**	
763.0	Fetus or newborn affected by breech delivery and extraction **171, 172**	
763.4	Fetus or newborn affected by cesarean delivery **163, 167**	
763.3	Fetus or newborn affected by delivery by vacuum extractor **171, 172**	
763.2	Fetus or newborn affected by forceps delivery **171, 172**	
762.6	Fetus or newborn affected by other and unspecified conditions of umbilical cord **171, 172**	
762.5	Fetus or newborn affected by other compression of umbilical cord **171, 172**	
763.1	Fetus or newborn affected by other malpresentation, malposition, and disproportion during labor and delivery **171, 172**	
763.6	Fetus or newborn affected by precipitate delivery **171, 172**	
762.4	Fetus or newborn affected by prolapsed cord **171, 172**	
780.61	Fever presenting with conditions classified elsewhere **184, 231**	
780.60	Fever, unspecified **184, 231**	
125*	Filarial infection and dracontiasis **186**	
915.1	Finger, abrasion or friction burn, infected **106**	
915.3	Finger, blister, infected **106**	
915.2	Finger, blister, without mention of infection **108**	
915.5	Finger, insect bite, nonvenomous, infected **106**	
915.4	Finger, insect bite, nonvenomous, without mention of infection **108**	
915.6	Finger, superficial foreign body (splinter), without major open wound and without mention of infection **107**	
915.7	Finger, superficial foreign body (splinter), without major open wound, infected **106**	
664.04	First-degree perineal laceration, postpartum condition or complication **152**	
664.00	First-degree perineal laceration, unspecified as to episode of care in pregnancy **137, 144, 150**	
664.01	First-degree perineal laceration, with delivery **137, 144, 150**	
569.81	Fistula of intestine, excluding rectum and anus **79**	
537.4	Fistula of stomach or duodenum **78**	
V52.0	Fitting and adjustment of artificial arm (complete) (partial) **99**	
V52.2	Fitting and adjustment of artificial eye **214**	
V52.1	Fitting and adjustment of artificial leg (complete) (partial) **99**	
V52.4	Fitting and adjustment of breast prosthesis and implant **214**	
V53.3*	Fitting and adjustment of cardiac device **69**	
V52.3	Fitting and adjustment of dental prosthetic device **214**	
V53.0*	Fitting and adjustment of devices related to nervous system and special senses **33**	
V53.2	Fitting and adjustment of hearing aid **214**	
V53.4	Fitting and adjustment of orthodontic devices **214**	
V53.7	Fitting and adjustment of orthopedic device **99**	
V53.9*	Fitting and adjustment of other and unspecified device **214**	
V53.5*	Fitting and adjustment of other gastrointestinal appliance and device **79**	

V52.8	Fitting and adjustment of other specified prosthetic device **213**	
V53.1	Fitting and adjustment of spectacles and contact lenses **214**	
V52.9	Fitting and adjustment of unspecified prosthetic device **213**	
V53.6	Fitting and adjustment of urinary device **120**	
V53.8	Fitting and adjustment of wheelchair **214**	
807.4	Flail chest **52, 221, 226**	
734	Flat foot **100**	
005.2	Food poisoning due to Clostridium perfringens (C. welchii) **75**	
005.3	Food poisoning due to other Clostridia **75**	
005.4	Food poisoning due to Vibrio parahaemolyticus **75**	
078.4	Foot and mouth disease **185**	
917.1	Foot and toe(s), abrasion or friction burn, infected **106**	
917.3	Foot and toe(s), blister, infected **106**	
917.2	Foot and toe(s), blister, without mention of infection **108**	
917.5	Foot and toe(s), insect bite, nonvenomous, infected **106**	
917.4	Foot and toe(s), insect bite, nonvenomous, without mention of infection **108**	
917.6	Foot and toe(s), superficial foreign body (splinter), without major open wound and without mention of infection **107**	
917.7	Foot and toe(s), superficial foreign body (splinter), without major open wound, infected **106**	
845.1*	Foot sprain and strain **100**	
669.51	Forceps or vacuum extractor delivery without mention of indication, delivered, with or without mention of antepartum condition **138, 145, 150**	
669.50	Forceps or vacuum extractor delivery without mention of indication, unspecified as to episode of care **138, 145, 150**	
998.4	Foreign body accidentally left during procedure, not elsewhere classified **167, 171, 204**	
728.82	Foreign body granuloma of muscle **99**	
937	Foreign body in anus and rectum **79**	
939.0	Foreign body in bladder and urethra **120**	
938	Foreign body in digestive system, unspecified **79**	
931	Foreign body in ear **48**	
935.1	Foreign body in esophagus **79**	
936	Foreign body in intestine and colon **79**	
934.1	Foreign body in main bronchus **54**	
935.0	Foreign body in mouth **4, 48**	
932	Foreign body in nose **48**	
934.8	Foreign body in other specified parts of trachea, bronchus, and lung **54**	
939.3	Foreign body in penis **124**	
933*	Foreign body in pharynx and larynx **4, 48**	
934.9	Foreign body in respiratory tree, unspecified **54**	
935.2	Foreign body in stomach **79**	
934.0	Foreign body in trachea **54**	
939.9	Foreign body in unspecified site in genitourinary tract **120**	
939.1	Foreign body in uterus, any part **128, 131**	
939.2	Foreign body in vulva and vagina **128, 131**	
930*	Foreign body on external eye **40**	
377.04	Foster-Kennedy syndrome **33**	
664.34	Fourth-degree perineal laceration, postpartum condition or complication **152**	
664.30	Fourth-degree perineal laceration, unspecified as to episode of care in pregnancy **137, 144, 150**	
664.31	Fourth-degree perineal laceration, with delivery **137, 144, 150**	
824*	Fracture of ankle **99**	
809.0	Fracture of bones of trunk, closed **101, 221**	
809.1	Fracture of bones of trunk, open **101, 221, 227**	
814*	Fracture of carpal bone(s) **99**	
810*	Fracture of clavicle **99**	

812*	Fracture of humerus **99**
815*	Fracture of metacarpal bone(s) **99**
820*	Fracture of neck of femur **96, 166, 170, 227**
826*	Fracture of one or more phalanges of foot **99**
816*	Fracture of one or more phalanges of hand **99**
821*	Fracture of other and unspecified parts of femur **96, 227**
822*	Fracture of patella **99**
808*	Fracture of pelvis **96, 227**
813*	Fracture of radius and ulna **99**
823*	Fracture of tibia and fibula **99**
829*	Fracture of unspecified bones **100**
806*	Fracture of vertebral column with spinal cord injury **19**
805*	Fracture of vertebral column without mention of spinal cord injury **98**
759.83	Fragile X syndrome **188**
788.4*	Frequency of urination and polyuria **119**
799.55	Frontal lobe and executive function deficit **188**
310.0	Frontal lobe syndrome **188**
331.1*	Frontotemporal dementia **19**
941.32	Full-thickness skin loss due to burn (third degree NOS) of eye (with other parts of face, head, and neck) **40**
941.3*	Full-thickness skin loss due to burn (third degree NOS) of face, head, and neck **206, 207, 208, 209**
945.3*	Full-thickness skin loss due to burn (third degree NOS) of lower limb(s) **206, 207, 208, 209**
946.3	Full-thickness skin loss due to burn (third degree NOS) of multiple specified sites **206, 207, 208, 209**
942.3*	Full-thickness skin loss due to burn (third degree NOS) of trunk **206, 207, 208, 209**
943.3*	Full-thickness skin loss due to burn (third degree NOS) of upper limb, except wrist and hand **206, 207, 208, 209**
944.3*	Full-thickness skin loss due to burn (third degree NOS) of wrist(s) and hand(s) **206, 207, 208, 209**
949.3	Full-thickness skin loss due to burn (third degree NOS), unspecified site **206, 207, 208, 209**
564.5	Functional diarrhea **78**
288.1	Functional disorders of polymorphonuclear neutrophils **175**
429.4	Functional disturbances following cardiac surgery **69, 165, 169**
780.72	Functional quadriplegia **19**
676.60	Galactorrhea associated with childbirth, unspecified as to episode of care **161**
676.63	Galactorrhea, antepartum condition or complication **156, 158**
676.64	Galactorrhea, postpartum condition or complication **153**
676.62	Galactorrhea, with delivery, with mention of postpartum complication **139, 145, 151**
676.61	Galactorrhea, with delivery, with or without mention of antepartum condition **139, 145, 151**
271.1	Galactosemia **113**
086.3	Gambian trypanosomiasis **185**
727.4*	Ganglion and cyst of synovium, tendon, and bursa **99**
102.5	Gangosa due to yaws **2, 47**
785.4	Gangrene **67, 166, 170**
040.0	Gas gangrene **164, 168, 185**
537.1	Gastric diverticulum **78**
535.21	Gastric mucosal hypertrophy with hemorrhage **76**
535.20	Gastric mucosal hypertrophy without mention of hemorrhage **78**
531.91	Gastric ulcer, unspecified as acute or chronic, without mention of hemorrhage or perforation, with obstruction **77**
531.90	Gastric ulcer, unspecified as acute or chronic, without mention of hemorrhage, perforation, or obstruction **77**
558.1	Gastroenteritis and colitis due to radiation **79, 230**
558.3	Gastroenteritis and colitis, allergic **78**
530.7	Gastroesophageal laceration-hemorrhage syndrome **75**
022.2	Gastrointestinal anthrax **75**
578*	Gastrointestinal hemorrhage **76, 166, 170**
306.4	Gastrointestinal malfunction arising from mental factors **78**
538	Gastrointestinal mucositis (ulcerative) **78**
863.90	Gastrointestinal tract injury, unspecified site, with open wound into cavity **79**
863.80	Gastrointestinal tract injury, unspecified site, without mention of open wound into cavity **79**
534.9*	Gastrojejunal ulcer, unspecified as acute or chronic, without mention of hemorrhage or perforation **77**
536.3	Gastroparesis **78**
537.5	Gastroptosis **78**
756.73	Gastroschisis **166, 170**
536.4*	Gastrostomy complications **78**
V25.0*	General counseling and advice for contraceptive management **214**
V70*	General medical examination **215**
094.1	General paresis **19**
440.9	Generalized and unspecified atherosclerosis **66**
368.45	Generalized contraction or constriction in visual field **38**
780.8	Generalized hyperhidrosis **108, 231**
659.33	Generalized infection during labor, antepartum **155, 158**
659.31	Generalized infection during labor, delivered **136, 140, 146**
659.30	Generalized infection during labor, unspecified as to episode of care **136, 143, 149**
999.0	Generalized vaccinia as complication of medical care, not elsewhere classified **185**
653.13	Generally contracted pelvis in pregnancy, antepartum **154, 157**
653.11	Generally contracted pelvis in pregnancy, delivered **135, 142, 148**
653.10	Generally contracted pelvis in pregnancy, unspecified as to episode of care in pregnancy **160**
288.2	Genetic anomalies of leukocytes **175**
V26.3*	Genetic counseling and testing **214**
V84.0*	Genetic susceptibility to malignant neoplasm **215**
V84.8*	Genetic susceptibility to other disease **215**
333.6	Genetic torsion dystonia **19**
053.11	Geniculate herpes zoster **21, 164, 168, 229**
618*	Genital prolapse **127, 130**
091.0	Genital syphilis (primary) **124, 127, 129**
619.2	Genital tract-skin fistula, female **127, 130**
016.9*	Genitourinary tuberculosis, unspecified **119**
736.5	Genu recurvatum (acquired) **100**
736.4*	Genu valgum or varum (acquired) **100**
446.5	Giant cell arteritis **97**
727.02	Giant cell tumor of tendon sheath **100**
523*	Gingival and periodontal diseases **3, 48**
024	Glanders **185**
365.4*	Glaucoma associated with congenital anomalies, dystrophies, and systemic syndromes **39**
365.5*	Glaucoma associated with disorders of the lens **39**
365.6*	Glaucoma associated with other ocular disorders **39**
365.7*	Glaucoma stage **39**
377.14	Glaucomatous atrophy (cupping) of optic disc **40**
271.0	Glycogenosis **113**
791.5	Glycosuria **113**
758.6	Gonadal dysgenesis **124, 127, 130**
098.50	Gonococcal arthritis **97**
098.52	Gonococcal bursitis **97**
098.15	Gonococcal cervicitis (acute) **127, 129**

*Code Range © 2013 OptumInsight, Inc.

098.35	Gonococcal cervicitis, chronic **127, 129**	V20*	Health supervision of infant or child **214**
098.11	Gonococcal cystitis (acute) **119**	V20.1	Health supervision of other healthy infant or child receiving care **172**
098.31	Gonococcal cystitis, chronic **119**	389*	Hearing loss **47**
098.84	Gonococcal endocarditis **65**	428*	Heart failure **66**
098.16	Gonococcal endometritis (acute) **127, 129**	861.1*	Heart injury, with open wound into thorax **69**
098.36	Gonococcal endometritis, chronic **127, 129**	861.0*	Heart injury, without mention of open wound into thorax **69**
098.13	Gonococcal epididymo-orchitis (acute) **124**	V43.2*	Heart replaced by other means **69**
098.33	Gonococcal epididymo-orchitis, chronic **124**	V42.1	Heart replaced by transplant **69**
098.0	Gonococcal infection (acute) of lower genitourinary tract **124, 127, 129**	V43.3	Heart valve replaced by other means **69**
098.10	Gonococcal infection (acute) of upper genitourinary tract, site unspecified **124, 127, 129**	V42.2	Heart valve replaced by transplant **69**
		228.04	Hemangioma of intra-abdominal structures **78**
098.7	Gonococcal infection of anus and rectum **78**	228.02	Hemangioma of intracranial structures **32**
098.4*	Gonococcal infection of eye **38**	228.09	Hemangioma of other sites **3, 68**
098.89	Gonococcal infection of other specified sites **185**	228.03	Hemangioma of retina **38**
098.6	Gonococcal infection of pharynx **2, 46**	228.01	Hemangioma of skin and subcutaneous tissue **3, 108**
098.2	Gonococcal infections, chronic, of lower genitourinary tract **124, 127, 129**	228.00	Hemangioma of unspecified site **3, 68**
		719.1*	Hemarthrosis **98**
098.81	Gonococcal keratosis (blennorrhagica) **38**	629.0	Hematocele, female, not elsewhere classified **130**
098.82	Gonococcal meningitis **9, 10, 33**	998.12	Hematoma complicating a procedure **167, 171**
098.83	Gonococcal pericarditis **68**	620.7	Hematoma of broad ligament **166, 170**
098.86	Gonococcal peritonitis **75**	599.7*	Hematuria **119, 166, 170**
098.12	Gonococcal prostatitis (acute) **124**	342*	Hemiplegia and hemiparesis **19**
098.32	Gonococcal prostatitis, chronic **124**	343.1	Hemiplegic infantile cerebral palsy **19**
098.37	Gonococcal salpingitis (chronic) **127, 129**	756.14	Hemivertebra **98**
098.17	Gonococcal salpingitis, specified as acute **127, 129**	282.47	Hemoglobin E-beta thalassemia **164, 169**
098.14	Gonococcal seminal vesiculitis (acute) **124**	791.2	Hemoglobinuria **120**
098.34	Gonococcal seminal vesiculitis, chronic **124**	283.2	Hemoglobinuria due to hemolysis from external causes **164, 169, 175**
098.53	Gonococcal spondylitis **96**		
098.51	Gonococcal synovitis and tenosynovitis **97**	773.2	Hemolytic disease due to other and unspecified isoimmunization of fetus or newborn **163, 167**
274.8*	Gout with other specified manifestations **98**		
274.9	Gout, unspecified **98**	999.83	Hemolytic transfusion reaction, incompatibility unspecified **176**
274.0*	Gouty arthropathy **98**	283.11	Hemolytic-uremic syndrome **175**
274.10	Gouty nephropathy, unspecified **120**	423.0	Hemopericardium **165, 169**
279.5*	Graft-versus-host disease **175**	568.81	Hemoperitoneum (nontraumatic) **166, 170**
659.43	Grand multiparity with current pregnancy, antepartum **155, 158**	288.4	Hemophagocytic syndromes **176**
		786.3*	Hemoptysis **54**
659.40	Grand multiparity with current pregnancy, unspecified as to episode of care **161**	246.3	Hemorrhage and infarction of thyroid **3**
		998.11	Hemorrhage complicating a procedure **167, 171**
659.41	Grand multiparity, delivered, with or without mention of antepartum condition **136, 143, 149**	641.13	Hemorrhage from placenta previa, antepartum **154, 157**
		641.10	Hemorrhage from placenta previa, unspecified as to episode of care **159**
099.2	Granuloma inguinale **124, 127, 130**		
102.4	Gummata and ulcers due to yaws **107**	641.11	Hemorrhage from placenta previa, with delivery **134, 140, 145**
780.1	Hallucinations **188**	784.8	Hemorrhage from throat **3, 47**
074.3	Hand, foot, and mouth disease **184**	596.7	Hemorrhage into bladder wall **166, 170**
914.1	Hand(s) except finger(s) alone, abrasion or friction burn, infected **106**	569.3	Hemorrhage of rectum and anus **76, 166, 170**
		998.1*	Hemorrhage or hematoma or seroma complicating procedure, not elsewhere classified **204**
914.0	Hand(s) except finger(s) alone, abrasion or friction burn, without mention of infection **107**		
		776.0	Hemorrhagic disease of newborn **163, 167**
914.3	Hand(s) except finger(s) alone, blister, infected **106**	078.6	Hemorrhagic nephrosonephritis **119**
914.2	Hand(s) except finger(s) alone, blister, without mention of infection **108**	455*	Hemorrhoids **78**
		289.84	Heparin-induced thrombocytopenia [HIT] **164, 169, 176, 230**
914.5	Hand(s) except finger(s) alone, insect bite, nonvenomous, infected **106**	572.2	Hepatic encephalopathy **166, 170**
		573.4	Hepatic infarction **83, 166, 170**
914.4	Hand(s) except finger(s) alone, insect bite, nonvenomous, without mention of infection **108**	130.5	Hepatitis due to toxoplasmosis **83, 164, 168**
		573.2	Hepatitis in other infectious diseases classified elsewhere **83**
914.7	Hand(s) except finger(s) alone, superficial foreign body (splinter) without major open wound, infected **106**	573.1	Hepatitis in viral diseases classified elsewhere **83**
		789.1	Hepatomegaly **83, 231**
914.6	Hand(s) except finger(s) alone, superficial foreign body (splinter), without major open wound and without mention of infection **107**	573.5	Hepatopulmonary syndrome **54**
		572.4	Hepatorenal syndrome **166, 170**
784.0	Headache **34**		
V61.4*	Health problems within family **214**		

655.23	Hereditary disease in family possibly affecting fetus, affecting management of mother, antepartum condition or complication **155, 157**
655.20	Hereditary disease in family possibly affecting fetus, affecting management of mother, unspecified as to episode of care in pregnancy **160**
655.21	Hereditary disease in family possibly affecting fetus, affecting management of mother, with delivery **135, 143, 148**
757.0	Hereditary edema of legs **108**
271.2	Hereditary fructose intolerance **78**
282*	Hereditary hemolytic anemias **175**
448.0	Hereditary hemorrhagic telangiectasia **66**
377.16	Hereditary optic atrophy **38**
356.0	Hereditary peripheral neuropathy **21**
359.1	Hereditary progressive muscular dystrophy **32**
362.7*	Hereditary retinal dystrophies **39**
356.2	Hereditary sensory neuropathy **21**
552.8	Hernia of other specified site, with obstruction **78, 166, 170**
553.8	Hernia of other specified sites of abdominal cavity without mention of obstruction or gangrene **79**
551.8	Hernia of other specified sites, with gangrene **166, 170**
553.9	Hernia of unspecified site of abdominal cavity without mention of obstruction or gangrene **79**
551.9	Hernia of unspecified site, with gangrene **166, 170**
552.9	Hernia of unspecified site, with obstruction **78, 166, 170**
074.0	Herpangina **2, 46**
054.41	Herpes simplex dermatitis of eyelid **229**
054.43	Herpes simplex disciform keratitis **229**
054.44	Herpes simplex iridocyclitis **229**
054.72	Herpes simplex meningitis **8, 10, 21, 164, 168, 229**
054.74	Herpes simplex myelitis **8, 10, 33**
054.73	Herpes simplex otitis externa **47, 164, 168, 229**
054.4*	Herpes simplex with ophthalmic complications **38, 164, 168**
054.49	Herpes simplex with other ophthalmic complications **229**
054.9	Herpes simplex without mention of complication **107, 229**
053.20	Herpes zoster dermatitis of eyelid **164, 168, 229**
053.22	Herpes zoster iridocyclitis **164, 168, 229**
053.21	Herpes zoster keratoconjunctivitis **164, 168, 229**
053.14	Herpes zoster myelitis **8, 10, 33**
053.0	Herpes zoster with meningitis **21, 164, 168, 229**
053.2*	Herpes zoster with ophthalmic complications **38**
053.10	Herpes zoster with unspecified nervous system complication **21, 164, 168, 229**
053.9	Herpes zoster without mention of complication **105, 164, 168, 229**
054.2	Herpetic gingivostomatitis **2, 48, 164, 168, 229**
054.13	Herpetic infection of penis **124, 229**
054.3	Herpetic meningoencephalitis **8, 10, 33, 164, 168, 229**
054.5	Herpetic septicemia **164, 168, 186, 229**
054.12	Herpetic ulceration of vulva **127, 129, 229**
054.11	Herpetic vulvovaginitis **127, 129, 229**
054.6	Herpetic whitlow **107, 229**
368.47	Heteronymous bilateral field defects in visual field **38**
378.4*	Heterophoria **40**
121.6	Heterophyiasis **185**
786.8	Hiccough **54**
327.22	High altitude periodic breathing **54**
652.53	High fetal head at term, antepartum **154, 157**
652.51	High fetal head at term, delivered **135, 142, 148**
652.50	High fetal head at term, unspecified as to episode of care **160**
238.73	High grade myelodysplastic syndrome lesions **175**

665.44	High vaginal laceration, postpartum condition or complication **152**
665.40	High vaginal laceration, unspecified as to episode of care in pregnancy **137, 144, 150**
665.41	High vaginal laceration, with delivery **137, 144, 150**
916.1	Hip, thigh, leg, and ankle, abrasion or friction burn, infected **106**
916.0	Hip, thigh, leg, and ankle, abrasion or friction burn, without mention of infection **107**
916.3	Hip, thigh, leg, and ankle, blister, infected **106**
916.2	Hip, thigh, leg, and ankle, blister, without mention of infection **108**
916.5	Hip, thigh, leg, and ankle, insect bite, nonvenomous, infected **106**
916.4	Hip, thigh, leg, and ankle, insect bite, nonvenomous, without mention of infection **108**
916.6	Hip, thigh, leg, and ankle, superficial foreign body (splinter), without major open wound and without mention of infection **107**
916.7	Hip, thigh, leg, and ankle, superficial foreign body (splinter), without major open wound, infected **106**
751.3	Hirschsprung's disease and other congenital functional disorders of colon **79**
115.04	Histoplasma capsulatum endocarditis **65, 164, 168**
115.01	Histoplasma capsulatum meningitis **9, 10, 34, 164, 168**
115.03	Histoplasma capsulatum pericarditis **68, 164, 168**
115.05	Histoplasma capsulatum pneumonia **51, 164, 168**
115.02	Histoplasma capsulatum retinitis **38, 164, 168**
115.09	Histoplasma capsulatum, with mention of other manifestation **185**
115.00	Histoplasma capsulatum, without mention of manifestation **185**
115.14	Histoplasma duboisii endocarditis **65, 164, 168**
115.11	Histoplasma duboisii meningitis **9, 10, 34, 164, 168**
115.13	Histoplasma duboisii pericarditis **68, 164, 168**
115.15	Histoplasma duboisii pneumonia **51, 164, 168**
115.12	Histoplasma duboisii retinitis **38, 164, 168**
115.19	Histoplasma duboisii with mention of other manifestation **185**
115.10	Histoplasma duboisii, without mention of manifestation **185**
115*	Histoplasmosis **230**
301.5*	Histrionic personality disorder **188**
201*	Hodgkin's disease **178, 181**
201.71	Hodgkin's disease, lymphocytic depletion, of lymph nodes of head, face, and neck **2**
201.41	Hodgkin's disease, lymphocytic-histiocytic predominance of lymph nodes of head, face, and neck **2**
201.61	Hodgkin's disease, mixed cellularity, involving lymph nodes of head, face, and neck **2**
201.51	Hodgkin's disease, nodular sclerosis, of lymph nodes of head, face, and neck **2**
201.91	Hodgkin's disease, unspecified type, of lymph nodes of head, face, and neck **2**
201.11	Hodgkin's granuloma of lymph nodes of head, face, and neck **2**
201.01	Hodgkin's paragranuloma of lymph nodes of head, face, and neck **2**
201.21	Hodgkin's sarcoma of lymph nodes of head, face, and neck **2**
V62.85	Homicidal ideation **214**
368.46	Homonymous bilateral field defects in visual field **38**
537.6	Hourglass stricture or stenosis of stomach **78**
V60*	Housing, household, and economic circumstances **214**
058.21	Human herpesvirus 6 encephalitis **9, 10, 33, 164, 168, 229**
042	Human immunodeficiency virus [HIV] **229, 230**
275.5	Hungry bone syndrome **113**
333.4	Huntington's chorea **19**
630	Hydatidiform mole **154, 157**

*Code Range

629.1	Hydrocele, canal of Nuck **130**
653.63	Hydrocephalic fetus causing disproportion, antepartum **154, 157**
653.61	Hydrocephalic fetus causing disproportion, delivered **135, 142, 148**
653.60	Hydrocephalic fetus causing disproportion, unspecified as to episode of care **160**
591	Hydronephrosis **119, 166, 170**
773.3	Hydrops fetalis due to isoimmunization **163, 167**
778.0	Hydrops fetalis not due to isoimmunization **163, 168**
593.5	Hydroureter **119, 166, 170**
123.6	Hymenolepiasis **75**
388.42	Hyperacusis **47**
278.3	Hypercarotinemia **113**
643.13	Hyperemesis gravidarum with metabolic disturbance, antepartum **154, 156**
643.11	Hyperemesis gravidarum with metabolic disturbance, delivered **134, 141, 147**
643.10	Hyperemesis gravidarum with metabolic disturbance, unspecified as to episode of care **156, 159**
102.3	Hyperkeratosis due to yaws **107**
429.82	Hyperkinetic heart disease **69, 165, 169**
314*	Hyperkinetic syndrome of childhood **189**
367.0	Hypermetropia **39**
728.5	Hypermobility syndrome **99**
733.3	Hyperostosis of skull **100**
374.52	Hyperpigmentation of eyelid **39**
600*	Hyperplasia of prostate **123**
447.3	Hyperplasia of renal artery **120**
446.2*	Hypersensitivity angiitis **97**
780.53	Hypersomnia with sleep apnea, unspecified **3, 47**
780.54	Hypersomnia, unspecified **189**
289.4	Hypersplenism **176, 230**
642.13	Hypertension secondary to renal disease, antepartum **154, 156**
642.14	Hypertension secondary to renal disease, complicating pregnancy, childbirth, and the puerperium, postpartum condition or complication **151**
642.10	Hypertension secondary to renal disease, complicating pregnancy, childbirth, and the puerperium, unspecified as to episode of care **159**
642.11	Hypertension secondary to renal disease, with delivery **134, 140, 145**
642.12	Hypertension secondary to renal disease, with delivery, with current postpartum complication **134, 140, 146**
403.10	Hypertensive chronic kidney disease, benign, with chronic kidney disease stage I through stage IV, or unspecified **118**
403.11	Hypertensive chronic kidney disease, benign, with chronic kidney disease stage V or end stage renal disease **2, 118**
403.00	Hypertensive chronic kidney disease, malignant, with chronic kidney disease stage I through stage IV, or unspecified **118**
403.01	Hypertensive chronic kidney disease, malignant, with chronic kidney disease stage V or end stage renal disease **2, 118**
403.90	Hypertensive chronic kidney disease, unspecified, with chronic kidney disease stage I through stage IV, or unspecified **118**
403.91	Hypertensive chronic kidney disease, unspecified, with chronic kidney disease stage V or end stage renal disease **2, 118**
437.2	Hypertensive encephalopathy **21**
404.13	Hypertensive heart and chronic kidney disease, benign, with heart failure and chronic kidney disease stage V or end stage renal disease **2, 56, 66, 165, 169**
404.11	Hypertensive heart and chronic kidney disease, benign, with heart failure and with chronic kidney disease stage I through stage IV, or unspecified **56, 66, 165, 169**

404.10	Hypertensive heart and chronic kidney disease, benign, without heart failure and with chronic kidney disease stage I through stage IV, or unspecified **67**
404.12	Hypertensive heart and chronic kidney disease, benign, without heart failure and with chronic kidney disease stage V or end stage renal disease **2, 118**
404.01	Hypertensive heart and chronic kidney disease, malignant, with heart failure and with chronic kidney disease stage I through stage IV, or unspecified **56, 66, 165, 169**
404.03	Hypertensive heart and chronic kidney disease, malignant, with heart failure and with chronic kidney disease stage V or end stage renal disease **2, 56, 66, 165, 169**
404.00	Hypertensive heart and chronic kidney disease, malignant, without heart failure and with chronic kidney disease stage I through stage IV, or unspecified **67**
404.02	Hypertensive heart and chronic kidney disease, malignant, without heart failure and with chronic kidney disease stage V or end stage renal disease **2, 118**
404.93	Hypertensive heart and chronic kidney disease, unspecified, with heart failure and chronic kidney disease stage V or end stage renal disease **2, 56, 66, 165, 169**
404.91	Hypertensive heart and chronic kidney disease, unspecified, with heart failure and with chronic kidney disease stage I through stage IV, or unspecified **56, 66, 165, 169**
404.90	Hypertensive heart and chronic kidney disease, unspecified, without heart failure and with chronic kidney disease stage I through stage IV, or unspecified **67**
404.92	Hypertensive heart and chronic kidney disease, unspecified, without heart failure and with chronic kidney disease stage V or end stage renal disease **2, 118**
402.91	Hypertensive heart disease, unspecified, with heart failure **56, 66, 165, 169**
661.43	Hypertonic, incoordinate, or prolonged uterine contractions, antepartum **155, 158**
661.40	Hypertonic, incoordinate, or prolonged uterine contractions, unspecified as to episode of care **136, 144, 149**
661.41	Hypertonic, incoordinate, or prolonged uterine contractions, with delivery **136, 144, 149**
374.54	Hypertrichosis of eyelid **39**
593.1	Hypertrophy of kidney **120**
478.0	Hypertrophy of nasal turbinates **47**
474.1*	Hypertrophy of tonsils and adenoids **47**
278.2	Hypervitaminosis A **113**
278.4	Hypervitaminosis D **113**
364.41	Hyphema **39**
775.4	Hypocalcemia and hypomagnesemia of newborn **163, 167**
300.7	Hypochondriasis **188**
251.2	Hypoglycemia, unspecified **113**
251.0	Hypoglycemic coma **113, 164, 168**
252.1	Hypoparathyroidism **164, 168**
374.53	Hypopigmentation of eyelid **39**
746.7	Hypoplastic left heart syndrome **68**
370.04	Hypopyon ulcer **38**
752.6*	Hypospadias and epispadias and other penile anomalies **124**
780.65	Hypothermia not associated with low environmental temperature **213**
360.3*	Hypotony of eye **39**
374.55	Hypotrichosis of eyelid **39**
300.10	Hysteria, unspecified **188**
277.83	Iatrogenic carnitine deficiency **114**
458.2*	Iatrogenic hypotension **68**
512.1	Iatrogenic pneumothorax **53**
757.1	Ichthyosis congenita **108**
516.30	Idiopathic interstitial pneumonia, not otherwise specified **230**

516.35	Idiopathic lymphoid interstitial pneumonia **230**
331.5	Idiopathic normal pressure hydrocephalus [INPH] **19**
356.4	Idiopathic progressive polyneuropathy **21**
327.24	Idiopathic sleep related nonobstructive alveolar hypoventilation **47**
341.22	Idiopathic transverse myelitis **10**
818.0	Ill-defined closed fractures of upper limb **221**
818*	Ill-defined fractures of upper limb **99**
009*	Ill-defined intestinal infections **77**, **230**
818.1	Ill-defined open fractures of upper limb **221**, **227**
636*	Illegally induced abortion **153**
V61.6	Illegitimacy or illegitimate pregnancy **156**, **159**
380.4	Impacted cerumen **47**
560.39	Impaction of intestine, other **166**, **170**
388.43	Impairment of auditory discrimination **47**
684	Impetigo **106**
694.3	Impetigo herpetiformis **108**
607.84	Impotence of organic origin **124**
312.30	Impulse control disorder, unspecified **189**
799.23	Impulsiveness **188**
752.7	Indeterminate sex and pseudohermaphroditism **124**, **127**, **130**
040.41	Infant botulism **164**, **168**, **185**
343.4	Infantile hemiplegia **19**
603.1	Infected hydrocele **124**
998.51	Infected postoperative seroma **167**, **171**, **184**
996.61	Infection and inflammatory reaction due to cardiac device, implant, and graft **69**
996.64	Infection and inflammatory reaction due to indwelling urinary catheter **120**
996.66	Infection and inflammatory reaction due to internal joint prosthesis **90**, **99**
996.63	Infection and inflammatory reaction due to nervous system device, implant, and graft **33**
996.65	Infection and inflammatory reaction due to other genitourinary device, implant, and graft **120**
996.67	Infection and inflammatory reaction due to other internal orthopedic device, implant, and graft **90**, **99**
996.69	Infection and inflammatory reaction due to other internal prosthetic device, implant, and graft **203**
996.62	Infection and inflammatory reaction due to other vascular device, implant, and graft **69**
996.68	Infection and inflammatory reaction due to peritoneal dialysis catheter **203**
996.60	Infection and inflammatory reaction due to unspecified device, implant, and graft **203**
658.43	Infection of amniotic cavity, antepartum **155**, **158**
658.41	Infection of amniotic cavity, delivered **136**, **143**, **149**
658.40	Infection of amniotic cavity, unspecified as to episode of care **136**, **143**, **149**
530.86	Infection of esophagostomy **78**
675.02	Infection of nipple associated with childbirth, delivered with mention of postpartum complication **139**, **141**, **147**
675.01	Infection of nipple associated with childbirth, delivered, with or without mention of antepartum condition **139**, **141**, **147**
675.00	Infection of nipple associated with childbirth, unspecified as to episode of care **161**
675.03	Infection of nipple, antepartum **156**, **158**
675.04	Infection of nipple, postpartum condition or complication **153**
V09*	Infection with drug-resistant microorganisms **186**
646.63	Infections of genitourinary tract antepartum **154**, **156**
646.64	Infections of genitourinary tract in pregnancy, postpartum condition or complication **152**

646.60	Infections of genitourinary tract in pregnancy, unspecified as to episode of care **156**, **159**
646.61	Infections of genitourinary tract in pregnancy, with delivery **134**, **141**, **147**
646.62	Infections of genitourinary tract in pregnancy, with delivery, with current postpartum complication **134**, **141**, **147**
590*	Infections of kidney **119**
323.61	Infectious acute disseminated encephalomyelitis [ADEM] **10**
075	Infectious mononucleosis **184**
728.0	Infective myositis **99**
380.1*	Infective otitis externa **47**
379.6*	Inflammation (infection) of postprocedural bleb **40**
373*	Inflammation of eyelids **39**
359.7*	Inflammatory and immune myopathies, NEC **97**
614*	Inflammatory disease of ovary, fallopian tube, pelvic cellular tissue, and peritoneum **127**
601*	Inflammatory diseases of prostate **124**
615*	Inflammatory diseases of uterus, except cervix **127**, **130**
488.19	Influenza due to identified 2009 H1N1 influenza virus with other manifestations **185**
488.12	Influenza due to identified 2009 H1N1 influenza virus with other respiratory manifestations **53**, **165**, **169**
488.11	Influenza due to identified 2009 H1N1 influenza virus with pneumonia **53**, **165**, **169**, **230**
488.09	Influenza due to identified avian influenza virus with other manifestations **185**
488.02	Influenza due to identified avian influenza virus with other respiratory manifestations **53**, **165**, **169**
488.01	Influenza due to identified avian influenza virus with pneumonia **53**, **165**, **169**, **230**
488.89	Influenza due to identified novel influenza A virus with other manifestations **185**
488.82	Influenza due to identified novel influenza A virus with other respiratory manifestations **53**, **165**, **169**
488.81	Influenza due to identified novel influenza A virus with pneumonia **53**, **165**, **169**, **230**
487.8	Influenza with other manifestations **185**
487.1	Influenza with other respiratory manifestations **46**
487.0	Influenza with pneumonia **51**, **53**
840.3	Infraspinatus (muscle) (tendon) sprain and strain **222**
550*	Inguinal hernia **78**
550.02	Inguinal hernia with gangrene, bilateral **166**, **170**
550.00	Inguinal hernia with gangrene, unilateral or unspecified, (not specified as recurrent) **166**, **170**
550.12	Inguinal hernia with obstruction, without mention gangrene, bilateral, (not specified as recurrent) **166**, **170**
550.10	Inguinal hernia with obstruction, without mention of gangrene, unilateral or unspecified, (not specified as recurrent) **166**, **170**
102.0	Initial lesions of yaws **107**
951.3	Injury to abducens nerve **21**
951.6	Injury to accessory nerve **21**
951.5	Injury to acoustic nerve **48**
955.0	Injury to axillary nerve **223**, **227**
902*	Injury to blood vessels of abdomen and pelvis **203**, **223**, **227**
900*	Injury to blood vessels of head and neck **203**
904*	Injury to blood vessels of lower extremity and unspecified sites **203**
901*	Injury to blood vessels of thorax **203**
903*	Injury to blood vessels of upper extremity **203**, **223**, **227**
904.9	Injury to blood vessels, unspecified site **223**
953.4	Injury to brachial plexus **166**, **170**, **223**, **227**
900.0*	Injury to carotid artery **166**, **170**, **223**

*Code Range

© 2013 OptumInsight, Inc.

954.0	Injury to cervical sympathetic nerve, excluding shoulder and pelvic girdles **223**
863.5*	Injury to colon or rectum with open wound into cavity **79**, **223**, **227**
956.4	Injury to cutaneous sensory nerve, lower limb **224**
955.5	Injury to cutaneous sensory nerve, upper limb **223**
955.6	Injury to digital nerve, upper limb **223**
953.1	Injury to dorsal nerve root **223**
951.4	Injury to facial nerve **21**
956.1	Injury to femoral nerve **224**, **227**
861*	Injury to heart and lung **222**, **226**
951.7	Injury to hypoglossal nerve **21**
866*	Injury to kidney **120**, **223**, **227**
864*	Injury to liver **83**, **227**
953.2	Injury to lumbar nerve root **223**
953.5	Injury to lumbosacral plexus **223**, **227**
955.1	Injury to median nerve **223**, **227**
862.9	Injury to multiple and unspecified intrathoracic organs with open wound into cavity **202**
862.8	Injury to multiple and unspecified intrathoracic organs without mention of open wound into cavity **202**
900.82	Injury to multiple blood vessels of head and neck **4**, **226**
901.83	Injury to multiple blood vessels of thorax **226**
956.8	Injury to multiple nerves of pelvic girdle and lower limb **224**, **228**
955.8	Injury to multiple nerves of shoulder girdle and upper limb **224**, **227**
953.8	Injury to multiple sites of nerve roots and spinal plexus **223**, **227**
955.4	Injury to musculocutaneous nerve **223**
953*	Injury to nerve roots and spinal plexus **21**, **223**
951.0	Injury to oculomotor nerve **21**
950.1	Injury to optic chiasm **33**
950*	Injury to optic nerve and pathways **223**
950.2	Injury to optic pathways **33**
868.09	Injury to other and multiple intra-abdominal organs without mention of open wound into cavity **202**, **227**
868.19	Injury to other and multiple intra-abdominal organs, with open wound into cavity **202**, **227**
863.99	Injury to other and unspecified gastrointestinal sites with open wound into cavity **79**
863.8*	Injury to other and unspecified gastrointestinal sites without mention of open wound into cavity **223**
863.89	Injury to other and unspecified gastrointestinal sites without mention of open wound into cavity **79**, **227**
863.9*	Injury to other and unspecified gastrointestinal sites, with open wound into cavity **223**, **227**
862*	Injury to other and unspecified intrathoracic organs **222**, **226**
957*	Injury to other and unspecified nerves **21**, **224**
951*	Injury to other cranial nerve(s) **223**
868.1*	Injury to other intra-abdominal organs with open wound into cavity **223**
868.0*	Injury to other intra-abdominal organs without mention of open wound into cavity **223**
954*	Injury to other nerve(s) of trunk, excluding shoulder and pelvic girdles **21**
900.8*	Injury to other specified blood vessels of head and neck **223**
900.89	Injury to other specified blood vessels of head and neck **4**
901.8*	Injury to other specified blood vessels of thorax **223**
951.8	Injury to other specified cranial nerves **21**
862.39	Injury to other specified intrathoracic organs with open wound into cavity **54**
862.29	Injury to other specified intrathoracic organs without mention of open wound into cavity **54**

956.5	Injury to other specified nerve(s) of pelvic girdle and lower limb **224**
955.7	Injury to other specified nerve(s) of shoulder girdle and upper limb **223**
954.8	Injury to other specified nerve(s) of trunk, excluding shoulder and pelvic girdles **223**, **227**
867.7	Injury to other specified pelvic organs with open wound into cavity **124**, **127**, **130**
867.6	Injury to other specified pelvic organs without mention of open wound into cavity **124**, **127**, **130**
954.1	Injury to other sympathetic nerve, excluding shoulder and pelvic girdles **223**
867*	Injury to pelvic organs **223**, **227**
956*	Injury to peripheral nerve(s) of pelvic girdle and lower limb **21**
955*	Injury to peripheral nerve(s) of shoulder girdle and upper limb **21**
956.3	Injury to peroneal nerve **224**, **228**
956.2	Injury to posterior tibial nerve **224**, **228**
955.3	Injury to radial nerve **223**, **227**
953.3	Injury to sacral nerve root **223**
956.0	Injury to sciatic nerve **224**, **227**
904.7	Injury to specified blood vessels of lower extremity, other **223**, **227**
901.89	Injury to specified blood vessels of thorax, other **226**
767.4	Injury to spine and spinal cord, birth trauma **163**, **167**
865*	Injury to spleen **166**, **170**, **176**, **223**, **227**
951.2	Injury to trigeminal nerve **21**
951.1	Injury to trochlear nerve **21**
955.2	Injury to ulnar nerve **223**, **227**
900.9	Injury to unspecified blood vessel of head and neck **4**, **223**
904.8	Injury to unspecified blood vessel of lower extremity **223**
901.9	Injury to unspecified blood vessel of thorax **223**, **226**
951.9	Injury to unspecified cranial nerve **21**
868.00	Injury to unspecified intra-abdominal organ without mention of open wound into cavity **79**
868.10	Injury to unspecified intra-abdominal organ, with open wound into cavity **79**
956.9	Injury to unspecified nerve of pelvic girdle and lower limb **224**, **228**
955.9	Injury to unspecified nerve of shoulder girdle and upper limb **224**
954.9	Injury to unspecified nerve of trunk, excluding shoulder and pelvic girdles **223**, **227**
950.9	Injury to unspecified optic nerve and pathways **33**
867.9	Injury to unspecified pelvic organ with open wound into cavity **124**, **127**, **130**
867.8	Injury to unspecified pelvic organ without mention of open wound into cavity **124**, **127**, **130**
953.9	Injury to unspecified site of nerve roots and spinal plexus **223**
950.3	Injury to visual cortex **33**
959*	Injury, other and unspecified **203**
959.3	Injury, other and unspecified, elbow, forearm, and wrist **224**
959.5	Injury, other and unspecified, finger **224**
959.4	Injury, other and unspecified, hand, except finger **224**
959.0*	Injury, other and unspecified, head, face, and neck **4**, **224**
959.6	Injury, other and unspecified, hip and thigh **224**
959.7	Injury, other and unspecified, knee, leg, ankle, and foot **224**
959.8	Injury, other and unspecified, other specified sites, including multiple **224**
959.2	Injury, other and unspecified, shoulder and upper arm **224**
959.1*	Injury, other and unspecified, trunk **224**
959.9	Injury, other and unspecified, unspecified site **224**
653.23	Inlet contraction of pelvis in pregnancy, antepartum **154**, **157**
653.21	Inlet contraction of pelvis in pregnancy, delivered **135**, **142**, **148**

653.20	Inlet contraction of pelvis in pregnancy, unspecified as to episode of care in pregnancy **160**	
901.1	Innominate and subclavian artery injury **166**, **170**, **223**, **226**	
901.3	Innominate and subclavian vein injury **166**, **170**, **223**, **226**	
V25.5	Insertion of implantable subdermal contraceptive **214**	
780.51	Insomnia with sleep apnea, unspecified **3**, **47**	
780.52	Insomnia, unspecified **189**	
798.1	Instantaneous death **66**	
V23.7	Insufficient prenatal care **161**	
411.1	Intermediate coronary syndrome **68**	
103.1	Intermediate lesions of pinta **107**	
376.34	Intermittent exophthalmos **38**	
312.34	Intermittent explosive disorder **188**	
378.2*	Intermittent heterotropia **40**	
900.03	Internal carotid artery injury **226**	
869*	Internal injury to unspecified or ill-defined organs **202**, **223**	
900.1	Internal jugular vein injury **166**, **170**, **223**, **226**	
378.86	Internuclear ophthalmoplegia **33**	
V62.81	Interpersonal problem, not elsewhere classified **214**	
518.1	Interstitial emphysema **53**, **165**, **170**	
770.2	Interstitial emphysema and related conditions of newborn **163**, **167**	
516.6*	Interstitial lung diseases of childhood **165**, **170**	
728.81	Interstitial myositis **99**	
722*	Intervertebral disc disorders **97**	
V45.3	Intestinal bypass or anastomosis status **214**	
271.3	Intestinal disaccharidase deficiencies and disaccharide malabsorption **78**	
008.2	Intestinal infection due to aerobacter aerogenes **75**	
008.1	Intestinal infection due to Arizona group of paracolon bacilli **75**	
008.04	Intestinal infection due to enterohemorrhagic E. coli **75**	
008.03	Intestinal infection due to enteroinvasive E. coli **75**	
008.01	Intestinal infection due to enteropathogenic E. coli **75**	
008.02	Intestinal infection due to enterotoxigenic E. coli **75**	
008.09	Intestinal infection due to other intestinal E. coli infections **75**	
008.8	Intestinal infection due to other organism, NEC **77**	
008.49	Intestinal infection due to other organisms **75**	
008.5	Intestinal infection due to unspecified bacterial enteritis **75**	
008.00	Intestinal infection due to unspecified E. coli **75**	
008.6*	Intestinal infection, enteritis due to specified virus **77**	
008.43	Intestinal infections due to campylobacter **75**	
008.45	Intestinal infections due to clostridium difficile **75**	
008.46	Intestinal infections due to other anaerobes **75**	
008.47	Intestinal infections due to other gram-negative bacteria **75**	
008.3	Intestinal infections due to proteus (mirabilis) (morganii) **75**	
008.42	Intestinal infections due to pseudomonas **75**	
008.41	Intestinal infections due to staphylococcus **75**	
008.44	Intestinal infections due to yersinia enterocolitica **75**	
579*	Intestinal malabsorption **78**	
560*	Intestinal obstruction without mention of hernia **77**	
596.1	Intestinovesical fistula **166**, **170**	
431	Intracerebral hemorrhage **8**, **9**, **10**, **20**, **165**, **169**	
324*	Intracranial and intraspinal abscess **9**, **10**, **33**, **165**, **169**	
854*	Intracranial injury of other and unspecified nature **222**, **226**	
854.1*	Intracranial injury of other and unspecified nature with open intracranial wound **9**, **11**	
854.12	Intracranial injury of other and unspecified nature, with open intracranial wound, brief (less than 1 hour) loss of consciousness **31**	

854.16	Intracranial injury of other and unspecified nature, with open intracranial wound, loss of consciousness of unspecified duration **27**
854.13	Intracranial injury of other and unspecified nature, with open intracranial wound, moderate (1-24 hours) loss of consciousness **27**
854.11	Intracranial injury of other and unspecified nature, with open intracranial wound, no loss of consciousness **31**
854.14	Intracranial injury of other and unspecified nature, with open intracranial wound, prolonged (more than 24 hours) loss of consciousness and return to pre-existing conscious level **27**
854.15	Intracranial injury of other and unspecified nature, with open intracranial wound, prolonged (more than 24 hours) loss of consciousness, without return to pre-existing conscious level **27**
854.10	Intracranial injury of other and unspecified nature, with open intracranial wound, unspecified state of consciousness **31**
854.19	Intracranial injury of other and unspecified nature, with open intracranial wound, with unspecified concussion **31**
854.02	Intracranial injury of other and unspecified nature, without mention of open intracranial wound, brief (less than 1 hour) loss of consciousness **31**
854.06	Intracranial injury of other and unspecified nature, without mention of open intracranial wound, loss of consciousness of unspecified duration **27**
854.03	Intracranial injury of other and unspecified nature, without mention of open intracranial wound, moderate (1-24 hours) loss of consciousness **27**
854.01	Intracranial injury of other and unspecified nature, without mention of open intracranial wound, no loss of consciousness **31**
854.04	Intracranial injury of other and unspecified nature, without mention of open intracranial wound, prolonged (more than 24 hours) loss of consciousness and return to pre-existing conscious level **27**
854.05	Intracranial injury of other and unspecified nature, without mention of open intracranial wound, prolonged (more than 24 hours) loss of consciousness, without return to pre-existing conscious level **27**
854.09	Intracranial injury of other and unspecified nature, without mention of open intracranial wound, unspecified concussion **31**
854.00	Intracranial injury of other and unspecified nature, without mention of open intracranial wound, unspecified state of consciousness **31**
656.43	Intrauterine death affecting management of mother, antepartum **155**, **157**
656.41	Intrauterine death affecting management of mother, delivered **136**, **143**, **149**
656.40	Intrauterine death affecting management of mother, unspecified as to episode of care **136**, **143**, **149**
772.1*	Intraventricular hemorrhage **163**, **167**
493.1*	Intrinsic asthma **53**
493.11	Intrinsic asthma with status asthmaticus **165**, **169**
560.0	Intussusception **166**, **170**
665.22	Inversion of uterus, delivered with postpartum complication **137**, **144**, **150**
665.24	Inversion of uterus, postpartum condition or complication **152**
665.20	Inversion of uterus, unspecified as to episode of care in pregnancy **137**, **144**, **150**
V26.2*	Investigation and testing for procreation management **214**
280*	Iron deficiency anemias **175**, **230**
595.82	Irradiation cystitis **120**
799.22	Irritability **188**
564.1	Irritable bowel syndrome **78**
656.23	Isoimmunization from other and unspecified blood-group incompatibility, affecting management of mother, antepartum **155**, **157**

*Code Range

© 2013 OptumInsight, Inc.

656.21	Isoimmunization from other and unspecified blood-group incompatibility, affecting management of mother, delivered **136, 143, 149**	905.5	Late effect of fracture of multiple and unspecified bones **99**
		905.3	Late effect of fracture of neck of femur **99**
656.20	Isoimmunization from other and unspecified blood-group incompatibility, unspecified as to episode of care in pregnancy **160**	905.0	Late effect of fracture of skull and face bones **33**
		905.1	Late effect of fracture of spine and trunk without mention of spinal cord lesion **98**
312.35	Isolated explosive disorder **188**	905.2	Late effect of fracture of upper extremities **99**
012.2*	Isolated tracheal or bronchial tuberculosis **51**	908.3	Late effect of injury to blood vessel of head, neck, and extremities **67**
782.4	Jaundice, unspecified, not of newborn **83**		
784.92	Jaw pain **3, 48**	908.4	Late effect of injury to blood vessel of thorax, abdomen, and pelvis **67**
V43.6*	Joint replaced by other means **101**		
714.3*	Juvenile chronic polyarthritis **97**	907.1	Late effect of injury to cranial nerve **33**
694.2	Juvenile dermatitis herpetiformis **108**	907.3	Late effect of injury to nerve root(s), spinal plexus(es), and other nerves of trunk **33**
090.4*	Juvenile neurosyphilis **34**		
732.0	Juvenile osteochondrosis of spine **87**	907.9	Late effect of injury to other and unspecified nerve **33**
176*	Kaposi's sarcoma **230**	907.5	Late effect of injury to peripheral nerve of pelvic girdle and lower limb **33**
176.3	Kaposi's sarcoma of gastrointestinal sites **76**		
176.4	Kaposi's sarcoma of lung **52**	907.4	Late effect of injury to peripheral nerve of shoulder girdle and upper limb **33**
176.5	Kaposi's sarcoma of lymph nodes **178, 181**		
176.8	Kaposi's sarcoma of other specified sites **108**	908.0	Late effect of internal injury to chest **54**
176.2	Kaposi's sarcoma of palate **2, 46**	908.1	Late effect of internal injury to intra-abdominal organs **79**
176.0	Kaposi's sarcoma of skin **108**	908.2	Late effect of internal injury to other internal organs **124, 127, 131**
176.1	Kaposi's sarcoma of soft tissue **108**		
176.9	Kaposi's sarcoma of unspecified site **108**	907.0	Late effect of intracranial injury without mention of skull fracture **33**
773.4	Kernicterus due to isoimmunization of fetus or newborn **163, 167**		
		907.2	Late effect of spinal cord injury **19**
774.7	Kernicterus of fetus or newborn not due to isoimmunization **163, 167**	905.7	Late effect of sprain and strain without mention of tendon injury **100**
V59.4	Kidney donor **120**	905.8	Late effect of tendon injury **99**
V42.0	Kidney replaced by transplant **2, 120**	905.9	Late effect of traumatic amputation **99**
312.32	Kleptomania **188**	908.9	Late effect of unspecified injury **203**
758.7	Klinefelter's syndrome **124**	138	Late effects of acute poliomyelitis **32**
756.16	Klippel-Feil syndrome **100**	137.1	Late effects of central nervous system tuberculosis **32**
260	Kwashiorkor **113, 230**	438*	Late effects of cerebrovascular disease **19**
737.3*	Kyphoscoliosis and scoliosis **87**	137.2	Late effects of genitourinary tuberculosis **119**
416.1	Kyphoscoliotic heart disease **69**	906*	Late effects of injuries to skin and subcutaneous tissues **107**
737.1*	Kyphosis (acquired) **87**	326	Late effects of intracranial abscess or pyogenic infection **32**
386.5*	Labyrinthine dysfunction **46**	909*	Late effects of other and unspecified external causes **204**
386.4*	Labyrinthine fistula **47**	139.8	Late effects of other and unspecified infectious and parasitic diseases **186**
386.3*	Labyrinthitis **46**		
665.34	Laceration of cervix, postpartum condition or complication **152**	137.0	Late effects of respiratory or unspecified tuberculosis **53**
665.30	Laceration of cervix, unspecified as to episode of care in pregnancy **137, 144, 150**	139.1	Late effects of trachoma **38**
		137.3	Late effects of tuberculosis of bones and joints **100**
665.31	Laceration of cervix, with delivery **137, 144, 150**	137.4	Late effects of tuberculosis of other specified organs **186**
781.3	Lack of coordination **33**	139.0	Late effects of viral encephalitis **32**
783.4*	Lack of expected normal physiological development **231**	766.2*	Late infant, not "heavy-for-dates" **171, 172**
374.2*	Lagophthalmos **39**	103.2	Late lesions of pinta **185**
358.3*	Lambert-Eaton syndrome **19**	775.7	Late metabolic acidosis of newborn **163, 167**
200.7*	Large cell lymphoma **230**	096	Late syphilis, latent **185**
032.3	Laryngeal diphtheria **2, 47**	643.23	Late vomiting of pregnancy, antepartum **154, 156**
478.75	Laryngeal spasm **47, 165, 169**	643.21	Late vomiting of pregnancy, delivered **134, 141, 147**
773.5	Late anemia due to isoimmunization of fetus or newborn **163, 167**	643.20	Late vomiting of pregnancy, unspecified as to episode of care **156, 159**
090.6	Late congenital syphilis, latent **185**	379.52	Latent nystagmus **38**
090.7	Late congenital syphilis, unspecified **185**	102.8	Latent yaws **185**
908.6	Late effect of certain complications of trauma **203**	376.36	Lateral displacement of globe of eye **38**
677	Late effect of complication of pregnancy, childbirth, and the puerperium **161**	728.4	Laxity of ligament **99**
		428.1	Left heart failure **57, 165, 169**
905.6	Late effect of dislocation **100**	V62.5	Legal circumstance **214**
908.5	Late effect of foreign body in orifice **203**	635*	Legally induced abortion **153**
905.4	Late effect of fracture of lower extremities **99**	482.84	Legionnaires' disease **51**
		V43.1	Lens replaced by other means **40**

030*	Leprosy **185**
100.0	Leptospirosis icterohemorrhagica **185**
765.21	Less than 24 completed weeks of gestation **163**
446.3	Lethal midline granuloma **97**
202.5*	Letterer-Siwe disease **180**, **181**
202.51	Letterer-Siwe disease of lymph nodes of head, face, and neck **3**
208*	Leukemia of unspecified cell type **178**
202.4*	Leukemic reticuloendotheliosis **178**, **181**
202.41	Leukemic reticuloendotheliosis of lymph nodes of head, face, and neck **3**
528.6	Leukoplakia of oral mucosa, including tongue **230**
607.0	Leukoplakia of penis **124**
697*	Lichen **108**
698.3	Lichenification and lichen simplex chronicus **108**
764.14	Light-for-dates with signs of fetal malnutrition, 1,000-1,249 grams **163**, **167**
764.15	Light-for-dates with signs of fetal malnutrition, 1,250-1,499 grams **163**, **167**
764.16	Light-for-dates with signs of fetal malnutrition, 1,500-1,749 grams **163**, **167**
764.17	Light-for-dates with signs of fetal malnutrition, 1,750-1,999 grams **163**, **167**
764.18	Light-for-dates with signs of fetal malnutrition, 2,000-2,499 grams **163**, **167**
764.12	Light-for-dates with signs of fetal malnutrition, 500-749 grams **163**, **167**
764.13	Light-for-dates with signs of fetal malnutrition, 750-999 grams **163**, **167**
764.11	Light-for-dates with signs of fetal malnutrition, less than 500 grams **163**, **167**
764.08	Light-for-dates without mention of fetal malnutrition, 2,000-2,499 grams **171**, **172**
764.09	Light-for-dates without mention of fetal malnutrition, 2,500 or more grams **171**, **172**
V43.7	Limb replaced by other means **101**
214.3	Lipoma of intra-abdominal organs **78**
214.2	Lipoma of intrathoracic organs **52**
214.1	Lipoma of other skin and subcutaneous tissue **108**
214.8	Lipoma of other specified sites **108**
214.0	Lipoma of skin and subcutaneous tissue of face **108**
214.4	Lipoma of spermatic cord **124**
214.9	Lipoma of unspecified site **108**
V39.01	Liveborn infant, unspecified whether single, twin, or multiple, born in hospital, delivered by cesarean **172**
V39.00	Liveborn infant, unspecified whether single, twin, or multiple, born in hospital, delivered without mention of cesarean delivery **172**
V39.1	Liveborn, unspecified whether single, twin or multiple, born before admission to hospital **172**
V39.2	Liveborn, unspecified whether single, twin or multiple, born outside hospital and not hospitalized **173**
572*	Liver abscess and sequelae of chronic liver disease **83**
646.73	Liver and biliary tract disorders in pregnancy, antepartum condition or complication **154**, **156**
646.71	Liver and biliary tract disorders in pregnancy, delivered, with or without mention of antepartum condition **134**, **142**, **147**
646.70	Liver and biliary tract disorders in pregnancy, unspecified as to episode of care or not applicable **156**, **159**
V59.6	Liver donor **83**
864.1*	Liver injury with open wound into cavity **223**
864.0*	Liver injury without mention of open wound into cavity **223**
V42.7	Liver replaced by transplant **83**
999.33	Local infection due to central venous catheter **69**

278.1	Localized adiposity **113**
003.2*	Localized salmonella infections **229**
782.2	Localized superficial swelling, mass, or lump **108**
660.50	Locked twins during labor and delivery, unspecified as to episode of care in pregnancy **136**, **143**, **149**
660.53	Locked twins, antepartum **155**, **158**
660.51	Locked twins, delivered **136**, **143**, **149**
V58.6*	Long-term (current) drug use **213**
718.1*	Loose body in joint **100**
717.6	Loose body in knee **100**
737.2*	Lordosis (acquired) **87**
781.91	Loss of height **33**
080	Louse-borne (epidemic) typhus **185**
238.72	Low grade myelodysplastic syndrome lesions **175**
365.12	Low tension open-angle glaucoma **38**
861.31	Lung contusion with open wound into thorax **54**
861.21	Lung contusion without mention of open wound into thorax **54**
517.8	Lung involvement in other diseases classified elsewhere **53**
517.2	Lung involvement in systemic sclerosis **53**
861.32	Lung laceration with open wound into thorax **52**
861.22	Lung laceration without mention of open wound into thorax **52**
V42.6	Lung replaced by transplant **54**
695.4	Lupus erythematosus **105**
289.3	Lymphadenitis, unspecified, except mesenteric **176**
228.1	Lymphangioma, any site **176**
457.2	Lymphangitis **106**, **165**, **169**
049.0	Lymphocytic choriomeningitis **21**
099.1	Lymphogranuloma venereum **124**, **127**, **130**
204*	Lymphoid leukemia **178**
200*	Lymphosarcoma and reticulosarcoma and other specified malignant tumors of lymphatic tissue **178**, **181**
200.11	Lymphosarcoma of lymph nodes of head, face, and neck **2**
744.81	Macrocheilia **48**
273.3	Macroglobulinemia **178**, **181**
744.83	Macrostomia **48**
039.4	Madura foot **107**
653.00	Major abnormality of bony pelvis, not further specified in pregnancy, unspecified as to episode of care **160**
653.03	Major abnormality of bony pelvis, not further specified, antepartum **154**, **157**
653.01	Major abnormality of bony pelvis, not further specified, delivered **135**, **142**, **148**
670.02	Major puerperal infection, unspecified, delivered, with mention of postpartum complication **138**, **141**, **146**
670.04	Major puerperal infection, unspecified, postpartum condition or complication **153**
670.00	Major puerperal infection, unspecified, unspecified as to episode of care or not applicable **161**
780.7*	Malaise and fatigue **231**
802.4	Malar and maxillary bones, closed fracture **3**, **48**, **221**
802.5	Malar and maxillary bones, open fracture **3**, **48**, **221**
084*	Malaria **185**
606*	Male infertility **124**
306.7	Malfunction of organs of special sense arising from mental factors **188**
209.25	Malignant carcinoid tumor of foregut, not otherwise specified **76**
209.27	Malignant carcinoid tumor of hindgut, not otherwise specified **76**
209.26	Malignant carcinoid tumor of midgut, not otherwise specified **76**
209.29	Malignant carcinoid tumor of other sites **180**, **181**
209.11	Malignant carcinoid tumor of the appendix **73**
209.21	Malignant carcinoid tumor of the bronchus and lung **52**

*Code Range

© 2013 OptumInsight, Inc.

209.24	Malignant carcinoid tumor of the kidney **116, 119**
209.23	Malignant carcinoid tumor of the stomach **76**
209.22	Malignant carcinoid tumor of the thymus **180, 181**
209.20	Malignant carcinoid tumor of unknown primary site **180, 181**
209.1*	Malignant carcinoid tumors of the appendix, large intestine, and rectum **76**
209.0*	Malignant carcinoid tumors of the small intestine **76**
202.3*	Malignant histiocytosis **178, 181**
202.31	Malignant histiocytosis of lymph nodes of head, face, and neck **3**
402.01	Malignant hypertensive heart disease with heart failure **56, 66, 165, 169**
402.00	Malignant hypertensive heart disease without heart failure **67**
202.6*	Malignant mast cell tumors **178, 181**
202.61	Malignant mast cell tumors of lymph nodes of head, face, and neck **3**
172.8	Malignant melanoma of other specified sites of skin **105**
172.2	Malignant melanoma of skin of ear and external auditory canal **105**
172.1	Malignant melanoma of skin of eyelid, including canthus **38**
172.0	Malignant melanoma of skin of lip **105**
172.7	Malignant melanoma of skin of lower limb, including hip **105**
172.3	Malignant melanoma of skin of other and unspecified parts of face **105**
172.4	Malignant melanoma of skin of scalp and neck **105**
172.5	Malignant melanoma of skin of trunk, except scrotum **105**
172.6	Malignant melanoma of skin of upper limb, including shoulder **105**
199.2	Malignant neoplasm associated with transplanted organ **180**
195.2	Malignant neoplasm of abdomen **76**
194.0	Malignant neoplasm of adrenal gland **114**
164.2	Malignant neoplasm of anterior mediastinum **52**
194.6	Malignant neoplasm of aortic body and other paraganglia **19**
153.5	Malignant neoplasm of appendix **73**
188*	Malignant neoplasm of bladder **116, 119**
182*	Malignant neoplasm of body of uterus **126, 129**
170*	Malignant neoplasm of bone and articular cartilage **97**
191*	Malignant neoplasm of brain **19**
194.5	Malignant neoplasm of carotid body **19**
180*	Malignant neoplasm of cervix uteri **126, 129**
153*	Malignant neoplasm of colon **76**
171*	Malignant neoplasm of connective and other soft tissue **97**
194.9	Malignant neoplasm of endocrine gland, site unspecified **114**
150*	Malignant neoplasm of esophagus **76**
190*	Malignant neoplasm of eye **38**
174*	Malignant neoplasm of female breast **104, 105**
144*	Malignant neoplasm of floor of mouth **2, 46**
156*	Malignant neoplasm of gallbladder and extrahepatic bile ducts **82**
143*	Malignant neoplasm of gum **2, 46**
195.0	Malignant neoplasm of head, face, and neck **2, 46**
164.1	Malignant neoplasm of heart **68**
148*	Malignant neoplasm of hypopharynx **2, 46**
159.9	Malignant neoplasm of ill-defined sites of digestive organs and peritoneum **76**
165.9	Malignant neoplasm of ill-defined sites within the respiratory system **52**
159.0	Malignant neoplasm of intestinal tract, part unspecified **76**
189*	Malignant neoplasm of kidney and other and unspecified urinary organs **116, 119**
161*	Malignant neoplasm of larynx **2, 46**
140*	Malignant neoplasm of lip **2, 46**
155*	Malignant neoplasm of liver and intrahepatic bile ducts **82**
195.5	Malignant neoplasm of lower limb **180, 181**
142*	Malignant neoplasm of major salivary glands **2, 46**
175*	Malignant neoplasm of male breast **104, 105**
170.1	Malignant neoplasm of mandible **2**
164.9	Malignant neoplasm of mediastinum, part unspecified **52**
160*	Malignant neoplasm of nasal cavities, middle ear, and accessory sinuses **2, 46**
147*	Malignant neoplasm of nasopharynx **2, 46**
146*	Malignant neoplasm of oropharynx **2, 46**
149*	Malignant neoplasm of other and ill-defined sites within the lip, oral cavity, and pharynx **2, 46**
184*	Malignant neoplasm of other and unspecified female genital organs **126, 129**
145*	Malignant neoplasm of other and unspecified parts of mouth **2, 46**
192*	Malignant neoplasm of other and unspecified parts of nervous system **19**
194.8	Malignant neoplasm of other endocrine glands and related structures **114**
164.8	Malignant neoplasm of other parts of mediastinum **52**
159.8	Malignant neoplasm of other sites of digestive system and intra-abdominal organs **76**
165.8	Malignant neoplasm of other sites within the respiratory system and intrathoracic organs **52**
195.8	Malignant neoplasm of other specified sites **180, 181**
183*	Malignant neoplasm of ovary and other uterine adnexa **126, 129**
157*	Malignant neoplasm of pancreas **82**
194.1	Malignant neoplasm of parathyroid gland **114**
195.3	Malignant neoplasm of pelvis **122, 123, 126, 129**
187*	Malignant neoplasm of penis and other male genital organs **122, 123**
158.9	Malignant neoplasm of peritoneum, unspecified **76**
194.4	Malignant neoplasm of pineal gland **19**
194.3	Malignant neoplasm of pituitary gland and craniopharyngeal duct **114**
181	Malignant neoplasm of placenta **126, 129**
163*	Malignant neoplasm of pleura **52**
164.3	Malignant neoplasm of posterior mediastinum **52**
185	Malignant neoplasm of prostate **122, 123**
154*	Malignant neoplasm of rectum, rectosigmoid junction, and anus **76**
158.0	Malignant neoplasm of retroperitoneum **180, 181**
152*	Malignant neoplasm of small intestine, including duodenum **76**
158.8	Malignant neoplasm of specified parts of peritoneum **76**
159.1	Malignant neoplasm of spleen, not elsewhere classified **178, 181**
151*	Malignant neoplasm of stomach **76**
186*	Malignant neoplasm of testis **122, 123**
195.1	Malignant neoplasm of thorax **52**
164.0	Malignant neoplasm of thymus **180, 181**
193	Malignant neoplasm of thyroid gland **2, 114**
141*	Malignant neoplasm of tongue **2, 46**
162*	Malignant neoplasm of trachea, bronchus, and lung **52**
195.4	Malignant neoplasm of upper limb **180, 181**
165.0	Malignant neoplasm of upper respiratory tract, part unspecified **2, 46**
179	Malignant neoplasm of uterus, part unspecified **126, 129**
170.2	Malignant neoplasm of vertebral column, excluding sacrum and coccyx **87**
199*	Malignant neoplasm without specification of site **181**
511.81	Malignant pleural effusion **52**

Alphabetic Index to Diseases

209.30	Malignant poorly differentiated neuroendocrine carcinoma, any site **180**, **181**
736.1	Mallet finger **100**
263.1	Malnutrition of mild degree **164**, **168**
263.0	Malnutrition of moderate degree **164**, **168**
733.8*	Malunion and nonunion of fracture **100**
802.2*	Mandible, closed fracture **3**, **48**, **221**
802.3*	Mandible, open fracture **3**, **48**, **221**
200.4*	Mantle cell lymphoma **230**
759.82	Marfan's syndrome **68**
370.01	Marginal corneal ulcer **39**
200.3*	Marginal zone lymphoma **230**
648.24	Maternal anemia complicating pregnancy, childbirth, or the puerperium, postpartum condition or complication **152**
648.20	Maternal anemia of mother, complicating pregnancy, childbirth, or the puerperium, unspecified as to episode of care **159**
648.22	Maternal anemia with delivery, with current postpartum complication **134**, **142**, **147**
648.23	Maternal anemia, antepartum **154**, **156**
648.21	Maternal anemia, with delivery **134**, **142**, **147**
679.03	Maternal complications from in utero procedure, antepartum condition or complication **156**, **158**
679.02	Maternal complications from in utero procedure, delivered, with mention of postpartum complication **139**, **141**, **147**
679.01	Maternal complications from in utero procedure, delivered, with or without mention of antepartum condition **139**, **141**, **147**
679.04	Maternal complications from in utero procedure, postpartum condition or complication **153**
679.00	Maternal complications from in utero procedure, unspecified as to episode of care or not applicable **139**, **145**, **151**
648.54	Maternal congenital cardiovascular disorders complicating pregnancy, childbirth, or the puerperium, postpartum condition or complication **152**
648.53	Maternal congenital cardiovascular disorders, antepartum **154**, **156**
648.50	Maternal congenital cardiovascular disorders, complicating pregnancy, childbirth, or the puerperium, unspecified as to episode of care **159**
648.51	Maternal congenital cardiovascular disorders, with delivery **134**, **140**, **146**
648.52	Maternal congenital cardiovascular disorders, with delivery, with current postpartum complication **134**, **140**, **146**
648.01	Maternal diabetes mellitus with delivery **134**, **140**, **146**
648.02	Maternal diabetes mellitus with delivery, with current postpartum complication **134**, **140**, **146**
648.03	Maternal diabetes mellitus, antepartum **154**, **156**
648.04	Maternal diabetes mellitus, complicating pregnancy, childbirth, or the puerperium, postpartum condition or complication **152**
648.00	Maternal diabetes mellitus, complicating pregnancy, childbirth, or the puerperium, unspecified as to episode of care **159**
669.03	Maternal distress complicating labor and delivery, antepartum condition or complication **155**, **158**
669.04	Maternal distress complicating labor and delivery, postpartum condition or complication **153**
669.00	Maternal distress complicating labor and delivery, unspecified as to episode of care **138**, **145**, **150**
669.02	Maternal distress, with delivery, with mention of postpartum complication **138**, **145**, **150**
669.01	Maternal distress, with delivery, with or without mention of antepartum condition **138**, **145**, **150**
648.34	Maternal drug dependence complicating pregnancy, childbirth, or the puerperium, postpartum condition or complication **152**
648.30	Maternal drug dependence complicating pregnancy, childbirth, or the puerperium, unspecified as to episode of care **159**

648.33	Maternal drug dependence, antepartum **154**, **156**
648.31	Maternal drug dependence, with delivery **134**, **142**, **147**
648.32	Maternal drug dependence, with delivery, with current postpartum complication **134**, **142**, **147**
647.10	Maternal gonorrhea complicating pregnancy, childbirth, or the puerperium, unspecified as to episode of care **159**
647.14	Maternal gonorrhea complicating pregnancy, childbrith, or the puerperium, postpartum condition or complication **152**
647.11	Maternal gonorrhea with delivery **134**, **140**, **146**
647.13	Maternal gonorrhea, antepartum **154**, **156**
647.12	Maternal gonorrhea, with delivery, with current postpartum complication **134**, **140**, **146**
669.20	Maternal hypotension syndrome complicating labor and delivery, unspecified as to episode of care **138**, **145**, **150**
669.23	Maternal hypotension syndrome, antepartum **155**, **158**
669.24	Maternal hypotension syndrome, postpartum condition or complication **153**
669.22	Maternal hypotension syndrome, with delivery, with mention of postpartum complication **138**, **145**, **150**
669.21	Maternal hypotension syndrome, with delivery, with or without mention of antepartum condition **138**, **145**, **150**
647.40	Maternal malaria complicating pregnancy, childbirth or the puerperium, unspecified as to episode of care **159**
647.41	Maternal malaria with delivery **134**, **140**, **146**
647.42	Maternal malaria with delivery, with current postpartum complication **134**, **140**, **146**
647.43	Maternal malaria, antepartum **154**, **156**
647.44	Maternal malaria, complicating pregnancy, childbirth, or the puerperium, postpartum condition or complication **152**
648.44	Maternal mental disorders complicating pregnancy, childbirth, or the puerperium, postpartum condition or complication **152**
648.43	Maternal mental disorders, antepartum **154**, **156**
648.40	Maternal mental disorders, complicating pregnancy, childbirth, or the puerperium, unspecified as to episode of care **159**
648.41	Maternal mental disorders, with delivery **134**, **142**, **147**
648.42	Maternal mental disorders, with delivery, with current postpartum complication **134**, **142**, **147**
647.54	Maternal rubella complicating pregnancy, childbirth, or the puerperium, postpartum condition or complication **152**
647.50	Maternal rubella complicating pregnancy, childbirth, or the puerperium, unspecified as to episode of care **159**
647.51	Maternal rubella with delivery **134**, **140**, **146**
647.52	Maternal rubella with delivery, with current postpartum complication **134**, **140**, **146**
647.53	Maternal rubella, antepartum **154**, **156**
647.04	Maternal syphilis complicating pregnancy, childbrith, or the puerperium, postpartum condition or complication **152**
647.03	Maternal syphilis, antepartum **154**, **156**
647.00	Maternal syphilis, complicating pregnancy, childbirth, or the puerperium, unspecified as to episode of care **159**
647.01	Maternal syphilis, complicating pregnancy, with delivery **134**, **140**, **146**
647.02	Maternal syphilis, complicating pregnancy, with delivery, with current postpartum complication **134**, **140**, **146**
648.14	Maternal thyroid dysfunction complicating pregnancy, childbirth, or the puerperium, postpartum condition or complication **152**
648.10	Maternal thyroid dysfunction complicating pregnancy, childbirth, or the puerperium, unspecified as to episode of care or not applicable **159**
648.12	Maternal thyroid dysfunction with delivery, with current postpartum complication **134**, **142**, **147**
648.11	Maternal thyroid dysfunction with delivery, with or without mention of antepartum condition **134**, **142**, **147**
648.13	Maternal thyroid dysfunction, antepartum condition or complication **154**, **156**

647.34	Maternal tuberculosis complicating pregnancy, childbirth, or the puerperium, postpartum condition or complication **152**
647.30	Maternal tuberculosis complicating pregnancy, childbirth, or the puerperium, unspecified as to episode of care **159**
647.31	Maternal tuberculosis with delivery **134, 140, 146**
647.32	Maternal tuberculosis with delivery, with current postpartum complication **134, 140, 146**
647.33	Maternal tuberculosis, antepartum **154, 156**
315.1	Mathematics disorder **189**
055.71	Measles keratoconjunctivitis **38**
055.9	Measles without mention of complication **184**
055.7*	Measles, with other specified complications **164, 168**
996.04	Mechanical complication due to automatic implantable cardiac defibrillator **68**
996.54	Mechanical complication due to breast prosthesis **106**
996.01	Mechanical complication due to cardiac pacemaker (electrode) **68**
996.51	Mechanical complication due to corneal graft **40**
996.03	Mechanical complication due to coronary bypass graft **69**
996.02	Mechanical complication due to heart valve prosthesis **68**
996.57	Mechanical complication due to insulin pump **203**
996.32	Mechanical complication due to intrauterine contraceptive device **128, 131**
996.53	Mechanical complication due to ocular lens prosthesis **40**
996.59	Mechanical complication due to other implant and internal device, not elsewhere classified **203**
996.52	Mechanical complication due to other tissue graft, not elsewhere classified **203**
996.31	Mechanical complication due to urethral (indwelling) catheter **120**
996.09	Mechanical complication of cardiac device, implant, and graft, other **69**
530.87	Mechanical complication of esophagostomy **78**
996.39	Mechanical complication of genitourinary device, implant, and graft, other **120**
996.4*	Mechanical complication of internal orthopedic device, implant, and graft **99**
996.2	Mechanical complication of nervous system device, implant, and graft **33**
996.1	Mechanical complication of other vascular device, implant, and graft **69**
996.00	Mechanical complication of unspecified cardiac device, implant, and graft **69**
996.30	Mechanical complication of unspecified genitourinary device, implant, and graft **120**
996.55	Mechanical complications due to artificial skin graft and decellularized allodermis **203**
996.56	Mechanical complications due to peritoneal dialysis catheter **203**
374.33	Mechanical ptosis **39**
378.6*	Mechanical strabismus **40**
751.0	Meckel's diverticulum **77**
519.2	Mediastinitis **51, 165, 170**
564.7	Megacolon, other than Hirschsprung's **79**
207.2*	Megakaryocytic leukemia **181**
172.9	Melanoma of skin, site unspecified **105**
025	Melioidosis **185**
386.0*	Meniere's disease **46**
781.6	Meningismus **33**
049.1	Meningitis due to adenovirus **21**
047*	Meningitis due to enterovirus **21**
321*	Meningitis due to other organisms **34, 164, 169**
321.3	Meningitis due to trypanosomiasis **9, 10**

321.2	Meningitis due to viruses not elsewhere classified **9, 10**
321.1	Meningitis in other fungal diseases **9, 10**
322*	Meningitis of unspecified cause **34**
036.82	Meningococcal arthropathy **97, 164, 168**
036.4*	Meningococcal carditis **164, 168**
036.40	Meningococcal carditis, unspecified **68**
036.1	Meningococcal encephalitis **8, 10, 33**
036.42	Meningococcal endocarditis **65**
036.0	Meningococcal meningitis **8, 10, 33**
036.43	Meningococcal myocarditis **68**
036.81	Meningococcal optic neuritis **38, 164, 168**
036.41	Meningococcal pericarditis **68**
036.2	Meningococcemia **186**
130.0	Meningoencephalitis due to toxoplasmosis **9, 10, 34, 164, 168**
627*	Menopausal and postmenopausal disorders **127, 130**
V25.3	Menstrual extraction **128, 131**
V40*	Mental and behavioral problems **214**
209.36	Merkel cell carcinoma of other sites **105**
209.31	Merkel cell carcinoma of the face **105**
209.34	Merkel cell carcinoma of the lower limb **105**
209.32	Merkel cell carcinoma of the scalp and neck **105**
209.35	Merkel cell carcinoma of the trunk **105**
209.33	Merkel cell carcinoma of the upper limb **105**
121.5	Metagonimiasis **185**
289.7	Methemoglobinemia **175**
482.42	Methicillin resistant pneumonia due to Staphylococcus aureus **51**
482.41	Methicillin susceptible pneumonia due to Staphylococcus aureus **51**
744.82	Microcheilia **48**
744.84	Microstomia **48**
346*	Migraine **34**
331.83	Mild cognitive impairment, so stated **19**
643.03	Mild hyperemesis gravidarum, antepartum **154, 156**
643.01	Mild hyperemesis gravidarum, delivered **134, 141, 147**
643.00	Mild hyperemesis gravidarum, unspecified as to episode of care **156, 159**
317	Mild intellectual disabilities **188**
768.6	Mild or moderate birth asphyxia **171, 172**
642.43	Mild or unspecified pre-eclampsia, antepartum **154, 156**
642.44	Mild or unspecified pre-eclampsia, postpartum condition or complication **151**
642.40	Mild or unspecified pre-eclampsia, unspecified as to episode of care **159**
642.41	Mild or unspecified pre-eclampsia, with delivery **134, 140, 146**
642.42	Mild or unspecified pre-eclampsia, with delivery, with current postpartum complication **134, 140, 146**
018*	Miliary tuberculosis **229**
379.42	Miosis (persistent), not due to miotics **38**
313.1	Misery and unhappiness disorder specific to childhood and adolescence **188**
632	Missed abortion **153**
625.2	Mittelschmerz **130**
315.5	Mixed development disorder **189**
312.4	Mixed disturbance of conduct and emotions **189**
127.8	Mixed intestinal helminthiasis **186**
103.3	Mixed lesions of pinta **107**
315.32	Mixed receptive-expressive language disorder **189**
768.72	Moderate hypoxic-ischemic encephalopathy **163, 167**
078.0	Molluscum contagiosum **107**
273.1	Monoclonal paraproteinemia **176**

206*	Monocytic leukemia **178**
355*	Mononeuritis of lower limb and unspecified site **21**
354*	Mononeuritis of upper limb and mononeuritis multiplex **21**
344.3*	Monoplegia of lower limb **32**
344.4*	Monoplegia of upper limb **32**
343.3	Monoplegic infantile cerebral palsy **32**
370.07	Mooren's ulcer **39**
278.01	Morbid obesity **113**
062*	Mosquito-borne viral encephalitis **9, 10, 33**
994.6	Motion sickness **46**
437.5	Moyamoya disease **33**
085.5	Mucocutaneous leishmaniasis, (American) **107**
277.5	Mucopolysaccharidosis **114**
491.1	Mucopurulent chronic bronchitis **53**
V61.5	Multiparity **128, 131**
894*	Multiple and unspecified open wound of lower limb **223**
894.1	Multiple and unspecified open wound of lower limb, complicated **203**
894.2	Multiple and unspecified open wound of lower limb, with tendon involvement **101**
894.0	Multiple and unspecified open wound of lower limb, without mention of complication **107**
884*	Multiple and unspecified open wound of upper limb **223**
884.1	Multiple and unspecified open wound of upper limb, complicated **203**
884.2	Multiple and unspecified open wound of upper limb, with tendon involvement **101**
884.0	Multiple and unspecified open wound of upper limb, without mention of complication **107**
828.0	Multiple closed fractures involving both lower limbs, lower with upper limb, and lower limb(s) with rib(s) and sternum **222**
819.0	Multiple closed fractures involving both upper limbs, and upper limb with rib(s) and sternum **221**
817.0	Multiple closed fractures of hand bones **221**
759.7	Multiple congenital anomalies, so described **101**
828*	Multiple fractures involving both lower limbs, lower with upper limb, and lower limb(s) with rib(s) and sternum **202, 227**
828.1	Multiple fractures involving both lower limbs, lower with upper limb, and lower limb(s) with rib(s) and sternum, open **222**
819*	Multiple fractures involving both upper limbs, and upper limb with rib(s) and sternum **202**
817*	Multiple fractures of hand bones **99**
651.73	Multiple gestation following (elective) fetal reduction, antepartum condition or complication **154, 157**
651.71	Multiple gestation following (elective) fetal reduction, delivered, with or without mention of antepartum condition **135, 142, 148**
651.70	Multiple gestation following (elective) fetal reduction, unspecified as to episode of care or not applicable **160**
652.63	Multiple gestation with malpresentation of one fetus or more, antepartum **154, 157**
652.61	Multiple gestation with malpresentation of one fetus or more, delivered **135, 142, 148**
652.60	Multiple gestation with malpresentation of one fetus or more, unspecified as to episode of care **160**
203*	Multiple myeloma and immunoproliferative neoplasms **178, 181**
819.1	Multiple open fractures involving both upper limbs, and upper limb with rib(s) and sternum **221, 226**
817.1	Multiple open fractures of hand bones **221**
102.1	Multiple papillomata and wet crab yaws due to yaws **107**
340	Multiple sclerosis **19**
130.8	Multisystemic disseminated toxoplasmosis **164, 168, 186**
072.2	Mumps encephalitis **9, 10, 34, 164, 168**
072.71	Mumps hepatitis **83**

072.1	Mumps meningitis **9, 10, 21, 164, 168**
072.0	Mumps orchitis **124, 164, 168**
072.3	Mumps pancreatitis **83, 164, 168**
072.72	Mumps polyneuropathy **21**
072.7*	Mumps with other specified complications **164, 168**
072.79	Mumps with other specified complications **184**
072.9	Mumps without mention of complication **184**
728.87	Muscle weakness (generalized) **98**
728.1*	Muscular calcification and ossification **99**
728.2	Muscular wasting and disuse atrophy, not elsewhere classified **99**
306.0	Musculoskeletal malfunction arising from mental factors **98**
358.0*	Myasthenia gravis **19**
358.1	Myasthenic syndromes in diseases classified elsewhere **19**
202.1*	Mycosis fungoides **178, 181**
202.11	Mycosis fungoides of lymph nodes of head, face, and neck **2**
370.05	Mycotic corneal ulcer **38**
117.4	Mycotic mycetomas **164, 168**
379.43	Mydriasis (persistent), not due to mydriatics **38**
323.52	Myelitis following immunization procedures **10**
323.02	Myelitis in viral diseases classified elsewhere **10**
238.74	Myelodysplastic syndrome with 5q deletion **175**
238.75	Myelodysplastic syndrome, unspecified **175**
289.83	Myelofibrosis **178, 181**
238.76	Myelofibrosis with myeloid metaplasia **178, 181**
205*	Myeloid leukemia **178**
205.3*	Myeloid sarcoma **181**
336.3	Myelopathy in other diseases classified elsewhere **32**
284.2	Myelophthisis **178, 181**
429.1	Myocardial degeneration **69**
130.3	Myocarditis due to toxoplasmosis **68, 164, 168**
333.2	Myoclonus **32**
374.32	Myogenic ptosis **38**
791.3	Myoglobinuria **213**
359.5	Myopathy in endocrine diseases classified elsewhere **32**
376.82	Myopathy of extraocular muscles **38**
367.1	Myopia **39**
359.22	Myotonia congenita **32**
359.23	Myotonic chondrodystrophy **32**
359.21	Myotonic muscular dystrophy **32**
802.0	Nasal bones, closed fracture **47, 221**
802.1	Nasal bones, open fracture **47, 221**
478.11	Nasal mucositis (ulcerative) **172**
471*	Nasal polyps **47**
032.1	Nasopharyngeal diphtheria **2, 47**
040.3	Necrobacillosis **185**
447.5	Necrosis of artery **66**
777.5*	Necrotizing enterocolitis in newborn **163, 168**
728.86	Necrotizing fasciitis **99**
V07*	Need for isolation and other prophylactic or treatment measures **214**
V05*	Need for other prophylactic vaccination and inoculation against single diseases **213**
V03*	Need for prophylactic vaccination and inoculation against bacterial diseases **213**
V04*	Need for prophylactic vaccination and inoculation against certain viral diseases **213**
V06*	Need for prophylactic vaccination and inoculation against combinations of diseases **213**
V05.8	Need for prophylactic vaccination and inoculation against other specified disease **172**

*Code Range

V05.4	Need for prophylactic vaccination and inoculation against varicella **172**	238.9	Neoplasm of uncertain behavior, site unspecified **180**, **182**
V05.3	Need for prophylactic vaccination and inoculation against viral hepatitis **172**	239.4	Neoplasm of unspecified nature of bladder **116**, **119**
		239.6	Neoplasm of unspecified nature of brain **19**
775.1	Neonatal diabetes mellitus **163**, **167**	239.3	Neoplasm of unspecified nature of breast **105**
775.6	Neonatal hypoglycemia **163**, **167**	239.0	Neoplasm of unspecified nature of digestive system **76**
771.5	Neonatal infective mastitis **163**, **167**	239.7	Neoplasm of unspecified nature of endocrine glands and other parts of nervous system **114**
777.2	Neonatal intestinal obstruction due to inspissated milk **163**, **168**		
774.3*	Neonatal jaundice due to delayed conjugation from other causes **171**, **172**	239.5	Neoplasm of unspecified nature of other genitourinary organs **116**, **119**
775.2	Neonatal myasthenia gravis **163**, **167**	239.8*	Neoplasm of unspecified nature of other specified sites **180**, **182**
775.3	Neonatal thyrotoxicosis **163**, **167**	239.1	Neoplasm of unspecified nature of respiratory system **52**
237.2	Neoplasm of uncertain behavior of adrenal gland **114**	239.9	Neoplasm of unspecified nature, site unspecified **180**, **182**
236.7	Neoplasm of uncertain behavior of bladder **116**, **119**	338.3	Neoplasm related pain (acute) (chronic) **213**
238.0	Neoplasm of uncertain behavior of bone and articular cartilage **87**, **97**	239.2	Neoplasms of unspecified nature of bone, soft tissue, and skin **87**, **100**
237.5	Neoplasm of uncertain behavior of brain and spinal cord **19**	583*	Nephritis and nephropathy, not specified as acute or chronic **120**, **230**
238.3	Neoplasm of uncertain behavior of breast **104**, **105**	593.0	Nephroptosis **120**
238.1	Neoplasm of uncertain behavior of connective and other soft tissue **100**	581*	Nephrotic syndrome **120**, **230**
238.5	Neoplasm of uncertain behavior of histiocytic and mast cells **178**, **181**	353*	Nerve root and plexus disorders **21**
		997.0*	Nervous system complications **33**, **167**, **171**
235.6	Neoplasm of uncertain behavior of larynx **3**, **46**	349.1	Nervous system complications from surgically implanted device **32**, **165**, **169**
235.1	Neoplasm of uncertain behavior of lip, oral cavity, and pharynx **3**, **46**	799.21	Nervousness **188**
235.3	Neoplasm of uncertain behavior of liver and biliary passages **83**	300.5	Neurasthenia **188**
235.0	Neoplasm of uncertain behavior of major salivary glands **3**, **46**	237.7*	Neurofibromatosis **32**
237.6	Neoplasm of uncertain behavior of meninges **19**	333.92	Neuroleptic malignant syndrome **32**
235.5	Neoplasm of uncertain behavior of other and unspecified digestive organs **76**	781.8	Neurological neglect syndrome **33**
		341.0	Neuromyelitis optica **19**
237.4	Neoplasm of uncertain behavior of other and unspecified endocrine glands **114**	288.0*	Neutropenia **175**, **230**
236.3	Neoplasm of uncertain behavior of other and unspecified female genital organs **126**, **129**	448.1	Nevus, non-neoplastic **108**
		V20.3*	Newborn health supervision **172**
236.6	Neoplasm of uncertain behavior of other and unspecified male genital organs **122**, **123**	279.13	Nezelof's syndrome **175**
		368.6*	Night blindness **39**
237.9	Neoplasm of uncertain behavior of other and unspecified parts of nervous system **19**	202.0*	Nodular lymphoma **178**, **181**
		202.01	Nodular lymphoma of lymph nodes of head, face, and neck **2**
235.9	Neoplasm of uncertain behavior of other and unspecified respiratory organs **52**	388.1*	Noise effects on inner ear **47**
236.9*	Neoplasm of uncertain behavior of other and unspecified urinary organs **116**, **119**	283.1*	Non-autoimmune hemolytic anemias **164**, **169**
		998.83	Non-healing surgical wound **204**
238.8	Neoplasm of uncertain behavior of other specified sites **180**, **182**	739.9	Nonallopathic lesion of abdomen and other sites, not elsewhere classified **98**
236.2	Neoplasm of uncertain behavior of ovary **126**, **129**	739.1	Nonallopathic lesion of cervical region, not elsewhere classified **97**
237.3	Neoplasm of uncertain behavior of paraganglia **19**		
237.1	Neoplasm of uncertain behavior of pineal gland **19**	739.0	Nonallopathic lesion of head region, not elsewhere classified **98**
237.0	Neoplasm of uncertain behavior of pituitary gland and craniopharyngeal duct **114**	739.6	Nonallopathic lesion of lower extremities, not elsewhere classified **98**
236.1	Neoplasm of uncertain behavior of placenta **126**, **129**	739.3	Nonallopathic lesion of lumbar region, not elsewhere classified **98**
238.6	Neoplasm of uncertain behavior of plasma cells **178**, **181**	739.5	Nonallopathic lesion of pelvic region, not elsewhere classified **98**
235.8	Neoplasm of uncertain behavior of pleura, thymus, and mediastinum **52**	739.8	Nonallopathic lesion of rib cage, not elsewhere classified **98**
238.4	Neoplasm of uncertain behavior of polycythemia vera **178**, **181**	739.4	Nonallopathic lesion of sacral region, not elsewhere classified **98**
236.5	Neoplasm of uncertain behavior of prostate **122**, **123**	739.2	Nonallopathic lesion of thoracic region, not elsewhere classified **97**
235.4	Neoplasm of uncertain behavior of retroperitoneum and peritoneum **76**	739.7	Nonallopathic lesion of upper extremities, not elsewhere classified **98**
238.2	Neoplasm of uncertain behavior of skin **108**	305.0*	Nondependent alcohol abuse **191**
235.2	Neoplasm of uncertain behavior of stomach, intestines, and rectum **76**	305.7*	Nondependent amphetamine or related acting sympathomimetic abuse **191**
236.4	Neoplasm of uncertain behavior of testis **122**, **123**	305.8*	Nondependent antidepressant type abuse **191**
235.7	Neoplasm of uncertain behavior of trachea, bronchus, and lung **52**	305.2*	Nondependent cannabis abuse **191**
		305.6*	Nondependent cocaine abuse **191**
236.0	Neoplasm of uncertain behavior of uterus **126**, **129**		

305.3*	Nondependent hallucinogen abuse **191**
305.5*	Nondependent opioid abuse **191**
305.4*	Nondependent sedative, hypnotic or anxiolytic abuse **191**
305.1	Nondependent tobacco use disorder **213**
380.3*	Noninfectious disorders of pinna **47**
622*	Noninflammatory disorders of cervix **127**, **130**
620*	Noninflammatory disorders of ovary, fallopian tube, and broad ligament **127**, **130**
623*	Noninflammatory disorders of vagina **127**, **130**
624*	Noninflammatory disorders of vulva and perineum **127**, **130**
675.23	Nonpurulent mastitis, antepartum **156**, **158**
675.22	Nonpurulent mastitis, delivered, with mention of postpartum complication **139**, **141**, **147**
675.21	Nonpurulent mastitis, delivered, with or without mention of antepartum condition **139**, **141**, **147**
675.24	Nonpurulent mastitis, postpartum condition or complication **153**
675.20	Nonpurulent mastitis, unspecified as to episode of prenatal or postnatal care **161**
322.0	Nonpyogenic meningitis **164**, **169**
437.6	Nonpyogenic thrombosis of intracranial venous sinus **33**
793.6	Nonspecific (abnormal) findings on radiological and other examination of abdominal area, including retroperitoneum **78**
793.3	Nonspecific (abnormal) findings on radiological and other examination of biliary tract **83**
793.4	Nonspecific (abnormal) findings on radiological and other examination of gastrointestinal tract **78**
793.5	Nonspecific (abnormal) findings on radiological and other examination of genitourinary organs **120**
793.7	Nonspecific (abnormal) findings on radiological and other examination of musculoskeletal system **101**
793.2	Nonspecific (abnormal) findings on radiological and other examination of other intrathoracic organs **67**
793.0	Nonspecific (abnormal) findings on radiological and other examination of skull and head **33**
794.15	Nonspecific abnormal auditory function studies **47**, **172**
794.12	Nonspecific abnormal electro-oculogram (EOG) **40**
794.31	Nonspecific abnormal electrocardiogram (ECG) (EKG) **69**
794.17	Nonspecific abnormal electromyogram (EMG) **101**
792.3	Nonspecific abnormal finding in amniotic fluid **156**, **159**
792.0	Nonspecific abnormal finding in cerebrospinal fluid **33**
792.4	Nonspecific abnormal finding in saliva **47**
792.2	Nonspecific abnormal finding in semen **124**
792.1	Nonspecific abnormal finding in stool contents **78**
795.2	Nonspecific abnormal findings on chromosomal analysis **213**
796.6	Nonspecific abnormal findings on neonatal screening **213**
793.8*	Nonspecific abnormal findings on radiological and other examinations of body structure, breast **106**
794.14	Nonspecific abnormal oculomotor studies **40**
794.10	Nonspecific abnormal response to unspecified nerve stimulation **33**
794.7	Nonspecific abnormal results of basal metabolism function study **114**
794.0*	Nonspecific abnormal results of function study of brain and central nervous system **33**
794.4	Nonspecific abnormal results of kidney function study **120**
794.8	Nonspecific abnormal results of liver function study **83**
794.6	Nonspecific abnormal results of other endocrine function study **114**
794.9	Nonspecific abnormal results of other specified function study **120**
794.2	Nonspecific abnormal results of pulmonary system function study **54**
794.5	Nonspecific abnormal results of thyroid function study **114**

794.11	Nonspecific abnormal retinal function studies **40**
796.0	Nonspecific abnormal toxicological findings **204**
794.30	Nonspecific abnormal unspecified cardiovascular function study **69**
794.16	Nonspecific abnormal vestibular function studies **47**
794.13	Nonspecific abnormal visually evoked potential **40**
790.4	Nonspecific elevation of levels of transaminase or lactic acid dehydrogenase (LDH) **213**
796.3	Nonspecific low blood pressure reading **69**
289.2	Nonspecific mesenteric lymphadenitis **78**
795.3*	Nonspecific positive culture findings **186**
795.5*	Nonspecific reaction to test for tuberculosis **51**
381.4	Nonsuppurative otitis media, not specified as acute or chronic **46**
241*	Nontoxic nodular goiter **114**
729.7*	Nontraumatic compartment syndrome **99**
596.6	Nontraumatic rupture of bladder **166**, **170**
650	Normal delivery **135**, **142**, **148**
V22*	Normal pregnancy **214**
832.2	Nursemaid's elbow **222**
261	Nutritional marasmus **113**, **164**, **168**, **230**
379.54	Nystagmus associated with disorders of the vestibular system **38**
379.57	Nystagmus with deficiencies of saccadic eye movements **38**
379.58	Nystagmus with deficiencies of smooth pursuit movements **38**
649.13	Obesity complicating pregnancy, childbirth, or the puerperium, antepartum condition or complication **154**, **157**
649.12	Obesity complicating pregnancy, childbirth, or the puerperium, delivered, with mention of postpartum complication **135**, **142**, **148**
649.11	Obesity complicating pregnancy, childbirth, or the puerperium, delivered, with or without mention of antepartum condition **135**, **142**, **148**
649.14	Obesity complicating pregnancy, childbirth, or the puerperium, postpartum condition or complication **152**
649.10	Obesity complicating pregnancy, childbirth, or the puerperium, unspecified as to episode of care or not applicable **160**
278.03	Obesity hypoventilation syndrome **54**
278.00	Obesity, unspecified **113**
V71.8*	Observation and evaluation for other specified suspected conditions **215**
V29*	Observation and evaluation of newborns and infants for suspected condition not found **172**, **214**
V71.3	Observation following accident at work **204**
V71.5	Observation following alleged rape or seduction **215**
V71.4	Observation following other accident **204**
V71.6	Observation following other inflicted injury **204**
V71.7	Observation for suspected cardiovascular disease **68**
V71.1	Observation for suspected malignant neoplasm **180**, **182**
V71.2	Observation for suspected tuberculosis **51**
V71.9	Observation for unspecified suspected condition **215**
V71.01	Observation of adult antisocial behavior **188**
V71.02	Observation of childhood or adolescent antisocial behavior **188**
V71.09	Observation of other suspected mental condition **189**
300.3	Obsessive-compulsive disorders **188**
301.4	Obsessive-compulsive personality disorder **188**
673.03	Obstetrical air embolism, antepartum condition or complication **156**, **158**
673.04	Obstetrical air embolism, postpartum condition or complication **153**
673.00	Obstetrical air embolism, unspecified as to episode of care **161**
673.02	Obstetrical air embolism, with delivery, with mention of postpartum complication **138**, **141**, **146**

673.01	Obstetrical air embolism, with delivery, with or without mention of antepartum condition **138**, **141**, **146**
673.23	Obstetrical blood-clot embolism, antepartum **156**, **158**
673.24	Obstetrical blood-clot embolism, postpartum condition or complication **153**
673.20	Obstetrical blood-clot embolism, unspecified as to episode of care **161**
673.21	Obstetrical blood-clot embolism, with delivery, with or without mention of antepartum condition **138**, **141**, **146**
673.22	Obstetrical blood-clot embolism, with mention of postpartum complication **138**, **141**, **146**
673.33	Obstetrical pyemic and septic embolism, antepartum **156**, **158**
673.34	Obstetrical pyemic and septic embolism, postpartum condition or complication **153**
673.30	Obstetrical pyemic and septic embolism, unspecified as to episode of care **161**
673.32	Obstetrical pyemic and septic embolism, with delivery, with mention of postpartum complication **138**, **141**, **147**
673.31	Obstetrical pyemic and septic embolism, with delivery, with or without mention of antepartum condition **138**, **141**, **147**
660.23	Obstruction by abnormal pelvic soft tissues during labor and delivery, antepartum **155**, **158**
660.21	Obstruction by abnormal pelvic soft tissues during labor and delivery, delivered **136**, **143**, **149**
660.20	Obstruction by abnormal pelvic soft tissues during labor and delivery, unspecified as to episode of care **136**, **143**, **149**
660.13	Obstruction by bony pelvis during labor and delivery, antepartum **155**, **158**
660.11	Obstruction by bony pelvis during labor and delivery, delivered **136**, **143**, **149**
660.10	Obstruction by bony pelvis during labor and delivery, unspecified as to episode of care **136**, **143**, **149**
660.03	Obstruction caused by malposition of fetus at onset of labor, antepartum **155**, **158**
660.01	Obstruction caused by malposition of fetus at onset of labor, delivered **136**, **143**, **149**
660.00	Obstruction caused by malposition of fetus at onset of labor, unspecified as to episode of care **136**, **143**, **149**
381.6*	Obstruction of Eustachian tube **47**
491.2*	Obstructive chronic bronchitis **53**
331.4	Obstructive hydrocephalus **19**
327.23	Obstructive sleep apnea (adult) (pediatric) **47**
433.01	Occlusion and stenosis of basilar artery with cerebral infarction **9**, **10**, **19**, **20**, **165**, **169**
433.00	Occlusion and stenosis of basilar artery without mention of cerebral infarction **20**
433.11	Occlusion and stenosis of carotid artery with cerebral infarction **9**, **10**, **19**, **20**, **165**, **169**
433.10	Occlusion and stenosis of carotid artery without mention of cerebral infarction **20**
433.31	Occlusion and stenosis of multiple and bilateral precerebral arteries with cerebral infarction **9**, **10**, **20**, **165**, **169**
433.30	Occlusion and stenosis of multiple and bilateral precerebral arteries without mention of cerebral infarction **20**
433.81	Occlusion and stenosis of other specified precerebral artery with cerebral infarction **9**, **10**, **20**, **165**, **169**
433.80	Occlusion and stenosis of other specified precerebral artery without mention of cerebral infarction **20**
433.91	Occlusion and stenosis of unspecified precerebral artery with cerebral infarction **9**, **10**, **20**, **165**, **169**
433.90	Occlusion and stenosis of unspecified precerebral artery without mention of cerebral infarction **20**
433.21	Occlusion and stenosis of vertebral artery with cerebral infarction **9**, **10**, **19**, **20**, **165**, **169**

433.20	Occlusion and stenosis of vertebral artery without mention of cerebral infarction **20**
434*	Occlusion of cerebral arteries **165**, **169**
V57.2*	Occupational therapy and vocational rehabilitation **213**
781.93	Ocular torticollis **98**
021.3	Oculoglandular tularemia **185**
717.0	Old bucket handle tear of medial meniscus **99**
412	Old myocardial infarction **67**
658.03	Oligohydramnios, antepartum **155**, **158**
658.01	Oligohydramnios, delivered **136**, **143**, **149**
658.00	Oligohydramnios, unspecified as to episode of care **160**
788.5	Oliguria and anuria **118**, **119**
771.4	Omphalitis of the newborn **163**, **167**
756.72	Omphalocele **166**, **170**
649.8*	Onset (spontaneous) of labor after 37 completed weeks of gestation but before 39 completed weeks gestation, with delivery by (planned) cesarean section **135**, **140**, **148**
649.82	Onset (spontaneous) of labor after 37 completed weeks of gestation but before 39 completed weeks gestation, with delivery by (planned) cesarean section, delivered, with mention of postpartum complication **142**
649.81	Onset (spontaneous) of labor after 37 completed weeks of gestation but before 39 completed weeks gestation, with delivery by (planned) cesarean section, delivered, with or without mention of antepartum condition **142**
824.5	Open bimalleolar fracture **222**
837.1	Open dislocation of ankle **222**, **227**
832.1*	Open dislocation of elbow **222**, **227**
834.1*	Open dislocation of finger **222**
838.1*	Open dislocation of foot **222**
835.1*	Open dislocation of hip **222**, **227**
830.1	Open dislocation of jaw **222**
836.4	Open dislocation of patella **222**
831.1*	Open dislocation of shoulder **222**, **227**
833.1*	Open dislocation of wrist **222**
839.1*	Open dislocation, cervical vertebra **98**, **222**, **227**
839.9	Open dislocation, multiple and ill-defined sites **100**, **222**
839.79	Open dislocation, other location **100**, **222**
839.59	Open dislocation, other vertebra **227**
839.5*	Open dislocation, other vertebra **98**, **222**
839.52	Open dislocation, sacrum **227**
839.71	Open dislocation, sternum **52**, **222**, **226**
839.3*	Open dislocation, thoracic and lumbar vertebra **98**, **222**
808.1	Open fracture of acetabulum **221**
811.11	Open fracture of acromial process of scapula **99**
801.6*	Open fracture of base of skull with cerebral laceration and contusion **221**, **225**
801.62	Open fracture of base of skull with cerebral laceration and contusion, brief (less than one hour) loss of consciousness **28**
801.66	Open fracture of base of skull with cerebral laceration and contusion, loss of consciousness of unspecified duration **23**
801.63	Open fracture of base of skull with cerebral laceration and contusion, moderate (1-24 hours) loss of consciousness **23**
801.61	Open fracture of base of skull with cerebral laceration and contusion, no loss of consciousness **28**
801.64	Open fracture of base of skull with cerebral laceration and contusion, prolonged (more than 24 hours) loss of consciousness and return to pre-existing conscious level **23**
801.65	Open fracture of base of skull with cerebral laceration and contusion, prolonged (more than 24 hours) loss of consciousness, without return to pre-existing conscious level **23**
801.69	Open fracture of base of skull with cerebral laceration and contusion, unspecified concussion **28**

Alphabetic Index to Diseases

801.60 Open fracture of base of skull with cerebral laceration and contusion, unspecified state of consciousness **28**

801.9* Open fracture of base of skull with intracranial injury of other and unspecified nature **221, 225**

801.92 Open fracture of base of skull with intracranial injury of other and unspecified nature, brief (less than one hour) loss of consciousness **29**

801.96 Open fracture of base of skull with intracranial injury of other and unspecified nature, loss of consciousness of unspecified duration **23**

801.93 Open fracture of base of skull with intracranial injury of other and unspecified nature, moderate (1-24 hours) loss of consciousness **23**

801.91 Open fracture of base of skull with intracranial injury of other and unspecified nature, no loss of consciousness **29**

801.94 Open fracture of base of skull with intracranial injury of other and unspecified nature, prolonged (more than 24 hours) loss of consciousness and return to pre-existing conscious level **23**

801.95 Open fracture of base of skull with intracranial injury of other and unspecified nature, prolonged (more than 24 hours) loss of consciousness, without return to pre-existing conscious level **23**

801.99 Open fracture of base of skull with intracranial injury of other and unspecified nature, unspecified concussion **29**

801.90 Open fracture of base of skull with intracranial injury of other and unspecified nature, unspecified state of consciousness **29**

801.8* Open fracture of base of skull with other and unspecified intracranial hemorrhage **221, 225**

801.82 Open fracture of base of skull with other and unspecified intracranial hemorrhage, brief (less than one hour) loss of consciousness **29**

801.86 Open fracture of base of skull with other and unspecified intracranial hemorrhage, loss of consciousness of unspecified duration **23**

801.83 Open fracture of base of skull with other and unspecified intracranial hemorrhage, moderate (1-24 hours) loss of consciousness **23**

801.81 Open fracture of base of skull with other and unspecified intracranial hemorrhage, no loss of consciousness **29**

801.84 Open fracture of base of skull with other and unspecified intracranial hemorrhage, prolonged (more than 24 hours) loss of consciousness and return to pre-existing conscious level **23**

801.85 Open fracture of base of skull with other and unspecified intracranial hemorrhage, prolonged (more than 24 hours) loss of consciousness, without return to pre-existing conscious level **23**

801.89 Open fracture of base of skull with other and unspecified intracranial hemorrhage, unspecified concussion **29**

801.80 Open fracture of base of skull with other and unspecified intracranial hemorrhage, unspecified state of consciousness **29**

801.7* Open fracture of base of skull with subarachnoid, subdural, and extradural hemorrhage **221, 225**

801.72 Open fracture of base of skull with subarachnoid, subdural, and extradural hemorrhage, brief (less than one hour) loss of consciousness **28**

801.76 Open fracture of base of skull with subarachnoid, subdural, and extradural hemorrhage, loss of consciousness of unspecified duration **23**

801.73 Open fracture of base of skull with subarachnoid, subdural, and extradural hemorrhage, moderate (1-24 hours) loss of consciousness **23**

801.71 Open fracture of base of skull with subarachnoid, subdural, and extradural hemorrhage, no loss of consciousness **28**

801.74 Open fracture of base of skull with subarachnoid, subdural, and extradural hemorrhage, prolonged (more than 24 hours) loss of consciousness and return to pre-existing conscious level **23**

801.75 Open fracture of base of skull with subarachnoid, subdural, and extradural hemorrhage, prolonged (more than 24 hours) loss of consciousness, without return to pre-existing conscious level **23**

801.79 Open fracture of base of skull with subarachnoid, subdural, and extradural hemorrhage, unspecified concussion **28**

801.70 Open fracture of base of skull with subarachnoid, subdural, and extradural hemorrhage, unspecified state of consciousness **28**

801.5* Open fracture of base of skull without mention of intracranial injury **220**

801.52 Open fracture of base of skull without mention of intracranial injury, brief (less than one hour) loss of consciousness **28, 225**

801.56 Open fracture of base of skull without mention of intracranial injury, loss of consciousness of unspecified duration **23**

801.53 Open fracture of base of skull without mention of intracranial injury, moderate (1-24 hours) loss of consciousness **23, 225**

801.51 Open fracture of base of skull without mention of intracranial injury, no loss of consciousness **28**

801.54 Open fracture of base of skull without mention of intracranial injury, prolonged (more than 24 hours) loss of consciousness and return to pre-existing conscious level **23, 225**

801.55 Open fracture of base of skull without mention of intracranial injury, prolonged (more than 24 hours) loss of consciousness, without return to pre-existing conscious level **23, 225**

801.59 Open fracture of base of skull without mention of intracranial injury, unspecified concussion **28**

801.50 Open fracture of base of skull without mention of intracranial injury, unspecified state of consciousness **28**

825.1 Open fracture of calcaneus **99, 222**

806.1* Open fracture of cervical vertebra with spinal cord injury **221, 227**

805.1* Open fracture of cervical vertebra without mention of spinal cord injury **221**

810.1* Open fracture of clavicle **221**

811.12 Open fracture of coracoid process **99**

805.3 Open fracture of dorsal (thoracic) vertebra without mention of spinal cord injury **221**

806.3* Open fracture of dorsal vertebra with spinal cord injury **221, 227**

807.18 Open fracture of eight or more ribs **226**

807.15 Open fracture of five ribs **226**

807.14 Open fracture of four ribs **226**

811.13 Open fracture of glenoid cavity and neck of scapula **99**

807.6 Open fracture of larynx and trachea **3, 47, 221, 226**

824.3 Open fracture of lateral malleolus **222**

821.3* Open fracture of lower end of femur **222**

812.5* Open fracture of lower end of humerus **221, 227**

813.5* Open fracture of lower end of radius and ulna **221, 227**

806.5 Open fracture of lumbar spine with spinal cord injury **221, 227**

805.5 Open fracture of lumbar vertebra without mention of spinal cord injury **221**

824.1 Open fracture of medial malleolus **222**

815.1* Open fracture of metacarpal bones **221**

807.19 Open fracture of multiple ribs, unspecified **226**

826.1 Open fracture of one or more phalanges of foot **222**

816.1* Open fracture of one or more phalanges of hand **221**

811.19 Open fracture of other part of scapula **101**

808.5* Open fracture of other specified part of pelvis **221**

825.3* Open fracture of other tarsal and metatarsal bones **99, 222**

822.1 Open fracture of patella **222**

808.3 Open fracture of pubis **221**

807.1* Open fracture of rib(s) **52, 221**

806.7* Open fracture of sacrum and coccyx with spinal cord injury **221, 227**

805.7 Open fracture of sacrum and coccyx without mention of spinal cord injury **221, 227**

811.1* Open fracture of scapula **221**

807.17 Open fracture of seven ribs **226**

812.31	Open fracture of shaft of humerus **227**	800.82	Open fracture of vault of skull with other and unspecified intracranial hemorrhage, brief (less than one hour) loss of consciousness **28**
813.3*	Open fracture of shaft of radius and ulna **221, 227**		
823.3*	Open fracture of shaft of tibia and fibula **222, 227**	800.86	Open fracture of vault of skull with other and unspecified intracranial hemorrhage, loss of consciousness of unspecified duration **22**
821.1*	Open fracture of shaft or unspecified part of femur **166, 170, 222**		
812.3*	Open fracture of shaft or unspecified part of humerus **221**	800.83	Open fracture of vault of skull with other and unspecified intracranial hemorrhage, moderate (1-24 hours) loss of consciousness **22**
807.16	Open fracture of six ribs **226**		
807.3	Open fracture of sternum **52, 221, 226**	800.81	Open fracture of vault of skull with other and unspecified intracranial hemorrhage, no loss of consciousness **28**
829.1	Open fracture of unspecified bone **222**		
812.30	Open fracture of unspecified part of humerus **227**	800.84	Open fracture of vault of skull with other and unspecified intracranial hemorrhage, prolonged (more than 24 hours) loss of consciousness and return to pre-existing conscious level **22**
820.9	Open fracture of unspecified part of neck of femur **222**		
813.9*	Open fracture of unspecified part of radius with ulna **221, 227**	800.85	Open fracture of vault of skull with other and unspecified intracranial hemorrhage, prolonged (more than 24 hours) loss of consciousness, without return to pre-existing conscious level **22**
811.10	Open fracture of unspecified part of scapula **99**		
823.9*	Open fracture of unspecified part of tibia and fibula **222, 227**	800.89	Open fracture of vault of skull with other and unspecified intracranial hemorrhage, unspecified concussion **28**
805.9	Open fracture of unspecified part of vertebral column without mention of spinal cord injury **221**		
		800.80	Open fracture of vault of skull with other and unspecified intracranial hemorrhage, unspecified state of consciousness **28**
806.9	Open fracture of unspecified vertebra with spinal cord injury **221, 227**		
		800.7*	Open fracture of vault of skull with subarachnoid, subdural, and extradural hemorrhage **220, 225**
812.1*	Open fracture of upper end of humerus **221, 227**		
813.1*	Open fracture of upper end of radius and ulna **221, 227**	800.72	Open fracture of vault of skull with subarachnoid, subdural, and extradural hemorrhage, brief (less than one hour) loss of consciousness **28**
823.1*	Open fracture of upper end of tibia and fibula **222, 227**		
800.6*	Open fracture of vault of skull with cerebral laceration and contusion **220, 225**	800.76	Open fracture of vault of skull with subarachnoid, subdural, and extradural hemorrhage, loss of consciousness of unspecified duration **22**
800.62	Open fracture of vault of skull with cerebral laceration and contusion, brief (less than one hour) loss of consciousness **28**		
		800.73	Open fracture of vault of skull with subarachnoid, subdural, and extradural hemorrhage, moderate (1-24 hours) loss of consciousness **22**
800.66	Open fracture of vault of skull with cerebral laceration and contusion, loss of consciousness of unspecified duration **22**		
		800.71	Open fracture of vault of skull with subarachnoid, subdural, and extradural hemorrhage, no loss of consciousness **28**
800.63	Open fracture of vault of skull with cerebral laceration and contusion, moderate (1-24 hours) loss of consciousness **22**		
800.61	Open fracture of vault of skull with cerebral laceration and contusion, no loss of consciousness **28**	800.74	Open fracture of vault of skull with subarachnoid, subdural, and extradural hemorrhage, prolonged (more than 24 hours) loss of consciousness and return to pre-existing conscious level **22**
800.64	Open fracture of vault of skull with cerebral laceration and contusion, prolonged (more than 24 hours) loss of consciousness and return to pre-existing conscious level **22**	800.75	Open fracture of vault of skull with subarachnoid, subdural, and extradural hemorrhage, prolonged (more than 24 hours) loss of consciousness, without return to pre-existing conscious level **22**
800.65	Open fracture of vault of skull with cerebral laceration and contusion, prolonged (more than 24 hours) loss of consciousness, without return to pre-existing conscious level **22**		
		800.79	Open fracture of vault of skull with subarachnoid, subdural, and extradural hemorrhage, unspecified concussion **28**
800.69	Open fracture of vault of skull with cerebral laceration and contusion, unspecified concussion **28**		
		800.70	Open fracture of vault of skull with subarachnoid, subdural, and extradural hemorrhage, unspecified state of consciousness **28**
800.60	Open fracture of vault of skull with cerebral laceration and contusion, unspecified state of consciousness **28**		
		800.5*	Open fracture of vault of skull without mention of intracranial injury **220**
800.9*	Open fracture of vault of skull with intracranial injury of other and unspecified nature **220, 225**		
		800.52	Open fracture of vault of skull without mention of intracranial injury, brief (less than one hour) loss of consciousness **28, 224**
800.92	Open fracture of vault of skull with intracranial injury of other and unspecified nature, brief (less than one hour) loss of consciousness **28**		
		800.56	Open fracture of vault of skull without mention of intracranial injury, loss of consciousness of unspecified duration **22**
800.96	Open fracture of vault of skull with intracranial injury of other and unspecified nature, loss of consciousness of unspecified duration **23**		
		800.53	Open fracture of vault of skull without mention of intracranial injury, moderate (1-24 hours) loss of consciousness **22, 225**
800.93	Open fracture of vault of skull with intracranial injury of other and unspecified nature, moderate (1-24 hours) loss of consciousness **22**		
		800.51	Open fracture of vault of skull without mention of intracranial injury, no loss of consciousness **28**
800.91	Open fracture of vault of skull with intracranial injury of other and unspecified nature, no loss of consciousness **28**		
		800.54	Open fracture of vault of skull without mention of intracranial injury, prolonged (more than 24 hours) loss of consciousness and return to pre-existing conscious level **22, 225**
800.94	Open fracture of vault of skull with intracranial injury of other and unspecified nature, prolonged (more than 24 hours) loss of consciousness and return to pre-existing conscious level **22**		
		800.55	Open fracture of vault of skull without mention of intracranial injury, prolonged (more than 24 hours) loss of consciousness, without return to pre-existing conscious level **22, 225**
800.95	Open fracture of vault of skull with intracranial injury of other and unspecified nature, prolonged (more than 24 hours) loss of consciousness, without return to pre-existing conscious level **22**		
		800.59	Open fracture of vault of skull without mention of intracranial injury, unspecified concussion **28**
800.99	Open fracture of vault of skull with intracranial injury of other and unspecified nature, unspecified concussion **28**		
		800.50	Open fracture of vault of skull without mention of intracranial injury, unspecified state of consciousness **28**
800.90	Open fracture of vault of skull with intracranial injury of other and unspecified nature, unspecified state of consciousness **28**		
		804.7*	Open fractures involving skull or face with other bones with subarachnoid, subdural, and extradural hemorrhage **221, 226**
800.8*	Open fracture of vault of skull with other and unspecified intracranial hemorrhage **220, 225**		

804.72 Open fractures involving skull or face with other bones with subarachnoid, subdural, and extradural hemorrhage, brief (less than one hour) loss of consciousness **30**

804.76 Open fractures involving skull or face with other bones with subarachnoid, subdural, and extradural hemorrhage, loss of consciousness of unspecified duration **25**

804.73 Open fractures involving skull or face with other bones with subarachnoid, subdural, and extradural hemorrhage, moderate (1-24 hours) loss of consciousness **25**

804.71 Open fractures involving skull or face with other bones with subarachnoid, subdural, and extradural hemorrhage, no loss of consciousness **30**

804.74 Open fractures involving skull or face with other bones with subarachnoid, subdural, and extradural hemorrhage, prolonged (more than 24 hours) loss of consciousness and return to pre-existing conscious level **25**

804.75 Open fractures involving skull or face with other bones with subarachnoid, subdural, and extradural hemorrhage, prolonged (more than 24 hours) loss of consciousness, without return to pre-existing conscious level **25**

804.79 Open fractures involving skull or face with other bones with subarachnoid, subdural, and extradural hemorrhage, unspecified concussion **30**

804.70 Open fractures involving skull or face with other bones with subarachnoid, subdural, and extradural hemorrhage, unspecified state of consciousness **30**

804.6* Open fractures involving skull or face with other bones, with cerebral laceration and contusion **221**

804.62 Open fractures involving skull or face with other bones, with cerebral laceration and contusion, brief (less than one hour) loss of consciousness **30, 226**

804.66 Open fractures involving skull or face with other bones, with cerebral laceration and contusion, loss of consciousness of unspecified duration **25, 226**

804.63 Open fractures involving skull or face with other bones, with cerebral laceration and contusion, moderate (1-24 hours) loss of consciousness **25, 226**

804.61 Open fractures involving skull or face with other bones, with cerebral laceration and contusion, no loss of consciousness **30, 226**

804.64 Open fractures involving skull or face with other bones, with cerebral laceration and contusion, prolonged (more than 24 hours) loss of consciousness and return to pre-existing conscious level **25, 226**

804.65 Open fractures involving skull or face with other bones, with cerebral laceration and contusion, prolonged (more than 24 hours) loss of consciousness, without return to pre-existing conscious level **25, 226**

804.69 Open fractures involving skull or face with other bones, with cerebral laceration and contusion, unspecified concussion **30**

804.60 Open fractures involving skull or face with other bones, with cerebral laceration and contusion, unspecified state of consciousness **30, 226**

804.9* Open fractures involving skull or face with other bones, with intracranial injury of other and unspecified nature **221, 226**

804.92 Open fractures involving skull or face with other bones, with intracranial injury of other and unspecified nature, brief (less than one hour) loss of consciousness **30**

804.96 Open fractures involving skull or face with other bones, with intracranial injury of other and unspecified nature, loss of consciousness of unspecified duration **25**

804.93 Open fractures involving skull or face with other bones, with intracranial injury of other and unspecified nature, moderate (1-24 hours) loss of consciousness **25**

804.91 Open fractures involving skull or face with other bones, with intracranial injury of other and unspecified nature, no loss of consciousness **30**

804.94 Open fractures involving skull or face with other bones, with intracranial injury of other and unspecified nature, prolonged (more than 24 hours) loss of consciousness and return to pre-existing conscious level **25**

804.95 Open fractures involving skull or face with other bones, with intracranial injury of other and unspecified nature, prolonged (more than 24 hours) loss of consciousness, without return to pre-existing level **25**

804.99 Open fractures involving skull or face with other bones, with intracranial injury of other and unspecified nature, unspecified concussion **30**

804.90 Open fractures involving skull or face with other bones, with intracranial injury of other and unspecified nature, unspecified state of consciousness **30**

804.8* Open fractures involving skull or face with other bones, with other and unspecified intracranial hemorrhage **221, 226**

804.82 Open fractures involving skull or face with other bones, with other and unspecified intracranial hemorrhage, brief (less than one hour) loss of consciousness **30**

804.86 Open fractures involving skull or face with other bones, with other and unspecified intracranial hemorrhage, loss of consciousness of unspecified duration **25**

804.83 Open fractures involving skull or face with other bones, with other and unspecified intracranial hemorrhage, moderate (1-24 hours) loss of consciousness **25**

804.81 Open fractures involving skull or face with other bones, with other and unspecified intracranial hemorrhage, no loss of consciousness **30**

804.84 Open fractures involving skull or face with other bones, with other and unspecified intracranial hemorrhage, prolonged (more than 24 hours) loss of consciousness and return to pre-existing conscious level **25**

804.85 Open fractures involving skull or face with other bones, with other and unspecified intracranial hemorrhage, prolonged (more than 24 hours) loss of consciousness, without return to pre-existing conscious level **25**

804.89 Open fractures involving skull or face with other bones, with other and unspecified intracranial hemorrhage, unspecified concussion **30**

804.80 Open fractures involving skull or face with other bones, with other and unspecified intracranial hemorrhage, unspecified state of consciousness **30**

804.5* Open fractures involving skull or face with other bones, without mention of intracranial injury **221**

804.52 Open fractures involving skull or face with other bones, without mention of intracranial injury, brief (less than one hour) loss of consciousness **30, 226**

804.56 Open fractures involving skull or face with other bones, without mention of intracranial injury, loss of consciousness of unspecified duration **25**

804.53 Open fractures involving skull or face with other bones, without mention of intracranial injury, moderate (1-24 hours) loss of consciousness **25, 226**

804.51 Open fractures involving skull or face with other bones, without mention of intracranial injury, no loss of consciousness **30**

804.54 Open fractures involving skull or face with other bones, without mention of intracranial injury, prolonged (more than 24 hours) loss of consciousness and return to pre-existing conscious level **25, 226**

804.55 Open fractures involving skull or face with other bones, without mention of intracranial injury, prolonged (more than 24 hours) loss of consciousness, without return to pre-existing conscious level **25, 226**

804.59 Open fractures involving skull or face with other bones, without mention of intracranial injury, unspecified concussion **30**

804.50 Open fractures involving skull or face with other bones, without mention of intracranial injury, unspecified state of consciousness **30**

814.1* Open fractures of carpal bones **221**

*Code Range

820.3*	Open pertrochanteric fracture of femur **222**
820.1*	Open transcervical fracture **222**
824.7	Open trimalleolar fracture **222**
879.3	Open wound of abdominal wall, anterior, complicated **202**
879.2	Open wound of abdominal wall, anterior, without mention of complication **106**
879.5	Open wound of abdominal wall, lateral, complicated **202**
879.4	Open wound of abdominal wall, lateral, without mention of complication **106**
876*	Open wound of back **106, 223**
879.1	Open wound of breast, complicated **106**
879.0	Open wound of breast, without mention of complication **106**
873.71	Open wound of buccal mucosa, complicated **3**
873.61	Open wound of buccal mucosa, without mention of complication **3**
877*	Open wound of buttock **106, 223**
873.51	Open wound of cheek, complicated **3, 106**
873.41	Open wound of cheek, without mention of complication **3, 106**
875*	Open wound of chest (wall) **223**
875.1	Open wound of chest (wall), complicated **202**
875.0	Open wound of chest (wall), without mention of complication **106**
872*	Open wound of ear **47, 223**
881*	Open wound of elbow, forearm, and wrist **223**
881.1*	Open wound of elbow, forearm, and wrist, complicated **202**
881.2*	Open wound of elbow, forearm, and wrist, with tendon involvement **101**
881.0*	Open wound of elbow, forearm, and wrist, without mention of complication **107**
871*	Open wound of eyeball **40, 223**
873.59	Open wound of face, other and multiple sites, complicated **106**
873.49	Open wound of face, other and multiple sites, without mention of complication **106**
873.50	Open wound of face, unspecified site, complicated **3, 106**
873.40	Open wound of face, unspecified site, without mention of complication **3, 106**
883*	Open wound of finger(s) **223**
883.1	Open wound of finger(s), complicated **202**
883.2	Open wound of finger(s), with tendon involvement **101**
883.0	Open wound of finger(s), without mention of complication **107**
892*	Open wound of foot except toe(s) alone **223**
892.1	Open wound of foot except toe(s) alone, complicated **203**
892.2	Open wound of foot except toe(s) alone, with tendon involvement **101**
892.0	Open wound of foot except toe(s) alone, without mention of complication **107**
873.52	Open wound of forehead, complicated **106**
873.42	Open wound of forehead, without mention of complication **106**
878*	Open wound of genital organs (external), including traumatic amputation **223**
873.72	Open wound of gum (alveolar process), complicated **4**
873.62	Open wound of gum (alveolar process), without mention of complication **3**
882*	Open wound of hand except finger(s) alone **223**
882.1	Open wound of hand except finger(s) alone, complicated **202**
882.2	Open wound of hand except finger(s) alone, with tendon involvement **101**
882.0	Open wound of hand except finger(s) alone, without mention of complication **107**
890*	Open wound of hip and thigh **223**
890.1	Open wound of hip and thigh, complicated **203**
890.2	Open wound of hip and thigh, with tendon involvement **101**

890.0	Open wound of hip and thigh, without mention of complication **107**
873.7*	Open wound of internal structure of mouth, complicated **48**
873.6*	Open wound of internal structures of mouth, without mention of complication **48**
873.54	Open wound of jaw, complicated **3, 48**
873.44	Open wound of jaw, without mention of complication **3, 48**
891*	Open wound of knee, leg (except thigh), and ankle **223**
891.1	Open wound of knee, leg (except thigh), and ankle, complicated **203**
891.2	Open wound of knee, leg (except thigh), and ankle, with tendon involvement **101**
891.0	Open wound of knee, leg (except thigh), and ankle, without mention of complication **107**
874.1*	Open wound of larynx and trachea, complicated **223**
874.0*	Open wound of larynx and trachea, without mention of complication **223**
874.10	Open wound of larynx with trachea, complicated **4, 48, 226**
874.00	Open wound of larynx with trachea, without mention of complication **4, 48**
874.11	Open wound of larynx, complicated **4, 48, 226**
874.01	Open wound of larynx, without mention of complication **4, 48**
873.53	Open wound of lip, complicated **3, 48**
873.43	Open wound of lip, without mention of complication **3, 48**
873.79	Open wound of mouth, other and multiple sites, complicated **4**
873.69	Open wound of mouth, other and multiple sites, without mention of complication **3**
873.70	Open wound of mouth, unspecified site, complicated **3**
873.60	Open wound of mouth, unspecified site, without mention of complication **3**
873.22	Open wound of nasal cavity, without mention of complication **47**
873.21	Open wound of nasal septum, without mention of complication **47**
873.23	Open wound of nasal sinus, without mention of complication **48**
873.3*	Open wound of nose, complicated **3, 48**
873.29	Open wound of nose, multiple sites, without mention of complication **48**
873.20	Open wound of nose, unspecified site, without mention of complication **47**
873.2*	Open wound of nose, without mention of complication **3**
870*	Open wound of ocular adnexa **40, 223**
878.9	Open wound of other and unspecified parts of genital organs, complicated **124, 127, 131**
878.8	Open wound of other and unspecified parts of genital organs, without mention of complication **124, 127, 130**
874.9	Open wound of other and unspecified parts of neck, complicated **4, 106, 223**
874.8	Open wound of other and unspecified parts of neck, without mention of complication **4, 106, 223**
879.7	Open wound of other and unspecified parts of trunk, complicated **202**
879.6	Open wound of other and unspecified parts of trunk, without mention of complication **106**
879*	Open wound of other and unspecified sites, except limbs **223**
873.75	Open wound of palate, complicated **4**
873.65	Open wound of palate, without mention of complication **3**
878.1	Open wound of penis, complicated **124**
878.0	Open wound of penis, without mention of complication **124**
874.5	Open wound of pharynx, complicated **4, 48, 223**
874.4	Open wound of pharynx, without mention of complication **4, 48, 223**
873.1	Open wound of scalp, complicated **106**
873.0	Open wound of scalp, without mention of complication **106**

878.3	Open wound of scrotum and testes, complicated **124**
878.2	Open wound of scrotum and testes, without mention of complication **124**
880*	Open wound of shoulder and upper arm **223**
880.1*	Open wound of shoulder and upper arm, complicated **202**
880.2*	Open wound of shoulder and upper arm, with tendon involvement **101**
880.0*	Open wound of shoulder and upper arm, without mention of complication **107**
874.3	Open wound of thyroid gland, complicated **4**, **114**, **223**
874.2	Open wound of thyroid gland, without mention of complication **4**, **114**, **223**
893*	Open wound of toe(s) **223**
893.1	Open wound of toe(s), complicated **203**
893.2	Open wound of toe(s), with tendon involvement **101**
893.0	Open wound of toe(s), without mention of complication **107**
873.74	Open wound of tongue and floor of mouth, complicated **4**
873.64	Open wound of tongue and floor of mouth, without mention of complication **3**
874.12	Open wound of trachea, complicated **4**, **52**, **226**
874.02	Open wound of trachea, without mention of complication **4**, **52**
878.7	Open wound of vagina, complicated **127**, **130**
878.6	Open wound of vagina, without mention of complication **127**, **130**
878.5	Open wound of vulva, complicated **127**, **130**
878.4	Open wound of vulva, without mention of complication **127**, **130**
879.9	Open wound(s) (multiple) of unspecified site(s), complicated **202**
879.8	Open wound(s) (multiple) of unspecified site(s), without mention of complication **107**
365.14	Open-angle glaucoma of childhood **39**
360.14	Ophthalmia nodosa **39**
121.0	Opisthorchiasis **83**
118	Opportunistic mycoses **164**, **168**, **185**, **230**
377.13	Optic atrophy associated with retinal dystrophies **40**
950.0	Optic nerve injury **40**
377.3*	Optic neuritis **38**
376.01	Orbital cellulitis **38**
376.81	Orbital cysts **40**
376.33	Orbital edema or congestion **39**
802.6	Orbital floor (blow-out), closed fracture **3**, **40**, **221**
802.7	Orbital floor (blow-out), open fracture **3**, **40**, **221**
376.32	Orbital hemorrhage **39**
376.03	Orbital osteomyelitis **38**
376.02	Orbital periostitis **38**
376.04	Orbital tenonitis **38**
604*	Orchitis and epididymitis **124**
V42.84	Organ or tissue replaced by transplant, intestines **214**
327.1*	Organic disorders of excessive somnolence [Organic hypersomnia] **189**
327.0*	Organic disorders of initiating and maintaining sleep [Organic insomnia] **189**
327.4*	Organic parasomnia **3**
327.40	Organic parasomnia, unspecified **47**
327.2*	Organic sleep apnea **3**
327.20	Organic sleep apnea, unspecified **47**
327.5*	Organic sleep related movement disorders **3**
333.84	Organic writers' cramp **32**
073.7	Ornithosis with other specified complications **184**
073.0	Ornithosis with pneumonia **51**
073.8	Ornithosis with unspecified complication **184**
333.82	Orofacial dyskinesia **32**

V58.5	Orthodontics aftercare **213**
V57.4	Orthoptic training **214**
458.0	Orthostatic hypotension **68**
V57.81	Orthotic training **214**
723.7	Ossification of posterior longitudinal ligament in cervical region **97**
733.5	Osteitis condensans **98**
731*	Osteitis deformans and osteopathies associated with other disorders classified elsewhere **98**
715*	Osteoarthrosis and allied disorders **98**
732*	Osteochondropathies **98**
756.51	Osteogenesis imperfecta **87**
268.2	Osteomalacia, unspecified **98**
730.7*	Osteopathy resulting from poliomyelitis **100**
733.0*	Osteoporosis **98**
745.61	Ostium primum defect **67**
745.5	Ostium secundum type atrial septal defect **67**
388.7*	Otalgia **47**
766.1	Other "heavy-for-dates" infants not related to gestation period **171**, **172**
388.44	Other abnormal auditory perception, recruitment **47**
790.6	Other abnormal blood chemistry **213**
796.4	Other abnormal clinical finding **172**, **213**
785.3	Other abnormal heart sounds **69**
631*	Other abnormal product of conception **154**, **157**
654.43	Other abnormalities in shape or position of gravid uterus and of neighboring structures, antepartum **154**, **157**
654.41	Other abnormalities in shape or position of gravid uterus and of neighboring structures, delivered **135**, **142**, **148**
654.42	Other abnormalities in shape or position of gravid uterus and of neighboring structures, delivered, with mention of postpartum complication **135**, **142**, **148**
654.44	Other abnormalities in shape or position of gravid uterus and of neighboring structures, postpartum condition or complication **152**
654.40	Other abnormalities in shape or position of gravid uterus and of neighboring structures, unspecified as to episode of care **160**
788.6*	Other abnormality of urination **119**
616.4	Other abscess of vulva **127**, **130**
V45.79	Other acquired absence of organ **214**
736.76	Other acquired calcaneus deformity **100**
736.2*	Other acquired deformities of finger **100**
736.09	Other acquired deformities of forearm, excluding fingers **100**
736.6	Other acquired deformities of knee **100**
736.79	Other acquired deformity of ankle and foot **100**
738.5	Other acquired deformity of back or spine **97**
738.1*	Other acquired deformity of head **100**
333.79	Other acquired torsion dystonia **32**
411.89	Other acute and subacute form of ischemic heart disease **68**
506.3	Other acute and subacute respiratory conditions due to fumes and vapors **54**
391.8	Other acute rheumatic heart disease **68**
995.7	Other adverse food reactions, not elsewhere classified **204**
726.2	Other affections of shoulder region, not elsewhere classified **98**
V58.4*	Other aftercare following surgery **213**
780.09	Other alteration of consciousness **21**
516*	Other alveolar and parietoalveolar pneumonopathy **53**
995.0	Other anaphylactic reaction **203**
848*	Other and ill-defined sprains and strains **222**
654.93	Other and unspecified abnormality of organs and soft tissues of pelvis, antepartum condition or complication **155**, **157**

*Code Range

© 2013 OptumInsight, Inc.

654.92   Other and unspecified abnormality of organs and soft tissues of pelvis, delivered, with mention of postpartum complication **135, 143, 148**

654.94   Other and unspecified abnormality of organs and soft tissues of pelvis, postpartum condition or complication **152**

654.90   Other and unspecified abnormality of organs and soft tissues of pelvis, unspecified as to episode of care in pregnancy **160**

654.91   Other and unspecified abnormality of organs and soft tissues of pelvis, with delivery **135, 143, 148**

422.9*   Other and unspecified acute myocarditis **230**

995.2*   Other and unspecified adverse effect of drug, medicinal and biological substance **203**

303.9*   Other and unspecified alcohol dependence **191**

285*   Other and unspecified anemias **175**

413.9   Other and unspecified angina pectoris **68**

716*   Other and unspecified arthropathies **98**

448.9   Other and unspecified capillary diseases **66**

779.1   Other and unspecified cerebral irritability in newborn **163, 168**

851.9*   Other and unspecified cerebral laceration and contusion, with open intracranial wound **9, 11, 222, 226**

851.92   Other and unspecified cerebral laceration and contusion, with open intracranial wound, brief (less than 1 hour) loss of consciousness **31**

851.96   Other and unspecified cerebral laceration and contusion, with open intracranial wound, loss of consciousness of unspecified duration **26**

851.93   Other and unspecified cerebral laceration and contusion, with open intracranial wound, moderate (1-24 hours) loss of consciousness **26**

851.91   Other and unspecified cerebral laceration and contusion, with open intracranial wound, no loss of consciousness **31**

851.94   Other and unspecified cerebral laceration and contusion, with open intracranial wound, prolonged (more than 24 hours) loss of consciousness and return to pre-existing conscious level **26**

851.95   Other and unspecified cerebral laceration and contusion, with open intracranial wound, prolonged (more than 24 hours) loss of consciousness, without return to pre-existing conscious level **26**

851.99   Other and unspecified cerebral laceration and contusion, with open intracranial wound, unspecified concussion **31**

851.90   Other and unspecified cerebral laceration and contusion, with open intracranial wound, unspecified state of consciousness **31**

851.8*   Other and unspecified cerebral laceration and contusion, without mention of open intracranial wound **9, 11, 222, 226**

851.82   Other and unspecified cerebral laceration and contusion, without mention of open intracranial wound, brief (less than 1 hour) loss of consciousness **31**

851.86   Other and unspecified cerebral laceration and contusion, without mention of open intracranial wound, loss of consciousness of unspecified duration **26**

851.83   Other and unspecified cerebral laceration and contusion, without mention of open intracranial wound, moderate (1-24 hours) loss of consciousness **26**

851.81   Other and unspecified cerebral laceration and contusion, without mention of open intracranial wound, no loss of consciousness **31**

851.84   Other and unspecified cerebral laceration and contusion, without mention of open intracranial wound, prolonged (more than 24 hours) loss of consciousness and return to preexisting conscious level **26**

851.85   Other and unspecified cerebral laceration and contusion, without mention of open intracranial wound, prolonged (more than 24 hours) loss of consciousness, without return to pre-existing conscious level **26**

851.89   Other and unspecified cerebral laceration and contusion, without mention of open intracranial wound, unspecified concussion **31**

851.80   Other and unspecified cerebral laceration and contusion, without mention of open intracranial wound, unspecified state of consciousness **31**

381.3   Other and unspecified chronic nonsuppurative otitis media **46**

286.9   Other and unspecified coagulation defects **176**

999.9   Other and unspecified complications of medical care, not elsewhere classified **204**

756.9   Other and unspecified congenital anomaly of musculoskeletal system **101**

663.23   Other and unspecified cord entanglement, with compression, complicating labor and delivery, antepartum **155, 158**

663.21   Other and unspecified cord entanglement, with compression, complicating labor and delivery, delivered **137, 144, 150**

663.20   Other and unspecified cord entanglement, with compression, complicating labor and delivery, unspecified as to episode of care **137, 144, 150**

663.33   Other and unspecified cord entanglement, without mention of compression, complicating labor and delivery, antepartum **155, 158**

663.31   Other and unspecified cord entanglement, without mention of compression, complicating labor and delivery, delivered **137, 144, 150**

663.30   Other and unspecified cord entanglement, without mention of compression, complicating labor and delivery, unspecified as to episode of care **137, 144, 150**

717.3   Other and unspecified derangement of medial meniscus **99**

478.9   Other and unspecified diseases of upper respiratory tract **3, 46**

676.33   Other and unspecified disorder of breast associated with childbirth, antepartum condition or complication **156, 158**

676.32   Other and unspecified disorder of breast associated with childbirth, delivered, with mention of postpartum complication **139, 145, 151**

676.31   Other and unspecified disorder of breast associated with childbirth, delivered, with or without mention of antepartum condition **139, 145, 151**

676.34   Other and unspecified disorder of breast associated with childbirth, postpartum condition or complication **153**

676.30   Other and unspecified disorder of breast associated with childbirth, unspecified as to episode of care **161**

724*   Other and unspecified disorders of back **97**

729.9*   Other and unspecified disorders of soft tissue **98**

122.9   Other and unspecified echinococcosis **186**

993.2   Other and unspecified effects of high altitude **204**

300.19   Other and unspecified factitious illness **188**

128*   Other and unspecified helminthiases **186**

378.3*   Other and unspecified heterotropia **40**

999.31   Other and unspecified infection due to central venous catheter **69**

999.8*   Other and unspecified infusion and transfusion reaction **167, 171**

432*   Other and unspecified intracranial hemorrhage **8, 20, 165, 169**

853*   Other and unspecified intracranial hemorrhage following injury **222, 226**

853.1*   Other and unspecified intracranial hemorrhage following injury with open intracranial wound **9, 11**

853.12   Other and unspecified intracranial hemorrhage following injury, with open intracranial wound, brief (less than 1 hour) loss of consciousness **31**

853.16   Other and unspecified intracranial hemorrhage following injury, with open intracranial wound, loss of consciousness of unspecified duration **27**

853.13   Other and unspecified intracranial hemorrhage following injury, with open intracranial wound, moderate (1-24 hours) loss of consciousness **27**

853.11   Other and unspecified intracranial hemorrhage following injury, with open intracranial wound, no loss of consciousness **31**

853.14   Other and unspecified intracranial hemorrhage following injury, with open intracranial wound, prolonged (more than 24 hours) loss of consciousness and return to pre-existing conscious level **27**

853.15	Other and unspecified intracranial hemorrhage following injury, with open intracranial wound, prolonged (more than 24 hours) loss of consciousness, without return to pre-existing conscious level **27**
853.19	Other and unspecified intracranial hemorrhage following injury, with open intracranial wound, unspecified concussion **31**
853.10	Other and unspecified intracranial hemorrhage following injury, with open intracranial wound, unspecified state of consciousness **31**
853.0*	Other and unspecified intracranial hemorrhage following injury, without mention of open intracranial wound **9, 11**
853.02	Other and unspecified intracranial hemorrhage following injury, without mention of open intracranial wound, brief (less than 1 hour) loss of consciousness **31**
853.06	Other and unspecified intracranial hemorrhage following injury, without mention of open intracranial wound, loss of consciousness of unspecified duration **27**
853.03	Other and unspecified intracranial hemorrhage following injury, without mention of open intracranial wound, moderate (1-24 hours) loss of consciousness **27**
853.01	Other and unspecified intracranial hemorrhage following injury, without mention of open intracranial wound, no loss of consciousness **31**
853.04	Other and unspecified intracranial hemorrhage following injury, without mention of open intracranial wound, prolonged (more than 24 hours) loss of consciousness and return to preexisting conscious level **27**
853.09	Other and unspecified intracranial hemorrhage following injury, without mention of open intracranial wound, unspecified concussion **31**
853.00	Other and unspecified intracranial hemorrhage following injury, without mention of open intracranial wound, unspecified state of consciousness **31**
853.05	Other and unspecified intracranial hemorrhage following injury. Without mention of open intracranial wound, prolonged (more than 24 hours) loss of consciousness, without return to pre-existing conscious level **27**
370.4*	Other and unspecified keratoconjunctivitis **39**
173.1*	Other and unspecified malignant neoplasm of eyelid, including canthus **38**
173.8*	Other and unspecified malignant neoplasm of other specified sites of skin **108**
173.4*	Other and unspecified malignant neoplasm of scalp and skin of neck **108**
173.2*	Other and unspecified malignant neoplasm of skin of ear and external auditory canal **108**
173.0*	Other and unspecified malignant neoplasm of skin of lip **2, 108**
173.7*	Other and unspecified malignant neoplasm of skin of lower limb, including hip **108**
173.3*	Other and unspecified malignant neoplasm of skin of other and unspecified parts of face **108**
173.5*	Other and unspecified malignant neoplasm of skin of trunk, except scrotum **108**
173.6*	Other and unspecified malignant neoplasm of skin of upper limb, including shoulder **108**
173.9*	Other and unspecified malignant neoplasm of skin, site unspecified **108**
202.9*	Other and unspecified malignant neoplasms of lymphoid and histiocytic tissue **178, 181**
202.91	Other and unspecified malignant neoplasms of lymphoid and histiocytic tissue of lymph nodes of head, face, and neck **3**
558.9	Other and unspecified noninfectious gastroenteritis and colitis **78, 230**
873.8	Other and unspecified open wound of head without mention of complication **106**
873.9	Other and unspecified open wound of head, complicated **106**
386.1*	Other and unspecified peripheral vertigo **46**
696.5	Other and unspecified pityriasis **108**
579.3	Other and unspecified postsurgical nonabsorption **166, 170**
263*	Other and unspecified protein-calorie malnutrition **113, 230**
298.8	Other and unspecified reactive psychosis **189**
398.99	Other and unspecified rheumatic heart diseases **68**
307.9	Other and unspecified special symptom or syndrome, not elsewhere classified **188**
913.9	Other and unspecified superficial injury of elbow, forearm, and wrist, infected **106**
913.8	Other and unspecified superficial injury of elbow, forearm, and wrist, without mention of infection **107**
910.9	Other and unspecified superficial injury of face, neck, and scalp, infected **106**
910.8	Other and unspecified superficial injury of face, neck, and scalp, without mention of infection **107**
915.8	Other and unspecified superficial injury of finger without mention of infection **107**
915.9	Other and unspecified superficial injury of finger, infected **106**
917.9	Other and unspecified superficial injury of foot and toes, infected **106**
917.8	Other and unspecified superficial injury of foot and toes, without mention of infection **107**
914.9	Other and unspecified superficial injury of hand(s) except finger(s) alone, infected **106**
914.8	Other and unspecified superficial injury of hand(s) except finger(s) alone, without mention of infection **107**
916.9	Other and unspecified superficial injury of hip, thigh, leg, and ankle, infected **106**
916.8	Other and unspecified superficial injury of hip, thigh, leg, and ankle, without mention of infection **107**
919.9	Other and unspecified superficial injury of other, multiple, and unspecified sites, infected **106**
919.8	Other and unspecified superficial injury of other, multiple, and unspecified sites, without mention of infection **107**
912.9	Other and unspecified superficial injury of shoulder and upper arm, infected **106**
912.8	Other and unspecified superficial injury of shoulder and upper arm, without mention of infection **107**
911.9	Other and unspecified superficial injury of trunk, infected **106**
911.8	Other and unspecified superficial injury of trunk, without mention of infection **107**
097*	Other and unspecified syphilis **185**
661.23	Other and unspecified uterine inertia, antepartum **155, 158**
661.20	Other and unspecified uterine inertia, unspecified as to episode of care **136, 144, 149**
661.21	Other and unspecified uterine inertia, with delivery **136, 144, 149**
442.9	Other aneurysm of unspecified site **66**
379.49	Other anomaly of pupillary function **38**
V28.2	Other antenatal screening based on amniocentesis **156, 159**
641.83	Other antepartum hemorrhage, antepartum **154, 157**
641.80	Other antepartum hemorrhage, unspecified as to episode of care **159**
641.81	Other antepartum hemorrhage, with delivery **134, 140, 145**
671.53	Other antepartum phlebitis and thrombosis **156, 158**
542	Other appendicitis **78**
088*	Other arthropod-borne diseases **185**
362.1*	Other background retinopathy and retinal vascular changes **39, 230**
005.8*	Other bacterial food poisoning **75**
482*	Other bacterial pneumonia **165, 169, 230**
215*	Other benign neoplasm of connective and other soft tissue **100**
219*	Other benign neoplasm of uterus **127, 130**

426.53	Other bilateral bundle branch block **165**, **169**
745.8	Other bulbus cordis anomalies and anomalies of cardiac septal closure **68**
727.3	Other bursitis disorders **99**
594.1	Other calculus in bladder **119**
112.89	Other candidiasis of other specified sites **185**
323.81	Other causes of encephalitis and encephalomyelitis **10**, **230**
323.8*	Other causes of encephalitis, myelitis, and encephalomyelitis **9**, **34**
323.82	Other causes of myelitis **10**, **230**
660.83	Other causes of obstructed labor, antepartum **155**, **158**
660.81	Other causes of obstructed labor, delivered **136**, **143**, **149**
660.80	Other causes of obstructed labor, unspecified as to episode of care **136**, **143**, **149**
791.7	Other cells and casts in urine **120**
682*	Other cellulitis and abscess **103**, **106**, **166**, **170**
331.89	Other cerebral degeneration **19**
429.79	Other certain sequelae of myocardial infarction, not elsewhere classified **69**
375.6*	Other changes of lacrimal passages **39**
333.5	Other choreas **19**
491.8	Other chronic bronchitis **53**
595.2	Other chronic cystitis **119**
474.8	Other chronic disease of tonsils and adenoids **47**
098.39	Other chronic gonococcal infections of upper genitourinary tract **124**, **127**, **129**
571.8	Other chronic nonalcoholic liver disease **83**
614.7	Other chronic pelvic peritonitis, female **130**
416.8	Other chronic pulmonary heart diseases **69**
836.5*	Other closed dislocation of knee **222**
803.1*	Other closed skull fracture with cerebral laceration and contusion **221**, **225**
803.12	Other closed skull fracture with cerebral laceration and contusion, brief (less than one hour) loss of consciousness **29**
803.16	Other closed skull fracture with cerebral laceration and contusion, loss of consciousness of unspecified duration **24**
803.13	Other closed skull fracture with cerebral laceration and contusion, moderate (1-24 hours) loss of consciousness **24**
803.11	Other closed skull fracture with cerebral laceration and contusion, no loss of consciousness **29**
803.14	Other closed skull fracture with cerebral laceration and contusion, prolonged (more than 24 hours) loss of consciousness and return to pre-existing conscious level **24**
803.15	Other closed skull fracture with cerebral laceration and contusion, prolonged (more than 24 hours) loss of consciousness, without return to pre-existing conscious level **24**
803.19	Other closed skull fracture with cerebral laceration and contusion, unspecified concussion **29**
803.10	Other closed skull fracture with cerebral laceration and contusion, unspecified state of consciousness **29**
803.4*	Other closed skull fracture with intracranial injury of other and unspecified nature **221**, **225**
803.42	Other closed skull fracture with intracranial injury of other and unspecified nature, brief (less than one hour) loss of consciousness **29**
803.46	Other closed skull fracture with intracranial injury of other and unspecified nature, loss of consciousness of unspecified duration **24**
803.43	Other closed skull fracture with intracranial injury of other and unspecified nature, moderate (1-24 hours) loss of consciousness **24**
803.41	Other closed skull fracture with intracranial injury of other and unspecified nature, no loss of consciousness **29**

803.44	Other closed skull fracture with intracranial injury of other and unspecified nature, prolonged (more than 24 hours) loss of consciousness and return to pre-existing conscious level **24**
803.45	Other closed skull fracture with intracranial injury of other and unspecified nature, prolonged (more than 24 hours) loss of consciousness, without return to pre-existing conscious level **24**
803.49	Other closed skull fracture with intracranial injury of other and unspecified nature, unspecified concussion **29**
803.40	Other closed skull fracture with intracranial injury of other and unspecified nature, unspecified state of consciousness **29**
803.32	Other closed skull fracture with other and unspecified intracranial hemorrhage, brief (less than one hour) loss of consciousness **29**
803.36	Other closed skull fracture with other and unspecified intracranial hemorrhage, loss of consciousness of unspecified duration **24**
803.33	Other closed skull fracture with other and unspecified intracranial hemorrhage, moderate (1-24 hours) loss of consciousness **24**
803.31	Other closed skull fracture with other and unspecified intracranial hemorrhage, no loss of consciousness **29**
803.34	Other closed skull fracture with other and unspecified intracranial hemorrhage, prolonged (more than 24 hours) loss of consciousness and return to pre-existing conscious level **24**
803.35	Other closed skull fracture with other and unspecified intracranial hemorrhage, prolonged (more than 24 hours) loss of consciousness, without return to pre-existing conscious level **24**
803.39	Other closed skull fracture with other and unspecified intracranial hemorrhage, unspecified concussion **29**
803.30	Other closed skull fracture with other and unspecified intracranial hemorrhage, unspecified state of unconsciousness **29**
803.2*	Other closed skull fracture with subarachnoid, subdural, and extradural hemorrhage **221**, **225**
803.22	Other closed skull fracture with subarachnoid, subdural, and extradural hemorrhage, brief (less than one hour) loss of consciousness **29**
803.26	Other closed skull fracture with subarachnoid, subdural, and extradural hemorrhage, loss of consciousness of unspecified duration **24**
803.23	Other closed skull fracture with subarachnoid, subdural, and extradural hemorrhage, moderate (1-24 hours) loss of consciousness **24**
803.21	Other closed skull fracture with subarachnoid, subdural, and extradural hemorrhage, no loss of consciousness **29**
803.24	Other closed skull fracture with subarachnoid, subdural, and extradural hemorrhage, prolonged (more than 24 hours) loss of consciousness and return to pre-existing conscious level **24**
803.25	Other closed skull fracture with subarachnoid, subdural, and extradural hemorrhage, prolonged (more than 24 hours) loss of consciousness, without return to pre-existing conscious level **24**
803.29	Other closed skull fracture with subarachnoid, subdural, and extradural hemorrhage, unspecified concussion **29**
803.20	Other closed skull fracture with subarachnoid, subdural, and extradural hemorrhage, unspecified state of consciousness **29**
803.0*	Other closed skull fracture without mention of intracranial injury **221**
803.02	Other closed skull fracture without mention of intracranial injury, brief (less than one hour) loss of consciousness **29**, **225**
803.06	Other closed skull fracture without mention of intracranial injury, loss of consciousness of unspecified duration **24**
803.03	Other closed skull fracture without mention of intracranial injury, moderate (1-24 hours) loss of consciousness **23**, **225**
803.01	Other closed skull fracture without mention of intracranial injury, no loss of consciousness **29**
803.04	Other closed skull fracture without mention of intracranial injury, prolonged (more than 24 hours) loss of consciousness and return to pre-existing conscious level **24**, **225**
803.05	Other closed skull fracture without mention of intracranial injury, prolonged (more than 24 hours) loss of consciousness, without return to pre-existing conscious level **24**, **225**

803.09	Other closed skull fracture without mention of intracranial injury, unspecified concussion **29**
803.00	Other closed skull fracture without mention of intracranial injury, unspecified state of consciousness **29**
368.59	Other color vision deficiencies **39**
669.83	Other complication of labor and delivery, antepartum condition or complication **156, 158**
669.82	Other complication of labor and delivery, delivered, with mention of postpartum complication **138, 145, 151**
669.81	Other complication of labor and delivery, delivered, with or without mention of antepartum condition **138, 145, 151**
669.84	Other complication of labor and delivery, postpartum condition or complication **153**
669.80	Other complication of labor and delivery, unspecified as to episode of care **138, 145, 151**
674.30	Other complication of obstetrical surgical wounds, unspecified as to episode of care **161**
674.32	Other complication of obstetrical surgical wounds, with delivery, with mention of postpartum complication **138, 141, 147**
674.80	Other complication of puerperium, unspecified as to episode of care **161**
674.82	Other complication of puerperium, with delivery, with mention of postpartum complication **138, 141, 147**
996.76	Other complications due to genitourinary device, implant, and graft **120**
996.71	Other complications due to heart valve prosthesis **69**
996.77	Other complications due to internal joint prosthesis **99**
996.75	Other complications due to nervous system device, implant, and graft **33**
996.72	Other complications due to other cardiac device, implant, and graft **69**
996.78	Other complications due to other internal orthopedic device, implant, and graft **99**
996.79	Other complications due to other internal prosthetic device, implant, and graft **203**
996.74	Other complications due to other vascular device, implant, and graft **69**
996.73	Other complications due to renal dialysis device, implant, and graft **69**
996.70	Other complications due to unspecified device, implant, and graft **203**
669.43	Other complications of obstetrical surgery and procedures, antepartum condition or complication **156, 158**
669.44	Other complications of obstetrical surgery and procedures, postpartum condition or complication **153**
669.40	Other complications of obstetrical surgery and procedures, unspecified as to episode of care **138, 145, 150**
669.42	Other complications of obstetrical surgery and procedures, with delivery, with mention of postpartum complication **138, 141, 146**
669.41	Other complications of obstetrical surgery and procedures, with delivery, with or without mention of antepartum condition **138, 141, 146**
674.34	Other complications of obstetrical surgical wounds, postpartum condition or complication **153**
674.84	Other complications of puerperium, postpartum condition or complication **153**
668.83	Other complications of the administration of anesthesia or other sedation in labor and delivery, antepartum **155, 158**
668.81	Other complications of the administration of anesthesia or other sedation in labor and delivery, delivered **137, 141, 146**
668.82	Other complications of the administration of anesthesia or other sedation in labor and delivery, delivered, with mention of postpartum complication **137, 141, 146**
668.84	Other complications of the administration of anesthesia or other sedation in labor and delivery, postpartum condition or complication **153**
668.80	Other complications of the administration of anesthesia or other sedation in labor and delivery, unspecified as to episode of care **137, 144, 150**
758.5	Other conditions due to autosomal anomalies **213**
758.8*	Other conditions due to chromosome anomalies **124, 127, 130**
348.89	Other conditions of brain **20**
751.5	Other congenital anomalies of intestine **79**
755*	Other congenital anomalies of limbs **100**
742*	Other congenital anomalies of nervous system **33, 166, 170**
750.1*	Other congenital anomalies of tongue **3, 48**
747.2*	Other congenital anomaly of aorta **68**
751.69	Other congenital anomaly of gallbladder, bile ducts, and liver **83**
748.3	Other congenital anomaly of larynx, trachea, and bronchus **3, 47**
748.69	Other congenital anomaly of lung **54**
748.1	Other congenital anomaly of nose **47**
747.6*	Other congenital anomaly of peripheral vascular system **67**
756.3	Other congenital anomaly of ribs and sternum **54**
756.19	Other congenital anomaly of spine **98**
752.3*	Other congenital anomaly of uterus **127, 130**
754.7*	Other congenital deformity of feet **100**
745.69	Other congenital endocardial cushion defect **67**
759.6	Other congenital hamartoses, not elsewhere classified **180, 182**
771.2	Other congenital infection specific to the perinatal period **163, 167**
654.63	Other congenital or acquired abnormality of cervix, antepartum condition or complication **154, 157**
654.62	Other congenital or acquired abnormality of cervix, delivered, with mention of postpartum complication **135, 143, 148**
654.64	Other congenital or acquired abnormality of cervix, postpartum condition or complication **152**
654.60	Other congenital or acquired abnormality of cervix, unspecified as to episode of care in pregnancy **160**
654.61	Other congenital or acquired abnormality of cervix, with delivery **135, 142, 148**
780.39	Other convulsions **166, 170**
767.7	Other cranial and peripheral nerve injuries, birth trauma **163, 167**
648.94	Other current maternal conditions classifiable elsewhere complicating pregnancy, childbirth, or the puerperium, postpartum condition or complication **152**
648.93	Other current maternal conditions classifiable elsewhere, antepartum **154, 156**
648.90	Other current maternal conditions classifiable elsewhere, complicating pregnancy, childbirth, or the puerperium, unspecified as to episode of care **159**
648.91	Other current maternal conditions classifiable elsewhere, with delivery **135, 142, 148**
648.92	Other current maternal conditions classifiable elsewhere, with delivery, with current postpartum complication **135, 142, 148**
737.8	Other curvatures of spine associated with other conditions **87**
277.6	Other deficiencies of circulating enzymes **114**
281*	Other deficiency anemias **175, 230**
279.19	Other deficiency of cell-mediated immunity **175**
333.0	Other degenerative diseases of the basal ganglia **19**
374.56	Other degenerative disorders of skin affecting eyelid **39**
341.8	Other demyelinating diseases of central nervous system **19**
V46*	Other dependence on machines and devices **214**
702*	Other dermatoses **108**
315.39	Other developmental speech or language disorder **189**
478.29	Other disease of pharynx or nasopharynx **47**

*Code Range

525*	Other diseases and conditions of the teeth and supporting structures **3, 48**	246*	Other disorders of thyroid **114**
543*	Other diseases of appendix **78**	378.87	Other dissociated deviation of eye movements **38**
077*	Other diseases of conjunctiva due to viruses and Chlamydiae **38**	995.27	Other drug allergy **166, 171**
424*	Other diseases of endocardium **67**	709.09	Other dyschromia **172**
478.79	Other diseases of larynx **47**	958.8	Other early complications of trauma **204, 224**
478.7*	Other diseases of larynx, not elsewhere classified **3**	102.2	Other early skin lesions due to yaws **107**
518.89	Other diseases of lung, not elsewhere classified **54**	122.3	Other echinococcus granulosus infection **186**
519.3	Other diseases of mediastinum, not elsewhere classified **54**	122.6	Other echinococcus multilocularis infection **186**

525* Other diseases and conditions of the teeth and supporting structures **3, 48**

543* Other diseases of appendix **78**

077* Other diseases of conjunctiva due to viruses and Chlamydiae **38**

424* Other diseases of endocardium **67**

478.79 Other diseases of larynx **47**

478.7* Other diseases of larynx, not elsewhere classified **3**

518.89 Other diseases of lung, not elsewhere classified **54**

519.3 Other diseases of mediastinum, not elsewhere classified **54**

478.19 Other diseases of nasal cavity and sinuses **172**

478.1* Other diseases of nasal cavity and sinuses **47**

423* Other diseases of pericardium **69**

478.2* Other diseases of pharynx, not elsewhere classified **3**

417* Other diseases of pulmonary circulation **69**

519.8 Other diseases of respiratory system, not elsewhere classified **54**

289.5* Other diseases of spleen **176**

519.19 Other diseases of trachea and bronchus **3**

519.1* Other diseases of trachea and bronchus, not elsewhere classified **54**

478.5 Other diseases of vocal cords **3, 47**

307.59 Other disorder of eating **189**

312.39 Other disorder of impulse control **188**

676.83 Other disorder of lactation, antepartum condition or complication **156, 158**

676.80 Other disorder of lactation, unspecified as to episode of care **161**

676.82 Other disorder of lactation, with delivery, with mention of postpartum complication **139, 145, 151**

676.81 Other disorder of lactation, with delivery, with or without mention of antepartum condition **139, 145, 151**

728.89 Other disorder of muscle, ligament, and fascia **99**

576* Other disorders of biliary tract **83**

368.3* Other disorders of binocular vision **39**

596* Other disorders of bladder **120**

733.99 Other disorders of bone and cartilage **100**

611* Other disorders of breast **106**

388.8 Other disorders of ear **47**

381.8* Other disorders of Eustachian tube **47**

380.8* Other disorders of external ear **47**

374.8* Other disorders of eyelid **39**

629* Other disorders of female genital organs **127**

575* Other disorders of gallbladder **83**

360.8* Other disorders of globe **39**

364.8* Other disorders of iris and ciliary body **39**

386.8 Other disorders of labyrinth **46**

375.1* Other disorders of lacrimal gland **39**

375.8* Other disorders of lacrimal system **39**

676.84 Other disorders of lactation, postpartum condition or complication **153**

383.8* Other disorders of mastoid **47**

385* Other disorders of middle ear and mastoid **47**

377.4* Other disorders of optic nerve **38**

429.81 Other disorders of papillary muscle **67, 165, 169**

568* Other disorders of peritoneum **79**

273.8 Other disorders of plasma protein metabolism **180, 182**

602* Other disorders of prostate **124**

277.2 Other disorders of purine and pyrimidine metabolism **114**

367.8* Other disorders of refraction and accommodation **39**

379.1* Other disorders of sclera **40**

709* Other disorders of skin and subcutaneous tissue **108**

727.8* Other disorders of synovium, tendon, and bursa **99**

246* Other disorders of thyroid **114**

378.87 Other dissociated deviation of eye movements **38**

995.27 Other drug allergy **166, 171**

709.09 Other dyschromia **172**

958.8 Other early complications of trauma **204, 224**

102.2 Other early skin lesions due to yaws **107**

122.3 Other echinococcus granulosus infection **186**

122.6 Other echinococcus multilocularis infection **186**

994.9 Other effects of external causes **204**

V50.8 Other elective surgery for purposes other than remedying health states **214**

492.8 Other emphysema **53**

323.41 Other encephalitis and encephalomyelitis due to other infections classified elsewhere **10**

323.4* Other encephalitis, myelitis, and encephalomyelitis due to other infections classified elsewhere **9, 34**

259* Other endocrine disorders **114**

360.19 Other endophthalmitis **38**

048 Other enterovirus diseases of central nervous system **21**

726.79 Other enthesopathy of ankle and tarsus **98**

333.99 Other extrapyramidal disease and abnormal movement disorder **19**

802.8 Other facial bones, closed fracture **3, 101, 221**

802.9 Other facial bones, open fracture **3, 101, 221**

653.73 Other fetal abnormality causing disproportion, antepartum **154, 157**

653.71 Other fetal abnormality causing disproportion, delivered **135, 142, 148**

653.70 Other fetal abnormality causing disproportion, unspecified as to episode of care **160**

728.7* Other fibromatoses of muscle, ligament, and fascia **99**

V67.5* Other follow-up examination **214**

493.8* Other forms of asthma **53**

370.8 Other forms of keratitis **39**

379.56 Other forms of nystagmus **40**

114.3 Other forms of progressive coccidioidomycosis **164, 168, 185**

361.8* Other forms of retinal detachment **39**

333.89 Other fragments of torsion dystonia **32**

V70.3 Other general medical exami for administrative purposes **173**

780.9* Other general symptoms **213**

437.1 Other generalized ischemic cerebrovascular disease **20**

V83.8* Other genetic carrier status **215**

054.19 Other genital herpes **124, 127, 129, 229**

306.59 Other genitourinary malfunction arising from mental factors **120**

098.85 Other gonococcal heart disease **68**

098.59 Other gonococcal infection of joint **97**

098.19 Other gonococcal infections (acute) of upper genitourinary tract **124, 127, 129**

274.19 Other gouty nephropathy **120**

339* Other headache syndromes **34**

286.59 Other hemorrhagic disorder due to intrinsic circulating anticoagulants, antibodies, or inhibitors **176**

551* Other hernia of abdominal cavity, with gangrene **78**

053.19 Other herpes zoster with nervous system complications **21, 164, 168, 229**

058.29 Other human herpesvirus encephalitis **9, 10, 33, 164, 168, 229**

058.8* Other human herpesvirus infections **107**

278.8 Other hyperalimentation **113**

701* Other hypertrophic and atrophic conditions of skin **108**

437.8 Other ill-defined cerebrovascular disease **21**

799.8* Other ill-defined conditions **213**

429.89	Other ill-defined heart disease **67**
666.14	Other immediate postpartum hemorrhage, postpartum condition or complication **152**
666.10	Other immediate postpartum hemorrhage, unspecified as to episode of care **161**
666.12	Other immediate postpartum hemorrhage, with delivery **137, 140, 146**
771.8*	Other infection specific to the perinatal period **163, 167**
730.8*	Other infections involving bone in diseases classified elsewhere **96**
134*	Other infestation **108**
357.8*	Other inflammatory and toxic neuropathy **21**
608.4	Other inflammatory disorder of male genital organs **124**
607.2	Other inflammatory disorders of penis **124**
720.8*	Other inflammatory spondylopathies **97**
999.88	Other infusion reaction **69**
665.54	Other injury to pelvic organs, postpartum condition or complication **152**
665.50	Other injury to pelvic organs, unspecified as to episode of care in pregnancy **137, 144, 150**
665.51	Other injury to pelvic organs, with delivery **137, 144, 150**
717.8*	Other internal derangement of knee **99**
370.59	Other interstitial and deep keratitis **39**
379.59	Other irregularities of eye movements **40**
718.8*	Other joint derangement, not elsewhere classified **100**
655.83	Other known or suspected fetal abnormality, not elsewhere classified, affecting management of mother, antepartum condition or complication **155, 157**
655.81	Other known or suspected fetal abnormality, not elsewhere classified, affecting management of mother, delivery **135, 143, 148**
655.80	Other known or suspected fetal abnormality, not elsewhere classified, affecting management of mother, unspecified as to episode of care **160**
090.5	Other late congenital syphilis, symptomatic **185**
208.8*	Other leukemia of unspecified cell type **181**
686*	Other local infection of skin and subcutaneous tissue **106**
003.29	Other localized salmonella infections **185**
368.44	Other localized visual field defect **38**
594.8	Other lower urinary tract calculus **119**
238.79	Other lymphatic and hematopoietic tissues **178, 181**
204.8*	Other lymphoid leukemia **181**
670.82	Other major puerperal infection, delivered, with mention of postpartum complication **138, 141, 146**
670.84	Other major puerperal infection, postpartum condition or complication **153**
670.80	Other major puerperal infection, unspecified as to episode of care or not applicable **161**
780.79	Other malaise and fatigue **213**
202.8*	Other malignant lymphomas **178, 181, 230**
202.81	Other malignant lymphomas of lymph nodes of head, face, and neck **3**
199.1	Other malignant neoplasm of unspecified site **180**
102.7	Other manifestations due to yaws **185**
264.8	Other manifestations of vitamin A deficiency **113**
648.64	Other maternal cardiovascular diseases complicating pregnancy, childbirth, or the puerperium, postpartum condition or complication **152**
648.60	Other maternal cardiovascular diseases complicating pregnancy, childbirth, or the puerperium, unspecified as to episode of care **159**
648.63	Other maternal cardiovascular diseases, antepartum **154, 156**
648.61	Other maternal cardiovascular diseases, with delivery **134, 140, 146**
648.62	Other maternal cardiovascular diseases, with delivery, with current postpartum complication **134, 140, 146**
647.21	Other maternal venereal diseases with delivery **134, 140, 146**
647.22	Other maternal venereal diseases with delivery, with current postpartum complication **134, 140, 146**
647.23	Other maternal venereal diseases, antepartum condition or complication **154, 156**
647.20	Other maternal venereal diseases, complicating pregnancy, childbirth, or the puerperium, unspecified as to episode of care **159**
647.60	Other maternal viral disease complicating pregnancy, childbirth, or the puerperium, unspecified as to episode of care **159**
647.61	Other maternal viral disease with delivery **134, 140, 146**
647.62	Other maternal viral disease with delivery, with current postpartum complication **134, 140, 146**
647.63	Other maternal viral disease, antepartum **154, 156**
647.64	Other maternal viral diseases complicating pregnancy, childbirth, or the puerperium, postpartum condition or complication **152**
206.8*	Other monocytic leukemia **181**
066.3	Other mosquito-borne fever **184**
V34.1	Other multiple birth (three or more), mates all liveborn, born before admission to hospital **171, 172**
V34.2	Other multiple birth (three or more), mates all liveborn, born outside hospital and not hospitalized **173**
V35.1	Other multiple birth (three or more), mates all stillborn, born before admission to hospital **171, 172**
V35.2	Other multiple birth (three or more), mates all stillborn, born outside of hospital and not hospitalized **173**
V36.1	Other multiple birth (three or more), mates liveborn and stillborn, born before admission to hospital **171, 172**
V36.2	Other multiple birth (three or more), mates liveborn and stillborn, born outside hospital and not hospitalized **173**
V37.1	Other multiple birth (three or more), unspecified whether mates liveborn or stillborn, born before admission to hospital **172**
V37.2	Other multiple birth (three or more), unspecified whether mates liveborn or stillborn, born outside of hospital **173**
651.63	Other multiple pregnancy with fetal loss and retention of one or more fetus(es), antepartum **154, 157**
651.61	Other multiple pregnancy with fetal loss and retention of one or more fetus(es), delivered **135, 142, 148**
651.60	Other multiple pregnancy with fetal loss and retention of one or more fetus(es), unspecified as to episode of care or not applicable **160**
V34.01	Other multiple, mates all liveborn, born in hospital, delivered by cesarean delivery **171, 172**
V34.00	Other multiple, mates all liveborn, born in hospital, delivered without mention of cesarean delivery **171, 172**
V35.01	Other multiple, mates all stillborn, born in hospital, delivered by cesarean delivery **171, 172**
V35.00	Other multiple, mates all stillborn, born in hospital, delivered without mention of cesarean delivery **171, 172**
V36.01	Other multiple, mates liveborn and stillborn, born in hospital, delivered by cesarean delivery **171, 172**
V36.00	Other multiple, mates liveborn and stillborn, born in hospital, delivered without mention of cesarean delivery **171, 172**
V37.01	Other multiple, unspecified whether mates stillborn or liveborn, born in hospital, delivered by cesarean delivery **172**
V37.00	Other multiple, unspecified whether mates stillborn or liveborn, born in hospital, delivered without mention of cesarean delivery **172**
729.89	Other musculoskeletal symptoms referable to limbs **98**
117*	Other mycoses **185**
323.42	Other myelitis due to other infections classified elsewhere **10**

205.8*	Other myeloid leukemia **181**
336.8	Other myelopathy **32**
359.89	Other myopathies **33**
200.8*	Other named variants of lymphosarcoma and reticulosarcoma **230**
200.81	Other named variants of lymphosarcoma and reticulosarcoma of lymph nodes of head, face, and neck **2**
056.09	Other neurological rubella complications **33**
283.19	Other non-autoimmune hemolytic anemias **175**
099.4*	Other nongonococcal urethritis (NGU) **124, 127, 130**
457.8	Other noninfectious disorders of lymphatic channels **176**
457.1	Other noninfectious lymphedema **108**
794.39	Other nonspecific abnormal cardiovascular system function study **69**
796.9	Other nonspecific abnormal finding **213**
792.9	Other nonspecific abnormal finding in body substances **213**
793.19	Other nonspecific abnormal finding of lung field **54**
793.9*	Other nonspecific abnormal findings on radiological and other examinations of body structure **213**
795.4	Other nonspecific abnormal histological findings **172, 213**
794.19	Other nonspecific abnormal result of function study of peripheral nervous system and special senses **33**
790.5	Other nonspecific abnormal serum enzyme levels **213**
791.9	Other nonspecific finding on examination of urine **120**
790.9*	Other nonspecific findings on examination of blood **213**
795.7*	Other nonspecific immunological findings **176**
269*	Other nutritional deficiencies **113, 230**
673.83	Other obstetrical pulmonary embolism, antepartum **156, 158**
673.84	Other obstetrical pulmonary embolism, postpartum condition or complication **153**
673.80	Other obstetrical pulmonary embolism, unspecified as to episode of care **161**
673.82	Other obstetrical pulmonary embolism, with delivery, with mention of postpartum complication **138, 141, 147**
673.81	Other obstetrical pulmonary embolism, with delivery, with or without mention of antepartum condition **138, 141, 147**
537.3	Other obstruction of duodenum **77**
V62.2*	Other occupational circumstances or maladjustment **214**
264.7	Other ocular manifestations of vitamin A deficiency **39**
836.6*	Other open dislocation of knee **222, 227**
803.6*	Other open skull fracture with cerebral laceration and contusion **221, 225**
803.62	Other open skull fracture with cerebral laceration and contusion, brief (less than one hour) loss of consciousness **29**
803.66	Other open skull fracture with cerebral laceration and contusion, loss of consciousness of unspecified duration **24**
803.63	Other open skull fracture with cerebral laceration and contusion, moderate (1-24 hours) loss of consciousness **24**
803.61	Other open skull fracture with cerebral laceration and contusion, no loss of consciousness **29**
803.64	Other open skull fracture with cerebral laceration and contusion, prolonged (more than 24 hours) loss of consciousness and return to pre-existing conscious level **24**
803.65	Other open skull fracture with cerebral laceration and contusion, prolonged (more than 24 hours) loss of consciousness, without return to pre-existing conscious level **24**
803.69	Other open skull fracture with cerebral laceration and contusion, unspecified concussion **29**
803.60	Other open skull fracture with cerebral laceration and contusion, unspecified state of consciousness **29**
803.9*	Other open skull fracture with intracranial injury of other and unspecified nature **221, 225**

803.92	Other open skull fracture with intracranial injury of other and unspecified nature, brief (less than one hour) loss of consciousness **29**
803.96	Other open skull fracture with intracranial injury of other and unspecified nature, loss of consciousness of unspecified duration **24**
803.93	Other open skull fracture with intracranial injury of other and unspecified nature, moderate (1-24 hours) loss of consciousness **24**
803.91	Other open skull fracture with intracranial injury of other and unspecified nature, no loss of consciousness **29**
803.94	Other open skull fracture with intracranial injury of other and unspecified nature, prolonged (more than 24 hours) loss of consciousness and return to pre-existing conscious level **24**
803.95	Other open skull fracture with intracranial injury of other and unspecified nature, prolonged (more than 24 hours) loss of consciousness, without return to pre-existing conscious level **24**
803.99	Other open skull fracture with intracranial injury of other and unspecified nature, unspecified concussion **29**
803.90	Other open skull fracture with intracranial injury of other and unspecified nature, unspecified state of consciousness **29**
803.8*	Other open skull fracture with other and unspecified intracranial hemorrhage **221, 225**
803.82	Other open skull fracture with other and unspecified intracranial hemorrhage, brief (less than one hour) loss of consciousness **29**
803.86	Other open skull fracture with other and unspecified intracranial hemorrhage, loss of consciousness of unspecified duration **24**
803.83	Other open skull fracture with other and unspecified intracranial hemorrhage, moderate (1-24 hours) loss of consciousness **24**
803.81	Other open skull fracture with other and unspecified intracranial hemorrhage, no loss of consciousness **29**
803.84	Other open skull fracture with other and unspecified intracranial hemorrhage, prolonged (more than 24 hours) loss of consciousness and return to pre-existing conscious level **24**
803.85	Other open skull fracture with other and unspecified intracranial hemorrhage, prolonged (more than 24 hours) loss of consciousness, without return to pre-existing conscious level **24**
803.89	Other open skull fracture with other and unspecified intracranial hemorrhage, unspecified concussion **29**
803.80	Other open skull fracture with other and unspecified intracranial hemorrhage, unspecified state of consciousness **29**
803.7*	Other open skull fracture with subarachnoid, subdural, and extradural hemorrhage **221, 225**
803.72	Other open skull fracture with subarachnoid, subdural, and extradural hemorrhage, brief (less than one hour) loss of consciousness **29**
803.76	Other open skull fracture with subarachnoid, subdural, and extradural hemorrhage, loss of consciousness of unspecified duration **24**
803.73	Other open skull fracture with subarachnoid, subdural, and extradural hemorrhage, moderate (1-24 hours) loss of consciousness **24**
803.71	Other open skull fracture with subarachnoid, subdural, and extradural hemorrhage, no loss of consciousness **29**
803.74	Other open skull fracture with subarachnoid, subdural, and extradural hemorrhage, prolonged (more than 24 hours) loss of consciousness and return to pre-existing conscious level **24**
803.75	Other open skull fracture with subarachnoid, subdural, and extradural hemorrhage, prolonged (more than 24 hours) loss of consciousness, without return to pre-existing conscious level **24**
803.79	Other open skull fracture with subarachnoid, subdural, and extradural hemorrhage, unspecified concussion **29**
803.70	Other open skull fracture with subarachnoid, subdural, and extradural hemorrhage, unspecified state of consciousness **29**
803.50	Other open skull fracture without mention of injury, state of consciousness unspecified **29**

803.5*	Other open skull fracture without mention of intracranial injury **221**
803.52	Other open skull fracture without mention of intracranial injury, brief (less than one hour) loss of consciousness **29**, **225**
803.56	Other open skull fracture without mention of intracranial injury, loss of consciousness of unspecified duration **24**
803.53	Other open skull fracture without mention of intracranial injury, moderate (1-24 hours) loss of consciousness **24**, **225**
803.51	Other open skull fracture without mention of intracranial injury, no loss of consciousness **29**
803.54	Other open skull fracture without mention of intracranial injury, prolonged (more than 24 hours) loss of consciousness and return to pre-existing conscious level **24**, **225**
803.55	Other open skull fracture without mention of intracranial injury, prolonged (more than 24 hours) loss of consciousness, without return to pre-existing conscious level **24**, **225**
803.59	Other open skull fracture without mention of intracranial injury, unspecified concussion **29**
873*	Other open wound of head **223**
053.29	Other ophthalmic herpes zoster complications **164**, **168**, **229**
313.8*	Other or mixed emotional disturbances of childhood or adolescence **189**
376.89	Other orbital disorder **40**
V43.89	Other organ or tissue replaced by other means **2**
V43.8*	Other organ or tissue replaced by other means **214**
V42.89	Other organ or tissue replaced by transplant **214**
327.49	Other organic parasomnia **47**
327.29	Other organic sleep apnea **47**
327.8	Other organic sleep disorders **3**, **47**
327.59	Other organic sleep related movement disorders **47**
V54.8*	Other orthopedic aftercare **99**
380.2*	Other otitis externa **47**
388.69	Other otorrhea **47**
307.89	Other pain disorder related to psychological factors **188**
273.2	Other paraproteinemias **178**, **181**
726.8	Other peripheral enthesopathies **98**
V15*	Other personal history presenting hazards to health **214**
301.8*	Other personality disorders **188**
V65*	Other persons seeking consultation **214**
671.50	Other phlebitis and thrombosis complicating pregnancy and the puerperium, unspecified as to episode of care **161**
671.52	Other phlebitis and thrombosis with delivery, with mention of postpartum complication **138**, **141**, **146**
671.51	Other phlebitis and thrombosis with delivery, with or without mention of antepartum condition **138**, **141**, **146**
671.54	Other phlebitis and thrombosis, postpartum condition or complication **153**
V57.1	Other physical therapy **213**
656.73	Other placental conditions affecting management of mother, antepartum **155**, **157**
656.71	Other placental conditions affecting management of mother, delivered **136**, **143**, **149**
656.70	Other placental conditions affecting management of mother, unspecified as to episode of care **160**
V50.1	Other plastic surgery for unacceptable cosmetic appearance **109**
512.8*	Other pneumothorax and air leak **53**
323.62	Other postinfectious encephalitis and encephalomyelitis **10**
564.4	Other postoperative functional disorders **78**
998.59	Other postoperative infection **167**, **171**, **184**
V45.8*	Other postprocedural status **214**
059*	Other poxvirus infections **184**
642.24	Other pre-existing hypertension complicating pregnancy, childbirth, and the puerperium, postpartum condition or complication **151**
642.20	Other pre-existing hypertension complicating pregnancy, childbirth, and the puerperium, unspecified as to episode of care **159**
642.23	Other pre-existing hypertension, antepartum **154**, **156**
642.21	Other pre-existing hypertension, with delivery **134**, **140**, **146**
642.22	Other pre-existing hypertension, with delivery, with current postpartum complication **134**, **140**, **146**
765.1*	Other preterm infants **163**, **167**
091.2	Other primary syphilis **185**
658.83	Other problem associated with amniotic cavity and membranes, antepartum **155**, **158**
658.81	Other problem associated with amniotic cavity and membranes, delivered **136**, **143**, **149**
658.80	Other problem associated with amniotic cavity and membranes, unspecified as to episode of care **160**
V47*	Other problems with internal organs **214**
362.2*	Other proliferative retinopathy **39**
V50.49	Other prophylactic organ removal **214**
263.8	Other protein-calorie malnutrition **164**, **168**
007*	Other protozoal intestinal diseases **75**
696.1	Other psoriasis **105**
V62.89	Other psychological or physical stress, not elsewhere classified **214**
518.82	Other pulmonary insufficiency, not elsewhere classified **54**
518.52	Other pulmonary insufficiency, not elsewhere classified, following trauma and surgery **165**, **170**
590.8*	Other pyelonephritis or pyonephrosis, not specified as acute or chronic **166**, **170**
012*	Other respiratory tuberculosis **229**
362.8*	Other retinal disorders **39**
714.2	Other rheumatoid arthritis with visceral or systemic involvement **97**
083*	Other rickettsioses **185**
277.84	Other secondary carnitine deficiency **114**
374.45	Other sensorimotor disorders of eyelid **38**
999.5*	Other serum reaction, not elsewhere classified **167**, **171**, **203**
262	Other severe protein-calorie malnutrition **113**, **164**, **168**, **230**
785.59	Other shock without mention of trauma **186**
799.59	Other signs and symptoms involving cognition **188**
799.29	Other signs and symptoms involving emotional state **188**
780.59	Other sleep disturbances **189**
315.2	Other specific developmental learning difficulties **189**
315.09	Other specific developmental reading disorder **189**
728.3	Other specific muscle disorders **99**
309.8*	Other specified adjustment reactions **188**
995.8*	Other specified adverse effects, not elsewhere classified **204**
V58.8*	Other specified aftercare **213**
516.8	Other specified alveolar and parietoalveolar pneumonopathies **230**
752.89	Other specified anomalies of genital organs **127**, **130**
284.8*	Other specified aplastic anemias **175**, **230**
066.8	Other specified arthropod-borne viral diseases **184**
040.89	Other specified bacterial diseases **185**
694.8	Other specified bullous dermatosis **105**
427.8*	Other specified cardiac dysrhythmias **68**
093.8*	Other specified cardiovascular syphilis **68**
123.8	Other specified cestode infection **75**
459.89	Other specified circulatory system disorders **67**

       *Code Range

646.80	Other specified complication of pregnancy, unspecified as to episode of care **156**, **159**	312.8*	Other specified disturbances of conduct, not elsewhere classified **189**
646.81	Other specified complication of pregnancy, with delivery **134**, **142**, **147**	993.8	Other specified effects of air pressure **204**
646.83	Other specified complication, antepartum **154**, **156**	695.89	Other specified erythematous condition **108**
998.89	Other specified complications **204**	V61.8	Other specified family circumstance **214**
646.84	Other specified complications of pregnancy, postpartum condition or complication **152**	656.83	Other specified fetal and placental problems affecting management of mother, antepartum **155**, **157**
646.82	Other specified complications of pregnancy, with delivery, with current postpartum complication **134**, **142**, **147**	656.81	Other specified fetal and placental problems affecting management of mother, delivered **136**, **143**, **149**
778.8	Other specified condition involving the integument of fetus and newborn **171**, **172**	656.80	Other specified fetal and placental problems affecting management of mother, unspecified as to episode of care **160**
426.89	Other specified conduction disorder **165**, **169**	619.8	Other specified fistula involving female genital tract **127**, **130**, **166**, **170**
751.8	Other specified congenital anomalies of digestive system **79**	414.8	Other specified forms of chronic ischemic heart disease **67**
744.2*	Other specified congenital anomalies of ear **47**	511.89	Other specified forms of effusion, except tuberculous **52**, **165**, **170**
752.8*	Other specified congenital anomalies of genital organs **124**		
750.26	Other specified congenital anomalies of mouth **3**, **48**	365.8*	Other specified forms of glaucoma **39**
756.8*	Other specified congenital anomalies of muscle, tendon, fascia, and connective tissue **100**	095.8	Other specified forms of late symptomatic syphilis **185**
		564.8*	Other specified functional disorders of intestine **78**
750.7	Other specified congenital anomalies of stomach **79**	535.41	Other specified gastritis with hemorrhage **76**
757.8	Other specified congenital anomalies of the integument **108**	535.40	Other specified gastritis without mention of hemorrhage **78**
750.8	Other specified congenital anomalies of upper alimentary tract **79**	640.83	Other specified hemorrhage in early pregnancy, antepartum **153**
747.89	Other specified congenital anomaly of circulatory system **67**	640.81	Other specified hemorrhage in early pregnancy, delivered **134**, **141**, **147**
750.4	Other specified congenital anomaly of esophagus **75**		
744.89	Other specified congenital anomaly of face and neck **47**	640.80	Other specified hemorrhage in early pregnancy, unspecified as to episode of care **153**
746.89	Other specified congenital anomaly of heart **68**	054.79	Other specified herpes simplex complications **164**, **168**, **184**, **229**
750.29	Other specified congenital anomaly of pharynx **3**, **47**		
748.8	Other specified congenital anomaly of respiratory system **54**	053.79	Other specified herpes zoster complications **164**, **168**, **184**, **229**
757.39	Other specified congenital anomaly of skin **108**, **172**	251.1	Other specified hypoglycemia **114**
V25.8	Other specified contraceptive management **214**	458.8	Other specified hypotension **69**
315.8	Other specified delay in development **189**	356.8	Other specified idiopathic peripheral neuropathy **21**
032.89	Other specified diphtheria **185**	659.83	Other specified indication for care or intervention related to labor and delivery, antepartum **155**, **158**
288.8	Other specified disease of white blood cells **176**		
078.88	Other specified diseases due to Chlamydiae **185**	659.81	Other specified indication for care or intervention related to labor and delivery, delivered **136**, **143**, **149**
074.8	Other specified diseases due to Coxsackievirus **184**		
031.8	Other specified diseases due to other mycobacteria **185**, **229**	659.80	Other specified indication for care or intervention related to labor and delivery, unspecified as to episode of care **136**, **143**, **149**
078.89	Other specified diseases due to viruses **185**		
289.89	Other specified diseases of blood and blood-forming organs **176**	343.8	Other specified infantile cerebral palsy **32**
569.89	Other specified disorder of intestines **79**	675.82	Other specified infection of the breast and nipple associated with childbirth, delivered, with mention of postpartum complication **139**, **145**, **151**
608.8*	Other specified disorder of male genital organs **124**		
349.89	Other specified disorder of nervous system **20**		
607.89	Other specified disorder of penis **124**	675.81	Other specified infection of the breast and nipple associated with childbirth, delivered, with or without mention of antepartum condition **139**, **145**, **151**
537.89	Other specified disorder of stomach and duodenum **78**		
530.89	Other specified disorder of the esophagus **78**		
599.8*	Other specified disorder of urethra and urinary tract **120**	675.80	Other specified infection of the breast and nipple associated with childbirth, unspecified as to episode of care **161**
279.8	Other specified disorders involving the immune mechanism **176**		
447.8	Other specified disorders of arteries and arterioles **66**	675.83	Other specified infection of the breast and nipple, antepartum **156**, **158**
271.8	Other specified disorders of carbohydrate transport and metabolism **113**	675.84	Other specified infections of the breast and nipple, postpartum condition or complication **153**
379.8	Other specified disorders of eye and adnexa **40**	136.8	Other specified infectious and parasitic diseases **186**, **230**
629.8*	Other specified disorders of female genital organs **130**	614.8	Other specified inflammatory disease of female pelvic organs and tissues **130**
719.8*	Other specified disorders of joint **98**		
593.8*	Other specified disorders of kidney and ureter **120**	616.8*	Other specified inflammatory diseases of cervix, vagina, and vulva **127**, **130**
573.8	Other specified disorders of liver **83**		
277.89	Other specified disorders of metabolism **114**	714.89	Other specified inflammatory polyarthropathies **97**
275.8	Other specified disorders of mineral metabolism **114**	318*	Other specified intellectual disabilities **188**
251.8	Other specified disorders of pancreatic internal secretion **114**	127.7	Other specified intestinal helminthiasis **78**
569.4*	Other specified disorders of rectum and anus **79**	560.89	Other specified intestinal obstruction **166**, **170**
246.8	Other specified disorders of thyroid **3**	100.8*	Other specified leptospiral infections **9**, **10**, **34**
384.8*	Other specified disorders of tympanic membrane **47**	207*	Other specified leukemia **178**
		207.8*	Other specified leukemia **181**

652.83	Other specified malposition or malpresentation of fetus, antepartum **154**, **157**
652.81	Other specified malposition or malpresentation of fetus, delivered **135**, **142**, **148**
652.80	Other specified malposition or malpresentation of fetus, unspecified as to episode of care **160**
022.8	Other specified manifestations of anthrax **185**
647.80	Other specified maternal infectious and parasitic disease complicating pregnancy, childbirth, or the puerperium, unspecified as to episode of care **159**
647.81	Other specified maternal infectious and parasitic disease with delivery **134**, **140**, **146**
647.82	Other specified maternal infectious and parasitic disease with delivery, with current postpartum complication **134**, **140**, **146**
647.83	Other specified maternal infectious and parasitic disease, antepartum **154**, **156**
647.84	Other specified maternal infectious and parasitic diseases complicating pregnancy, childbirth, or the puerperium, postpartum condition or complication **152**
055.79	Other specified measles complications **184**
036.89	Other specified meningococcal infections **186**
018.8*	Other specified miliary tuberculosis **185**
759.89	Other specified multiple congenital anomalies, so described **101**
V91.9*	Other specified multiple gestation placenta status **215**
651.83	Other specified multiple gestation, antepartum **154**, **157**
651.81	Other specified multiple gestation, delivered **135**, **142**, **148**
651.80	Other specified multiple gestation, unspecified as to episode of care **160**
358.8	Other specified myoneural disorders **21**
359.29	Other specified myotonic disorder **32**
094.89	Other specified neurosyphilis **19**
049.8	Other specified non-arthropod-borne viral diseases of central nervous system **33**, **229**
623.8	Other specified noninflammatory disorder of vagina **172**
310.8*	Other specified nonpsychotic mental disorder following organic brain damage **19**
754.89	Other specified nonteratogenic anomalies **100**
665.83	Other specified obstetrical trauma, antepartum **155**, **158**
665.82	Other specified obstetrical trauma, delivered, with postpartum **137**, **144**, **150**
665.84	Other specified obstetrical trauma, postpartum condition or complication **152**
665.80	Other specified obstetrical trauma, unspecified as to episode of care **137**, **144**, **150**
665.81	Other specified obstetrical trauma, with delivery **137**, **144**, **150**
344.8*	Other specified paralytic syndromes **32**
443.8*	Other specified peripheral vascular diseases **66**
567.89	Other specified peritonitis **76**
299.8*	Other specified pervasive developmental disorders **189**
046.7*	Other specified prion diseases of central nervous system **229**
V26.8*	Other specified procreative management **214**
698.8	Other specified pruritic conditions **108**
306.8	Other specified psychophysiological malfunction **189**
V57.89	Other specified rehabilitation procedure **213**
012.8*	Other specified respiratory tuberculosis **51**
V90.8*	Other specified retained foreign body **215**
003.8	Other specified salmonella infections **185**, **229**
120.8	Other specified schistosomiasis **185**
848.8	Other specified sites of sprains and strains **100**
046.8	Other specified slow virus infection of central nervous system **229**
625.8	Other specified symptom associated with female genital organs **130**
293.8*	Other specified transient mental disorders due to conditions classified elsewhere **188**
664.84	Other specified trauma to perineum and vulva, postpartum condition or complication **152**
664.80	Other specified trauma to perineum and vulva, unspecified as to episode of care in pregnancy **137**, **144**, **150**
664.81	Other specified trauma to perineum and vulva, with delivery **137**, **144**, **150**
121.8	Other specified trematode infections **185**
021.8	Other specified tularemia **185**
603.8	Other specified type of hydrocele **124**
595.89	Other specified types of cystitis **119**, **166**, **170**
020.8	Other specified types of plague **185**
099.8	Other specified venereal diseases **124**, **127**, **130**
070.4*	Other specified viral hepatitis with hepatic coma **164**, **168**
070.5*	Other specified viral hepatitis without mention of hepatic coma **164**, **168**
368.8	Other specified visual disturbances **39**
784.5*	Other speech disturbance **33**
104*	Other spirochetal infection **185**
482.49	Other Staphylococcus pneumonia **51**
V45.69	Other states following surgery of eye and adnexa **214**
567.2*	Other suppurative peritonitis **76**
784.69	Other symbolic dysfunction **189**
789.9	Other symptoms involving abdomen and pelvis **78**
785.9	Other symptoms involving cardiovascular system **69**
784.99	Other symptoms involving head and neck **47**
781.99	Other symptoms involving nervous and musculoskeletal systems **33**
786.9	Other symptoms involving respiratory system and chest **54**
782.9	Other symptoms involving skin and integumentary tissues **108**
788.9*	Other symptoms involving urinary system **119**
719.6*	Other symptoms referable to joint **98**
723.8	Other syndromes affecting cervical region **97**
727.09	Other synovitis and tenosynovitis **99**
836.2	Other tear of cartilage or meniscus of knee, current **222**
727.05	Other tenosynovitis of hand and wrist **99**
282.49	Other thalassemia **164**, **169**
644.13	Other threatened labor, antepartum **153**
644.10	Other threatened labor, unspecified as to episode of care **153**
999.89	Other transfusion reaction **176**
776.3	Other transient neonatal disorders of coagulation **163**, **168**
775.5	Other transitory neonatal electrolyte disturbances **163**, **167**
081*	Other typhus **185**
663.83	Other umbilical cord complications during labor and delivery, antepartum **155**, **158**
663.81	Other umbilical cord complications during labor and delivery, delivered **137**, **144**, **150**
663.80	Other umbilical cord complications during labor and delivery, unspecified as to episode of care **137**, **144**, **150**
799.9	Other unknown and unspecified cause of morbidity or mortality **213**
V61.7	Other unwanted pregnancy **153**
593.4	Other ureteric obstruction **119**
131.09	Other urogenital trichomoniasis **124**, **127**, **130**
999.2	Other vascular complications of medical care, not elsewhere classified **69**, **167**, **171**
647.24	Other venereal diseases complicating pregnancy, childbirth, or the puerperium, postpartum condition or complication **152**
671.80	Other venous complication of pregnancy and the puerperium, unspecified as to episode of care **161**
671.83	Other venous complication, antepartum **156**, **158**

*Code Range   © 2013 OptumInsight, Inc.

671.82	Other venous complication, with delivery, with mention of postpartum complication **138, 145, 151**
671.81	Other venous complication, with delivery, with or without mention of antepartum condition **138, 145, 151**
671.84	Other venous complications, postpartum condition or complication **153**
453.2	Other venous embolism and thrombosis, of inferior vena cava **66, 165, 169**
057*	Other viral exanthemata **184**
368.15	Other visual distortions and entoptic phenomena **39**
643.83	Other vomiting complicating pregnancy, antepartum **154, 156**
643.81	Other vomiting complicating pregnancy, delivered **134, 141, 147**
643.80	Other vomiting complicating pregnancy, unspecified as to episode of care **156, 159**
779.33	Other vomiting in newborn **171**
625.79	Other vulvodynia **130**
027*	Other zoonotic bacterial diseases **185**
305.9*	Other, mixed, or unspecified nondependent drug abuse **191**
827.0	Other, multiple and ill-defined closed fractures of lower limb **222**
827.1	Other, multiple and ill-defined open fractures of lower limb **222**
827*	Other, multiple, and ill-defined fractures of lower limb **99**
919.1	Other, multiple, and unspecified sites, abrasion or friction burn, infected **106**
919.3	Other, multiple, and unspecified sites, blister, infected **106**
919.2	Other, multiple, and unspecified sites, blister, without mention of infection **108**
919.5	Other, multiple, and unspecified sites, insect bite, nonvenomous, infected **106**
919.4	Other, multiple, and unspecified sites, insect bite, nonvenomous, without mention of infection **109**
919.6	Other, multiple, and unspecified sites, superficial foreign body (splinter), without major open wound and without mention of infection **107**
919.7	Other, multiple, and unspecified sites, superficial foreign body (splinter), without major open wound, infected **106**
053.71	Otitis externa due to herpes zoster **47, 164, 168, 229**
387*	Otosclerosis **47**
V27*	Outcome of delivery **214**
653.33	Outlet contraction of pelvis in pregnancy, antepartum **154, 157**
653.31	Outlet contraction of pelvis in pregnancy, delivered **135, 142, 148**
653.30	Outlet contraction of pelvis in pregnancy, unspecified as to episode of care in pregnancy **160**
256*	Ovarian dysfunction **127, 130**
313.0	Overanxious disorder specific to childhood and adolescence **188**
278.02	Overweight **113**
625*	Pain and other symptoms associated with female genital organs **127**
719.4*	Pain in joint **98**
729.5	Pain in soft tissues of limb **98**
786.52	Painful respiration **54**
719.3*	Palindromic rheumatism **98**
782.6*	Pallor and flushing **213**
785.1	Palpitations **68**
378.81	Palsy of conjugate gaze **40**
863.92	Pancreas body injury with open wound into cavity **83**
863.82	Pancreas body injury without mention of open wound into cavity **83, 227**
863.91	Pancreas head injury with open wound into cavity **83**
863.81	Pancreas head injury without mention of open wound into cavity **83, 227**

863.94	Pancreas injury, multiple and unspecified sites, with open wound into cavity **83**
863.84	Pancreas injury, multiple and unspecified sites, without mention of open wound into cavity **83, 227**
V42.83	Pancreas replaced by transplant **83**
863.93	Pancreas tail injury with open wound into cavity **83**
863.83	Pancreas tail injury without mention of open wound into cavity **83, 227**
284.1*	Pancytopenia **175**
723.6	Panniculitis specified as affecting neck **108**
360.02	Panophthalmitis **38**
360.12	Panuveitis **39**
377.02	Papilledema associated with decreased ocular pressure **40, 165, 169**
377.01	Papilledema associated with increased intracranial pressure **33, 165, 169**
377.03	Papilledema associated with retinal disorder **40**
646.03	Papyraceous fetus, antepartum **154, 157**
646.01	Papyraceous fetus, delivered, with or without mention of antepartum condition **134, 141, 147**
646.00	Papyraceous fetus, unspecified as to episode of care **134, 141, 147**
116.1	Paracoccidioidomycosis **164, 168**
121.2	Paragonimiasis **51**
478.3*	Paralysis of vocal cords or larynx **3, 47, 165, 169**
560.1	Paralytic ileus **166, 170**
374.31	Paralytic ptosis **38**
378.5*	Paralytic strabismus **38**
301.0	Paranoid personality disorder **188**
478.22	Parapharyngeal abscess **46, 165, 169**
344.1	Paraplegia **19**
696.2	Parapsoriasis **105**
360.13	Parasitic endophthalmitis NOS **38**
327.44	Parasomnia in conditions classified elsewhere **47**
V61.2*	Parent-child problems **214**
367.51	Paresis of accommodation **39**
332*	Parkinson's disease **19**
427.0	Paroxysmal supraventricular tachycardia **68**
427.1	Paroxysmal ventricular tachycardia **68, 165, 169**
377.15	Partial optic atrophy **38**
758.1	Patau's syndrome **188**
747.0	Patent ductus arteriosus **68**
733.1*	Pathologic fracture **97, 166, 170**
733.13	Pathologic fracture of vertebrae **87**
718.27	Pathological dislocation of ankle and foot joint **99**
718.23	Pathological dislocation of forearm joint **99**
718.24	Pathological dislocation of hand joint **99**
718.29	Pathological dislocation of joint of multiple sites **100**
718.28	Pathological dislocation of joint of other specified site **100**
718.20	Pathological dislocation of joint, site unspecified **99**
718.26	Pathological dislocation of lower leg joint **99**
718.25	Pathological dislocation of pelvic region and thigh joint **100**
718.21	Pathological dislocation of shoulder joint **99**
718.22	Pathological dislocation of upper arm joint **99**
312.31	Pathological gambling **188**
381.7	Patulous Eustachian tube **47**
754.82	Pectus carinatum **54**
754.81	Pectus excavatum **54**
132*	Pediculosis and phthirus infestation **107**
625.5	Pelvic congestion syndrome **130**

665.72	Pelvic hematoma, delivered with postpartum complication **137, 144, 150**
665.74	Pelvic hematoma, postpartum condition or complication **152**
665.70	Pelvic hematoma, unspecified as to episode of care **137, 144, 150**
665.71	Pelvic hematoma, with delivery **137, 144, 150**
614.6	Pelvic peritoneal adhesions, female (postoperative) (postinfection) **130**
848.5	Pelvic sprain and strains **96**
456.5	Pelvic varices **124, 127, 130**
694.5	Pemphigoid **105**
694.4	Pemphigus **105**
533.91	Peptic ulcer, unspecified site, unspecified as acute or chronic, without mention of hemorrhage or perforation, with obstruction **77**
533.90	Peptic ulcer, unspecified site, unspecified as acute or chronic, without mention of hemorrhage, perforation, or obstruction **77**
370.06	Perforated corneal ulcer **38**
530.4	Perforation of esophagus **75, 165, 170**
569.83	Perforation of intestine **79, 166, 170**
384.2*	Perforation of tympanic membrane **47**
777.6	Perinatal intestinal perforation **163, 168**
774.4	Perinatal jaundice due to hepatocellular damage **163, 167**
774.5	Perinatal jaundice from other causes **171, 172**
327.51	Periodic limb movement disorder **32**
359.3	Periodic paralysis **32**
730.37	Periostitis, without mention of osteomyelitis, ankle and foot **100**
730.33	Periostitis, without mention of osteomyelitis, forearm **98**
730.34	Periostitis, without mention of osteomyelitis, hand **98**
730.36	Periostitis, without mention of osteomyelitis, lower leg **98**
730.39	Periostitis, without mention of osteomyelitis, multiple sites **100**
730.38	Periostitis, without mention of osteomyelitis, other specified sites **100**
730.35	Periostitis, without mention of osteomyelitis, pelvic region and thigh **98**
730.31	Periostitis, without mention of osteomyelitis, shoulder region **98**
730.30	Periostitis, without mention of osteomyelitis, unspecified site **98**
730.32	Periostitis, without mention of osteomyelitis, upper arm **98**
674.53	Peripartum cardiomyopathy, antepartum condition or complication **156, 158**
674.52	Peripartum cardiomyopathy, delivered, with mention of postpartum condition **138, 141, 147**
674.51	Peripartum cardiomyopathy, delivered, with or without mention of antepartum condition **138, 141, 147**
674.54	Peripartum cardiomyopathy, postpartum condition or complication **153**
674.50	Peripartum cardiomyopathy, unspecified as to episode of care or not applicable **161**
646.43	Peripheral neuritis antepartum **154, 156**
646.44	Peripheral neuritis in pregnancy, postpartum condition or complication **151**
646.40	Peripheral neuritis in pregnancy, unspecified as to episode of care **159**
646.41	Peripheral neuritis in pregnancy, with delivery **134, 141, 147**
646.42	Peripheral neuritis in pregnancy, with delivery, with current postpartum complication **134, 141, 147**
362.6*	Peripheral retinal degenerations **39**
V42.82	Peripheral stem cells replaced by transplant **176**
202.7*	Peripheral T-cell lymphoma **178, 181, 230**
997.2	Peripheral vascular complications **67, 167, 171**
868.13	Peritoneum injury with open wound into cavity **79, 227**
868.03	Peritoneum injury without mention of open wound into cavity **79, 227**
567*	Peritonitis and retroperitoneal infections **166, 170**
567.0	Peritonitis in infectious diseases classified elsewhere **76**
475	Peritonsillar abscess **3, 46**
779.7	Periventricular leukomalacia **33, 166, 170**
356.1	Peroneal muscular atrophy **21**
277.86	Peroxisomal disorders **114**
747.83	Persistent fetal circulation **163, 167**
294*	Persistent mental disorders due to conditions classified elsewhere **188**
998.6	Persistent postoperative fistula, not elsewhere classified **167, 171, 204**
780.03	Persistent vegetative state **21, 166, 170**
536.2	Persistent vomiting **78**
V14*	Personal history of allergy to medicinal agents **214**
V13.4	Personal history of arthritis **214**
V12*	Personal history of certain other diseases **214**
V13.22	Personal history of cervical dysplasia **180, 182**
V13.6*	Personal history of congenital (corrected) malformations **214**
V13.3	Personal history of diseases of skin and subcutaneous tissue **214**
V13.0*	Personal history of disorders of urinary system **214**
V87.4*	Personal history of drug therapy **213**
V10*	Personal history of malignant neoplasm **180, 182**
V10.21	Personal history of malignant neoplasm of larynx **4**
V10.02	Personal history of malignant neoplasm of other and unspecified parts of oral cavity and pharynx **4**
V10.01	Personal history of malignant neoplasm of tongue **4**
V11*	Personal history of mental disorder **214**
V13.29	Personal history of other genital system and obstetric disorders **214**
V13.5*	Personal history of other musculoskeletal disorders **214**
V13.8*	Personal history of other specified diseases **214**
V13.7	Personal history of perinatal problems **214**
V13.21	Personal history of pre-term labor **214**
V13.1	Personal history of trophoblastic disease **214**
V13.9	Personal history of unspecified disease **214**
V13.23	Personal history of vaginal dysplasia **214**
V13.24	Personal history of vulvar dysplasia **214**
310.1	Personality change due to conditions classified elsewhere **188**
V64*	Persons encountering health services for specific procedures, not carried out **214**
383.2*	Petrositis **46**
607.85	Peyronie's disease **124**
451.1*	Phlebitis and thrombophlebitis of deep veins of lower extremities **66, 165, 169**
451.83	Phlebitis and thrombophlebitis of deep veins of upper extremities **67**
451.81	Phlebitis and thrombophlebitis of iliac vein **66, 165, 169**
325	Phlebitis and thrombophlebitis of intracranial venous sinuses **9, 10, 32**
451.2	Phlebitis and thrombophlebitis of lower extremities, unspecified **66, 165, 169**
451.89	Phlebitis and thrombophlebitis of other site **67**
451.82	Phlebitis and thrombophlebitis of superficial veins of upper extremities **67**
451.0	Phlebitis and thrombophlebitis of superficial vessels of lower extremities **67**
451.9	Phlebitis and thrombophlebitis of unspecified site **67**
451.84	Phlebitis and thrombophlebitis of upper extremities, unspecified **67**
066.0	Phlebotomus fever **184**

375.33	Phlegmonous dacryocystitis **39**
300.2*	Phobic disorders **188**
307.52	Pica **189**
365.13	Pigmentary open-angle glaucoma **39**
685*	Pilonidal cyst **106**
696.3	Pityriasis rosea **108**
696.4	Pityriasis rubra pilaris **108**
641.03	Placenta previa without hemorrhage, antepartum **154**, **157**
641.00	Placenta previa without hemorrhage, unspecified as to episode of care **159**
641.01	Placenta previa without hemorrhage, with delivery **134**, **140**, **145**
674.44	Placental polyp, postpartum condition or complication **153**
674.40	Placental polyp, unspecified as to episode of care **161**
674.42	Placental polyp, with delivery, with mention of postpartum complication **138**, **145**, **151**
511.1	Pleurisy with effusion, with mention of bacterial cause other than tuberculosis **51**, **165**, **170**
511.0	Pleurisy without mention of effusion or current tuberculosis **53**
567.1	Pneumococcal peritonitis **76**
481	Pneumococcal pneumonia (streptococcus pneumoniae pneumonia) **53**, **165**, **169**, **230**
503	Pneumoconiosis due to other inorganic dust **53**
502	Pneumoconiosis due to other silica or silicates **53**
136.3	Pneumocystosis **51**, **164**, **168**, **230**
482.81	Pneumonia due to anaerobes **51**
482.82	Pneumonia due to Escherichia coli (E. coli) **51**
482.2	Pneumonia due to Hemophilus influenzae (H. influenzae) **53**
482.0	Pneumonia due to Klebsiella pneumoniae **51**
482.83	Pneumonia due to other gram-negative bacteria **51**
482.8*	Pneumonia due to other specified bacteria **51**
482.89	Pneumonia due to other specified bacteria **51**
483*	Pneumonia due to other specified organism **53**, **165**, **169**
480.8	Pneumonia due to other virus not elsewhere classified **230**
482.1	Pneumonia due to Pseudomonas **51**
480.3	Pneumonia due to SARS-associated coronavirus **230**
482.4*	Pneumonia due to Staphylococcus **51**
482.40	Pneumonia due to Staphylococcus, unspecified **51**
482.3*	Pneumonia due to Streptococcus **53**
484*	Pneumonia in infectious diseases classified elsewhere **51**
486	Pneumonia, organism unspecified **53**, **165**, **169**, **230**
020.5	Pneumonic plague, unspecified **51**
507.0	Pneumonitis due to inhalation of food or vomitus **165**, **169**
507.8	Pneumonitis due to other solids and liquids **165**, **169**
507*	Pneumonitis due to solids and liquids **51**
130.4	Pneumonitis due to toxoplasmosis **51**, **164**, **168**
504	Pneumonopathy due to inhalation of other dust **53**
975*	Poisoning by agents primarily acting on the smooth and skeletal muscles and respiratory system **203**
964*	Poisoning by agents primarily affecting blood constituents **203**
972*	Poisoning by agents primarily affecting the cardiovascular system **203**
973*	Poisoning by agents primarily affecting the gastrointestinal system **203**
965*	Poisoning by analgesics, antipyretics, and antirheumatics **203**
976.6	Poisoning by anti-infectives and other drugs and preparations for ear, nose, and throat **203**
960*	Poisoning by antibiotics **203**
966*	Poisoning by anticonvulsants and anti-Parkinsonism drugs **203**
976.1	Poisoning by antipruritics **203**
978*	Poisoning by bacterial vaccines **203**

970*	Poisoning by central nervous system stimulants **203**
976.7	Poisoning by dental drugs topically applied **203**
971*	Poisoning by drugs primarily affecting the autonomic nervous system **203**
976.3	Poisoning by emollients, demulcents, and protectants **203**
976.5	Poisoning by eye anti-infectives and other eye drugs **40**
962*	Poisoning by hormones and synthetic substitutes **203**
976.4	Poisoning by keratolytics, keratoplastics, other hair treatment drugs and preparations **203**
976.0	Poisoning by local anti-infectives and anti-inflammatory drugs **203**
976.2	Poisoning by local astringents and local detergents **203**
976.8	Poisoning by other agents primarily affecting skin and mucous membrane **203**
977*	Poisoning by other and unspecified drugs and medicinal substances **203**
961*	Poisoning by other anti-infectives **203**
968*	Poisoning by other central nervous system depressants and anesthetics **203**
979*	Poisoning by other vaccines and biological substances **203**
963*	Poisoning by primarily systemic agents **203**
969*	Poisoning by psychotropic agents **203**
967*	Poisoning by sedatives and hypnotics **203**
976.9	Poisoning by unspecified agent primarily affecting skin and mucous membrane **203**
974*	Poisoning by water, mineral, and uric acid metabolism drugs **203**
446.0	Polyarteritis nodosa **97**
273.0	Polyclonal hypergammaglobulinemia **176**
289.0	Polycythemia, secondary **176**
258*	Polyglandular dysfunction and related disorders **114**
657.03	Polyhydramnios, antepartum complication **155**, **158**
657.00	Polyhydramnios, unspecified as to episode of care **160**
657.01	Polyhydramnios, with delivery **136**, **143**, **149**
725	Polymyalgia rheumatica **97**
357.6	Polyneuropathy due to drugs **21**
357.7	Polyneuropathy due to other toxic agents **21**
357.1	Polyneuropathy in collagen vascular disease **21**
357.2	Polyneuropathy in diabetes **21**
357.3	Polyneuropathy in malignant disease **21**
357.4	Polyneuropathy in other diseases classified elsewhere **21**
478.4	Polyp of vocal cord or larynx **3**, **47**
656.53	Poor fetal growth, affecting management of mother, antepartum condition or complication **155**, **157**
656.51	Poor fetal growth, affecting management of mother, delivered **136**, **143**, **149**
656.50	Poor fetal growth, affecting management of mother, unspecified as to episode of care **160**
904.4*	Popliteal blood vessel vein **223**, **227**
572.1	Portal pyemia **166**, **170**
452	Portal vein thrombosis **83**
645.13	Post term pregnancy, antepartum condition or complication **154**, **157**
645.11	Post term pregnancy, delivered, with or without mention of antepartum condition **134**, **141**, **147**
645.10	Post term pregnancy, unspecified as to episode of care or not applicable **159**
238.77	Post-transplant lymphoproliferative disorder [PTLD] **203**
383.81	Postauricular fistula **165**, **169**
310.2	Postconcussion syndrome **34**
711.3*	Postdysenteric arthropathy **98**
564.2	Postgastric surgery syndromes **78**
053.13	Postherpetic polyneuropathy **21**, **164**, **168**, **229**

053.12	Postherpetic trigeminal neuralgia **21, 164, 168, 229**	
323.6*	Postinfectious encephalitis, myelitis, and encephalomyelitis **9, 34**	
323.63	Postinfectious myelitis **10**	
377.12	Postinflammatory optic atrophy **38**	
515	Postinflammatory pulmonary fibrosis **53**	
457.0	Postmastectomy lymphedema syndrome **106**	
055.0	Postmeasles encephalitis **9, 10, 33, 164, 168**	
055.2	Postmeasles otitis media **46, 164, 168**	
055.1	Postmeasles pneumonia **51, 164, 168**	
411.0	Postmyocardial infarction syndrome **69**	
784.91	Postnasal drip **47**	
512.2	Postoperative air leak **53**	
998.5*	Postoperative infection, not elsewhere classified **184**	
998.0*	Postoperative shock **167, 171, 204**	
V24.0	Postpartum care and examination immediately after delivery **153**	
V24.1	Postpartum care and examination of lactating mother **214**	
666.34	Postpartum coagulation defects, postpartum condition or complication **152**	
666.30	Postpartum coagulation defects, unspecified as to episode of care **161**	
666.32	Postpartum coagulation defects, with delivery **137, 140, 146**	
459.1*	Postphlebitic syndrome **67**	
780.62	Postprocedural fever **184, 231**	
V45.0*	Postsurgical cardiac pacemaker in situ **214**	
251.3	Postsurgical hypoinsulinemia **2, 113**	
958.3	Posttraumatic wound infection not elsewhere classified **166, 171, 184, 224**	
593.6	Postural proteinuria **120**	
780.63	Postvaccination fever **184, 231**	
052.0	Postvaricella encephalitis **33, 164, 168**	
052.2	Postvaricella myelitis **8, 10, 33**	
759.81	Prader-Willi syndrome **101**	
642.73	Pre-eclampsia or eclampsia superimposed on pre-existing hypertension, antepartum **154, 156**	
642.70	Pre-eclampsia or eclampsia superimposed on pre-existing hypertension, complicating pregnancy, childbirth, or the puerperium, unspecified as to episode of care **156, 159**	
642.74	Pre-eclampsia or eclampsia superimposed on pre-existing hypertension, postpartum condition or complication **151**	
642.71	Pre-eclampsia or eclampsia superimposed on pre-existing hypertension, with delivery **134, 140, 146**	
642.72	Pre-eclampsia or eclampsia superimposed on pre-existing hypertension, with delivery, with current postpartum complication **134, 140, 146**	
661.33	Precipitate labor, antepartum **155, 158**	
661.30	Precipitate labor, unspecified as to episode of care **136, 144, 149**	
661.31	Precipitate labor, with delivery **136, 144, 149**	
786.51	Precordial pain **68**	
309.2*	Predominant disturbance of other emotions as adjustment reaction **188**	
646.33	Pregnancy complication, recurrent pregnancy loss, antepartum condition or complication **154, 157**	
646.30	Pregnancy complication, recurrent pregnancy loss, unspecified as to episode of care **159**	
646.31	Pregnancy complication, recurrent pregnancy loss, with or without mention of antepartum condition **134, 141, 147**	
V23.3	Pregnancy with grand multiparity **161**	
V23.2	Pregnancy with history of abortion **161**	
V23.0	Pregnancy with history of infertility **161**	
V23.1	Pregnancy with history of trophoblastic disease **161**	
V23.4*	Pregnancy with other poor obstetric history **161**	
V23.5	Pregnancy with other poor reproductive history **161**	

427.6*	Premature beats **68**
658.13	Premature rupture of membranes in pregnancy, antepartum **155, 158**
658.11	Premature rupture of membranes in pregnancy, delivered **136, 143, 149**
658.10	Premature rupture of membranes in pregnancy, unspecified as to episode of care **136, 143, 149**
641.23	Premature separation of placenta, antepartum **154, 157**
641.20	Premature separation of placenta, unspecified as to episode of care **159**
641.21	Premature separation of placenta, with delivery **134, 140, 145**
625.4	Premenstrual tension syndromes **130**
367.4	Presbyopia **39**
V45.2	Presence of cerebrospinal fluid drainage device **214**
V45.5*	Presence of contraceptive device **214**
290.1*	Presenile dementia **230**
654.23	Previous cesarean delivery, antepartum condition or complication **154, 157**
654.21	Previous cesarean delivery, delivered, with or without mention of antepartum condition **135, 142, 148**
654.20	Previous cesarean delivery, unspecified as to episode of care or not applicable **160**
607.3	Priapism **124**
091.1	Primary anal syphilis **78**
365.2*	Primary angle-closure glaucoma **39**
770.4	Primary atelectasis of newborn **163, 167**
277.81	Primary carnitine deficiency **114**
200.5*	Primary central nervous system lymphoma **230**
327.21	Primary central sleep apnea **32**
114.0	Primary coccidioidomycosis (pulmonary) **51**
114.1	Primary extrapulmonary coccidioidomycosis **107**
289.81	Primary hypercoagulable state **176**
103.0	Primary lesions of pinta **107**
365.11	Primary open-angle glaucoma **39**
377.11	Primary optic atrophy **38**
020.3	Primary pneumonic plague **51**
416.0	Primary pulmonary hypertension **69**
010*	Primary tuberculous infection **51, 229**
661.03	Primary uterine inertia, antepartum **155, 158**
661.00	Primary uterine inertia, unspecified as to episode of care **136, 143, 149**
661.01	Primary uterine inertia, with delivery **136, 143, 149**
413.1	Prinzmetal angina **68**
V69*	Problems related to lifestyle **215**
V61.3	Problems with aged parents or in-laws **214**
V48*	Problems with head, neck, and trunk **214**
V49*	Problems with limbs and other problems **214**
V41*	Problems with special senses and other special functions **214**
V64.3	Procedure not carried out for other reasons **173**
V26.4*	Procreative management, general counseling and advice **214**
378.72	Progressive external ophthalmoplegia **38**
046.3	Progressive multifocal leukoencephalopathy **229**
663.03	Prolapse of cord, complicating labor and delivery, antepartum **155, 158**
663.01	Prolapse of cord, complicating labor and delivery, delivered **137, 144, 149**
663.00	Prolapse of cord, complicating labor and delivery, unspecified as to episode of care **136, 144, 149**
652.73	Prolapsed arm of fetus, antepartum condition or complication **154, 157**
652.71	Prolapsed arm of fetus, delivered **135, 142, 148**

*Code Range

652.70	Prolapsed arm of fetus, unspecified as to episode of care **160**
599.5	Prolapsed urethral mucosa **120**
309.1	Prolonged depressive reaction as adjustment reaction **188**
662.03	Prolonged first stage of labor, antepartum **155**, **158**
662.01	Prolonged first stage of labor, delivered **136**, **144**, **149**
662.00	Prolonged first stage of labor, unspecified as to episode of care **136**, **144**, **149**
645.23	Prolonged pregnancy, antepartum condition or complication **154**, **157**
645.21	Prolonged pregnancy, delivered, with or without mention of antepartum condition **134**, **141**, **147**
645.20	Prolonged pregnancy, unspecified as to episode of care or not applicable **159**
662.23	Prolonged second stage of labor, antepartum **155**, **158**
662.21	Prolonged second stage of labor, delivered **136**, **144**, **149**
662.20	Prolonged second stage of labor, unspecified as to episode of care **136**, **144**, **149**
V50.41	Prophylactic breast removal **106**
V50.42	Prophylactic ovary removal **128**, **131**
368.51	Protan defect in color vision **39**
791.0	Proteinuria **119**
698.2	Prurigo **108**
698.0	Pruritus ani **108**
698.1	Pruritus of genital organs **124**, **127**, **130**
051.1	Pseudocowpox **107**
377.24	Pseudopapilledema **38**
696.8	Psoriasis related disease NEC **108**
696.0	Psoriatic arthropathy **97**
136.4	Psorospermiasis **186**
316	Psychic factors associated with diseases classified elsewhere **188**
306.52	Psychogenic dysmenorrhea **127**, **130**
306.53	Psychogenic dysuria **120**
306.50	Psychogenic genitourinary malfunction, unspecified **120**
307.80	Psychogenic pain, site unspecified **188**
298.4	Psychogenic paranoid psychosis **189**
306.51	Psychogenic vaginismus **127**, **130**
307.54	Psychogenic vomiting **188**
799.54	Psychomotor deficit **188**
368.16	Psychophysical visual disturbances **39**
V67.3	Psychotherapy and other treatment for mental disorder follow-up examination **214**
670.12	Puerperal endometritis, delivered, with mention of postpartum complication **138**, **141**, **146**
670.14	Puerperal endometritis, postpartum condition or complication **153**
670.10	Puerperal endometritis, unspecified as to episode of care or not applicable **161**
672.02	Puerperal pyrexia of unknown origin, delivered, with mention of postpartum complication **138**, **141**, **146**
672.04	Puerperal pyrexia of unknown origin, postpartum condition or complication **153**
672.00	Puerperal pyrexia of unknown origin, unspecified as to episode of care **161**
670.22	Puerperal sepsis, delivered, with mention of postpartum complication **138**, **141**, **146**
670.24	Puerperal sepsis, postpartum condition or complication **153**
670.20	Puerperal sepsis, unspecified as to episode of care or not applicable **161**
670.32	Puerperal septic thrombophlebitis, delivered, with mention of postpartum complication **138**, **141**, **146**
670.34	Puerperal septic thrombophlebitis, postpartum condition or complication **153**
670.30	Puerperal septic thrombophlebitis, unspecified as to episode of care or not applicable **161**
039.1	Pulmonary actinomycotic infection **51**
022.1	Pulmonary anthrax **51**
901.41	Pulmonary artery injury **166**, **170**
901.4*	Pulmonary blood vessel injury **223**, **226**
518.0	Pulmonary collapse **54**, **165**, **170**
668.03	Pulmonary complications of the administration of anesthesia or other sedation in labor and delivery, antepartum **155**, **158**
668.01	Pulmonary complications of the administration of anesthesia or other sedation in labor and delivery, delivered **137**, **140**, **146**
668.02	Pulmonary complications of the administration of anesthesia or other sedation in labor and delivery, delivered, with mention of postpartum complication **137**, **140**, **146**
668.04	Pulmonary complications of the administration of anesthesia or other sedation in labor and delivery, postpartum condition or complication **152**
668.00	Pulmonary complications of the administration of anesthesia or other sedation in labor and delivery, unspecified as to episode of care **137**, **144**, **150**
514	Pulmonary congestion and hypostasis **52**
031.0	Pulmonary diseases due to other mycobacteria **51**
415.1*	Pulmonary embolism and infarction **51**
518.3	Pulmonary eosinophilia **53**
770.3	Pulmonary hemorrhage of fetus or newborn **163**, **167**
518.5*	Pulmonary insufficiency following trauma and surgery **52**, **207**
011*	Pulmonary tuberculosis **51**, **229**
021.2	Pulmonary tularemia **51**
901.42	Pulmonary vein injury **166**, **170**
376.35	Pulsating exophthalmos **38**
287*	Purpura and other hemorrhagic conditions **176**
590.3	Pyeloureteritis cystica **166**, **170**
537.81	Pylorospasm **78**
711.0*	Pyogenic arthritis **97**, **230**
711.06	Pyogenic arthritis, lower leg **90**
312.33	Pyromania **189**
344.0*	Quadriplegia and quadriparesis **19**
343.2	Quadriplegic infantile cerebral palsy **19**
V91.2*	Quadruplet gestation placenta status **215**
651.53	Quadruplet pregnancy with fetal loss and retention of one or more, antepartum **154**, **157**
651.51	Quadruplet pregnancy with fetal loss and retention of one or more, delivered **135**, **142**, **148**
651.50	Quadruplet pregnancy with fetal loss and retention of one or more, unspecified as to episode of care or not applicable **160**
651.23	Quadruplet pregnancy, antepartum **154**, **157**
651.21	Quadruplet pregnancy, delivered **135**, **142**, **148**
651.20	Quadruplet pregnancy, unspecified as to episode of care **160**
071	Rabies **9**, **10**, **34**
727.04	Radial styloid tenosynovitis **99**
V58.0	Radiotherapy **180**, **182**
V67.1	Radiotherapy follow-up examination **180**, **182**
782.1	Rash and other nonspecific skin eruption **108**, **231**
026*	Rat-bite fever **185**
443.0	Raynaud's syndrome **97**
349.0	Reaction to spinal or lumbar puncture **34**, **165**, **169**
298.2	Reactive confusion **189**
569.1	Rectal prolapse **79**
718.37	Recurrent dislocation of ankle and foot joint **99**
718.33	Recurrent dislocation of forearm joint **99**
718.34	Recurrent dislocation of hand joint **99**

718.39	Recurrent dislocation of joint of multiple sites **100**	
718.38	Recurrent dislocation of joint of other specified site **100**	
718.30	Recurrent dislocation of joint, site unspecified **100**	
718.36	Recurrent dislocation of lower leg joint **99**	
718.35	Recurrent dislocation of pelvic region and thigh joint **100**	
718.31	Recurrent dislocation of shoulder joint **99**	
718.32	Recurrent dislocation of upper arm joint **99**	
327.43	Recurrent isolated sleep paralysis **32**	
605	Redundant prepuce and phimosis **124, 172**	
356.3	Refsum's disease **32**	
V62.6	Refusal of treatment for reasons of religion or conscience **214**	
555*	Regional enteritis **77**	
099.3	Reiter's disease **97**	
087*	Relapsing fever **185**	
313.3	Relationship problems specific to childhood and adolescence **189**	
327.42	REM sleep behavior disorder **47**	
590.2	Renal and perinephric abscess **166, 170**	
788.0	Renal colic **119**	
V45.1*	Renal dialysis status **214**	
271.4	Renal glycosuria **113**	
729.6	Residual foreign body in soft tissue **100**	
365.15	Residual stage of open angle glaucoma **39**	
799.1	Respiratory arrest **54, 166, 170**	
997.3*	Respiratory complications **54, 167, 171**	
508.8	Respiratory conditions due to other specified external agents **54**	
508.2	Respiratory conditions due to smoke inhalation **54, 207**	
508.9	Respiratory conditions due to unspecified external agent **54**	
769	Respiratory distress syndrome in newborn **163**	
770.84	Respiratory failure of newborn **163, 167**	
306.1	Respiratory malfunction arising from mental factors **54**	
079.6	Respiratory syncytial virus (RSV) **164, 168**	
333.94	Restless legs syndrome [RLS] **19**	
376.6	Retained (old) foreign body following penetrating wound of orbit **40**	
360.5*	Retained (old) intraocular foreign body, magnetic **39**	
360.6*	Retained (old) intraocular foreign body, nonmagnetic **39**	
V90.9	Retained foreign body, unspecified material **215**	
V90.1*	Retained metal fragments **215**	
V90.3*	Retained organic fragments **215**	
667.04	Retained placenta without hemorrhage, postpartum condition or complication **152**	
667.00	Retained placenta without hemorrhage, unspecified as to episode of care **161**	
667.02	Retained placenta without hemorrhage, with delivery, with mention of postpartum complication **137, 140, 146**	
V90.2	Retained plastic fragments **215**	
667.12	Retained portions of placenta or membranes, without hemorrhage, delivered, with mention of postpartum complication **137, 140, 146**	
667.14	Retained portions of placenta or membranes, without hemorrhage, postpartum condition or complication **152**	
667.10	Retained portions of placenta or membranes, without hemorrhage, unspecified as to episode of care **161**	
V90.0*	Retained radioactive fragment **215**	
788.2*	Retention of urine **119, 166, 170**	
200.0*	Reticulosarcoma **230**	
200.01	Reticulosarcoma of lymph nodes of head, face, and neck **2**	
361.3*	Retinal defects without detachment **39**	
361.0*	Retinal detachment with retinal defect **39**	
362.3*	Retinal vascular occlusion **38**	

361.1*	Retinoschisis and retinal cysts **39**
676.03	Retracted nipple, antepartum condition or complication **156, 158**
676.02	Retracted nipple, delivered, with mention of postpartum complication **139, 145, 151**
676.01	Retracted nipple, delivered, with or without mention of antepartum condition **139, 145, 151**
676.04	Retracted nipple, postpartum condition or complication **153**
676.00	Retracted nipple, unspecified as to prenatal or postnatal episode of care **161**
567.3*	Retroperitoneal infections **76**
868.14	Retroperitoneum injury with open wound into cavity **120, 227**
868.04	Retroperitoneum injury without mention of open wound into cavity **120, 227**
478.24	Retropharyngeal abscess **46, 165, 169**
654.33	Retroverted and incarcerated gravid uterus, antepartum **154, 157**
654.31	Retroverted and incarcerated gravid uterus, delivered **135, 142, 148**
654.32	Retroverted and incarcerated gravid uterus, delivered, with mention of postpartum complication **135, 142, 148**
654.34	Retroverted and incarcerated gravid uterus, postpartum condition or complication **152**
654.30	Retroverted and incarcerated gravid uterus, unspecified as to episode of care **160**
331.81	Reye's syndrome **32**
999.7*	Rh and other non-ABO incompatibility reaction due to transfusion of blood or blood products **167, 171, 176**
728.88	Rhabdomyolysis **99**
656.13	Rhesus isoimmunization affecting management of mother, antepartum condition **155, 157**
656.11	Rhesus isoimmunization affecting management of mother, delivered **136, 143, 149**
656.10	Rhesus isoimmunization unspecified as to episode of care in pregnancy **160**
392*	Rheumatic chorea **68**
390	Rheumatic fever without mention of heart involvement **97**
398.91	Rheumatic heart failure (congestive) **56, 66, 165, 169**
398.0	Rheumatic myocarditis **68**
517.1	Rheumatic pneumonia **53**
729.0	Rheumatism, unspecified and fibrositis **98**
714.0	Rheumatoid arthritis **97**
714.81	Rheumatoid lung **53**
040.1	Rhinoscleroma **185**
086.4	Rhodesian trypanosomiasis **185**
268.0	Rickets, active **98**
268.1	Rickets, late effect **98**
370.02	Ring corneal ulcer **39**
695.81	Ritter's disease **105**
695.3	Rosacea **108**
058.11	Roseola infantum due to human herpesvirus 6 **164, 168, 184**
058.12	Roseola infantum due to human herpesvirus 7 **164, 168, 184**
058.10	Roseola infantum, unspecified **164, 168, 184**
840.4	Rotator cuff (capsule) sprain and strain **222**
726.1*	Rotator cuff syndrome of shoulder and allied disorders **98**
V20.2	Routine infant or child health check **172**
V50.2	Routine or ritual circumcision **124, 173**
V24.2	Routine postpartum follow-up **214**
056.0*	Rubella with neurological complications **164, 168**
056.7*	Rubella with other specified complications **164, 168**
056.79	Rubella with other specified complications **184**
056.9	Rubella without mention of complication **184**

*Code Range

364.42	Rubeosis iridis **39**	249.6*	Secondary diabetes mellitus with neurological manifestations **21**
307.53	Rumination disorder **188**	249.5*	Secondary diabetes mellitus with ophthalmic manifestations **38**
447.2	Rupture of artery **66**	249.3*	Secondary diabetes mellitus with other coma **113**
429.5	Rupture of chordae tendineae **67**	249.8*	Secondary diabetes mellitus with other specified manifestations **113**
728.83	Rupture of muscle, nontraumatic **99**		
429.6	Rupture of papillary muscle **67**	249.7*	Secondary diabetes mellitus with peripheral circulatory disorders **66**
727.5*	Rupture of synovium **99**		
727.6*	Rupture of tendon, nontraumatic **99**	249.4*	Secondary diabetes mellitus with renal manifestations **120**
665.03	Rupture of uterus before onset of labor, antepartum **155, 158**	249.9*	Secondary diabetes mellitus with unspecified complication **113**
665.00	Rupture of uterus before onset of labor, unspecified as to episode of care **137, 144, 150**	249.0*	Secondary diabetes mellitus without mention of complication **113**
665.01	Rupture of uterus before onset of labor, with delivery **137, 144, 150**	289.82	Secondary hypercoagulable state **176**
		405*	Secondary hypertension **67**
665.10	Rupture of uterus during labor, unspecified as to episode **137, 144, 150**	198.7	Secondary malignant neoplasm of adrenal gland **114**
		198.5	Secondary malignant neoplasm of bone and bone marrow **87, 97**
665.11	Rupture of uterus during labor, with delivery **137, 144, 150**	198.3	Secondary malignant neoplasm of brain and spinal cord **19**
720.2	Sacroiliitis, not elsewhere classified **97**	198.81	Secondary malignant neoplasm of breast **104, 105**
003.23	Salmonella arthritis **97**	198.82	Secondary malignant neoplasm of genital organs **122, 123, 126, 129**
003.0	Salmonella gastroenteritis **75**		
003.21	Salmonella meningitis **8, 10, 33**	198.0	Secondary malignant neoplasm of kidney **116, 119**
003.24	Salmonella osteomyelitis **96**	197.5	Secondary malignant neoplasm of large intestine and rectum **76**
003.22	Salmonella pneumonia **51**	197.7	Secondary malignant neoplasm of liver **82**
003.1	Salmonella septicemia **186, 229**	197.0	Secondary malignant neoplasm of lung **52**
614.2	Salpingitis and oophoritis not specified as acute, subacute, or chronic **130**	197.1	Secondary malignant neoplasm of mediastinum **52**
		197.8	Secondary malignant neoplasm of other digestive organs and spleen **76**
904.3	Saphenous vein injury **223**		
135	Sarcoidosis **53**	198.4	Secondary malignant neoplasm of other parts of nervous system **19**
136.5	Sarcosporidiosis **186**		
034.1	Scarlet fever **185**	197.3	Secondary malignant neoplasm of other respiratory organs **52**
341.1	Schilder's disease **19**	198.89	Secondary malignant neoplasm of other specified sites **180, 181**
120.0	Schistosomiasis due to schistosoma haematobium **119**	198.1	Secondary malignant neoplasm of other urinary organs **116, 119**
120.2	Schistosomiasis due to schistosoma japonicum **185**	198.6	Secondary malignant neoplasm of ovary **126, 129**
120.1	Schistosomiasis due to schistosoma mansoni **83**	197.2	Secondary malignant neoplasm of pleura **52**
301.2*	Schizoid personality disorder **188**	197.6	Secondary malignant neoplasm of retroperitoneum and peritoneum **76**
295*	Schizophrenic disorders **189**		
379.0*	Scleritis and episcleritis **40**	198.2	Secondary malignant neoplasm of skin **104, 105**
370.54	Sclerosing keratitis **39**	197.4	Secondary malignant neoplasm of small intestine including duodenum **76**
567.82	Sclerosing mesenteritis **79**		
368.41	Scotoma involving central area in visual field **38**	209.75	Secondary Merkel cell carcinoma **180, 182**
368.42	Scotoma of blind spot area in visual field **39**	209.73	Secondary neuroendocrine tumor of bone **87, 97**
V28.0	Screening for chromosomal anomalies by amniocentesis **156, 159**	209.71	Secondary neuroendocrine tumor of distant lymph nodes **178, 181**
V77.3	Screening for phenylketonuria (PKU) **173**	209.72	Secondary neuroendocrine tumor of liver **82**
V28.1	Screening for raised alpha-fetoprotein levels in amniotic fluid **156, 159**	209.79	Secondary neuroendocrine tumor of other sites **180, 182**
		209.74	Secondary neuroendocrine tumor of peritoneum **76**
V28.6	Screening of Streptococcus B **214**	209.70	Secondary neuroendocrine tumor, unspecified site **180, 182**
456.4	Scrotal varices **124**	020.4	Secondary pneumonic plague **51**
664.14	Second-degree perineal laceration, postpartum condition or complication **152**	091.3	Secondary syphilis of skin or mucous membranes **107**
664.10	Second-degree perineal laceration, unspecified as to episode of care in pregnancy **137, 144, 150**	287.4*	Secondary thrombocytopenia **164, 169, 230**
		661.13	Secondary uterine inertia, antepartum **155, 158**
664.11	Second-degree perineal laceration, with delivery **137, 144, 150**	661.10	Secondary uterine inertia, unspecified as to episode of care **136, 144, 149**
958.2	Secondary and recurrent hemorrhage as an early complication of trauma **166, 171, 204, 224**	661.11	Secondary uterine inertia, with delivery **136, 144, 149**
		368.43	Sector or arcuate defects in visual field **38**
196*	Secondary and unspecified malignant neoplasm of lymph nodes **178, 181**	608.0	Seminal vesiculitis **124**
		331.2	Senile degeneration of brain **19**
196.0	Secondary and unspecified malignant neoplasm of lymph nodes of head, face, and neck **2**	797	Senility without mention of psychosis **188**
		313.2*	Sensitivity, shyness, and social withdrawal disorder specific to childhood and adolescence **189**
249*	Secondary diabetes mellitus **1, 2**		
249.2*	Secondary diabetes mellitus with hyperosmolarity **113**	374.44	Sensory disorders of eyelid **39**
249.1*	Secondary diabetes mellitus with ketoacidosis **113**	362.4*	Separation of retinal layers **39**

449	Septic arterial embolism **67, 165, 169**	
422.92	Septic myocarditis **165, 169**	
785.52	Septic shock **186**	
038*	Septicemia **164, 168, 186, 229**	
020.2	Septicemic plague **186**	
998.13	Seroma complicating a procedure **167, 171**	
361.2	Serous retinal detachment **39**	
768.5	Severe birth asphyxia **163, 167**	
768.73	Severe hypoxic-ischemic encephalopathy **163, 167**	
642.53	Severe pre-eclampsia, antepartum **154, 156**	
642.54	Severe pre-eclampsia, postpartum condition or complication **151**	
642.50	Severe pre-eclampsia, unspecified as to episode of care **156, 159**	
642.51	Severe pre-eclampsia, with delivery **134, 140, 146**	
642.52	Severe pre-eclampsia, with delivery, with current postpartum complication **134, 140, 146**	
302*	Sexual and gender identity disorders **189**	
202.2*	Sezary's disease **178, 181**	
202.21	Sezary's disease of lymph nodes of head, face, and neck **3**	
004*	Shigellosis **75**	
995.4	Shock due to anesthesia not elsewhere classified **166, 171, 204**	
669.13	Shock during or following labor and delivery, antepartum shock **155, 158**	
669.14	Shock during or following labor and delivery, postpartum condition or complication **153**	
669.10	Shock during or following labor and delivery, unspecified as to episode of care **138, 145, 150**	
669.12	Shock during or following labor and delivery, with delivery, with mention of postpartum complication **138, 141, 146**	
669.11	Shock during or following labor and delivery, with delivery, with or without mention of antepartum condition **138, 141, 146**	
663.43	Short cord complicating labor and delivery, antepartum **155, 158**	
663.41	Short cord complicating labor and delivery, delivered **137, 144, 150**	
663.40	Short cord complicating labor and delivery, unspecified as to episode of care **137, 144, 150**	
660.41	Shoulder (girdle) dystocia during labor and deliver, delivered **136, 143, 149**	
660.43	Shoulder (girdle) dystocia during labor and delivery, antepartum **155, 158**	
660.40	Shoulder (girdle) dystocia during labor and delivery, unspecified as to episode of care **136, 143, 149**	
912.1	Shoulder and upper arm, abrasion or friction burn, infected **106**	
912.0	Shoulder and upper arm, abrasion or friction burn, without mention of infection **107**	
912.3	Shoulder and upper arm, blister, infected **106**	
912.2	Shoulder and upper arm, blister, without mention of infection **107**	
912.5	Shoulder and upper arm, insect bite, nonvenomous, infected **106**	
912.4	Shoulder and upper arm, insect bite, nonvenomous, without mention of infection **108**	
912.6	Shoulder and upper arm, superficial foreign body (splinter), without major open wound and without mention of infection **107**	
912.7	Shoulder and upper arm, superficial foreign body (splinter), without major open wound, infected **106**	
282.42	Sickle-cell thalassemia with crisis **164, 168**	
282.41	Sickle-cell thalassemia without crisis **164, 168**	
240*	Simple and unspecified goiter **114**	
491.0	Simple chronic bronchitis **53**	
V30.1	Single liveborn, born before admission to hospital **171, 172**	
V30.01	Single liveborn, born in hospital, delivered by cesarean delivery **171, 172**	

V30.00	Single liveborn, born in hospital, delivered without mention of cesarean delivery **171, 172**	
V30.2	Single liveborn, born outside hospital and not hospitalized **173**	
759.3	Situs inversus **79**	
V59.1	Skin donor **109**	
306.3	Skin malfunction arising from mental factors **108**	
V42.3	Skin replaced by transplant **109**	
327.53	Sleep related bruxism **47**	
327.26	Sleep related hypoventilation/hypoxemia in conditions classifiable elsewhere **47**	
327.52	Sleep related leg cramps **32**	
780.58	Sleep related movement disorder, unspecified **189**	
046*	Slow virus infections and prion diseases of central nervous system **19**	
863.3*	Small intestine injury with open wound into cavity **79, 223, 227**	
863.2*	Small intestine injury without mention of open wound into cavity **79, 222, 227**	
589*	Small kidney of unknown cause **120**	
050*	Smallpox **184**	
V62.4	Social maladjustment **214**	
312.2*	Socialized conduct disorder **189**	
793.11	Solitary pulmonary nodule **54**	
300.8*	Somatoform disorders **188**	
123.5	Sparganosis (larval diphyllobothriasis) **75**	
367.53	Spasm of accommodation **39**	
378.82	Spasm of conjugate gaze **40**	
728.85	Spasm of muscle **98**	
333.83	Spasmodic torticollis **32**	
V72*	Special investigations and examinations **215**	
V74*	Special screening examination for bacterial and spirochetal diseases **215**	
V75*	Special screening examination for other infectious diseases **215**	
V73*	Special screening examination for viral and chlamydial diseases **215**	
V81*	Special screening for cardiovascular, respiratory, and genitourinary diseases **215**	
V78*	Special screening for disorders of blood and blood-forming organs **215**	
V77*	Special screening for endocrine, nutritional, metabolic, and immunity disorders **215**	
V76*	Special screening for malignant neoplasms **215**	
V79*	Special screening for mental disorders and developmental handicaps **215**	
V80*	Special screening for neurological, eye, and ear diseases **215**	
V82*	Special screening for other condition **215**	
727.2	Specific bursitides often of occupational origin **99**	
307.4*	Specific disorders of sleep of nonorganic origin **189**	
136.2*	Specific infections by free-living amebae **186**	
757.6	Specified congenital anomalies of breast **106**	
757.4	Specified congenital anomalies of hair **108**	
757.5	Specified congenital anomalies of nails **108**	
315.34	Speech and language developmental delay due to hearing loss **189**	
608.1	Spermatocele **124**	
741*	Spina bifida **33, 166, 170**	
756.17	Spina bifida occulta **33**	
952*	Spinal cord injury without evidence of spinal bone injury **19, 223, 227**	
720.1	Spinal enthesopathy **97**	
723.0	Spinal stenosis in cervical region **97**	
334*	Spinocerebellar disease **19**	

*Code Range

789.2	Splenomegaly **176**, **231**	
721*	Spondylosis and allied disorders **97**	
634*	Spontaneous abortion **153**	
782.7	Spontaneous ecchymoses **176**	
512.0	Spontaneous tension pneumothorax **53**	
649.53	Spotting complicating pregnancy, antepartum condition or complication **154**, **157**	
649.51	Spotting complicating pregnancy, delivered, with or without mention of antepartum condition **135**, **142**, **148**	
649.50	Spotting complicating pregnancy, unspecified as to episode of care or not applicable **160**	
848.1	Sprain and strain of jaw **48**	
840.8	Sprain and strain of other specified sites of shoulder and upper arm **222**	
848.3	Sprain and strain of ribs **54**	
848.0	Sprain and strain of septal cartilage of nose **101**	
848.4*	Sprain and strain of sternum **54**	
848.2	Sprain and strain of thyroid region **101**	
840.9	Sprain and strain of unspecified site of shoulder and upper arm **222**	
845*	Sprains and strains of ankle and foot **222**	
841*	Sprains and strains of elbow and forearm **100**, **222**	
843*	Sprains and strains of hip and thigh **96**, **222**	
844*	Sprains and strains of knee and leg **100**, **222**	
847*	Sprains and strains of other and unspecified parts of back **98**, **222**	
846*	Sprains and strains of sacroiliac region **98**, **222**	
840*	Sprains and strains of shoulder and upper arm **100**	
842*	Sprains and strains of wrist and hand **100**, **222**	
005.0	Staphylococcal food poisoning **75**	
V45.88	Status post administration of tPA (rtPA) in a different facility within the last 24 hours prior to admission to current facility **20**	
375.5*	Stenosis and insufficiency of lacrimal passages **39**	
478.74	Stenosis of larynx **47**	
569.2	Stenosis of rectum and anus **79**	
307.3	Stereotypic movement disorder **189**	
V25.2	Sterilization **124**, **128**, **131**	
V26.5*	Sterilization status **214**	
333.91	Stiff-man syndrome **32**	
719.5*	Stiffness of joint, not elsewhere classified **98**	
863.1	Stomach injury with open wound into cavity **79**, **222**, **227**	
863.0	Stomach injury without mention of open wound into cavity **79**, **222**, **227**	
378.73	Strabismus in other neuromuscular disorders **38**	
034.0	Streptococcal sore throat **2**, **46**	
733.96	Stress fracture of femoral neck **97**	
733.95	Stress fracture of other bone **97**	
733.98	Stress fracture of pelvis **97**	
733.97	Stress fracture of shaft of femur **97**	
733.94	Stress fracture of the metatarsals **97**	
733.93	Stress fracture of tibia or fibula **97**	
530.3	Stricture and stenosis of esophagus **78**	
447.1	Stricture of artery **66**	
593.3	Stricture or kinking of ureter **119**	
786.1	Stridor **54**	
127.2	Strongyloidiasis **78**, **230**	
336.2	Subacute combined degeneration of spinal cord in diseases classified elsewhere **32**	
293.1	Subacute delirium **188**	
333.85	Subacute dyskinesia due to drugs **32**	
208.2*	Subacute leukemia of unspecified cell type **181**	

204.2*	Subacute lymphoid leukemia **181**
206.2*	Subacute monocytic leukemia **181**
205.2*	Subacute myeloid leukemia **181**
046.2	Subacute sclerosing panencephalitis **164**, **168**
430	Subarachnoid hemorrhage **8**, **9**, **10**, **20**, **165**, **169**
852.0*	Subarachnoid hemorrhage following injury without mention of open intracranial wound **9**, **11**
852.1*	Subarachnoid hemorrhage following injury, with open intracranial wound **9**, **11**
852.12	Subarachnoid hemorrhage following injury, with open intracranial wound, brief (less than 1 hour) loss of consciousness **31**
852.16	Subarachnoid hemorrhage following injury, with open intracranial wound, loss of consciousness of unspecified duration **26**
852.13	Subarachnoid hemorrhage following injury, with open intracranial wound, moderate (1-24 hours) loss of consciousness **26**
852.11	Subarachnoid hemorrhage following injury, with open intracranial wound, no loss of consciousness **31**
852.14	Subarachnoid hemorrhage following injury, with open intracranial wound, prolonged (more than 24 hours) loss of consciousness and return to pre-existing conscious level **26**
852.15	Subarachnoid hemorrhage following injury, with open intracranial wound, prolonged (more than 24 hours) loss of consciousness, without return to pre-existing conscious level **26**
852.19	Subarachnoid hemorrhage following injury, with open intracranial wound, unspecified concussion **31**
852.10	Subarachnoid hemorrhage following injury, with open intracranial wound, unspecified state of consciousness **31**
852.02	Subarachnoid hemorrhage following injury, without mention of open intracranial wound, brief (less than 1 hour) loss of consciousness **31**
852.06	Subarachnoid hemorrhage following injury, without mention of open intracranial wound, loss of consciousness of unspecified duration **26**
852.03	Subarachnoid hemorrhage following injury, without mention of open intracranial wound, moderate (1-24 hours) loss of consciousness **26**
852.01	Subarachnoid hemorrhage following injury, without mention of open intracranial wound, no loss of consciousness **31**
852.04	Subarachnoid hemorrhage following injury, without mention of open intracranial wound, prolonged (more than 24 hours) loss of consciousness and return to pre-existing conscious level **26**
852.05	Subarachnoid hemorrhage following injury, without mention of open intracranial wound, prolonged (more than 24 hours) loss of consciousness, without return to pre-existing conscious level **26**
852.09	Subarachnoid hemorrhage following injury, without mention of open intracranial wound, unspecified concussion **31**
852.00	Subarachnoid hemorrhage following injury, without mention of open intracranial wound, unspecified state of consciousness **31**
852*	Subarachnoid, subdural, and extradural hemorrhage, following injury **222**, **226**
694.1	Subcorneal pustular dermatosis **108**
767.0	Subdural and cerebral hemorrhage, birth trauma **163**, **167**
852.3*	Subdural hemorrhage following injury, with open intracranial wound **9**, **11**
852.32	Subdural hemorrhage following injury, with open intracranial wound, brief (less than 1 hour) loss of consciousness **31**
852.36	Subdural hemorrhage following injury, with open intracranial wound, loss of consciousness of unspecified duration **27**
852.33	Subdural hemorrhage following injury, with open intracranial wound, moderate (1-24 hours) loss of consciousness **27**
852.31	Subdural hemorrhage following injury, with open intracranial wound, no loss of consciousness **31**

852.34	Subdural hemorrhage following injury, with open intracranial wound, prolonged (more than 24 hours) loss of consciousness and return to pre-existing conscious level **27**
852.35	Subdural hemorrhage following injury, with open intracranial wound, prolonged (more than 24 hours) loss of consciousness, without return to pre-existing conscious level **27**
852.30	Subdural hemorrhage following injury, with open intracranial wound, state of consciousness unspecified **31**
852.39	Subdural hemorrhage following injury, with open intracranial wound, unspecified concussion **31**
852.22	Subdural hemorrhage following injury, without mention of open intracranial wound, brief (less than one hour) loss of consciousness **31**
852.26	Subdural hemorrhage following injury, without mention of open intracranial wound, loss of consciousness of unspecified duration **27**
852.23	Subdural hemorrhage following injury, without mention of open intracranial wound, moderate (1-24 hours) loss of consciousness **26**
852.21	Subdural hemorrhage following injury, without mention of open intracranial wound, no loss of consciousness **31**
852.24	Subdural hemorrhage following injury, without mention of open intracranial wound, prolonged (more than 24 hours) loss of consciousness and return to pre-existing conscious level **27**
852.25	Subdural hemorrhage following injury, without mention of open intracranial wound, prolonged (more than 24 hours) loss of consciousness, without return to pre-existing conscious level **27**
852.29	Subdural hemorrhage following injury, without mention of open intracranial wound, unspecified concussion **31**
852.20	Subdural hemorrhage following injury, without mention of open intracranial wound, unspecified state of consciousness **31**
456.3	Sublingual varices **67**
383.01	Subperiosteal abscess of mastoid **165**, **169**
840.5	Subscapularis (muscle) sprain and strain **222**
798.0	Sudden infant death syndrome **33**
368.11	Sudden visual loss **38**
V62.84	Suicidal ideation **188**
904.1	Superficial femoral artery injury **223**, **227**
913*	Superficial injury of elbow, forearm, and wrist **223**
918*	Superficial injury of eye and adnexa **40**, **223**
910*	Superficial injury of face, neck, and scalp, except eye **223**
915*	Superficial injury of finger(s) **223**
917*	Superficial injury of foot and toe(s) **223**
914*	Superficial injury of hand(s) except finger(s) alone **223**
916*	Superficial injury of hip, thigh, leg, and ankle **223**
919*	Superficial injury of other, multiple, and unspecified sites **223**
912*	Superficial injury of shoulder and upper arm **223**
911*	Superficial injury of trunk **223**
370.2*	Superficial keratitis without conjunctivitis **39**
671.20	Superficial thrombophlebitis complicating pregnancy and the puerperium, unspecified as to episode of care **161**
671.22	Superficial thrombophlebitis with delivery, with mention of postpartum complication **138**, **145**, **151**
671.21	Superficial thrombophlebitis with delivery, with or without mention of antepartum condition **138**, **145**, **151**
671.23	Superficial thrombophlebitis, antepartum **156**, **158**
671.24	Superficial thrombophlebitis, postpartum condition or complication **153**
840.7	Superior glenoid labrum lesions (SLAP) **222**
901.2	Superior vena cava injury **166**, **170**, **223**, **226**
V23.8*	Supervision of other high-risk pregnancy **161**
676.53	Suppressed lactation, antepartum condition or complication **156**, **158**
676.54	Suppressed lactation, postpartum condition or complication **153**
676.50	Suppressed lactation, unspecified as to episode of care **161**
676.52	Suppressed lactation, with delivery, with mention of postpartum complication **139**, **145**, **151**
676.51	Suppressed lactation, with delivery, with or without mention of antepartum condition **139**, **145**, **151**
382*	Suppurative and unspecified otitis media **46**
840.6	Supraspinatus (muscle) (tendon) sprain and strain **222**
V67.0*	Surgery follow-up examination **213**
V64.1	Surgical or other procedure not carried out because of contraindication **173**
V64.2	Surgical or other procedure not carried out because of patient's decision **173**
V25.4*	Surveillance of previously prescribed contraceptive methods **214**
655.53	Suspected damage to fetus from drugs, affecting management of mother, antepartum **155**, **157**
655.51	Suspected damage to fetus from drugs, affecting management of mother, delivered **135**, **143**, **148**
655.50	Suspected damage to fetus from drugs, affecting management of mother, unspecified as to episode of care **160**
655.43	Suspected damage to fetus from other disease in mother, affecting management of mother, antepartum condition or complication **155**, **157**
655.40	Suspected damage to fetus from other disease in mother, affecting management of mother, unspecified as to episode of care in pregnancy **160**
655.41	Suspected damage to fetus from other disease in mother, affecting management of mother, with delivery **135**, **143**, **148**
655.63	Suspected damage to fetus from radiation, affecting management of mother, antepartum condition or complication **155**, **157**
655.61	Suspected damage to fetus from radiation, affecting management of mother, delivered **135**, **143**, **148**
655.60	Suspected damage to fetus from radiation, affecting management of mother, unspecified as to episode of care **160**
655.33	Suspected damage to fetus from viral disease in mother, affecting management of mother, antepartum condition or complication **155**, **157**
655.30	Suspected damage to fetus from viral disease in mother, affecting management of mother, unspecified as to episode of care in pregnancy **160**
655.31	Suspected damage to fetus from viral disease in mother, affecting management of mother, with delivery **135**, **143**, **148**
V89.0*	Suspected maternal and fetal conditions not found **215**
078.2	Sweating fever **185**
729.81	Swelling of limb **98**
786.6	Swelling, mass, or lump in chest **54**
784.2	Swelling, mass, or lump in head and neck **108**
784.60	Symbolic dysfunction, unspecified **189**
360.11	Sympathetic uveitis **39**
V83.02	Symptomatic hemophilia A carrier **215**
359.6	Symptomatic inflammatory myopathy in diseases classified elsewhere **33**
783*	Symptoms concerning nutrition, metabolism, and development **113**
787*	Symptoms involving digestive system **78**
780.2	Syncope and collapse **68**
727.01	Synovitis and tenosynovitis in diseases classified elsewhere **98**
095.5	Syphilis of bone **96**
095.4	Syphilis of kidney **119**
095.3	Syphilis of liver **83**
095.1	Syphilis of lung **51**
095.6	Syphilis of muscle **98**
095.7	Syphilis of synovium, tendon, and bursa **98**
094.86	Syphilitic acoustic neuritis **47**

*Code Range

093.1	Syphilitic aortitis **67**		446.6	Thrombotic microangiopathy **97**
094.83	Syphilitic disseminated retinochoroiditis **38**		245*	Thyroiditis **3**, **114**
094.81	Syphilitic encephalitis **9**, **10**, **34**		242*	Thyrotoxicosis with or without goiter **3**, **114**
093.22	Syphilitic endocarditis, aortic valve **67**		904.5*	Tibial blood vessel(s) injury **223**, **227**
093.21	Syphilitic endocarditis, mitral valve **67**		726.72	Tibialis tendinitis **98**
093.24	Syphilitic endocarditis, pulmonary valve **67**		066.1	Tick-borne fever **184**
093.23	Syphilitic endocarditis, tricuspid valve **67**		082*	Tick-borne rickettsioses **185**
095.0	Syphilitic episcleritis **38**		063*	Tick-borne viral encephalitis **9**, **10**, **33**
090.3	Syphilitic interstitial keratitis **38**		307.2*	Tics **32**
094.2	Syphilitic meningitis **9**, **10**, **34**		333.3	Tics of organic origin **32**
094.84	Syphilitic optic atrophy **38**		733.6	Tietze's disease **54**
094.82	Syphilitic Parkinsonism **19**		388.3*	Tinnitus **47**
095.2	Syphilitic peritonitis **75**		649.03	Tobacco use disorder complicating pregnancy, childbirth, or the puerperium, antepartum condition or complication **154**, **157**
094.85	Syphilitic retrobulbar neuritis **19**			
094.87	Syphilitic ruptured cerebral aneurysm **8**, **32**		649.02	Tobacco use disorder complicating pregnancy, childbirth, or the puerperium, delivered, with mention of postpartum complication **135**, **142**, **148**
336.0	Syringomyelia and syringobulbia **19**			
995.9*	Systemic inflammatory response syndrome (SIRS) **186**			
428.2*	Systolic heart failure **57**, **165**, **169**		649.01	Tobacco use disorder complicating pregnancy, childbirth, or the puerperium, delivered, with or without mention of antepartum condition **135**, **142**, **148**
094.0	Tabes dorsalis **19**			
123.2	Taenia saginata infection **77**			
123.0	Taenia solium infection, intestinal form **77**		649.04	Tobacco use disorder complicating pregnancy, childbirth, or the puerperium, postpartum condition or complication **152**
123.3	Taeniasis, unspecified **77**			
446.7	Takayasu's disease **97**		649.00	Tobacco use disorder complicating pregnancy, childbirth, or the puerperium, unspecified as to episode of care or not applicable **159**
429.83	Takotsubo syndrome **69**			
836.1	Tear of lateral cartilage or meniscus of knee, current **222**			
836.0	Tear of medial cartilage or meniscus of knee, current **222**		750.0	Tongue tie **3**, **48**
348.81	Temporal sclerosis **20**		379.46	Tonic pupillary reaction **38**
727.06	Tenosynovitis of foot and ankle **99**		608.2*	Torsion of testis **124**
307.81	Tension headache **34**		723.5	Torticollis, unspecified **97**
257*	Testicular dysfunction **114**		823.4*	Torus fracture of tibia and fibula **222**, **227**
037	Tetanus **164**, **168**, **185**		367.52	Total or complete internal ophthalmoplegia **38**
781.7	Tetany **113**, **166**, **170**		980*	Toxic effect of alcohol **203**
745.2	Tetralogy of Fallot **67**		986	Toxic effect of carbon monoxide **203**
282.40	Thalassemia, unspecified **164**, **168**		983*	Toxic effect of corrosive aromatics, acids, and caustic alkalis **203**
265*	Thiamine and niacin deficiency states **113**, **230**		984*	Toxic effect of lead and its compounds (including fumes) **203**
664.24	Third-degree perineal laceration, postpartum condition or complication **152**		988*	Toxic effect of noxious substances eaten as food **203**
			987*	Toxic effect of other gases, fumes, or vapors **203**
664.20	Third-degree perineal laceration, unspecified as to episode of care in pregnancy **137**, **144**, **150**		985*	Toxic effect of other metals **203**
			989*	Toxic effect of other substances, chiefly nonmedicinal as to source **203**
664.21	Third-degree perineal laceration, with delivery **137**, **144**, **150**			
666.04	Third-stage postpartum hemorrhage, postpartum condition or complication **152**		981	Toxic effect of petroleum products **203**
			982*	Toxic effect of solvents other than petroleum-based **203**
666.00	Third-stage postpartum hemorrhage, unspecified as to episode of care **161**		987.9	Toxic effect of unspecified gas, fume, or vapor **207**
			323.71	Toxic encephalitis and encephalomyelitis **10**, **32**
666.02	Third-stage postpartum hemorrhage, with delivery **137**, **140**, **146**		323.7*	Toxic encephalitis, myelitis, and encephalomyelitis **9**
			349.82	Toxic encephalopathy **32**, **165**, **169**
441.2	Thoracic aneurysm without mention of rupture **66**		695.0	Toxic erythema **105**, **166**, **170**
441.1	Thoracic aneurysm, ruptured **66**		558.2	Toxic gastroenteritis and colitis **79**, **166**, **170**, **230**
901.0	Thoracic aorta injury **166**, **170**, **223**, **226**		323.72	Toxic myelitis **10**, **32**
441.7	Thoracoabdominal aneurysm without mention of rupture **66**		358.2	Toxic myoneural disorders **21**
441.6	Thoracoabdominal aneurysm, ruptured **66**		359.4	Toxic myopathy **32**
640.03	Threatened abortion, antepartum **153**		040.82	Toxic shock syndrome **185**
640.01	Threatened abortion, delivered **134**, **141**, **147**		130*	Toxoplasmosis **230**
640.00	Threatened abortion, unspecified as to episode of care **153**		130.7	Toxoplasmosis of other specified sites **164**, **168**, **186**
644.03	Threatened premature labor, antepartum **153**		530.84	Tracheoesophageal fistula **75**, **165**, **170**
644.00	Threatened premature labor, unspecified as to episode of care **153**		519.0*	Tracheostomy complications **3**, **54**
			076*	Trachoma **38**
784.1	Throat pain **47**		999.80	Transfusion reaction, unspecified **176**
443.1	Thromboangiitis obliterans (Buerger's disease) **66**		518.7	Transfusion related acute lung injury [TRALI] **54**
453.1	Thrombophlebitis migrans **67**		780.02	Transient alteration of awareness **188**
			435*	Transient cerebral ischemia **20**

437.7	Transient global amnesia **21**
642.33	Transient hypertension of pregnancy, antepartum **154**, **157**
642.34	Transient hypertension of pregnancy, postpartum condition or complication **151**
642.30	Transient hypertension of pregnancy, unspecified as to episode of care **159**
642.31	Transient hypertension of pregnancy, with delivery **134**, **141**, **147**
642.32	Transient hypertension of pregnancy, with delivery, with current postpartum complication **134**, **141**, **147**
776.1	Transient neonatal thrombocytopenia **163**, **167**
781.4	Transient paralysis of limb **33**
368.12	Transient visual loss **38**
745.1*	Transposition of great vessels **67**
652.33	Transverse or oblique fetal presentation, antepartum **154**, **157**
652.31	Transverse or oblique fetal presentation, delivered **135**, **142**, **148**
652.30	Transverse or oblique fetal presentation, unspecified as to episode of care **160**
887*	Traumatic amputation of arm and hand (complete) (partial) **203**, **223**, **227**
896*	Traumatic amputation of foot (complete) (partial) **203**, **223**, **227**
897*	Traumatic amputation of leg(s) (complete) (partial) **203**, **223**, **227**
886*	Traumatic amputation of other finger(s) (complete) (partial) **203**, **223**
885*	Traumatic amputation of thumb (complete) (partial) **203**, **223**
895*	Traumatic amputation of toe(s) (complete) (partial) **203**, **223**
958.5	Traumatic anuria **118**, **119**, **166**, **171**, **224**
958.9*	Traumatic compartment syndrome **204**
958.93	Traumatic compartment syndrome of abdomen **224**, **227**
958.92	Traumatic compartment syndrome of lower extremity **224**, **228**
958.99	Traumatic compartment syndrome of other sites **224**
958.91	Traumatic compartment syndrome of upper extremity **224**, **227**
860*	Traumatic pneumothorax and hemothorax **53**, **166**, **170**, **222**, **226**
958.4	Traumatic shock **166**, **171**, **204**, **224**
958.7	Traumatic subcutaneous emphysema **53**, **166**, **171**, **224**
V67.4	Treatment of healed fracture follow-up examination **213**
124	Trichinosis **186**
131.03	Trichomonal prostatitis **124**
131.02	Trichomonal urethritis **124**, **127**, **130**
131.01	Trichomonal vulvovaginitis **127**, **130**
131.8	Trichomoniasis of other specified sites **186**
127.6	Trichostrongyliasis **78**
127.3	Trichuriasis **78**
426.54	Trifascicular block **165**, **169**
350*	Trigeminal nerve disorders **21**
727.03	Trigger finger (acquired) **99**
595.3	Trigonitis **119**
V91.1*	Triplet gestation placenta status **215**
651.43	Triplet pregnancy with fetal loss and retention of one or more, antepartum **154**, **157**
651.41	Triplet pregnancy with fetal loss and retention of one or more, delivered **135**, **142**, **148**
651.40	Triplet pregnancy with fetal loss and retention of one or more, unspecified as to episode of care or not applicable **160**
651.13	Triplet pregnancy, antepartum **154**, **157**
651.11	Triplet pregnancy, delivered **135**, **142**, **148**
651.10	Triplet pregnancy, unspecified as to episode of care **160**
368.53	Tritan defect in color vision **39**
040.81	Tropical pyomyositis **98**

911.1	Trunk abrasion or friction burn, infected **106**
911.0	Trunk abrasion or friction burn, without mention of infection **107**
911.3	Trunk blister, infected **106**
911.2	Trunk blister, without mention of infection **108**
911.5	Trunk, insect bite, nonvenomous, infected **106**
911.4	Trunk, insect bite, nonvenomous, without mention of infection **108**
911.6	Trunk, superficial foreign body (splinter), without major open wound and without mention of infection **107**
911.7	Trunk, superficial foreign body (splinter), without major open wound, infected **106**
017.6*	Tuberculosis of adrenal glands **114**
016.1*	Tuberculosis of bladder **119**
015*	Tuberculosis of bones and joints **229**
017.4*	Tuberculosis of ear **47**
016.4*	Tuberculosis of epididymis **123**
017.8*	Tuberculosis of esophagus **75**
017.3*	Tuberculosis of eye **38**
016*	Tuberculosis of genitourinary system **229**
015.1*	Tuberculosis of hip **97**
014*	Tuberculosis of intestines, peritoneum, and mesenteric glands **75**, **229**
012.1*	Tuberculosis of intrathoracic lymph nodes **51**
016.0*	Tuberculosis of kidney **119**
015.2*	Tuberculosis of knee **97**
015.5*	Tuberculosis of limb bones **96**
015.6*	Tuberculosis of mastoid **47**
013*	Tuberculosis of meninges and central nervous system **8**, **10**, **33**, **229**
016.7*	Tuberculosis of other female genital organs **127**, **129**
016.5*	Tuberculosis of other male genital organs **123**
017*	Tuberculosis of other organs **229**
015.7*	Tuberculosis of other specified bone **96**
015.8*	Tuberculosis of other specified joint **97**
017.9*	Tuberculosis of other specified organs **185**
016.3*	Tuberculosis of other urinary organs **119**
017.2*	Tuberculosis of peripheral lymph nodes **176**
017.0*	Tuberculosis of skin and subcutaneous cellular tissue **107**
017.7*	Tuberculosis of spleen **176**
017.5*	Tuberculosis of thyroid gland **114**
015.9*	Tuberculosis of unspecified bones and joints **97**
016.2*	Tuberculosis of ureter **119**
015.0*	Tuberculosis of vertebral column **96**
015.02	Tuberculosis of vertebral column, bacteriological or histological examination unknown (at present) **87**
015.04	Tuberculosis of vertebral column, tubercle bacilli not found (in sputum) by microscopy, but found by bacterial culture **87**
015.05	Tuberculosis of vertebral column, tubercle bacilli not found by bacteriological examination, but tuberculosis confirmed histologically **87**
012.3*	Tuberculous laryngitis **2**, **47**
016.6*	Tuberculous oophoritis and salpingitis **127**, **129**
012.0*	Tuberculous pleurisy **51**
759.5	Tuberous sclerosis **33**
V26.0	Tuboplasty or vasoplasty after previous sterilization **124**, **128**, **131**
277.88	Tumor lysis syndrome **118**, **164**, **168**
654.10	Tumors of body of pregnant uterus, unspecified as to episode of care in pregnancy **160**
654.13	Tumors of body of uterus, antepartum condition or complication **154**, **157**

*Code Range

654.11	Tumors of body of uterus, delivered **135, 142, 148**	
654.12	Tumors of body of uterus, delivered, with mention of postpartum complication **135, 142, 148**	
654.14	Tumors of body of uterus, postpartum condition or complication **152**	
V31.1	Twin birth, mate liveborn, born before admission to hospital **171, 172**	
V31.2	Twin birth, mate liveborn, born outside hospital and not hospitalized **173**	
V32.1	Twin birth, mate stillborn, born before admission to hospital **171, 172**	
V32.2	Twin birth, mate stillborn, born outside hospital and not hospitalized **173**	
V33.1	Twin birth, unspecified whether mate liveborn or stillborn, born before admission to hospital **171, 172**	
V33.2	Twin birth, unspecified whether mate liveborn or stillborn, born outside hospital and not hospitalized **173**	
V91.0*	Twin gestation placenta status **215**	
651.33	Twin pregnancy with fetal loss and retention of one fetus, antepartum **154, 157**	
651.31	Twin pregnancy with fetal loss and retention of one fetus, delivered **135, 142, 148**	
651.30	Twin pregnancy with fetal loss and retention of one fetus, unspecified as to episode of care or not applicable **160**	
651.03	Twin pregnancy, antepartum **154, 157**	
651.01	Twin pregnancy, delivered **135, 142, 148**	
651.00	Twin pregnancy, unspecified as to episode of care **160**	
V31.01	Twin, mate liveborn, born in hospital, delivered by cesarean delivery **171, 172**	
V31.00	Twin, mate liveborn, born in hospital, delivered without mention of cesarean delivery **171, 172**	
V32.01	Twin, mate stillborn, born in hospital, delivered by cesarean delivery **171, 172**	
V32.00	Twin, mate stillborn, born in hospital, delivered without mention of cesarean delivery **171, 172**	
V33.01	Twin, unspecified whether mate stillborn or liveborn, born in hospital, delivered by cesarean delivery **171, 172**	
V33.00	Twin, unspecified whether mate stillborn or liveborn, born in hospital, delivered without mention of cesarean delivery **171, 172**	
002*	Typhoid and paratyphoid fevers **185**	
530.2*	Ulcer of esophagus **77**	
569.82	Ulceration of intestine **79**	
616.5*	Ulceration of vulva **127, 130**	
556*	Ulcerative colitis **77**	
021.0	Ulceroglandular tularemia **185**	
551.1	Umbilical hernia with gangrene **166, 170**	
552.1	Umbilical hernia with obstruction **78, 166, 170**	
553.1	Umbilical hernia without mention of obstruction or gangrene **79**	
798.9	Unattended death **213**	
V63*	Unavailability of other medical facilities for care **214**	
312.0*	Undersocialized conduct disorder, aggressive type **189**	
312.1*	Undersocialized conduct disorder, unaggressive type **189**	
752.5*	Undescended and retractile testicle **124, 172**	
785.2	Undiagnosed cardiac murmurs **68**	
V62.0	Unemployment **214**	
552.00	Unilateral or unspecified femoral hernia with obstruction **166, 170**	
388.40	Unspecified abnormal auditory perception **47**	
379.40	Unspecified abnormal pupillary function **38**	
661.93	Unspecified abnormality of labor, antepartum **155, 158**	
661.90	Unspecified abnormality of labor, unspecified as to episode of care **136, 144, 149**	

661.91	Unspecified abnormality of labor, with delivery **136, 144, 149**
518.4	Unspecified acute edema of lung **52, 165, 170**
421.9	Unspecified acute endocarditis **65, 230**
376.00	Unspecified acute inflammation of orbit **39**
391.9	Unspecified acute rheumatic heart disease **68**
309.9	Unspecified adjustment reaction **188**
995.22	Unspecified adverse effect of anesthesia **166, 171**
995.23	Unspecified adverse effect of insulin **166, 171**
995.29	Unspecified adverse effect of other drug, medicinal and biological substance **166, 171**
995.20	Unspecified adverse effect of unspecified drug, medicinal and biological substance **166, 171**
V58.9	Unspecified aftercare **213**
571.3	Unspecified alcoholic liver damage **82**
006.9	Unspecified amebiasis **185**
285.9	Unspecified anemia **230**
V28.9	Unspecified antenatal screening **214**
641.93	Unspecified antepartum hemorrhage, antepartum **154, 157**
641.90	Unspecified antepartum hemorrhage, unspecified as to episode of care **159**
641.91	Unspecified antepartum hemorrhage, with delivery **134, 140, 145**
646.23	Unspecified antepartum renal disease **154, 156**
022.9	Unspecified anthrax **185**
284.9	Unspecified aplastic anemia **175, 230**
447.6	Unspecified arteritis **97**
716.9*	Unspecified arthropathy **230**
066.9	Unspecified arthropod-borne viral disease **184**
493.9*	Unspecified asthma **54**
482.9	Unspecified bacterial pneumonia **53**
694.9	Unspecified bullous dermatosis **105**
594.9	Unspecified calculus of lower urinary tract **119**
427.9	Unspecified cardiac dysrhythmia **68**
429.2	Unspecified cardiovascular disease **67**
093.9	Unspecified cardiovascular syphilis **68**
323.9	Unspecified causes of encephalitis, myelitis, and encephalomyelitis **9, 10, 34, 230**
434.91	Unspecified cerebral artery occlusion with cerebral infarction **9, 11, 20**
434.90	Unspecified cerebral artery occlusion without mention of cerebral infarction **20**
331.9	Unspecified cerebral degeneration **19**
437.9	Unspecified cerebrovascular disease **21**
123.9	Unspecified cestode infection **76**
491.9	Unspecified chronic bronchitis **53**
474.9	Unspecified chronic disease of tonsils and adenoids **47**
414.9	Unspecified chronic ischemic heart disease **67**
571.9	Unspecified chronic liver disease without mention of alcohol **83**
416.9	Unspecified chronic pulmonary heart disease **69**
459.9	Unspecified circulatory system disorder **67**
824.8	Unspecified closed fracture of ankle **222**
808.8	Unspecified closed fracture of pelvis **221**
114.9	Unspecified coccidioidomycosis **185**
763.9	Unspecified complication of labor and delivery affecting fetus or newborn **171, 172**
669.93	Unspecified complication of labor and delivery, antepartum condition or complication **156, 158**
669.94	Unspecified complication of labor and delivery, postpartum condition or complication **153**
669.90	Unspecified complication of labor and delivery, unspecified as to episode of care **138, 145, 151**

669.92	Unspecified complication of labor and delivery, with delivery, with mention of postpartum complication **138**, **145**, **151**
669.91	Unspecified complication of labor and delivery, with delivery, with or without mention of antepartum condition **138**, **145**, **151**
646.93	Unspecified complication of pregnancy, antepartum **154**, **157**
646.90	Unspecified complication of pregnancy, unspecified as to episode of care **159**
646.91	Unspecified complication of pregnancy, with delivery **134**, **142**, **147**
998.9	Unspecified complication of procedure, not elsewhere classified **167**, **171**, **204**
668.93	Unspecified complication of the administration of anesthesia or other sedation in labor and delivery, antepartum **155**, **158**
668.91	Unspecified complication of the administration of anesthesia or other sedation in labor and delivery, delivered **138**, **141**, **146**
668.92	Unspecified complication of the administration of anesthesia or other sedation in labor and delivery, delivered, with mention of postpartum complication **138**, **141**, **146**
668.94	Unspecified complication of the administration of anesthesia or other sedation in labor and delivery, postpartum condition or complication **153**
668.90	Unspecified complication of the administration of anesthesia or other sedation in labor and delivery, unspecified as to episode of care **138**, **144**, **150**
674.94	Unspecified complications of puerperium, postpartum condition or complication **153**
674.90	Unspecified complications of puerperium, unspecified as to episode of care **161**
674.92	Unspecified complications of puerperium, with delivery, with mention of postpartum complication **138**, **145**, **151**
850.9	Unspecified concussion **222**
348.9	Unspecified condition of brain **20**, **230**
759.9	Unspecified congenital anomaly **213**
747.9	Unspecified congenital anomaly of circulatory system **67**
751.9	Unspecified congenital anomaly of digestive system **79**
744.3	Unspecified congenital anomaly of ear **47**
744.9	Unspecified congenital anomaly of face and neck **108**
751.60	Unspecified congenital anomaly of gallbladder, bile ducts, and liver **83**
752.9	Unspecified congenital anomaly of genital organs **124**, **127**, **130**
746.9	Unspecified congenital anomaly of heart **68**
748.60	Unspecified congenital anomaly of lung **54**
748.9	Unspecified congenital anomaly of respiratory system **54**
757.9	Unspecified congenital anomaly of the integument **108**
750.9	Unspecified congenital anomaly of upper alimentary tract **79**
745.9	Unspecified congenital defect of septal closure **68**
V25.9	Unspecified contraceptive management **214**
921.9	Unspecified contusion of eye **40**
370.00	Unspecified corneal ulcer **38**
737.9	Unspecified curvature of spine associated with other condition **87**
595.9	Unspecified cystitis **119**, **166**, **170**
375.00	Unspecified dacryoadenitis **39**
375.30	Unspecified dacryocystitis **39**
799.3	Unspecified debility **213**
736.70	Unspecified deformity of ankle and foot, acquired **100**
736.00	Unspecified deformity of forearm, excluding fingers **100**
374.50	Unspecified degenerative disorder of eyelid **39**
315.9	Unspecified delay in development **189**
341.9	Unspecified demyelinating disease of central nervous system **19**, **230**
718.9*	Unspecified derangement of joint **100**
032.9	Unspecified diphtheria **185**
478.70	Unspecified disease of larynx **47**
478.20	Unspecified disease of pharynx **47**
519.9	Unspecified disease of respiratory system **54**
336.9	Unspecified disease of spinal cord **32**, **230**
527.9	Unspecified disease of the salivary glands **230**
288.9	Unspecified disease of white blood cells **176**
031.9	Unspecified diseases due to mycobacteria **185**, **229**
289.9	Unspecified diseases of blood and blood-forming organs **176**, **230**
271.9	Unspecified disorder of carbohydrate transport and metabolism **113**
388.9	Unspecified disorder of ear **47**
530.9	Unspecified disorder of esophagus **78**
380.9	Unspecified disorder of external ear **47**
379.9*	Unspecified disorder of eye and adnexa **40**
378.9	Unspecified disorder of eye movements **40**
374.9	Unspecified disorder of eyelid **39**
629.9	Unspecified disorder of female genital organs **130**
360.9	Unspecified disorder of globe **39**
279.9	Unspecified disorder of immune mechanism **176**
569.9	Unspecified disorder of intestine **79**
364.9	Unspecified disorder of iris and ciliary body **39**
719.9*	Unspecified disorder of joint **98**
593.9	Unspecified disorder of kidney and ureter **120**
375.9	Unspecified disorder of lacrimal system **39**
676.93	Unspecified disorder of lactation, antepartum condition or complication **156**, **158**
676.94	Unspecified disorder of lactation, postpartum condition or complication **153**
676.90	Unspecified disorder of lactation, unspecified as to episode of care **161**
676.92	Unspecified disorder of lactation, with delivery, with mention of postpartum complication **139**, **145**, **151**
676.91	Unspecified disorder of lactation, with delivery, with or without mention of antepartum condition **139**, **145**, **151**
573.9	Unspecified disorder of liver **83**
608.9	Unspecified disorder of male genital organs **124**
277.9	Unspecified disorder of metabolism **114**
275.9	Unspecified disorder of mineral metabolism **114**
728.9	Unspecified disorder of muscle, ligament, and fascia **99**
377.9	Unspecified disorder of optic nerve and visual pathways **33**
376.9	Unspecified disorder of orbit **40**
251.9	Unspecified disorder of pancreatic internal secretion **114**
607.9	Unspecified disorder of penis **124**
273.9	Unspecified disorder of plasma protein metabolism **180**, **182**
367.9	Unspecified disorder of refraction and accommodation **39**
709.9	Unspecified disorder of skin and subcutaneous tissue **230**
537.9	Unspecified disorder of stomach and duodenum **78**
727.9	Unspecified disorder of synovium, tendon, and bursa **99**
246.9	Unspecified disorder of thyroid **3**
384.9	Unspecified disorder of tympanic membrane **47**
599.9	Unspecified disorder of urethra and urinary tract **120**
447.9	Unspecified disorders of arteries and arterioles **66**
349.9	Unspecified disorders of nervous system **20**, **230**
312.9	Unspecified disturbance of conduct **189**
090.2	Unspecified early congenital syphilis **185**
122.4	Unspecified echinococcus granulosus infection **186**
122.7	Unspecified echinococcus multilocularis infection **186**
122.8	Unspecified echinococcus of liver **83**
993.9	Unspecified effect of air pressure **204**

*Code Range

V50.9	Unspecified elective surgery for purposes other than remedying health states **214**
313.9	Unspecified emotional disturbance of childhood or adolescence **189**
726.9*	Unspecified enthesopathy **98**
726.70	Unspecified enthesopathy of ankle and tarsus **98**
695.9	Unspecified erythematous condition **108**
401.9	Unspecified essential hypertension **67**
381.9	Unspecified Eustachian tube disorder **47**
376.30	Unspecified exophthalmos **39**
333.90	Unspecified extrapyramidal disease and abnormal movement disorder **19**
660.71	Unspecified failed forceps or vacuum extractor, delivered **136, 143, 149**
660.70	Unspecified failed forceps or vacuum extractor, unspecified as to episode of care **136, 143, 149**
660.63	Unspecified failed trial of labor, antepartum **155, 158**
660.61	Unspecified failed trial of labor, delivered **136, 143, 149**
660.60	Unspecified failed trial of labor, unspecified as to episode **136, 143, 149**
V61.9	Unspecified family circumstance **214**
729.4	Unspecified fasciitis **99**
655.93	Unspecified fetal abnormality affecting management of mother, antepartum condition or complication **155, 157**
655.91	Unspecified fetal abnormality affecting management of mother, delivery **136, 143, 149**
655.90	Unspecified fetal abnormality affecting management of mother, unspecified as to episode of care **160**
774.6	Unspecified fetal and neonatal jaundice **171, 172**
656.93	Unspecified fetal and placental problem affecting management of mother, antepartum **155, 158**
656.91	Unspecified fetal and placental problem affecting management of mother, delivered **136, 143, 149**
656.90	Unspecified fetal and placental problem affecting management of mother, unspecified as to episode of care **160**
653.93	Unspecified fetal disproportion, antepartum **154, 157**
653.91	Unspecified fetal disproportion, delivered **135, 142, 148**
653.90	Unspecified fetal disproportion, unspecified as to episode of care **160**
764.98	Unspecified fetal growth retardation, 2,000-2,499 grams **171, 172**
764.99	Unspecified fetal growth retardation, 2,500 or more grams **171, 172**
619.9	Unspecified fistula involving female genital tract **127, 130**
V67.9	Unspecified follow-up examination **215**
005.9	Unspecified food poisoning **77**
564.9	Unspecified functional disorder of intestine **78**
536.9	Unspecified functional disorder of stomach **78**
535.51	Unspecified gastritis and gastroduodenitis with hemorrhage **76**
535.50	Unspecified gastritis and gastroduodenitis without mention of hemorrhage **78**
054.10	Unspecified genital herpes **123, 127, 129, 229**
365.9	Unspecified glaucoma **39**
429.9	Unspecified heart disease **67**
428.9	Unspecified heart failure **57, 165, 169**
459.0	Unspecified hemorrhage **69, 165, 169**
640.93	Unspecified hemorrhage in early pregnancy, antepartum **153**
640.91	Unspecified hemorrhage in early pregnancy, delivered **134, 141, 147**
640.90	Unspecified hemorrhage in early pregnancy, unspecified as to episode of care **153**
573.3	Unspecified hepatitis **83, 166, 170**
356.9	Unspecified hereditary and idiopathic peripheral neuropathy **21**
054.8	Unspecified herpes simplex complication **164, 168, 184, 229**
053.8	Unspecified herpes zoster complication **164, 168, 184, 229**
V23.9	Unspecified high-risk pregnancy **161**
115.94	Unspecified Histoplasmosis endocarditis **65, 164, 168**
115.91	Unspecified Histoplasmosis meningitis **9, 10, 34, 164, 168**
115.93	Unspecified Histoplasmosis pericarditis **68, 164, 168**
115.95	Unspecified Histoplasmosis pneumonia **51, 164, 168**
115.92	Unspecified Histoplasmosis retinitis **38, 164, 168**
115.99	Unspecified Histoplasmosis with mention of other manifestation **185**
115.90	Unspecified Histoplasmosis without mention of manifestation **185**
603.9	Unspecified hydrocele **124**
642.93	Unspecified hypertension antepartum **154, 156**
642.94	Unspecified hypertension complicating pregnancy, childbirth, or the puerperium, postpartum condition or complication **151**
642.90	Unspecified hypertension complicating pregnancy, childbirth, or the puerperium, unspecified as to episode of care **159**
642.91	Unspecified hypertension, with delivery **134, 140, 146**
642.92	Unspecified hypertension, with delivery, with current postpartum complication **134, 140, 146**
402.90	Unspecified hypertensive heart disease without heart failure **67**
458.9	Unspecified hypotension **69**
279.3	Unspecified immunity deficiency **176**
279.10	Unspecified immunodeficiency with predominant T-cell defect **176**
560.30	Unspecified impaction of intestine **166, 170**
659.93	Unspecified indication for care or intervention related to labor and delivery, antepartum **155, 158**
659.91	Unspecified indication for care or intervention related to labor and delivery, delivered **136, 143, 149**
659.90	Unspecified indication for care or intervention related to labor and delivery, unspecified as to episode of care **136, 143, 149**
343.9	Unspecified infantile cerebral palsy **32**
730.9*	Unspecified infection of bone **96**
590.9	Unspecified infection of kidney **166, 170**
675.93	Unspecified infection of the breast and nipple, antepartum **156, 158**
675.92	Unspecified infection of the breast and nipple, delivered, with mention of postpartum complication **139, 145, 151**
675.91	Unspecified infection of the breast and nipple, delivered, with or without mention of antepartum condition **139, 145, 151**
675.94	Unspecified infection of the breast and nipple, postpartum condition or complication **153**
675.90	Unspecified infection of the breast and nipple, unspecified as to prenatal or postnatal episode of care **161**
136.9	Unspecified infectious and parasitic diseases **186**
711.9*	Unspecified infective arthritis **97, 230**
902.10	Unspecified inferior vena cava injury **166, 170**
357.9	Unspecified inflammatory and toxic neuropathy **21, 230**
616.9	Unspecified inflammatory disease of cervix, vagina, and vulva **127, 130**
614.9	Unspecified inflammatory disease of female pelvic organs and tissues **130**
714.9	Unspecified inflammatory polyarthropathy **98**
720.9	Unspecified inflammatory spondylopathy **97**
319	Unspecified intellectual disabilities **188**
717.9	Unspecified internal derangement of knee **99**
370.50	Unspecified interstitial keratitis **39**
127.9	Unspecified intestinal helminthiasis **78**
579.9	Unspecified intestinal malabsorption **230**
560.9	Unspecified intestinal obstruction **166, 170**

129	Unspecified intestinal parasitism **78**
432.9	Unspecified intracranial hemorrhage **9**, **10**
718.65	Unspecified intrapelvic protrusion acetabulum, pelvic region and thigh **100**
364.3	Unspecified iridocyclitis **39**
370.9	Unspecified keratitis **39**
095.9	Unspecified late symptomatic syphilis **185**
085.9	Unspecified leishmaniasis **185**
100.9	Unspecified leptospirosis **185**
208.9*	Unspecified leukemia **181**
686.9	Unspecified local infection of skin and subcutaneous tissue **172**
003.20	Unspecified localized salmonella infection **185**
861.30	Unspecified lung injury with open wound into thorax **54**
861.20	Unspecified lung injury without mention of open wound into thorax **54**
204.9*	Unspecified lymphoid leukemia **181**
652.93	Unspecified malposition or malpresentation of fetus, antepartum **154**, **157**
652.91	Unspecified malposition or malpresentation of fetus, delivered **135**, **142**, **148**
652.90	Unspecified malposition or malpresentation of fetus, unspecified as to episode of care **160**
383.9	Unspecified mastoiditis **46**
647.94	Unspecified maternal infection or infestation complicating pregnancy, childbirth, or the puerperium, postpartum condition or complication **152**
647.90	Unspecified maternal infection or infestation complicating pregnancy, childbirth, or the puerperium, unspecified as to episode of care **159**
647.91	Unspecified maternal infection or infestation with delivery **134**, **140**, **146**
647.92	Unspecified maternal infection or infestation with delivery, with current postpartum complication **134**, **140**, **146**
647.93	Unspecified maternal infection or infestation, antepartum **154**, **156**
659.21	Unspecified maternal pyrexia during labor, delivered **136**, **140**, **146**
659.20	Unspecified maternal pyrexia during labor, unspecified as to episode of care **136**, **143**, **149**
659.23	Unspecified maternal pyrexia, antepartum **155**, **158**
055.8	Unspecified measles complication **164**, **168**, **184**
322.9	Unspecified meningitis **165**, **169**
036.9	Unspecified meningococcal infection **186**
018.9*	Unspecified miliary tuberculosis **185**
206.9*	Unspecified monocytic leukemia **181**
344.5	Unspecified monoplegia **32**
651.93	Unspecified multiple gestation, antepartum **154**, **157**
651.91	Unspecified multiple gestation, delivered **135**, **142**, **148**
651.90	Unspecified multiple gestation, unspecified as to episode of care **160**
072.8	Unspecified mumps complication **164**, **168**, **184**
723.9	Unspecified musculoskeletal disorders and symptoms referable to neck **97**
729.1	Unspecified myalgia and myositis **98**
205.9*	Unspecified myeloid leukemia **181**
429.0	Unspecified myocarditis **69**
358.9	Unspecified myoneural disorders **21**
359.9	Unspecified myopathy **33**
729.2	Unspecified neuralgia, neuritis, and radiculitis **21**, **230**
094.9	Unspecified neurosyphilis **19**
049.9	Unspecified non-arthropod-borne viral disease of central nervous system **33**, **229**
283.10	Unspecified non-autoimmune hemolytic anemia **175**
457.9	Unspecified noninfectious disorder of lymphatic channels **176**
300.9	Unspecified nonpsychotic mental disorder **188**
310.9	Unspecified nonpsychotic mental disorder following organic brain damage **188**, **230**
379.50	Unspecified nystagmus **38**
665.93	Unspecified obstetrical trauma, antepartum **155**, **158**
665.92	Unspecified obstetrical trauma, delivered, with postpartum complication **137**, **144**, **150**
665.94	Unspecified obstetrical trauma, postpartum condition or complication **152**
665.90	Unspecified obstetrical trauma, unspecified as to episode of care **137**, **144**, **150**
665.91	Unspecified obstetrical trauma, with delivery **137**, **144**, **150**
660.93	Unspecified obstructed labor, antepartum **155**, **158**
660.90	Unspecified obstructed labor, unspecified as to episode of care **136**, **143**, **149**
660.91	Unspecified obstructed labor, with delivery **136**, **143**, **149**
824.9	Unspecified open fracture of ankle **222**
808.9	Unspecified open fracture of pelvis **221**
365.10	Unspecified open-angle glaucoma **39**
054.40	Unspecified ophthalmic complication herpes simplex **229**
377.10	Unspecified optic atrophy **38**
V42.9	Unspecified organ or tissue replaced by transplant **214**
073.9	Unspecified ornithosis **184**
V54.9	Unspecified orthopedic aftercare **99**
730.2*	Unspecified osteomyelitis **96**
730.26	Unspecified osteomyelitis, lower leg **90**
730.28	Unspecified osteomyelitis, other specified sites **87**
388.60	Unspecified otorrhea **47**
729.3*	Unspecified panniculitis **108**
377.00	Unspecified papilledema **33**, **165**, **169**
344.9	Unspecified paralysis **32**
051.9	Unspecified paravaccinia **184**
427.2	Unspecified paroxysmal tachycardia **68**
380.00	Unspecified perichondritis of pinna **46**
664.44	Unspecified perineal laceration, postpartum condition or complication **152**
664.40	Unspecified perineal laceration, unspecified as to episode of care in pregnancy **137**, **144**, **150**
664.41	Unspecified perineal laceration, with delivery **137**, **144**, **150**
443.9	Unspecified peripheral vascular disease **66**
567.9	Unspecified peritonitis **76**
294.9	Unspecified persistent mental disorders due to conditions classified elsewhere **230**
301.9	Unspecified personality disorder **188**
299.9*	Unspecified pervasive developmental disorder **189**
103.9	Unspecified pinta **185**
020.9	Unspecified plague **185**
511.9	Unspecified pleural effusion **52**, **165**, **170**
505	Unspecified pneumoconiosis **53**
658.93	Unspecified problem associated with amniotic cavity and membranes, antepartum **155**, **158**
658.91	Unspecified problem associated with amniotic cavity and membranes, delivered **136**, **143**, **149**
658.90	Unspecified problem associated with amniotic cavity and membranes, unspecified as to episode of care **161**
V26.9	Unspecified procreative management **214**
662.13	Unspecified prolonged labor, antepartum **155**, **158**
662.11	Unspecified prolonged labor, delivered **136**, **144**, **149**

*Code Range

© 2013 OptumInsight, Inc.

662.10	Unspecified prolonged labor, unspecified as to episode of care **136, 144, 149**	663.91	Unspecified umbilical cord complication during labor and delivery, delivered **137, 144, 150**
263.9	Unspecified protein-calorie malnutrition **164, 168**	663.90	Unspecified umbilical cord complication during labor and delivery, unspecified as to episode of care **137, 144, 150**
698.9	Unspecified pruritic disorder **108**	131.00	Unspecified urogenital trichomoniasis **124, 127, 130**
306.9	Unspecified psychophysiological malfunction **188**	099.9	Unspecified venereal disease **124, 127, 130**
298.9	Unspecified psychosis **189, 230**	459.81	Unspecified venous (peripheral) insufficiency **67**
V62.9	Unspecified psychosocial circumstance **214**	671.90	Unspecified venous complication of pregnancy and the puerperium, unspecified as to episode of care **161**
374.30	Unspecified ptosis of eyelid **38**	671.93	Unspecified venous complication, antepartum **156, 158**
114.5	Unspecified pulmonary coccidioidomycosis **51**	671.94	Unspecified venous complication, postpartum condition or complication **153**
360.00	Unspecified purulent endophthalmitis **38**		
V57.9	Unspecified rehabilitation procedure **213**	671.92	Unspecified venous complication, with delivery, with mention of postpartum complication **138, 145, 151**
646.20	Unspecified renal disease in pregnancy, unspecified as to episode of care **156, 159**	671.91	Unspecified venous complication, with delivery, with or **without** mention of antepartum condition **138, 145, 151**
646.21	Unspecified renal disease in pregnancy, with delivery **134, 141, 147**	386.9	Unspecified vertiginous syndromes and labyrinthine disorders **46**
646.22	Unspecified renal disease in pregnancy, with delivery, with current postpartum complication **134, 141, 147**	079.9*	Unspecified viral and chlamydial infections, in conditions classified elsewhere and of unspecified site **230**
646.24	Unspecified renal disease in pregnancy, without mention of hypertension, postpartum condition or complication **151**	070.6	Unspecified viral hepatitis with hepatic coma **164, 168**
586	Unspecified renal failure **118, 119**	070.9	Unspecified viral hepatitis without mention of hepatic coma **164, 168**
587	Unspecified renal sclerosis **120**	047.9	Unspecified viral meningitis **230**
506.9	Unspecified respiratory conditions due to fumes and vapors **53**	480.9	Unspecified viral pneumonia **230**
361.9	Unspecified retinal detachment **39**	790.8	Unspecified viremia **185**
362.9	Unspecified retinal disorder **39**	368.9	Unspecified visual disturbance **39**
398.90	Unspecified rheumatic heart disease **68**	368.40	Unspecified visual field defect **38**
056.8	Unspecified rubella complications **164, 168, 184**	264.9	Unspecified vitamin A deficiency **113**
056.00	Unspecified rubella neurological complication **21**	268.9	Unspecified vitamin D deficiency **113**
003.9	Unspecified salmonella infection **185, 229**	643.93	Unspecified vomiting of pregnancy, antepartum **154, 156**
120.9	Unspecified schistosomiasis **185**	643.91	Unspecified vomiting of pregnancy, delivered **134, 141, 147**
425.9	Unspecified secondary cardiomyopathy **230**	643.90	Unspecified vomiting of pregnancy, unspecified as to episode of care **156, 159**
785.50	Unspecified shock **57, 66, 166, 170**	765.20	Unspecified weeks of gestation **171, 172**
848.9	Unspecified site of sprain and strain **100**	102.9	Unspecified yaws **185**
780.57	Unspecified sleep apnea **3, 47**	652.03	Unstable lie of fetus, antepartum **154, 157**
780.50	Unspecified sleep disturbance **189**	652.01	Unstable lie of fetus, delivered **135, 142, 148**
046.9	Unspecified slow virus infection of central nervous system **229**	652.00	Unstable lie of fetus, unspecified as to episode of care **160**
368.10	Unspecified subjective visual disturbance **39**	653.53	Unusually large fetus causing disproportion, antepartum **154, 157**
388.2	Unspecified sudden hearing loss **47**		
464.51	Unspecified supraglottis, with obstruction **3, 46**	653.51	Unusually large fetus causing disproportion, delivered **135, 142, 148**
464.50	Unspecified supraglottis, without mention of obstruction **3, 46**		
625.9	Unspecified symptom associated with female genital organs **130**	653.50	Unusually large fetus causing disproportion, unspecified as to episode of care **160**
727.00	Unspecified synovitis and tenosynovitis **98**	506.2	Upper respiratory inflammation due to fumes and vapors **54**
093.20	Unspecified syphilitic endocarditis of valve **65**	478.8	Upper respiratory tract hypersensitivity reaction, site unspecified **3, 46**
785.0	Unspecified tachycardia **68, 166, 170**	867.3	Ureter injury with open wound into cavity **120**
287.5	Unspecified thrombocytopenia **230**	867.2	Ureter injury without mention of open wound into cavity **120**
130.9	Unspecified toxoplasmosis **186**	597.0	Urethral abscess **166, 170**
293.9	Unspecified transient mental disorder in conditions classified elsewhere **188**	599.3	Urethral caruncle **120**
664.94	Unspecified trauma to perineum and vulva, postpartum condition or complication **152**	788.7	Urethral discharge **119**
		599.2	Urethral diverticulum **120**
664.90	Unspecified trauma to perineum and vulva, unspecified as to episode of care in pregnancy **137, 144, 150**	599.4	Urethral false passage **120**
		599.1	Urethral fistula **120**
664.91	Unspecified trauma to perineum and vulva, with delivery **137, 144, 150**	598*	Urethral stricture **120**
121.9	Unspecified trematode infection **186**	597*	Urethritis, not sexually transmitted, and urethral syndrome **119**
131.9	Unspecified trichomoniasis **186**	274.11	Uric acid nephrolithiasis **119**
086.9	Unspecified trypanosomiasis **185**	997.5	Urinary complications **120, 167, 171**
021.9	Unspecified tularemia **185**	788.3*	Urinary incontinence **119**
745.60	Unspecified type congenital endocardial cushion defect **67**	599.6*	Urinary obstruction **120, 166, 170**
663.93	Unspecified umbilical cord complication during labor and delivery, antepartum **155, 158**	599.0	Urinary tract infection, site not specified **119, 166, 170**

619.0	Urinary-genital tract fistula, female **127**, **130**
708*	Urticaria **108**
218*	Uterine leiomyoma **127**, **130**
649.63	Uterine size date discrepancy, antepartum condition or complication **154**, **157**
649.62	Uterine size date discrepancy, delivered, with mention of postpartum complication **135**, **142**, **148**
649.61	Uterine size date discrepancy, delivered, with or without mention of antepartum condition **135**, **142**, **148**
649.64	Uterine size date discrepancy, postpartum condition or complication **152**
649.60	Uterine size date discrepancy, unspecified as to episode of care or not applicable **160**
867.5	Uterus injury with open wound into cavity **127**, **130**
867.4	Uterus injury without mention of open wound into cavity **127**, **130**
V64.0*	Vaccination not carried out **173**
625.1	Vaginismus **130**
616.1*	Vaginitis and vulvovaginitis **127**, **130**
736.03	Valgus deformity of wrist (acquired) **100**
052.1	Varicella (hemorrhagic) pneumonitis **51**, **164**, **168**
052.9	Varicella without mention of complication **164**, **168**, **184**
456.8	Varices of other sites **67**
671.00	Varicose veins of legs complicating pregnancy and the puerperium, unspecified as to episode of care **161**
671.03	Varicose veins of legs, antepartum **156**, **158**
671.04	Varicose veins of legs, postpartum condition or complication **153**
671.02	Varicose veins of legs, with delivery, with mention of postpartum complication **138**, **145**, **151**
671.01	Varicose veins of legs, with delivery, with or without mention of antepartum condition **138**, **145**, **151**
454.1	Varicose veins of lower extremities with inflammation **67**
454.0	Varicose veins of lower extremities with ulcer **67**
454.2	Varicose veins of lower extremities with ulcer and inflammation **67**
454.8	Varicose veins of the lower extremities with other complications **67**
671.10	Varicose veins of vulva and perineum complicating pregnancy and the puerperium, unspecified as to episode of care **161**
671.13	Varicose veins of vulva and perineum, antepartum **156**, **158**
671.14	Varicose veins of vulva and perineum, postpartum condition or complication **153**
671.12	Varicose veins of vulva and perineum, with delivery, with mention of postpartum complication **138**, **145**, **151**
671.11	Varicose veins of vulva and perineum, with delivery, with or without mention of antepartum condition **138**, **145**, **151**
736.04	Varus deformity of wrist (acquired) **100**
663.53	Vasa previa complicating labor and delivery, antepartum **155**, **158**
663.51	Vasa previa complicating labor and delivery, delivered **137**, **144**, **150**
663.50	Vasa previa complicating labor and delivery, unspecified as to episode of care **137**, **144**, **150**
997.71	Vascular complications of mesenteric artery **79**, **167**, **171**
997.79	Vascular complications of other vessels **67**, **167**, **171**
997.72	Vascular complications of renal artery **120**, **167**, **171**
607.82	Vascular disorders of penis **124**
557*	Vascular insufficiency of intestine **79**
663.63	Vascular lesions of cord complicating labor and delivery, antepartum **155**, **158**
663.61	Vascular lesions of cord complicating labor and delivery, delivered **137**, **144**, **150**
663.60	Vascular lesions of cord complicating labor and delivery, unspecified as to episode of care **137**, **144**, **150**
336.1	Vascular myelopathies **32**
066.2	Venezuelan equine fever **9**, **10**, **34**
453.6	Venous embolism and thrombosis of superficial vessels of lower extremity **67**
551.2*	Ventral hernia with gangrene **166**, **170**
552.2*	Ventral hernia with obstruction **78**, **166**, **170**
553.2*	Ventral hernia without mention of obstruction or gangrene **79**
427.4*	Ventricular fibrillation and flutter **68**, **165**, **169**
745.4	Ventricular septal defect **67**, **166**, **170**
386.2	Vertigo of central origin **46**
596.2	Vesical fistula, not elsewhere classified **166**, **170**
593.7*	Vesicoureteral reflux **120**
719.2*	Villonodular synovitis **98**
101	Vincent's angina **2**, **46**
079*	Viral and chlamydial infection in conditions classified elsewhere and of unspecified site **185**
064	Viral encephalitis transmitted by other and unspecified arthropods **9**, **10**, **34**
070*	Viral hepatitis **83**
070.2*	Viral hepatitis B with hepatic coma **164**, **168**
070.3*	Viral hepatitis B without mention of hepatic coma **164**, **168**
480*	Viral pneumonia **53**
078.1*	Viral warts **107**
054.71	Visceral herpes simplex **78**, **164**, **168**, **229**
085.0	Visceral leishmaniasis (kala-azar) **185**
379.53	Visual deprivation nystagmus **40**
368.13	Visual discomfort **39**
368.14	Visual distortions of shape and size **39**
799.53	Visuospatial deficit **33**
264*	Vitamin A deficiency **230**
264.0	Vitamin A deficiency with conjunctival xerosis **38**
264.1	Vitamin A deficiency with conjunctival xerosis and Bitot's spot **38**
264.3	Vitamin A deficiency with corneal ulceration and xerosis **39**
264.2	Vitamin A deficiency with corneal xerosis **38**
264.4	Vitamin A deficiency with keratomalacia **39**
264.5	Vitamin A deficiency with night blindness **39**
264.6	Vitamin A deficiency with xerophthalmic scars of cornea **39**
268*	Vitamin D deficiency **230**
709.01	Vitiligo **172**
360.04	Vitreous abscess **38**
784.4*	Voice and resonance disorders **47**
958.6	Volkmann's ischemic contracture **101**, **224**, **227**
276.5*	Volume depletion **230**
560.2	Volvulus **166**, **170**
564.3	Vomiting following gastrointestinal surgery **78**
569.87	Vomiting of fecal matter **79**
286.4	Von Willebrand's disease **176**
456.6	Vulval varices **127**, **130**
664.54	Vulvar and perineal hematoma, postpartum condition or complication **152**
664.50	Vulvar and perineal hematoma, unspecified as to episode of care in pregnancy **137**, **144**, **150**
664.51	Vulvar and perineal hematoma, with delivery **137**, **144**, **150**
625.71	Vulvar vestibulitis **130**
625.70	Vulvodynia, unspecified **130**
036.3	Waterhouse-Friderichsen syndrome, meningococcal **164**, **168**, **186**
446.4	Wegener's granulomatosis **97**

066.4*	West Nile fever **184**	
040.2	Whipple's disease **78**	
033*	Whooping cough **53**	
279.12	Wiskott-Aldrich syndrome **175**	
040.42	Wound botulism **185**	
736.05	Wrist drop (acquired) **21**	
374.51	Xanthelasma of eyelid **108**	
060*	Yellow fever **184**	
117.7	Zygomycosis (Phycomycosis or Mucormycosis) **164**, **168**	

Numeric Index to Diseases

001*	Cholera **75**
002*	Typhoid and paratyphoid fevers **185**
003.0	Salmonella gastroenteritis **75**
003.1	Salmonella septicemia **186, 229**
003.2*	Localized salmonella infections **229**
003.20	Unspecified localized salmonella infection **185**
003.21	Salmonella meningitis **8, 10, 33**
003.22	Salmonella pneumonia **51**
003.23	Salmonella arthritis **97**
003.24	Salmonella osteomyelitis **96**
003.29	Other localized salmonella infections **185**
003.8	Other specified salmonella infections **185, 229**
003.9	Unspecified salmonella infection **185, 229**
004*	Shigellosis **75**
005.0	Staphylococcal food poisoning **75**
005.1	Botulism food poisoning **185**
005.2	Food poisoning due to Clostridium perfringens (C. welchii) **75**
005.3	Food poisoning due to other Clostridia **75**
005.4	Food poisoning due to Vibrio parahaemolyticus **75**
005.8*	Other bacterial food poisoning **75**
005.9	Unspecified food poisoning **77**
006.0	Acute amebic dysentery without mention of abscess **75**
006.1	Chronic intestinal amebiasis without mention of abscess **75**
006.2	Amebic nondysenteric colitis **75**
006.3	Amebic liver abscess **83**
006.4	Amebic lung abscess **51**
006.5	Amebic brain abscess **8, 10, 33**
006.6	Amebic skin ulceration **107**
006.8	Amebic infection of other sites **185**
006.9	Unspecified amebiasis **185**
007.2	Coccidiosis **229**
007*	Other protozoal intestinal diseases **75**
008.00	Intestinal infection due to unspecified E. coli **75**
008.01	Intestinal infection due to enteropathogenic E. coli **75**
008.02	Intestinal infection due to enterotoxigenic E. coli **75**
008.03	Intestinal infection due to enteroinvasive E. coli **75**
008.04	Intestinal infection due to enterohemorrhagic E. coli **75**
008.09	Intestinal infection due to other intestinal E. coli infections **75**
008.1	Intestinal infection due to Arizona group of paracolon bacilli **75**
008.2	Intestinal infection due to aerobacter aerogenes **75**
008.3	Intestinal infections due to proteus (mirabilis) (morganii) **75**
008.41	Intestinal infections due to staphylococcus **75**
008.42	Intestinal infections due to pseudomonas **75**
008.43	Intestinal infections due to campylobacter **75**
008.44	Intestinal infections due to yersinia enterocolitica **75**
008.45	Intestinal infections due to clostridium difficile **75**
008.46	Intestinal infections due to other anaerobes **75**
008.47	Intestinal infections due to other gram-negative bacteria **75**
008.49	Intestinal infection due to other organisms **75**
008.5	Intestinal infection due to unspecified bacterial enteritis **75**
008.6*	Intestinal infection, enteritis due to specified virus **77**
008.8	Intestinal infection due to other organism, NEC **77**
009*	Ill-defined intestinal infections **77, 230**
010*	Primary tuberculous infection **51, 229**
011*	Pulmonary tuberculosis **51, 229**
012.0*	Tuberculous pleurisy **51**
012.1*	Tuberculosis of intrathoracic lymph nodes **51**
012.2*	Isolated tracheal or bronchial tuberculosis **51**
012.3*	Tuberculous laryngitis **2, 47**
012.8*	Other specified respiratory tuberculosis **51**
012*	Other respiratory tuberculosis **229**
013*	Tuberculosis of meninges and central nervous system **8, 10, 33, 229**
014*	Tuberculosis of intestines, peritoneum, and mesenteric glands **75, 229**
015.0*	Tuberculosis of vertebral column **96**
015.02	Tuberculosis of vertebral column, bacteriological or histological examination unknown (at present) **87**
015.04	Tuberculosis of vertebral column, tubercle bacilli not found (in sputum) by microscopy, but found by bacterial culture **87**
015.05	Tuberculosis of vertebral column, tubercle bacilli not found by bacteriological examination, but tuberculosis confirmed histologically **87**
015.1*	Tuberculosis of hip **97**
015.2*	Tuberculosis of knee **97**
015.5*	Tuberculosis of limb bones **96**
015.6*	Tuberculosis of mastoid **47**
015.7*	Tuberculosis of other specified bone **96**
015.8*	Tuberculosis of other specified joint **97**
015.9*	Tuberculosis of unspecified bones and joints **97**
015*	Tuberculosis of bones and joints **229**
016.0*	Tuberculosis of kidney **119**
016.1*	Tuberculosis of bladder **119**
016.2*	Tuberculosis of ureter **119**
016.3*	Tuberculosis of other urinary organs **119**
016.4*	Tuberculosis of epididymis **123**
016.5*	Tuberculosis of other male genital organs **123**
016.6*	Tuberculous oophoritis and salpingitis **127, 129**
016.7*	Tuberculosis of other female genital organs **127, 129**
016.9*	Genitourinary tuberculosis, unspecified **119**
016*	Tuberculosis of genitourinary system **229**
017.0*	Tuberculosis of skin and subcutaneous cellular tissue **107**
017.1*	Erythema nodosum with hypersensitivity reaction in tuberculosis **105**
017.2*	Tuberculosis of peripheral lymph nodes **176**
017.3*	Tuberculosis of spleen **176**
017.3*	Tuberculosis of eye **38**
017.4*	Tuberculosis of ear **47**
017.5*	Tuberculosis of thyroid gland **114**
017.6*	Tuberculosis of adrenal glands **114**
017.7*	Tuberculosis of spleen **176**
017.8*	Tuberculosis of esophagus **75**
017.9*	Tuberculosis of other specified organs **185**
017*	Tuberculosis of other organs **229**
018.0*	Acute miliary tuberculosis **185**
018.8*	Other specified miliary tuberculosis **185**
018.9*	Unspecified miliary tuberculosis **185**
018*	Miliary tuberculosis **229**
020.0	Bubonic plague **185**
020.1	Cellulocutaneous plague **185**
020.2	Septicemic plague **186**

020.3	Primary pneumonic plague **51**	
020.4	Secondary pneumonic plague **51**	
020.5	Pneumonic plague, unspecified **51**	
020.8	Other specified types of plague **185**	
020.9	Unspecified plague **185**	
021.0	Ulceroglandular tularemia **185**	
021.1	Enteric tularemia **75**	
021.2	Pulmonary tularemia **51**	
021.3	Oculoglandular tularemia **185**	
021.8	Other specified tularemia **185**	
021.9	Unspecified tularemia **185**	
022.0	Cutaneous anthrax **107**	
022.1	Pulmonary anthrax **51**	
022.2	Gastrointestinal anthrax **75**	
022.3	Anthrax septicemia **186**	
022.8	Other specified manifestations of anthrax **185**	
022.9	Unspecified anthrax **185**	
023*	Brucellosis **185**	
024	Glanders **185**	
025	Melioidosis **185**	
026*	Rat-bite fever **185**	
027*	Other zoonotic bacterial diseases **185**	
030*	Leprosy **185**	
031.0	Pulmonary diseases due to other mycobacteria **51**	
031.1	Cutaneous diseases due to other mycobacteria **107**	
031.2	Disseminated diseases due to other mycobacteria **185, 229**	
031.8	Other specified diseases due to other mycobacteria **185, 229**	
031.9	Unspecified diseases due to mycobacteria **185, 229**	
032.0	Faucial diphtheria **2, 47**	
032.1	Nasopharyngeal diphtheria **2, 47**	
032.2	Anterior nasal diphtheria **2, 47**	
032.3	Laryngeal diphtheria **2, 47**	
032.81	Conjunctival diphtheria **38**	
032.82	Diphtheritic myocarditis **68**	
032.83	Diphtheritic peritonitis **75**	
032.84	Diphtheritic cystitis **119**	
032.85	Cutaneous diphtheria **107**	
032.89	Other specified diphtheria **185**	
032.9	Unspecified diphtheria **185**	
033*	Whooping cough **53**	
034.0	Streptococcal sore throat **2, 46**	
034.1	Scarlet fever **185**	
035	Erysipelas **106**	
036.0	Meningococcal meningitis **8, 10, 33**	
036.1	Meningococcal encephalitis **8, 10, 33**	
036.2	Meningococcemia **186**	
036.3	Waterhouse-Friderichsen syndrome, meningococcal **164, 168, 186**	
036.4*	Meningococcal carditis **164, 168**	
036.40	Meningococcal carditis, unspecified **68**	
036.41	Meningococcal pericarditis **68**	
036.42	Meningococcal endocarditis **65**	
036.43	Meningococcal myocarditis **68**	
036.81	Meningococcal optic neuritis **38, 164, 168**	
036.82	Meningococcal arthropathy **97, 164, 168**	
036.89	Other specified meningococcal infections **186**	
036.9	Unspecified meningococcal infection **186**	
037	Tetanus **164, 168, 185**	
038*	Septicemia **164, 168, 186, 229**	

039.0	Cutaneous actinomycotic infection **107**
039.1	Pulmonary actinomycotic infection **51**
039.2	Abdominal actinomycotic infection **75**
039.3	Cervicofacial actinomycotic infection **107**
039.4	Madura foot **107**
039.8	Actinomycotic infection of other specified sites **185**
039.9	Actinomycotic infection of unspecified site **185**
039*	Actinomycotic infections **229**
040.0	Gas gangrene **164, 168, 185**
040.1	Rhinoscleroma **185**
040.2	Whipple's disease **78**
040.3	Necrobacillosis **185**
040.41	Infant botulism **164, 168, 185**
040.42	Wound botulism **185**
040.81	Tropical pyomyositis **98**
040.82	Toxic shock syndrome **185**
040.89	Other specified bacterial diseases **185**
041*	Bacterial infection in conditions classified elsewhere and of unspecified site **185**
042	Human immunodeficiency virus [HIV] **229, 230**
045.0*	Acute paralytic poliomyelitis specified as bulbar **8, 10, 33**
045.1*	Acute poliomyelitis with other paralysis **8, 10, 33**
045.2*	Acute nonparalytic poliomyelitis **184**
045.9*	Acute unspecified poliomyelitis **8, 10, 33**
046.2	Subacute sclerosing panencephalitis **164, 168**
046.3	Progressive multifocal leukoencephalopathy **229**
046.7*	Other specified prion diseases of central nervous system **229**
046.8	Other specified slow virus infection of central nervous system **229**
046.9	Unspecified slow virus infection of central nervous system **229**
046*	Slow virus infections and prion diseases of central nervous system **19**
047.9	Unspecified viral meningitis **230**
047*	Meningitis due to enterovirus **21**
048	Other enterovirus diseases of central nervous system **21**
049.0	Lymphocytic choriomeningitis **21**
049.1	Meningitis due to adenovirus **21**
049.8	Other specified non-arthropod-borne viral diseases of central nervous system **33, 229**
049.9	Unspecified non-arthropod-borne viral disease of central nervous system **33, 229**
050*	Smallpox **184**
051.0*	Cowpox and vaccinia not from vaccination **184**
051.1	Pseudocowpox **107**
051.2	Contagious pustular dermatitis **107**
051.9	Unspecified paravaccinia **184**
052.0	Postvaricella encephalitis **33, 164, 168**
052.1	Varicella (hemorrhagic) pneumonitis **51, 164, 168**
052.2	Postvaricella myelitis **8, 10, 33**
052.7	Chickenpox with other specified complications **164, 168, 184**
052.8	Chickenpox with unspecified complication **164, 168, 184**
052.9	Varicella without mention of complication **164, 168, 184**
053.0	Herpes zoster with meningitis **21, 164, 168, 229**
053.10	Herpes zoster with unspecified nervous system complication **21, 164, 168, 229**
053.11	Geniculate herpes zoster **21, 164, 168, 229**
053.12	Postherpetic trigeminal neuralgia **21, 164, 168, 229**
053.13	Postherpetic polyneuropathy **21, 164, 168, 229**
053.14	Herpes zoster myelitis **8, 10, 33**
053.19	Other herpes zoster with nervous system complications **21, 164, 168, 229**

*Code Range

© 2013 OptumInsight, Inc.

053.2*	Herpes zoster with ophthalmic complications **38**	
053.20	Herpes zoster dermatitis of eyelid **164, 168, 229**	
053.21	Herpes zoster keratoconjunctivitis **164, 168, 229**	
053.22	Herpes zoster iridocyclitis **164, 168, 229**	
053.29	Other ophthalmic herpes zoster complications **164, 168, 229**	
053.71	Otitis externa due to herpes zoster **47, 164, 168, 229**	
053.79	Other specified herpes zoster complications **164, 168, 184, 229**	
053.8	Unspecified herpes zoster complication **164, 168, 184, 229**	
053.9	Herpes zoster without mention of complication **105, 164, 168, 229**	
054.0	Eczema herpeticum **107, 164, 168, 229**	
054.10	Unspecified genital herpes **123, 127, 129, 229**	
054.11	Herpetic vulvovaginitis **127, 129, 229**	
054.12	Herpetic ulceration of vulva **127, 129, 229**	
054.13	Herpetic infection of penis **124, 229**	
054.19	Other genital herpes **124, 127, 129, 229**	
054.2	Herpetic gingivostomatitis **2, 48, 164, 168, 229**	
054.3	Herpetic meningoencephalitis **8, 10, 33, 164, 168, 229**	
054.4*	Herpes simplex with ophthalmic complications **38, 164, 168**	
054.40	Unspecified ophthalmic complication herpes simplex **229**	
054.41	Herpes simplex dermatitis of eyelid **229**	
054.42	Dendritic keratitis **229**	
054.43	Herpes simplex disciform keratitis **229**	
054.44	Herpes simplex iridocyclitis **229**	
054.49	Herpes simplex with other ophthalmic complications **229**	
054.5	Herpetic septicemia **164, 168, 186, 229**	
054.6	Herpetic whitlow **107, 229**	
054.71	Visceral herpes simplex **78, 164, 168, 229**	
054.72	Herpes simplex meningitis **8, 10, 21, 164, 168, 229**	
054.73	Herpes simplex otitis externa **47, 164, 168, 229**	
054.74	Herpes simplex myelitis **8, 10, 33**	
054.79	Other specified herpes simplex complications **164, 168, 184, 229**	
054.8	Unspecified herpes simplex complication **164, 168, 184, 229**	
054.9	Herpes simplex without mention of complication **107, 229**	
055.0	Postmeasles encephalitis **9, 10, 33, 164, 168**	
055.1	Postmeasles pneumonia **51, 164, 168**	
055.2	Postmeasles otitis media **46, 164, 168**	
055.7*	Measles, with other specified complications **164, 168**	
055.71	Measles keratoconjunctivitis **38**	
055.79	Other specified measles complications **184**	
055.8	Unspecified measles complication **164, 168, 184**	
055.9	Measles without mention of complication **184**	
056.0*	Rubella with neurological complications **164, 168**	
056.00	Unspecified rubella neurological complication **21**	
056.01	Encephalomyelitis due to rubella **33**	
056.09	Other neurological rubella complications **33**	
056.7*	Rubella with other specified complications **164, 168**	
056.71	Arthritis due to rubella **98**	
056.79	Rubella with other specified complications **184**	
056.8	Unspecified rubella complications **164, 168, 184**	
056.9	Rubella without mention of complication **184**	
057*	Other viral exanthemata **184**	
058.10	Roseola infantum, unspecified **164, 168, 184**	
058.11	Roseola infantum due to human herpesvirus 6 **164, 168, 184**	
058.12	Roseola infantum due to human herpesvirus 7 **164, 168, 184**	
058.21	Human herpesvirus 6 encephalitis **9, 10, 33, 164, 168, 229**	
058.29	Other human herpesvirus encephalitis **9, 10, 33, 164, 168, 229**	
058.8*	Other human herpesvirus infections **107**	

059*	Other poxvirus infections **184**	
060*	Yellow fever **184**	
061	Dengue **184**	
062*	Mosquito-borne viral encephalitis **9, 10, 33**	
063*	Tick-borne viral encephalitis **9, 10, 33**	
064	Viral encephalitis transmitted by other and unspecified arthropods **9, 10, 34**	
065*	Arthropod-borne hemorrhagic fever **184**	
066.0	Phlebotomus fever **184**	
066.1	Tick-borne fever **184**	
066.2	Venezuelan equine fever **9, 10, 34**	
066.3	Other mosquito-borne fever **184**	
066.4*	West Nile fever **184**	
066.8	Other specified arthropod-borne viral diseases **184**	
066.9	Unspecified arthropod-borne viral disease **184**	
070.2*	Viral hepatitis B with hepatic coma **164, 168**	
070.3*	Viral hepatitis B without mention of hepatic coma **164, 168**	
070.4*	Other specified viral hepatitis with hepatic coma **164, 168**	
070.5*	Other specified viral hepatitis without mention of hepatic coma **164, 168**	
070.6	Unspecified viral hepatitis with hepatic coma **164, 168**	
070.9	Unspecified viral hepatitis without mention of hepatic coma **164, 168**	
070*	Viral hepatitis **83**	
071	Rabies **9, 10, 34**	
072.0	Mumps orchitis **124, 164, 168**	
072.1	Mumps meningitis **9, 10, 21, 164, 168**	
072.2	Mumps encephalitis **9, 10, 34, 164, 168**	
072.3	Mumps pancreatitis **83, 164, 168**	
072.7*	Mumps with other specified complications **164, 168**	
072.71	Mumps hepatitis **83**	
072.72	Mumps polyneuropathy **21**	
072.79	Mumps with other specified complications **184**	
072.8	Unspecified mumps complication **164, 168, 184**	
072.9	Mumps without mention of complication **184**	
073.0	Ornithosis with pneumonia **51**	
073.7	Ornithosis with other specified complications **184**	
073.8	Ornithosis with unspecified complication **184**	
073.9	Unspecified ornithosis **184**	
074.0	Herpangina **2, 46**	
074.1	Epidemic pleurodynia **53**	
074.20	Coxsackie carditis, unspecified **68**	
074.21	Coxsackie pericarditis **68**	
074.22	Coxsackie endocarditis **67**	
074.23	Coxsackie myocarditis **68**	
074.3	Hand, foot, and mouth disease **184**	
074.8	Other specified diseases due to Coxsackievirus **184**	
075	Infectious mononucleosis **184**	
076*	Trachoma **38**	
077*	Other diseases of conjunctiva due to viruses and Chlamydiae **38**	
078.0	Molluscum contagiosum **107**	
078.1*	Viral warts **107**	
078.2	Sweating fever **185**	
078.3	Cat-scratch disease **176**	
078.4	Foot and mouth disease **185**	
078.5	Cytomegaloviral disease **185, 230**	
078.6	Hemorrhagic nephrosonephritis **119**	
078.7	Arenaviral hemorrhagic fever **185**	
078.81	Epidemic vertigo **32**	

078.82	Epidemic vomiting syndrome **77**	
078.88	Other specified diseases due to Chlamydiae **185**	
078.89	Other specified diseases due to viruses **185**	
079.6	Respiratory syncytial virus (RSV) **164**, **168**	
079.9*	Unspecified viral and chlamydial infections, in conditions classified elsewhere and of unspecified site **230**	
079*	Viral and chlamydial infection in conditions classified elsewhere and of unspecified site **185**	
080	Louse-borne (epidemic) typhus **185**	
081*	Other typhus **185**	
082*	Tick-borne rickettsioses **185**	
083*	Other rickettsioses **185**	
084*	Malaria **185**	
085.0	Visceral leishmaniasis (kala-azar) **185**	
085.1	Cutaneous leishmaniasis, urban **107**	
085.2	Cutaneous leishmaniasis, Asian desert **107**	
085.3	Cutaneous leishmaniasis, Ethiopian **107**	
085.4	Cutaneous leishmaniasis, American **107**	
085.5	Mucocutaneous leishmaniasis, (American) **107**	
085.9	Unspecified leishmaniasis **185**	
086.0	Chagas' disease with heart involvement **68**	
086.1	Chagas' disease with other organ involvement **185**	
086.2	Chagas' disease without mention of organ involvement **185**	
086.3	Gambian trypanosomiasis **185**	
086.4	Rhodesian trypanosomiasis **185**	
086.5	African trypanosomiasis, unspecified **185**	
086.9	Unspecified trypanosomiasis **185**	
087*	Relapsing fever **185**	
088*	Other arthropod-borne diseases **185**	
090.0	Early congenital syphilis, symptomatic **185**	
090.1	Early congenital syphilis, latent **185**	
090.2	Unspecified early congenital syphilis **185**	
090.3	Syphilitic interstitial keratitis **38**	
090.4*	Juvenile neurosyphilis **34**	
090.5	Other late congenital syphilis, symptomatic **185**	
090.6	Late congenital syphilis, latent **185**	
090.7	Late congenital syphilis, unspecified **185**	
090.9	Congenital syphilis, unspecified **185**	
091.0	Genital syphilis (primary) **124**, **127**, **129**	
091.1	Primary anal syphilis **78**	
091.2	Other primary syphilis **185**	
091.3	Secondary syphilis of skin or mucous membranes **107**	
091.4	Adenopathy due to secondary syphilis **176**	
091.5*	Early syphilis, uveitis due to secondary syphilis **38**	
091.61	Early syphilis, secondary syphilitic periostitis **96**	
091.62	Early syphilis, secondary syphilitic hepatitis **83**	
091.69	Early syphilis, secondary syphilis of other viscera **78**	
091.7	Early syphilis, secondary syphilis, relapse **185**	
091.81	Early syphilis, acute syphilitic meningitis (secondary) **9**, **10**, **34**	
091.82	Early syphilis, syphilitic alopecia **107**	
091.89	Early syphilis, other forms of secondary syphilis **185**	
091.9	Early syphilis, unspecified secondary syphilis **185**	
092*	Early syphilis, latent **185**	
093.0	Aneurysm of aorta, specified as syphilitic **67**	
093.1	Syphilitic aortitis **67**	
093.20	Unspecified syphilitic endocarditis of valve **65**	
093.21	Syphilitic endocarditis, mitral valve **67**	
093.22	Syphilitic endocarditis, aortic valve **67**	
093.23	Syphilitic endocarditis, tricuspid valve **67**	

093.24	Syphilitic endocarditis, pulmonary valve **67**
093.8*	Other specified cardiovascular syphilis **68**
093.9	Unspecified cardiovascular syphilis **68**
094.0	Tabes dorsalis **19**
094.1	General paresis **19**
094.2	Syphilitic meningitis **9**, **10**, **34**
094.3	Asymptomatic neurosyphilis **34**
094.81	Syphilitic encephalitis **9**, **10**, **34**
094.82	Syphilitic Parkinsonism **19**
094.83	Syphilitic disseminated retinochoroiditis **38**
094.84	Syphilitic optic atrophy **38**
094.85	Syphilitic retrobulbar neuritis **19**
094.86	Syphilitic acoustic neuritis **47**
094.87	Syphilitic ruptured cerebral aneurysm **8**, **32**
094.89	Other specified neurosyphilis **19**
094.9	Unspecified neurosyphilis **19**
095.0	Syphilitic episcleritis **38**
095.1	Syphilis of lung **51**
095.2	Syphilitic peritonitis **75**
095.3	Syphilis of liver **83**
095.4	Syphilis of kidney **119**
095.5	Syphilis of bone **96**
095.6	Syphilis of muscle **98**
095.7	Syphilis of synovium, tendon, and bursa **98**
095.8	Other specified forms of late symptomatic syphilis **185**
095.9	Unspecified late symptomatic syphilis **185**
096	Late syphilis, latent **185**
097*	Other and unspecified syphilis **185**
098.0	Gonococcal infection (acute) of lower genitourinary tract **124**, **127**, **129**
098.10	Gonococcal infection (acute) of upper genitourinary tract, site unspecified **124**, **127**, **129**
098.11	Gonococcal cystitis (acute) **119**
098.12	Gonococcal prostatitis (acute) **124**
098.13	Gonococcal epididymo-orchitis (acute) **124**
098.14	Gonococcal seminal vesiculitis (acute) **124**
098.15	Gonococcal cervicitis (acute) **127**, **129**
098.16	Gonococcal endometritis (acute) **127**, **129**
098.17	Gonococcal salpingitis, specified as acute **127**, **129**
098.19	Other gonococcal infections (acute) of upper genitourinary tract **124**, **127**, **129**
098.2	Gonococcal infections, chronic, of lower genitourinary tract **124**, **127**, **129**
098.30	Chronic gonococcal infection of upper genitourinary tract, site unspecified **119**
098.31	Gonococcal cystitis, chronic **119**
098.32	Gonococcal prostatitis, chronic **124**
098.33	Gonococcal epididymo-orchitis, chronic **124**
098.34	Gonococcal seminal vesiculitis, chronic **124**
098.35	Gonococcal cervicitis, chronic **127**, **129**
098.36	Gonococcal endometritis, chronic **127**, **129**
098.37	Gonococcal salpingitis (chronic) **127**, **129**
098.39	Other chronic gonococcal infections of upper genitourinary tract **124**, **127**, **129**
098.4*	Gonococcal infection of eye **38**
098.50	Gonococcal arthritis **97**
098.51	Gonococcal synovitis and tenosynovitis **97**
098.52	Gonococcal bursitis **97**
098.53	Gonococcal spondylitis **96**
098.59	Other gonococcal infection of joint **97**

*Code Range

098.6	Gonococcal infection of pharynx **2, 46**
098.7	Gonococcal infection of anus and rectum **78**
098.81	Gonococcal keratosis (blennorrhagica) **38**
098.82	Gonococcal meningitis **9, 10, 33**
098.83	Gonococcal pericarditis **68**
098.84	Gonococcal endocarditis **65**
098.85	Other gonococcal heart disease **68**
098.86	Gonococcal peritonitis **75**
098.89	Gonococcal infection of other specified sites **185**
099.0	Chancroid **124, 127, 130**
099.1	Lymphogranuloma venereum **124, 127, 130**
099.2	Granuloma inguinale **124, 127, 130**
099.3	Reiter's disease **97**
099.4*	Other nongonococcal urethritis (NGU) **124, 127, 130**
099.50	Chlamydia trachomatis infection of unspecified site **124, 127, 130**
099.51	Chlamydia trachomatis infection of pharynx **2, 46**
099.52	Chlamydia trachomatis infection of anus and rectum **78**
099.53	Chlamydia trachomatis infection of lower genitourinary sites **124, 127, 130**
099.54	Chlamydia trachomatis infection of other genitourinary sites **119**
099.55	Chlamydia trachomatis infection of unspecified genitourinary site **124, 127, 130**
099.56	Chlamydia trachomatis infection of peritoneum **78**
099.59	Chlamydia trachomatis infection of other specified site **124, 127, 130**
099.8	Other specified venereal diseases **124, 127, 130**
099.9	Unspecified venereal disease **124, 127, 130**
100.0	Leptospirosis icterohemorrhagica **185**
100.8*	Other specified leptospiral infections **9, 10, 34**
100.9	Unspecified leptospirosis **185**
101	Vincent's angina **2, 46**
102.0	Initial lesions of yaws **107**
102.1	Multiple papillomata and wet crab yaws due to yaws **107**
102.2	Other early skin lesions due to yaws **107**
102.3	Hyperkeratosis due to yaws **107**
102.4	Gummata and ulcers due to yaws **107**
102.5	Gangosa due to yaws **2, 47**
102.6	Bone and joint lesions due to yaws **97**
102.7	Other manifestations due to yaws **185**
102.8	Latent yaws **185**
102.9	Unspecified yaws **185**
103.0	Primary lesions of pinta **107**
103.1	Intermediate lesions of pinta **107**
103.2	Late lesions of pinta **185**
103.3	Mixed lesions of pinta **107**
103.9	Unspecified pinta **185**
104*	Other spirochetal infection **185**
110*	Dermatophytosis **107, 230**
111*	Dermatomycosis, other and unspecified **107, 230**
112.0	Candidiasis of mouth **2, 48, 230**
112.1	Candidiasis of vulva and vagina **127, 130**
112.2	Candidiasis of other urogenital sites **124, 127, 130**
112.3	Candidiasis of skin and nails **107, 230**
112.4	Candidiasis of lung **51, 164, 168, 230**
112.5	Disseminated candidiasis **164, 168, 185, 230**
112.8*	Candidiasis of other specified sites **230**
112.81	Candidal endocarditis **65, 164, 168**
112.82	Candidal otitis externa **47, 164, 168**
112.83	Candidal meningitis **9, 10, 34, 164, 168**

112.84	Candidiasis of the esophagus **75, 164, 168**
112.85	Candidiasis of the intestine **77, 164, 168**
112.89	Other candidiasis of other specified sites **185**
112.9	Candidiasis of unspecified site **185, 230**
114.0	Primary coccidioidomycosis (pulmonary) **51**
114.1	Primary extrapulmonary coccidioidomycosis **107**
114.2	Coccidioidal meningitis **9, 10, 34, 164, 168**
114.3	Other forms of progressive coccidioidomycosis **164, 168, 185**
114.4	Chronic pulmonary coccidioidomycosis **51**
114.5	Unspecified pulmonary coccidioidomycosis **51**
114.9	Unspecified coccidioidomycosis **185**
114*	Coccidioidomycosis **230**
115.00	Histoplasma capsulatum, without mention of manifestation **185**
115.01	Histoplasma capsulatum meningitis **9, 10, 34, 164, 168**
115.02	Histoplasma capsulatum retinitis **38, 164, 168**
115.03	Histoplasma capsulatum pericarditis **68, 164, 168**
115.04	Histoplasma capsulatum endocarditis **65, 164, 168**
115.05	Histoplasma capsulatum pneumonia **51, 164, 168**
115.09	Histoplasma capsulatum, with mention of other manifestation **185**
115.10	Histoplasma duboisii, without mention of manifestation **185**
115.11	Histoplasma duboisii meningitis **9, 10, 34, 164, 168**
115.12	Histoplasma duboisii retinitis **38, 164, 168**
115.13	Histoplasma duboisii pericarditis **68, 164, 168**
115.14	Histoplasma duboisii endocarditis **65, 164, 168**
115.15	Histoplasma duboisii pneumonia **51, 164, 168**
115.19	Histoplasma duboisii with mention of other manifestation **185**
115.90	Unspecified Histoplasmosis without mention of manifestation **185**
115.91	Unspecified Histoplasmosis meningitis **9, 10, 34, 164, 168**
115.92	Unspecified Histoplasmosis retinitis **38, 164, 168**
115.93	Unspecified Histoplasmosis pericarditis **68, 164, 168**
115.94	Unspecified Histoplasmosis endocarditis **65, 164, 168**
115.95	Unspecified Histoplasmosis pneumonia **51, 164, 168**
115.99	Unspecified Histoplasmosis with mention of other manifestation **185**
115*	Histoplasmosis **230**
116.0	Blastomycosis **164, 168**
116.1	Paracoccidioidomycosis **164, 168**
116*	Blastomycotic infection **185**
117.3	Aspergillosis **164, 168**
117.4	Mycotic mycetomas **164, 168**
117.5	Cryptococcosis **164, 168, 230**
117.6	Allescheriosis (Petriellidiosis) **164, 168**
117.7	Zygomycosis (Phycomycosis or Mucormycosis) **164, 168**
117*	Other mycoses **185**
118	Opportunistic mycoses **164, 168, 185, 230**
120.0	Schistosomiasis due to schistosoma haematobium **119**
120.1	Schistosomiasis due to schistosoma mansoni **83**
120.2	Schistosomiasis due to schistosoma japonicum **185**
120.3	Cutaneous schistosomiasis **107**
120.8	Other specified schistosomiasis **185**
120.9	Unspecified schistosomiasis **185**
121.0	Opisthorchiasis **83**
121.1	Clonorchiasis **83**
121.2	Paragonimiasis **51**
121.3	Fascioliasis **83**
121.4	Fasciolopsiasis **83**
121.5	Metagonimiasis **185**

*Code Range

*Code Range

© 2013 OptumInsight, Inc.

165.0	Malignant neoplasm of upper respiratory tract, part unspecified **2, 46**	186*	Malignant neoplasm of testis **122, 123**
165.8	Malignant neoplasm of other sites within the respiratory system and intrathoracic organs **52**	187*	Malignant neoplasm of penis and other male genital organs **122, 123**
165.9	Malignant neoplasm of ill-defined sites within the respiratory system **52**	188*	Malignant neoplasm of bladder **116, 119**
170.1	Malignant neoplasm of mandible **2**	189*	Malignant neoplasm of kidney and other and unspecified urinary organs **116, 119**
170.2	Malignant neoplasm of vertebral column, excluding sacrum and coccyx **87**	190*	Malignant neoplasm of eye **38**
170*	Malignant neoplasm of bone and articular cartilage **97**	191*	Malignant neoplasm of brain **19**
171*	Malignant neoplasm of connective and other soft tissue **97**	192*	Malignant neoplasm of other and unspecified parts of nervous system **19**
172.0	Malignant melanoma of skin of lip **105**	193	Malignant neoplasm of thyroid gland **2, 114**
172.1	Malignant melanoma of skin of eyelid, including canthus **38**	194.0	Malignant neoplasm of adrenal gland **114**
172.2	Malignant melanoma of skin of ear and external auditory canal **105**	194.1	Malignant neoplasm of parathyroid gland **114**
172.3	Malignant melanoma of skin of other and unspecified parts of face **105**	194.3	Malignant neoplasm of pituitary gland and craniopharyngeal duct **114**
172.4	Malignant melanoma of skin of scalp and neck **105**	194.4	Malignant neoplasm of pineal gland **19**
172.5	Malignant melanoma of skin of trunk, except scrotum **105**	194.5	Malignant neoplasm of carotid body **19**
172.6	Malignant melanoma of skin of upper limb, including shoulder **105**	194.6	Malignant neoplasm of aortic body and other paraganglia **19**
172.7	Malignant melanoma of skin of lower limb, including hip **105**	194.8	Malignant neoplasm of other endocrine glands and related structures **114**
172.8	Malignant melanoma of other specified sites of skin **105**	194.9	Malignant neoplasm of endocrine gland, site unspecified **114**
172.9	Melanoma of skin, site unspecified **105**	195.0	Malignant neoplasm of head, face, and neck **2, 46**
173.0*	Other and unspecified malignant neoplasm of skin of lip **2, 108**	195.1	Malignant neoplasm of thorax **52**
173.1*	Other and unspecified malignant neoplasm of eyelid, including canthus **38**	195.2	Malignant neoplasm of abdomen **76**
173.2*	Other and unspecified malignant neoplasm of skin of ear and external auditory canal **108**	195.3	Malignant neoplasm of pelvis **122, 123, 126, 129**
173.3*	Other and unspecified malignant neoplasm of skin of other and unspecified parts of face **108**	195.4	Malignant neoplasm of upper limb **180, 181**
173.4*	Other and unspecified malignant neoplasm of scalp and skin of neck **108**	195.5	Malignant neoplasm of lower limb **180, 181**
173.5*	Other and unspecified malignant neoplasm of skin of trunk, except scrotum **108**	195.8	Malignant neoplasm of other specified sites **180, 181**
173.6*	Other and unspecified malignant neoplasm of skin of upper limb, including shoulder **108**	196.0	Secondary and unspecified malignant neoplasm of lymph nodes of head, face, and neck **2**
173.7*	Other and unspecified malignant neoplasm of skin of lower limb, including hip **108**	196*	Secondary and unspecified malignant neoplasm of lymph nodes **178, 181**
173.8*	Other and unspecified malignant neoplasm of other specified sites of skin **108**	197.0	Secondary malignant neoplasm of lung **52**
173.9*	Other and unspecified malignant neoplasm of skin, site unspecified **108**	197.1	Secondary malignant neoplasm of mediastinum **52**
		197.2	Secondary malignant neoplasm of pleura **52**
174*	Malignant neoplasm of female breast **104, 105**	197.3	Secondary malignant neoplasm of other respiratory organs **52**
175*	Malignant neoplasm of male breast **104, 105**	197.4	Secondary malignant neoplasm of small intestine including duodenum **76**
176.0	Kaposi's sarcoma of skin **108**	197.5	Secondary malignant neoplasm of large intestine and rectum **76**
176.1	Kaposi's sarcoma of soft tissue **108**	197.6	Secondary malignant neoplasm of retroperitoneum and peritoneum **76**
176.2	Kaposi's sarcoma of palate **2, 46**	197.7	Secondary malignant neoplasm of liver **82**
176.3	Kaposi's sarcoma of gastrointestinal sites **76**	197.8	Secondary malignant neoplasm of other digestive organs and spleen **76**
176.4	Kaposi's sarcoma of lung **52**	198.0	Secondary malignant neoplasm of kidney **116, 119**
176.5	Kaposi's sarcoma of lymph nodes **178, 181**	198.1	Secondary malignant neoplasm of other urinary organs **116, 119**
176.8	Kaposi's sarcoma of other specified sites **108**	198.2	Secondary malignant neoplasm of skin **104, 105**
176.9	Kaposi's sarcoma of unspecified site **108**	198.3	Secondary malignant neoplasm of brain and spinal cord **19**
176*	Kaposi's sarcoma **230**	198.4	Secondary malignant neoplasm of other parts of nervous system **19**
179	Malignant neoplasm of uterus, part unspecified **126, 129**	198.5	Secondary malignant neoplasm of bone and bone marrow **87, 97**
180*	Malignant neoplasm of cervix uteri **126, 129**	198.6	Secondary malignant neoplasm of ovary **126, 129**
181	Malignant neoplasm of placenta **126, 129**	198.7	Secondary malignant neoplasm of adrenal gland **114**
182*	Malignant neoplasm of body of uterus **126, 129**	198.81	Secondary malignant neoplasm of breast **104, 105**
183*	Malignant neoplasm of ovary and other uterine adnexa **126, 129**	198.82	Secondary malignant neoplasm of genital organs **122, 123, 126, 129**
184*	Malignant neoplasm of other and unspecified female genital organs **126, 129**	198.89	Secondary malignant neoplasm of other specified sites **180, 181**
		199.0	Disseminated malignant neoplasm **180**
185	Malignant neoplasm of prostate **122, 123**	199.1	Other malignant neoplasm of unspecified site **180**
		199.2	Malignant neoplasm associated with transplanted organ **180**
		199*	Malignant neoplasm without specification of site **181**

200.0*	Reticulosarcoma **230**	204*	Lymphoid leukemia **178**
200.01	Reticulosarcoma of lymph nodes of head, face, and neck **2**	205.0*	Acute myeloid leukemia **180, 181**
200.11	Lymphosarcoma of lymph nodes of head, face, and neck **2**	205.1*	Chronic myeloid leukemia **181**
200.2*	Burkitt's tumor or lymphoma **230**	205.2*	Subacute myeloid leukemia **181**
200.21	Burkitt's tumor or lymphoma of lymph nodes of head, face, and neck **2**	205.3*	Myeloid sarcoma **181**
		205.8*	Other myeloid leukemia **181**
200.3*	Marginal zone lymphoma **230**	205.9*	Unspecified myeloid leukemia **181**
200.4*	Mantle cell lymphoma **230**	205*	Myeloid leukemia **178**
200.5*	Primary central nervous system lymphoma **230**	206.0*	Acute monocytic leukemia **180, 181**
200.6*	Anaplastic large cell lymphoma **230**	206.1*	Chronic monocytic leukemia **181**
200.7*	Large cell lymphoma **230**	206.2*	Subacute monocytic leukemia **181**
200.8*	Other named variants of lymphosarcoma and reticulosarcoma **230**	206.8*	Other monocytic leukemia **181**
		206.9*	Unspecified monocytic leukemia **181**
200.81	Other named variants of lymphosarcoma and reticulosarcoma of lymph nodes of head, face, and neck **2**	206*	Monocytic leukemia **178**
		207.0*	Acute erythremia and erythroleukemia **180, 181**
200*	Lymphosarcoma and reticulosarcoma and other specified malignant tumors of lymphatic tissue **178, 181**	207.1*	Chronic erythremia **181**
		207.2*	Megakaryocytic leukemia **181**
201.01	Hodgkin's paragranuloma of lymph nodes of head, face, and neck **2**	207.8*	Other specified leukemia **181**
		207*	Other specified leukemia **178**
201.11	Hodgkin's granuloma of lymph nodes of head, face, and neck **2**	208.0*	Acute leukemia of unspecified cell type **180, 181**
201.21	Hodgkin's sarcoma of lymph nodes of head, face, and neck **2**	208.1*	Chronic leukemia of unspecified cell type **181**
201.41	Hodgkin's disease, lymphocytic-histiocytic predominance of lymph nodes of head, face, and neck **2**	208.2*	Subacute leukemia of unspecified cell type **181**
		208.8*	Other leukemia of unspecified cell type **181**
201.51	Hodgkin's disease, nodular sclerosis, of lymph nodes of head, face, and neck **2**	208.9*	Unspecified leukemia **181**
		208*	Leukemia of unspecified cell type **178**
201.61	Hodgkin's disease, mixed cellularity, involving lymph nodes of head, face, and neck **2**	209.0*	Malignant carcinoid tumors of the small intestine **76**
201.71	Hodgkin's disease, lymphocytic depletion, of lymph nodes of head, face, and neck **2**	209.1*	Malignant carcinoid tumors of the appendix, large intestine, and rectum **76**
201.91	Hodgkin's disease, unspecified type, of lymph nodes of head, face, and neck **2**	209.11	Malignant carcinoid tumor of the appendix **73**
		209.20	Malignant carcinoid tumor of unknown primary site **180, 181**
201*	Hodgkin's disease **178, 181**	209.21	Malignant carcinoid tumor of the bronchus and lung **52**
202.0*	Nodular lymphoma **178, 181**	209.22	Malignant carcinoid tumor of the thymus **180, 181**
202.01	Nodular lymphoma of lymph nodes of head, face, and neck **2**	209.23	Malignant carcinoid tumor of the stomach **76**
202.1*	Mycosis fungoides **178, 181**	209.24	Malignant carcinoid tumor of the kidney **116, 119**
202.11	Mycosis fungoides of lymph nodes of head, face, and neck **2**	209.25	Malignant carcinoid tumor of foregut, not otherwise specified **76**
202.2*	Sezary's disease **178, 181**	209.26	Malignant carcinoid tumor of midgut, not otherwise specified **76**
202.21	Sezary's disease of lymph nodes of head, face, and neck **3**	209.27	Malignant carcinoid tumor of hindgut, not otherwise specified **76**
202.3*	Malignant histiocytosis **178, 181**	209.29	Malignant carcinoid tumor of other sites **180, 181**
202.31	Malignant histiocytosis of lymph nodes of head, face, and neck **3**	209.30	Malignant poorly differentiated neuroendocrine carcinoma, any site **180, 181**
202.4*	Leukemic reticuloendotheliosis **178, 181**		
202.41	Leukemic reticuloendotheliosis of lymph nodes of head, face, and neck **3**	209.31	Merkel cell carcinoma of the face **105**
		209.32	Merkel cell carcinoma of the scalp and neck **105**
202.5*	Letterer-Siwe disease **180, 181**	209.33	Merkel cell carcinoma of the upper limb **105**
202.51	Letterer-Siwe disease of lymph nodes of head, face, and neck **3**	209.34	Merkel cell carcinoma of the lower limb **105**
202.6*	Malignant mast cell tumors **178, 181**	209.35	Merkel cell carcinoma of the trunk **105**
202.61	Malignant mast cell tumors of lymph nodes of head, face, and neck **3**	209.36	Merkel cell carcinoma of other sites **105**
		209.4*	Benign carcinoid tumors of the small intestine **78**
202.7*	Peripheral T-cell lymphoma **178, 181, 230**	209.5*	Benign carcinoid tumors of the appendix, large intestine, and rectum **78**
202.8*	Other malignant lymphomas **178, 181, 230**		
202.81	Other malignant lymphomas of lymph nodes of head, face, and neck **3**	209.60	Benign carcinoid tumor of unknown primary site **180, 181**
		209.61	Benign carcinoid tumor of the bronchus and lung **52**
202.9*	Other and unspecified malignant neoplasms of lymphoid and histiocytic tissue **178, 181**	209.62	Benign carcinoid tumor of the thymus **176**
		209.63	Benign carcinoid tumor of the stomach **78**
202.91	Other and unspecified malignant neoplasms of lymphoid and histiocytic tissue of lymph nodes of head, face, and neck **3**	209.64	Benign carcinoid tumor of the kidney **116, 119**
		209.65	Benign carcinoid tumor of foregut, not otherwise specified **78**
203*	Multiple myeloma and immunoproliferative neoplasms **178, 181**	209.66	Benign carcinoid tumor of midgut, not otherwise specified **78**
204.0*	Acute lymphoid leukemia **180, 181**	209.67	Benign carcinoid tumor of hindgut, not otherwise specified **78**
204.1*	Chronic lymphoid leukemia **181**	209.69	Benign carcinoid tumor of other sites **180, 181**
204.2*	Subacute lymphoid leukemia **181**	209.70	Secondary neuroendocrine tumor, unspecified site **180, 182**
204.8*	Other lymphoid leukemia **181**		
204.9*	Unspecified lymphoid leukemia **181**		

*Code Range

209.71	Secondary neuroendocrine tumor of distant lymph nodes **178**, **181**
209.72	Secondary neuroendocrine tumor of liver **82**
209.73	Secondary neuroendocrine tumor of bone **87**, **97**
209.74	Secondary neuroendocrine tumor of peritoneum **76**
209.75	Secondary Merkel cell carcinoma **180**, **182**
209.79	Secondary neuroendocrine tumor of other sites **180**, **182**
210.0	Benign neoplasm of lip **48**
210.1	Benign neoplasm of tongue **48**
210.2	Benign neoplasm of major salivary glands **47**
210.3	Benign neoplasm of floor of mouth **48**
210.4	Benign neoplasm of other and unspecified parts of mouth **48**
210.5	Benign neoplasm of tonsil **47**
210.6	Benign neoplasm of other parts of oropharynx **47**
210.7	Benign neoplasm of nasopharynx **47**
210.8	Benign neoplasm of hypopharynx **47**
210.9	Benign neoplasm of pharynx, unspecified **47**
210*	Benign neoplasm of lip, oral cavity, and pharynx **3**
211.0	Benign neoplasm of esophagus **78**
211.1	Benign neoplasm of stomach **78**
211.2	Benign neoplasm of duodenum, jejunum, and ileum **78**
211.3	Benign neoplasm of colon **78**
211.4	Benign neoplasm of rectum and anal canal **78**
211.5	Benign neoplasm of liver and biliary passages **83**
211.6	Benign neoplasm of pancreas, except islets of Langerhans **83**
211.7	Benign neoplasm of islets of Langerhans **114**
211.8	Benign neoplasm of retroperitoneum and peritoneum **78**
211.9	Benign neoplasm of other and unspecified site of the digestive system **78**
212.0	Benign neoplasm of nasal cavities, middle ear, and accessory sinuses **3**, **47**
212.1	Benign neoplasm of larynx **3**, **47**
212.2	Benign neoplasm of trachea **52**
212.3	Benign neoplasm of bronchus and lung **52**
212.4	Benign neoplasm of pleura **52**
212.5	Benign neoplasm of mediastinum **52**
212.6	Benign neoplasm of thymus **176**
212.7	Benign neoplasm of heart **68**
212.8	Benign neoplasm of other specified sites of respiratory and intrathoracic organs **52**
212.9	Benign neoplasm of respiratory and intrathoracic organs, site unspecified **52**
213.0	Benign neoplasm of bones of skull and face **3**, **100**
213.1	Benign neoplasm of lower jaw bone **3**, **48**
213.2	Benign neoplasm of vertebral column, excluding sacrum and coccyx **87**, **100**
213.3	Benign neoplasm of ribs, sternum, and clavicle **52**
213.4	Benign neoplasm of scapula and long bones of upper limb **100**
213.5	Benign neoplasm of short bones of upper limb **100**
213.6	Benign neoplasm of pelvic bones, sacrum, and coccyx **100**
213.7	Benign neoplasm of long bones of lower limb **100**
213.8	Benign neoplasm of short bones of lower limb **100**
213.9	Benign neoplasm of bone and articular cartilage, site unspecified **100**
214.0	Lipoma of skin and subcutaneous tissue of face **108**
214.1	Lipoma of other skin and subcutaneous tissue **108**
214.2	Lipoma of intrathoracic organs **52**
214.3	Lipoma of intra-abdominal organs **78**
214.4	Lipoma of spermatic cord **124**
214.8	Lipoma of other specified sites **108**
214.9	Lipoma of unspecified site **108**
215*	Other benign neoplasm of connective and other soft tissue **100**
216.0	Benign neoplasm of skin of lip **108**
216.1	Benign neoplasm of eyelid, including canthus **38**
216.2	Benign neoplasm of ear and external auditory canal **108**
216.3	Benign neoplasm of skin of other and unspecified parts of face **108**
216.4	Benign neoplasm of scalp and skin of neck **108**
216.5	Benign neoplasm of skin of trunk, except scrotum **108**
216.6	Benign neoplasm of skin of upper limb, including shoulder **108**
216.7	Benign neoplasm of skin of lower limb, including hip **108**
216.8	Benign neoplasm of other specified sites of skin **108**
216.9	Benign neoplasm of skin, site unspecified **108**
217	Benign neoplasm of breast **108**
218*	Uterine leiomyoma **127**, **130**
219*	Other benign neoplasm of uterus **127**, **130**
220	Benign neoplasm of ovary **127**, **130**
221*	Benign neoplasm of other female genital organs **127**, **130**
222*	Benign neoplasm of male genital organs **124**
223*	Benign neoplasm of kidney and other urinary organs **116**, **119**
224*	Benign neoplasm of eye **38**
225*	Benign neoplasm of brain and other parts of nervous system **19**
226	Benign neoplasm of thyroid glands **3**, **114**
227.0	Benign neoplasm of adrenal gland **114**
227.1	Benign neoplasm of parathyroid gland **114**
227.3	Benign neoplasm of pituitary gland and craniopharyngeal duct (pouch) **114**
227.4	Benign neoplasm of pineal gland **19**
227.5	Benign neoplasm of carotid body **19**
227.6	Benign neoplasm of aortic body and other paraganglia **19**
227.8	Benign neoplasm of other endocrine glands and related structures **114**
227.9	Benign neoplasm of endocrine gland, site unspecified **114**
228.00	Hemangioma of unspecified site **3**, **68**
228.01	Hemangioma of skin and subcutaneous tissue **3**, **108**
228.02	Hemangioma of intracranial structures **32**
228.03	Hemangioma of retina **38**
228.04	Hemangioma of intra-abdominal structures **78**
228.09	Hemangioma of other sites **3**, **68**
228.1	Lymphangioma, any site **176**
229.0	Benign neoplasm of lymph nodes **176**
229.8	Benign neoplasm of other specified sites **180**, **182**
229.9	Benign neoplasm of unspecified site **180**, **182**
230.0	Carcinoma in situ of lip, oral cavity, and pharynx **3**, **46**
230.1	Carcinoma in situ of esophagus **76**
230.2	Carcinoma in situ of stomach **76**
230.3	Carcinoma in situ of colon **76**
230.4	Carcinoma in situ of rectum **76**
230.5	Carcinoma in situ of anal canal **76**
230.6	Carcinoma in situ of anus, unspecified **76**
230.7	Carcinoma in situ of other and unspecified parts of intestine **76**
230.8	Carcinoma in situ of liver and biliary system **83**
230.9	Carcinoma in situ of other and unspecified digestive organs **76**
231.0	Carcinoma in situ of larynx **3**, **46**
231.1	Carcinoma in situ of trachea **52**
231.2	Carcinoma in situ of bronchus and lung **52**
231.8	Carcinoma in situ of other specified parts of respiratory system **52**
231.9	Carcinoma in situ of respiratory system, part unspecified **52**
232.0	Carcinoma in situ of skin of lip **108**

232.1 Carcinoma in situ of eyelid, including canthus **38**

232.2 Carcinoma in situ of skin of ear and external auditory canal **108**

232.3 Carcinoma in situ of skin of other and unspecified parts of face **108**

232.4 Carcinoma in situ of scalp and skin of neck **108**

232.5 Carcinoma in situ of skin of trunk, except scrotum **108**

232.6 Carcinoma in situ of skin of upper limb, including shoulder **108**

232.7 Carcinoma in situ of skin of lower limb, including hip **108**

232.8 Carcinoma in situ of other specified sites of skin **108**

232.9 Carcinoma in situ of skin, site unspecified **108**

233.0 Carcinoma in situ of breast **104, 105**

233.1 Carcinoma in situ of cervix uteri **126, 129**

233.2 Carcinoma in situ of other and unspecified parts of uterus **126, 129**

233.3* Carcinoma in situ, other and unspecified female genital organs **126, 129**

233.4 Carcinoma in situ of prostate **122, 123**

233.5 Carcinoma in situ of penis **122, 123**

233.6 Carcinoma in situ of other and unspecified male genital organs **122, 123**

233.7 Carcinoma in situ of bladder **116, 119**

233.9 Carcinoma in situ of other and unspecified urinary organs **116, 119**

234.0 Carcinoma in situ of eye **38**

234.8 Carcinoma in situ of other specified sites **180, 182**

234.9 Carcinoma in situ, site unspecified **180, 182**

235.0 Neoplasm of uncertain behavior of major salivary glands **3, 46**

235.1 Neoplasm of uncertain behavior of lip, oral cavity, and pharynx **3, 46**

235.2 Neoplasm of uncertain behavior of stomach, intestines, and rectum **76**

235.3 Neoplasm of uncertain behavior of liver and biliary passages **83**

235.4 Neoplasm of uncertain behavior of retroperitoneum and peritoneum **76**

235.5 Neoplasm of uncertain behavior of other and unspecified digestive organs **76**

235.6 Neoplasm of uncertain behavior of larynx **3, 46**

235.7 Neoplasm of uncertain behavior of trachea, bronchus, and lung **52**

235.8 Neoplasm of uncertain behavior of pleura, thymus, and mediastinum **52**

235.9 Neoplasm of uncertain behavior of other and unspecified respiratory organs **52**

236.0 Neoplasm of uncertain behavior of uterus **126, 129**

236.1 Neoplasm of uncertain behavior of placenta **126, 129**

236.2 Neoplasm of uncertain behavior of ovary **126, 129**

236.3 Neoplasm of uncertain behavior of other and unspecified female genital organs **126, 129**

236.4 Neoplasm of uncertain behavior of testis **122, 123**

236.5 Neoplasm of uncertain behavior of prostate **122, 123**

236.6 Neoplasm of uncertain behavior of other and unspecified male genital organs **122, 123**

236.7 Neoplasm of uncertain behavior of bladder **116, 119**

236.9* Neoplasm of uncertain behavior of other and unspecified urinary organs **116, 119**

237.0 Neoplasm of uncertain behavior of pituitary gland and craniopharyngeal duct **114**

237.1 Neoplasm of uncertain behavior of pineal gland **19**

237.2 Neoplasm of uncertain behavior of adrenal gland **114**

237.3 Neoplasm of uncertain behavior of paraganglia **19**

237.4 Neoplasm of uncertain behavior of other and unspecified endocrine glands **114**

237.5 Neoplasm of uncertain behavior of brain and spinal cord **19**

237.6 Neoplasm of uncertain behavior of meninges **19**

237.7* Neurofibromatosis **32**

237.9 Neoplasm of uncertain behavior of other and unspecified parts of nervous system **19**

238.0 Neoplasm of uncertain behavior of bone and articular cartilage **87, 97**

238.1 Neoplasm of uncertain behavior of connective and other soft tissue **100**

238.2 Neoplasm of uncertain behavior of skin **108**

238.3 Neoplasm of uncertain behavior of breast **104, 105**

238.4 Neoplasm of uncertain behavior of polycythemia vera **178, 181**

238.5 Neoplasm of uncertain behavior of histiocytic and mast cells **178, 181**

238.6 Neoplasm of uncertain behavior of plasma cells **178, 181**

238.71 Essential thrombocythemia **176**

238.72 Low grade myelodysplastic syndrome lesions **175**

238.73 High grade myelodysplastic syndrome lesions **175**

238.74 Myelodysplastic syndrome with 5q deletion **175**

238.75 Myelodysplastic syndrome, unspecified **175**

238.76 Myelofibrosis with myeloid metaplasia **178, 181**

238.77 Post-transplant lymphoproliferative disorder [PTLD] **203**

238.79 Other lymphatic and hematopoietic tissues **178, 181**

238.8 Neoplasm of uncertain behavior of other specified sites **180, 182**

238.9 Neoplasm of uncertain behavior, site unspecified **180, 182**

239.0 Neoplasm of unspecified nature of digestive system **76**

239.1 Neoplasm of unspecified nature of respiratory system **52**

239.2 Neoplasms of unspecified nature of bone, soft tissue, and skin **87, 100**

239.3 Neoplasm of unspecified nature of breast **105**

239.4 Neoplasm of unspecified nature of bladder **116, 119**

239.5 Neoplasm of unspecified nature of other genitourinary organs **116, 119**

239.6 Neoplasm of unspecified nature of brain **19**

239.7 Neoplasm of unspecified nature of endocrine glands and other parts of nervous system **114**

239.8* Neoplasm of unspecified nature of other specified sites **180, 182**

239.9 Neoplasm of unspecified nature, site unspecified **180, 182**

240* Simple and unspecified goiter **114**

241* Nontoxic nodular goiter **114**

242* Thyrotoxicosis with or without goiter **3, 114**

243 Congenital hypothyroidism **114**

244* Acquired hypothyroidism **114**

245* Thyroiditis **3, 114**

246.2 Cyst of thyroid **3**

246.3 Hemorrhage and infarction of thyroid **3**

246.8 Other specified disorders of thyroid **3**

246.9 Unspecified disorder of thyroid **3**

246* Other disorders of thyroid **114**

249.0* Secondary diabetes mellitus without mention of complication **113**

249.1* Secondary diabetes mellitus with ketoacidosis **113**

249.2* Secondary diabetes mellitus with hyperosmolarity **113**

249.3* Secondary diabetes mellitus with other coma **113**

249.4* Secondary diabetes mellitus with renal manifestations **120**

249.5* Secondary diabetes mellitus with ophthalmic manifestations **38**

249.6* Secondary diabetes mellitus with neurological manifestations **21**

249.7* Secondary diabetes mellitus with peripheral circulatory disorders **66**

249.8* Secondary diabetes mellitus with other specified manifestations **113**

*Code Range

249.9*	Secondary diabetes mellitus with unspecified complication **113**	
249*	Secondary diabetes mellitus **1**, **2**	
250.0*	Diabetes mellitus without mention of complication **1**, **2**, **113**	
250.1*	Diabetes with ketoacidosis **1**, **2**, **113**	
250.2*	Diabetes with hyperosmolarity **1**, **2**, **113**	
250.3*	Diabetes with other coma **1**, **2**, **113**	
250.4*	Diabetes with renal manifestations **1**, **2**, **120**	
250.41	Diabetes with renal manifestations, type I [juvenile type], not stated as uncontrolled **118**	
250.43	Diabetes with renal manifestations, type I [juvenile type], uncontrolled **118**	
250.5*	Diabetes with ophthalmic manifestations **1**, **2**, **38**	
250.6*	Diabetes with neurological manifestations **1**, **2**, **21**	
250.7*	Diabetes with peripheral circulatory disorders **1**, **2**, **66**	
250.8*	Diabetes with other specified manifestations **1**, **2**, **113**	
250.9*	Diabetes with unspecified complication **2**, **113**	
251.0	Hypoglycemic coma **113**, **164**, **168**	
251.1	Other specified hypoglycemia **114**	
251.2	Hypoglycemia, unspecified **113**	
251.3	Postsurgical hypoinsulinemia **2**, **113**	
251.4	Abnormality of secretion of glucagon **114**	
251.5	Abnormality of secretion of gastrin **77**	
251.8	Other specified disorders of pancreatic internal secretion **114**	
251.9	Unspecified disorder of pancreatic internal secretion **114**	
252.1	Hypoparathyroidism **164**, **168**	
252*	Disorders of parathyroid gland **114**	
253.5	Diabetes insipidus **164**, **168**	
253*	Disorders of the pituitary gland and its hypothalamic control **114**	
254.1	Abscess of thymus **164**, **168**	
254*	Diseases of thymus gland **176**	
255*	Disorders of adrenal glands **114**	
256*	Ovarian dysfunction **127**, **130**	
257*	Testicular dysfunction **114**	
258*	Polyglandular dysfunction and related disorders **114**	
259*	Other endocrine disorders **114**	
260	Kwashiorkor **113**, **230**	
261	Nutritional marasmus **113**, **164**, **168**, **230**	
262	Other severe protein-calorie malnutrition **113**, **164**, **168**, **230**	
263.0	Malnutrition of moderate degree **164**, **168**	
263.1	Malnutrition of mild degree **164**, **168**	
263.8	Other protein-calorie malnutrition **164**, **168**	
263.9	Unspecified protein-calorie malnutrition **164**, **168**	
263*	Other and unspecified protein-calorie malnutrition **113**, **230**	
264.0	Vitamin A deficiency with conjunctival xerosis **38**	
264.1	Vitamin A deficiency with conjunctival xerosis and Bitot's spot **38**	
264.2	Vitamin A deficiency with corneal xerosis **38**	
264.3	Vitamin A deficiency with corneal ulceration and xerosis **39**	
264.4	Vitamin A deficiency with keratomalacia **39**	
264.5	Vitamin A deficiency with night blindness **39**	
264.6	Vitamin A deficiency with xerophthalmic scars of cornea **39**	
264.7	Other ocular manifestations of vitamin A deficiency **39**	
264.8	Other manifestations of vitamin A deficiency **113**	
264.9	Unspecified vitamin A deficiency **113**	
264*	Vitamin A deficiency **230**	
265*	Thiamine and niacin deficiency states **113**, **230**	
266*	Deficiency of B-complex components **113**, **230**	
267	Ascorbic acid deficiency **113**, **230**	
268.0	Rickets, active **98**	
268.1	Rickets, late effect **98**	

268.2	Osteomalacia, unspecified **98**	
268.9	Unspecified vitamin D deficiency **113**	
268*	Vitamin D deficiency **230**	
269*	Other nutritional deficiencies **113**, **230**	
270*	Disorders of amino-acid transport and metabolism **113**	
271.0	Glycogenosis **113**	
271.1	Galactosemia **113**	
271.2	Hereditary fructose intolerance **78**	
271.3	Intestinal disaccharidase deficiencies and disaccharide malabsorption **78**	
271.4	Renal glycosuria **113**	
271.8	Other specified disorders of carbohydrate transport and metabolism **113**	
271.9	Unspecified disorder of carbohydrate transport and metabolism **113**	
272*	Disorders of lipoid metabolism **113**	
273.0	Polyclonal hypergammaglobulinemia **176**	
273.1	Monoclonal paraproteinemia **176**	
273.2	Other paraproteinemias **178**, **181**	
273.3	Macroglobulinemia **178**, **181**	
273.4	Alpha-1-antitrypsin deficiency **114**	
273.8	Other disorders of plasma protein metabolism **180**, **182**	
273.9	Unspecified disorder of plasma protein metabolism **180**, **182**	
274.0*	Gouty arthropathy **98**	
274.10	Gouty nephropathy, unspecified **120**	
274.11	Uric acid nephrolithiasis **119**	
274.19	Other gouty nephropathy **120**	
274.8*	Gout with other specified manifestations **98**	
274.9	Gout, unspecified **98**	
275.0*	Disorders of iron metabolism **114**	
275.1	Disorders of copper metabolism **114**	
275.2	Disorders of magnesium metabolism **113**	
275.3	Disorders of phosphorus metabolism **114**	
275.4*	Disorders of calcium metabolism **113**	
275.5	Hungry bone syndrome **113**	
275.8	Other specified disorders of mineral metabolism **114**	
275.9	Unspecified disorder of mineral metabolism **114**	
276.5*	Volume depletion **230**	
276*	Disorders of fluid, electrolyte, and acid-base balance **113**, **164**, **168**	
277.00	Cystic fibrosis without mention of meconium ileus **113**	
277.01	Cystic fibrosis with meconium ileus **163**, **167**	
277.02	Cystic fibrosis with pulmonary manifestations **51**	
277.03	Cystic fibrosis with gastrointestinal manifestations **78**	
277.09	Cystic fibrosis with other manifestations **113**	
277.1	Disorders of porphyrin metabolism **114**	
277.2	Other disorders of purine and pyrimidine metabolism **114**	
277.3*	Amyloidosis **97**	
277.4	Disorders of bilirubin excretion **83**	
277.5	Mucopolysaccharidosis **114**	
277.6	Other deficiencies of circulating enzymes **114**	
277.7	Dysmetabolic Syndrome X **114**	
277.81	Primary carnitine deficiency **114**	
277.82	Carnitine deficiency due to inborn errors of metabolism **114**	
277.83	Iatrogenic carnitine deficiency **114**	
277.84	Other secondary carnitine deficiency **114**	
277.85	Disorders of fatty acid oxidation **114**	
277.86	Peroxisomal disorders **114**	
277.87	Disorders of mitochondrial metabolism **114**	
277.88	Tumor lysis syndrome **118**, **164**, **168**	

Numeric Index to Diseases

277.89	Other specified disorders of metabolism **114**	
277.9	Unspecified disorder of metabolism **114**	
278.00	Obesity, unspecified **113**	
278.01	Morbid obesity **113**	
278.02	Overweight **113**	
278.03	Obesity hypoventilation syndrome **54**	
278.1	Localized adiposity **113**	
278.2	Hypervitaminosis A **113**	
278.3	Hypercarotinemia **113**	
278.4	Hypervitaminosis D **113**	
278.8	Other hyperalimentation **113**	
279.0*	Deficiency of humoral immunity **176**	
279.10	Unspecified immunodeficiency with predominant T-cell defect **176**	
279.11	DiGeorge's syndrome **175**	
279.12	Wiskott-Aldrich syndrome **175**	
279.13	Nezelof's syndrome **175**	
279.19	Other deficiency of cell-mediated immunity **175**	
279.2	Combined immunity deficiency **175**	
279.3	Unspecified immunity deficiency **176**	
279.4*	Autoimmune disease, not elsewhere classified **97**	
279.5*	Graft-versus-host disease **175**	
279.8	Other specified disorders involving the immune mechanism **176**	
279.9	Unspecified disorder of immune mechanism **176**	
279*	Disorders involving the immune mechanism **230**	
280*	Iron deficiency anemias **175**, **230**	
281*	Other deficiency anemias **175**, **230**	
282.40	Thalassemia, unspecified **164**, **168**	
282.41	Sickle-cell thalassemia without crisis **164**, **168**	
282.42	Sickle-cell thalassemia with crisis **164**, **168**	
282.43	Alpha thalassemia **164**, **169**	
282.44	Beta thalassemia **164**, **169**	
282.45	Delta-beta thalassemia **164**, **169**	
282.47	Hemoglobin E-beta thalassemia **164**, **169**	
282.49	Other thalassemia **164**, **169**	
282*	Hereditary hemolytic anemias **175**	
283.0	Autoimmune hemolytic anemias **175**	
283.1*	Non-autoimmune hemolytic anemias **164**, **169**	
283.10	Unspecified non-autoimmune hemolytic anemia **175**	
283.11	Hemolytic-uremic syndrome **175**	
283.19	Other non-autoimmune hemolytic anemias **175**	
283.2	Hemoglobinuria due to hemolysis from external causes **164**, **169**, **175**	
283.9	Acquired hemolytic anemia, unspecified **164**, **169**, **175**	
283*	Acquired hemolytic anemias **230**	
284.0*	Constitutional aplastic anemia **175**	
284.1*	Pancytopenia **175**	
284.2	Myelophthisis **178**, **181**	
284.8*	Other specified aplastic anemias **175**, **230**	
284.9	Unspecified aplastic anemia **175**, **230**	
285.1	Acute posthemorrhagic anemia **164**, **169**	
285.9	Unspecified anemia **230**	
285*	Other and unspecified anemias **175**	
286.0	Congenital factor VIII disorder **176**	
286.1	Congenital factor IX disorder **176**	
286.2	Congenital factor XI deficiency **176**	
286.3	Congenital deficiency of other clotting factors **176**	
286.4	Von Willebrand's disease **176**	
286.52	Acquired hemophilia **176**	

286.53	Antiphospholipid antibody with hemorrhagic disorder **176**
286.59	Other hemorrhagic disorder due to intrinsic circulating anticoagulants, antibodies, or inhibitors **176**
286.6	Defibrination syndrome **164**, **169**, **176**
286.7	Acquired coagulation factor deficiency **176**
286.9	Other and unspecified coagulation defects **176**
287.4*	Secondary thrombocytopenia **164**, **169**, **230**
287.5	Unspecified thrombocytopenia **230**
287*	Purpura and other hemorrhagic conditions **176**
288.0*	Neutropenia **175**, **230**
288.1	Functional disorders of polymorphonuclear neutrophils **175**
288.2	Genetic anomalies of leukocytes **175**
288.3	Eosinophilia **176**
288.4	Hemophagocytic syndromes **176**
288.5*	Decreased white blood cell count **176**
288.6*	Elevated white blood cell count **176**
288.8	Other specified disease of white blood cells **176**
288.9	Unspecified disease of white blood cells **176**
289.0	Polycythemia, secondary **176**
289.1	Chronic lymphadenitis **176**
289.2	Nonspecific mesenteric lymphadenitis **78**
289.3	Lymphadenitis, unspecified, except mesenteric **176**
289.4	Hypersplenism **176**, **230**
289.5*	Other diseases of spleen **176**
289.6	Familial polycythemia **176**
289.7	Methemoglobinemia **175**
289.81	Primary hypercoagulable state **176**
289.82	Secondary hypercoagulable state **176**
289.83	Myelofibrosis **178**, **181**
289.84	Heparin-induced thrombocytopenia [HIT] **164**, **169**, **176**, **230**
289.89	Other specified diseases of blood and blood-forming organs **176**
289.9	Unspecified diseases of blood and blood-forming organs **176**, **230**
290.1*	Presenile dementia **230**
290*	Dementias **188**
291*	Alcohol-induced mental disorders **191**
292.0	Drug withdrawal **164**, **169**
292*	Drug-induced mental disorders **191**
293.0	Delirium due to conditions classified elsewhere **188**
293.1	Subacute delirium **188**
293.8*	Other specified transient mental disorders due to conditions classified elsewhere **188**
293.9	Unspecified transient mental disorder in conditions classified elsewhere **188**
294.9	Unspecified persistent mental disorders due to conditions classified elsewhere **230**
294*	Persistent mental disorders due to conditions classified elsewhere **188**
295*	Schizophrenic disorders **189**
296*	Episodic mood disorders **189**
297*	Delusional disorders **189**
298.0	Depressive type psychosis **189**
298.1	Excitative type psychosis **189**
298.2	Reactive confusion **189**
298.3	Acute paranoid reaction **189**
298.4	Psychogenic paranoid psychosis **189**
298.8	Other and unspecified reactive psychosis **189**
298.9	Unspecified psychosis **189**, **230**
299.0*	Autistic disorder **188**
299.1*	Childhood disintegrative disorder **188**

*Code Range

299.8*	Other specified pervasive developmental disorders **189**	
299.9*	Unspecified pervasive developmental disorder **189**	
300.0*	Anxiety states **188**	
300.10	Hysteria, unspecified **188**	
300.11	Conversion disorder **188**	
300.12	Dissociative amnesia **188**	
300.13	Dissociative fugue **188**	
300.14	Dissociative identity disorder **188**	
300.15	Dissociative disorder or reaction, unspecified **188**	
300.16	Factitious disorder with predominantly psychological signs and symptoms **188**	
300.19	Other and unspecified factitious illness **188**	
300.2*	Phobic disorders **188**	
300.3	Obsessive-compulsive disorders **188**	
300.4	Dysthymic disorder **188**	
300.5	Neurasthenia **188**	
300.6	Depersonalization disorder **188**	
300.7	Hypochondriasis **188**	
300.8*	Somatoform disorders **188**	
300.9	Unspecified nonpsychotic mental disorder **188**	
301.0	Paranoid personality disorder **188**	
301.10	Affective personality disorder, unspecified **188**	
301.11	Chronic hypomanic personality disorder **188**	
301.12	Chronic depressive personality disorder **188**	
301.13	Cyclothymic disorder **188**	
301.2*	Schizoid personality disorder **188**	
301.3	Explosive personality disorder **188**	
301.4	Obsessive-compulsive personality disorder **188**	
301.5*	Histrionic personality disorder **188**	
301.6	Dependent personality disorder **188**	
301.7	Antisocial personality disorder **188**	
301.8*	Other personality disorders **188**	
301.9	Unspecified personality disorder **188**	
302*	Sexual and gender identity disorders **189**	
303.0*	Acute alcoholic intoxication **191**	
303.9*	Other and unspecified alcohol dependence **191**	
304*	Drug dependence **191**	
305.0*	Nondependent alcohol abuse **191**	
305.1	Nondependent tobacco use disorder **213**	
305.2*	Nondependent cannabis abuse **191**	
305.3*	Nondependent hallucinogen abuse **191**	
305.4*	Nondependent sedative, hypnotic or anxiolytic abuse **191**	
305.5*	Nondependent opioid abuse **191**	
305.6*	Nondependent cocaine abuse **191**	
305.7*	Nondependent amphetamine or related acting sympathomimetic abuse **191**	
305.8*	Nondependent antidepressant type abuse **191**	
305.9*	Other, mixed, or unspecified nondependent drug abuse **191**	
306.0	Musculoskeletal malfunction arising from mental factors **98**	
306.1	Respiratory malfunction arising from mental factors **54**	
306.2	Cardiovascular malfunction arising from mental factors **68**	
306.3	Skin malfunction arising from mental factors **108**	
306.4	Gastrointestinal malfunction arising from mental factors **78**	
306.50	Psychogenic genitourinary malfunction, unspecified **120**	
306.51	Psychogenic vaginismus **127, 130**	
306.52	Psychogenic dysmenorrhea **127, 130**	
306.53	Psychogenic dysuria **120**	
306.59	Other genitourinary malfunction arising from mental factors **120**	
306.6	Endocrine malfunction arising from mental factors **114**	

306.7	Malfunction of organs of special sense arising from mental factors **188**
306.8	Other specified psychophysiological malfunction **189**
306.9	Unspecified psychophysiological malfunction **188**
307.0	Adult onset fluency disorder **189**
307.1	Anorexia nervosa **188**
307.2*	Tics **32**
307.3	Stereotypic movement disorder **189**
307.4*	Specific disorders of sleep of nonorganic origin **189**
307.50	Eating disorder, unspecified **189**
307.51	Bulimia nervosa **189**
307.52	Pica **189**
307.53	Rumination disorder **188**
307.54	Psychogenic vomiting **188**
307.59	Other disorder of eating **189**
307.6	Enuresis **189**
307.7	Encopresis **189**
307.80	Psychogenic pain, site unspecified **188**
307.81	Tension headache **34**
307.89	Other pain disorder related to psychological factors **188**
307.9	Other and unspecified special symptom or syndrome, not elsewhere classified **188**
308*	Acute reaction to stress **188**
309.0	Adjustment disorder with depressed mood **188**
309.1	Prolonged depressive reaction as adjustment reaction **188**
309.2*	Predominant disturbance of other emotions as adjustment reaction **188**
309.3	Adjustment disorder with disturbance of conduct **188**
309.4	Adjustment disorder with mixed disturbance of emotions and conduct **188**
309.8*	Other specified adjustment reactions **188**
309.9	Unspecified adjustment reaction **188**
310.0	Frontal lobe syndrome **188**
310.1	Personality change due to conditions classified elsewhere **188**
310.2	Postconcussion syndrome **34**
310.8*	Other specified nonpsychotic mental disorder following organic brain damage **19**
310.9	Unspecified nonpsychotic mental disorder following organic brain damage **188, 230**
311	Depressive disorder, not elsewhere classified **188**
312.0*	Undersocialized conduct disorder, aggressive type **189**
312.1*	Undersocialized conduct disorder, unaggressive type **189**
312.2*	Socialized conduct disorder **189**
312.30	Impulse control disorder, unspecified **189**
312.31	Pathological gambling **188**
312.32	Kleptomania **188**
312.33	Pyromania **189**
312.34	Intermittent explosive disorder **188**
312.35	Isolated explosive disorder **188**
312.39	Other disorder of impulse control **188**
312.4	Mixed disturbance of conduct and emotions **189**
312.8*	Other specified disturbances of conduct, not elsewhere classified **189**
312.9	Unspecified disturbance of conduct **189**
313.0	Overanxious disorder specific to childhood and adolescence **188**
313.1	Misery and unhappiness disorder specific to childhood and adolescence **188**
313.2*	Sensitivity, shyness, and social withdrawal disorder specific to childhood and adolescence **189**
313.3	Relationship problems specific to childhood and adolescence **189**

Numeric Index to Diseases

313.8*	Other or mixed emotional disturbances of childhood or adolescence **189**	
313.9	Unspecified emotional disturbance of childhood or adolescence **189**	
314*	Hyperkinetic syndrome of childhood **189**	
315.00	Developmental reading disorder, unspecified **189**	
315.01	Alexia **189**	
315.02	Developmental dyslexia **189**	
315.09	Other specific developmental reading disorder **189**	
315.1	Mathematics disorder **189**	
315.2	Other specific developmental learning difficulties **189**	
315.31	Expressive language disorder **189**	
315.32	Mixed receptive-expressive language disorder **189**	
315.34	Speech and language developmental delay due to hearing loss **189**	
315.35	Childhood onset fluency disorder **32**	
315.39	Other developmental speech or language disorder **189**	
315.4	Developmental coordination disorder **189**	
315.5	Mixed development disorder **189**	
315.8	Other specified delay in development **189**	
315.9	Unspecified delay in development **189**	
316	Psychic factors associated with diseases classified elsewhere **188**	
317	Mild intellectual disabilities **188**	
318*	Other specified intellectual disabilities **188**	
319	Unspecified intellectual disabilities **188**	
320*	Bacterial meningitis **9, 10, 33, 164, 169**	
321.0	Cryptococcal meningitis **9, 10**	
321.1	Meningitis in other fungal diseases **9, 10**	
321.2	Meningitis due to viruses not elsewhere classified **9, 10**	
321.3	Meningitis due to trypanosomiasis **9, 10**	
321*	Meningitis due to other organisms **34, 164, 169**	
322.0	Nonpyogenic meningitis **164, 169**	
322.1	Eosinophilic meningitis **165, 169**	
322.9	Unspecified meningitis **165, 169**	
322*	Meningitis of unspecified cause **34**	
323.0*	Encephalitis, myelitis, and encephalomyelitis in viral diseases classified elsewhere **9, 34**	
323.01	Encephalitis and encephalomyelitis in viral diseases classified elsewhere **10**	
323.02	Myelitis in viral diseases classified elsewhere **10**	
323.1	Encephalitis, myelitis, and encephalomyelitis in rickettsial diseases classified elsewhere **9, 10, 34**	
323.2	Encephalitis, myelitis, and encephalomyelitis in protozoal diseases classified elsewhere **9, 10, 34**	
323.4*	Other encephalitis, myelitis, and encephalomyelitis due to other infections classified elsewhere **9, 34**	
323.41	Other encephalitis and encephalomyelitis due to other infections classified elsewhere **10**	
323.42	Other myelitis due to other infections classified elsewhere **10**	
323.5*	Encephalitis, myelitis, and encephalomyelitis following immunization procedures **9, 34**	
323.51	Encephalitis and encephalomyelitis following immunization procedures **10**	
323.52	Myelitis following immunization procedures **10**	
323.6*	Postinfectious encephalitis, myelitis, and encephalomyelitis **9, 34**	
323.61	Infectious acute disseminated encephalomyelitis [ADEM] **10**	
323.62	Other postinfectious encephalitis and encephalomyelitis **10**	
323.63	Postinfectious myelitis **10**	
323.7*	Toxic encephalitis, myelitis, and encephalomyelitis **9**	
323.71	Toxic encephalitis and encephalomyelitis **10, 32**	
323.72	Toxic myelitis **10, 32**	

323.8*	Other causes of encephalitis, myelitis, and encephalomyelitis **9, 34**
323.81	Other causes of encephalitis and encephalomyelitis **10, 230**
323.82	Other causes of myelitis **10, 230**
323.9	Unspecified causes of encephalitis, myelitis, and encephalomyelitis **9, 10, 34, 230**
324*	Intracranial and intraspinal abscess **9, 10, 33, 165, 169**
325	Phlebitis and thrombophlebitis of intracranial venous sinuses **9, 10, 32**
326	Late effects of intracranial abscess or pyogenic infection **32**
327.0*	Organic disorders of initiating and maintaining sleep [Organic insomnia] **189**
327.1*	Organic disorders of excessive somnolence [Organic hypersomnia] **189**
327.2*	Organic sleep apnea **3**
327.20	Organic sleep apnea, unspecified **47**
327.21	Primary central sleep apnea **32**
327.22	High altitude periodic breathing **54**
327.23	Obstructive sleep apnea (adult) (pediatric) **47**
327.24	Idiopathic sleep related nonobstructive alveolar hypoventilation **47**
327.25	Congenital central alveolar hypoventilation syndrome **32**
327.26	Sleep related hypoventilation/hypoxemia in conditions classifiable elsewhere **47**
327.27	Central sleep apnea in conditions classified elsewhere **32**
327.29	Other organic sleep apnea **47**
327.3*	Circadian rhythm sleep disorder **3, 32**
327.4*	Organic parasomnia **3**
327.40	Organic parasomnia, unspecified **47**
327.41	Confusional arousals **32**
327.42	REM sleep behavior disorder **47**
327.43	Recurrent isolated sleep paralysis **32**
327.44	Parasomnia in conditions classified elsewhere **47**
327.49	Other organic parasomnia **47**
327.5*	Organic sleep related movement disorders **3**
327.51	Periodic limb movement disorder **32**
327.52	Sleep related leg cramps **32**
327.53	Sleep related bruxism **47**
327.59	Other organic sleep related movement disorders **47**
327.8	Other organic sleep disorders **3, 47**
330*	Cerebral degenerations usually manifest in childhood **19**
331.0	Alzheimer's disease **19**
331.1*	Frontotemporal dementia **19**
331.2	Senile degeneration of brain **19**
331.3	Communicating hydrocephalus **19**
331.4	Obstructive hydrocephalus **19**
331.5	Idiopathic normal pressure hydrocephalus [INPH] **19**
331.6	Corticobasal degeneration **19**
331.7	Cerebral degeneration in diseases classified elsewhere **19**
331.81	Reye's syndrome **32**
331.82	Dementia with Lewy bodies **19**
331.83	Mild cognitive impairment, so stated **19**
331.89	Other cerebral degeneration **19**
331.9	Unspecified cerebral degeneration **19**
332*	Parkinson's disease **19**
333.0	Other degenerative diseases of the basal ganglia **19**
333.1	Essential and other specified forms of tremor **32**
333.2	Myoclonus **32**
333.3	Tics of organic origin **32**
333.4	Huntington's chorea **19**

333.5	Other choreas **19**	
333.6	Genetic torsion dystonia **19**	
333.71	Athetoid cerebral palsy **19**	
333.72	Acute dystonia due to drugs **32**	
333.79	Other acquired torsion dystonia **32**	
333.81	Blepharospasm **39**	
333.82	Orofacial dyskinesia **32**	
333.83	Spasmodic torticollis **32**	
333.84	Organic writers' cramp **32**	
333.85	Subacute dyskinesia due to drugs **32**	
333.89	Other fragments of torsion dystonia **32**	
333.90	Unspecified extrapyramidal disease and abnormal movement disorder **19**	
333.91	Stiff-man syndrome **32**	
333.92	Neuroleptic malignant syndrome **32**	
333.93	Benign shuddering attacks **32**	
333.94	Restless legs syndrome [RLS] **19**	
333.99	Other extrapyramidal disease and abnormal movement disorder **19**	
334*	Spinocerebellar disease **19**	
335*	Anterior horn cell disease **19**	
336.0	Syringomyelia and syringobulbia **19**	
336.1	Vascular myelopathies **32**	
336.2	Subacute combined degeneration of spinal cord in diseases classified elsewhere **32**	
336.3	Myelopathy in other diseases classified elsewhere **32**	
336.8	Other myelopathy **32**	
336.9	Unspecified disease of spinal cord **32, 230**	
337*	Disorders of the autonomic nervous system **21**	
338.0	Central pain syndrome **32**	
338.1*	Acute pain **213**	
338.2*	Chronic pain **32**	
338.3	Neoplasm related pain (acute) (chronic) **213**	
338.4	Chronic pain syndrome **32**	
339*	Other headache syndromes **34**	
340	Multiple sclerosis **19**	
341.0	Neuromyelitis optica **19**	
341.1	Schilder's disease **19**	
341.2*	Acute (transverse) myelitis **9, 34**	
341.20	Acute (transverse) myelitis NOS **10**	
341.21	Acute (transverse) myelitis in conditions classified elsewhere **10**	
341.22	Idiopathic transverse myelitis **10**	
341.8	Other demyelinating diseases of central nervous system **19**	
341.9	Unspecified demyelinating disease of central nervous system **19, 230**	
342*	Hemiplegia and hemiparesis **19**	
343.0	Diplegic infantile cerebral palsy **19**	
343.1	Hemiplegic infantile cerebral palsy **19**	
343.2	Quadriplegic infantile cerebral palsy **19**	
343.3	Monoplegic infantile cerebral palsy **32**	
343.4	Infantile hemiplegia **19**	
343.8	Other specified infantile cerebral palsy **32**	
343.9	Unspecified infantile cerebral palsy **32**	
344.0*	Quadriplegia and quadriparesis **19**	
344.1	Paraplegia **19**	
344.2	Diplegia of upper limbs **19**	
344.3*	Monoplegia of lower limb **32**	
344.4*	Monoplegia of upper limb **32**	
344.5	Unspecified monoplegia **32**	

344.60	Cauda equina syndrome without mention of neurogenic bladder **21**
344.61	Cauda equina syndrome with neurogenic bladder **120**
344.8*	Other specified paralytic syndromes **32**
344.9	Unspecified paralysis **32**
345*	Epilepsy and recurrent seizures **34**
346*	Migraine **34**
347*	Cataplexy and narcolepsy **32**
348.0	Cerebral cysts **32**
348.1	Anoxic brain damage **32, 165, 169**
348.2	Benign intracranial hypertension **34**
348.3*	Encephalopathy, not elsewhere classified **20, 230**
348.4	Compression of brain **21**
348.5	Cerebral edema **21**
348.81	Temporal sclerosis **20**
348.82	Brain death **21**
348.89	Other conditions of brain **20**
348.9	Unspecified condition of brain **20, 230**
349.0	Reaction to spinal or lumbar puncture **34, 165, 169**
349.1	Nervous system complications from surgically implanted device **32, 165, 169**
349.2	Disorders of meninges, not elsewhere classified **32**
349.3*	Dural tear **165, 169, 203**
349.81	Cerebrospinal fluid rhinorrhea **32, 165, 169**
349.82	Toxic encephalopathy **32, 165, 169**
349.89	Other specified disorder of nervous system **20**
349.9	Unspecified disorders of nervous system **20, 230**
350*	Trigeminal nerve disorders **21**
351*	Facial nerve disorders **21**
352*	Disorders of other cranial nerves **21**
353*	Nerve root and plexus disorders **21**
354*	Mononeuritis of upper limb and mononeuritis multiplex **21**
355*	Mononeuritis of lower limb and unspecified site **21**
356.0	Hereditary peripheral neuropathy **21**
356.1	Peroneal muscular atrophy **21**
356.2	Hereditary sensory neuropathy **21**
356.3	Refsum's disease **32**
356.4	Idiopathic progressive polyneuropathy **21**
356.8	Other specified idiopathic peripheral neuropathy **21**
356.9	Unspecified hereditary and idiopathic peripheral neuropathy **21**
357.0	Acute infective polyneuritis **33, 230**
357.1	Polyneuropathy in collagen vascular disease **21**
357.2	Polyneuropathy in diabetes **21**
357.3	Polyneuropathy in malignant disease **21**
357.4	Polyneuropathy in other diseases classified elsewhere **21**
357.5	Alcoholic polyneuropathy **21**
357.6	Polyneuropathy due to drugs **21**
357.7	Polyneuropathy due to other toxic agents **21**
357.8*	Other inflammatory and toxic neuropathy **21**
357.9	Unspecified inflammatory and toxic neuropathy **21, 230**
358.0*	Myasthenia gravis **19**
358.1	Myasthenic syndromes in diseases classified elsewhere **19**
358.2	Toxic myoneural disorders **21**
358.3*	Lambert-Eaton syndrome **19**
358.8	Other specified myoneural disorders **21**
358.9	Unspecified myoneural disorders **21**
359.0	Congenital hereditary muscular dystrophy **32**
359.1	Hereditary progressive muscular dystrophy **32**
359.21	Myotonic muscular dystrophy **32**

Numeric Index to Diseases

359.22	Myotonia congenita	**32**
359.23	Myotonic chondrodystrophy	**32**
359.24	Drug-induced myotonia	**32**
359.29	Other specified myotonic disorder	**32**
359.3	Periodic paralysis	**32**
359.4	Toxic myopathy	**32**
359.5	Myopathy in endocrine diseases classified elsewhere	**32**
359.6	Symptomatic inflammatory myopathy in diseases classified elsewhere	**33**
359.7*	Inflammatory and immune myopathies, NEC	**97**
359.81	Critical illness myopathy	**33**
359.89	Other myopathies	**33**
359.9	Unspecified myopathy	**33**
360.00	Unspecified purulent endophthalmitis	**38**
360.01	Acute endophthalmitis	**38**
360.02	Panophthalmitis	**38**
360.03	Chronic endophthalmitis	**39**
360.04	Vitreous abscess	**38**
360.11	Sympathetic uveitis	**39**
360.12	Panuveitis	**39**
360.13	Parasitic endophthalmitis NOS	**38**
360.14	Ophthalmia nodosa	**39**
360.19	Other endophthalmitis	**38**
360.2*	Degenerative disorders of globe	**39**
360.3*	Hypotony of eye	**39**
360.4*	Degenerated conditions of globe	**39**
360.5*	Retained (old) intraocular foreign body, magnetic	**39**
360.6*	Retained (old) intraocular foreign body, nonmagnetic	**39**
360.8*	Other disorders of globe	**39**
360.9	Unspecified disorder of globe	**39**
361.0*	Retinal detachment with retinal defect	**39**
361.1*	Retinoschisis and retinal cysts	**39**
361.2	Serous retinal detachment	**39**
361.3*	Retinal defects without detachment	**39**
361.8*	Other forms of retinal detachment	**39**
361.9	Unspecified retinal detachment	**39**
362.0*	Diabetic retinopathy	**39**
362.1*	Other background retinopathy and retinal vascular changes	**39**, **230**
362.2*	Other proliferative retinopathy	**39**
362.3*	Retinal vascular occlusion	**38**
362.4*	Separation of retinal layers	**39**
362.5*	Degeneration of macula and posterior pole of retina	**39**
362.6*	Peripheral retinal degenerations	**39**
362.7*	Hereditary retinal dystrophies	**39**
362.8*	Other retinal disorders	**39**
362.9	Unspecified retinal disorder	**39**
363*	Chorioretinal inflammations, scars, and other disorders of choroid	**39**
364.0*	Acute and subacute iridocyclitis	**39**
364.1*	Chronic iridocyclitis	**39**
364.2*	Certain types of iridocyclitis	**39**
364.3	Unspecified iridocyclitis	**39**
364.41	Hyphema	**39**
364.42	Rubeosis iridis	**39**
364.5*	Degenerations of iris and ciliary body	**39**
364.6*	Cysts of iris, ciliary body, and anterior chamber	**39**
364.7*	Adhesions and disruptions of iris and ciliary body	**39**
364.8*	Other disorders of iris and ciliary body	**39**

364.9	Unspecified disorder of iris and ciliary body	**39**
365.0*	Borderline glaucoma (glaucoma suspect)	**39**
365.10	Unspecified open-angle glaucoma	**39**
365.11	Primary open-angle glaucoma	**39**
365.12	Low tension open-angle glaucoma	**38**
365.13	Pigmentary open-angle glaucoma	**39**
365.14	Open-angle glaucoma of childhood	**39**
365.15	Residual stage of open angle glaucoma	**39**
365.2*	Primary angle-closure glaucoma	**39**
365.3*	Corticosteroid-induced glaucoma	**39**
365.4*	Glaucoma associated with congenital anomalies, dystrophies, and systemic syndromes	**39**
365.5*	Glaucoma associated with disorders of the lens	**39**
365.6*	Glaucoma associated with other ocular disorders	**39**
365.7*	Glaucoma stage	**39**
365.8*	Other specified forms of glaucoma	**39**
365.9	Unspecified glaucoma	**39**
366*	Cataract	**39**
367.0	Hypermetropia	**39**
367.1	Myopia	**39**
367.2*	Astigmatism	**39**
367.3*	Anisometropia and aniseikonia	**39**
367.4	Presbyopia	**39**
367.51	Paresis of accommodation	**39**
367.52	Total or complete internal ophthalmoplegia	**38**
367.53	Spasm of accommodation	**39**
367.8*	Other disorders of refraction and accommodation	**39**
367.9	Unspecified disorder of refraction and accommodation	**39**
368.0*	Amblyopia ex anopsia	**39**
368.10	Unspecified subjective visual disturbance	**39**
368.11	Sudden visual loss	**38**
368.12	Transient visual loss	**38**
368.13	Visual discomfort	**39**
368.14	Visual distortions of shape and size	**39**
368.15	Other visual distortions and entoptic phenomena	**39**
368.16	Psychophysical visual disturbances	**39**
368.2	Diplopia	**38**
368.3*	Other disorders of binocular vision	**39**
368.40	Unspecified visual field defect	**38**
368.41	Scotoma involving central area in visual field	**38**
368.42	Scotoma of blind spot area in visual field	**39**
368.43	Sector or arcuate defects in visual field	**38**
368.44	Other localized visual field defect	**38**
368.45	Generalized contraction or constriction in visual field	**38**
368.46	Homonymous bilateral field defects in visual field	**38**
368.47	Heteronymous bilateral field defects in visual field	**38**
368.51	Protan defect in color vision	**39**
368.52	Deutan defect in color vision	**39**
368.53	Tritan defect in color vision	**39**
368.54	Achromatopsia	**39**
368.55	Acquired color vision deficiencies	**38**
368.59	Other color vision deficiencies	**39**
368.6*	Night blindness	**39**
368.8	Other specified visual disturbances	**39**
368.9	Unspecified visual disturbance	**39**
369*	Blindness and low vision	**39**, **230**
370.00	Unspecified corneal ulcer	**38**
370.01	Marginal corneal ulcer	**39**
370.02	Ring corneal ulcer	**39**

*Code Range

370.03	Central corneal ulcer **38**	376.03	Orbital osteomyelitis **38**
370.04	Hypopyon ulcer **38**	376.04	Orbital tenonitis **38**
370.05	Mycotic corneal ulcer **38**	376.1*	Chronic inflammatory disorders of orbit **39**
370.06	Perforated corneal ulcer **38**	376.2*	Endocrine exophthalmos **39**
370.07	Mooren's ulcer **39**	376.30	Unspecified exophthalmos **39**
370.2*	Superficial keratitis without conjunctivitis **39**	376.31	Constant exophthalmos **39**
370.3*	Certain types of keratoconjunctivitis **39**	376.32	Orbital hemorrhage **39**
370.4*	Other and unspecified keratoconjunctivitis **39**	376.33	Orbital edema or congestion **39**
370.50	Unspecified interstitial keratitis **39**	376.34	Intermittent exophthalmos **38**
370.52	Diffuse interstitial keratitis **39**	376.35	Pulsating exophthalmos **38**
370.54	Sclerosing keratitis **39**	376.36	Lateral displacement of globe of eye **38**
370.55	Corneal abscess **38**	376.4*	Deformity of orbit **39**
370.59	Other interstitial and deep keratitis **39**	376.5*	Enophthalmos **40**
370.6*	Corneal neovascularization **39**	376.6	Retained (old) foreign body following penetrating wound of orbit **40**
370.8	Other forms of keratitis **39**		
370.9	Unspecified keratitis **39**	376.81	Orbital cysts **40**
371*	Corneal opacity and other disorders of cornea **39**	376.82	Myopathy of extraocular muscles **38**
372*	Disorders of conjunctiva **39**	376.89	Other orbital disorder **40**
373*	Inflammation of eyelids **39**	376.9	Unspecified disorder of orbit **40**
374.0*	Entropion and trichiasis of eyelid **39**	377.00	Unspecified papilledema **33**, **165**, **169**
374.1*	Ectropion **39**	377.01	Papilledema associated with increased intracranial pressure **33**, **165**, **169**
374.2*	Lagophthalmos **39**		
374.30	Unspecified ptosis of eyelid **38**	377.02	Papilledema associated with decreased ocular pressure **40**, **165**, **169**
374.31	Paralytic ptosis **38**		
374.32	Myogenic ptosis **38**	377.03	Papilledema associated with retinal disorder **40**
374.33	Mechanical ptosis **39**	377.04	Foster-Kennedy syndrome **33**
374.34	Blepharochalasis **39**	377.10	Unspecified optic atrophy **38**
374.41	Eyelid retraction or lag **39**	377.11	Primary optic atrophy **38**
374.43	Abnormal innervation syndrome of eyelid **39**	377.12	Postinflammatory optic atrophy **38**
374.44	Sensory disorders of eyelid **39**	377.13	Optic atrophy associated with retinal dystrophies **40**
374.45	Other sensorimotor disorders of eyelid **38**	377.14	Glaucomatous atrophy (cupping) of optic disc **40**
374.46	Blepharophimosis **39**	377.15	Partial optic atrophy **38**
374.50	Unspecified degenerative disorder of eyelid **39**	377.16	Hereditary optic atrophy **38**
374.51	Xanthelasma of eyelid **108**	377.21	Drusen of optic disc **38**
374.52	Hyperpigmentation of eyelid **39**	377.22	Crater-like holes of optic disc **40**
374.53	Hypopigmentation of eyelid **39**	377.23	Coloboma of optic disc **40**
374.54	Hypertrichosis of eyelid **39**	377.24	Pseudopapilledema **38**
374.55	Hypotrichosis of eyelid **39**	377.3*	Optic neuritis **38**
374.56	Other degenerative disorders of skin affecting eyelid **39**	377.4*	Other disorders of optic nerve **38**
374.8*	Other disorders of eyelid **39**	377.5*	Disorders of optic chiasm **33**
374.9	Unspecified disorder of eyelid **39**	377.6*	Disorders of other visual pathways **33**
375.00	Unspecified dacryoadenitis **39**	377.7*	Disorders of visual cortex **33**
375.01	Acute dacryoadenitis **38**	377.9	Unspecified disorder of optic nerve and visual pathways **33**
375.02	Chronic dacryoadenitis **39**	378.0*	Esotropia **40**
375.03	Chronic enlargement of lacrimal gland **39**	378.1*	Exotropia **40**
375.1*	Other disorders of lacrimal gland **39**	378.2*	Intermittent heterotropia **40**
375.2*	Epiphora **39**	378.3*	Other and unspecified heterotropia **40**
375.30	Unspecified dacryocystitis **39**	378.4*	Heterophoria **40**
375.31	Acute canaliculitis, lacrimal **38**	378.5*	Paralytic strabismus **38**
375.32	Acute dacryocystitis **38**	378.6*	Mechanical strabismus **40**
375.33	Phlegmonous dacryocystitis **39**	378.71	Duane's syndrome **40**
375.4*	Chronic inflammation of lacrimal passages **39**	378.72	Progressive external ophthalmoplegia **38**
375.5*	Stenosis and insufficiency of lacrimal passages **39**	378.73	Strabismus in other neuromuscular disorders **38**
375.6*	Other changes of lacrimal passages **39**	378.81	Palsy of conjugate gaze **40**
375.8*	Other disorders of lacrimal system **39**	378.82	Spasm of conjugate gaze **40**
375.9	Unspecified disorder of lacrimal system **39**	378.83	Convergence insufficiency or palsy in binocular eye movement **40**
376.00	Unspecified acute inflammation of orbit **39**	378.84	Convergence excess or spasm in binocular eye movement **40**
376.01	Orbital cellulitis **38**	378.85	Anomalies of divergence in binocular eye movement **40**
376.02	Orbital periostitis **38**	378.86	Internuclear ophthalmoplegia **33**

378.87	Other dissociated deviation of eye movements **38**	
378.9	Unspecified disorder of eye movements **40**	
379.0*	Scleritis and episcleritis **40**	
379.1*	Other disorders of sclera **40**	
379.2*	Disorders of vitreous body **40**	
379.3*	Aphakia and other disorders of lens **40**	
379.40	Unspecified abnormal pupillary function **38**	
379.41	Anisocoria **38**	
379.42	Miosis (persistent), not due to miotics **38**	
379.43	Mydriasis (persistent), not due to mydriatics **38**	
379.45	Argyll Robertson pupil, atypical **19**	
379.46	Tonic pupillary reaction **38**	
379.49	Other anomaly of pupillary function **38**	
379.50	Unspecified nystagmus **38**	
379.51	Congenital nystagmus **40**	
379.52	Latent nystagmus **38**	
379.53	Visual deprivation nystagmus **40**	
379.54	Nystagmus associated with disorders of the vestibular system **38**	
379.55	Dissociated nystagmus **38**	
379.56	Other forms of nystagmus **40**	
379.57	Nystagmus with deficiencies of saccadic eye movements **38**	
379.58	Nystagmus with deficiencies of smooth pursuit movements **38**	
379.59	Other irregularities of eye movements **40**	
379.6*	Inflammation (infection) of postprocedural bleb **40**	
379.8	Other specified disorders of eye and adnexa **40**	
379.9*	Unspecified disorder of eye and adnexa **40**	
380.00	Unspecified perichondritis of pinna **46**	
380.01	Acute perichondritis of pinna **100**	
380.02	Chronic perichondritis of pinna **100**	
380.03	Chondritis of pinna **100**	
380.1*	Infective otitis externa **47**	
380.2*	Other otitis externa **47**	
380.3*	Noninfectious disorders of pinna **47**	
380.4	Impacted cerumen **47**	
380.5*	Acquired stenosis of external ear canal **47**	
380.8*	Other disorders of external ear **47**	
380.9	Unspecified disorder of external ear **47**	
381.0*	Acute nonsuppurative otitis media **46**	
381.1*	Chronic serous otitis media **46**	
381.2*	Chronic mucoid otitis media **46**	
381.3	Other and unspecified chronic nonsuppurative otitis media **46**	
381.4	Nonsuppurative otitis media, not specified as acute or chronic **46**	
381.5*	Eustachian salpingitis **46**	
381.6*	Obstruction of Eustachian tube **47**	
381.7	Patulous Eustachian tube **47**	
381.8*	Other disorders of Eustachian tube **47**	
381.9	Unspecified Eustachian tube disorder **47**	
382*	Suppurative and unspecified otitis media **46**	
383.0*	Acute mastoiditis **46**	
383.01	Subperiosteal abscess of mastoid **165, 169**	
383.1	Chronic mastoiditis **46**	
383.2*	Petrositis **46**	
383.3*	Complications following mastoidectomy **47**	
383.8*	Other disorders of mastoid **47**	
383.81	Postauricular fistula **165, 169**	
383.9	Unspecified mastoiditis **46**	
384.0*	Acute myringitis without mention of otitis media **46**	
384.1	Chronic myringitis without mention of otitis media **46**	
384.2*	Perforation of tympanic membrane **47**	

384.8*	Other specified disorders of tympanic membrane **47**	
384.9	Unspecified disorder of tympanic membrane **47**	
385*	Other disorders of middle ear and mastoid **47**	
386.0*	Meniere's disease **46**	
386.1*	Other and unspecified peripheral vertigo **46**	
386.2	Vertigo of central origin **46**	
386.3*	Labyrinthitis **46**	
386.4*	Labyrinthine fistula **47**	
386.5*	Labyrinthine dysfunction **46**	
386.8	Other disorders of labyrinth **46**	
386.9	Unspecified vertiginous syndromes and labyrinthine disorders **46**	
387*	Otosclerosis **47**	
388.0*	Degenerative and vascular disorders of ear **47**	
388.1*	Noise effects on inner ear **47**	
388.2	Unspecified sudden hearing loss **47**	
388.3*	Tinnitus **47**	
388.40	Unspecified abnormal auditory perception **47**	
388.41	Diplacusis **47**	
388.42	Hyperacusis **47**	
388.43	Impairment of auditory discrimination **47**	
388.44	Other abnormal auditory perception, recruitment **47**	
388.45	Acquired auditory processing disorder **189**	
388.5	Disorders of acoustic nerve **47**	
388.60	Unspecified otorrhea **47**	
388.61	Cerebrospinal fluid otorrhea **33**	
388.69	Other otorrhea **47**	
388.7*	Otalgia **47**	
388.8	Other disorders of ear **47**	
388.9	Unspecified disorder of ear **47**	
389*	Hearing loss **47**	
390	Rheumatic fever without mention of heart involvement **97**	
391.0	Acute rheumatic pericarditis **68**	
391.1	Acute rheumatic endocarditis **67**	
391.2	Acute rheumatic myocarditis **68**	
391.8	Other acute rheumatic heart disease **68**	
391.9	Unspecified acute rheumatic heart disease **68**	
392*	Rheumatic chorea **68**	
393	Chronic rheumatic pericarditis **68**	
394*	Diseases of mitral valve **67**	
395*	Diseases of aortic valve **67**	
396*	Diseases of mitral and aortic valves **67**	
397*	Diseases of other endocardial structures **67**	
398.0	Rheumatic myocarditis **68**	
398.90	Unspecified rheumatic heart disease **68**	
398.91	Rheumatic heart failure (congestive) **56, 66, 165, 169**	
398.99	Other and unspecified rheumatic heart diseases **68**	
401.0	Essential hypertension, malignant **67**	
401.1	Essential hypertension, benign **67**	
401.9	Unspecified essential hypertension **67**	
402.00	Malignant hypertensive heart disease without heart failure **67**	
402.01	Malignant hypertensive heart disease with heart failure **56, 66, 165, 169**	
402.10	Benign hypertensive heart disease without heart failure **67**	
402.11	Benign hypertensive heart disease with heart failure **56, 66, 165, 169**	
402.90	Unspecified hypertensive heart disease without heart failure **67**	
402.91	Hypertensive heart disease, unspecified, with heart failure **56, 66, 165, 169**	
403.00	Hypertensive chronic kidney disease, malignant, with chronic kidney disease stage I through stage IV, or unspecified **118**	

403.01	Hypertensive chronic kidney disease, malignant, with chronic kidney disease stage V or end stage renal disease **2**, **118**
403.10	Hypertensive chronic kidney disease, benign, with chronic kidney disease stage I through stage IV, or unspecified **118**
403.11	Hypertensive chronic kidney disease, benign, with chronic kidney disease stage V or end stage renal disease **2**, **118**
403.90	Hypertensive chronic kidney disease, unspecified, with chronic kidney disease stage I through stage IV, or unspecified **118**
403.91	Hypertensive chronic kidney disease, unspecified, with chronic kidney disease stage V or end stage renal disease **2**, **118**
404.00	Hypertensive heart and chronic kidney disease, malignant, without heart failure and with chronic kidney disease stage I through stage IV, or unspecified **67**
404.01	Hypertensive heart and chronic kidney disease, malignant, with heart failure and with chronic kidney disease stage I through stage IV, or unspecified **56**, **66**, **165**, **169**
404.02	Hypertensive heart and chronic kidney disease, malignant, without heart failure and with chronic kidney disease stage V or end stage renal disease **2**, **118**
404.03	Hypertensive heart and chronic kidney disease, malignant, with heart failure and with chronic kidney disease stage V or end stage renal disease **2**, **56**, **66**, **165**, **169**
404.10	Hypertensive heart and chronic kidney disease, benign, without heart failure and with chronic kidney disease stage I through stage IV, or unspecified **67**
404.11	Hypertensive heart and chronic kidney disease, benign, with heart failure and with chronic kidney disease stage I through stage IV, or unspecified **56**, **66**, **165**, **169**
404.12	Hypertensive heart and chronic kidney disease, benign, without heart failure and with chronic kidney disease stage V or end stage renal disease **2**, **118**
404.13	Hypertensive heart and chronic kidney disease, benign, with heart failure and chronic kidney disease stage V or end stage renal disease **2**, **56**, **66**, **165**, **169**
404.90	Hypertensive heart and chronic kidney disease, unspecified, without heart failure and with chronic kidney disease stage I through stage IV, or unspecified **67**
404.91	Hypertensive heart and chronic kidney disease, unspecified, with heart failure and with chronic kidney disease stage I through stage IV, or unspecified **56**, **66**, **165**, **169**
404.92	Hypertensive heart and chronic kidney disease, unspecified, without heart failure and with chronic kidney disease stage V or end stage renal disease **2**, **118**
404.93	Hypertensive heart and chronic kidney disease, unspecified, with heart failure and chronic kidney disease stage V or end stage renal disease **2**, **56**, **66**, **165**, **169**
405*	Secondary hypertension **67**
410.00	Acute myocardial infarction of anterolateral wall, episode of care unspecified **68**
410.01	Acute myocardial infarction of anterolateral wall, initial episode of care **56**, **65**
410.02	Acute myocardial infarction of anterolateral wall, subsequent episode of care **68**
410.10	Acute myocardial infarction of other anterior wall, episode of care unspecified **68**
410.11	Acute myocardial infarction of other anterior wall, initial episode of care **56**, **65**
410.12	Acute myocardial infarction of other anterior wall, subsequent episode of care **68**
410.20	Acute myocardial infarction of inferolateral wall, episode of care unspecified **69**
410.21	Acute myocardial infarction of inferolateral wall, initial episode of care **56**, **65**
410.22	Acute myocardial infarction of inferolateral wall, subsequent episode of care **69**
410.30	Acute myocardial infarction of inferoposterior wall, episode of care unspecified **69**

410.31	Acute myocardial infarction of inferoposterior wall, initial episode of care **56**, **65**
410.32	Acute myocardial infarction of inferoposterior wall, subsequent episode of care **69**
410.40	Acute myocardial infarction of other inferior wall, episode of care unspecified **69**
410.41	Acute myocardial infarction of other inferior wall, initial episode of care **56**, **65**
410.42	Acute myocardial infarction of other inferior wall, subsequent episode of care **69**
410.50	Acute myocardial infarction of other lateral wall, episode of care unspecified **69**
410.51	Acute myocardial infarction of other lateral wall, initial episode of care **56**, **65**
410.52	Acute myocardial infarction of other lateral wall, subsequent episode of care **69**
410.60	Acute myocardial infarction, true posterior wall infarction, episode of care unspecified **69**
410.61	Acute myocardial infarction, true posterior wall infarction, initial episode of care **57**, **65**
410.62	Acute myocardial infarction, true posterior wall infarction, subsequent episode of care **69**
410.70	Acute myocardial infarction, subendocardial infarction, episode of care unspecified **69**
410.71	Acute myocardial infarction, subendocardial infarction, initial episode of care **57**, **65**
410.72	Acute myocardial infarction, subendocardial infarction, subsequent episode of care **69**
410.80	Acute myocardial infarction of other specified sites, episode of care unspecified **69**
410.81	Acute myocardial infarction of other specified sites, initial episode of care **57**, **65**
410.82	Acute myocardial infarction of other specified sites, subsequent episode of care **69**
410.90	Acute myocardial infarction, unspecified site, episode of care unspecified **69**
410.91	Acute myocardial infarction, unspecified site, initial episode of care **57**, **65**
410.92	Acute myocardial infarction, unspecified site, subsequent episode of care **69**
411.0	Postmyocardial infarction syndrome **69**
411.1	Intermediate coronary syndrome **68**
411.81	Acute coronary occlusion without myocardial infarction **68**
411.89	Other acute and subacute form of ischemic heart disease **68**
412	Old myocardial infarction **67**
413.0	Angina decubitus **68**
413.1	Prinzmetal angina **68**
413.9	Other and unspecified angina pectoris **68**
414.0*	Coronary atherosclerosis **67**
414.1*	Aneurysm and dissection of heart **69**
414.10	Aneurysm of heart **165**, **169**
414.2	Chronic total occlusion of coronary artery **67**
414.3	Coronary atherosclerosis due to lipid rich plaque **67**
414.4	Coronary atherosclerosis due to calcified coronary lesion **67**
414.8	Other specified forms of chronic ischemic heart disease **67**
414.9	Unspecified chronic ischemic heart disease **67**
415.0	Acute cor pulmonale **69**
415.1*	Pulmonary embolism and infarction **51**
415*	Acute pulmonary heart disease **165**, **169**
416.0	Primary pulmonary hypertension **69**
416.1	Kyphoscoliotic heart disease **69**
416.2	Chronic pulmonary embolism **51**, **165**, **169**
416.8	Other chronic pulmonary heart diseases **69**

416.9	Unspecified chronic pulmonary heart disease	**69**
417*	Other diseases of pulmonary circulation	**69**
420.0	Acute pericarditis in diseases classified elsewhere	**165, 169**
420*	Acute pericarditis	**69**
421.0	Acute and subacute bacterial endocarditis	**65, 230**
421.1	Acute and subacute infective endocarditis in diseases classified elsewhere	**65**
421.9	Unspecified acute endocarditis	**65, 230**
421*	Acute and subacute endocarditis	**165, 169**
422.0	Acute myocarditis in diseases classified elsewhere	**165, 169**
422.9*	Other and unspecified acute myocarditis	**230**
422.92	Septic myocarditis	**165, 169**
422*	Acute myocarditis	**69**
423.0	Hemopericardium	**165, 169**
423*	Other diseases of pericardium	**69**
424.9*	Endocarditis, valve unspecified	**165, 169**
424*	Other diseases of endocardium	**67**
425.8	Cardiomyopathy in other diseases classified elsewhere	**165, 169**
425.9	Unspecified secondary cardiomyopathy	**230**
425*	Cardiomyopathy	**69**
426.0	Atrioventricular block, complete	**165, 169**
426.53	Other bilateral bundle branch block	**165, 169**
426.54	Trifascicular block	**165, 169**
426.7	Anomalous atrioventricular excitation	**165, 169**
426.89	Other specified conduction disorder	**165, 169**
426*	Conduction disorders	**68**
427.0	Paroxysmal supraventricular tachycardia	**68**
427.1	Paroxysmal ventricular tachycardia	**68, 165, 169**
427.2	Unspecified paroxysmal tachycardia	**68**
427.3*	Atrial fibrillation and flutter	**68, 165, 169**
427.4*	Ventricular fibrillation and flutter	**68, 165, 169**
427.5	Cardiac arrest	**66, 165, 169**
427.6*	Premature beats	**68**
427.8*	Other specified cardiac dysrhythmias	**68**
427.9	Unspecified cardiac dysrhythmia	**68**
428.0	Congestive heart failure, unspecified	**57, 165, 169**
428.1	Left heart failure	**57, 165, 169**
428.2*	Systolic heart failure	**57, 165, 169**
428.3*	Diastolic heart failure	**57, 165, 169**
428.4*	Combined systolic and diastolic heart failure	**57, 165, 169**
428.9	Unspecified heart failure	**57, 165, 169**
428*	Heart failure	**66**
429.0	Unspecified myocarditis	**69**
429.1	Myocardial degeneration	**69**
429.2	Unspecified cardiovascular disease	**67**
429.3	Cardiomegaly	**67**
429.4	Functional disturbances following cardiac surgery	**69, 165, 169**
429.5	Rupture of chordae tendineae	**67**
429.6	Rupture of papillary muscle	**67**
429.71	Acquired cardiac septal defect	**69**
429.79	Other certain sequelae of myocardial infarction, not elsewhere classified	**69**
429.81	Other disorders of papillary muscle	**67, 165, 169**
429.82	Hyperkinetic heart disease	**69, 165, 169**
429.83	Takotsubo syndrome	**69**
429.89	Other ill-defined heart disease	**67**
429.9	Unspecified heart disease	**67**
430	Subarachnoid hemorrhage	**8, 9, 10, 20, 165, 169**
431	Intracerebral hemorrhage	**8, 9, 10, 20, 165, 169**

432.9	Unspecified intracranial hemorrhage	**9, 10**
432*	Other and unspecified intracranial hemorrhage	**8, 20, 165, 169**
433.00	Occlusion and stenosis of basilar artery without mention of cerebral infarction	**20**
433.01	Occlusion and stenosis of basilar artery with cerebral infarction	**9, 10, 19, 20, 165, 169**
433.10	Occlusion and stenosis of carotid artery without mention of cerebral infarction	**20**
433.11	Occlusion and stenosis of carotid artery with cerebral infarction	**9, 10, 19, 20, 165, 169**
433.20	Occlusion and stenosis of vertebral artery without mention of cerebral infarction	**20**
433.21	Occlusion and stenosis of vertebral artery with cerebral infarction	**9, 10, 19, 20, 165, 169**
433.30	Occlusion and stenosis of multiple and bilateral precerebral arteries without mention of cerebral infarction	**20**
433.31	Occlusion and stenosis of multiple and bilateral precerebral arteries with cerebral infarction	**9, 10, 20, 165, 169**
433.80	Occlusion and stenosis of other specified precerebral artery without mention of cerebral infarction	**20**
433.81	Occlusion and stenosis of other specified precerebral artery with cerebral infarction	**9, 10, 20, 165, 169**
433.90	Occlusion and stenosis of unspecified precerebral artery without mention of cerebral infarction	**20**
433.91	Occlusion and stenosis of unspecified precerebral artery with cerebral infarction	**9, 10, 20, 165, 169**
434.00	Cerebral thrombosis without mention of cerebral infarction	**20**
434.01	Cerebral thrombosis with cerebral infarction	**9, 10, 20**
434.10	Cerebral embolism without mention of cerebral infarction	**20**
434.11	Cerebral embolism with cerebral infarction	**9, 10, 20**
434.90	Unspecified cerebral artery occlusion without mention of cerebral infarction	**20**
434.91	Unspecified cerebral artery occlusion with cerebral infarction	**9, 11, 20**
434*	Occlusion of cerebral arteries	**165, 169**
435*	Transient cerebral ischemia	**20**
436	Acute, but ill-defined, cerebrovascular disease	**20, 165, 169**
437.0	Cerebral atherosclerosis	**20**
437.1	Other generalized ischemic cerebrovascular disease	**20**
437.2	Hypertensive encephalopathy	**21**
437.3	Cerebral aneurysm, nonruptured	**33**
437.4	Cerebral arteritis	**34**
437.5	Moyamoya disease	**33**
437.6	Nonpyogenic thrombosis of intracranial venous sinus	**33**
437.7	Transient global amnesia	**21**
437.8	Other ill-defined cerebrovascular disease	**21**
437.9	Unspecified cerebrovascular disease	**21**
438*	Late effects of cerebrovascular disease	**19**
440.0	Atherosclerosis of aorta	**66**
440.1	Atherosclerosis of renal artery	**120**
440.2*	Atherosclerosis of native arteries of the extremities	**66**
440.24	Atherosclerosis of native arteries of the extremities with gangrene	**165, 169**
440.3*	Atherosclerosis of bypass graft of extremities	**66**
440.4	Chronic total occlusion of artery of the extremities	**66**
440.8	Atherosclerosis of other specified arteries	**66**
440.9	Generalized and unspecified atherosclerosis	**66**
441.0*	Dissection of aorta	**66**
441.1	Thoracic aneurysm, ruptured	**66**
441.2	Thoracic aneurysm without mention of rupture	**66**
441.3	Abdominal aneurysm, ruptured	**66**
441.4	Abdominal aneurysm without mention of rupture	**66**

*Code Range

441.5	Aortic aneurysm of unspecified site, ruptured **66**	
441.6	Thoracoabdominal aneurysm, ruptured **66**	
441.7	Thoracoabdominal aneurysm without mention of rupture **66**	
441.9	Aortic aneurysm of unspecified site without mention of rupture **66**	
442.0	Aneurysm of artery of upper extremity **66**	
442.1	Aneurysm of renal artery **120**	
442.2	Aneurysm of iliac artery **66**	
442.3	Aneurysm of artery of lower extremity **66**	
442.8*	Aneurysm of other specified artery **66**	
442.9	Other aneurysm of unspecified site **66**	
443.0	Raynaud's syndrome **97**	
443.1	Thromboangiitis obliterans (Buerger's disease) **66**	
443.21	Dissection of carotid artery **66**	
443.22	Dissection of iliac artery **66**	
443.23	Dissection of renal artery **120**	
443.24	Dissection of vertebral artery **66**	
443.29	Dissection of other artery **66**	
443.8*	Other specified peripheral vascular diseases **66**	
443.9	Unspecified peripheral vascular disease **66**	
444.0*	Arterial embolism and thrombosis of abdominal aorta **66**	
444.1	Embolism and thrombosis of thoracic aorta **66**	
444.2*	Embolism and thrombosis of arteries of the extremities **66**	
444.8*	Embolism and thrombosis of other specified artery **66**	
444.9	Embolism and thrombosis of unspecified artery **66**	
444*	Arterial embolism and thrombosis **165, 169**	
445.0*	Atheroembolism of extremities **66**	
445.81	Atheroembolism of kidney **120**	
445.89	Atheroembolism of other site **66**	
446.0	Polyarteritis nodosa **97**	
446.1	Acute febrile mucocutaneous lymph node syndrome (MCLS) **97**	
446.2*	Hypersensitivity angiitis **97**	
446.3	Lethal midline granuloma **97**	
446.4	Wegener's granulomatosis **97**	
446.5	Giant cell arteritis **97**	
446.6	Thrombotic microangiopathy **97**	
446.7	Takayasu's disease **97**	
447.0	Arteriovenous fistula, acquired **66**	
447.1	Stricture of artery **66**	
447.2	Rupture of artery **66**	
447.3	Hyperplasia of renal artery **120**	
447.4	Celiac artery compression syndrome **78**	
447.5	Necrosis of artery **66**	
447.6	Unspecified arteritis **97**	
447.7*	Aortic ectasia **66**	
447.8	Other specified disorders of arteries and arterioles **66**	
447.9	Unspecified disorders of arteries and arterioles **66**	
448.0	Hereditary hemorrhagic telangiectasia **66**	
448.1	Nevus, non-neoplastic **108**	
448.9	Other and unspecified capillary diseases **66**	
449	Septic arterial embolism **67, 165, 169**	
451.0	Phlebitis and thrombophlebitis of superficial vessels of lower extremities **67**	
451.1*	Phlebitis and thrombophlebitis of deep veins of lower extremities **66, 165, 169**	
451.2	Phlebitis and thrombophlebitis of lower extremities, unspecified **66, 165, 169**	
451.81	Phlebitis and thrombophlebitis of iliac vein **66, 165, 169**	
451.82	Phlebitis and thrombophlebitis of superficial veins of upper extremities **67**	

451.83	Phlebitis and thrombophlebitis of deep veins of upper extremities **67**
451.84	Phlebitis and thrombophlebitis of upper extremities, unspecified **67**
451.89	Phlebitis and thrombophlebitis of other site **67**
451.9	Phlebitis and thrombophlebitis of unspecified site **67**
452	Portal vein thrombosis **83**
453.0	Budd-Chiari syndrome **83**
453.1	Thrombophlebitis migrans **67**
453.2	Other venous embolism and thrombosis, of inferior vena cava **66, 165, 169**
453.3	Embolism and thrombosis of renal vein **120**
453.4*	Acute venous embolism and thrombosis of deep vessels of lower extremity **67**
453.5*	Chronic venous embolism and thrombosis of deep vessels of lower extremity **67**
453.6	Venous embolism and thrombosis of superficial vessels of lower extremity **67**
453.7*	Chronic venous embolism and thrombosis of other specified vessels **67**
453.8*	Acute venous embolism and thrombosis of other specified veins **67**
453.9	Embolism and thrombosis of unspecified site **67**
454.0	Varicose veins of lower extremities with ulcer **67**
454.1	Varicose veins of lower extremities with inflammation **67**
454.2	Varicose veins of lower extremities with ulcer and inflammation **67**
454.8	Varicose veins of the lower extremities with other complications **67**
454.9	Asymptomatic varicose veins **67**
455*	Hemorrhoids **78**
456.0	Esophageal varices with bleeding **75**
456.1	Esophageal varices without mention of bleeding **75**
456.20	Esophageal varices with bleeding in diseases classified elsewhere **75**
456.21	Esophageal varices without mention of bleeding in diseases classified elsewhere **78**
456.3	Sublingual varices **67**
456.4	Scrotal varices **124**
456.5	Pelvic varices **124, 127, 130**
456.6	Vulval varices **127, 130**
456.8	Varices of other sites **67**
457.0	Postmastectomy lymphedema syndrome **106**
457.1	Other noninfectious lymphedema **108**
457.2	Lymphangitis **106, 165, 169**
457.8	Other noninfectious disorders of lymphatic channels **176**
457.9	Unspecified noninfectious disorder of lymphatic channels **176**
458.0	Orthostatic hypotension **68**
458.1	Chronic hypotension **69**
458.2*	Iatrogenic hypotension **68**
458.8	Other specified hypotension **69**
458.9	Unspecified hypotension **69**
459.0	Unspecified hemorrhage **69, 165, 169**
459.1*	Postphlebitic syndrome **67**
459.2	Compression of vein **67**
459.3*	Chronic venous hypertension **67**
459.81	Unspecified venous (peripheral) insufficiency **67**
459.89	Other specified circulatory system disorders **67**
459.9	Unspecified circulatory system disorder **67**
460	Acute nasopharyngitis (common cold) **3, 46**
461*	Acute sinusitis **46**

462	Acute pharyngitis **3**, **46**
463	Acute tonsillitis **3**, **46**
464.00	Acute laryngitis, without mention of obstruction **3**, **46**
464.01	Acute laryngitis, with obstruction **3**, **46**
464.1*	Acute tracheitis **53**
464.2*	Acute laryngotracheitis **3**, **46**
464.3*	Acute epiglottitis **3**, **46**
464.4	Croup **3**, **46**
464.50	Unspecified supraglottis, without mention of obstruction **3**, **46**
464.51	Unspecified supraglottis, with obstruction **3**, **46**
465*	Acute upper respiratory infections of multiple or unspecified sites **3**, **46**
466*	Acute bronchitis and bronchiolitis **53**
470	Deviated nasal septum **3**, **47**
471*	Nasal polyps **47**
472.1	Chronic pharyngitis **3**
472.2	Chronic nasopharyngitis **3**
472*	Chronic pharyngitis and nasopharyngitis **46**
473*	Chronic sinusitis **46**
474.00	Chronic tonsillitis **46**
474.01	Chronic adenoiditis **46**
474.02	Chronic tonsillitis and adenoiditis **46**
474.1*	Hypertrophy of tonsils and adenoids **47**
474.2	Adenoid vegetations **47**
474.8	Other chronic disease of tonsils and adenoids **47**
474.9	Unspecified chronic disease of tonsils and adenoids **47**
474*	Chronic disease of tonsils and adenoids **3**
475	Peritonsillar abscess **3**, **46**
476.0	Chronic laryngitis **3**
476.1	Chronic laryngotracheitis **3**
476*	Chronic laryngitis and laryngotracheitis **46**
477*	Allergic rhinitis **46**
478.0	Hypertrophy of nasal turbinates **47**
478.1*	Other diseases of nasal cavity and sinuses **47**
478.11	Nasal mucositis (ulcerative) **172**
478.19	Other diseases of nasal cavity and sinuses **172**
478.2*	Other diseases of pharynx, not elsewhere classified **3**
478.20	Unspecified disease of pharynx **47**
478.21	Cellulitis of pharynx or nasopharynx **46**
478.22	Parapharyngeal abscess **46**, **165**, **169**
478.24	Retropharyngeal abscess **46**, **165**, **169**
478.25	Edema of pharynx or nasopharynx **47**
478.26	Cyst of pharynx or nasopharynx **47**
478.29	Other disease of pharynx or nasopharynx **47**
478.3*	Paralysis of vocal cords or larynx **3**, **47**, **165**, **169**
478.4	Polyp of vocal cord or larynx **3**, **47**
478.5	Other diseases of vocal cords **3**, **47**
478.6	Edema of larynx **3**, **47**
478.7*	Other diseases of larynx, not elsewhere classified **3**
478.70	Unspecified disease of larynx **47**
478.71	Cellulitis and perichondritis of larynx **46**
478.74	Stenosis of larynx **47**
478.75	Laryngeal spasm **47**, **165**, **169**
478.79	Other diseases of larynx **47**
478.8	Upper respiratory tract hypersensitivity reaction, site unspecified **3**, **46**
478.9	Other and unspecified diseases of upper respiratory tract **3**, **46**
480.3	Pneumonia due to SARS-associated coronavirus **230**
480.8	Pneumonia due to other virus not elsewhere classified **230**

480.9	Unspecified viral pneumonia **230**
480*	Viral pneumonia **53**
481	Pneumococcal pneumonia (streptococcus pneumoniae pneumonia) **53**, **165**, **169**, **230**
482.0	Pneumonia due to Klebsiella pneumoniae **51**
482.1	Pneumonia due to Pseudomonas **51**
482.2	Pneumonia due to Hemophilus influenzae (H. influenzae) **53**
482.3*	Pneumonia due to Streptococcus **53**
482.4*	Pneumonia due to Staphylococcus **51**
482.40	Pneumonia due to Staphylococcus, unspecified **51**
482.41	Methicillin susceptible pneumonia due to Staphylococcus aureus **51**
482.42	Methicillin resistant pneumonia due to Staphylococcus aureus **51**
482.49	Other Staphylococcus pneumonia **51**
482.8*	Pneumonia due to other specified bacteria **51**
482.81	Pneumonia due to anaerobes **51**
482.82	Pneumonia due to Escherichia coli (E. coli) **51**
482.83	Pneumonia due to other gram-negative bacteria **51**
482.84	Legionnaires' disease **51**
482.89	Pneumonia due to other specified bacteria **51**
482.9	Unspecified bacterial pneumonia **53**
482*	Other bacterial pneumonia **165**, **169**, **230**
483*	Pneumonia due to other specified organism **53**, **165**, **169**
484*	Pneumonia in infectious diseases classified elsewhere **51**
485	Bronchopneumonia, organism unspecified **53**, **165**, **169**
486	Pneumonia, organism unspecified **53**, **165**, **169**, **230**
487.0	Influenza with pneumonia **51**, **53**
487.1	Influenza with other respiratory manifestations **46**
487.8	Influenza with other manifestations **185**
488.01	Influenza due to identified avian influenza virus with pneumonia **53**, **165**, **169**, **230**
488.02	Influenza due to identified avian influenza virus with other respiratory manifestations **53**, **165**, **169**
488.09	Influenza due to identified avian influenza virus with other manifestations **185**
488.11	Influenza due to identified 2009 H1N1 influenza virus with pneumonia **53**, **165**, **169**, **230**
488.12	Influenza due to identified 2009 H1N1 influenza virus with other respiratory manifestations **53**, **165**, **169**
488.19	Influenza due to identified 2009 H1N1 influenza virus with other manifestations **185**
488.81	Influenza due to identified novel influenza A virus with pneumonia **53**, **165**, **169**, **230**
488.82	Influenza due to identified novel influenza A virus with other respiratory manifestations **53**, **165**, **169**
488.89	Influenza due to identified novel influenza A virus with other manifestations **185**
490	Bronchitis, not specified as acute or chronic **53**
491.0	Simple chronic bronchitis **53**
491.1	Mucopurulent chronic bronchitis **53**
491.2*	Obstructive chronic bronchitis **53**
491.8	Other chronic bronchitis **53**
491.9	Unspecified chronic bronchitis **53**
492.0	Emphysematous bleb **53**
492.8	Other emphysema **53**
493.0*	Extrinsic asthma **53**
493.01	Extrinsic asthma with status asthmaticus **165**, **169**
493.1*	Intrinsic asthma **53**
493.11	Intrinsic asthma with status asthmaticus **165**, **169**
493.20	Chronic obstructive asthma, unspecified **53**
493.21	Chronic obstructive asthma with status asthmaticus **53**

493.22	Chronic obstructive asthma, with (acute) exacerbation **53**	
493.8*	Other forms of asthma **53**	
493.9*	Unspecified asthma **54**	
493.91	Asthma, unspecified with status asthmaticus **165**, **169**	
494*	Bronchiectasis **53**	
495*	Extrinsic allergic alveolitis **53**	
496	Chronic airway obstruction, not elsewhere classified **53**	
500	Coal workers' pneumoconiosis **53**	
501	Asbestosis **53**	
502	Pneumoconiosis due to other silica or silicates **53**	
503	Pneumoconiosis due to other inorganic dust **53**	
504	Pneumonopathy due to inhalation of other dust **53**	
505	Unspecified pneumoconiosis **53**	
506.0	Bronchitis and pneumonitis due to fumes and vapors **54**	
506.1	Acute pulmonary edema due to fumes and vapors **52**	
506.2	Upper respiratory inflammation due to fumes and vapors **54**	
506.3	Other acute and subacute respiratory conditions due to fumes and vapors **54**	
506.4	Chronic respiratory conditions due to fumes and vapors **53**	
506.9	Unspecified respiratory conditions due to fumes and vapors **53**	
507.0	Pneumonitis due to inhalation of food or vomitus **165**, **169**	
507.8	Pneumonitis due to other solids and liquids **165**, **169**	
507*	Pneumonitis due to solids and liquids **51**	
508.0	Acute pulmonary manifestations due to radiation **54**, **165**, **169**	
508.1	Chronic and other pulmonary manifestations due to radiation **53**	
508.2	Respiratory conditions due to smoke inhalation **54**, **207**	
508.8	Respiratory conditions due to other specified external agents **54**	
508.9	Respiratory conditions due to unspecified external agent **54**	
510*	Empyema **51**, **165**, **169**	
511.0	Pleurisy without mention of effusion or current tuberculosis **53**	
511.1	Pleurisy with effusion, with mention of bacterial cause other than tuberculosis **51**, **165**, **170**	
511.81	Malignant pleural effusion **52**	
511.89	Other specified forms of effusion, except tuberculous **52**, **165**, **170**	
511.9	Unspecified pleural effusion **52**, **165**, **170**	
512.0	Spontaneous tension pneumothorax **53**	
512.1	Iatrogenic pneumothorax **53**	
512.2	Postoperative air leak **53**	
512.8*	Other pneumothorax and air leak **53**	
513*	Abscess of lung and mediastinum **51**, **165**, **170**	
514	Pulmonary congestion and hypostasis **52**	
515	Postinflammatory pulmonary fibrosis **53**	
516.30	Idiopathic interstitial pneumonia, not otherwise specified **230**	
516.35	Idiopathic lymphoid interstitial pneumonia **230**	
516.36	Cryptogenic organizing pneumonia **230**	
516.37	Desquamative interstitial pneumonia **230**	
516.6*	Interstitial lung diseases of childhood **165**, **170**	
516.8	Other specified alveolar and parietoalveolar pneumonopathies **230**	
516*	Other alveolar and parietoalveolar pneumonopathy **53**	
517.1	Rheumatic pneumonia **53**	
517.2	Lung involvement in systemic sclerosis **53**	
517.3	Acute chest syndrome **53**	
517.8	Lung involvement in other diseases classified elsewhere **53**	
518.0	Pulmonary collapse **54**, **165**, **170**	
518.1	Interstitial emphysema **53**, **165**, **170**	
518.2	Compensatory emphysema **54**	
518.3	Pulmonary eosinophilia **53**	
518.4	Unspecified acute edema of lung **52**, **165**, **170**	

518.5*	Pulmonary insufficiency following trauma and surgery **52**, **207**
518.52	Other pulmonary insufficiency, not elsewhere classified, following trauma and surgery **165**, **170**
518.6	Allergic bronchopulmonary aspergillosis **53**
518.7	Transfusion related acute lung injury [TRALI] **54**
518.81	Acute respiratory failure **52**, **207**
518.82	Other pulmonary insufficiency, not elsewhere classified **54**
518.83	Chronic respiratory failure **52**
518.84	Acute and chronic respiratory failure **52**, **207**
518.89	Other diseases of lung, not elsewhere classified **54**
519.0*	Tracheostomy complications **3**, **54**
519.1*	Other diseases of trachea and bronchus, not elsewhere classified **54**
519.11	Acute bronchospasm **3**
519.19	Other diseases of trachea and bronchus **3**
519.2	Mediastinitis **51**, **165**, **170**
519.3	Other diseases of mediastinum, not elsewhere classified **54**
519.4	Disorders of diaphragm **54**
519.8	Other diseases of respiratory system, not elsewhere classified **54**
519.9	Unspecified disease of respiratory system **54**
520.6	Disturbances in tooth eruption **172**
520*	Disorders of tooth development and eruption **3**, **48**
521*	Diseases of hard tissues of teeth **3**, **48**
522*	Diseases of pulp and periapical tissues **3**, **48**
523*	Gingival and periodontal diseases **3**, **48**
524*	Dentofacial anomalies, including malocclusion **3**, **48**
525*	Other diseases and conditions of the teeth and supporting structures **3**, **48**
526*	Diseases of the jaws **3**, **48**
527.9	Unspecified disease of the salivary glands **230**
527*	Diseases of the salivary glands **3**, **47**
528.6	Leukoplakia of oral mucosa, including tongue **230**
528*	Diseases of the oral soft tissues, excluding lesions specific for gingiva and tongue **3**, **48**
529*	Diseases and other conditions of the tongue **3**, **48**
530.0	Achalasia and cardiospasm **78**
530.1*	Esophagitis **78**
530.2*	Ulcer of esophagus **77**
530.3	Stricture and stenosis of esophagus **78**
530.4	Perforation of esophagus **75**, **165**, **170**
530.5	Dyskinesia of esophagus **78**
530.6	Diverticulum of esophagus, acquired **78**
530.7	Gastroesophageal laceration-hemorrhage syndrome **75**
530.81	Esophageal reflux **78**
530.82	Esophageal hemorrhage **75**
530.83	Esophageal leukoplakia **78**
530.84	Tracheoesophageal fistula **75**, **165**, **170**
530.85	Barrett's esophagus **77**
530.86	Infection of esophagostomy **78**
530.87	Mechanical complication of esophagostomy **78**
530.89	Other specified disorder of the esophagus **78**
530.9	Unspecified disorder of esophagus **78**
531.0*	Acute gastric ulcer with hemorrhage **76**
531.1*	Acute gastric ulcer with perforation **77**
531.2*	Acute gastric ulcer with hemorrhage and perforation **76**
531.30	Acute gastric ulcer without mention of hemorrhage, perforation, or obstruction **77**
531.31	Acute gastric ulcer without mention of hemorrhage or perforation, with obstruction **77**
531.4*	Chronic or unspecified gastric ulcer with hemorrhage **76**

531.5* Chronic or unspecified gastric ulcer with perforation **77**

531.6* Chronic or unspecified gastric ulcer with hemorrhage and perforation **76**

531.70 Chronic gastric ulcer without mention of hemorrhage, perforation, without mention of obstruction **77**

531.71 Chronic gastric ulcer without mention of hemorrhage or perforation, with obstruction **77**

531.90 Gastric ulcer, unspecified as acute or chronic, without mention of hemorrhage, perforation, or obstruction **77**

531.91 Gastric ulcer, unspecified as acute or chronic, without mention of hemorrhage or perforation, with obstruction **77**

532.0* Acute duodenal ulcer with hemorrhage **76**

532.1* Acute duodenal ulcer with perforation **77**

532.2* Acute duodenal ulcer with hemorrhage and perforation **76**

532.30 Acute duodenal ulcer without mention of hemorrhage, perforation, or obstruction **77**

532.31 Acute duodenal ulcer without mention of hemorrhage or perforation, with obstruction **77**

532.4* Chronic or unspecified duodenal ulcer with hemorrhage **76**

532.5* Chronic or unspecified duodenal ulcer with perforation **77**

532.6* Chronic or unspecified duodenal ulcer with hemorrhage and perforation **76**

532.70 Chronic duodenal ulcer without mention of hemorrhage, perforation, or obstruction **77**

532.71 Chronic duodenal ulcer without mention of hemorrhage or perforation, with obstruction **77**

532.90 Duodenal ulcer, unspecified as acute or chronic, without hemorrhage, perforation, or obstruction **77**

532.91 Duodenal ulcer, unspecified as acute or chronic, without mention of hemorrhage or perforation, with obstruction **77**

533.0* Acute peptic ulcer, unspecified site, with hemorrhage **76**

533.1* Acute peptic ulcer, unspecified site, with perforation **77**

533.2* Acute peptic ulcer, unspecified site, with hemorrhage and perforation **76**

533.30 Acute peptic ulcer, unspecified site, without mention of hemorrhage, perforation, or obstruction **77**

533.31 Acute peptic ulcer, unspecified site, without mention of hemorrhage and perforation, with obstruction **77**

533.4* Chronic or unspecified peptic ulcer, unspecified site, with hemorrhage **76**

533.5* Chronic or unspecified peptic ulcer, unspecified site, with perforation **77**

533.6* Chronic or unspecified peptic ulcer, unspecified site, with hemorrhage and perforation **76**

533.70 Chronic peptic ulcer, unspecified site, without mention of hemorrhage, perforation, or obstruction **77**

533.71 Chronic peptic ulcer of unspecified site without mention of hemorrhage or perforation, with obstruction **77**

533.90 Peptic ulcer, unspecified site, unspecified as acute or chronic, without mention of hemorrhage, perforation, or obstruction **77**

533.91 Peptic ulcer, unspecified site, unspecified as acute or chronic, without mention of hemorrhage or perforation, with obstruction **77**

534.0* Acute gastrojejunal ulcer with hemorrhage **76**

534.1* Acute gastrojejunal ulcer with perforation **77**

534.2* Acute gastrojejunal ulcer with hemorrhage and perforation **76**

534.3* Acute gastrojejunal ulcer without mention of hemorrhage or perforation **77**

534.4* Chronic or unspecified gastrojejunal ulcer with hemorrhage **76**

534.5* Chronic or unspecified gastrojejunal ulcer with perforation **77**

534.6* Chronic or unspecified gastrojejunal ulcer with hemorrhage and perforation **76**

534.7* Chronic gastrojejunal ulcer without mention of hemorrhage or perforation **77**

534.9* Gastrojejunal ulcer, unspecified as acute or chronic, without mention of hemorrhage or perforation **77**

535.00 Acute gastritis without mention of hemorrhage **78**

535.01 Acute gastritis with hemorrhage **76**

535.10 Atrophic gastritis without mention of hemorrhage **78**

535.11 Atrophic gastritis with hemorrhage **76**

535.20 Gastric mucosal hypertrophy without mention of hemorrhage **78**

535.21 Gastric mucosal hypertrophy with hemorrhage **76**

535.30 Alcoholic gastritis without mention of hemorrhage **78**

535.31 Alcoholic gastritis with hemorrhage **76**

535.40 Other specified gastritis without mention of hemorrhage **78**

535.41 Other specified gastritis with hemorrhage **76**

535.50 Unspecified gastritis and gastroduodenitis without mention of hemorrhage **78**

535.51 Unspecified gastritis and gastroduodenitis with hemorrhage **76**

535.60 Duodenitis without mention of hemorrhage **78**

535.61 Duodenitis with hemorrhage **76**

535.70 Eosinophilic gastritis without mention of hemorrhage **78**

535.71 Eosinophilic gastritis with hemorrhage **76**

536.0 Achlorhydria **78**

536.1 Acute dilatation of stomach **78, 165, 170**

536.2 Persistent vomiting **78**

536.3 Gastroparesis **78**

536.4* Gastrostomy complications **78**

536.8 Dyspepsia and other specified disorders of function of stomach **78**

536.9 Unspecified functional disorder of stomach **78**

537.0 Acquired hypertrophic pyloric stenosis **77**

537.1 Gastric diverticulum **78**

537.2 Chronic duodenal ileus **78**

537.3 Other obstruction of duodenum **77**

537.4 Fistula of stomach or duodenum **78**

537.5 Gastroptosis **78**

537.6 Hourglass stricture or stenosis of stomach **78**

537.81 Pylorospasm **78**

537.82 Angiodysplasia of stomach and duodenum (without mention of hemorrhage) **78**

537.83 Angiodysplasia of stomach and duodenum with hemorrhage **76**

537.84 Dieulafoy lesion (hemorrhagic) of stomach and duodenum **76**

537.89 Other specified disorder of stomach and duodenum **78**

537.9 Unspecified disorder of stomach and duodenum **78**

538 Gastrointestinal mucositis (ulcerative) **78**

539* Complications of bariatric procedures **78**

540.0 Acute appendicitis with generalized peritonitis **73, 76**

540.1 Acute appendicitis with peritoneal abscess **73, 76**

540.9 Acute appendicitis without mention of peritonitis **78**

541 Appendicitis, unqualified **78**

542 Other appendicitis **78**

543* Other diseases of appendix **78**

550.00 Inguinal hernia with gangrene, unilateral or unspecified, (not specified as recurrent) **166, 170**

550.02 Inguinal hernia with gangrene, bilateral **166, 170**

550.10 Inguinal hernia with obstruction, without mention of gangrene, unilateral or unspecified, (not specified as recurrent) **166, 170**

550.12 Inguinal hernia with obstruction, without mention gangrene, bilateral, (not specified as recurrent) **166, 170**

550* Inguinal hernia **78**

551.00 Femoral hernia with gangrene, unilateral or unspecified (not specified as recurrent) **166, 170**

551.02 Femoral hernia with gangrene, bilateral, (not specified as recurrent) **166, 170**

551.1	Umbilical hernia with gangrene **166, 170**
551.2*	Ventral hernia with gangrene **166, 170**
551.3	Diaphragmatic hernia with gangrene **166, 170**
551.8	Hernia of other specified sites, with gangrene **166, 170**
551.9	Hernia of unspecified site, with gangrene **166, 170**
551*	Other hernia of abdominal cavity, with gangrene **78**
552.0*	Femoral hernia with obstruction **78**
552.00	Unilateral or unspecified femoral hernia with obstruction **166, 170**
552.02	Bilateral femoral hernia with obstruction **166, 170**
552.1	Umbilical hernia with obstruction **78, 166, 170**
552.2*	Ventral hernia with obstruction **78, 166, 170**
552.3	Diaphragmatic hernia with obstruction **78, 166, 170**
552.8	Hernia of other specified site, with obstruction **78, 166, 170**
552.9	Hernia of unspecified site, with obstruction **78, 166, 170**
553.0*	Femoral hernia without mention of obstruction or gangrene **79**
553.1	Umbilical hernia without mention of obstruction or gangrene **79**
553.2*	Ventral hernia without mention of obstruction or gangrene **79**
553.3	Diaphragmatic hernia without mention of obstruction or gangrene **78**
553.8	Hernia of other specified sites of abdominal cavity without mention of obstruction or gangrene **79**
553.9	Hernia of unspecified site of abdominal cavity without mention of obstruction or gangrene **79**
555*	Regional enteritis **77**
556*	Ulcerative colitis **77**
557.0	Acute vascular insufficiency of intestine **166, 170**
557*	Vascular insufficiency of intestine **79**
558.1	Gastroenteritis and colitis due to radiation **79, 230**
558.2	Toxic gastroenteritis and colitis **79, 166, 170, 230**
558.3	Gastroenteritis and colitis, allergic **78**
558.4*	Eosinophilic gastroenteritis and colitis **78, 230**
558.9	Other and unspecified noninfectious gastroenteritis and colitis **78, 230**
560.0	Intussusception **166, 170**
560.1	Paralytic ileus **166, 170**
560.2	Volvulus **166, 170**
560.30	Unspecified impaction of intestine **166, 170**
560.32	Fecal impaction **166, 170**
560.39	Impaction of intestine, other **166, 170**
560.89	Other specified intestinal obstruction **166, 170**
560.9	Unspecified intestinal obstruction **166, 170**
560*	Intestinal obstruction without mention of hernia **77**
562.00	Diverticulosis of small intestine (without mention of hemorrhage) **78**
562.01	Diverticulitis of small intestine (without mention of hemorrhage) **78**
562.02	Diverticulosis of small intestine with hemorrhage **76**
562.03	Diverticulitis of small intestine with hemorrhage **76**
562.10	Diverticulosis of colon (without mention of hemorrhage) **78**
562.11	Diverticulitis of colon (without mention of hemorrhage) **78**
562.12	Diverticulosis of colon with hemorrhage **76**
562.13	Diverticulitis of colon with hemorrhage **76**
564.0*	Constipation **78**
564.1	Irritable bowel syndrome **78**
564.2	Postgastric surgery syndromes **78**
564.3	Vomiting following gastrointestinal surgery **78**
564.4	Other postoperative functional disorders **78**
564.5	Functional diarrhea **78**
564.6	Anal spasm **78**

564.7	Megacolon, other than Hirschsprung's **79**
564.8*	Other specified functional disorders of intestine **78**
564.9	Unspecified functional disorder of intestine **78**
565*	Anal fissure and fistula **79**
566	Abscess of anal and rectal regions **79, 166, 170**
567.0	Peritonitis in infectious diseases classified elsewhere **76**
567.1	Pneumococcal peritonitis **76**
567.2*	Other suppurative peritonitis **76**
567.3*	Retroperitoneal infections **76**
567.81	Choleperitonitis **79**
567.82	Sclerosing mesenteritis **79**
567.89	Other specified peritonitis **76**
567.9	Unspecified peritonitis **76**
567*	Peritonitis and retroperitoneal infections **166, 170**
568.81	Hemoperitoneum (nontraumatic) **166, 170**
568*	Other disorders of peritoneum **79**
569.0	Anal and rectal polyp **79**
569.1	Rectal prolapse **79**
569.2	Stenosis of rectum and anus **79**
569.3	Hemorrhage of rectum and anus **76, 166, 170**
569.4*	Other specified disorders of rectum and anus **79**
569.5	Abscess of intestine **76**
569.6*	Colostomy and enterostomy complications **79**
569.7*	Complications of intestinal pouch **79, 166, 170**
569.81	Fistula of intestine, excluding rectum and anus **79**
569.82	Ulceration of intestine **79**
569.83	Perforation of intestine **79, 166, 170**
569.84	Angiodysplasia of intestine (without mention of hemorrhage) **79**
569.85	Angiodysplasia of intestine with hemorrhage **76**
569.86	Dieulafoy lesion (hemorrhagic) of intestine **79**
569.87	Vomiting of fecal matter **79**
569.89	Other specified disorder of intestines **79**
569.9	Unspecified disorder of intestine **79**
570	Acute and subacute necrosis of liver **83, 166, 170**
571.0	Alcoholic fatty liver **83**
571.1	Acute alcoholic hepatitis **82**
571.2	Alcoholic cirrhosis of liver **82**
571.3	Unspecified alcoholic liver damage **82**
571.4*	Chronic hepatitis **83**
571.5	Cirrhosis of liver without mention of alcohol **82**
571.6	Biliary cirrhosis **82**
571.8	Other chronic nonalcoholic liver disease **83**
571.9	Unspecified chronic liver disease without mention of alcohol **83**
572.0	Abscess of liver **166, 170**
572.1	Portal pyemia **166, 170**
572.2	Hepatic encephalopathy **166, 170**
572.4	Hepatorenal syndrome **166, 170**
572*	Liver abscess and sequelae of chronic liver disease **83**
573.0	Chronic passive congestion of liver **83**
573.1	Hepatitis in viral diseases classified elsewhere **83**
573.2	Hepatitis in other infectious diseases classified elsewhere **83**
573.3	Unspecified hepatitis **83, 166, 170**
573.4	Hepatic infarction **83, 166, 170**
573.5	Hepatopulmonary syndrome **54**
573.8	Other specified disorders of liver **83**
573.9	Unspecified disorder of liver **83**
574*	Cholelithiasis **83**
575*	Other disorders of gallbladder **83**
576.1	Cholangitis **166, 170**

576*	Other disorders of biliary tract **83**	
577.0	Acute pancreatitis **166**, **170**	
577.2	Cyst and pseudocyst of pancreas **166**, **170**	
577*	Diseases of pancreas **83**	
578*	Gastrointestinal hemorrhage **76**, **166**, **170**	
579.3	Other and unspecified postsurgical nonabsorption **166**, **170**	
579.9	Unspecified intestinal malabsorption **230**	
579*	Intestinal malabsorption **78**	
580*	Acute glomerulonephritis **120**, **166**, **170**, **230**	
581*	Nephrotic syndrome **120**, **230**	
582*	Chronic glomerulonephritis **120**, **230**	
583*	Nephritis and nephropathy, not specified as acute or chronic **120**, **230**	
584.5	Acute kidney failure with lesion of tubular necrosis **118**	
584.6	Acute kidney failure with lesion of renal cortical necrosis **118**	
584.7	Acute kidney failure with lesion of medullary [papillary] necrosis **118**	
584.8	Acute kidney failure with other specified pathological lesion in kidney **118**	
584.9	Acute kidney failure, unspecified **118**	
584*	Acute kidney failure **166**, **170**	
585*	Chronic kidney disease (CKD) **2**, **118**	
586	Unspecified renal failure **118**, **119**	
587	Unspecified renal sclerosis **120**	
588*	Disorders resulting from impaired renal function **120**	
589*	Small kidney of unknown cause **120**	
590.1*	Acute pyelonephritis **166**, **170**	
590.2	Renal and perinephric abscess **166**, **170**	
590.3	Pyeloureteritis cystica **166**, **170**	
590.8*	Other pyelonephritis or pyonephrosis, not specified as acute or chronic **166**, **170**	
590.9	Unspecified infection of kidney **166**, **170**	
590*	Infections of kidney **119**	
591	Hydronephrosis **119**, **166**, **170**	
592*	Calculus of kidney and ureter **119**	
593.0	Nephroptosis **120**	
593.1	Hypertrophy of kidney **120**	
593.2	Acquired cyst of kidney **120**	
593.3	Stricture or kinking of ureter **119**	
593.4	Other ureteric obstruction **119**	
593.5	Hydroureter **119**, **166**, **170**	
593.6	Postural proteinuria **120**	
593.7*	Vesicoureteral reflux **120**	
593.8*	Other specified disorders of kidney and ureter **120**	
593.9	Unspecified disorder of kidney and ureter **120**	
594.0	Calculus in diverticulum of bladder **120**	
594.1	Other calculus in bladder **119**	
594.2	Calculus in urethra **119**	
594.8	Other lower urinary tract calculus **119**	
594.9	Unspecified calculus of lower urinary tract **119**	
595.0	Acute cystitis **119**, **166**, **170**	
595.1	Chronic interstitial cystitis **119**	
595.2	Other chronic cystitis **119**	
595.3	Trigonitis **119**	
595.4	Cystitis in diseases classified elsewhere **119**, **166**, **170**	
595.81	Cystitis cystica **119**, **166**, **170**	
595.82	Irradiation cystitis **120**	
595.89	Other specified types of cystitis **119**, **166**, **170**	
595.9	Unspecified cystitis **119**, **166**, **170**	
596.0	Bladder neck obstruction **166**, **170**	

596.1	Intestinovesical fistula **166**, **170**
596.2	Vesical fistula, not elsewhere classified **166**, **170**
596.4	Atony of bladder **166**, **170**
596.6	Nontraumatic rupture of bladder **166**, **170**
596.7	Hemorrhage into bladder wall **166**, **170**
596*	Other disorders of bladder **120**
597.0	Urethral abscess **166**, **170**
597*	Urethritis, not sexually transmitted, and urethral syndrome **119**
598*	Urethral stricture **120**
599.0	Urinary tract infection, site not specified **119**, **166**, **170**
599.1	Urethral fistula **120**
599.2	Urethral diverticulum **120**
599.3	Urethral caruncle **120**
599.4	Urethral false passage **120**
599.5	Prolapsed urethral mucosa **120**
599.6*	Urinary obstruction **120**, **166**, **170**
599.7*	Hematuria **119**, **166**, **170**
599.8*	Other specified disorder of urethra and urinary tract **120**
599.9	Unspecified disorder of urethra and urinary tract **120**
600*	Hyperplasia of prostate **123**
601*	Inflammatory diseases of prostate **124**
602*	Other disorders of prostate **124**
603.0	Encysted hydrocele **124**
603.1	Infected hydrocele **124**
603.8	Other specified type of hydrocele **124**
603.9	Unspecified hydrocele **124**
604*	Orchitis and epididymitis **124**
605	Redundant prepuce and phimosis **124**, **172**
606*	Male infertility **124**
607.0	Leukoplakia of penis **124**
607.1	Balanoposthitis **124**
607.2	Other inflammatory disorders of penis **124**
607.3	Priapism **124**
607.81	Balanitis xerotica obliterans **124**
607.82	Vascular disorders of penis **124**
607.83	Edema of penis **124**
607.84	Impotence of organic origin **124**
607.85	Peyronie's disease **124**
607.89	Other specified disorder of penis **124**
607.9	Unspecified disorder of penis **124**
608.0	Seminal vesiculitis **124**
608.1	Spermatocele **124**
608.2*	Torsion of testis **124**
608.3	Atrophy of testis **124**
608.4	Other inflammatory disorder of male genital organs **124**
608.8*	Other specified disorder of male genital organs **124**
608.9	Unspecified disorder of male genital organs **124**
610*	Benign mammary dysplasias **106**
611*	Other disorders of breast **106**
612*	Deformity and disproportion of reconstructed breast **106**
614.0	Acute salpingitis and oophoritis **130**
614.1	Chronic salpingitis and oophoritis **130**
614.2	Salpingitis and oophoritis not specified as acute, subacute, or chronic **130**
614.3	Acute parametritis and pelvic cellulitis **130**
614.4	Chronic or unspecified parametritis and pelvic cellulitis **130**
614.5	Acute or unspecified pelvic peritonitis, female **130**
614.6	Pelvic peritoneal adhesions, female (postoperative) (postinfection) **130**

614.7	Other chronic pelvic peritonitis, female **130**	
614.8	Other specified inflammatory disease of female pelvic organs and tissues **130**	
614.9	Unspecified inflammatory disease of female pelvic organs and tissues **130**	
614*	Inflammatory disease of ovary, fallopian tube, pelvic cellular tissue, and peritoneum **127**	
615*	Inflammatory diseases of uterus, except cervix **127**, **130**	
616.0	Cervicitis and endocervicitis **127**, **130**	
616.1*	Vaginitis and vulvovaginitis **127**, **130**	
616.2	Cyst of Bartholin's gland **127**, **130**	
616.3	Abscess of Bartholin's gland **127**, **130**	
616.4	Other abscess of vulva **127**, **130**	
616.5*	Ulceration of vulva **127**, **130**	
616.8*	Other specified inflammatory diseases of cervix, vagina, and vulva **127**, **130**	
616.9	Unspecified inflammatory disease of cervix, vagina, and vulva **127**, **130**	
617.0	Endometriosis of uterus **127**, **130**	
617.1	Endometriosis of ovary **127**, **130**	
617.2	Endometriosis of fallopian tube **127**, **130**	
617.3	Endometriosis of pelvic peritoneum **127**, **130**	
617.4	Endometriosis of rectovaginal septum and vagina **127**, **130**	
617.5	Endometriosis of intestine **78**	
617.6	Endometriosis in scar of skin **108**	
617.8	Endometriosis of other specified sites **127**, **130**	
617.9	Endometriosis, site unspecified **127**, **130**	
618*	Genital prolapse **127**, **130**	
619.0	Urinary-genital tract fistula, female **127**, **130**	
619.1	Digestive-genital tract fistula, female **79**, **166**, **170**	
619.2	Genital tract-skin fistula, female **127**, **130**	
619.8	Other specified fistula involving female genital tract **127**, **130**, **166**, **170**	
619.9	Unspecified fistula involving female genital tract **127**, **130**	
620.7	Hematoma of broad ligament **166**, **170**	
620*	Noninflammatory disorders of ovary, fallopian tube, and broad ligament **127**, **130**	
621*	Disorders of uterus, not elsewhere classified **127**, **130**	
622*	Noninflammatory disorders of cervix **127**, **130**	
623.8	Other specified noninflammatory disorder of vagina **172**	
623*	Noninflammatory disorders of vagina **127**, **130**	
624*	Noninflammatory disorders of vulva and perineum **127**, **130**	
625.0	Dyspareunia **130**	
625.1	Vaginismus **130**	
625.2	Mittelschmerz **130**	
625.3	Dysmenorrhea **130**	
625.4	Premenstrual tension syndromes **130**	
625.5	Pelvic congestion syndrome **130**	
625.6	Female stress incontinence **130**	
625.70	Vulvodynia, unspecified **130**	
625.71	Vulvar vestibulitis **130**	
625.79	Other vulvodynia **130**	
625.8	Other specified symptom associated with female genital organs **130**	
625.9	Unspecified symptom associated with female genital organs **130**	
625*	Pain and other symptoms associated with female genital organs **127**	
626*	Disorders of menstruation and other abnormal bleeding from female genital tract **127**, **130**	
627*	Menopausal and postmenopausal disorders **127**, **130**	
628*	Female infertility **127**, **130**	

629.0	Hematocele, female, not elsewhere classified **130**
629.1	Hydrocele, canal of Nuck **130**
629.2*	Female genital mutilation status **130**
629.3*	Complication of implanted vaginal mesh and other prosthetic materials **130**
629.8*	Other specified disorders of female genital organs **130**
629.9	Unspecified disorder of female genital organs **130**
629*	Other disorders of female genital organs **127**
630	Hydatidiform mole **154**, **157**
631*	Other abnormal product of conception **154**, **157**
632	Missed abortion **153**
633*	Ectopic pregnancy **153**
634*	Spontaneous abortion **153**
635*	Legally induced abortion **153**
636*	Illegally induced abortion **153**
637*	Abortion, unspecified as to legality **153**
638*	Failed attempted abortion **153**
639*	Complications following abortion or ectopic and molar pregnancies **151**
640.00	Threatened abortion, unspecified as to episode of care **153**
640.01	Threatened abortion, delivered **134**, **141**, **147**
640.03	Threatened abortion, antepartum **153**
640.80	Other specified hemorrhage in early pregnancy, unspecified as to episode of care **153**
640.81	Other specified hemorrhage in early pregnancy, delivered **134**, **141**, **147**
640.83	Other specified hemorrhage in early pregnancy, antepartum **153**
640.90	Unspecified hemorrhage in early pregnancy, unspecified as to episode of care **153**
640.91	Unspecified hemorrhage in early pregnancy, delivered **134**, **141**, **147**
640.93	Unspecified hemorrhage in early pregnancy, antepartum **153**
641.00	Placenta previa without hemorrhage, unspecified as to episode of care **159**
641.01	Placenta previa without hemorrhage, with delivery **134**, **140**, **145**
641.03	Placenta previa without hemorrhage, antepartum **154**, **157**
641.10	Hemorrhage from placenta previa, unspecified as to episode of care **159**
641.11	Hemorrhage from placenta previa, with delivery **134**, **140**, **145**
641.13	Hemorrhage from placenta previa, antepartum **154**, **157**
641.20	Premature separation of placenta, unspecified as to episode of care **159**
641.21	Premature separation of placenta, with delivery **134**, **140**, **145**
641.23	Premature separation of placenta, antepartum **154**, **157**
641.30	Antepartum hemorrhage associated with coagulation defects, unspecified as to episode of care **156**, **159**
641.31	Antepartum hemorrhage associated with coagulation defects, with delivery **134**, **140**, **145**
641.33	Antepartum hemorrhage associated with coagulation defect, antepartum **154**, **156**
641.80	Other antepartum hemorrhage, unspecified as to episode of care **159**
641.81	Other antepartum hemorrhage, with delivery **134**, **140**, **145**
641.83	Other antepartum hemorrhage, antepartum **154**, **157**
641.90	Unspecified antepartum hemorrhage, unspecified as to episode of care **159**
641.91	Unspecified antepartum hemorrhage, with delivery **134**, **140**, **145**
641.93	Unspecified antepartum hemorrhage, antepartum **154**, **157**
642.00	Benign essential hypertension complicating pregnancy, childbirth, and the puerperium, unspecified as to episode of care **159**

642.01	Benign essential hypertension with delivery **134**, **140**, **145**
642.02	Benign essential hypertension, with delivery, with current postpartum complication **134**, **140**, **145**
642.03	Benign essential hypertension antepartum **154**, **156**
642.04	Benign essential hypertension, complicating pregnancy, childbirth, and the puerperium, postpartum condition or complication **151**
642.10	Hypertension secondary to renal disease, complicating pregnancy, childbirth, and the puerperium, unspecified as to episode of care **159**
642.11	Hypertension secondary to renal disease, with delivery **134**, **140**, **145**
642.12	Hypertension secondary to renal disease, with delivery, with current postpartum complication **134**, **140**, **146**
642.13	Hypertension secondary to renal disease, antepartum **154**, **156**
642.14	Hypertension secondary to renal disease, complicating pregnancy, childbirth, and the puerperium, postpartum condition or complication **151**
642.20	Other pre-existing hypertension complicating pregnancy, childbirth, and the puerperium, unspecified as to episode of care **159**
642.21	Other pre-existing hypertension, with delivery **134**, **140**, **146**
642.22	Other pre-existing hypertension, with delivery, with current postpartum complication **134**, **140**, **146**
642.23	Other pre-existing hypertension, antepartum **154**, **156**
642.24	Other pre-existing hypertension complicating pregnancy, childbirth, and the puerperium, postpartum condition or complication **151**
642.30	Transient hypertension of pregnancy, unspecified as to episode of care **159**
642.31	Transient hypertension of pregnancy, with delivery **134**, **141**, **147**
642.32	Transient hypertension of pregnancy, with delivery, with current postpartum complication **134**, **141**, **147**
642.33	Transient hypertension of pregnancy, antepartum **154**, **157**
642.34	Transient hypertension of pregnancy, postpartum condition or complication **151**
642.40	Mild or unspecified pre-eclampsia, unspecified as to episode of care **159**
642.41	Mild or unspecified pre-eclampsia, with delivery **134**, **140**, **146**
642.42	Mild or unspecified pre-eclampsia, with delivery, with current postpartum complication **134**, **140**, **146**
642.43	Mild or unspecified pre-eclampsia, antepartum **154**, **156**
642.44	Mild or unspecified pre-eclampsia, postpartum condition or complication **151**
642.50	Severe pre-eclampsia, unspecified as to episode of care **156**, **159**
642.51	Severe pre-eclampsia, with delivery **134**, **140**, **146**
642.52	Severe pre-eclampsia, with delivery, with current postpartum complication **134**, **140**, **146**
642.53	Severe pre-eclampsia, antepartum **154**, **156**
642.54	Severe pre-eclampsia, postpartum condition or complication **151**
642.60	Eclampsia complicating pregnancy, childbirth or the puerperium, unspecified as to episode of care **156**, **159**
642.61	Eclampsia, with delivery **134**, **140**, **146**
642.62	Eclampsia, with delivery, with current postpartum complication **134**, **140**, **146**
642.63	Eclampsia, antepartum **154**, **156**
642.64	Eclampsia, postpartum condition or complication **151**
642.70	Pre-eclampsia or eclampsia superimposed on pre-existing hypertension, complicating pregnancy, childbirth, or the puerperium, unspecified as to episode of care **156**, **159**
642.71	Pre-eclampsia or eclampsia superimposed on pre-existing hypertension, with delivery **134**, **140**, **146**
642.72	Pre-eclampsia or eclampsia superimposed on pre-existing hypertension, with delivery, with current postpartum complication **134**, **140**, **146**
642.73	Pre-eclampsia or eclampsia superimposed on pre-existing hypertension, antepartum **154**, **156**
642.74	Pre-eclampsia or eclampsia superimposed on pre-existing hypertension, postpartum condition or complication **151**
642.90	Unspecified hypertension complicating pregnancy, childbirth, or the puerperium, unspecified as to episode of care **159**
642.91	Unspecified hypertension, with delivery **134**, **140**, **146**
642.92	Unspecified hypertension, with delivery, with current postpartum complication **134**, **140**, **146**
642.93	Unspecified hypertension antepartum **154**, **156**
642.94	Unspecified hypertension complicating pregnancy, childbirth, or the puerperium, postpartum condition or complication **151**
643.00	Mild hyperemesis gravidarum, unspecified as to episode of care **156**, **159**
643.01	Mild hyperemesis gravidarum, delivered **134**, **141**, **147**
643.03	Mild hyperemesis gravidarum, antepartum **154**, **156**
643.10	Hyperemesis gravidarum with metabolic disturbance, unspecified as to episode of care **156**, **159**
643.11	Hyperemesis gravidarum with metabolic disturbance, delivered **134**, **141**, **147**
643.13	Hyperemesis gravidarum with metabolic disturbance, antepartum **154**, **156**
643.20	Late vomiting of pregnancy, unspecified as to episode of care **156**, **159**
643.21	Late vomiting of pregnancy, delivered **134**, **141**, **147**
643.23	Late vomiting of pregnancy, antepartum **154**, **156**
643.80	Other vomiting complicating pregnancy, unspecified as to episode of care **156**, **159**
643.81	Other vomiting complicating pregnancy, delivered **134**, **141**, **147**
643.83	Other vomiting complicating pregnancy, antepartum **154**, **156**
643.90	Unspecified vomiting of pregnancy, unspecified as to episode of care **156**, **159**
643.91	Unspecified vomiting of pregnancy, delivered **134**, **141**, **147**
643.93	Unspecified vomiting of pregnancy, antepartum **154**, **156**
644.00	Threatened premature labor, unspecified as to episode of care **153**
644.03	Threatened premature labor, antepartum **153**
644.10	Other threatened labor, unspecified as to episode of care **153**
644.13	Other threatened labor, antepartum **153**
644.20	Early onset of delivery, unspecified as to episode of care **154**, **157**
644.21	Early onset of delivery, delivered, with or without mention of antepartum condition **134**, **141**, **147**
645.10	Post term pregnancy, unspecified as to episode of care or not applicable **159**
645.11	Post term pregnancy, delivered, with or without mention of antepartum condition **134**, **141**, **147**
645.13	Post term pregnancy, antepartum condition or complication **154**, **157**
645.20	Prolonged pregnancy, unspecified as to episode of care or not applicable **159**
645.21	Prolonged pregnancy, delivered, with or without mention of antepartum condition **134**, **141**, **147**
645.23	Prolonged pregnancy, antepartum condition or complication **154**, **157**
646.00	Papyraceous fetus, unspecified as to episode of care **134**, **141**, **147**
646.01	Papyraceous fetus, delivered, with or without mention of antepartum condition **134**, **141**, **147**
646.03	Papyraceous fetus, antepartum **154**, **157**

646.10	Edema or excessive weight gain in pregnancy, unspecified as to episode of care **156**, **159**
646.11	Edema or excessive weight gain in pregnancy, with delivery, with or without mention of antepartum complication **134**, **141**, **147**
646.12	Edema or excessive weight gain in pregnancy, with delivery, with current postpartum complication **134**, **141**, **147**
646.13	Edema or excessive weight gain, antepartum **154**, **156**
646.14	Edema or excessive weight gain in pregnancy, without mention of hypertension, postpartum condition or complication **151**
646.20	Unspecified renal disease in pregnancy, unspecified as to episode of care **156**, **159**
646.21	Unspecified renal disease in pregnancy, with delivery **134**, **141**, **147**
646.22	Unspecified renal disease in pregnancy, with delivery, with current postpartum complication **134**, **141**, **147**
646.23	Unspecified antepartum renal disease **154**, **156**
646.24	Unspecified renal disease in pregnancy, without mention of hypertension, postpartum condition or complication **151**
646.30	Pregnancy complication, recurrent pregnancy loss, unspecified as to episode of care **159**
646.31	Pregnancy complication, recurrent pregnancy loss, with or without mention of antepartum condition **134**, **141**, **147**
646.33	Pregnancy complication, recurrent pregnancy loss, antepartum condition or complication **154**, **157**
646.40	Peripheral neuritis in pregnancy, unspecified as to episode of care **159**
646.41	Peripheral neuritis in pregnancy, with delivery **134**, **141**, **147**
646.42	Peripheral neuritis in pregnancy, with delivery, with current postpartum complication **134**, **141**, **147**
646.43	Peripheral neuritis antepartum **154**, **156**
646.44	Peripheral neuritis in pregnancy, postpartum condition or complication **151**
646.50	Asymptomatic bacteriuria in pregnancy, unspecified as to episode of care **159**
646.51	Asymptomatic bacteriuria in pregnancy, with delivery **134**, **141**, **147**
646.52	Asymptomatic bacteriuria in pregnancy, with delivery, with current postpartum complication **134**, **141**, **147**
646.53	Asymptomatic bacteriuria antepartum **154**, **157**
646.54	Asymptomatic bacteriuria in pregnancy, postpartum condition or complication **151**
646.60	Infections of genitourinary tract in pregnancy, unspecified as to episode of care **156**, **159**
646.61	Infections of genitourinary tract in pregnancy, with delivery **134**, **141**, **147**
646.62	Infections of genitourinary tract in pregnancy, with delivery, with current postpartum complication **134**, **141**, **147**
646.63	Infections of genitourinary tract antepartum **154**, **156**
646.64	Infections of genitourinary tract in pregnancy, postpartum condition or complication **152**
646.70	Liver and biliary tract disorders in pregnancy, unspecified as to episode of care or not applicable **156**, **159**
646.71	Liver and biliary tract disorders in pregnancy, delivered, with or without mention of antepartum condition **134**, **142**, **147**
646.73	Liver and biliary tract disorders in pregnancy, antepartum condition or complication **154**, **156**
646.80	Other specified complication of pregnancy, unspecified as to episode of care **156**, **159**
646.81	Other specified complication of pregnancy, with delivery **134**, **142**, **147**
646.82	Other specified complications of pregnancy, with delivery, with current postpartum complication **134**, **142**, **147**
646.83	Other specified complication, antepartum **154**, **156**
646.84	Other specified complications of pregnancy, postpartum condition or complication **152**
646.90	Unspecified complication of pregnancy, unspecified as to episode of care **159**
646.91	Unspecified complication of pregnancy, with delivery **134**, **142**, **147**
646.93	Unspecified complication of pregnancy, antepartum **154**, **157**
647.00	Maternal syphilis, complicating pregnancy, childbirth, or the puerperium, unspecified as to episode of care **159**
647.01	Maternal syphilis, complicating pregnancy, with delivery **134**, **140**, **146**
647.02	Maternal syphilis, complicating pregnancy, with delivery, with current postpartum complication **134**, **140**, **146**
647.03	Maternal syphilis, antepartum **154**, **156**
647.04	Maternal syphilis complicating pregnancy, childbrith, or the puerperium, postpartum condition or complication **152**
647.10	Maternal gonorrhea complicating pregnancy, childbirth, or the puerperium, unspecified as to episode of care **159**
647.11	Maternal gonorrhea with delivery **134**, **140**, **146**
647.12	Maternal gonorrhea, with delivery, with current postpartum complication **134**, **140**, **146**
647.13	Maternal gonorrhea, antepartum **154**, **156**
647.14	Maternal gonorrhea complicating pregnancy, childbrith, or the puerperium, postpartum condition or complication **152**
647.20	Other maternal venereal diseases, complicating pregnancy, childbirth, or the puerperium, unspecified as to episode of care **159**
647.21	Other maternal venereal diseases with delivery **134**, **140**, **146**
647.22	Other maternal venereal diseases with delivery, with current postpartum complication **134**, **140**, **146**
647.23	Other maternal venereal diseases, antepartum condition or complication **154**, **156**
647.24	Other venereal diseases complicating pregnancy, childbrith, or the puerperium, postpartum condition or complication **152**
647.30	Maternal tuberculosis complicating pregnancy, childbirth, or the puerperium, unspecified as to episode of care **159**
647.31	Maternal tuberculosis with delivery **134**, **140**, **146**
647.32	Maternal tuberculosis with delivery, with current postpartum complication **134**, **140**, **146**
647.33	Maternal tuberculosis, antepartum **154**, **156**
647.34	Maternal tuberculosis complicating pregnancy, childbirth, or the puerperium, postpartum condition or complication **152**
647.40	Maternal malaria complicating pregnancy, childbirth or the puerperium, unspecified as to episode of care **159**
647.41	Maternal malaria with delivery **134**, **140**, **146**
647.42	Maternal malaria with delivery, with current postpartum complication **134**, **140**, **146**
647.43	Maternal malaria, antepartum **154**, **156**
647.44	Maternal malaria, complicating pregnancy, childbirth, or the puerperium, postpartum condition or complication **152**
647.50	Maternal rubella complicating pregnancy, childbirth, or the puerperium, unspecified as to episode of care **159**
647.51	Maternal rubella with delivery **134**, **140**, **146**
647.52	Maternal rubella with delivery, with current postpartum complication **134**, **140**, **146**
647.53	Maternal rubella, antepartum **154**, **156**
647.54	Maternal rubella complicating pregnancy, childbirth, or the puerperium, postpartum condition or complication **152**
647.60	Other maternal viral disease complicating pregnancy, childbirth, or the puerperium, unspecified as to episode of care **159**
647.61	Other maternal viral disease with delivery **134**, **140**, **146**
647.62	Other maternal viral disease with delivery, with current postpartum complication **134**, **140**, **146**
647.63	Other maternal viral disease, antepartum **154**, **156**
647.64	Other maternal viral diseases complicating pregnancy, childbirth, or the puerperium, postpartum condition or complication **152**

647.80 Other specified maternal infectious and parasitic disease complicating pregnancy, childbirth, or the puerperium, unspecified as to episode of care **159**

647.81 Other specified maternal infectious and parasitic disease with delivery **134**, **140**, **146**

647.82 Other specified maternal infectious and parasitic disease with delivery, with current postpartum complication **134**, **140**, **146**

647.83 Other specified maternal infectious and parasitic disease, antepartum **154**, **156**

647.84 Other specified maternal infectious and parasitic diseases complicating pregnancy, childbirth, or the puerperium, postpartum condition or complication **152**

647.90 Unspecified maternal infection or infestation complicating pregnancy, childbirth, or the puerperium, unspecified as to episode of care **159**

647.91 Unspecified maternal infection or infestation with delivery **134**, **140**, **146**

647.92 Unspecified maternal infection or infestation with delivery, with current postpartum complication **134**, **140**, **146**

647.93 Unspecified maternal infection or infestation, antepartum **154**, **156**

647.94 Unspecified maternal infection or infestation complicating pregnancy, childbirth, or the puerperium, postpartum condition or complication **152**

648.00 Maternal diabetes mellitus, complicating pregnancy, childbirth, or the puerperium, unspecified as to episode of care **159**

648.01 Maternal diabetes mellitus with delivery **134**, **140**, **146**

648.02 Maternal diabetes mellitus with delivery, with current postpartum complication **134**, **140**, **146**

648.03 Maternal diabetes mellitus, antepartum **154**, **156**

648.04 Maternal diabetes mellitus, complicating pregnancy, childbirth, or the puerperium, postpartum condition or complication **152**

648.10 Maternal thyroid dysfunction complicating pregnancy, childbirth, or the puerperium, unspecified as to episode of care or not applicable **159**

648.11 Maternal thyroid dysfunction with delivery, with or without mention of antepartum condition **134**, **142**, **147**

648.12 Maternal thyroid dysfunction with delivery, with current postpartum complication **134**, **142**, **147**

648.13 Maternal thyroid dysfunction, antepartum condition or complication **154**, **156**

648.14 Maternal thyroid dysfunction complicating pregnancy, childbirth, or the puerperium, postpartum condition or complication **152**

648.20 Maternal anemia of mother, complicating pregnancy, childbirth, or the puerperium, unspecified as to episode of care **159**

648.21 Maternal anemia, with delivery **134**, **142**, **147**

648.22 Maternal anemia with delivery, with current postpartum complication **134**, **142**, **147**

648.23 Maternal anemia, antepartum **154**, **156**

648.24 Maternal anemia complicating pregnancy, childbirth, or the puerperium, postpartum condition or complication **152**

648.30 Maternal drug dependence complicating pregnancy, childbirth, or the puerperium, unspecified as to episode of care **159**

648.31 Maternal drug dependence, with delivery **134**, **142**, **147**

648.32 Maternal drug dependence, with delivery, with current postpartum complication **134**, **142**, **147**

648.33 Maternal drug dependence, antepartum **154**, **156**

648.34 Maternal drug dependence complicating pregnancy, childbirth, or the puerperium, postpartum condition or complication **152**

648.40 Maternal mental disorders, complicating pregnancy, childbirth, or the puerperium, unspecified as to episode of care **159**

648.41 Maternal mental disorders, with delivery **134**, **142**, **147**

648.42 Maternal mental disorders, with delivery, with current postpartum complication **134**, **142**, **147**

648.43 Maternal mental disorders, antepartum **154**, **156**

648.44 Maternal mental disorders complicating pregnancy, childbirth, or the puerperium, postpartum condition or complication **152**

648.50 Maternal congenital cardiovascular disorders, complicating pregnancy, childbirth, or the puerperium, unspecified as to episode of care **159**

648.51 Maternal congenital cardiovascular disorders, with delivery **134**, **140**, **146**

648.52 Maternal congenital cardiovascular disorders, with delivery, with current postpartum complication **134**, **140**, **146**

648.53 Maternal congenital cardiovascular disorders, antepartum **154**, **156**

648.54 Maternal congenital cardiovascular disorders complicating pregnancy, childbirth, or the puerperium, postpartum condition or complication **152**

648.60 Other maternal cardiovascular diseases complicating pregnancy, childbirth, or the puerperium, unspecified as to episode of care **159**

648.61 Other maternal cardiovascular diseases, with delivery **134**, **140**, **146**

648.62 Other maternal cardiovascular diseases, with delivery, with current postpartum complication **134**, **140**, **146**

648.63 Other maternal cardiovascular diseases, antepartum **154**, **156**

648.64 Other maternal cardiovascular diseases complicating pregnancy, childbirth, or the puerperium, postpartum condition or complication **152**

648.70 Bone and joint disorders of maternal back, pelvis, and lower limbs, complicating pregnancy, childbirth, or the puerperium, unspecified as to episode of care **159**

648.71 Bone and joint disorders of maternal back, pelvis, and lower limbs, with delivery **134**, **142**, **147**

648.72 Bone and joint disorders of maternal back, pelvis, and lower limbs, with delivery, with current postpartum complication **134**, **142**, **147**

648.73 Bone and joint disorders of maternal back, pelvis, and lower limbs, antepartum **154**, **156**

648.74 Bone and joint disorders of maternal back, pelvis, and lower limbs complicating pregnancy, childbirth, or the puerperium, postpartum condition or complication **152**

648.80 Abnormal maternal glucose tolerance, complicating pregnancy, childbirth, or the puerperium, unspecified as to episode of care **159**

648.81 Abnormal maternal glucose tolerance, with delivery **134**, **142**, **148**

648.82 Abnormal maternal glucose tolerance, with delivery, with current postpartum complication **135**, **142**, **148**

648.83 Abnormal maternal glucose tolerance, antepartum **154**, **156**

648.84 Abnormal maternal glucose tolerance complicating pregnancy, childbirth, or the puerperium, postpartum condition or complication **152**

648.90 Other current maternal conditions classifiable elsewhere, complicating pregnancy, childbirth, or the puerperium, unspecified as to episode of care **159**

648.91 Other current maternal conditions classifiable elsewhere, with delivery **135**, **142**, **148**

648.92 Other current maternal conditions classifiable elsewhere, with delivery, with current postpartum complication **135**, **142**, **148**

648.93 Other current maternal conditions classifiable elsewhere, antepartum **154**, **156**

648.94 Other current maternal conditions classifiable elsewhere complicating pregnancy, childbirth, or the puerperium, postpartum condition or complication **152**

649.00 Tobacco use disorder complicating pregnancy, childbirth, or the puerperium, unspecified as to episode of care or not applicable **159**

649.01 Tobacco use disorder complicating pregnancy, childbirth, or the puerperium, delivered, with or without mention of antepartum condition **135**, **142**, **148**

*Code Range

649.02	Tobacco use disorder complicating pregnancy, childbirth, or the puerperium, delivered, with mention of postpartum complication **135**, **142**, **148**
649.03	Tobacco use disorder complicating pregnancy, childbirth, or the puerperium, antepartum condition or complication **154**, **157**
649.04	Tobacco use disorder complicating pregnancy, childbirth, or the puerperium, postpartum condition or complication **152**
649.10	Obesity complicating pregnancy, childbirth, or the puerperium, unspecified as to episode of care or not applicable **160**
649.11	Obesity complicating pregnancy, childbirth, or the puerperium, delivered, with or without mention of antepartum condition **135**, **142**, **148**
649.12	Obesity complicating pregnancy, childbirth, or the puerperium, delivered, with mention of postpartum complication **135**, **142**, **148**
649.13	Obesity complicating pregnancy, childbirth, or the puerperium, antepartum condition or complication **154**, **157**
649.14	Obesity complicating pregnancy, childbirth, or the puerperium, postpartum condition or complication **152**
649.20	Bariatric surgery status complicating pregnancy, childbirth, or the puerperium, unspecified as to episode of care or not applicable **160**
649.21	Bariatric surgery status complicating pregnancy, childbirth, or the puerperium, delivered, with or without mention of antepartum condition **135**, **142**, **148**
649.22	Bariatric surgery status complicating pregnancy, childbirth, or the puerperium, delivered, with mention of postpartum complication **135**, **142**, **148**
649.23	Bariatric surgery status complicating pregnancy, childbirth, or the puerperium, antepartum condition or complication **154**, **157**
649.24	Bariatric surgery status complicating pregnancy, childbirth, or the puerperium, postpartum condition or complication **152**
649.30	Coagulation defects complicating pregnancy, childbirth, or the puerperium, unspecified as to episode of care or not applicable **160**
649.31	Coagulation defects complicating pregnancy, childbirth, or the puerperium, delivered, with or without mention of antepartum condition **135**, **142**, **148**
649.32	Coagulation defects complicating pregnancy, childbirth, or the puerperium, delivered, with mention of postpartum complication **135**, **142**, **148**
649.33	Coagulation defects complicating pregnancy, childbirth, or the puerperium, antepartum condition or complication **154**, **157**
649.34	Coagulation defects complicating pregnancy, childbirth, or the puerperium, postpartum condition or complication **152**
649.40	Epilepsy complicating pregnancy, childbirth, or the puerperium, unspecified as to episode of care or not applicable **160**
649.41	Epilepsy complicating pregnancy, childbirth, or the puerperium, delivered, with or without mention of antepartum condition **135**, **142**, **148**
649.42	Epilepsy complicating pregnancy, childbirth, or the puerperium, delivered, with mention of postpartum complication **135**, **142**, **148**
649.43	Epilepsy complicating pregnancy, childbirth, or the puerperium, antepartum condition or complication **154**, **157**
649.44	Epilepsy complicating pregnancy, childbirth, or the puerperium, postpartum condition or complication **152**
649.50	Spotting complicating pregnancy, unspecified as to episode of care or not applicable **160**
649.51	Spotting complicating pregnancy, delivered, with or without mention of antepartum condition **135**, **142**, **148**
649.53	Spotting complicating pregnancy, antepartum condition or complication **154**, **157**
649.60	Uterine size date discrepancy, unspecified as to episode of care or not applicable **160**
649.61	Uterine size date discrepancy, delivered, with or without mention of antepartum condition **135**, **142**, **148**

649.62	Uterine size date discrepancy, delivered, with mention of postpartum complication **135**, **142**, **148**
649.63	Uterine size date discrepancy, antepartum condition or complication **154**, **157**
649.64	Uterine size date discrepancy, postpartum condition or complication **152**
649.70	Cervical shortening, unspecified as to episode of care or not applicable **160**
649.71	Cervical shortening, delivered, with or without mention of antepartum condition **135**, **142**, **148**
649.73	Cervical shortening, antepartum condition or complication **154**, **157**
649.8*	Onset (spontaneous) of labor after 37 completed weeks of gestation but before 39 completed weeks gestation, with delivery by (planned) cesarean section **135**, **140**, **148**
649.81	Onset (spontaneous) of labor after 37 completed weeks of gestation but before 39 completed weeks gestation, with delivery by (planned) cesarean section, delivered, with or without mention of antepartum condition **142**
649.82	Onset (spontaneous) of labor after 37 completed weeks of gestation but before 39 completed weeks gestation, with delivery by (planned) cesarean section, delivered, with mention of postpartum complication **142**
650	Normal delivery **135**, **142**, **148**
651.00	Twin pregnancy, unspecified as to episode of care **160**
651.01	Twin pregnancy, delivered **135**, **142**, **148**
651.03	Twin pregnancy, antepartum **154**, **157**
651.10	Triplet pregnancy, unspecified as to episode of care **160**
651.11	Triplet pregnancy, delivered **135**, **142**, **148**
651.13	Triplet pregnancy, antepartum **154**, **157**
651.20	Quadruplet pregnancy, unspecified as to episode of care **160**
651.21	Quadruplet pregnancy, delivered **135**, **142**, **148**
651.23	Quadruplet pregnancy, antepartum **154**, **157**
651.30	Twin pregnancy with fetal loss and retention of one fetus, unspecified as to episode of care or not applicable **160**
651.31	Twin pregnancy with fetal loss and retention of one fetus, delivered **135**, **142**, **148**
651.33	Twin pregnancy with fetal loss and retention of one fetus, antepartum **154**, **157**
651.40	Triplet pregnancy with fetal loss and retention of one or more, unspecified as to episode of care or not applicable **160**
651.41	Triplet pregnancy with fetal loss and retention of one or more, delivered **135**, **142**, **148**
651.43	Triplet pregnancy with fetal loss and retention of one or more, antepartum **154**, **157**
651.50	Quadruplet pregnancy with fetal loss and retention of one or more, unspecified as to episode of care or not applicable **160**
651.51	Quadruplet pregnancy with fetal loss and retention of one or more, delivered **135**, **142**, **148**
651.53	Quadruplet pregnancy with fetal loss and retention of one or more, antepartum **154**, **157**
651.60	Other multiple pregnancy with fetal loss and retention of one or more fetus(es), unspecified as to episode of care or not applicable **160**
651.61	Other multiple pregnancy with fetal loss and retention of one or more fetus(es), delivered **135**, **142**, **148**
651.63	Other multiple pregnancy with fetal loss and retention of one or more fetus(es), antepartum **154**, **157**
651.70	Multiple gestation following (elective) fetal reduction, unspecified as to episode of care or not applicable **160**
651.71	Multiple gestation following (elective) fetal reduction, delivered, with or without mention of antepartum condition **135**, **142**, **148**
651.73	Multiple gestation following (elective) fetal reduction, antepartum condition or complication **154**, **157**

*Code Range

651.80 Other specified multiple gestation, unspecified as to episode of care **160**

651.81 Other specified multiple gestation, delivered **135**, **142**, **148**

651.83 Other specified multiple gestation, antepartum **154**, **157**

651.90 Unspecified multiple gestation, unspecified as to episode of care **160**

651.91 Unspecified multiple gestation, delivered **135**, **142**, **148**

651.93 Unspecified multiple gestation, antepartum **154**, **157**

652.00 Unstable lie of fetus, unspecified as to episode of care **160**

652.01 Unstable lie of fetus, delivered **135**, **142**, **148**

652.03 Unstable lie of fetus, antepartum **154**, **157**

652.10 Breech or other malpresentation successfully converted to cephalic presentation, unspecified as to episode of care **160**

652.11 Breech or other malpresentation successfully converted to cephalic presentation, delivered **135**, **142**, **148**

652.13 Breech or other malpresentation successfully converted to cephalic presentation, antepartum **154**, **157**

652.20 Breech presentation without mention of version, unspecified as to episode of care **160**

652.21 Breech presentation without mention of version, delivered **135**, **142**, **148**

652.23 Breech presentation without mention of version, antepartum **154**, **157**

652.30 Transverse or oblique fetal presentation, unspecified as to episode of care **160**

652.31 Transverse or oblique fetal presentation, delivered **135**, **142**, **148**

652.33 Transverse or oblique fetal presentation, antepartum **154**, **157**

652.40 Fetal face or brow presentation, unspecified as to episode of care **160**

652.41 Fetal face or brow presentation, delivered **135**, **142**, **148**

652.43 Fetal face or brow presentation, antepartum **154**, **157**

652.50 High fetal head at term, unspecified as to episode of care **160**

652.51 High fetal head at term, delivered **135**, **142**, **148**

652.53 High fetal head at term, antepartum **154**, **157**

652.60 Multiple gestation with malpresentation of one fetus or more, unspecified as to episode of care **160**

652.61 Multiple gestation with malpresentation of one fetus or more, delivered **135**, **142**, **148**

652.63 Multiple gestation with malpresentation of one fetus or more, antepartum **154**, **157**

652.70 Prolapsed arm of fetus, unspecified as to episode of care **160**

652.71 Prolapsed arm of fetus, delivered **135**, **142**, **148**

652.73 Prolapsed arm of fetus, antepartum condition or complication **154**, **157**

652.80 Other specified malposition or malpresentation of fetus, unspecified as to episode of care **160**

652.81 Other specified malposition or malpresentation of fetus, delivered **135**, **142**, **148**

652.83 Other specified malposition or malpresentation of fetus, antepartum **154**, **157**

652.90 Unspecified malposition or malpresentation of fetus, unspecified as to episode of care **160**

652.91 Unspecified malposition or malpresentation of fetus, delivered **135**, **142**, **148**

652.93 Unspecified malposition or malpresentation of fetus, antepartum **154**, **157**

653.00 Major abnormality of bony pelvis, not further specified in pregnancy, unspecified as to episode of care **160**

653.01 Major abnormality of bony pelvis, not further specified, delivered **135**, **142**, **148**

653.03 Major abnormality of bony pelvis, not further specified, antepartum **154**, **157**

653.10 Generally contracted pelvis in pregnancy, unspecified as to episode of care in pregnancy **160**

653.11 Generally contracted pelvis in pregnancy, delivered **135**, **142**, **148**

653.13 Generally contracted pelvis in pregnancy, antepartum **154**, **157**

653.20 Inlet contraction of pelvis in pregnancy, unspecified as to episode of care in pregnancy **160**

653.21 Inlet contraction of pelvis in pregnancy, delivered **135**, **142**, **148**

653.23 Inlet contraction of pelvis in pregnancy, antepartum **154**, **157**

653.30 Outlet contraction of pelvis in pregnancy, unspecified as to episode of care in pregnancy **160**

653.31 Outlet contraction of pelvis in pregnancy, delivered **135**, **142**, **148**

653.33 Outlet contraction of pelvis in pregnancy, antepartum **154**, **157**

653.40 Fetopelvic disproportion, unspecified as to episode of care **160**

653.41 Fetopelvic disproportion, delivered **135**, **142**, **148**

653.43 Fetopelvic disproportion, antepartum **154**, **157**

653.50 Unusually large fetus causing disproportion, unspecified as to episode of care **160**

653.51 Unusually large fetus causing disproportion, delivered **135**, **142**, **148**

653.53 Unusually large fetus causing disproportion, antepartum **154**, **157**

653.60 Hydrocephalic fetus causing disproportion, unspecified as to episode of care **160**

653.61 Hydrocephalic fetus causing disproportion, delivered **135**, **142**, **148**

653.63 Hydrocephalic fetus causing disproportion, antepartum **154**, **157**

653.70 Other fetal abnormality causing disproportion, unspecified as to episode of care **160**

653.71 Other fetal abnormality causing disproportion, delivered **135**, **142**, **148**

653.73 Other fetal abnormality causing disproportion, antepartum **154**, **157**

653.80 Fetal disproportion of other origin, unspecified as to episode of care **160**

653.81 Fetal disproportion of other origin, delivered **135**, **142**, **148**

653.83 Fetal disproportion of other origin, antepartum **154**, **157**

653.90 Unspecified fetal disproportion, unspecified as to episode of care **160**

653.91 Unspecified fetal disproportion, delivered **135**, **142**, **148**

653.93 Unspecified fetal disproportion, antepartum **154**, **157**

654.00 Congenital abnormalities of pregnant uterus, unspecified as to episode of care **160**

654.01 Congenital abnormalities of pregnant uterus, delivered **135**, **142**, **148**

654.02 Congenital abnormalities of pregnant uterus, delivered, with mention of postpartum complication **135**, **142**, **148**

654.03 Congenital abnormalities of pregnant uterus, antepartum **154**, **157**

654.04 Congenital abnormalities of uterus, postpartum condition or complication **152**

654.10 Tumors of body of pregnant uterus, unspecified as to episode of care in pregnancy **160**

654.11 Tumors of body of uterus, delivered **135**, **142**, **148**

654.12 Tumors of body of uterus, delivered, with mention of postpartum complication **135**, **142**, **148**

654.13 Tumors of body of uterus, antepartum condition or complication **154**, **157**

654.14 Tumors of body of uterus, postpartum condition or complication **152**

654.20 Previous cesarean delivery, unspecified as to episode of care or not applicable **160**

654.21 Previous cesarean delivery, delivered, with or without mention of antepartum condition **135**, **142**, **148**

654.23   Previous cesarean delivery, antepartum condition or complication **154**, **157**

654.30   Retroverted and incarcerated gravid uterus, unspecified as to episode of care **160**

654.31   Retroverted and incarcerated gravid uterus, delivered **135**, **142**, **148**

654.32   Retroverted and incarcerated gravid uterus, delivered, with mention of postpartum complication **135**, **142**, **148**

654.33   Retroverted and incarcerated gravid uterus, antepartum **154**, **157**

654.34   Retroverted and incarcerated gravid uterus, postpartum condition or complication **152**

654.40   Other abnormalities in shape or position of gravid uterus and of neighboring structures, unspecified as to episode of care **160**

654.41   Other abnormalities in shape or position of gravid uterus and of neighboring structures, delivered **135**, **142**, **148**

654.42   Other abnormalities in shape or position of gravid uterus and of neighboring structures, delivered, with mention of postpartum complication **135**, **142**, **148**

654.43   Other abnormalities in shape or position of gravid uterus and of neighboring structures, antepartum **154**, **157**

654.44   Other abnormalities in shape or position of gravid uterus and of neighboring structures, postpartum condition or complication **152**

654.50   Cervical incompetence, unspecified as to episode of care in pregnancy **160**

654.51   Cervical incompetence, delivered **135**, **142**, **148**

654.52   Cervical incompetence, delivered, with mention of postpartum complication **135**, **142**, **148**

654.53   Cervical incompetence, antepartum condition or complication **154**, **157**

654.54   Cervical incompetence, postpartum condition or complication **152**

654.60   Other congenital or acquired abnormality of cervix, unspecified as to episode of care in pregnancy **160**

654.61   Other congenital or acquired abnormality of cervix, with delivery **135**, **142**, **148**

654.62   Other congenital or acquired abnormality of cervix, delivered, with mention of postpartum complication **135**, **143**, **148**

654.63   Other congenital or acquired abnormality of cervix, antepartum condition or complication **154**, **157**

654.64   Other congenital or acquired abnormality of cervix, postpartum condition or complication **152**

654.70   Congenital or acquired abnormality of vagina, unspecified as to episode of care in pregnancy **160**

654.71   Congenital or acquired abnormality of vagina, with delivery **135**, **143**, **148**

654.72   Congenital or acquired abnormality of vagina, delivered, with mention of postpartum complication **135**, **143**, **148**

654.73   Congenital or acquired abnormality of vagina, antepartum condition or complication **155**, **157**

654.74   Congenital or acquired abnormality of vagina, postpartum condition or complication **152**

654.80   Congenital or acquired abnormality of vulva, unspecified as to episode of care in pregnancy **160**

654.81   Congenital or acquired abnormality of vulva, with delivery **135**, **143**, **148**

654.82   Congenital or acquired abnormality of vulva, delivered, with mention of postpartum complication **135**, **143**, **148**

654.83   Congenital or acquired abnormality of vulva, antepartum condition or complication **155**, **157**

654.84   Congenital or acquired abnormality of vulva, postpartum condition or complication **152**

654.90   Other and unspecified abnormality of organs and soft tissues of pelvis, unspecified as to episode of care in pregnancy **160**

654.91   Other and unspecified abnormality of organs and soft tissues of pelvis, with delivery **135**, **143**, **148**

654.92   Other and unspecified abnormality of organs and soft tissues of pelvis, delivered, with mention of postpartum complication **135**, **143**, **148**

654.93   Other and unspecified abnormality of organs and soft tissues of pelvis, antepartum condition or complication **155**, **157**

654.94   Other and unspecified abnormality of organs and soft tissues of pelvis, postpartum condition or complication **152**

655.00   Central nervous system malformation in fetus, unspecified as to episode of care in pregnancy **160**

655.01   Central nervous system malformation in fetus, with delivery **135**, **143**, **148**

655.03   Central nervous system malformation in fetus, antepartum **155**, **157**

655.10   Chromosomal abnormality in fetus, affecting management of mother, unspecified as to episode of care in pregnancy **160**

655.11   Chromosomal abnormality in fetus, affecting management of mother, with delivery **135**, **143**, **148**

655.13   Chromosomal abnormality in fetus, affecting management of mother, antepartum **155**, **157**

655.20   Hereditary disease in family possibly affecting fetus, affecting management of mother, unspecified as to episode of care in pregnancy **160**

655.21   Hereditary disease in family possibly affecting fetus, affecting management of mother, with delivery **135**, **143**, **148**

655.23   Hereditary disease in family possibly affecting fetus, affecting management of mother, antepartum condition or complication **155**, **157**

655.30   Suspected damage to fetus from viral disease in mother, affecting management of mother, unspecified as to episode of care in pregnancy **160**

655.31   Suspected damage to fetus from viral disease in mother, affecting management of mother, with delivery **135**, **143**, **148**

655.33   Suspected damage to fetus from viral disease in mother, affecting management of mother, antepartum condition or complication **155**, **157**

655.40   Suspected damage to fetus from other disease in mother, affecting management of mother, unspecified as to episode of care in pregnancy **160**

655.41   Suspected damage to fetus from other disease in mother, affecting management of mother, with delivery **135**, **143**, **148**

655.43   Suspected damage to fetus from other disease in mother, affecting management of mother, antepartum condition or complication **155**, **157**

655.50   Suspected damage to fetus from drugs, affecting management of mother, unspecified as to episode of care **160**

655.51   Suspected damage to fetus from drugs, affecting management of mother, delivered **135**, **143**, **148**

655.53   Suspected damage to fetus from drugs, affecting management of mother, antepartum **155**, **157**

655.60   Suspected damage to fetus from radiation, affecting management of mother, unspecified as to episode of care **160**

655.61   Suspected damage to fetus from radiation, affecting management of mother, delivered **135**, **143**, **148**

655.63   Suspected damage to fetus from radiation, affecting management of mother, antepartum condition or complication **155**, **157**

655.70   Decreased fetal movements, unspecified as to episode of care **160**

655.71   Decreased fetal movements, affecting management of mother, delivered **135**, **143**, **148**

655.73   Decreased fetal movements, affecting management of mother, antepartum condition or complication **155**, **157**

655.80   Other known or suspected fetal abnormality, not elsewhere classified, affecting management of mother, unspecified as to episode of care **160**

655.81	Other known or suspected fetal abnormality, not elsewhere classified, affecting management of mother, delivery **135**, **143**, **148**
655.83	Other known or suspected fetal abnormality, not elsewhere classified, affecting management of mother, antepartum condition or complication **155**, **157**
655.90	Unspecified fetal abnormality affecting management of mother, unspecified as to episode of care **160**
655.91	Unspecified fetal abnormality affecting management of mother, delivery **136**, **143**, **149**
655.93	Unspecified fetal abnormality affecting management of mother, antepartum condition or complication **155**, **157**
656.00	Fetal-maternal hemorrhage, unspecified as to episode of care in pregnancy **160**
656.01	Fetal-maternal hemorrhage, with delivery **136**, **143**, **149**
656.03	Fetal-maternal hemorrhage, antepartum condition or complication **155**, **157**
656.10	Rhesus isoimmunization unspecified as to episode of care in pregnancy **160**
656.11	Rhesus isoimmunization affecting management of mother, delivered **136**, **143**, **149**
656.13	Rhesus isoimmunization affecting management of mother, antepartum condition **155**, **157**
656.20	Isoimmunization from other and unspecified blood-group incompatibility, unspecified as to episode of care in pregnancy **160**
656.21	Isoimmunization from other and unspecified blood-group incompatibility, affecting management of mother, delivered **136**, **143**, **149**
656.23	Isoimmunization from other and unspecified blood-group incompatibility, affecting management of mother, antepartum **155**, **157**
656.30	Fetal distress affecting management of mother, unspecified as to episode of care **136**, **143**, **149**
656.31	Fetal distress affecting management of mother, delivered **136**, **143**, **149**
656.33	Fetal distress affecting management of mother, antepartum **155**, **157**
656.40	Intrauterine death affecting management of mother, unspecified as to episode of care **136**, **143**, **149**
656.41	Intrauterine death affecting management of mother, delivered **136**, **143**, **149**
656.43	Intrauterine death affecting management of mother, antepartum **155**, **157**
656.50	Poor fetal growth, affecting management of mother, unspecified as to episode of care **160**
656.51	Poor fetal growth, affecting management of mother, delivered **136**, **143**, **149**
656.53	Poor fetal growth, affecting management of mother, antepartum condition or complication **155**, **157**
656.60	Excessive fetal growth affecting management of mother, unspecified as to episode of care **160**
656.61	Excessive fetal growth affecting management of mother, delivered **136**, **143**, **149**
656.63	Excessive fetal growth affecting management of mother, antepartum **155**, **157**
656.70	Other placental conditions affecting management of mother, unspecified as to episode of care **160**
656.71	Other placental conditions affecting management of mother, delivered **136**, **143**, **149**
656.73	Other placental conditions affecting management of mother, antepartum **155**, **157**
656.80	Other specified fetal and placental problems affecting management of mother, unspecified as to episode of care **160**
656.81	Other specified fetal and placental problems affecting management of mother, delivered **136**, **143**, **149**
656.83	Other specified fetal and placental problems affecting management of mother, antepartum **155**, **157**
656.90	Unspecified fetal and placental problem affecting management of mother, unspecified as to episode of care **160**
656.91	Unspecified fetal and placental problem affecting management of mother, delivered **136**, **143**, **149**
656.93	Unspecified fetal and placental problem affecting management of mother, antepartum **155**, **158**
657.00	Polyhydramnios, unspecified as to episode of care **160**
657.01	Polyhydramnios, with delivery **136**, **143**, **149**
657.03	Polyhydramnios, antepartum complication **155**, **158**
658.00	Oligohydramnios, unspecified as to episode of care **160**
658.01	Oligohydramnios, delivered **136**, **143**, **149**
658.03	Oligohydramnios, antepartum **155**, **158**
658.10	Premature rupture of membranes in pregnancy, unspecified as to episode of care **136**, **143**, **149**
658.11	Premature rupture of membranes in pregnancy, delivered **136**, **143**, **149**
658.13	Premature rupture of membranes in pregnancy, antepartum **155**, **158**
658.20	Delayed delivery after spontaneous or unspecified rupture of membranes, unspecified as to episode of care **136**, **143**, **149**
658.21	Delayed delivery after spontaneous or unspecified rupture of membranes, delivered **136**, **143**, **149**
658.23	Delayed delivery after spontaneous or unspecified rupture of membranes, antepartum **155**, **158**
658.30	Delayed delivery after artificial rupture of membranes, unspecified as to episode of care **136**, **143**, **149**
658.31	Delayed delivery after artificial rupture of membranes, delivered **136**, **143**, **149**
658.33	Delayed delivery after artificial rupture of membranes, antepartum **155**, **158**
658.40	Infection of amniotic cavity, unspecified as to episode of care **136**, **143**, **149**
658.41	Infection of amniotic cavity, delivered **136**, **143**, **149**
658.43	Infection of amniotic cavity, antepartum **155**, **158**
658.80	Other problem associated with amniotic cavity and membranes, unspecified as to episode of care **160**
658.81	Other problem associated with amniotic cavity and membranes, delivered **136**, **143**, **149**
658.83	Other problem associated with amniotic cavity and membranes, antepartum **155**, **158**
658.90	Unspecified problem associated with amniotic cavity and membranes, unspecified as to episode of care **161**
658.91	Unspecified problem associated with amniotic cavity and membranes, delivered **136**, **143**, **149**
658.93	Unspecified problem associated with amniotic cavity and membranes, antepartum **155**, **158**
659.00	Failed mechanical induction of labor, unspecified as to episode of care **136**, **143**, **149**
659.01	Failed mechanical induction of labor, delivered **136**, **143**, **149**
659.03	Failed mechanical induction of labor, antepartum **155**, **158**
659.10	Failed medical or unspecified induction of labor, unspecified as to episode of care **136**, **143**, **149**
659.11	Failed medical or unspecified induction of labor, delivered **136**, **143**, **149**
659.13	Failed medical or unspecified induction of labor, antepartum **155**, **158**
659.20	Unspecified maternal pyrexia during labor, unspecified as to episode of care **136**, **143**, **149**
659.21	Unspecified maternal pyrexia during labor, delivered **136**, **140**, **146**
659.23	Unspecified maternal pyrexia, antepartum **155**, **158**
659.30	Generalized infection during labor, unspecified as to episode of care **136**, **143**, **149**

*Code Range

© 2013 OptumInsight, Inc.

659.31	Generalized infection during labor, delivered **136**, **140**, **146**	
659.33	Generalized infection during labor, antepartum **155**, **158**	
659.40	Grand multiparity with current pregnancy, unspecified as to episode of care **161**	
659.41	Grand multiparity, delivered, with or without mention of antepartum condition **136**, **143**, **149**	
659.43	Grand multiparity with current pregnancy, antepartum **155**, **158**	
659.50	Elderly primigravida, unspecified as to episode of care **136**, **143**, **149**	
659.51	Elderly primigravida, delivered **136**, **143**, **149**	
659.53	Elderly primigravida, antepartum **155**, **158**	
659.60	Elderly multigravida, unspecified as to episode of care or not applicable **136**, **143**, **149**	
659.61	Elderly multigravida, delivered, with mention of antepartum condition **136**, **143**, **149**	
659.63	Elderly multigravida, with antepartum condition or complication **155**, **158**	
659.70	Abnormality in fetal heart rate or rhythm, unspecified as to episode of care or not applicable **136**, **143**, **149**	
659.71	Abnormality in fetal heart rate or rhythm, delivered, with or without mention of antepartum condition **136**, **143**, **149**	
659.73	Abnormality in fetal heart rate or rhythm, antepartum condition or complication **155**, **158**	
659.80	Other specified indication for care or intervention related to labor and delivery, unspecified as to episode of care **136**, **143**, **149**	
659.81	Other specified indication for care or intervention related to labor and delivery, delivered **136**, **143**, **149**	
659.83	Other specified indication for care or intervention related to labor and delivery, antepartum **155**, **158**	
659.90	Unspecified indication for care or intervention related to labor and delivery, unspecified as to episode of care **136**, **143**, **149**	
659.91	Unspecified indication for care or intervention related to labor and delivery, delivered **136**, **143**, **149**	
659.93	Unspecified indication for care or intervention related to labor and delivery, antepartum **155**, **158**	
660.00	Obstruction caused by malposition of fetus at onset of labor, unspecified as to episode of care **136**, **143**, **149**	
660.01	Obstruction caused by malposition of fetus at onset of labor, delivered **136**, **143**, **149**	
660.03	Obstruction caused by malposition of fetus at onset of labor, antepartum **155**, **158**	
660.10	Obstruction by bony pelvis during labor and delivery, unspecified as to episode of care **136**, **143**, **149**	
660.11	Obstruction by bony pelvis during labor and delivery, delivered **136**, **143**, **149**	
660.13	Obstruction by bony pelvis during labor and delivery, antepartum **155**, **158**	
660.20	Obstruction by abnormal pelvic soft tissues during labor and delivery, unspecified as to episode of care **136**, **143**, **149**	
660.21	Obstruction by abnormal pelvic soft tissues during labor and delivery, delivered **136**, **143**, **149**	
660.23	Obstruction by abnormal pelvic soft tissues during labor and delivery, antepartum **155**, **158**	
660.30	Deep transverse arrest and persistent occipitoposterior position during labor and delivery, unspecified as to episode of care **136**, **143**, **149**	
660.31	Deep transverse arrest and persistent occipitoposterior position during labor and deliver, delivered **136**, **143**, **149**	
660.33	Deep transverse arrest and persistent occipitoposterior position during labor and delivery, antepartum **155**, **158**	
660.40	Shoulder (girdle) dystocia during labor and delivery, unspecified as to episode of care **136**, **143**, **149**	
660.41	Shoulder (girdle) dystocia during labor and deliver, delivered **136**, **143**, **149**	

660.43	Shoulder (girdle) dystocia during labor and delivery, antepartum **155**, **158**
660.50	Locked twins during labor and delivery, unspecified as to episode of care in pregnancy **136**, **143**, **149**
660.51	Locked twins, delivered **136**, **143**, **149**
660.53	Locked twins, antepartum **155**, **158**
660.60	Unspecified failed trial of labor, unspecified as to episode **136**, **143**, **149**
660.61	Unspecified failed trial of labor, delivered **136**, **143**, **149**
660.63	Unspecified failed trial of labor, antepartum **155**, **158**
660.70	Unspecified failed forceps or vacuum extractor, unspecified as to episode of care **136**, **143**, **149**
660.71	Unspecified failed forceps or vacuum extractor, delivered **136**, **143**, **149**
660.73	Failed forceps or vacuum extractor, unspecified, antepartum **155**, **158**
660.80	Other causes of obstructed labor, unspecified as to episode of care **136**, **143**, **149**
660.81	Other causes of obstructed labor, delivered **136**, **143**, **149**
660.83	Other causes of obstructed labor, antepartum **155**, **158**
660.90	Unspecified obstructed labor, unspecified as to episode of care **136**, **143**, **149**
660.91	Unspecified obstructed labor, with delivery **136**, **143**, **149**
660.93	Unspecified obstructed labor, antepartum **155**, **158**
661.00	Primary uterine inertia, unspecified as to episode of care **136**, **143**, **149**
661.01	Primary uterine inertia, with delivery **136**, **143**, **149**
661.03	Primary uterine inertia, antepartum **155**, **158**
661.10	Secondary uterine inertia, unspecified as to episode of care **136**, **144**, **149**
661.11	Secondary uterine inertia, with delivery **136**, **144**, **149**
661.13	Secondary uterine inertia, antepartum **155**, **158**
661.20	Other and unspecified uterine inertia, unspecified as to episode of care **136**, **144**, **149**
661.21	Other and unspecified uterine inertia, with delivery **136**, **144**, **149**
661.23	Other and unspecified uterine inertia, antepartum **155**, **158**
661.30	Precipitate labor, unspecified as to episode of care **136**, **144**, **149**
661.31	Precipitate labor, with delivery **136**, **144**, **149**
661.33	Precipitate labor, antepartum **155**, **158**
661.40	Hypertonic, incoordinate, or prolonged uterine contractions, unspecified as to episode of care **136**, **144**, **149**
661.41	Hypertonic, incoordinate, or prolonged uterine contractions, with delivery **136**, **144**, **149**
661.43	Hypertonic, incoordinate, or prolonged uterine contractions, antepartum **155**, **158**
661.90	Unspecified abnormality of labor, unspecified as to episode of care **136**, **144**, **149**
661.91	Unspecified abnormality of labor, with delivery **136**, **144**, **149**
661.93	Unspecified abnormality of labor, antepartum **155**, **158**
662.00	Prolonged first stage of labor, unspecified as to episode of care **136**, **144**, **149**
662.01	Prolonged first stage of labor, delivered **136**, **144**, **149**
662.03	Prolonged first stage of labor, antepartum **155**, **158**
662.10	Unspecified prolonged labor, unspecified as to episode of care **136**, **144**, **149**
662.11	Unspecified prolonged labor, delivered **136**, **144**, **149**
662.13	Unspecified prolonged labor, antepartum **155**, **158**
662.20	Prolonged second stage of labor, unspecified as to episode of care **136**, **144**, **149**
662.21	Prolonged second stage of labor, delivered **136**, **144**, **149**
662.23	Prolonged second stage of labor, antepartum **155**, **158**

662.30   Delayed delivery of second twin, triplet, etc., unspecified as to episode of care **136**, **144**, **149**

662.31   Delayed delivery of second twin, triplet, etc., delivered **136**, **144**, **149**

662.33   Delayed delivery of second twin, triplet, etc., antepartum **155**, **158**

663.00   Prolapse of cord, complicating labor and delivery, unspecified as to episode of care **136**, **144**, **149**

663.01   Prolapse of cord, complicating labor and delivery, delivered **137**, **144**, **149**

663.03   Prolapse of cord, complicating labor and delivery, antepartum **155**, **158**

663.10   Cord around neck, with compression, complicating labor and delivery, unspecified as to episode of care **137**, **144**, **150**

663.11   Cord around neck, with compression, complicating labor and delivery, delivered **137**, **144**, **150**

663.13   Cord around neck, with compression, complicating labor and delivery, antepartum **155**, **158**

663.20   Other and unspecified cord entanglement, with compression, complicating labor and delivery, unspecified as to episode of care **137**, **144**, **150**

663.21   Other and unspecified cord entanglement, with compression, complicating labor and delivery, delivered **137**, **144**, **150**

663.23   Other and unspecified cord entanglement, with compression, complicating labor and delivery, antepartum **155**, **158**

663.30   Other and unspecified cord entanglement, without mention of compression, complicating labor and delivery, unspecified as to episode of care **137**, **144**, **150**

663.31   Other and unspecified cord entanglement, without mention of compression, complicating labor and delivery, delivered **137**, **144**, **150**

663.33   Other and unspecified cord entanglement, without mention of compression, complicating labor and delivery, antepartum **155**, **158**

663.40   Short cord complicating labor and delivery, unspecified as to episode of care **137**, **144**, **150**

663.41   Short cord complicating labor and delivery, delivered **137**, **144**, **150**

663.43   Short cord complicating labor and delivery, antepartum **155**, **158**

663.50   Vasa previa complicating labor and delivery, unspecified as to episode of care **137**, **144**, **150**

663.51   Vasa previa complicating labor and delivery, delivered **137**, **144**, **150**

663.53   Vasa previa complicating labor and delivery, antepartum **155**, **158**

663.60   Vascular lesions of cord complicating labor and delivery, unspecified as to episode of care **137**, **144**, **150**

663.61   Vascular lesions of cord complicating labor and delivery, delivered **137**, **144**, **150**

663.63   Vascular lesions of cord complicating labor and delivery, antepartum **155**, **158**

663.80   Other umbilical cord complications during labor and delivery, unspecified as to episode of care **137**, **144**, **150**

663.81   Other umbilical cord complications during labor and delivery, delivered **137**, **144**, **150**

663.83   Other umbilical cord complications during labor and delivery, antepartum **155**, **158**

663.90   Unspecified umbilical cord complication during labor and delivery, unspecified as to episode of care **137**, **144**, **150**

663.91   Unspecified umbilical cord complication during labor and delivery, delivered **137**, **144**, **150**

663.93   Unspecified umbilical cord complication during labor and delivery, antepartum **155**, **158**

664.00   First-degree perineal laceration, unspecified as to episode of care in pregnancy **137**, **144**, **150**

664.01   First-degree perineal laceration, with delivery **137**, **144**, **150**

664.04   First-degree perineal laceration, postpartum condition or complication **152**

664.10   Second-degree perineal laceration, unspecified as to episode of care in pregnancy **137**, **144**, **150**

664.11   Second-degree perineal laceration, with delivery **137**, **144**, **150**

664.14   Second-degree perineal laceration, postpartum condition or complication **152**

664.20   Third-degree perineal laceration, unspecified as to episode of care in pregnancy **137**, **144**, **150**

664.21   Third-degree perineal laceration, with delivery **137**, **144**, **150**

664.24   Third-degree perineal laceration, postpartum condition or complication **152**

664.30   Fourth-degree perineal laceration, unspecified as to episode of care in pregnancy **137**, **144**, **150**

664.31   Fourth-degree perineal laceration, with delivery **137**, **144**, **150**

664.34   Fourth-degree perineal laceration, postpartum condition or complication **152**

664.40   Unspecified perineal laceration, unspecified as to episode of care in pregnancy **137**, **144**, **150**

664.41   Unspecified perineal laceration, with delivery **137**, **144**, **150**

664.44   Unspecified perineal laceration, postpartum condition or complication **152**

664.50   Vulvar and perineal hematoma, unspecified as to episode of care in pregnancy **137**, **144**, **150**

664.51   Vulvar and perineal hematoma, with delivery **137**, **144**, **150**

664.54   Vulvar and perineal hematoma, postpartum condition or complication **152**

664.60   Anal sphincter tear complicating delivery, not associated with third-degree perineal laceration, unspecified as to episode of care or not applicable **137**, **144**, **150**

664.61   Anal sphincter tear complicating delivery, not associated with third-degree perineal laceration, delivered, with or without mention of antepartum condition **137**, **144**, **150**

664.64   Anal sphincter tear complicating delivery, not associated with third-degree perineal laceration, postpartum condition or complication **152**

664.80   Other specified trauma to perineum and vulva, unspecified as to episode of care in pregnancy **137**, **144**, **150**

664.81   Other specified trauma to perineum and vulva, with delivery **137**, **144**, **150**

664.84   Other specified trauma to perineum and vulva, postpartum condition or complication **152**

664.90   Unspecified trauma to perineum and vulva, unspecified as to episode of care in pregnancy **137**, **144**, **150**

664.91   Unspecified trauma to perineum and vulva, with delivery **137**, **144**, **150**

664.94   Unspecified trauma to perineum and vulva, postpartum condition or complication **152**

665.00   Rupture of uterus before onset of labor, unspecified as to episode of care **137**, **144**, **150**

665.01   Rupture of uterus before onset of labor, with delivery **137**, **144**, **150**

665.03   Rupture of uterus before onset of labor, antepartum **155**, **158**

665.10   Rupture of uterus during labor, unspecified as to episode **137**, **144**, **150**

665.11   Rupture of uterus during labor, with delivery **137**, **144**, **150**

665.20   Inversion of uterus, unspecified as to episode of care in pregnancy **137**, **144**, **150**

665.22   Inversion of uterus, delivered with postpartum complication **137**, **144**, **150**

665.24   Inversion of uterus, postpartum condition or complication **152**

665.30   Laceration of cervix, unspecified as to episode of care in pregnancy **137**, **144**, **150**

665.31   Laceration of cervix, with delivery **137**, **144**, **150**

665.34   Laceration of cervix, postpartum condition or complication **152**

*Code Range

665.40 High vaginal laceration, unspecified as to episode of care in pregnancy **137, 144, 150**

665.41 High vaginal laceration, with delivery **137, 144, 150**

665.44 High vaginal laceration, postpartum condition or complication **152**

665.50 Other injury to pelvic organs, unspecified as to episode of care in pregnancy **137, 144, 150**

665.51 Other injury to pelvic organs, with delivery **137, 144, 150**

665.54 Other injury to pelvic organs, postpartum condition or complication **152**

665.60 Damage to pelvic joints and ligaments, unspecified as to episode of care in pregnancy **137, 144, 150**

665.61 Damage to pelvic joints and ligaments, with delivery **137, 144, 150**

665.64 Damage to pelvic joints and ligaments, postpartum condition or complication **152**

665.70 Pelvic hematoma, unspecified as to episode of care **137, 144, 150**

665.71 Pelvic hematoma, with delivery **137, 144, 150**

665.72 Pelvic hematoma, delivered with postpartum complication **137, 144, 150**

665.74 Pelvic hematoma, postpartum condition or complication **152**

665.80 Other specified obstetrical trauma, unspecified as to episode of care **137, 144, 150**

665.81 Other specified obstetrical trauma, with delivery **137, 144, 150**

665.82 Other specified obstetrical trauma, delivered, with postpartum **137, 144, 150**

665.83 Other specified obstetrical trauma, antepartum **155, 158**

665.84 Other specified obstetrical trauma, postpartum condition or complication **152**

665.90 Unspecified obstetrical trauma, unspecified as to episode of care **137, 144, 150**

665.91 Unspecified obstetrical trauma, with delivery **137, 144, 150**

665.92 Unspecified obstetrical trauma, delivered, with postpartum complication **137, 144, 150**

665.93 Unspecified obstetrical trauma, antepartum **155, 158**

665.94 Unspecified obstetrical trauma, postpartum condition or complication **152**

666.00 Third-stage postpartum hemorrhage, unspecified as to episode of care **161**

666.02 Third-stage postpartum hemorrhage, with delivery **137, 140, 146**

666.04 Third-stage postpartum hemorrhage, postpartum condition or complication **152**

666.10 Other immediate postpartum hemorrhage, unspecified as to episode of care **161**

666.12 Other immediate postpartum hemorrhage, with delivery **137, 140, 146**

666.14 Other immediate postpartum hemorrhage, postpartum condition or complication **152**

666.20 Delayed and secondary postpartum hemorrhage, unspecified as to episode of care **161**

666.22 Delayed and secondary postpartum hemorrhage, with delivery **137, 140, 146**

666.24 Delayed and secondary postpartum hemorrhage, postpartum condition or complication **152**

666.30 Postpartum coagulation defects, unspecified as to episode of care **161**

666.32 Postpartum coagulation defects, with delivery **137, 140, 146**

666.34 Postpartum coagulation defects, postpartum condition or complication **152**

667.00 Retained placenta without hemorrhage, unspecified as to episode of care **161**

667.02 Retained placenta without hemorrhage, with delivery, with mention of postpartum complication **137, 140, 146**

667.04 Retained placenta without hemorrhage, postpartum condition or complication **152**

667.10 Retained portions of placenta or membranes, without hemorrhage, unspecified as to episode of care **161**

667.12 Retained portions of placenta or membranes, without hemorrhage, delivered, with mention of postpartum complication **137, 140, 146**

667.14 Retained portions of placenta or membranes, without hemorrhage, postpartum condition or complication **152**

668.00 Pulmonary complications of the administration of anesthesia or other sedation in labor and delivery, unspecified as to episode of care **137, 144, 150**

668.01 Pulmonary complications of the administration of anesthesia or other sedation in labor and delivery, delivered **137, 140, 146**

668.02 Pulmonary complications of the administration of anesthesia or other sedation in labor and delivery, delivered, with mention of postpartum complication **137, 140, 146**

668.03 Pulmonary complications of the administration of anesthesia or other sedation in labor and delivery, antepartum **155, 158**

668.04 Pulmonary complications of the administration of anesthesia or other sedation in labor and delivery, postpartum condition or complication **152**

668.10 Cardiac complications of the administration of anesthesia or other sedation in labor and delivery, unspecified as to episode of care **137, 144, 150**

668.11 Cardiac complications of the administration of anesthesia or other sedation in labor and delivery, delivered **137, 140, 146**

668.12 Cardiac complications of the administration of anesthesia or other sedation in labor and delivery, delivered, with mention of postpartum complication **137, 140, 146**

668.13 Cardiac complications of the administration of anesthesia or other sedation in labor and delivery, antepartum **155, 158**

668.14 Cardiac complications of the administration of anesthesia or other sedation in labor and delivery, postpartum condition or complication **152**

668.20 Central nervous system complications of the administration of anesthesia or other sedation in labor and delivery, unspecified as to episode of care **137, 144, 150**

668.21 Central nervous system complications of the administration of anesthesia or other sedation in labor and delivery, delivered **137, 141, 146**

668.22 Central nervous system complications of the administration of anesthesia or other sedation in labor and delivery, delivered, with mention of postpartum complication **137, 141, 146**

668.23 Central nervous system complications of the administration of anesthesia or other sedation in labor and delivery, antepartum **155, 158**

668.24 Central nervous system complications of the administration of anesthesia or other sedation in labor and delivery, postpartum condition or complication **152**

668.80 Other complications of the administration of anesthesia or other sedation in labor and delivery, unspecified as to episode of care **137, 144, 150**

668.81 Other complications of the administration of anesthesia or other sedation in labor and delivery, delivered **137, 141, 146**

668.82 Other complications of the administration of anesthesia or other sedation in labor and delivery, delivered, with mention of postpartum complication **137, 141, 146**

668.83 Other complications of the administration of anesthesia or other sedation in labor and delivery, antepartum **155, 158**

668.84 Other complications of the administration of anesthesia or other sedation in labor and delivery, postpartum condition or complication **153**

668.90 Unspecified complication of the administration of anesthesia or other sedation in labor and delivery, unspecified as to episode of care **138, 144, 150**

668.91 Unspecified complication of the administration of anesthesia or other sedation in labor and delivery, delivered **138, 141, 146**

668.92	Unspecified complication of the administration of anesthesia or other sedation in labor and delivery, delivered, with mention of postpartum complication **138**, **141**, **146**
668.93	Unspecified complication of the administration of anesthesia or other sedation in labor and delivery, antepartum **155**, **158**
668.94	Unspecified complication of the administration of anesthesia or other sedation in labor and delivery, postpartum condition or complication **153**
669.00	Maternal distress complicating labor and delivery, unspecified as to episode of care **138**, **145**, **150**
669.01	Maternal distress, with delivery, with or without mention of antepartum condition **138**, **145**, **150**
669.02	Maternal distress, with delivery, with mention of postpartum complication **138**, **145**, **150**
669.03	Maternal distress complicating labor and delivery, antepartum condition or complication **155**, **158**
669.04	Maternal distress complicating labor and delivery, postpartum condition or complication **153**
669.10	Shock during or following labor and delivery, unspecified as to episode of care **138**, **145**, **150**
669.11	Shock during or following labor and delivery, with delivery, with or without mention of antepartum condition **138**, **141**, **146**
669.12	Shock during or following labor and delivery, with delivery, with mention of postpartum complication **138**, **141**, **146**
669.13	Shock during or following labor and delivery, antepartum shock **155**, **158**
669.14	Shock during or following labor and delivery, postpartum condition or complication **153**
669.20	Maternal hypotension syndrome complicating labor and delivery, unspecified as to episode of care **138**, **145**, **150**
669.21	Maternal hypotension syndrome, with delivery, with or without mention of antepartum condition **138**, **145**, **150**
669.22	Maternal hypotension syndrome, with delivery, with mention of postpartum complication **138**, **145**, **150**
669.23	Maternal hypotension syndrome, antepartum **155**, **158**
669.24	Maternal hypotension syndrome, postpartum condition or complication **153**
669.30	Acute kidney failure following labor and delivery, unspecified as to episode of care or not applicable **138**, **145**, **150**
669.32	Acute kidney failure following labor and delivery, delivered, with mention of postpartum complication **138**, **141**, **146**
669.34	Acute kidney failure following labor and delivery, postpartum condition or complication **153**
669.40	Other complications of obstetrical surgery and procedures, unspecified as to episode of care **138**, **145**, **150**
669.41	Other complications of obstetrical surgery and procedures, with delivery, with or without mention of antepartum condition **138**, **141**, **146**
669.42	Other complications of obstetrical surgery and procedures, with delivery, with mention of postpartum complication **138**, **141**, **146**
669.43	Other complications of obstetrical surgery and procedures, antepartum condition or complication **156**, **158**
669.44	Other complications of obstetrical surgery and procedures, postpartum condition or complication **153**
669.50	Forceps or vacuum extractor delivery without mention of indication, unspecified as to episode of care **138**, **145**, **150**
669.51	Forceps or vacuum extractor delivery without mention of indication, delivered, with or without mention of antepartum condition **138**, **145**, **150**
669.60	Breech extraction, without mention of indication, unspecified as to episode of care **138**, **145**, **150**
669.61	Breech extraction, without mention of indication, delivered, with or without mention of antepartum condition **138**, **145**, **150**
669.70	Cesarean delivery, without mention of indication, unspecified as to episode of care **138**, **145**, **150**
669.71	Cesarean delivery, without mention of indication, delivered, with or without mention of antepartum condition **138**, **145**, **151**
669.80	Other complication of labor and delivery, unspecified as to episode of care **138**, **145**, **151**
669.81	Other complication of labor and delivery, delivered, with or without mention of antepartum condition **138**, **145**, **151**
669.82	Other complication of labor and delivery, delivered, with mention of postpartum complication **138**, **145**, **151**
669.83	Other complication of labor and delivery, antepartum condition or complication **156**, **158**
669.84	Other complication of labor and delivery, postpartum condition or complication **153**
669.90	Unspecified complication of labor and delivery, unspecified as to episode of care **138**, **145**, **151**
669.91	Unspecified complication of labor and delivery, with delivery, with or without mention of antepartum condition **138**, **145**, **151**
669.92	Unspecified complication of labor and delivery, with delivery, with mention of postpartum complication **138**, **145**, **151**
669.93	Unspecified complication of labor and delivery, antepartum condition or complication **156**, **158**
669.94	Unspecified complication of labor and delivery, postpartum condition or complication **153**
670.00	Major puerperal infection, unspecified, unspecified as to episode of care or not applicable **161**
670.02	Major puerperal infection, unspecified, delivered, with mention of postpartum complication **138**, **141**, **146**
670.04	Major puerperal infection, unspecified, postpartum condition or complication **153**
670.10	Puerperal endometritis, unspecified as to episode of care or not applicable **161**
670.12	Puerperal endometritis, delivered, with mention of postpartum complication **138**, **141**, **146**
670.14	Puerperal endometritis, postpartum condition or complication **153**
670.20	Puerperal sepsis, unspecified as to episode of care or not applicable **161**
670.22	Puerperal sepsis, delivered, with mention of postpartum complication **138**, **141**, **146**
670.24	Puerperal sepsis, postpartum condition or complication **153**
670.30	Puerperal septic thrombophlebitis, unspecified as to episode of care or not applicable **161**
670.32	Puerperal septic thrombophlebitis, delivered, with mention of postpartum complication **138**, **141**, **146**
670.34	Puerperal septic thrombophlebitis, postpartum condition or complication **153**
670.80	Other major puerperal infection, unspecified as to episode of care or not applicable **161**
670.82	Other major puerperal infection, delivered, with mention of postpartum complication **138**, **141**, **146**
670.84	Other major puerperal infection, postpartum condition or complication **153**
671.00	Varicose veins of legs complicating pregnancy and the puerperium, unspecified as to episode of care **161**
671.01	Varicose veins of legs, with delivery, with or without mention of antepartum condition **138**, **145**, **151**
671.02	Varicose veins of legs, with delivery, with mention of postpartum complication **138**, **145**, **151**
671.03	Varicose veins of legs, antepartum **156**, **158**
671.04	Varicose veins of legs, postpartum condition or complication **153**
671.10	Varicose veins of vulva and perineum complicating pregnancy and the puerperium, unspecified as to episode of care **161**
671.11	Varicose veins of vulva and perineum, with delivery, with or without mention of antepartum condition **138**, **145**, **151**
671.12	Varicose veins of vulva and perineum, with delivery, with mention of postpartum complication **138**, **145**, **151**

*Code Range

671.13	Varicose veins of vulva and perineum, antepartum **156**, **158**	
671.14	Varicose veins of vulva and perineum, postpartum condition or complication **153**	
671.20	Superficial thrombophlebitis complicating pregnancy and the puerperium, unspecified as to episode of care **161**	
671.21	Superficial thrombophlebitis with delivery, with or without mention of antepartum condition **138**, **145**, **151**	
671.22	Superficial thrombophlebitis with delivery, with mention of postpartum complication **138**, **145**, **151**	
671.23	Superficial thrombophlebitis, antepartum **156**, **158**	
671.24	Superficial thrombophlebitis, postpartum condition or complication **153**	
671.30	Deep phlebothrombosis, antepartum, unspecified as to episode of care **161**	
671.31	Deep phlebothrombosis, antepartum, with delivery **138**, **141**, **146**	
671.33	Deep phlebothrombosis, antepartum **156**, **158**	
671.40	Deep phlebothrombosis, postpartum, unspecified as to episode of care **161**	
671.42	Deep phlebothrombosis, postpartum, with delivery **138**, **141**, **146**	
671.44	Deep phlebothrombosis, postpartum condition or complication **153**	
671.50	Other phlebitis and thrombosis complicating pregnancy and the puerperium, unspecified as to episode of care **161**	
671.51	Other phlebitis and thrombosis with delivery, with or without mention of antepartum condition **138**, **141**, **146**	
671.52	Other phlebitis and thrombosis with delivery, with mention of postpartum complication **138**, **141**, **146**	
671.53	Other antepartum phlebitis and thrombosis **156**, **158**	
671.54	Other phlebitis and thrombosis, postpartum condition or complication **153**	
671.80	Other venous complication of pregnancy and the puerperium, unspecified as to episode of care **161**	
671.81	Other venous complication, with delivery, with or without mention of antepartum condition **138**, **145**, **151**	
671.82	Other venous complication, with delivery, with mention of postpartum complication **138**, **145**, **151**	
671.83	Other venous complication, antepartum **156**, **158**	
671.84	Other venous complications, postpartum condition or complication **153**	
671.90	Unspecified venous complication of pregnancy and the puerperium, unspecified as to episode of care **161**	
671.91	Unspecified venous complication, with delivery, with or without mention of antepartum condition **138**, **145**, **151**	
671.92	Unspecified venous complication, with delivery, with mention of postpartum complication **138**, **145**, **151**	
671.93	Unspecified venous complication, antepartum **156**, **158**	
671.94	Unspecified venous complication, postpartum condition or complication **153**	
672.00	Puerperal pyrexia of unknown origin, unspecified as to episode of care **161**	
672.02	Puerperal pyrexia of unknown origin, delivered, with mention of postpartum complication **138**, **141**, **146**	
672.04	Puerperal pyrexia of unknown origin, postpartum condition or complication **153**	
673.00	Obstetrical air embolism, unspecified as to episode of care **161**	
673.01	Obstetrical air embolism, with delivery, with or without mention of antepartum condition **138**, **141**, **146**	
673.02	Obstetrical air embolism, with delivery, with mention of postpartum complication **138**, **141**, **146**	
673.03	Obstetrical air embolism, antepartum condition or complication **156**, **158**	
673.04	Obstetrical air embolism, postpartum condition or complication **153**	

673.10	Amniotic fluid embolism, unspecified as to episode of care **161**
673.11	Amniotic fluid embolism, with delivery, with or without mention of antepartum condition **138**, **141**, **146**
673.12	Amniotic fluid embolism, with delivery, with mention of postpartum complication **138**, **141**, **146**
673.13	Amniotic fluid embolism, antepartum condition or complication **156**, **158**
673.14	Amniotic fluid embolism, postpartum condition or complication **153**
673.20	Obstetrical blood-clot embolism, unspecified as to episode of care **161**
673.21	Obstetrical blood-clot embolism, with delivery, with or without mention of antepartum condition **138**, **141**, **146**
673.22	Obstetrical blood-clot embolism, with mention of postpartum complication **138**, **141**, **146**
673.23	Obstetrical blood-clot embolism, antepartum **156**, **158**
673.24	Obstetrical blood-clot embolism, postpartum condition or complication **153**
673.30	Obstetrical pyemic and septic embolism, unspecified as to episode of care **161**
673.31	Obstetrical pyemic and septic embolism, with delivery, with or without mention of antepartum condition **138**, **141**, **147**
673.32	Obstetrical pyemic and septic embolism, with delivery, with mention of postpartum complication **138**, **141**, **147**
673.33	Obstetrical pyemic and septic embolism, antepartum **156**, **158**
673.34	Obstetrical pyemic and septic embolism, postpartum condition or complication **153**
673.80	Other obstetrical pulmonary embolism, unspecified as to episode of care **161**
673.81	Other obstetrical pulmonary embolism, with delivery, with or without mention of antepartum condition **138**, **141**, **147**
673.82	Other obstetrical pulmonary embolism, with delivery, with mention of postpartum complication **138**, **141**, **147**
673.83	Other obstetrical pulmonary embolism, antepartum **156**, **158**
673.84	Other obstetrical pulmonary embolism, postpartum condition or complication **153**
674.00	Cerebrovascular disorder occurring in pregnancy, childbirth, or the puerperium, unspecified as to episode of care **161**
674.01	Cerebrovascular disorder, with delivery, with or without mention of antepartum condition **138**, **141**, **147**
674.02	Cerebrovascular disorder, with delivery, with mention of postpartum complication **138**, **141**, **147**
674.03	Cerebrovascular disorder, antepartum **156**, **158**
674.04	Cerebrovascular disorders in the puerperium, postpartum condition or complication **153**
674.10	Disruption of cesarean wound, unspecified as to episode of care **161**
674.12	Disruption of cesarean wound, with delivery, with mention of postpartum complication **138**, **141**, **147**
674.14	Disruption of cesarean wound, postpartum condition or complication **153**
674.20	Disruption of perineal wound, unspecified as to episode of care in pregnancy **161**
674.22	Disruption of perineal wound, with delivery, with mention of postpartum complication **138**, **141**, **147**
674.24	Disruption of perineal wound, postpartum condition or complication **153**
674.30	Other complication of obstetrical surgical wounds, unspecified as to episode of care **161**
674.32	Other complication of obstetrical surgical wounds, with delivery, with mention of postpartum complication **138**, **141**, **147**
674.34	Other complications of obstetrical surgical wounds, postpartum condition or complication **153**
674.40	Placental polyp, unspecified as to episode of care **161**

674.42	Placental polyp, with delivery, with mention of postpartum complication **138**, **145**, **151**	675.92	Unspecified infection of the breast and nipple, delivered, with mention of postpartum complication **139**, **145**, **151**
674.44	Placental polyp, postpartum condition or complication **153**	675.93	Unspecified infection of the breast and nipple, antepartum **156**, **158**
674.50	Peripartum cardiomyopathy, unspecified as to episode of care or not applicable **161**	675.94	Unspecified infection of the breast and nipple, postpartum condition or complication **153**
674.51	Peripartum cardiomyopathy, delivered, with or without mention of antepartum condition **138**, **141**, **147**	676.00	Retracted nipple, unspecified as to prenatal or postnatal episode of care **161**
674.52	Peripartum cardiomyopathy, delivered, with mention of postpartum condition **138**, **141**, **147**	676.01	Retracted nipple, delivered, with or without mention of antepartum condition **139**, **145**, **151**
674.53	Peripartum cardiomyopathy, antepartum condition or complication **156**, **158**	676.02	Retracted nipple, delivered, with mention of postpartum complication **139**, **145**, **151**
674.54	Peripartum cardiomyopathy, postpartum condition or complication **153**	676.03	Retracted nipple, antepartum condition or complication **156**, **158**
674.80	Other complication of puerperium, unspecified as to episode of care **161**	676.04	Retracted nipple, postpartum condition or complication **153**
674.82	Other complication of puerperium, with delivery, with mention of postpartum complication **138**, **141**, **147**	676.10	Cracked nipple, unspecified as to prenatal or postnatal episode of care **161**
674.84	Other complications of puerperium, postpartum condition or complication **153**	676.11	Cracked nipple, delivered, with or without mention of antepartum condition **139**, **145**, **151**
674.90	Unspecified complications of puerperium, unspecified as to episode of care **161**	676.12	Cracked nipple, delivered, with mention of postpartum complication **139**, **145**, **151**
674.92	Unspecified complications of puerperium, with delivery, with mention of postpartum complication **138**, **145**, **151**	676.13	Cracked nipple, antepartum condition or complication **156**, **158**
		676.14	Cracked nipple, postpartum condition or complication **153**
674.94	Unspecified complications of puerperium, postpartum condition or complication **153**	676.20	Engorgement of breasts, unspecified as to prenatal or postnatal episode of care **161**
675.00	Infection of nipple associated with childbirth, unspecified as to episode of care **161**	676.21	Engorgement of breasts, delivered, with or without mention of antepartum condition **139**, **145**, **151**
675.01	Infection of nipple associated with childbirth, delivered, with or without mention of antepartum condition **139**, **141**, **147**	676.22	Engorgement of breasts, delivered, with mention of postpartum complication **139**, **145**, **151**
675.02	Infection of nipple associated with childbirth, delivered with mention of postpartum complication **139**, **141**, **147**	676.23	Engorgement of breast, antepartum **156**, **158**
		676.24	Engorgement of breasts, postpartum condition or complication **153**
675.03	Infection of nipple, antepartum **156**, **158**	676.30	Other and unspecified disorder of breast associated with childbirth, unspecified as to episode of care **161**
675.04	Infection of nipple, postpartum condition or complication **153**		
675.10	Abscess of breast associated with childbirth, unspecified as to episode of care **161**	676.31	Other and unspecified disorder of breast associated with childbirth, delivered, with or without mention of antepartum condition **139**, **145**, **151**
675.11	Abscess of breast associated with childbirth, delivered, with or without mention of antepartum condition **139**, **141**, **147**	676.32	Other and unspecified disorder of breast associated with childbirth, delivered, with mention of postpartum complication **139**, **145**, **151**
675.12	Abscess of breast associated with childbirth, delivered, with mention of postpartum complication **139**, **141**, **147**	676.33	Other and unspecified disorder of breast associated with childbirth, antepartum condition or complication **156**, **158**
675.13	Abscess of breast, antepartum **156**, **158**		
675.14	Abscess of breast, postpartum condition or complication **153**	676.34	Other and unspecified disorder of breast associated with childbirth, postpartum condition or complication **153**
675.20	Nonpurulent mastitis, unspecified as to episode of prenatal or postnatal care **161**	676.40	Failure of lactation, unspecified as to episode of care **161**
675.21	Nonpurulent mastitis, delivered, with or without mention of antepartum condition **139**, **141**, **147**	676.41	Failure of lactation, with delivery, with or without mention of antepartum condition **139**, **145**, **151**
675.22	Nonpurulent mastitis, delivered, with mention of postpartum complication **139**, **141**, **147**	676.42	Failure of lactation, with delivery, with mention of postpartum complication **139**, **145**, **151**
675.23	Nonpurulent mastitis, antepartum **156**, **158**	676.43	Failure of lactation, antepartum condition or complication **156**, **158**
675.24	Nonpurulent mastitis, postpartum condition or complication **153**	676.44	Failure of lactation, postpartum condition or complication **153**
675.80	Other specified infection of the breast and nipple associated with childbirth, unspecified as to episode of care **161**	676.50	Suppressed lactation, unspecified as to episode of care **161**
		676.51	Suppressed lactation, with delivery, with or without mention of antepartum condition **139**, **145**, **151**
675.81	Other specified infection of the breast and nipple associated with childbirth, delivered, with or without mention of antepartum condition **139**, **145**, **151**	676.52	Suppressed lactation, with delivery, with mention of postpartum complication **139**, **145**, **151**
675.82	Other specified infection of the breast and nipple associated with childbirth, delivered, with mention of postpartum complication **139**, **145**, **151**	676.53	Suppressed lactation, antepartum condition or complication **156**, **158**
		676.54	Suppressed lactation, postpartum condition or complication **153**
675.83	Other specified infection of the breast and nipple, antepartum **156**, **158**	676.60	Galactorrhea associated with childbirth, unspecified as to episode of care **161**
675.84	Other specified infections of the breast and nipple, postpartum condition or complication **153**		
675.90	Unspecified infection of the breast and nipple, unspecified as to prenatal or postnatal episode of care **161**	676.61	Galactorrhea, with delivery, with or without mention of antepartum condition **139**, **145**, **151**
675.91	Unspecified infection of the breast and nipple, delivered, with or without mention of antepartum condition **139**, **145**, **151**		

*Code Range

© 2013 OptumInsight, Inc.

676.62	Galactorrhea, with delivery, with mention of postpartum complication **139, 145, 151**
676.63	Galactorrhea, antepartum condition or complication **156, 158**
676.64	Galactorrhea, postpartum condition or complication **153**
676.80	Other disorder of lactation, unspecified as to episode of care **161**
676.81	Other disorder of lactation, with delivery, with or without mention of antepartum condition **139, 145, 151**
676.82	Other disorder of lactation, with delivery, with mention of postpartum complication **139, 145, 151**
676.83	Other disorder of lactation, antepartum condition or complication **156, 158**
676.84	Other disorders of lactation, postpartum condition or complication **153**
676.90	Unspecified disorder of lactation, unspecified as to episode of care **161**
676.91	Unspecified disorder of lactation, with delivery, with or without mention of antepartum condition **139, 145, 151**
676.92	Unspecified disorder of lactation, with delivery, with mention of postpartum complication **139, 145, 151**
676.93	Unspecified disorder of lactation, antepartum condition or complication **156, 158**
676.94	Unspecified disorder of lactation, postpartum condition or complication **153**
677	Late effect of complication of pregnancy, childbirth, and the puerperium **161**
678.00	Fetal hematologic conditions, unspecified as to episode of care or not applicable **161**
678.01	Fetal hematologic conditions, delivered, with or without mention of antepartum condition **139, 145, 151**
678.03	Fetal hematologic conditions, antepartum condition or complication **156, 158**
678.10	Fetal conjoined twins, unspecified as to episode of care or not applicable **161**
678.11	Fetal conjoined twins, delivered, with or without mention of antepartum condition **139, 145, 151**
678.13	Fetal conjoined twins, antepartum condition or complication **156, 158**
679.00	Maternal complications from in utero procedure, unspecified as to episode of care or not applicable **139, 145, 151**
679.01	Maternal complications from in utero procedure, delivered, with or without mention of antepartum condition **139, 141, 147**
679.02	Maternal complications from in utero procedure, delivered, with mention of postpartum complication **139, 141, 147**
679.03	Maternal complications from in utero procedure, antepartum condition or complication **156, 158**
679.04	Maternal complications from in utero procedure, postpartum condition or complication **153**
679.10	Fetal complications from in utero procedure, unspecified as to episode of care or not applicable **161**
679.11	Fetal complications from in utero procedure, delivered, with or without mention of antepartum condition **139, 145, 151**
679.12	Fetal complications from in utero procedure, delivered, with mention of postpartum complication **139, 145, 151**
679.13	Fetal complications from in utero procedure, antepartum condition or complication **156, 159**
679.14	Fetal complications from in utero procedure, postpartum condition or complication **153**
680*	Carbuncle and furuncle **106**
681*	Cellulitis and abscess of finger and toe **103, 106**
682.0	Cellulitis and abscess of face **3**
682.1	Cellulitis and abscess of neck **3**
682*	Other cellulitis and abscess **103, 106, 166, 170**
683	Acute lymphadenitis **166, 170, 176, 230**
684	Impetigo **106**
685*	Pilonidal cyst **106**

686.9	Unspecified local infection of skin and subcutaneous tissue **172**
686*	Other local infection of skin and subcutaneous tissue **106**
690*	Erythematosquamous dermatosis **108**
691.0	Diaper or napkin rash **172**
691*	Atopic dermatitis and related conditions **108**
692*	Contact dermatitis and other eczema **108**
693.0	Dermatitis due to drugs and medicines taken internally **166, 170**
693*	Dermatitis due to substances taken internally **108**
694.0	Dermatitis herpetiformis **108**
694.1	Subcorneal pustular dermatosis **108**
694.2	Juvenile dermatitis herpetiformis **108**
694.3	Impetigo herpetiformis **108**
694.4	Pemphigus **105**
694.5	Pemphigoid **105**
694.60	Benign mucous membrane pemphigoid without mention of ocular involvement **105**
694.61	Benign mucous membrane pemphigoid with ocular involvement **40**
694.8	Other specified bullous dermatosis **105**
694.9	Unspecified bullous dermatosis **105**
695.0	Toxic erythema **105, 166, 170**
695.1*	Erythema multiforme **105**
695.2	Erythema nodosum **105**
695.3	Rosacea **108**
695.4	Lupus erythematosus **105**
695.5*	Exfoliation due to erythematous conditions according to extent of body surface involved **108**
695.81	Ritter's disease **105**
695.89	Other specified erythematous condition **108**
695.9	Unspecified erythematous condition **108**
696.0	Psoriatic arthropathy **97**
696.1	Other psoriasis **105**
696.2	Parapsoriasis **105**
696.3	Pityriasis rosea **108**
696.4	Pityriasis rubra pilaris **108**
696.5	Other and unspecified pityriasis **108**
696.8	Psoriasis related disease NEC **108**
697*	Lichen **108**
698.0	Pruritus ani **108**
698.1	Pruritus of genital organs **124, 127, 130**
698.2	Prurigo **108**
698.3	Lichenification and lichen simplex chronicus **108**
698.4	Dermatitis factitia (artefacta) **108**
698.8	Other specified pruritic conditions **108**
698.9	Unspecified pruritic disorder **108**
700	Corns and callosities **108**
701*	Other hypertrophic and atrophic conditions of skin **108**
702*	Other dermatoses **108**
703*	Diseases of nail **108**
704*	Diseases of hair and hair follicles **108**
705*	Disorders of sweat glands **108**
706*	Diseases of sebaceous glands **108**
707*	Chronic ulcer of skin **103, 105**
708.0	Allergic urticaria **166, 170**
708*	Urticaria **108**
709.00	Dyschromia, unspecified **172**
709.01	Vitiligo **172**
709.09	Other dyschromia **172**
709.9	Unspecified disorder of skin and subcutaneous tissue **230**

709*	Other disorders of skin and subcutaneous tissue **108**	718.30	Recurrent dislocation of joint, site unspecified **100**
710*	Diffuse diseases of connective tissue **97**	718.31	Recurrent dislocation of shoulder joint **99**
711.0*	Pyogenic arthritis **97, 230**	718.32	Recurrent dislocation of upper arm joint **99**
711.06	Pyogenic arthritis, lower leg **90**	718.33	Recurrent dislocation of forearm joint **99**
711.1*	Arthropathy associated with Reiter's disease and nonspecific urethritis **97**	718.34	Recurrent dislocation of hand joint **99**
		718.35	Recurrent dislocation of pelvic region and thigh joint **100**
711.2*	Arthropathy in Behcet's syndrome **97**	718.36	Recurrent dislocation of lower leg joint **99**
711.3*	Postdysenteric arthropathy **98**	718.37	Recurrent dislocation of ankle and foot joint **99**
711.4*	Arthropathy associated with other bacterial diseases **97**	718.38	Recurrent dislocation of joint of other specified site **100**
711.5*	Arthropathy associated with other viral diseases **98**	718.39	Recurrent dislocation of joint of multiple sites **100**
711.6*	Arthropathy associated with mycoses **97**	718.4*	Contracture of joint **100**
711.7*	Arthropathy associated with helminthiasis **97**	718.5*	Ankylosis of joint **98**
711.8*	Arthropathy associated with other infectious and parasitic diseases **97**	718.65	Unspecified intrapelvic protrusion acetabulum, pelvic region and thigh **100**
711.9*	Unspecified infective arthritis **97, 230**	718.7*	Developmental dislocation of joint **100**
712*	Crystal arthropathies **98**	718.8*	Other joint derangement, not elsewhere classified **100**
713*	Arthropathy associated with other disorders classified elsewhere **98**	718.9*	Unspecified derangement of joint **100**
		719.0*	Effusion of joint **100**
714.0	Rheumatoid arthritis **97**	719.1*	Hemarthrosis **98**
714.1	Felty's syndrome **97**	719.2*	Villonodular synovitis **98**
714.2	Other rheumatoid arthritis with visceral or systemic involvement **97**	719.3*	Palindromic rheumatism **98**
		719.4*	Pain in joint **98**
714.3*	Juvenile chronic polyarthritis **97**	719.5*	Stiffness of joint, not elsewhere classified **98**
714.4	Chronic postrheumatic arthropathy **98**	719.6*	Other symptoms referable to joint **98**
714.81	Rheumatoid lung **53**	719.7	Difficulty in walking **98**
714.89	Other specified inflammatory polyarthropathies **97**	719.8*	Other specified disorders of joint **98**
714.9	Unspecified inflammatory polyarthropathy **98**	719.9*	Unspecified disorder of joint **98**
715*	Osteoarthrosis and allied disorders **98**	720.0	Ankylosing spondylitis **97**
716.9*	Unspecified arthropathy **230**	720.1	Spinal enthesopathy **97**
716*	Other and unspecified arthropathies **98**	720.2	Sacroiliitis, not elsewhere classified **97**
717.0	Old bucket handle tear of medial meniscus **99**	720.8*	Other inflammatory spondylopathies **97**
717.1	Derangement of anterior horn of medial meniscus **99**	720.9	Unspecified inflammatory spondylopathy **97**
717.2	Derangement of posterior horn of medial meniscus **99**	721*	Spondylosis and allied disorders **97**
717.3	Other and unspecified derangement of medial meniscus **99**	722*	Intervertebral disc disorders **97**
717.4*	Derangement of lateral meniscus **99**	723.0	Spinal stenosis in cervical region **97**
717.5	Derangement of meniscus, not elsewhere classified **99**	723.1	Cervicalgia **97**
717.6	Loose body in knee **100**	723.2	Cervicocranial syndrome **21**
717.7	Chondromalacia of patella **99**	723.3	Cervicobrachial syndrome (diffuse) **21**
717.8*	Other internal derangement of knee **99**	723.4	Brachial neuritis or radiculitis NOS **21**
717.9	Unspecified internal derangement of knee **99**	723.5	Torticollis, unspecified **97**
718.00	Articular cartilage disorder, site unspecified **100**	723.6	Panniculitis specified as affecting neck **108**
718.01	Articular cartilage disorder, shoulder region **99**	723.7	Ossification of posterior longitudinal ligament in cervical region **97**
718.02	Articular cartilage disorder, upper arm **99**		
718.03	Articular cartilage disorder, forearm **99**	723.8	Other syndromes affecting cervical region **97**
718.04	Articular cartilage disorder, hand **99**	723.9	Unspecified musculoskeletal disorders and symptoms referable to neck **97**
718.05	Articular cartilage disorder, pelvic region and thigh **100**		
718.07	Articular cartilage disorder, ankle and foot **99**	724*	Other and unspecified disorders of back **97**
718.08	Articular cartilage disorder, other specified site **100**	725	Polymyalgia rheumatica **97**
718.09	Articular cartilage disorder, multiple sites **100**	726.0	Adhesive capsulitis of shoulder **98**
718.1*	Loose body in joint **100**	726.1*	Rotator cuff syndrome of shoulder and allied disorders **98**
718.20	Pathological dislocation of joint, site unspecified **99**	726.2	Other affections of shoulder region, not elsewhere classified **98**
718.21	Pathological dislocation of shoulder joint **99**	726.3*	Enthesopathy of elbow region **98**
718.22	Pathological dislocation of upper arm joint **99**	726.4	Enthesopathy of wrist and carpus **98**
718.23	Pathological dislocation of forearm joint **99**	726.5	Enthesopathy of hip region **98**
718.24	Pathological dislocation of hand joint **99**	726.6*	Enthesopathy of knee **98**
718.25	Pathological dislocation of pelvic region and thigh joint **100**	726.70	Unspecified enthesopathy of ankle and tarsus **98**
718.26	Pathological dislocation of lower leg joint **99**	726.71	Achilles bursitis or tendinitis **98**
718.27	Pathological dislocation of ankle and foot joint **99**	726.72	Tibialis tendinitis **98**
718.28	Pathological dislocation of joint of other specified site **100**	726.73	Calcaneal spur **100**
718.29	Pathological dislocation of joint of multiple sites **100**		

*Code Range

726.79	Other enthesopathy of ankle and tarsus **98**	730.31	Periostitis, without mention of osteomyelitis, shoulder region **98**
726.8	Other peripheral enthesopathies **98**	730.32	Periostitis, without mention of osteomyelitis, upper arm **98**
726.9*	Unspecified enthesopathy **98**	730.33	Periostitis, without mention of osteomyelitis, forearm **98**
727.00	Unspecified synovitis and tenosynovitis **98**	730.34	Periostitis, without mention of osteomyelitis, hand **98**
727.01	Synovitis and tenosynovitis in diseases classified elsewhere **98**	730.35	Periostitis, without mention of osteomyelitis, pelvic region and thigh **98**
727.02	Giant cell tumor of tendon sheath **100**	730.36	Periostitis, without mention of osteomyelitis, lower leg **98**
727.03	Trigger finger (acquired) **99**	730.37	Periostitis, without mention of osteomyelitis, ankle and foot **100**
727.04	Radial styloid tenosynovitis **99**	730.38	Periostitis, without mention of osteomyelitis, other specified sites **100**
727.05	Other tenosynovitis of hand and wrist **99**	730.39	Periostitis, without mention of osteomyelitis, multiple sites **100**
727.06	Tenosynovitis of foot and ankle **99**	730.7*	Osteopathy resulting from poliomyelitis **100**
727.09	Other synovitis and tenosynovitis **99**	730.8*	Other infections involving bone in diseases classified elsewhere **96**
727.1	Bunion **100**	730.9*	Unspecified infection of bone **96**
727.2	Specific bursitides often of occupational origin **99**	731*	Osteitis deformans and osteopathies associated with other disorders classified elsewhere **98**
727.3	Other bursitis disorders **99**	732.0	Juvenile osteochondrosis of spine **87**
727.4*	Ganglion and cyst of synovium, tendon, and bursa **99**	732*	Osteochondropathies **98**
727.5*	Rupture of synovium **99**	733.0*	Osteoporosis **98**
727.6*	Rupture of tendon, nontraumatic **99**	733.1*	Pathologic fracture **97, 166, 170**
727.8*	Other disorders of synovium, tendon, and bursa **99**	733.13	Pathologic fracture of vertebrae **87**
727.9	Unspecified disorder of synovium, tendon, and bursa **99**	733.2*	Cyst of bone **98**
728.0	Infective myositis **99**	733.3	Hyperostosis of skull **100**
728.1*	Muscular calcification and ossification **99**	733.4*	Aseptic necrosis of bone **98**
728.2	Muscular wasting and disuse atrophy, not elsewhere classified **99**	733.5	Osteitis condensans **98**
728.3	Other specific muscle disorders **99**	733.6	Tietze's disease **54**
728.4	Laxity of ligament **99**	733.7	Algoneurodystrophy **100**
728.5	Hypermobility syndrome **99**	733.8*	Malunion and nonunion of fracture **100**
728.6	Contracture of palmar fascia **99**	733.90	Disorder of bone and cartilage, unspecified **100**
728.7*	Other fibromatoses of muscle, ligament, and fascia **99**	733.91	Arrest of bone development or growth **100**
728.81	Interstitial myositis **99**	733.92	Chondromalacia **98**
728.82	Foreign body granuloma of muscle **99**	733.93	Stress fracture of tibia or fibula **97**
728.83	Rupture of muscle, nontraumatic **99**	733.94	Stress fracture of the metatarsals **97**
728.84	Diastasis of muscle **99**	733.95	Stress fracture of other bone **97**
728.85	Spasm of muscle **98**	733.96	Stress fracture of femoral neck **97**
728.86	Necrotizing fasciitis **99**	733.97	Stress fracture of shaft of femur **97**
728.87	Muscle weakness (generalized) **98**	733.98	Stress fracture of pelvis **97**
728.88	Rhabdomyolysis **99**	733.99	Other disorders of bone and cartilage **100**
728.89	Other disorder of muscle, ligament, and fascia **99**	734	Flat foot **100**
728.9	Unspecified disorder of muscle, ligament, and fascia **99**	735*	Acquired deformities of toe **100**
729.0	Rheumatism, unspecified and fibrositis **98**	736.00	Unspecified deformity of forearm, excluding fingers **100**
729.1	Unspecified myalgia and myositis **98**	736.01	Cubitus valgus (acquired) **100**
729.2	Unspecified neuralgia, neuritis, and radiculitis **21, 230**	736.02	Cubitus varus (acquired) **100**
729.3*	Unspecified panniculitis **108**	736.03	Valgus deformity of wrist (acquired) **100**
729.4	Unspecified fasciitis **99**	736.04	Varus deformity of wrist (acquired) **100**
729.5	Pain in soft tissues of limb **98**	736.05	Wrist drop (acquired) **21**
729.6	Residual foreign body in soft tissue **100**	736.06	Claw hand (acquired) **21**
729.7*	Nontraumatic compartment syndrome **99**	736.07	Club hand, acquired **21**
729.81	Swelling of limb **98**	736.09	Other acquired deformities of forearm, excluding fingers **100**
729.82	Cramp of limb **98**	736.1	Mallet finger **100**
729.89	Other musculoskeletal symptoms referable to limbs **98**	736.2*	Other acquired deformities of finger **100**
729.9*	Other and unspecified disorders of soft tissue **98**	736.3*	Acquired deformities of hip **100**
730.0*	Acute osteomyelitis **96**	736.4*	Genu valgum or varum (acquired) **100**
730.06	Acute osteomyelitis, lower leg **90**	736.5	Genu recurvatum (acquired) **100**
730.08	Acute osteomyelitis, other specified site **87**	736.6	Other acquired deformities of knee **100**
730.1*	Chronic osteomyelitis **96**	736.70	Unspecified deformity of ankle and foot, acquired **100**
730.16	Chronic osteomyelitis, lower leg **90**	736.71	Acquired equinovarus deformity **100**
730.18	Chronic osteomyelitis, other specified sites **87**	736.72	Equinus deformity of foot, acquired **100**
730.2*	Unspecified osteomyelitis **96**	736.73	Cavus deformity of foot, acquired **100**
730.26	Unspecified osteomyelitis, lower leg **90**		
730.28	Unspecified osteomyelitis, other specified sites **87**		
730.30	Periostitis, without mention of osteomyelitis, unspecified site **98**		

736.74	Claw foot, acquired **21**	
736.75	Cavovarus deformity of foot, acquired **100**	
736.76	Other acquired calcaneus deformity **100**	
736.79	Other acquired deformity of ankle and foot **100**	
736.8*	Acquired deformities of other parts of limbs **100**	
736.9	Acquired deformity of limb, site unspecified **100**	
737.0	Adolescent postural kyphosis **87**	
737.1*	Kyphosis (acquired) **87**	
737.2*	Lordosis (acquired) **87**	
737.3*	Kyphoscoliosis and scoliosis **87**	
737.4*	Curvature of spine associated with other conditions **87**	
737.8	Other curvatures of spine associated with other conditions **87**	
737.9	Unspecified curvature of spine associated with other condition **87**	
737*	Curvature of spine **97**	
738.0	Acquired deformity of nose **47**	
738.1*	Other acquired deformity of head **100**	
738.2	Acquired deformity of neck **100**	
738.3	Acquired deformity of chest and rib **100**	
738.4	Acquired spondylolisthesis **97**	
738.5	Other acquired deformity of back or spine **97**	
738.6	Acquired deformity of pelvis **100**	
738.7	Cauliflower ear **47**	
738.8	Acquired musculoskeletal deformity of other specified site **100**	
738.9	Acquired musculoskeletal deformity of unspecified site **100**	
739.0	Nonallopathic lesion of head region, not elsewhere classified **98**	
739.1	Nonallopathic lesion of cervical region, not elsewhere classified **97**	
739.2	Nonallopathic lesion of thoracic region, not elsewhere classified **97**	
739.3	Nonallopathic lesion of lumbar region, not elsewhere classified **98**	
739.4	Nonallopathic lesion of sacral region, not elsewhere classified **98**	
739.5	Nonallopathic lesion of pelvic region, not elsewhere classified **98**	
739.6	Nonallopathic lesion of lower extremities, not elsewhere classified **98**	
739.7	Nonallopathic lesion of upper extremities, not elsewhere classified **98**	
739.8	Nonallopathic lesion of rib cage, not elsewhere classified **98**	
739.9	Nonallopathic lesion of abdomen and other sites, not elsewhere classified **98**	
740*	Anencephalus and similar anomalies **33, 166, 170**	
741*	Spina bifida **33, 166, 170**	
742*	Other congenital anomalies of nervous system **33, 166, 170**	
743*	Congenital anomalies of eye **40**	
744.0*	Congenital anomalies of ear causing impairment of hearing **47**	
744.1	Congenital anomalies of accessory auricle **47, 172**	
744.2*	Other specified congenital anomalies of ear **47**	
744.3	Unspecified congenital anomaly of ear **47**	
744.4*	Congenital branchial cleft cyst or fistula; preauricular sinus **47**	
744.5	Congenital webbing of neck **108**	
744.81	Macrocheilia **48**	
744.82	Microcheilia **48**	
744.83	Macrostomia **48**	
744.84	Microstomia **48**	
744.89	Other specified congenital anomaly of face and neck **47**	
744.9	Unspecified congenital anomaly of face and neck **108**	
745.0	Bulbus cordis anomalies and anomalies of cardiac septal closure, common truncus **67**	
745.1*	Transposition of great vessels **67**	
745.2	Tetralogy of Fallot **67**	

745.3	Bulbus cordis anomalies and anomalies of cardiac septal closure, common ventricle **67**
745.4	Ventricular septal defect **67, 166, 170**
745.5	Ostium secundum type atrial septal defect **67**
745.60	Unspecified type congenital endocardial cushion defect **67**
745.61	Ostium primum defect **67**
745.69	Other congenital endocardial cushion defect **67**
745.7	Cor biloculare **68**
745.8	Other bulbus cordis anomalies and anomalies of cardiac septal closure **68**
745.9	Unspecified congenital defect of septal closure **68**
746.0*	Congenital anomalies of pulmonary valve **68**
746.1	Congenital tricuspid atresia and stenosis **68**
746.2	Ebstein's anomaly **68**
746.3	Congenital stenosis of aortic valve **68**
746.4	Congenital insufficiency of aortic valve **68**
746.5	Congenital mitral stenosis **68**
746.6	Congenital mitral insufficiency **68**
746.7	Hypoplastic left heart syndrome **68**
746.81	Congenital subaortic stenosis **68**
746.82	Cor triatriatum **68**
746.83	Congenital infundibular pulmonic stenosis **68**
746.84	Congenital obstructive anomalies of heart, not elsewhere classified **68**
746.85	Congenital coronary artery anomaly **68**
746.86	Congenital heart block **68**
746.87	Congenital malposition of heart and cardiac apex **68**
746.89	Other specified congenital anomaly of heart **68**
746.9	Unspecified congenital anomaly of heart **68**
747.0	Patent ductus arteriosus **68**
747.1*	Coarctation of aorta **68**
747.2*	Other congenital anomaly of aorta **68**
747.3*	Anomalies of pulmonary artery **68**
747.4*	Congenital anomalies of great veins **68**
747.5	Congenital absence or hypoplasia of umbilical artery **67**
747.6*	Other congenital anomaly of peripheral vascular system **67**
747.81	Congenital anomaly of cerebrovascular system **33**
747.82	Congenital spinal vessel anomaly **33**
747.83	Persistent fetal circulation **163, 167**
747.89	Other specified congenital anomaly of circulatory system **67**
747.9	Unspecified congenital anomaly of circulatory system **67**
748.0	Congenital choanal atresia **47**
748.1	Other congenital anomaly of nose **47**
748.2	Congenital web of larynx **3, 47**
748.3	Other congenital anomaly of larynx, trachea, and bronchus **3, 47**
748.4	Congenital cystic lung **54**
748.5	Congenital agenesis, hypoplasia, and dysplasia of lung **54**
748.60	Unspecified congenital anomaly of lung **54**
748.61	Congenital bronchiectasis **53**
748.69	Other congenital anomaly of lung **54**
748.8	Other specified congenital anomaly of respiratory system **54**
748.9	Unspecified congenital anomaly of respiratory system **54**
749.0*	Cleft palate **3**
749.1*	Cleft lip **3**
749.2*	Cleft palate with cleft lip **3**
749*	Cleft palate and cleft lip **48**
750.0	Tongue tie **3, 48**
750.1*	Other congenital anomalies of tongue **3, 48**
750.21	Congenital absence of salivary gland **3, 47**

750.22	Congenital accessory salivary gland **3, 47**	
750.23	Congenital atresia, salivary duct **3, 47**	
750.24	Congenital fistula of salivary gland **3, 47**	
750.25	Congenital fistula of lip **3, 48**	
750.26	Other specified congenital anomalies of mouth **3, 48**	
750.27	Congenital diverticulum of pharynx **3, 47**	
750.29	Other specified congenital anomaly of pharynx **3, 47**	
750.3	Congenital tracheoesophageal fistula, esophageal atresia and stenosis **75**	
750.4	Other specified congenital anomaly of esophagus **75**	
750.5	Congenital hypertrophic pyloric stenosis **79**	
750.6	Congenital hiatus hernia **79**	
750.7	Other specified congenital anomalies of stomach **79**	
750.8	Other specified congenital anomalies of upper alimentary tract **79**	
750.9	Unspecified congenital anomaly of upper alimentary tract **79**	
751.0	Meckel's diverticulum **77**	
751.1	Congenital atresia and stenosis of small intestine **79**	
751.2	Congenital atresia and stenosis of large intestine, rectum, and anal canal **79**	
751.3	Hirschsprung's disease and other congenital functional disorders of colon **79**	
751.4	Congenital anomalies of intestinal fixation **79**	
751.5	Other congenital anomalies of intestine **79**	
751.60	Unspecified congenital anomaly of gallbladder, bile ducts, and liver **83**	
751.61	Congenital biliary atresia **83**	
751.62	Congenital cystic disease of liver **83**	
751.69	Other congenital anomaly of gallbladder, bile ducts, and liver **83**	
751.7	Congenital anomalies of pancreas **83**	
751.8	Other specified congenital anomalies of digestive system **79**	
751.9	Unspecified congenital anomaly of digestive system **79**	
752.0	Congenital anomalies of ovaries **127, 130**	
752.1*	Congenital anomalies of fallopian tubes and broad ligaments **127, 130**	
752.2	Congenital doubling of uterus **127, 130**	
752.3*	Other congenital anomaly of uterus **127, 130**	
752.4*	Congenital anomalies of cervix, vagina, and external female genitalia **127, 130**	
752.5*	Undescended and retractile testicle **124, 172**	
752.6*	Hypospadias and epispadias and other penile anomalies **124**	
752.7	Indeterminate sex and pseudohermaphroditism **124, 127, 130**	
752.8*	Other specified congenital anomalies of genital organs **124**	
752.89	Other specified anomalies of genital organs **127, 130**	
752.9	Unspecified congenital anomaly of genital organs **124, 127, 130**	
753*	Congenital anomalies of urinary system **120**	
754.0	Congenital musculoskeletal deformities of skull, face, and jaw **100**	
754.1	Congenital musculoskeletal deformity of sternocleidomastoid muscle **100**	
754.2	Congenital musculoskeletal deformity of spine **87, 100**	
754.3*	Congenital dislocation of hip **100**	
754.40	Congenital genu recurvatum **100**	
754.41	Congenital dislocation of knee (with genu recurvatum) **99**	
754.42	Congenital bowing of femur **100**	
754.43	Congenital bowing of tibia and fibula **100**	
754.44	Congenital bowing of unspecified long bones of leg **100**	
754.5*	Congenital varus deformities of feet **100**	
754.6*	Congenital valgus deformities of feet **100**	
754.61	Congenital pes planus **172**	
754.7*	Other congenital deformity of feet **100**	

754.81	Pectus excavatum **54**	
754.82	Pectus carinatum **54**	
754.89	Other specified nonteratogenic anomalies **100**	
755*	Other congenital anomalies of limbs **100**	
756.0	Congenital anomalies of skull and face bones **100**	
756.10	Congenital anomaly of spine, unspecified **98**	
756.11	Congenital spondylolysis, lumbosacral region **98**	
756.12	Congenital spondylolisthesis **98**	
756.13	Congenital absence of vertebra **98**	
756.14	Hemivertebra **98**	
756.15	Congenital fusion of spine (vertebra) **98**	
756.16	Klippel-Feil syndrome **100**	
756.17	Spina bifida occulta **33**	
756.19	Other congenital anomaly of spine **98**	
756.2	Cervical rib **100**	
756.3	Other congenital anomaly of ribs and sternum **54**	
756.4	Chondrodystrophy **100**	
756.5*	Congenital osteodystrophies **100**	
756.51	Osteogenesis imperfecta **87**	
756.6	Congenital anomaly of diaphragm **54**	
756.7*	Congenital anomaly of abdominal wall **79**	
756.72	Omphalocele **166, 170**	
756.73	Gastroschisis **166, 170**	
756.8*	Other specified congenital anomalies of muscle, tendon, fascia, and connective tissue **100**	
756.9	Other and unspecified congenital anomaly of musculoskeletal system **101**	
757.0	Hereditary edema of legs **108**	
757.1	Ichthyosis congenita **108**	
757.2	Dermatoglyphic anomalies **108**	
757.31	Congenital ectodermal dysplasia **108**	
757.32	Congenital vascular hamartomas **108**	
757.33	Congenital pigmentary anomaly of skin **108, 172**	
757.39	Other specified congenital anomaly of skin **108, 172**	
757.4	Specified congenital anomalies of hair **108**	
757.5	Specified congenital anomalies of nails **108**	
757.6	Specified congenital anomalies of breast **106**	
757.8	Other specified congenital anomalies of the integument **108**	
757.9	Unspecified congenital anomaly of the integument **108**	
758.0	Down's syndrome **188**	
758.1	Patau's syndrome **188**	
758.2	Edwards' syndrome **188**	
758.3*	Autosomal deletion syndromes **188**	
758.4	Balanced autosomal translocation in normal individual **213**	
758.5	Other conditions due to autosomal anomalies **213**	
758.6	Gonadal dysgenesis **124, 127, 130**	
758.7	Klinefelter's syndrome **124**	
758.8*	Other conditions due to chromosome anomalies **124, 127, 130**	
758.9	Conditions due to anomaly of unspecified chromosome **213**	
759.0	Congenital anomalies of spleen **176**	
759.1	Congenital anomalies of adrenal gland **114**	
759.2	Congenital anomalies of other endocrine glands **114**	
759.3	Situs inversus **79**	
759.4	Conjoined twins **79, 166, 170**	
759.5	Tuberous sclerosis **33**	
759.6	Other congenital hamartoses, not elsewhere classified **180, 182**	
759.7	Multiple congenital anomalies, so described **101**	
759.81	Prader-Willi syndrome **101**	
759.82	Marfan's syndrome **68**	

759.83	Fragile X syndrome **188**	
759.89	Other specified multiple congenital anomalies, so described **101**	
759.9	Unspecified congenital anomaly **213**	
762.4	Fetus or newborn affected by prolapsed cord **171**, **172**	
762.5	Fetus or newborn affected by other compression of umbilical cord **171**, **172**	
762.6	Fetus or newborn affected by other and unspecified conditions of umbilical cord **171**, **172**	
763.0	Fetus or newborn affected by breech delivery and extraction **171**, **172**	
763.1	Fetus or newborn affected by other malpresentation, malposition, and disproportion during labor and delivery **171**, **172**	
763.2	Fetus or newborn affected by forceps delivery **171**, **172**	
763.3	Fetus or newborn affected by delivery by vacuum extractor **171**, **172**	
763.4	Fetus or newborn affected by cesarean delivery **163**, **167**	
763.6	Fetus or newborn affected by precipitate delivery **171**, **172**	
763.9	Unspecified complication of labor and delivery affecting fetus or newborn **171**, **172**	
764.08	Light-for-dates without mention of fetal malnutrition, 2,000-2,499 grams **171**, **172**	
764.09	Light-for-dates without mention of fetal malnutrition, 2,500 or more grams **171**, **172**	
764.11	Light-for-dates with signs of fetal malnutrition, less than 500 grams **163**, **167**	
764.12	Light-for-dates with signs of fetal malnutrition, 500-749 grams **163**, **167**	
764.13	Light-for-dates with signs of fetal malnutrition, 750-999 grams **163**, **167**	
764.14	Light-for-dates with signs of fetal malnutrition, 1,000-1,249 grams **163**, **167**	
764.15	Light-for-dates with signs of fetal malnutrition, 1,250-1,499 grams **163**, **167**	
764.16	Light-for-dates with signs of fetal malnutrition, 1,500-1,749 grams **163**, **167**	
764.17	Light-for-dates with signs of fetal malnutrition, 1,750-1,999 grams **163**, **167**	
764.18	Light-for-dates with signs of fetal malnutrition, 2,000-2,499 grams **163**, **167**	
764.21	Fetal malnutrition without mention of "light-for-dates", less than 500 grams **163**, **167**	
764.22	Fetal malnutrition without mention of "light-for-dates", 500-749 grams **163**, **167**	
764.23	Fetal malnutrition without mention of "light-for-dates", 750-999 grams **163**, **167**	
764.24	Fetal malnutrition without mention of "light-for-dates", 1,000-1,249 grams **163**, **167**	
764.25	Fetal malnutrition without mention of "light-for-dates", 1,250-1,499 grams **163**, **167**	
764.26	Fetal malnutrition without mention of "light-for-dates", 1,500-1,749 grams **163**, **167**	
764.27	Fetal malnutrition without mention of "light-for-dates", 1,750-1,999 grams **163**, **167**	
764.28	Fetal malnutrition without mention of "light-for-dates", 2,000-2,499 grams **163**, **167**	
764.98	Unspecified fetal growth retardation, 2,000-2,499 grams **171**, **172**	
764.99	Unspecified fetal growth retardation, 2,500 or more grams **171**, **172**	
765.00	Extreme fetal immaturity, unspecified (weight) **163**, **167**	
765.01	Extreme fetal immaturity, less than 500 grams **163**	
765.02	Extreme fetal immaturity, 500-749 grams **163**	
765.03	Extreme fetal immaturity, 750-999 grams **163**	
765.04	Extreme fetal immaturity, 1,000-1,249 grams **163**	

765.05	Extreme fetal immaturity, 1,250-1,499 grams **163**	
765.06	Extreme fetal immaturity, 1,500-1,749 grams **163**, **167**	
765.07	Extreme fetal immaturity, 1,750-1,999 grams **163**, **167**	
765.08	Extreme fetal immaturity, 2,000-2,499 grams **163**, **167**	
765.1*	Other preterm infants **163**, **167**	
765.20	Unspecified weeks of gestation **171**, **172**	
765.21	Less than 24 completed weeks of gestation **163**	
765.22	24 completed weeks of gestation **163**	
765.23	25-26 completed weeks of gestation **163**	
765.24	27-28 completed weeks of gestation **163**, **167**	
765.25	29-30 completed weeks of gestation **163**, **167**	
765.26	31-32 completed weeks of gestation **163**, **167**	
765.27	33-34 completed weeks of gestation **163**, **167**	
765.28	35-36 completed weeks of gestation **163**, **167**	
765.29	37 or more completed weeks of gestation **171**, **172**	
766.0	Exceptionally large baby relating to long gestation **171**, **172**	
766.1	Other "heavy-for-dates" infants not related to gestation period **171**, **172**	
766.2*	Late infant, not "heavy-for-dates" **171**, **172**	
767.0	Subdural and cerebral hemorrhage, birth trauma **163**, **167**	
767.11	Birth trauma, epicranial subaponeurotic hemorrhage (massive) **163**, **167**	
767.19	Birth trauma, other injuries to scalp **171**, **172**	
767.4	Injury to spine and spinal cord, birth trauma **163**, **167**	
767.7	Other cranial and peripheral nerve injuries, birth trauma **163**, **167**	
768.5	Severe birth asphyxia **163**, **167**	
768.6	Mild or moderate birth asphyxia **171**, **172**	
768.72	Moderate hypoxic-ischemic encephalopathy **163**, **167**	
768.73	Severe hypoxic-ischemic encephalopathy **163**, **167**	
769	Respiratory distress syndrome in newborn **163**	
770.0	Congenital pneumonia **163**, **167**	
770.1*	Fetal and newborn aspiration **163**, **167**	
770.2	Interstitial emphysema and related conditions of newborn **163**, **167**	
770.3	Pulmonary hemorrhage of fetus or newborn **163**, **167**	
770.4	Primary atelectasis of newborn **163**, **167**	
770.7	Chronic respiratory disease arising in the perinatal period **53**	
770.84	Respiratory failure of newborn **163**, **167**	
770.85	Aspiration of postnatal stomach contents without respiratory symptoms **163**, **167**	
770.86	Aspiration of postnatal stomach contents with respiratory symptoms **163**, **167**	
771.0	Congenital rubella **163**, **167**	
771.1	Congenital cytomegalovirus infection **163**, **167**	
771.2	Other congenital infection specific to the perinatal period **163**, **167**	
771.4	Omphalitis of the newborn **163**, **167**	
771.5	Neonatal infective mastitis **163**, **167**	
771.8*	Other infection specific to the perinatal period **163**, **167**	
772.0	Fetal blood loss affecting newborn **163**, **167**	
772.1*	Intraventricular hemorrhage **163**, **167**	
772.2	Fetal and neonatal subarachnoid hemorrhage of newborn **163**, **167**	
772.4	Fetal and neonatal gastrointestinal hemorrhage **163**, **167**	
772.5	Fetal and neonatal adrenal hemorrhage **163**, **167**	
772.6	Fetal and neonatal cutaneous hemorrhage **171**, **172**	
773.2	Hemolytic disease due to other and unspecified isoimmunization of fetus or newborn **163**, **167**	
773.3	Hydrops fetalis due to isoimmunization **163**, **167**	
773.4	Kernicterus due to isoimmunization of fetus or newborn **163**, **167**	

*Code Range

773.5	Late anemia due to isoimmunization of fetus or newborn **163, 167**	
774.3*	Neonatal jaundice due to delayed conjugation from other causes **171, 172**	
774.4	Perinatal jaundice due to hepatocellular damage **163, 167**	
774.5	Perinatal jaundice from other causes **171, 172**	
774.6	Unspecified fetal and neonatal jaundice **171, 172**	
774.7	Kernicterus of fetus or newborn not due to isoimmunization **163, 167**	

780.58 Sleep related movement disorder, unspecified **189**
780.59 Other sleep disturbances **189**
780.60 Fever, unspecified **184, 231**
780.61 Fever presenting with conditions classified elsewhere **184, 231**
780.62 Postprocedural fever **184, 231**
780.63 Postvaccination fever **184, 231**
780.64 Chills (without fever) **213**
780.65 Hypothermia not associated with low environmental temperature **213**
780.66 Febrile nonhemolytic transfusion reaction **184, 231**
780.7* Malaise and fatigue **231**
780.71 Chronic fatigue syndrome **213**
780.72 Functional quadriplegia **19**
780.79 Other malaise and fatigue **213**
780.8 Generalized hyperhidrosis **108, 231**
780.9* Other general symptoms **213**

775.1 Neonatal diabetes mellitus **163, 167**
775.2 Neonatal myasthenia gravis **163, 167**
775.3 Neonatal thyrotoxicosis **163, 167**
775.4 Hypocalcemia and hypomagnesemia of newborn **163, 167**
775.5 Other transitory neonatal electrolyte disturbances **163, 167**
775.6 Neonatal hypoglycemia **163, 167**
775.7 Late metabolic acidosis of newborn **163, 167**
776.0 Hemorrhagic disease of newborn **163, 167**
776.1 Transient neonatal thrombocytopenia **163, 167**
776.2 Disseminated intravascular coagulation in newborn **163, 167**
776.3 Other transient neonatal disorders of coagulation **163, 168**
776.6 Anemia of neonatal prematurity **163, 168**
777.1 Fetal and newborn meconium obstruction **163, 168**
777.2 Neonatal intestinal obstruction due to inspissated milk **163, 168**
777.5* Necrotizing enterocolitis in newborn **163, 168**
777.6 Perinatal intestinal perforation **163, 168**
778.0 Hydrops fetalis not due to isoimmunization **163, 168**
778.8 Other specified condition involving the integument of fetus and newborn **171, 172**
779.0 Convulsions in newborn **163, 168**
779.1 Other and unspecified cerebral irritability in newborn **163, 168**
779.2 Cerebral depression, coma, and other abnormal cerebral signs in fetus or newborn **163, 168**
779.31 Feeding problems in newborn **171**
779.32 Bilious vomiting in newborn **163, 168**
779.33 Other vomiting in newborn **171**
779.34 Failure to thrive in newborn **113, 231**
779.4 Drug reactions and intoxications specific to newborn **163, 168**
779.5 Drug withdrawal syndrome in newborn **163, 168**
779.7 Periventricular leukomalacia **33, 166, 170**
779.83 Delayed separation of umbilical cord **171**
779.85 Cardiac arrest of newborn **163, 168**
780.01 Coma **21, 166, 170**
780.02 Transient alteration of awareness **188**
780.03 Persistent vegetative state **21, 166, 170**
780.09 Other alteration of consciousness **21**
780.1 Hallucinations **188**
780.2 Syncope and collapse **68**
780.3* Convulsions **34**
780.31 Febrile convulsions (simple), unspecified **166, 170**
780.39 Other convulsions **166, 170**
780.4 Dizziness and giddiness **46**
780.50 Unspecified sleep disturbance **189**
780.51 Insomnia with sleep apnea, unspecified **3, 47**
780.52 Insomnia, unspecified **189**
780.53 Hypersomnia with sleep apnea, unspecified **3, 47**
780.54 Hypersomnia, unspecified **189**
780.55 Disruption of 24 hour sleep wake cycle, unspecified **189**
780.56 Dysfunctions associated with sleep stages or arousal from sleep **189**
780.57 Unspecified sleep apnea **3, 47**

781.0 Abnormal involuntary movements **33**
781.1 Disturbances of sensation of smell and taste **33**
781.2 Abnormality of gait **33**
781.3 Lack of coordination **33**
781.4 Transient paralysis of limb **33**
781.5 Clubbing of fingers **54**
781.6 Meningismus **33**
781.7 Tetany **113, 166, 170**
781.8 Neurological neglect syndrome **33**
781.91 Loss of height **33**
781.92 Abnormal posture **33**
781.93 Ocular torticollis **98**
781.94 Facial weakness **33**
781.99 Other symptoms involving nervous and musculoskeletal systems **33**
782.0 Disturbance of skin sensation **33**
782.1 Rash and other nonspecific skin eruption **108, 231**
782.2 Localized superficial swelling, mass, or lump **108**
782.3 Edema **213**
782.4 Jaundice, unspecified, not of newborn **83**
782.5 Cyanosis **213**
782.6* Pallor and flushing **213**
782.7 Spontaneous ecchymoses **176**
782.8 Changes in skin texture **108**
782.9 Other symptoms involving skin and integumentary tissues **108**
783.2* Abnormal loss of weight **231**
783.4* Lack of expected normal physiological development **231**
783* Symptoms concerning nutrition, metabolism, and development **113**
784.0 Headache **34**
784.1 Throat pain **47**
784.2 Swelling, mass, or lump in head and neck **108**
784.3 Aphasia **33**
784.4* Voice and resonance disorders **47**
784.5* Other speech disturbance **33**
784.60 Symbolic dysfunction, unspecified **189**
784.61 Alexia and dyslexia **189**
784.69 Other symbolic dysfunction **189**
784.7 Epistaxis **46**
784.8 Hemorrhage from throat **3, 47**
784.91 Postnasal drip **47**
784.92 Jaw pain **3, 48**
784.99 Other symptoms involving head and neck **47**

*Code Range   **359**

Numeric Index to Diseases

785.0	Unspecified tachycardia **68, 166, 170**	
785.1	Palpitations **68**	
785.2	Undiagnosed cardiac murmurs **68**	
785.3	Other abnormal heart sounds **69**	
785.4	Gangrene **67, 166, 170**	
785.50	Unspecified shock **57, 66, 166, 170**	
785.51	Cardiogenic shock **57, 66**	
785.52	Septic shock **186**	
785.59	Other shock without mention of trauma **186**	
785.6	Enlargement of lymph nodes **176, 231**	
785.9	Other symptoms involving cardiovascular system **69**	
786.0*	Dyspnea and respiratory abnormalities **54, 231**	
786.1	Stridor **54**	
786.2	Cough **54**	
786.3*	Hemoptysis **54**	
786.4	Abnormal sputum **54**	
786.50	Chest pain, unspecified **68**	
786.51	Precordial pain **68**	
786.52	Painful respiration **54**	
786.59	Chest pain, other **68**	
786.6	Swelling, mass, or lump in chest **54**	
786.7	Abnormal chest sounds **54**	
786.8	Hiccough **54**	
786.9	Other symptoms involving respiratory system and chest **54**	
787*	Symptoms involving digestive system **78**	
788.0	Renal colic **119**	
788.1	Dysuria **119**	
788.2*	Retention of urine **119, 166, 170**	
788.3*	Urinary incontinence **119**	
788.4*	Frequency of urination and polyuria **119**	
788.5	Oliguria and anuria **118, 119**	
788.6*	Other abnormality of urination **119**	
788.7	Urethral discharge **119**	
788.8	Extravasation of urine **119**	
788.9*	Other symptoms involving urinary system **119**	
789.0*	Abdominal pain **78**	
789.1	Hepatomegaly **83, 231**	
789.2	Splenomegaly **176, 231**	
789.3*	Abdominal or pelvic swelling, mass, or lump **78**	
789.4*	Abdominal rigidity **79**	
789.5*	Ascites **213**	
789.6*	Abdominal tenderness **78**	
789.7	Colic **78**	
789.9	Other symptoms involving abdomen and pelvis **78**	
790.0*	Abnormality of red blood cells **175**	
790.1	Elevated sedimentation rate **213**	
790.2*	Abnormal glucose **113**	
790.3	Excessive blood level of alcohol **191**	
790.4	Nonspecific elevation of levels of transaminase or lactic acid dehydrogenase (LDH) **213**	
790.5	Other nonspecific abnormal serum enzyme levels **213**	
790.6	Other abnormal blood chemistry **213**	
790.7	Bacteremia **166, 170, 186**	
790.8	Unspecified viremia **185**	
790.9*	Other nonspecific findings on examination of blood **213**	
791.0	Proteinuria **119**	
791.1	Chyluria **119, 166, 170**	
791.2	Hemoglobinuria **120**	
791.3	Myoglobinuria **213**	

791.4	Biliuria **83**
791.5	Glycosuria **113**
791.6	Acetonuria **113**
791.7	Other cells and casts in urine **120**
791.9	Other nonspecific finding on examination of urine **120**
792.0	Nonspecific abnormal finding in cerebrospinal fluid **33**
792.1	Nonspecific abnormal finding in stool contents **78**
792.2	Nonspecific abnormal finding in semen **124**
792.3	Nonspecific abnormal finding in amniotic fluid **156, 159**
792.4	Nonspecific abnormal finding in saliva **47**
792.5	Cloudy (hemodialysis) (peritoneal) dialysis affluent **213**
792.9	Other nonspecific abnormal finding in body substances **213**
793.0	Nonspecific (abnormal) findings on radiological and other examination of skull and head **33**
793.11	Solitary pulmonary nodule **54**
793.19	Other nonspecific abnormal finding of lung field **54**
793.2	Nonspecific (abnormal) findings on radiological and other examination of other intrathoracic organs **67**
793.3	Nonspecific (abnormal) findings on radiological and other examination of biliary tract **83**
793.4	Nonspecific (abnormal) findings on radiological and other examination of gastrointestinal tract **78**
793.5	Nonspecific (abnormal) findings on radiological and other examination of genitourinary organs **120**
793.6	Nonspecific (abnormal) findings on radiological and other examination of abdominal area, including retroperitoneum **78**
793.7	Nonspecific (abnormal) findings on radiological and other examination of musculoskeletal system **101**
793.8*	Nonspecific abnormal findings on radiological and other examinations of body structure, breast **106**
793.9*	Other nonspecific abnormal findings on radiological and other examinations of body structure **213**
794.0*	Nonspecific abnormal results of function study of brain and central nervous system **33**
794.10	Nonspecific abnormal response to unspecified nerve stimulation **33**
794.11	Nonspecific abnormal retinal function studies **40**
794.12	Nonspecific abnormal electro-oculogram (EOG) **40**
794.13	Nonspecific abnormal visually evoked potential **40**
794.14	Nonspecific abnormal oculomotor studies **40**
794.15	Nonspecific abnormal auditory function studies **47, 172**
794.16	Nonspecific abnormal vestibular function studies **47**
794.17	Nonspecific abnormal electromyogram (EMG) **101**
794.19	Other nonspecific abnormal result of function study of peripheral nervous system and special senses **33**
794.2	Nonspecific abnormal results of pulmonary system function study **54**
794.30	Nonspecific abnormal unspecified cardiovascular function study **69**
794.31	Nonspecific abnormal electrocardiogram (ECG) (EKG) **69**
794.39	Other nonspecific abnormal cardiovascular system function study **69**
794.4	Nonspecific abnormal results of kidney function study **120**
794.5	Nonspecific abnormal results of thyroid function study **114**
794.6	Nonspecific abnormal results of other endocrine function study **114**
794.7	Nonspecific abnormal results of basal metabolism function study **114**
794.8	Nonspecific abnormal results of liver function study **83**
794.9	Nonspecific abnormal results of other specified function study **120**
795.0*	Abnormal Papanicolaou smear of cervix and cervical HPV **127, 130**

*Code Range

© 2013 OptumInsight, Inc.

795.1*	Abnormal Papanicolaou smear of vagina and vaginal HPV **127, 130**	
795.2	Nonspecific abnormal findings on chromosomal analysis **213**	
795.3*	Nonspecific positive culture findings **186**	
795.4	Other nonspecific abnormal histological findings **172, 213**	
795.5*	Nonspecific reaction to test for tuberculosis **51**	
795.6	False positive serological test for syphilis **97**	
795.7*	Other nonspecific immunological findings **176**	
795.8*	Abnormal tumor markers **213**	
796.0	Nonspecific abnormal toxicological findings **204**	
796.1	Abnormal reflex **33**	
796.2	Elevated blood pressure reading without diagnosis of hypertension **69**	
796.3	Nonspecific low blood pressure reading **69**	
796.4	Other abnormal clinical finding **172, 213**	
796.5	Abnormal finding on antenatal screening **156, 159**	
796.6	Nonspecific abnormal findings on neonatal screening **213**	
796.7*	Abnormal cytologic smear of anus and anal HPV **79**	
796.9	Other nonspecific abnormal finding **213**	
797	Senility without mention of psychosis **188**	
798.0	Sudden infant death syndrome **33**	
798.1	Instantaneous death **66**	
798.2	Death occurring in less than 24 hours from onset of symptoms, not otherwise explained **66**	
798.9	Unattended death **213**	
799.0*	Asphyxia and hypoxemia **54**	
799.1	Respiratory arrest **54, 166, 170**	
799.21	Nervousness **188**	
799.22	Irritability **188**	
799.23	Impulsiveness **188**	
799.24	Emotional lability **188**	
799.25	Demoralization and apathy **188**	
799.29	Other signs and symptoms involving emotional state **188**	
799.3	Unspecified debility **213**	
799.4	Cachexia **213, 231**	
799.51	Attention or concentration deficit **189**	
799.52	Cognitive communication deficit **188**	
799.53	Visuospatial deficit **33**	
799.54	Psychomotor deficit **188**	
799.55	Frontal lobe and executive function deficit **188**	
799.59	Other signs and symptoms involving cognition **188**	
799.8*	Other ill-defined conditions **213**	
799.9	Other unknown and unspecified cause of morbidity or mortality **213**	
800.0*	Closed fracture of vault of skull without mention of intracranial injury **220**	
800.00	Closed fracture of vault of skull without mention of intracranial injury, unspecified state of consciousness **27**	
800.01	Closed fracture of vault of skull without mention of intracranial injury, no loss of consciousness **27**	
800.02	Closed fracture of vault of skull without mention of intracranial injury, brief (less than one hour) loss of consciousness **27, 224**	
800.03	Closed fracture of vault of skull without mention of intracranial injury, moderate (1-24 hours) loss of consciousness **22, 224**	
800.04	Closed fracture of vault of skull without mention of intracranial injury, prolonged (more than 24 hours) loss of consciousness and return to pre-existing conscious level **22, 224**	
800.05	Closed fracture of vault of skull without mention of intracranial injury, prolonged (more than 24 hours) loss of consciousness, without return to pre-existing conscious level **22, 224**	
800.06	Closed fracture of vault of skull without mention of intracranial injury, loss of consciousness of unspecified duration **22**	

800.09	Closed fracture of vault of skull without mention of intracranial injury, unspecified concussion **27**
800.1*	Closed fracture of vault of skull with cerebral laceration and contusion **220**
800.10	Closed fracture of vault of skull with cerebral laceration and contusion, unspecified state of consciousness **27, 224**
800.11	Closed fracture of vault of skull with cerebral laceration and contusion, no loss of consciousness **27**
800.12	Closed fracture of vault of skull with cerebral laceration and contusion, brief (less than one hour) loss of consciousness **27, 224**
800.13	Closed fracture of vault of skull with cerebral laceration and contusion, moderate (1-24 hours) loss of consciousness **22, 224**
800.14	Closed fracture of vault of skull with cerebral laceration and contusion, prolonged (more than 24 hours) loss of consciousness and return to pre-existing conscious level **22, 224**
800.15	Closed fracture of vault of skull with cerebral laceration and contusion, prolonged (more than 24 hours) loss of consciousness, without return to pre-existing conscious level **22, 224**
800.16	Closed fracture of vault of skull with cerebral laceration and contusion, loss of consciousness of unspecified duration **22, 224**
800.19	Closed fracture of vault of skull with cerebral laceration and contusion, unspecified concussion **27, 224**
800.2*	Closed fracture of vault of skull with subarachnoid, subdural, and extradural hemorrhage **220**
800.20	Closed fracture of vault of skull with subarachnoid, subdural, and extradural hemorrhage, unspecified state of consciousness **27, 224**
800.21	Closed fracture of vault of skull with subarachnoid, subdural, and extradural hemorrhage, no loss of consciousness **27**
800.22	Closed fracture of vault of skull with subarachnoid, subdural, and extradural hemorrhage, brief (less than one hour) loss of consciousness **27, 224**
800.23	Closed fracture of vault of skull with subarachnoid, subdural, and extradural hemorrhage, moderate (1-24 hours) loss of consciousness **22, 224**
800.24	Closed fracture of vault of skull with subarachnoid, subdural, and extradural hemorrhage, prolonged (more than 24 hours) loss of consciousness and return to pre-existing conscious level **22, 224**
800.25	Closed fracture of vault of skull with subarachnoid, subdural, and extradural hemorrhage, prolonged (more than 24 hours) loss of consciousness, without return to pre-existing conscious level **22, 224**
800.26	Closed fracture of vault of skull with subarachnoid, subdural, and extradural hemorrhage, loss of consciousness of unspecified duration **22, 224**
800.29	Closed fracture of vault of skull with subarachnoid, subdural, and extradural hemorrhage, unspecified concussion **27, 224**
800.3*	Closed fracture of vault of skull with other and unspecified intracranial hemorrhage **220**
800.30	Closed fracture of vault of skull with other and unspecified intracranial hemorrhage, unspecified state of consciousness **28, 224**
800.31	Closed fracture of vault of skull with other and unspecified intracranial hemorrhage, no loss of consciousness **28**
800.32	Closed fracture of vault of skull with other and unspecified intracranial hemorrhage, brief (less than one hour) loss of consciousness **28, 224**
800.33	Closed fracture of vault of skull with other and unspecified intracranial hemorrhage, moderate (1-24 hours) loss of consciousness **22, 224**
800.34	Closed fracture of vault of skull with other and unspecified intracranial hemorrhage, prolonged (more than 24 hours) loss of consciousness and return to pre-existing conscious level **22, 224**
800.35	Closed fracture of vault of skull with other and unspecified intracranial hemorrhage, prolonged (more than 24 hours) loss of consciousness, without return to pre-existing conscious level **22, 224**

800.36   Closed fracture of vault of skull with other and unspecified intracranial hemorrhage, loss of consciousness of unspecified duration **22**, **224**

800.39   Closed fracture of vault of skull with other and unspecified intracranial hemorrhage, unspecified concussion **28**, **224**

800.4*   Closed fracture of vault of skull with intercranial injury of other and unspecified nature **220**

800.40   Closed fracture of vault of skull with intracranial injury of other and unspecified nature, unspecified state of consciousness **28**, **224**

800.41   Closed fracture of vault of skull with intracranial injury of other and unspecified nature, no loss of consciousness **28**

800.42   Closed fracture of vault of skull with intracranial injury of other and unspecified nature, brief (less than one hour) loss of consciousness **28**, **224**

800.43   Closed fracture of vault of skull with intracranial injury of other and unspecified nature, moderate (1-24 hours) loss of consciousness **22**, **224**

800.44   Closed fracture of vault of skull with intracranial injury of other and unspecified nature, prolonged (more than 24 hours) loss of consciousness and return to pre-existing conscious level **22**, **224**

800.45   Closed fracture of vault of skull with intracranial injury of other and unspecified nature, prolonged (more than 24 hours) loss of consciousness, without return to pre-existing conscious level **22**, **224**

800.46   Closed fracture of vault of skull with intracranial injury of other and unspecified nature, loss of consciousness of unspecified duration **22**, **224**

800.49   Closed fracture of vault of skull with intracranial injury of other and unspecified nature, unspecified concussion **28**, **224**

800.5*   Open fracture of vault of skull without mention of intracranial injury **220**

800.50   Open fracture of vault of skull without mention of intracranial injury, unspecified state of consciousness **28**

800.51   Open fracture of vault of skull without mention of intracranial injury, no loss of consciousness **28**

800.52   Open fracture of vault of skull without mention of intracranial injury, brief (less than one hour) loss of consciousness **28**, **224**

800.53   Open fracture of vault of skull without mention of intracranial injury, moderate (1-24 hours) loss of consciousness **22**, **225**

800.54   Open fracture of vault of skull without mention of intracranial injury, prolonged (more than 24 hours) loss of consciousness and return to pre-existing conscious level **22**, **225**

800.55   Open fracture of vault of skull without mention of intracranial injury, prolonged (more than 24 hours) loss of consciousness, without return to pre-existing conscious level **22**, **225**

800.56   Open fracture of vault of skull without mention of intracranial injury, loss of consciousness of unspecified duration **22**

800.59   Open fracture of vault of skull without mention of intracranial injury, unspecified concussion **28**

800.6*   Open fracture of vault of skull with cerebral laceration and contusion **220**, **225**

800.60   Open fracture of vault of skull with cerebral laceration and contusion, unspecified state of consciousness **28**

800.61   Open fracture of vault of skull with cerebral laceration and contusion, no loss of consciousness **28**

800.62   Open fracture of vault of skull with cerebral laceration and contusion, brief (less than one hour) loss of consciousness **28**

800.63   Open fracture of vault of skull with cerebral laceration and contusion, moderate (1-24 hours) loss of consciousness **22**

800.64   Open fracture of vault of skull with cerebral laceration and contusion, prolonged (more than 24 hours) loss of consciousness and return to pre-existing conscious level **22**

800.65   Open fracture of vault of skull with cerebral laceration and contusion, prolonged (more than 24 hours) loss of consciousness, without return to pre-existing conscious level **22**

800.66   Open fracture of vault of skull with cerebral laceration and contusion, loss of consciousness of unspecified duration **22**

800.69   Open fracture of vault of skull with cerebral laceration and contusion, unspecified concussion **28**

800.7*   Open fracture of vault of skull with subarachnoid, subdural, and extradural hemorrhage **220**, **225**

800.70   Open fracture of vault of skull with subarachnoid, subdural, and extradural hemorrhage, unspecified state of consciousness **28**

800.71   Open fracture of vault of skull with subarachnoid, subdural, and extradural hemorrhage, no loss of consciousness **28**

800.72   Open fracture of vault of skull with subarachnoid, subdural, and extradural hemorrhage, brief (less than one hour) loss of consciousness **28**

800.73   Open fracture of vault of skull with subarachnoid, subdural, and extradural hemorrhage, moderate (1-24 hours) loss of consciousness **22**

800.74   Open fracture of vault of skull with subarachnoid, subdural, and extradural hemorrhage, prolonged (more than 24 hours) loss of consciousness and return to pre-existing conscious level **22**

800.75   Open fracture of vault of skull with subarachnoid, subdural, and extradural hemorrhage, prolonged (more than 24 hours) loss of consciousness, without return to pre-existing conscious level **22**

800.76   Open fracture of vault of skull with subarachnoid, subdural, and extradural hemorrhage, loss of consciousness of unspecified duration **22**

800.79   Open fracture of vault of skull with subarachnoid, subdural, and extradural hemorrhage, unspecified concussion **28**

800.8*   Open fracture of vault of skull with other and unspecified intracranial hemorrhage **220**, **225**

800.80   Open fracture of vault of skull with other and unspecified intracranial hemorrhage, unspecified state of consciousness **28**

800.81   Open fracture of vault of skull with other and unspecified intracranial hemorrhage, no loss of consciousness **28**

800.82   Open fracture of vault of skull with other and unspecified intracranial hemorrhage, brief (less than one hour) loss of consciousness **28**

800.83   Open fracture of vault of skull with other and unspecified intracranial hemorrhage, moderate (1-24 hours) loss of consciousness **22**

800.84   Open fracture of vault of skull with other and unspecified intracranial hemorrhage, prolonged (more than 24 hours) loss of consciousness and return to pre-existing conscious level **22**

800.85   Open fracture of vault of skull with other and unspecified intracranial hemorrhage, prolonged (more than 24 hours) loss of consciousness, without return to pre-existing conscious level **22**

800.86   Open fracture of vault of skull with other and unspecified intracranial hemorrhage, loss of consciousness of unspecified duration **22**

800.89   Open fracture of vault of skull with other and unspecified intracranial hemorrhage, unspecified concussion **28**

800.9*   Open fracture of vault of skull with intracranial injury of other and unspecified nature **220**, **225**

800.90   Open fracture of vault of skull with intracranial injury of other and unspecified nature, unspecified state of consciousness **28**

800.91   Open fracture of vault of skull with intracranial injury of other and unspecified nature, no loss of consciousness **28**

800.92   Open fracture of vault of skull with intracranial injury of other and unspecified nature, brief (less than one hour) loss of consciousness **28**

800.93   Open fracture of vault of skull with intracranial injury of other and unspecified nature, moderate (1-24 hours) loss of consciousness **22**

800.94   Open fracture of vault of skull with intracranial injury of other and unspecified nature, prolonged (more than 24 hours) loss of consciousness and return to pre-existing conscious level **22**

800.95   Open fracture of vault of skull with intracranial injury of other and unspecified nature, prolonged (more than 24 hours) loss of consciousness, without return to pre-existing conscious level **22**

*Code Range

800.96	Open fracture of vault of skull with intracranial injury of other and unspecified nature, loss of consciousness of unspecified duration **23**
800.99	Open fracture of vault of skull with intracranial injury of other and unspecified nature, unspecified concussion **28**
801.0*	Closed fracture of base of skull without mention of intracranial injury **220**
801.00	Closed fracture of base of skull without mention of intracranial injury, unspecified state of consciousness **28**
801.01	Closed fracture of base of skull without mention of intracranial injury, no loss of consciousness **28**
801.02	Closed fracture of base of skull without mention of intracranial injury, brief (less than one hour) loss of consciousness **28, 225**
801.03	Closed fracture of base of skull without mention of intracranial injury, moderate (1-24 hours) loss of consciousness **23, 225**
801.04	Closed fracture of base of skull without mention of intracranial injury, prolonged (more than 24 hours) loss of consciousness and return to pre-existing conscious level **23, 225**
801.05	Closed fracture of base of skull without mention of intracranial injury, prolonged (more than 24 hours) loss of consciousness, without return to pre-existing conscious level **23, 225**
801.06	Closed fracture of base of skull without mention of intracranial injury, loss of consciousness of unspecified duration **23**
801.09	Closed fracture of base of skull without mention of intracranial injury, unspecified concussion **28**
801.1*	Closed fracture of base of skull with cerebral laceration and contusion **220, 225**
801.10	Closed fracture of base of skull with cerebral laceration and contusion, unspecified state of consciousness **28**
801.11	Closed fracture of base of skull with cerebral laceration and contusion, no loss of consciousness **28**
801.12	Closed fracture of base of skull with cerebral laceration and contusion, brief (less than one hour) loss of consciousness **28**
801.13	Closed fracture of base of skull with cerebral laceration and contusion, moderate (1-24 hours) loss of consciousness **23**
801.14	Closed fracture of base of skull with cerebral laceration and contusion, prolonged (more than 24 hours) loss of consciousness and return to pre-existing conscious level **23**
801.15	Closed fracture of base of skull with cerebral laceration and contusion, prolonged (more than 24 hours) loss of consciousness, without return to pre-existing conscious level **23**
801.16	Closed fracture of base of skull with cerebral laceration and contusion, loss of consciousness of unspecified duration **23**
801.19	Closed fracture of base of skull with cerebral laceration and contusion, unspecified concussion **28**
801.2*	Closed fracture of base of skull with subarachnoid, subdural, and extradural hemorrhage **220, 225**
801.20	Closed fracture of base of skull with subarachnoid, subdural, and extradural hemorrhage, unspecified state of consciousness **28**
801.21	Closed fracture of base of skull with subarachnoid, subdural, and extradural hemorrhage, no loss of consciousness **28**
801.22	Closed fracture of base of skull with subarachnoid, subdural, and extradural hemorrhage, brief (less than one hour) loss of consciousness **28**
801.23	Closed fracture of base of skull with subarachnoid, subdural, and extradural hemorrhage, moderate (1-24 hours) loss of consciousness **23**
801.24	Closed fracture of base of skull with subarachnoid, subdural, and extradural hemorrhage, prolonged (more than 24 hours) loss of consciousness and return to pre-existing conscious level **23**
801.25	Closed fracture of base of skull with subarachnoid, subdural, and extradural hemorrhage, prolonged (more than 24 hours) loss of consciousness, without return to pre-existing conscious level **23**
801.26	Closed fracture of base of skull with subarachnoid, subdural, and extradural hemorrhage, loss of consciousness of unspecified duration **23**
801.29	Closed fracture of base of skull with subarachnoid, subdural, and extradural hemorrhage, unspecified concussion **28**
801.3*	Closed fracture of base of skull with other and unspecified intracranial hemorrhage **220, 225**
801.30	Closed fracture of base of skull with other and unspecified intracranial hemorrhage, unspecified state of consciousness **28**
801.31	Closed fracture of base of skull with other and unspecified intracranial hemorrhage, no loss of consciousness **28**
801.32	Closed fracture of base of skull with other and unspecified intracranial hemorrhage, brief (less than one hour) loss of consciousness **28**
801.33	Closed fracture of base of skull with other and unspecified intracranial hemorrhage, moderate (1-24 hours) loss of consciousness **23**
801.34	Closed fracture of base of skull with other and unspecified intracranial hemorrhage, prolonged (more than 24 hours) loss of consciousness and return to pre-existing conscious level **23**
801.35	Closed fracture of base of skull with other and unspecified intracranial hemorrhage, prolonged (more than 24 hours) loss of consciousness, without return to pre-existing conscious level **23**
801.36	Closed fracture of base of skull with other and unspecified intracranial hemorrhage, loss of consciousness of unspecified duration **23**
801.39	Closed fracture of base of skull with other and unspecified intracranial hemorrhage, unspecified concussion **28**
801.4*	Closed fracture of base of skull with intracranial injury of other and unspecified nature **220, 225**
801.40	Closed fracture of base of skull with intracranial injury of other and unspecified nature, unspecified state of consciousness **28**
801.41	Closed fracture of base of skull with intracranial injury of other and unspecified nature, no loss of consciousness **28**
801.42	Closed fracture of base of skull with intracranial injury of other and unspecified nature, brief (less than one hour) loss of consciousness **28**
801.43	Closed fracture of base of skull with intracranial injury of other and unspecified nature, moderate (1-24 hours) loss of consciousness **23**
801.44	Closed fracture of base of skull with intracranial injury of other and unspecified nature, prolonged (more than 24 hours) loss of consciousness and return to pre-existing conscious level **23**
801.45	Closed fracture of base of skull with intracranial injury of other and unspecified nature, prolonged (more than 24 hours) loss of consciousness, without return to pre-existing conscious level **23**
801.46	Closed fracture of base of skull with intracranial injury of other and unspecified nature, loss of consciousness of unspecified duration **23**
801.49	Closed fracture of base of skull with intracranial injury of other and unspecified nature, unspecified concussion **28**
801.5*	Open fracture of base of skull without mention of intracranial injury **220**
801.50	Open fracture of base of skull without mention of intracranial injury, unspecified state of consciousness **28**
801.51	Open fracture of base of skull without mention of intracranial injury, no loss of consciousness **28**
801.52	Open fracture of base of skull without mention of intracranial injury, brief (less than one hour) loss of consciousness **28, 225**
801.53	Open fracture of base of skull without mention of intracranial injury, moderate (1-24 hours) loss of consciousness **23, 225**
801.54	Open fracture of base of skull without mention of intracranial injury, prolonged (more than 24 hours) loss of consciousness and return to pre-existing conscious level **23, 225**
801.55	Open fracture of base of skull without mention of intracranial injury, prolonged (more than 24 hours) loss of consciousness, without return to pre-existing conscious level **23, 225**
801.56	Open fracture of base of skull without mention of intracranial injury, loss of consciousness of unspecified duration **23**

801.59 Open fracture of base of skull without mention of intracranial injury, unspecified concussion **28**

801.6★ Open fracture of base of skull with cerebral laceration and contusion **221**, **225**

801.60 Open fracture of base of skull with cerebral laceration and contusion, unspecified state of consciousness **28**

801.61 Open fracture of base of skull with cerebral laceration and contusion, no loss of consciousness **28**

801.62 Open fracture of base of skull with cerebral laceration and contusion, brief (less than one hour) loss of consciousness **28**

801.63 Open fracture of base of skull with cerebral laceration and contusion, moderate (1-24 hours) loss of consciousness **23**

801.64 Open fracture of base of skull with cerebral laceration and contusion, prolonged (more than 24 hours) loss of consciousness and return to pre-existing conscious level **23**

801.65 Open fracture of base of skull with cerebral laceration and contusion, prolonged (more than 24 hours) loss of consciousness, without return to pre-existing conscious level **23**

801.66 Open fracture of base of skull with cerebral laceration and contusion, loss of consciousness of unspecified duration **23**

801.69 Open fracture of base of skull with cerebral laceration and contusion, unspecified concussion **28**

801.7★ Open fracture of base of skull with subarachnoid, subdural, and extradural hemorrhage **221**, **225**

801.70 Open fracture of base of skull with subarachnoid, subdural, and extradural hemorrhage, unspecified state of consciousness **28**

801.71 Open fracture of base of skull with subarachnoid, subdural, and extradural hemorrhage, no loss of consciousness **28**

801.72 Open fracture of base of skull with subarachnoid, subdural, and extradural hemorrhage, brief (less than one hour) loss of consciousness **28**

801.73 Open fracture of base of skull with subarachnoid, subdural, and extradural hemorrhage, moderate (1-24 hours) loss of consciousness **23**

801.74 Open fracture of base of skull with subarachnoid, subdural, and extradural hemorrhage, prolonged (more than 24 hours) loss of consciousness and return to pre-existing conscious level **23**

801.75 Open fracture of base of skull with subarachnoid, subdural, and extradural hemorrhage, prolonged (more than 24 hours) loss of consciousness, without return to pre-existing conscious level **23**

801.76 Open fracture of base of skull with subarachnoid, subdural, and extradural hemorrhage, loss of consciousness of unspecified duration **23**

801.79 Open fracture of base of skull with subarachnoid, subdural, and extradural hemorrhage, unspecified concussion **28**

801.8★ Open fracture of base of skull with other and unspecified intracranial hemorrhage **221**, **225**

801.80 Open fracture of base of skull with other and unspecified intracranial hemorrhage, unspecified state of consciousness **29**

801.81 Open fracture of base of skull with other and unspecified intracranial hemorrhage, no loss of consciousness **29**

801.82 Open fracture of base of skull with other and unspecified intracranial hemorrhage, brief (less than one hour) loss of consciousness **29**

801.83 Open fracture of base of skull with other and unspecified intracranial hemorrhage, moderate (1-24 hours) loss of consciousness **23**

801.84 Open fracture of base of skull with other and unspecified intracranial hemorrhage, prolonged (more than 24 hours) loss of consciousness and return to pre-existing conscious level **23**

801.85 Open fracture of base of skull with other and unspecified intracranial hemorrhage, prolonged (more than 24 hours) loss of consciousness, without return to pre-existing conscious level **23**

801.86 Open fracture of base of skull with other and unspecified intracranial hemorrhage, loss of consciousness of unspecified duration **23**

801.89 Open fracture of base of skull with other and unspecified intracranial hemorrhage, unspecified concussion **29**

801.9★ Open fracture of base of skull with intracranial injury of other and unspecified nature **221**, **225**

801.90 Open fracture of base of skull with intracranial injury of other and unspecified nature, unspecified state of consciousness **29**

801.91 Open fracture of base of skull with intracranial injury of other and unspecified nature, no loss of consciousness **29**

801.92 Open fracture of base of skull with intracranial injury of other and unspecified nature, brief (less than one hour) loss of consciousness **29**

801.93 Open fracture of base of skull with intracranial injury of other and unspecified nature, moderate (1-24 hours) loss of consciousness **23**

801.94 Open fracture of base of skull with intracranial injury of other and unspecified nature, prolonged (more than 24 hours) loss of consciousness and return to pre-existing conscious level **23**

801.95 Open fracture of base of skull with intracranial injury of other and unspecified nature, prolonged (more than 24 hours) loss of consciousness, without return to pre-existing conscious level **23**

801.96 Open fracture of base of skull with intracranial injury of other and unspecified nature, loss of consciousness of unspecified duration **23**

801.99 Open fracture of base of skull with intracranial injury of other and unspecified nature, unspecified concussion **29**

802.0 Nasal bones, closed fracture **47**, **221**

802.1 Nasal bones, open fracture **47**, **221**

802.2★ Mandible, closed fracture **3**, **48**, **221**

802.3★ Mandible, open fracture **3**, **48**, **221**

802.4 Malar and maxillary bones, closed fracture **3**, **48**, **221**

802.5 Malar and maxillary bones, open fracture **3**, **48**, **221**

802.6 Orbital floor (blow-out), closed fracture **3**, **40**, **221**

802.7 Orbital floor (blow-out), open fracture **3**, **40**, **221**

802.8 Other facial bones, closed fracture **3**, **101**, **221**

802.9 Other facial bones, open fracture **3**, **101**, **221**

803.0★ Other closed skull fracture without mention of intracranial injury **221**

803.00 Other closed skull fracture without mention of intracranial injury, unspecified state of consciousness **29**

803.01 Other closed skull fracture without mention of intracranial injury, no loss of consciousness **29**

803.02 Other closed skull fracture without mention of intracranial injury, brief (less than one hour) loss of consciousness **29**, **225**

803.03 Other closed skull fracture without mention of intracranial injury, moderate (1-24 hours) loss of consciousness **23**, **225**

803.04 Other closed skull fracture without mention of intracranial injury, prolonged (more than 24 hours) loss of consciousness and return to pre-existing conscious level **24**, **225**

803.05 Other closed skull fracture without mention of intracranial injury, prolonged (more than 24 hours) loss of consciousness, without return to pre-existing conscious level **24**, **225**

803.06 Other closed skull fracture without mention of intracranial injury, loss of consciousness of unspecified duration **24**

803.09 Other closed skull fracture without mention of intracranial injury, unspecified concussion **29**

803.1★ Other closed skull fracture with cerebral laceration and contusion **221**, **225**

803.10 Other closed skull fracture with cerebral laceration and contusion, unspecified state of consciousness **29**

803.11 Other closed skull fracture with cerebral laceration and contusion, no loss of consciousness **29**

803.12 Other closed skull fracture with cerebral laceration and contusion, brief (less than one hour) loss of consciousness **29**

803.13 Other closed skull fracture with cerebral laceration and contusion, moderate (1-24 hours) loss of consciousness **24**

*Code Range

803.14   Other closed skull fracture with cerebral laceration and contusion, prolonged (more than 24 hours) loss of consciousness and return to pre-existing conscious level **24**

803.15   Other closed skull fracture with cerebral laceration and contusion, prolonged (more than 24 hours) loss of consciousness, without return to pre-existing conscious level **24**

803.16   Other closed skull fracture with cerebral laceration and contusion, loss of consciousness of unspecified duration **24**

803.19   Other closed skull fracture with cerebral laceration and contusion, unspecified concussion **29**

803.2*   Other closed skull fracture with subarachnoid, subdural, and extradural hemorrhage **221, 225**

803.20   Other closed skull fracture with subarachnoid, subdural, and extradural hemorrhage, unspecified state of consciousness **29**

803.21   Other closed skull fracture with subarachnoid, subdural, and extradural hemorrhage, no loss of consciousness **29**

803.22   Other closed skull fracture with subarachnoid, subdural, and extradural hemorrhage, brief (less than one hour) loss of consciousness **29**

803.23   Other closed skull fracture with subarachnoid, subdural, and extradural hemorrhage, moderate (1-24 hours) loss of consciousness **24**

803.24   Other closed skull fracture with subarachnoid, subdural, and extradural hemorrhage, prolonged (more than 24 hours) loss of consciousness and return to pre-existing conscious level **24**

803.25   Other closed skull fracture with subarachnoid, subdural, and extradural hemorrhage, prolonged (more than 24 hours) loss of consciousness, without return to pre-existing conscious level **24**

803.26   Other closed skull fracture with subarachnoid, subdural, and extradural hemorrhage, loss of consciousness of unspecified duration **24**

803.29   Other closed skull fracture with subarachnoid, subdural, and extradural hemorrhage, unspecified concussion **29**

803.3*   Closed skull fracture with other and unspecified intracranial hemorrhage **221, 225**

803.30   Other closed skull fracture with other and unspecified intracranial hemorrhage, unspecified state of unconsciousness **29**

803.31   Other closed skull fracture with other and unspecified intracranial hemorrhage, no loss of consciousness **29**

803.32   Other closed skull fracture with other and unspecified intracranial hemorrhage, brief (less than one hour) loss of consciousness **29**

803.33   Other closed skull fracture with other and unspecified intracranial hemorrhage, moderate (1-24 hours) loss of consciousness **24**

803.34   Other closed skull fracture with other and unspecified intracranial hemorrhage, prolonged (more than 24 hours) loss of consciousness and return to pre-existing conscious level **24**

803.35   Other closed skull fracture with other and unspecified intracranial hemorrhage, prolonged (more than 24 hours) loss of consciousness, without return to pre-existing conscious level **24**

803.36   Other closed skull fracture with other and unspecified intracranial hemorrhage, loss of consciousness of unspecified duration **24**

803.39   Other closed skull fracture with other and unspecified intracranial hemorrhage, unspecified concussion **29**

803.4*   Other closed skull fracture with intracranial injury of other and unspecified nature **221, 225**

803.40   Other closed skull fracture with intracranial injury of other and unspecified nature, unspecified state of consciousness **29**

803.41   Other closed skull fracture with intracranial injury of other and unspecified nature, no loss of consciousness **29**

803.42   Other closed skull fracture with intracranial injury of other and unspecified nature, brief (less than one hour) loss of consciousness **29**

803.43   Other closed skull fracture with intracranial injury of other and unspecified nature, moderate (1-24 hours) loss of consciousness **24**

803.44   Other closed skull fracture with intracranial injury of other and unspecified nature, prolonged (more than 24 hours) loss of consciousness and return to pre-existing conscious level **24**

803.45   Other closed skull fracture with intracranial injury of other and unspecified nature, prolonged (more than 24 hours) loss of consciousness, without return to pre-existing conscious level **24**

803.46   Other closed skull fracture with intracranial injury of other and unspecified nature, loss of consciousness of unspecified duration **24**

803.49   Other closed skull fracture with intracranial injury of other and unspecified nature, unspecified concussion **29**

803.5*   Other open skull fracture without mention of intracranial injury **221**

803.50   Other open skull fracture without mention of injury, state of consciousness unspecified **29**

803.51   Other open skull fracture without mention of intracranial injury, no loss of consciousness **29**

803.52   Other open skull fracture without mention of intracranial injury, brief (less than one hour) loss of consciousness **29, 225**

803.53   Other open skull fracture without mention of intracranial injury, moderate (1-24 hours) loss of consciousness **24, 225**

803.54   Other open skull fracture without mention of intracranial injury, prolonged (more than 24 hours) loss of consciousness and return to pre-existing conscious level **24, 225**

803.55   Other open skull fracture without mention of intracranial injury, prolonged (more than 24 hours) loss of consciousness, without return to pre-existing conscious level **24, 225**

803.56   Other open skull fracture without mention of intracranial injury, loss of consciousness of unspecified duration **24**

803.59   Other open skull fracture without mention of intracranial injury, unspecified concussion **29**

803.6*   Other open skull fracture with cerebral laceration and contusion **221, 225**

803.60   Other open skull fracture with cerebral laceration and contusion, unspecified state of consciousness **29**

803.61   Other open skull fracture with cerebral laceration and contusion, no loss of consciousness **29**

803.62   Other open skull fracture with cerebral laceration and contusion, brief (less than one hour) loss of consciousness **29**

803.63   Other open skull fracture with cerebral laceration and contusion, moderate (1-24 hours) loss of consciousness **24**

803.64   Other open skull fracture with cerebral laceration and contusion, prolonged (more than 24 hours) loss of consciousness and return to pre-existing conscious level **24**

803.65   Other open skull fracture with cerebral laceration and contusion, prolonged (more than 24 hours) loss of consciousness, without return to pre-existing conscious level **24**

803.66   Other open skull fracture with cerebral laceration and contusion, loss of consciousness of unspecified duration **24**

803.69   Other open skull fracture with cerebral laceration and contusion, unspecified concussion **29**

803.7*   Other open skull fracture with subarachnoid, subdural, and extradural hemorrhage **221, 225**

803.70   Other open skull fracture with subarachnoid, subdural, and extradural hemorrhage, unspecified state of consciousness **29**

803.71   Other open skull fracture with subarachnoid, subdural, and extradural hemorrhage, no loss of consciousness **29**

803.72   Other open skull fracture with subarachnoid, subdural, and extradural hemorrhage, brief (less than one hour) loss of consciousness **29**

803.73   Other open skull fracture with subarachnoid, subdural, and extradural hemorrhage, moderate (1-24 hours) loss of consciousness **24**

803.74   Other open skull fracture with subarachnoid, subdural, and extradural hemorrhage, prolonged (more than 24 hours) loss of consciousness and return to pre-existing conscious level **24**

803.75   Other open skull fracture with subarachnoid, subdural, and extradural hemorrhage, prolonged (more than 24 hours) loss of consciousness, without return to pre-existing conscious level **24**

803.76   Other open skull fracture with subarachnoid, subdural, and extradural hemorrhage, loss of consciousness of unspecified duration **24**

803.79   Other open skull fracture with subarachnoid, subdural, and extradural hemorrhage, unspecified concussion **29**

803.8*   Other open skull fracture with other and unspecified intracranial hemorrhage **221, 225**

803.80   Other open skull fracture with other and unspecified intracranial hemorrhage, unspecified state of consciousness **29**

803.81   Other open skull fracture with other and unspecified intracranial hemorrhage, no loss of consciousness **29**

803.82   Other open skull fracture with other and unspecified intracranial hemorrhage, brief (less than one hour) loss of consciousness **29**

803.83   Other open skull fracture with other and unspecified intracranial hemorrhage, moderate (1-24 hours) loss of consciousness **24**

803.84   Other open skull fracture with other and unspecified intracranial hemorrhage, prolonged (more than 24 hours) loss of consciousness and return to pre-existing conscious level **24**

803.85   Other open skull fracture with other and unspecified intracranial hemorrhage, prolonged (more than 24 hours) loss of consciousness, without return to pre-existing conscious level **24**

803.86   Other open skull fracture with other and unspecified intracranial hemorrhage, loss of consciousness of unspecified duration **24**

803.89   Other open skull fracture with other and unspecified intracranial hemorrhage, unspecified concussion **29**

803.9*   Other open skull fracture with intracranial injury of other and unspecified nature **221, 225**

803.90   Other open skull fracture with intracranial injury of other and unspecified nature, unspecified state of consciousness **29**

803.91   Other open skull fracture with intracranial injury of other and unspecified nature, no loss of consciousness **29**

803.92   Other open skull fracture with intracranial injury of other and unspecified nature, brief (less than one hour) loss of consciousness **29**

803.93   Other open skull fracture with intracranial injury of other and unspecified nature, moderate (1-24 hours) loss of consciousness **24**

803.94   Other open skull fracture with intracranial injury of other and unspecified nature, prolonged (more than 24 hours) loss of consciousness and return to pre-existing conscious level **24**

803.95   Other open skull fracture with intracranial injury of other and unspecified nature, prolonged (more than 24 hours) loss of consciousness, without return to pre-existing conscious level **24**

803.96   Other open skull fracture with intracranial injury of other and unspecified nature, loss of consciousness of unspecified duration **24**

803.99   Other open skull fracture with intracranial injury of other and unspecified nature, unspecified concussion **29**

804.0*   Closed fractures involving skull or face with other bones, without mention of intracranial injury **221**

804.00   Closed fractures involving skull or face with other bones, without mention of intracranial injury, unspecified state of consciousness **29**

804.01   Closed fractures involving skull or face with other bones, without mention of intracranial injury, no loss of consciousness **29**

804.02   Closed fractures involving skull or face with other bones, without mention of intracranial injury, brief (less than one hour) loss of consciousness **29, 225**

804.03   Closed fractures involving skull or face with other bones, without mention of intracranial injury, moderate (1-24 hours) loss of consciousness **24, 225**

804.04   Closed fractures involving skull or face with other bones, without mention or intracranial injury, prolonged (more than 24 hours) loss of consciousness and return to pre-existing conscious level **24, 225**

804.05   Closed fractures involving skull of face with other bones, without mention of intracranial injury, prolonged (more than 24 hours) loss of consciousness, without return to pre-existing conscious level **24, 225**

804.06   Closed fractures involving skull of face with other bones, without mention of intracranial injury, loss of consciousness of unspecified duration **24, 225**

804.09   Closed fractures involving skull of face with other bones, without mention of intracranial injury, unspecified concussion **29**

804.1*   Closed fractures involving skull or face with other bones, with cerebral laceration and contusion **221, 225**

804.10   Closed fractures involving skull or face with other bones, with cerebral laceration and contusion, unspecified state of consciousness **29**

804.11   Closed fractures involving skull or face with other bones, with cerebral laceration and contusion, no loss of consciousness **29**

804.12   Closed fractures involving skull or face with other bones, with cerebral laceration and contusion, brief (less than one hour) loss of consciousness **29**

804.13   Closed fractures involving skull or face with other bones, with cerebral laceration and contusion, moderate (1-24 hours) loss of consciousness **25**

804.14   Closed fractures involving skull or face with other bones, with cerebral laceration and contusion, prolonged (more than 24 hours) loss of consciousness and return to pre-existing conscious level **25**

804.15   Closed fractures involving skull or face with other bones, with cerebral laceration and contusion, prolonged (more than 24 hours) loss of consciousness, without return to pre-existing conscious level **25**

804.16   Closed fractures involving skull or face with other bones, with cerebral laceration and contusion, loss of consciousness of unspecified duration **25**

804.19   Closed fractures involving skull or face with other bones, with cerebral laceration and contusion, unspecified concussion **29**

804.2*   Closed fractures involving skull or face with other bones with subarachnoid, subdural, and extradural hemorrhage **221, 225**

804.20   Closed fractures involving skull or face with other bones with subarachnoid, subdural, and extradural hemorrhage, unspecified state of consciousness **29**

804.21   Closed fractures involving skull or face with other bones with subarachnoid, subdural, and extradural hemorrhage, no loss of consciousness **29**

804.22   Closed fractures involving skull or face with other bones with subarachnoid, subdural, and extradural hemorrhage, brief (less than one hour) loss of consciousness **29**

804.23   Closed fractures involving skull or face with other bones with subarachnoid, subdural, and extradural hemorrhage, moderate (1-24 hours) loss of consciousness **25**

804.24   Closed fractures involving skull or face with other bones with subarachnoid, subdural, and extradural hemorrhage, prolonged (more than 24 hours) loss of consciousness and return to pre-existing conscious level **25**

804.25   Closed fractures involving skull or face with other bones with subarachnoid, subdural, and extradural hemorrhage, prolonged (more than 24 hours) loss of consciousness, without return to pre-existing conscious level **25**

804.26   Closed fractures involving skull or face with other bones with subarachnoid, subdural, and extradural hemorrhage, loss of consciousness of unspecified duration **25**

804.29   Closed fractures involving skull or face with other bones with subarachnoid, subdural, and extradural hemorrhage, unspecified concussion **30**

804.3*   Closed fractures involving skull or face with other bones, with other and unspecified intracranial hemorrhage **221, 225**

804.30   Closed fractures involving skull or face with other bones, with other and unspecified intracranial hemorrhage, unspecified state of consciousness **30**

804.31   Closed fractures involving skull or face with other bones, with other and unspecified intracranial hemorrhage, no loss of consciousness **30**

804.32   Closed fractures involving skull or face with other bones, with other and unspecified intracranial hemorrhage, brief (less than one hour) loss of consciousness **30**

804.33   Closed fractures involving skull or face with other bones, with other and unspecified intracranial hemorrhage, moderate (1-24 hours) loss of consciousness **25**

804.34   Closed fractures involving skull or face with other bones, with other and unspecified intracranial hemorrhage, prolonged (more than 24 hours) loss of consciousness and return to preexisting conscious level **25**

804.35   Closed fractures involving skull or face with other bones, with other and unspecified intracranial hemorrhage, prolonged (more than 24 hours) loss of consciousness, without return to pre-existing conscious level **25**

804.36   Closed fractures involving skull or face with other bones, with other and unspecified intracranial hemorrhage, loss of consciousness of unspecified duration **25**

804.39   Closed fractures involving skull or face with other bones, with other and unspecified intracranial hemorrhage, unspecified concussion **30**

804.4*   Closed fractures involving skull or face with other bones, with intracranial injury of other and unspecified nature **221**

804.40   Closed fractures involving skull or face with other bones, with intracranial injury of other and unspecified nature, unspecified state of consciousness **30, 225**

804.41   Closed fractures involving skull or face with other bones, with intracranial injury of other and unspecified nature, no loss of consciousness **30, 225**

804.42   Closed fractures involving skull or face with other bones, with intracranial injury of other and unspecified nature, brief (less than one hour) loss of consciousness **30, 225**

804.43   Closed fractures involving skull or face with other bones, with intracranial injury of other and unspecified nature, moderate (1-24 hours) loss of consciousness **25, 225**

804.44   Closed fractures involving skull or face with other bones, with intracranial injury of other and unspecified nature, prolonged (more than 24 hours) loss of consciousness and return to pre-existing conscious level **25, 225**

804.45   Closed fractures involving skull or face with other bones, with intracranial injury of other and unspecified nature, prolonged (more than 24 hours) loss of consciousness, without return to pre-existing conscious level **25, 226**

804.46   Closed fractures involving skull or face with other bones, with intracranial injury of other and unspecified nature, loss of consciousness of unspecified duration **25, 226**

804.49   Closed fractures involving skull or face with other bones, with intracranial injury of other and unspecified nature, unspecified concussion **30**

804.5*   Open fractures involving skull or face with other bones, without mention of intracranial injury **221**

804.50   Open fractures involving skull or face with other bones, without mention of intracranial injury, unspecified state of consciousness **30**

804.51   Open fractures involving skull or face with other bones, without mention of intracranial injury, no loss of consciousness **30**

804.52   Open fractures involving skull or face with other bones, without mention of intracranial injury, brief (less than one hour) loss of consciousness **30, 226**

804.53   Open fractures involving skull or face with other bones, without mention of intracranial injury, moderate (1-24 hours) loss of consciousness **25, 226**

804.54   Open fractures involving skull or face with other bones, without mention of intracranial injury, prolonged (more than 24 hours) loss of consciousness and return to pre-existing conscious level **25, 226**

804.55   Open fractures involving skull or face with other bones, without mention of intracranial injury, prolonged (more than 24 hours) loss of consciousness, without return to pre-existing conscious level **25, 226**

804.56   Open fractures involving skull or face with other bones, without mention of intracranial injury, loss of consciousness of unspecified duration **25**

804.59   Open fractures involving skull or face with other bones, without mention of intracranial injury, unspecified concussion **30**

804.6*   Open fractures involving skull or face with other bones, with cerebral laceration and contusion **221**

804.60   Open fractures involving skull or face with other bones, with cerebral laceration and contusion, unspecified state of consciousness **30, 226**

804.61   Open fractures involving skull or face with other bones, with cerebral laceration and contusion, no loss of consciousness **30, 226**

804.62   Open fractures involving skull or face with other bones, with cerebral laceration and contusion, brief (less than one hour) loss of consciousness **30, 226**

804.63   Open fractures involving skull or face with other bones, with cerebral laceration and contusion, moderate (1-24 hours) loss of consciousness **25, 226**

804.64   Open fractures involving skull or face with other bones, with cerebral laceration and contusion, prolonged (more than 24 hours) loss of consciousness and return to pre-existing conscious level **25, 226**

804.65   Open fractures involving skull or face with other bones, with cerebral laceration and contusion, prolonged (more than 24 hours) loss of consciousness, without return to pre-existing conscious level **25, 226**

804.66   Open fractures involving skull or face with other bones, with cerebral laceration and contusion, loss of consciousness of unspecified duration **25, 226**

804.69   Open fractures involving skull or face with other bones, with cerebral laceration and contusion, unspecified concussion **30**

804.7*   Open fractures involving skull or face with other bones with subarachnoid, subdural, and extradural hemorrhage **221, 226**

804.70   Open fractures involving skull or face with other bones with subarachnoid, subdural, and extradural hemorrhage, unspecified state of consciousness **30**

804.71   Open fractures involving skull or face with other bones with subarachnoid, subdural, and extradural hemorrhage, no loss of consciousness **30**

804.72   Open fractures involving skull or face with other bones with subarachnoid, subdural, and extradural hemorrhage, brief (less than one hour) loss of consciousness **30**

804.73   Open fractures involving skull or face with other bones with subarachnoid, subdural, and extradural hemorrhage, moderate (1-24 hours) loss of consciousness **25**

804.74   Open fractures involving skull or face with other bones with subarachnoid, subdural, and extradural hemorrhage, prolonged (more than 24 hours) loss of consciousness and return to pre-existing conscious level **25**

804.75   Open fractures involving skull or face with other bones with subarachnoid, subdural, and extradural hemorrhage, prolonged (more than 24 hours) loss of consciousness, without return to pre-existing conscious level **25**

804.76   Open fractures involving skull or face with other bones with subarachnoid, subdural, and extradural hemorrhage, loss of consciousness of unspecified duration **25**

804.79   Open fractures involving skull or face with other bones with subarachnoid, subdural, and extradural hemorrhage, unspecified concussion **30**

804.8*   Open fractures involving skull or face with other bones, with other and unspecified intracranial hemorrhage **221, 226**

804.80   Open fractures involving skull or face with other bones, with other and unspecified intracranial hemorrhage, unspecified state of consciousness **30**

804.81 Open fractures involving skull or face with other bones, with other and unspecified intracranial hemorrhage, no loss of consciousness **30**

804.82 Open fractures involving skull or face with other bones, with other and unspecified intracranial hemorrhage, brief (less than one hour) loss of consciousness **30**

804.83 Open fractures involving skull or face with other bones, with other and unspecified intracranial hemorrhage, moderate (1-24 hours) loss of consciousness **25**

804.84 Open fractures involving skull or face with other bones, with other and unspecified intracranial hemorrhage, prolonged (more than 24 hours) loss of consciousness and return to pre-existing conscious level **25**

804.85 Open fractures involving skull or face with other bones, with other and unspecified intracranial hemorrhage, prolonged (more than 24 hours) loss of consciousness, without return to pre-existing conscious level **25**

804.86 Open fractures involving skull or face with other bones, with other and unspecified intracranial hemorrhage, loss of consciousness of unspecified duration **25**

804.89 Open fractures involving skull or face with other bones, with other and unspecified intracranial hemorrhage, unspecified concussion **30**

804.9* Open fractures involving skull or face with other bones, with intracranial injury of other and unspecified nature **221, 226**

804.90 Open fractures involving skull or face with other bones, with intracranial injury of other and unspecified nature, unspecified state of consciousness **30**

804.91 Open fractures involving skull or face with other bones, with intracranial injury of other and unspecified nature, no loss of consciousness **30**

804.92 Open fractures involving skull or face with other bones, with intracranial injury of other and unspecified nature, brief (less than one hour) loss of consciousness **30**

804.93 Open fractures involving skull or face with other bones, with intracranial injury of other and unspecified nature, moderate (1-24 hours) loss of consciousness **25**

804.94 Open fractures involving skull or face with other bones, with intracranial injury of other and unspecified nature, prolonged (more than 24 hours) loss of consciousness and return to pre-existing conscious level **25**

804.95 Open fractures involving skull or face with other bones, with intracranial injury of other and unspecified nature, prolonged (more than 24 hours) loss of consciousness, without return to pre-existing level **25**

804.96 Open fractures involving skull or face with other bones, with intracranial injury of other and unspecified nature, loss of consciousness of unspecified duration **25**

804.99 Open fractures involving skull or face with other bones, with intracranial injury of other and unspecified nature, unspecified concussion **30**

805.0* Closed fracture of cervical vertebra without mention of spinal cord injury **221**

805.1* Open fracture of cervical vertebra without mention of spinal cord injury **221**

805.2 Closed fracture of dorsal (thoracic) vertebra without mention of spinal cord injury **221**

805.3 Open fracture of dorsal (thoracic) vertebra without mention of spinal cord injury **221**

805.4 Closed fracture of lumbar vertebra without mention of spinal cord injury **221**

805.5 Open fracture of lumbar vertebra without mention of spinal cord injury **221**

805.6 Closed fracture of sacrum and coccyx without mention of spinal cord injury **221, 227**

805.7 Open fracture of sacrum and coccyx without mention of spinal cord injury **221, 227**

805.8 Closed fracture of unspecified part of vertebral column without mention of spinal cord injury **221**

805.9 Open fracture of unspecified part of vertebral column without mention of spinal cord injury **221**

805* Fracture of vertebral column without mention of spinal cord injury **98**

806.0* Closed fracture of cervical vertebra with spinal cord injury **221, 227**

806.1* Open fracture of cervical vertebra with spinal cord injury **221, 227**

806.2* Closed fracture of dorsal (thoracic) vertebra with spinal cord injury **221, 227**

806.3* Open fracture of dorsal vertebra with spinal cord injury **221, 227**

806.4 Closed fracture of lumbar spine with spinal cord injury **221, 227**

806.5 Open fracture of lumbar spine with spinal cord injury **221, 227**

806.6* Closed fracture of sacrum and coccyx with spinal cord injury **221**

806.60 Closed fracture of sacrum and coccyx with unspecified spinal cord injury **227**

806.7* Open fracture of sacrum and coccyx with spinal cord injury **221, 227**

806.8 Closed fracture of unspecified vertebra with spinal cord injury **221, 227**

806.9 Open fracture of unspecified vertebra with spinal cord injury **221, 227**

806* Fracture of vertebral column with spinal cord injury **19**

807.0* Closed fracture of rib(s) **221**

807.00 Closed fracture of rib(s), unspecified **54**

807.01 Closed fracture of one rib **54**

807.02 Closed fracture of two ribs **54**

807.03 Closed fracture of three ribs **52**

807.04 Closed fracture of four ribs **52**

807.05 Closed fracture of five ribs **52**

807.06 Closed fracture of six ribs **52**

807.07 Closed fracture of seven ribs **52, 226**

807.08 Closed fracture of eight or more ribs **52, 226**

807.09 Closed fracture of multiple ribs, unspecified **52**

807.1* Open fracture of rib(s) **52, 221**

807.14 Open fracture of four ribs **226**

807.15 Open fracture of five ribs **226**

807.16 Open fracture of six ribs **226**

807.17 Open fracture of seven ribs **226**

807.18 Open fracture of eight or more ribs **226**

807.19 Open fracture of multiple ribs, unspecified **226**

807.2 Closed fracture of sternum **52, 221**

807.3 Open fracture of sternum **52, 221, 226**

807.4 Flail chest **52, 221, 226**

807.5 Closed fracture of larynx and trachea **3, 47, 221, 226**

807.6 Open fracture of larynx and trachea **3, 47, 221, 226**

808.0 Closed fracture of acetabulum **221**

808.1 Open fracture of acetabulum **221**

808.2 Closed fracture of pubis **221**

808.3 Open fracture of pubis **221**

808.4* Closed fracture of other specified part of pelvis **221**

808.5* Open fracture of other specified part of pelvis **221**

808.8 Unspecified closed fracture of pelvis **221**

808.9 Unspecified open fracture of pelvis **221**

808* Fracture of pelvis **96, 227**

809.0 Fracture of bones of trunk, closed **101, 221**

809.1 Fracture of bones of trunk, open **101, 221, 227**

810.0* Closed fracture of clavicle **221**

810.1* Open fracture of clavicle **221**

810*	Fracture of clavicle **99**
811.0*	Closed fracture of scapula **221**
811.00	Closed fracture of unspecified part of scapula **99**
811.01	Closed fracture of acromial process of scapula **99**
811.02	Closed fracture of coracoid process of scapula **99**
811.03	Closed fracture of glenoid cavity and neck of scapula **99**
811.09	Closed fracture of other part of scapula **101**
811.1*	Open fracture of scapula **221**
811.10	Open fracture of unspecified part of scapula **99**
811.11	Open fracture of acromial process of scapula **99**
811.12	Open fracture of coracoid process **99**
811.13	Open fracture of glenoid cavity and neck of scapula **99**
811.19	Open fracture of other part of scapula **101**
812.0*	Closed fracture of upper end of humerus **221**
812.1*	Open fracture of upper end of humerus **221, 227**
812.2*	Closed fracture of shaft or unspecified part of humerus **221**
812.3*	Open fracture of shaft or unspecified part of humerus **221**
812.30	Open fracture of unspecified part of humerus **227**
812.31	Open fracture of shaft of humerus **227**
812.4*	Closed fracture of lower end of humerus **221**
812.5*	Open fracture of lower end of humerus **221, 227**
812*	Fracture of humerus **99**
813.0*	Closed fracture of upper end of radius and ulna **221**
813.1*	Open fracture of upper end of radius and ulna **221, 227**
813.2*	Closed fracture of shaft of radius and ulna **221**
813.3*	Open fracture of shaft of radius and ulna **221, 227**
813.4*	Closed fracture of lower end of radius and ulna **221**
813.5*	Open fracture of lower end of radius and ulna **221, 227**
813.8*	Closed fracture of unspecified part of radius with ulna **221**
813.9*	Open fracture of unspecified part of radius with ulna **221, 227**
813*	Fracture of radius and ulna **99**
814.0*	Closed fractures of carpal bones **221**
814.1*	Open fractures of carpal bones **221**
814*	Fracture of carpal bone(s) **99**
815.0*	Closed fracture of metacarpal bones **221**
815.1*	Open fracture of metacarpal bones **221**
815*	Fracture of metacarpal bone(s) **99**
816.0*	Closed fracture of one or more phalanges of hand **221**
816.1*	Open fracture of one or more phalanges of hand **221**
816*	Fracture of one or more phalanges of hand **99**
817.0	Multiple closed fractures of hand bones **221**
817.1	Multiple open fractures of hand bones **221**
817*	Multiple fractures of hand bones **99**
818.0	Ill-defined closed fractures of upper limb **221**
818.1	Ill-defined open fractures of upper limb **221, 227**
818*	Ill-defined fractures of upper limb **99**
819.0	Multiple closed fractures involving both upper limbs, and upper limb with rib(s) and sternum **221**
819.1	Multiple open fractures involving both upper limbs, and upper limb with rib(s) and sternum **221, 226**
819*	Multiple fractures involving both upper limbs, and upper limb with rib(s) and sternum **202**
820.0*	Closed transcervical fracture **221**
820.1*	Open transcervical fracture **222**
820.2*	Closed pertrochanteric fracture of femur **222**
820.3*	Open pertrochanteric fracture of femur **222**
820.8	Closed fracture of unspecified part of neck of femur **222**
820.9	Open fracture of unspecified part of neck of femur **222**
820*	Fracture of neck of femur **96, 166, 170, 227**

821.0*	Closed fracture of shaft or unspecified part of femur **166, 170, 222**
821.1*	Open fracture of shaft or unspecified part of femur **166, 170, 222**
821.2*	Closed fracture of lower end of femur **222**
821.3*	Open fracture of lower end of femur **222**
821*	Fracture of other and unspecified parts of femur **96, 227**
822.0	Closed fracture of patella **222**
822.1	Open fracture of patella **222**
822*	Fracture of patella **99**
823.0*	Closed fracture of upper end of tibia and fibula **222**
823.1*	Open fracture of upper end of tibia and fibula **222, 227**
823.2*	Closed fracture of shaft of tibia and fibula **222**
823.3*	Open fracture of shaft of tibia and fibula **222, 227**
823.4*	Torus fracture of tibia and fibula **222, 227**
823.8*	Closed fracture of unspecified part of tibia and fibula **222**
823.9*	Open fracture of unspecified part of tibia and fibula **222, 227**
823*	Fracture of tibia and fibula **99**
824.0	Closed fracture of medial malleolus **222**
824.1	Open fracture of medial malleolus **222**
824.2	Closed fracture of lateral malleolus **222**
824.3	Open fracture of lateral malleolus **222**
824.4	Closed bimalleolar fracture **222**
824.5	Open bimalleolar fracture **222**
824.6	Closed trimalleolar fracture **222**
824.7	Open trimalleolar fracture **222**
824.8	Unspecified closed fracture of ankle **222**
824.9	Unspecified open fracture of ankle **222**
824*	Fracture of ankle **99**
825.0	Closed fracture of calcaneus **99, 222**
825.1	Open fracture of calcaneus **99, 222**
825.2*	Closed fracture of other tarsal and metatarsal bones **99, 222**
825.3*	Open fracture of other tarsal and metatarsal bones **99, 222**
826.0	Closed fracture of one or more phalanges of foot **222**
826.1	Open fracture of one or more phalanges of foot **222**
826*	Fracture of one or more phalanges of foot **99**
827.0	Other, multiple and ill-defined closed fractures of lower limb **222**
827.1	Other, multiple and ill-defined open fractures of lower limb **222**
827*	Other, multiple, and ill-defined fractures of lower limb **99**
828.0	Multiple closed fractures involving both lower limbs, lower with upper limb, and lower limb(s) with rib(s) and sternum **222**
828.1	Multiple fractures involving both lower limbs, lower with upper limb, and lower limb(s) with rib(s) and sternum, open **222**
828*	Multiple fractures involving both lower limbs, lower with upper limb, and lower limb(s) with rib(s) and sternum **202, 227**
829.0	Closed fracture of unspecified bone **222**
829.1	Open fracture of unspecified bone **222**
829*	Fracture of unspecified bones **100**
830.0	Closed dislocation of jaw **222**
830.1	Open dislocation of jaw **222**
830*	Dislocation of jaw **3, 48**
831.0*	Closed dislocation of shoulder, unspecified **222**
831.1*	Open dislocation of shoulder **222, 227**
831*	Dislocation of shoulder **100**
832.0*	Closed dislocation of elbow **222**
832.1*	Open dislocation of elbow **222, 227**
832.2	Nursemaid's elbow **222**
832*	Dislocation of elbow **100**
833.0*	Closed dislocation of wrist **222**
833.1*	Open dislocation of wrist **222**
833*	Dislocation of wrist **100**

Numeric Index to Diseases

834.0*	Closed dislocation of finger **222**	
834.1*	Open dislocation of finger **222**	
834*	Dislocation of finger **100**	
835.0*	Closed dislocation of hip **222**	
835.1*	Open dislocation of hip **222, 227**	
835*	Dislocation of hip **96**	
836.0	Tear of medial cartilage or meniscus of knee, current **222**	
836.1	Tear of lateral cartilage or meniscus of knee, current **222**	
836.2	Other tear of cartilage or meniscus of knee, current **222**	
836.3	Closed dislocation of patella **222**	
836.4	Open dislocation of patella **222**	
836.5*	Other closed dislocation of knee **222**	
836.6*	Other open dislocation of knee **222, 227**	
836*	Dislocation of knee **100**	
837.0	Closed dislocation of ankle **222**	
837.1	Open dislocation of ankle **222, 227**	
837*	Dislocation of ankle **100**	
838.0*	Closed dislocation of foot **222**	
838.1*	Open dislocation of foot **222**	
838*	Dislocation of foot **100**	
839.0*	Closed dislocation, cervical vertebra **98, 222, 227**	
839.1*	Open dislocation, cervical vertebra **98, 222, 227**	
839.2*	Closed dislocation, thoracic and lumbar vertebra **98, 222**	
839.3*	Open dislocation, thoracic and lumbar vertebra **98, 222**	
839.4*	Closed dislocation, other vertebra **98, 222**	
839.5*	Open dislocation, other vertebra **98, 222**	
839.52	Open dislocation, sacrum **227**	
839.59	Open dislocation, other vertebra **227**	
839.6*	Closed dislocation, other location **222**	
839.61	Closed dislocation, sternum **52**	
839.69	Closed dislocation, other location **100**	
839.71	Open dislocation, sternum **52, 222, 226**	
839.79	Open dislocation, other location **100, 222**	
839.8	Closed dislocation, multiple and ill-defined sites **100, 222**	
839.9	Open dislocation, multiple and ill-defined sites **100, 222**	
840.0	Acromioclavicular (joint) (ligament) sprain and strain **222**	
840.1	Coracoclavicular (ligament) sprain and strain **222**	
840.2	Coracohumeral (ligament) sprain and strain **222**	
840.3	Infraspinatus (muscle) (tendon) sprain and strain **222**	
840.4	Rotator cuff (capsule) sprain and strain **222**	
840.5	Subscapularis (muscle) sprain and strain **222**	
840.6	Supraspinatus (muscle) (tendon) sprain and strain **222**	
840.7	Superior glenoid labrum lesions (SLAP) **222**	
840.8	Sprain and strain of other specified sites of shoulder and upper arm **222**	
840.9	Sprain and strain of unspecified site of shoulder and upper arm **222**	
840*	Sprains and strains of shoulder and upper arm **100**	
841*	Sprains and strains of elbow and forearm **100, 222**	
842*	Sprains and strains of wrist and hand **100, 222**	
843*	Sprains and strains of hip and thigh **96, 222**	
844*	Sprains and strains of knee and leg **100, 222**	
845.0*	Ankle sprain and strain **100**	
845.1*	Foot sprain and strain **100**	
845*	Sprains and strains of ankle and foot **222**	
846*	Sprains and strains of sacroiliac region **98, 222**	
847*	Sprains and strains of other and unspecified parts of back **98, 222**	
848.0	Sprain and strain of septal cartilage of nose **101**	
848.1	Sprain and strain of jaw **48**	

848.2	Sprain and strain of thyroid region **101**
848.3	Sprain and strain of ribs **54**
848.4*	Sprain and strain of sternum **54**
848.5	Pelvic sprain and strains **96**
848.8	Other specified sites of sprains and strains **100**
848.9	Unspecified site of sprain and strain **100**
848*	Other and ill-defined sprains and strains **222**
850.0	Concussion with no loss of consciousness **222**
850.1*	Concussion with brief (less than one hour) loss of consciousness **222**
850.2	Concussion with moderate (1-24 hours) loss of consciousness **222, 226**
850.3	Concussion with prolonged (more than 24 hours) loss of consciousness and return to pre-existing conscious level **222, 226**
850.4	Concussion with prolonged (more than 24 hours) loss of consciousness, without return to pre-existing conscious level **222, 226**
850.5	Concussion with loss of consciousness of unspecified duration **222**
850.9	Unspecified concussion **222**
850*	Concussion **32**
851.0*	Cortex (cerebral) contusion without mention of open intracranial wound **222**
851.00	Cortex (cerebral) contusion without mention of open intracranial wound, state of consciousness unspecified **30, 226**
851.01	Cortex (cerebral) contusion without mention of open intracranial wound, no loss of consciousness **30, 226**
851.02	Cortex (cerebral) contusion without mention of open intracranial wound, brief (less than 1 hour) loss of consciousness **30, 226**
851.03	Cortex (cerebral) contusion without mention of open intracranial wound, moderate (1-24 hours) loss of consciousness **25, 226**
851.04	Cortex (cerebral) contusion without mention of open intracranial wound, prolonged (more than 24 hours) loss of consciousness and return to pre-existing conscious level **25, 226**
851.05	Cortex (cerebral) contusion without mention of open intracranial wound, prolonged (more than 24 hours) loss of consciousness, without return to pre-existing conscious level **25, 226**
851.06	Cortex (cerebral) contusion without mention of open intracranial wound, loss of consciousness of unspecified duration **25, 226**
851.09	Cortex (cerebral) contusion without mention of open intracranial wound, unspecified concussion **30, 226**
851.1*	Cortex (cerebral) contusion with open intracranial wound **9, 11, 222, 226**
851.10	Cortex (cerebral) contusion with open intracranial wound, unspecified state of consciousness **30**
851.11	Cortex (cerebral) contusion with open intracranial wound, no loss of consciousness **30**
851.12	Cortex (cerebral) contusion with open intracranial wound, brief (less than 1 hour) loss of consciousness **30**
851.13	Cortex (cerebral) contusion with open intracranial wound, moderate (1-24 hours) loss of consciousness **26**
851.14	Cortex (cerebral) contusion with open intracranial wound, prolonged (more than 24 hours) loss of consciousness and return to pre-existing conscious level **26**
851.15	Cortex (cerebral) contusion with open intracranial wound, prolonged (more than 24 hours) loss of consciousness, without return to pre-existing conscious level **26**
851.16	Cortex (cerebral) contusion with open intracranial wound, loss of consciousness of unspecified duration **26**
851.19	Cortex (cerebral) contusion with open intracranial wound, unspecified concussion **30**
851.2*	Cortex (cerebral) laceration without mention of open intracranial wound **9, 11, 222, 226**

*Code Range

© 2013 OptumInsight, Inc.

851.20 Cortex (cerebral) laceration without mention of open intracranial wound, unspecified state of consciousness **30**

851.21 Cortex (cerebral) laceration without mention of open intracranial wound, no loss of consciousness **30**

851.22 Cortex (cerebral) laceration without mention of open intracranial wound, brief (less than 1 hour) loss of consciousness **30**

851.23 Cortex (cerebral) laceration without mention of open intracranial wound, moderate (1-24 hours) loss of consciousness **26**

851.24 Cortex (cerebral) laceration without mention of open intracranial wound, prolonged (more than 24 hours) loss of consciousness and return to pre-existing conscious level **26**

851.25 Cortex (cerebral) laceration without mention of open intracranial wound, prolonged (more than 24 hours) loss of consciousness, without return to pre-existing conscious level **26**

851.26 Cortex (cerebral) laceration without mention of open intracranial wound, loss of consciousness of unspecified duration **26**

851.29 Cortex (cerebral) laceration without mention of open intracranial wound, unspecified concussion **30**

851.3* Cortex (cerebral) laceration with open intracranial wound **9, 11, 222, 226**

851.30 Cortex (cerebral) laceration with open intracranial wound, unspecified state of consciousness **30**

851.31 Cortex (cerebral) laceration with open intracranial wound, no loss of consciousness **30**

851.32 Cortex (cerebral) laceration with open intracranial wound, brief (less than 1 hour) loss of consciousness **30**

851.33 Cortex (cerebral) laceration with open intracranial wound, moderate (1-24 hours) loss of consciousness **26**

851.34 Cortex (cerebral) laceration with open intracranial wound, prolonged (more than 24 hours) loss of consciousness and return to pre-existing conscious level **26**

851.35 Cortex (cerebral) laceration with open intracranial wound, prolonged (more than 24 hours) loss of consciousness, without return to pre-existing conscious level **26**

851.36 Cortex (cerebral) laceration with open intracranial wound, loss of consciousness of unspecified duration **26**

851.39 Cortex (cerebral) laceration with open intracranial wound, unspecified concussion **30**

851.4* Cerebellar or brain stem contusion without mention of open intracranial wound **222, 226**

851.40 Cerebellar or brain stem contusion without mention of open intracranial wound, unspecified state of consciousness **30**

851.41 Cerebellar or brain stem contusion without mention of open intracranial wound, no loss of consciousness **30**

851.42 Cerebellar or brain stem contusion without mention of open intracranial wound, brief (less than 1 hour) loss of consciousness **30**

851.43 Cerebellar or brain stem contusion without mention of open intracranial wound, moderate (1-24 hours) loss of consciousness **26**

851.44 Cerebellar or brain stem contusion without mention of open intracranial wound, prolonged (more than 24 hours) loss consciousness and return to pre-existing conscious level **26**

851.45 Cerebellar or brain stem contusion without mention of open intracranial wound, prolonged (more than 24 hours) loss of consciousness, without return to pre-existing conscious level **26**

851.46 Cerebellar or brain stem contusion without mention of open intracranial wound, loss of consciousness of unspecified duration **26**

851.49 Cerebellar or brain stem contusion without mention of open intracranial wound, unspecified concussion **30**

851.5* Cerebellar or brain stem contusion with open intracranial wound **9, 11, 222, 226**

851.50 Cerebellar or brain stem contusion with open intracranial wound, unspecified state of consciousness **30**

851.51 Cerebellar or brain stem contusion with open intracranial wound, no loss of consciousness **30**

851.52 Cerebellar or brain stem contusion with open intracranial wound, brief (less than 1 hour) loss of consciousness **30**

851.53 Cerebellar or brain stem contusion with open intracranial wound, moderate (1-24 hours) loss of consciousness **26**

851.54 Cerebellar or brain stem contusion with open intracranial wound, prolonged (more than 24 hours) loss of consciousness and return to pre-existing conscious level **26**

851.55 Cerebellar or brain stem contusion with open intracranial wound, prolonged (more than 24 hours) loss of consciousness, without return to pre-existing conscious level **26**

851.56 Cerebellar or brain stem contusion with open intracranial wound, loss of consciousness of unspecified duration **26**

851.59 Cerebellar or brain stem contusion with open intracranial wound, unspecified concussion **30**

851.6* Cerebellar or brain stem laceration without mention of open intracranial wound **9, 11, 222, 226**

851.60 Cerebellar or brain stem laceration without mention of open intracranial wound, unspecified state of consciousness **30**

851.61 Cerebellar or brain stem laceration without mention of open intracranial wound, no loss of consciousness **30**

851.62 Cerebellar or brain stem laceration without mention of open intracranial wound, brief (less than 1 hour) loss of consciousness **31**

851.63 Cerebellar or brain stem laceration without mention of open intracranial wound, moderate (1-24 hours) loss of consciousness **26**

851.64 Cerebellar or brain stem laceration without mention of open intracranial wound, prolonged (more than 24 hours) loss of consciousness and return to pre-existing conscious level **26**

851.65 Cerebellar or brain stem laceration without mention of open intracranial wound, prolonged (more than 24 hours) loss of consciousness, without return to pre-existing conscious level **26**

851.66 Cerebellar or brain stem laceration without mention of open intracranial wound, loss of consciousness of unspecified duration **26**

851.69 Cerebellar or brain stem laceration without mention of open intracranial wound, unspecified concussion **31**

851.7* Cerebellar or brain stem laceration with open intracranial wound **9, 11, 222, 226**

851.70 Cerebellar or brain stem laceration with open intracranial wound, state of consciousness unspecified **31**

851.71 Cerebellar or brain stem laceration with open intracranial wound, no loss of consciousness **31**

851.72 Cerebellar or brain stem laceration with open intracranial wound, brief (less than one hour) loss of consciousness **31**

851.73 Cerebellar or brain stem laceration with open intracranial wound, moderate (1-24 hours) loss of consciousness **26**

851.74 Cerebellar or brain stem laceration with open intracranial wound, prolonged (more than 24 hours) loss of consciousness and return to pre-existing conscious level **26**

851.75 Cerebellar or brain stem laceration with open intracranial wound, prolonged (more than 24 hours) loss of consciousness, without return to pre-existing conscious level **26**

851.76 Cerebellar or brain stem laceration with open intracranial wound, loss of consciousness of unspecified duration **26**

851.79 Cerebellar or brain stem laceration with open intracranial wound, unspecified concussion **31**

851.8* Other and unspecified cerebral laceration and contusion, without mention of open intracranial wound **9, 11, 222, 226**

851.80 Other and unspecified cerebral laceration and contusion, without mention of open intracranial wound, unspecified state of consciousness **31**

851.81 Other and unspecified cerebral laceration and contusion, without mention of open intracranial wound, no loss of consciousness **31**

851.82 Other and unspecified cerebral laceration and contusion, without mention of open intracranial wound, brief (less than 1 hour) loss of consciousness **31**

851.83 Other and unspecified cerebral laceration and contusion, without mention of open intracranial wound, moderate (1-24 hours) loss of consciousness **26**

851.84 Other and unspecified cerebral laceration and contusion, without mention of open intracranial wound, prolonged (more than 24 hours) loss of consciousness and return to preexisting conscious level **26**

851.85 Other and unspecified cerebral laceration and contusion, without mention of open intracranial wound, prolonged (more than 24 hours) loss of consciousness, without return to pre-existing conscious level **26**

851.86 Other and unspecified cerebral laceration and contusion, without mention of open intracranial wound, loss of consciousness of unspecified duration **26**

851.89 Other and unspecified cerebral laceration and contusion, without mention of open intracranial wound, unspecified concussion **31**

851.9* Other and unspecified cerebral laceration and contusion, with open intracranial wound **9, 11, 222, 226**

851.90 Other and unspecified cerebral laceration and contusion, with open intracranial wound, unspecified state of consciousness **31**

851.91 Other and unspecified cerebral laceration and contusion, with open intracranial wound, no loss of consciousness **31**

851.92 Other and unspecified cerebral laceration and contusion, with open intracranial wound, brief (less than 1 hour) loss of consciousness **31**

851.93 Other and unspecified cerebral laceration and contusion, with open intracranial wound, moderate (1-24 hours) loss of consciousness **26**

851.94 Other and unspecified cerebral laceration and contusion, with open intracranial wound, prolonged (more than 24 hours) loss of consciousness and return to pre-existing conscious level **26**

851.95 Other and unspecified cerebral laceration and contusion, with open intracranial wound, prolonged (more than 24 hours) loss of consciousness, without return to pre-existing conscious level **26**

851.96 Other and unspecified cerebral laceration and contusion, with open intracranial wound, loss of consciousness of unspecified duration **26**

851.99 Other and unspecified cerebral laceration and contusion, with open intracranial wound, unspecified concussion **31**

852.0* Subarachnoid hemorrhage following injury without mention of open intracranial wound **9, 11**

852.00 Subarachnoid hemorrhage following injury, without mention of open intracranial wound, unspecified state of consciousness **31**

852.01 Subarachnoid hemorrhage following injury, without mention of open intracranial wound, no loss of consciousness **31**

852.02 Subarachnoid hemorrhage following injury, without mention of open intracranial wound, brief (less than 1 hour) loss of consciousness **31**

852.03 Subarachnoid hemorrhage following injury, without mention of open intracranial wound, moderate (1-24 hours) loss of consciousness **26**

852.04 Subarachnoid hemorrhage following injury, without mention of open intracranial wound, prolonged (more than 24 hours) loss of consciousness and return to pre-existing conscious level **26**

852.05 Subarachnoid hemorrhage following injury, without mention of open intracranial wound, prolonged (more than 24 hours) loss of consciousness, without return to pre-existing conscious level **26**

852.06 Subarachnoid hemorrhage following injury, without mention of open intracranial wound, loss of consciousness of unspecified duration **26**

852.09 Subarachnoid hemorrhage following injury, without mention of open intracranial wound, unspecified concussion **31**

852.1* Subarachnoid hemorrhage following injury, with open intracranial wound **9, 11**

852.10 Subarachnoid hemorrhage following injury, with open intracranial wound, unspecified state of consciousness **31**

852.11 Subarachnoid hemorrhage following injury, with open intracranial wound, no loss of consciousness **31**

852.12 Subarachnoid hemorrhage following injury, with open intracranial wound, brief (less than 1 hour) loss of consciousness **31**

852.13 Subarachnoid hemorrhage following injury, with open intracranial wound, moderate (1-24 hours) loss of consciousness **26**

852.14 Subarachnoid hemorrhage following injury, with open intracranial wound, prolonged (more than 24 hours) loss of consciousness and return to pre-existing conscious level **26**

852.15 Subarachnoid hemorrhage following injury, with open intracranial wound, prolonged (more than 24 hours) loss of consciousness, without return to pre-existing conscious level **26**

852.16 Subarachnoid hemorrhage following injury, with open intracranial wound, loss of consciousness of unspecified duration **26**

852.19 Subarachnoid hemorrhage following injury, with open intracranial wound, unspecified concussion **31**

852.20 Subdural hemorrhage following injury, without mention of open intracranial wound, unspecified state of consciousness **31**

852.21 Subdural hemorrhage following injury, without mention of open intracranial wound, no loss of consciousness **31**

852.22 Subdural hemorrhage following injury, without mention of open intracranial wound, brief (less than one hour) loss of consciousness **31**

852.23 Subdural hemorrhage following injury, without mention of open intracranial wound, moderate (1-24 hours) loss of consciousness **26**

852.24 Subdural hemorrhage following injury, without mention of open intracranial wound, prolonged (more than 24 hours) loss of consciousness and return to pre-existing conscious level **27**

852.25 Subdural hemorrhage following injury, without mention of open intracranial wound, prolonged (more than 24 hours) loss of consciousness, without return to pre-existing conscious level **27**

852.26 Subdural hemorrhage following injury, without mention of open intracranial wound, loss of consciousness of unspecified duration **27**

852.29 Subdural hemorrhage following injury, without mention of open intracranial wound, unspecified concussion **31**

852.3* Subdural hemorrhage following injury, with open intracranial wound **9, 11**

852.30 Subdural hemorrhage following injury, with open intracranial wound, state of consciousness unspecified **31**

852.31 Subdural hemorrhage following injury, with open intracranial wound, no loss of consciousness **31**

852.32 Subdural hemorrhage following injury, with open intracranial wound, brief (less than 1 hour) loss of consciousness **31**

852.33 Subdural hemorrhage following injury, with open intracranial wound, moderate (1-24 hours) loss of consciousness **27**

852.34 Subdural hemorrhage following injury, with open intracranial wound, prolonged (more than 24 hours) loss of consciousness and return to pre-existing conscious level **27**

852.35 Subdural hemorrhage following injury, with open intracranial wound, prolonged (more than 24 hours) loss of consciousness, without return to pre-existing conscious level **27**

852.36 Subdural hemorrhage following injury, with open intracranial wound, loss of consciousness of unspecified duration **27**

852.39 Subdural hemorrhage following injury, with open intracranial wound, unspecified concussion **31**

852.40 Extradural hemorrhage following injury, without mention of open intracranial wound, unspecified state of consciousness **31**

852.41 Extradural hemorrhage following injury, without mention of open intracranial wound, no loss of consciousness **31**

852.42 Extradural hemorrhage following injury, without mention of open intracranial wound, brief (less than 1 hour) loss of consciousness **31**

852.43 Extradural hemorrhage following injury, without mention of open intracranial wound, moderate (1-24 hours) loss of consciousness **27**

852.44 Extradural hemorrhage following injury, without mention of open intracranial wound, prolonged (more than 24 hours) loss of consciousness and return to pre-existing conscious level **27**

852.45 Extradural hemorrhage following injury, without mention of open intracranial wound, prolonged (more than 24 hours) loss of consciousness, without return to pre-existing conscious level **27**

852.46 Extradural hemorrhage following injury, without mention of open intracranial wound, loss of consciousness of unspecified duration **27**

852.49 Extradural hemorrhage following injury, without mention of open intracranial wound, unspecified concussion **31**

852.50 Extradural hemorrhage following injury, with open intracranial wound, state of consciousness unspecified **31**

852.51 Extradural hemorrhage following injury, with open intracranial wound, no loss of consciousness **31**

852.52 Extradural hemorrhage following injury, with open intracranial wound, brief (less than 1 hour) loss of consciousness **31**

852.53 Extradural hemorrhage following injury, with open intracranial wound, moderate (1-24 hours) loss of consciousness **27**

852.54 Extradural hemorrhage following injury, with open intracranial wound, prolonged (more than 24 hours) loss of consciousness and return to pre-existing conscious level **27**

852.55 Extradural hemorrhage following injury, with open intracranial wound, prolonged (more than 24 hours) loss of consciousness, without return to pre-existing conscious level **27**

852.56 Extradural hemorrhage following injury, with open intracranial wound, loss of consciousness of unspecified duration **27**

852.59 Extradural hemorrhage following injury, with open intracranial wound, unspecified concussion **31**

852* Subarachnoid, subdural, and extradural hemorrhage, following injury **222, 226**

853.0* Other and unspecified intracranial hemorrhage following injury, without mention of open intracranial wound **9, 11**

853.00 Other and unspecified intracranial hemorrhage following injury, without mention of open intracranial wound, unspecified state of consciousness **31**

853.01 Other and unspecified intracranial hemorrhage following injury, without mention of open intracranial wound, no loss of consciousness **31**

853.02 Other and unspecified intracranial hemorrhage following injury, without mention of open intracranial wound, brief (less than 1 hour) loss of consciousness **31**

853.03 Other and unspecified intracranial hemorrhage following injury, without mention of open intracranial wound, moderate (1-24 hours) loss of consciousness **27**

853.04 Other and unspecified intracranial hemorrhage following injury, without mention of open intracranial wound, prolonged (more than 24 hours) loss of consciousness and return to preexisting conscious level **27**

853.05 Other and unspecified intracranial hemorrhage following injury. Without mention of open intracranial wound, prolonged (more than 24 hours) loss of consciousness, without return to pre-existing conscious level **27**

853.06 Other and unspecified intracranial hemorrhage following injury, without mention of open intracranial wound, loss of consciousness of unspecified duration **27**

853.09 Other and unspecified intracranial hemorrhage following injury, without mention of open intracranial wound, unspecified concussion **31**

853.1* Other and unspecified intracranial hemorrhage following injury with open intracranial wound **9, 11**

853.10 Other and unspecified intracranial hemorrhage following injury, with open intracranial wound, unspecified state of consciousness **31**

853.11 Other and unspecified intracranial hemorrhage following injury, with open intracranial wound, no loss of consciousness **31**

853.12 Other and unspecified intracranial hemorrhage following injury, with open intracranial wound, brief (less than 1 hour) loss of consciousness **31**

853.13 Other and unspecified intracranial hemorrhage following injury, with open intracranial wound, moderate (1-24 hours) loss of consciousness **27**

853.14 Other and unspecified intracranial hemorrhage following injury, with open intracranial wound, prolonged (more than 24 hours) loss of consciousness and return to pre-existing conscious level **27**

853.15 Other and unspecified intracranial hemorrhage following injury, with open intracranial wound, prolonged (more than 24 hours) loss of consciousness, without return to pre-existing conscious level **27**

853.16 Other and unspecified intracranial hemorrhage following injury, with open intracranial wound, loss of consciousness of unspecified duration **27**

853.19 Other and unspecified intracranial hemorrhage following injury, with open intracranial wound, unspecified concussion **31**

853* Other and unspecified intracranial hemorrhage following injury **222, 226**

854.00 Intracranial injury of other and unspecified nature, without mention of open intracranial wound, unspecified state of consciousness **31**

854.01 Intracranial injury of other and unspecified nature, without mention of open intracranial wound, no loss of consciousness **31**

854.02 Intracranial injury of other and unspecified nature, without mention of open intracranial wound, brief (less than 1 hour) loss of consciousness **31**

854.03 Intracranial injury of other and unspecified nature, without mention of open intracranial wound, moderate (1-24 hours) loss of consciousness **27**

854.04 Intracranial injury of other and unspecified nature, without mention of open intracranial wound, prolonged (more than 24 hours) loss of consciousness and return to pre-existing conscious level **27**

854.05 Intracranial injury of other and unspecified nature, without mention of open intracranial wound, prolonged (more than 24 hours) loss of consciousness, without return to pre-existing conscious level **27**

854.06 Intracranial injury of other and unspecified nature, without mention of open intracranial wound, loss of consciousness of unspecified duration **27**

854.09 Intracranial injury of other and unspecified nature, without mention of open intracranial wound, unspecified concussion **31**

854.1* Intracranial injury of other and unspecified nature with open intracranial wound **9, 11**

854.10 Intracranial injury of other and unspecified nature, with open intracranial wound, unspecified state of consciousness **31**

854.11 Intracranial injury of other and unspecified nature, with open intracranial wound, no loss of consciousness **31**

854.12 Intracranial injury of other and unspecified nature, with open intracranial wound, brief (less than 1 hour) loss of consciousness **31**

854.13 Intracranial injury of other and unspecified nature, with open intracranial wound, moderate (1-24 hours) loss of consciousness **27**

854.14 Intracranial injury of other and unspecified nature, with open intracranial wound, prolonged (more than 24 hours) loss of consciousness and return to pre-existing conscious level **27**

854.15 Intracranial injury of other and unspecified nature, with open intracranial wound, prolonged (more than 24 hours) loss of consciousness, without return to pre-existing conscious level **27**

854.16 Intracranial injury of other and unspecified nature, with open intracranial wound, loss of consciousness of unspecified duration **27**

854.19 Intracranial injury of other and unspecified nature, with open intracranial wound, with unspecified concussion **31**

854*	Intracranial injury of other and unspecified nature **222**, **226**	
860*	Traumatic pneumothorax and hemothorax **53**, **166**, **170**, **222**, **226**	
861.0*	Heart injury, without mention of open wound into thorax **69**	
861.1*	Heart injury, with open wound into thorax **69**	
861.20	Unspecified lung injury without mention of open wound into thorax **54**	
861.21	Lung contusion without mention of open wound into thorax **54**	
861.22	Lung laceration without mention of open wound into thorax **52**	
861.30	Unspecified lung injury with open wound into thorax **54**	
861.31	Lung contusion with open wound into thorax **54**	
861.32	Lung laceration with open wound into thorax **52**	
861*	Injury to heart and lung **222**, **226**	
862.0	Diaphragm injury without mention of open wound into cavity **52**	
862.1	Diaphragm injury with open wound into cavity **52**	
862.21	Bronchus injury without mention of open wound into cavity **52**	
862.22	Esophagus injury without mention of open wound into cavity **75**	
862.29	Injury to other specified intrathoracic organs without mention of open wound into cavity **54**	
862.31	Bronchus injury with open wound into cavity **52**	
862.32	Esophagus injury with open wound into cavity **79**	
862.39	Injury to other specified intrathoracic organs with open wound into cavity **54**	
862.8	Injury to multiple and unspecified intrathoracic organs without mention of open wound into cavity **202**	
862.9	Injury to multiple and unspecified intrathoracic organs with open wound into cavity **202**	
862*	Injury to other and unspecified intrathoracic organs **222**, **226**	
863.0	Stomach injury without mention of open wound into cavity **79**, **222**, **227**	
863.1	Stomach injury with open wound into cavity **79**, **222**, **227**	
863.2*	Small intestine injury without mention of open wound into cavity **79**, **222**, **227**	
863.3*	Small intestine injury with open wound into cavity **79**, **223**, **227**	
863.4*	Colon or rectal injury without mention of open wound into cavity **79**, **223**, **227**	
863.5*	Injury to colon or rectum with open wound into cavity **79**, **223**, **227**	
863.8*	Injury to other and unspecified gastrointestinal sites without mention of open wound into cavity **223**	
863.80	Gastrointestinal tract injury, unspecified site, without mention of open wound into cavity **79**	
863.81	Pancreas head injury without mention of open wound into cavity **83**, **227**	
863.82	Pancreas body injury without mention of open wound into cavity **83**, **227**	
863.83	Pancreas tail injury without mention of open wound into cavity **83**, **227**	
863.84	Pancreas injury, multiple and unspecified sites, without mention of open wound into cavity **83**, **227**	
863.85	Appendix injury without mention of open wound into cavity **79**, **227**	
863.89	Injury to other and unspecified gastrointestinal sites without mention of open wound into cavity **79**, **227**	
863.9*	Injury to other and unspecified gastrointestinal sites, with open wound into cavity **223**, **227**	
863.90	Gastrointestinal tract injury, unspecified site, with open wound into cavity **79**	
863.91	Pancreas head injury with open wound into cavity **83**	
863.92	Pancreas body injury with open wound into cavity **83**	
863.93	Pancreas tail injury with open wound into cavity **83**	
863.94	Pancreas injury, multiple and unspecified sites, with open wound into cavity **83**	

863.95	Appendix injury with open wound into cavity **79**
863.99	Injury to other and unspecified gastrointestinal sites with open wound into cavity **79**
864.0*	Liver injury without mention of open wound into cavity **223**
864.1*	Liver injury with open wound into cavity **223**
864*	Injury to liver **83**, **227**
865*	Injury to spleen **166**, **170**, **176**, **223**, **227**
866*	Injury to kidney **120**, **223**, **227**
867.0	Bladder and urethra injury without mention of open wound into cavity **120**
867.1	Bladder and urethra injury with open wound into cavity **120**
867.2	Ureter injury without mention of open wound into cavity **120**
867.3	Ureter injury with open wound into cavity **120**
867.4	Uterus injury without mention of open wound into cavity **127**, **130**
867.5	Uterus injury with open wound into cavity **127**, **130**
867.6	Injury to other specified pelvic organs without mention of open wound into cavity **124**, **127**, **130**
867.7	Injury to other specified pelvic organs with open wound into cavity **124**, **127**, **130**
867.8	Injury to unspecified pelvic organ without mention of open wound into cavity **124**, **127**, **130**
867.9	Injury to unspecified pelvic organ with open wound into cavity **124**, **127**, **130**
867*	Injury to pelvic organs **223**, **227**
868.0*	Injury to other intra-abdominal organs without mention of open wound into cavity **223**
868.00	Injury to unspecified intra-abdominal organ without mention of open wound into cavity **79**
868.01	Adrenal gland injury without mention of open wound into cavity **114**, **227**
868.02	Bile duct and gallbladder injury without mention of open wound into cavity **83**, **227**
868.03	Peritoneum injury without mention of open wound into cavity **79**, **227**
868.04	Retroperitoneum injury without mention of open wound into cavity **120**, **227**
868.09	Injury to other and multiple intra-abdominal organs without mention of open wound into cavity **202**, **227**
868.1*	Injury to other intra-abdominal organs with open wound into cavity **223**
868.10	Injury to unspecified intra-abdominal organ, with open wound into cavity **79**
868.11	Adrenal gland injury, with open wound into cavity **114**, **227**
868.12	Bile duct and gallbladder injury, with open wound into cavity **83**, **227**
868.13	Peritoneum injury with open wound into cavity **79**, **227**
868.14	Retroperitoneum injury with open wound into cavity **120**, **227**
868.19	Injury to other and multiple intra-abdominal organs, with open wound into cavity **202**, **227**
869*	Internal injury to unspecified or ill-defined organs **202**, **223**
870*	Open wound of ocular adnexa **40**, **223**
871*	Open wound of eyeball **40**, **223**
872*	Open wound of ear **47**, **223**
873.0	Open wound of scalp, without mention of complication **106**
873.1	Open wound of scalp, complicated **106**
873.2*	Open wound of nose, without mention of complication **3**
873.20	Open wound of nose, unspecified site, without mention of complication **47**
873.21	Open wound of nasal septum, without mention of complication **47**
873.22	Open wound of nasal cavity, without mention of complication **47**
873.23	Open wound of nasal sinus, without mention of complication **48**

*Code Range

873.29	Open wound of nose, multiple sites, without mention of complication **48**	
873.3*	Open wound of nose, complicated **3, 48**	
873.40	Open wound of face, unspecified site, without mention of complication **3, 106**	
873.41	Open wound of cheek, without mention of complication **3, 106**	
873.42	Open wound of forehead, without mention of complication **106**	
873.43	Open wound of lip, without mention of complication **3, 48**	
873.44	Open wound of jaw, without mention of complication **3, 48**	
873.49	Open wound of face, other and multiple sites, without mention of complication **106**	
873.50	Open wound of face, unspecified site, complicated **3, 106**	
873.51	Open wound of cheek, complicated **3, 106**	
873.52	Open wound of forehead, complicated **106**	
873.53	Open wound of lip, complicated **3, 48**	
873.54	Open wound of jaw, complicated **3, 48**	
873.59	Open wound of face, other and multiple sites, complicated **106**	
873.6*	Open wound of internal structures of mouth, without mention of complication **48**	
873.60	Open wound of mouth, unspecified site, without mention of complication **3**	
873.61	Open wound of buccal mucosa, without mention of complication **3**	
873.62	Open wound of gum (alveolar process), without mention of complication **3**	
873.64	Open wound of tongue and floor of mouth, without mention of complication **3**	
873.65	Open wound of palate, without mention of complication **3**	
873.69	Open wound of mouth, other and multiple sites, without mention of complication **3**	
873.7*	Open wound of internal structure of mouth, complicated **48**	
873.70	Open wound of mouth, unspecified site, complicated **3**	
873.71	Open wound of buccal mucosa, complicated **3**	
873.72	Open wound of gum (alveolar process), complicated **4**	
873.74	Open wound of tongue and floor of mouth, complicated **4**	
873.75	Open wound of palate, complicated **4**	
873.79	Open wound of mouth, other and multiple sites, complicated **4**	
873.8	Other and unspecified open wound of head without mention of complication **106**	
873.9	Other and unspecified open wound of head, complicated **106**	
873*	Other open wound of head **223**	
874.0*	Open wound of larynx and trachea, without mention of complication **223**	
874.00	Open wound of larynx with trachea, without mention of complication **4, 48**	
874.01	Open wound of larynx, without mention of complication **4, 48**	
874.02	Open wound of trachea, without mention of complication **4, 52**	
874.1*	Open wound of larynx and trachea, complicated **223**	
874.10	Open wound of larynx with trachea, complicated **4, 48, 226**	
874.11	Open wound of larynx, complicated **4, 48, 226**	
874.12	Open wound of trachea, complicated **4, 52, 226**	
874.2	Open wound of thyroid gland, without mention of complication **4, 114, 223**	
874.3	Open wound of thyroid gland, complicated **4, 114, 223**	
874.4	Open wound of pharynx, without mention of complication **4, 48, 223**	
874.5	Open wound of pharynx, complicated **4, 48, 223**	
874.8	Open wound of other and unspecified parts of neck, without mention of complication **4, 106, 223**	
874.9	Open wound of other and unspecified parts of neck, complicated **4, 106, 223**	

875.0	Open wound of chest (wall), without mention of complication **106**
875.1	Open wound of chest (wall), complicated **202**
875*	Open wound of chest (wall) **223**
876*	Open wound of back **106, 223**
877*	Open wound of buttock **106, 223**
878.0	Open wound of penis, without mention of complication **124**
878.1	Open wound of penis, complicated **124**
878.2	Open wound of scrotum and testes, without mention of complication **124**
878.3	Open wound of scrotum and testes, complicated **124**
878.4	Open wound of vulva, without mention of complication **127, 130**
878.5	Open wound of vulva, complicated **127, 130**
878.6	Open wound of vagina, without mention of complication **127, 130**
878.7	Open wound of vagina, complicated **127, 130**
878.8	Open wound of other and unspecified parts of genital organs, without mention of complication **124, 127, 130**
878.9	Open wound of other and unspecified parts of genital organs, complicated **124, 127, 131**
878*	Open wound of genital organs (external), including traumatic amputation **223**
879.0	Open wound of breast, without mention of complication **106**
879.1	Open wound of breast, complicated **106**
879.2	Open wound of abdominal wall, anterior, without mention of complication **106**
879.3	Open wound of abdominal wall, anterior, complicated **202**
879.4	Open wound of abdominal wall, lateral, without mention of complication **106**
879.5	Open wound of abdominal wall, lateral, complicated **202**
879.6	Open wound of other and unspecified parts of trunk, without mention of complication **106**
879.7	Open wound of other and unspecified parts of trunk, complicated **202**
879.8	Open wound(s) (multiple) of unspecified site(s), without mention of complication **107**
879.9	Open wound(s) (multiple) of unspecified site(s), complicated **202**
879*	Open wound of other and unspecified sites, except limbs **223**
880.0*	Open wound of shoulder and upper arm, without mention of complication **107**
880.1*	Open wound of shoulder and upper arm, complicated **202**
880.2*	Open wound of shoulder and upper arm, with tendon involvement **101**
880*	Open wound of shoulder and upper arm **223**
881.0*	Open wound of elbow, forearm, and wrist, without mention of complication **107**
881.1*	Open wound of elbow, forearm, and wrist, complicated **202**
881.2*	Open wound of elbow, forearm, and wrist, with tendon involvement **101**
881*	Open wound of elbow, forearm, and wrist **223**
882.0	Open wound of hand except finger(s) alone, without mention of complication **107**
882.1	Open wound of hand except finger(s) alone, complicated **202**
882.2	Open wound of hand except finger(s) alone, with tendon involvement **101**
882*	Open wound of hand except finger(s) alone **223**
883.0	Open wound of finger(s), without mention of complication **107**
883.1	Open wound of finger(s), complicated **202**
883.2	Open wound of finger(s), with tendon involvement **101**
883*	Open wound of finger(s) **223**
884.0	Multiple and unspecified open wound of upper limb, without mention of complication **107**

884.1	Multiple and unspecified open wound of upper limb, complicated **203**
884.2	Multiple and unspecified open wound of upper limb, with tendon involvement **101**
884*	Multiple and unspecified open wound of upper limb **223**
885*	Traumatic amputation of thumb (complete) (partial) **203**, **223**
886*	Traumatic amputation of other finger(s) (complete) (partial) **203**, **223**
887*	Traumatic amputation of arm and hand (complete) (partial) **203**, **223**, **227**
890.0	Open wound of hip and thigh, without mention of complication **107**
890.1	Open wound of hip and thigh, complicated **203**
890.2	Open wound of hip and thigh, with tendon involvement **101**
890*	Open wound of hip and thigh **223**
891.0	Open wound of knee, leg (except thigh), and ankle, without mention of complication **107**
891.1	Open wound of knee, leg (except thigh), and ankle, complicated **203**
891.2	Open wound of knee, leg (except thigh), and ankle, with tendon involvement **101**
891*	Open wound of knee, leg (except thigh), and ankle **223**
892.0	Open wound of foot except toe(s) alone, without mention of complication **107**
892.1	Open wound of foot except toe(s) alone, complicated **203**
892.2	Open wound of foot except toe(s) alone, with tendon involvement **101**
892*	Open wound of foot except toe(s) alone **223**
893.0	Open wound of toe(s), without mention of complication **107**
893.1	Open wound of toe(s), complicated **203**
893.2	Open wound of toe(s), with tendon involvement **101**
893*	Open wound of toe(s) **223**
894.0	Multiple and unspecified open wound of lower limb, without mention of complication **107**
894.1	Multiple and unspecified open wound of lower limb, complicated **203**
894.2	Multiple and unspecified open wound of lower limb, with tendon involvement **101**
894*	Multiple and unspecified open wound of lower limb **223**
895*	Traumatic amputation of toe(s) (complete) (partial) **203**, **223**
896*	Traumatic amputation of foot (complete) (partial) **203**, **223**, **227**
897*	Traumatic amputation of leg(s) (complete) (partial) **203**, **223**, **227**
900.0*	Injury to carotid artery **166**, **170**, **223**
900.01	Common carotid artery injury **226**
900.02	External carotid artery injury **226**
900.03	Internal carotid artery injury **226**
900.1	Internal jugular vein injury **166**, **170**, **223**, **226**
900.8*	Injury to other specified blood vessels of head and neck **223**
900.81	External jugular vein injury **166**, **170**, **226**
900.82	Injury to multiple blood vessels of head and neck **4**, **226**
900.89	Injury to other specified blood vessels of head and neck **4**
900.9	Injury to unspecified blood vessel of head and neck **4**, **223**
900*	Injury to blood vessels of head and neck **203**
901.0	Thoracic aorta injury **166**, **170**, **223**, **226**
901.1	Innominate and subclavian artery injury **166**, **170**, **223**, **226**
901.2	Superior vena cava injury **166**, **170**, **223**, **226**
901.3	Innominate and subclavian vein injury **166**, **170**, **223**, **226**
901.4*	Pulmonary blood vessel injury **223**, **226**
901.41	Pulmonary artery injury **166**, **170**
901.42	Pulmonary vein injury **166**, **170**
901.8*	Injury to other specified blood vessels of thorax **223**
901.83	Injury to multiple blood vessels of thorax **226**
901.89	Injury to specified blood vessels of thorax, other **226**
901.9	Injury to unspecified blood vessel of thorax **223**, **226**
901*	Injury to blood vessels of thorax **203**
902.0	Abdominal aorta injury **166**, **170**
902.10	Unspecified inferior vena cava injury **166**, **170**
902*	Injury to blood vessels of abdomen and pelvis **203**, **223**, **227**
903*	Injury to blood vessels of upper extremity **203**, **223**, **227**
904.0	Common femoral artery injury **223**, **227**
904.1	Superficial femoral artery injury **223**, **227**
904.2	Femoral vein injury **223**, **227**
904.3	Saphenous vein injury **223**
904.4*	Popliteal blood vessel vein **223**, **227**
904.5*	Tibial blood vessel(s) injury **223**, **227**
904.6	Deep plantar blood vessels injury **223**
904.7	Injury to specified blood vessels of lower extremity, other **223**, **227**
904.8	Injury to unspecified blood vessel of lower extremity **223**
904.9	Injury to blood vessels, unspecified site **223**
904*	Injury to blood vessels of lower extremity and unspecified sites **203**
905.0	Late effect of fracture of skull and face bones **33**
905.1	Late effect of fracture of spine and trunk without mention of spinal cord lesion **98**
905.2	Late effect of fracture of upper extremities **99**
905.3	Late effect of fracture of neck of femur **99**
905.4	Late effect of fracture of lower extremities **99**
905.5	Late effect of fracture of multiple and unspecified bones **99**
905.6	Late effect of dislocation **100**
905.7	Late effect of sprain and strain without mention of tendon injury **100**
905.8	Late effect of tendon injury **99**
905.9	Late effect of traumatic amputation **99**
906*	Late effects of injuries to skin and subcutaneous tissues **107**
907.0	Late effect of intracranial injury without mention of skull fracture **33**
907.1	Late effect of injury to cranial nerve **33**
907.2	Late effect of spinal cord injury **19**
907.3	Late effect of injury to nerve root(s), spinal plexus(es), and other nerves of trunk **33**
907.4	Late effect of injury to peripheral nerve of shoulder girdle and upper limb **33**
907.5	Late effect of injury to peripheral nerve of pelvic girdle and lower limb **33**
907.9	Late effect of injury to other and unspecified nerve **33**
908.0	Late effect of internal injury to chest **54**
908.1	Late effect of internal injury to intra-abdominal organs **79**
908.2	Late effect of internal injury to other internal organs **124**, **127**, **131**
908.3	Late effect of injury to blood vessel of head, neck, and extremities **67**
908.4	Late effect of injury to blood vessel of thorax, abdomen, and pelvis **67**
908.5	Late effect of foreign body in orifice **203**
908.6	Late effect of certain complications of trauma **203**
908.9	Late effect of unspecified injury **203**
909*	Late effects of other and unspecified external causes **204**
910.0	Face, neck, and scalp, except eye, abrasion or friction burn, without mention of infection **107**
910.1	Face, neck, and scalp except eye, abrasion or friction burn, infected **106**

910.2   Face, neck, and scalp except eye, blister, without mention of infection **108**

910.3   Face, neck, and scalp except eye, blister, infected **108**

910.4   Face, neck, and scalp except eye, insect bite, nonvenomous, without mention of infection **108**

910.5   Face, neck, and scalp except eye, insect bite, nonvenomous, infected **106**

910.6   Face, neck, and scalp, except eye, superficial foreign body (splinter), without major open wound or mention of infection **107**

910.7   Face, neck, and scalp except eye, superficial foreign body (splinter), without major open wound, infected **106**

910.8   Other and unspecified superficial injury of face, neck, and scalp, without mention of infection **107**

910.9   Other and unspecified superficial injury of face, neck, and scalp, infected **106**

910*   Superficial injury of face, neck, and scalp, except eye **223**

911.0   Trunk abrasion or friction burn, without mention of infection **107**

911.1   Trunk abrasion or friction burn, infected **106**

911.2   Trunk blister, without mention of infection **108**

911.3   Trunk blister, infected **106**

911.4   Trunk, insect bite, nonvenomous, without mention of infection **108**

911.5   Trunk, insect bite, nonvenomous, infected **106**

911.6   Trunk, superficial foreign body (splinter), without major open wound and without mention of infection **107**

911.7   Trunk, superficial foreign body (splinter), without major open wound, infected **106**

911.8   Other and unspecified superficial injury of trunk, without mention of infection **107**

911.9   Other and unspecified superficial injury of trunk, infected **106**

911*   Superficial injury of trunk **223**

912.0   Shoulder and upper arm, abrasion or friction burn, without mention of infection **107**

912.1   Shoulder and upper arm, abrasion or friction burn, infected **106**

912.2   Shoulder and upper arm, blister, without mention of infection **107**

912.3   Shoulder and upper arm, blister, infected **106**

912.4   Shoulder and upper arm, insect bite, nonvenomous, without mention of infection **108**

912.5   Shoulder and upper arm, insect bite, nonvenomous, infected **106**

912.6   Shoulder and upper arm, superficial foreign body (splinter), without major open wound and without mention of infection **107**

912.7   Shoulder and upper arm, superficial foreign body (splinter), without major open wound, infected **106**

912.8   Other and unspecified superficial injury of shoulder and upper arm, without mention of infection **107**

912.9   Other and unspecified superficial injury of shoulder and upper arm, infected **106**

912*   Superficial injury of shoulder and upper arm **223**

913.0   Elbow, forearm, and wrist, abrasion or friction burn, without mention of infection **107**

913.1   Elbow, forearm, and wrist, abrasion or friction burn, infected **106**

913.2   Elbow, forearm, and wrist, blister, without mention of infection **108**

913.3   Elbow, forearm, and wrist, blister infected **106**

913.4   Elbow, forearm, and wrist, insect bite, nonvenomous, without mention of infection **108**

913.5   Elbow, forearm, and wrist, insect bite, nonvenomous, infected **106**

913.6   Elbow, forearm, and wrist, superficial foreign body (splinter), without major open wound and without mention of infection **107**

913.7   Elbow, forearm, and wrist, superficial foreign body (splinter), without major open wound, infected **106**

913.8   Other and unspecified superficial injury of elbow, forearm, and wrist, without mention of infection **107**

913.9   Other and unspecified superficial injury of elbow, forearm, and wrist, infected **106**

913*   Superficial injury of elbow, forearm, and wrist **223**

914.0   Hand(s) except finger(s) alone, abrasion or friction burn, without mention of infection **107**

914.1   Hand(s) except finger(s) alone, abrasion or friction burn, infected **106**

914.2   Hand(s) except finger(s) alone, blister, without mention of infection **108**

914.3   Hand(s) except finger(s) alone, blister, infected **106**

914.4   Hand(s) except finger(s) alone, insect bite, nonvenomous, without mention of infection **108**

914.5   Hand(s) except finger(s) alone, insect bite, nonvenomous, infected **106**

914.6   Hand(s) except finger(s) alone, superficial foreign body (splinter), without major open wound and without mention of infection **107**

914.7   Hand(s) except finger(s) alone, superficial foreign body (splinter) without major open wound, infected **106**

914.8   Other and unspecified superficial injury of hand(s) except finger(s) alone, without mention of infection **107**

914.9   Other and unspecified superficial injury of hand(s) except finger(s) alone, infected **106**

914*   Superficial injury of hand(s) except finger(s) alone **223**

915.0   Abrasion or friction burn of finger, without mention of infection **107**

915.1   Finger, abrasion or friction burn, infected **106**

915.2   Finger, blister, without mention of infection **108**

915.3   Finger, blister, infected **106**

915.4   Finger, insect bite, nonvenomous, without mention of infection **108**

915.5   Finger, insect bite, nonvenomous, infected **106**

915.6   Finger, superficial foreign body (splinter), without major open wound and without mention of infection **107**

915.7   Finger, superficial foreign body (splinter), without major open wound, infected **106**

915.8   Other and unspecified superficial injury of finger without mention of infection **107**

915.9   Other and unspecified superficial injury of finger, infected **106**

915*   Superficial injury of finger(s) **223**

916.0   Hip, thigh, leg, and ankle, abrasion or friction burn, without mention of infection **107**

916.1   Hip, thigh, leg, and ankle, abrasion or friction burn, infected **106**

916.2   Hip, thigh, leg, and ankle, blister, without mention of infection **108**

916.3   Hip, thigh, leg, and ankle, blister, infected **106**

916.4   Hip, thigh, leg, and ankle, insect bite, nonvenomous, without mention of infection **108**

916.5   Hip, thigh, leg, and ankle, insect bite, nonvenomous, infected **106**

916.6   Hip, thigh, leg, and ankle, superficial foreign body (splinter), without major open wound and without mention of infection **107**

916.7   Hip, thigh, leg, and ankle, superficial foreign body (splinter), without major open wound, infected **106**

916.8   Other and unspecified superficial injury of hip, thigh, leg, and ankle, without mention of infection **107**

916.9   Other and unspecified superficial injury of hip, thigh, leg, and ankle, infected **106**

916*   Superficial injury of hip, thigh, leg, and ankle **223**

917.0   Abrasion or friction burn of foot and toe(s), without mention of infection **107**

917.1	Foot and toe(s), abrasion or friction burn, infected **106**	926.19	Crushing injury of other specified sites of trunk **227**
917.2	Foot and toe(s), blister, without mention of infection **108**	926.8	Crushing injury of multiple sites of trunk **203, 223, 227**
917.3	Foot and toe(s), blister, infected **106**	926.9	Crushing injury of unspecified site of trunk **203, 223, 227**
917.4	Foot and toe(s), insect bite, nonvenomous, without mention of infection **108**	927.0*	Crushing injury of shoulder and upper arm **223, 227**
917.5	Foot and toe(s), insect bite, nonvenomous, infected **106**	927.01	Crushing injury of scapular region **226**
917.6	Foot and toe(s), superficial foreign body (splinter), without major open wound and without mention of infection **107**	927.1*	Crushing injury of elbow and forearm **223, 227**
		927.2*	Crushing injury of wrist and hand(s), except finger(s) alone **223**
917.7	Foot and toe(s), superficial foreign body (splinter), without major open wound, infected **106**	927.3	Crushing injury of finger(s) **223**
		927.8	Crushing injury of multiple sites of upper limb **223, 227**
917.8	Other and unspecified superficial injury of foot and toes, without mention of infection **107**	927.9	Crushing injury of unspecified site of upper limb **223, 227**
917.9	Other and unspecified superficial injury of foot and toes, infected **106**	927*	Crushing injury of upper limb **203**
		928.0*	Crushing injury of hip and thigh **223, 227**
917*	Superficial injury of foot and toe(s) **223**	928.1*	Crushing injury of knee and lower leg **223, 227**
918*	Superficial injury of eye and adnexa **40, 223**	928.2*	Crushing injury of ankle and foot, excluding toe(s) alone **223**
919.0	Abrasion or friction burn of other, multiple, and unspecified sites, without mention of infection **107**	928.3	Crushing injury of toe(s) **223**
919.1	Other, multiple, and unspecified sites, abrasion or friction burn, infected **106**	928.8	Crushing injury of multiple sites of lower limb **223, 227**
		928.9	Crushing injury of unspecified site of lower limb **223, 227**
919.2	Other, multiple, and unspecified sites, blister, without mention of infection **108**	928*	Crushing injury of lower limb **203**
919.3	Other, multiple, and unspecified sites, blister, infected **106**	929*	Crushing injury of multiple and unspecified sites **203, 223**
919.4	Other, multiple, and unspecified sites, insect bite, nonvenomous, without mention of infection **109**	930*	Foreign body on external eye **40**
		931	Foreign body in ear **48**
919.5	Other, multiple, and unspecified sites, insect bite, nonvenomous, infected **106**	932	Foreign body in nose **48**
		933*	Foreign body in pharynx and larynx **4, 48**
919.6	Other, multiple, and unspecified sites, superficial foreign body (splinter), without major open wound and without mention of infection **107**	934.0	Foreign body in trachea **54**
		934.1	Foreign body in main bronchus **54**
919.7	Other, multiple, and unspecified sites, superficial foreign body (splinter), without major open wound, infected **106**	934.8	Foreign body in other specified parts of trachea, bronchus, and lung **54**
		934.9	Foreign body in respiratory tree, unspecified **54**
919.8	Other and unspecified superficial injury of other, multiple, and unspecified sites, without mention of infection **107**	935.0	Foreign body in mouth **4, 48**
		935.1	Foreign body in esophagus **79**
919.9	Other and unspecified superficial injury of other, multiple, and unspecified sites, infected **106**	935.2	Foreign body in stomach **79**
		936	Foreign body in intestine and colon **79**
919*	Superficial injury of other, multiple, and unspecified sites **223**	937	Foreign body in anus and rectum **79**
920	Contusion of face, scalp, and neck except eye(s) **107, 223**	938	Foreign body in digestive system, unspecified **79**
921.0	Black eye, not otherwise specified **40**	939.0	Foreign body in bladder and urethra **120**
921.1	Contusion of eyelids and periocular area **40**	939.1	Foreign body in uterus, any part **128, 131**
921.2	Contusion of orbital tissues **40**	939.2	Foreign body in vulva and vagina **128, 131**
921.3	Contusion of eyeball **40**	939.3	Foreign body in penis **124**
921.9	Unspecified contusion of eye **40**	939.9	Foreign body in unspecified site in genitourinary tract **120**
921*	Contusion of eye and adnexa **223**	940*	Burn confined to eye and adnexa **40**
922.0	Contusion of breast **107**	941.00	Burn of unspecified degree of unspecified site of face and head **209**
922.1	Contusion of chest wall **107**		
922.2	Contusion of abdominal wall **107**	941.01	Burn of unspecified degree of ear (any part) **209**
922.3*	Contusion of trunk **107**	941.02	Burn of unspecified degree of eye (with other parts of face, head, and neck) **40**
922.4	Contusion of genital organs **124, 127, 131**		
922.8	Contusion of multiple sites of trunk **107**	941.03	Burn of unspecified degree of lip(s) **209**
922.9	Contusion of unspecified part of trunk **107**	941.04	Burn of unspecified degree of chin **209**
922*	Contusion of trunk **223**	941.05	Burn of unspecified degree of nose (septum) **209**
923*	Contusion of upper limb **107, 223**	941.06	Burn of unspecified degree of scalp (any part) **209**
924*	Contusion of lower limb and of other and unspecified sites **107, 223**	941.07	Burn of unspecified degree of forehead and cheek **209**
		941.08	Burn of unspecified degree of neck **209**
925.1	Crushing injury of face and scalp **226**	941.09	Burn of unspecified degree of multiple sites (except with eye) of face, head, and neck **209**
925.2	Crushing injury of neck **226**		
925*	Crushing injury of face, scalp, and neck **4, 203, 223**	941.10	Erythema due to burn (first degree) of unspecified site of face and head **209**
926.0	Crushing injury of external genitalia **124, 127, 131, 223**		
926.1*	Crushing injury of other specified sites of trunk **203, 223**	941.11	Erythema due to burn (first degree) of ear (any part) **209**
		941.12	Erythema due to burn (first degree) of eye (with other parts face, head, and neck) **40**
926.11	Crushing injury of back **227**		
926.12	Crushing injury of buttock **227**	941.13	Erythema due to burn (first degree) of lip(s) **209**
		941.14	Erythema due to burn (first degree) of chin **209**

*Code Range

941.15	Erythema due to burn (first degree) of nose (septum) **209**
941.16	Erythema due to burn (first degree) of scalp (any part) **209**
941.17	Erythema due to burn (first degree) of forehead and cheek **209**
941.18	Erythema due to burn (first degree) of neck **209**
941.19	Erythema due to burn (first degree) of multiple sites (except with eye) of face, head, and neck **209**
941.20	Blisters, with epidermal loss due to burn (second degree) of face and head, unspecified site **209**
941.21	Blisters, with epidermal loss due to burn (second degree) of ear (any part) **209**
941.22	Blisters, with epidermal loss due to burn (second degree) of eye (with other parts of face, head, and neck) **40**
941.23	Blisters, with epidermal loss due to burn (second degree) of lip(s) **209**
941.24	Blisters, with epidermal loss due to burn (second degree) of chin **209**
941.25	Blisters, with epidermal loss due to burn (second degree) of nose (septum) **209**
941.26	Blisters, with epidermal loss due to burn (second degree) of scalp (any part) **209**
941.27	Blisters, with epidermal loss due to burn (second degree) of forehead and cheek **209**
941.28	Blisters, with epidermal loss due to burn (second degree) of neck **209**
941.29	Blisters, with epidermal loss due to burn (second degree) of multiple sites (except with eye) of face, head, and neck **209**
941.3*	Full-thickness skin loss due to burn (third degree NOS) of face, head, and neck **206, 207, 208, 209**
941.32	Full-thickness skin loss due to burn (third degree NOS) of eye (with other parts of face, head, and neck) **40**
941.4*	Deep necrosis of underlying tissues due to burn (deep third degree) of face, head, and neck without mention of loss of a body part **206, 207, 208, 209**
941.42	Deep necrosis of underlying tissues due to burn (deep third degree) of eye (with other parts of face, head, and neck), without mention of loss of a body part **40**
941.5*	Deep necrosis of underlying tissues due to burn (deep third degree) of face, head, and neck with loss of a body part **206, 207, 208, 209**
941.52	Deep necrosis of underlying tissues due to burn (deep third degree) of eye (with other parts of face, head, and neck), with loss of a body part **40**
942.0*	Burn of trunk, unspecified degree **209**
942.1*	Erythema due to burn (first degree) of trunk **209**
942.2*	Blisters with epidermal loss due to burn (second degree) of trunk **209**
942.3*	Full-thickness skin loss due to burn (third degree NOS) of trunk **206, 207, 208, 209**
942.4*	Deep necrosis of underlying tissues due to burn (deep third degree) of trunk without mention of loss of a body part **206, 207, 208, 209**
942.5*	Deep necrosis of underlying tissues due to burn (deep third degree) of trunk with loss of a body part **206, 207, 208, 209**
943.0*	Burn of upper limb, except wrist and hand, unspecified degree **209**
943.1*	Erythema due to burn (first degree) of upper limb, except wrist and hand **209**
943.2*	Blisters with epidermal loss due to burn (second degree) of upper limb, except wrist and hand **210**
943.3*	Full-thickness skin loss due to burn (third degree NOS) of upper limb, except wrist and hand **206, 207, 208, 209**
943.4*	Deep necrosis of underlying tissues due to burn (deep third degree) of upper limb, except wrist and hand, without mention of loss of a body part **206, 207, 208, 209**

943.5*	Deep necrosis of underlying tissues due to burn (deep third degree) of upper limb, except wrist and hand, with loss of a body part **206, 207, 208, 209**
944.0*	Burn of wrist(s) and hand(s), unspecified degree **210**
944.1*	Erythema due to burn (first degree) of wrist(s) and hand(s) **210**
944.2*	Blisters with epidermal loss due to burn (second degree) of wrist(s) and hand(s) **210**
944.3*	Full-thickness skin loss due to burn (third degree NOS) of wrist(s) and hand(s) **206, 207, 208, 209**
944.4*	Deep necrosis of underlying tissues due to burn (deep third degree) of wrist(s) and hand(s), without mention of loss of a body part **206, 207, 208, 209**
944.5*	Deep necrosis of underlying tissues due to burn (deep third degree) of wrist(s) and hand(s), with loss of a body part **206, 207, 208, 209**
945.0*	Burn of lower limb(s), unspecified degree **210**
945.1*	Erythema due to burn (first degree) of lower limb(s) **210**
945.2*	Blisters with epidermal loss due to burn (second degree) of lower limb(s) **210**
945.3*	Full-thickness skin loss due to burn (third degree NOS) of lower limb(s) **206, 207, 208, 209**
945.4*	Deep necrosis of underlying tissues due to burn (deep third degree) of lower limb(s) without mention of loss of a body part **206, 207, 208, 209**
945.5*	Deep necrosis of underlying tissues due to burn (deep third degree) of lower limb(s) with loss of a body part **206, 207, 208, 209**
946.0	Burns of multiple specified sites, unspecified degree **210**
946.1	Erythema due to burn (first degree) of multiple specified sites **210**
946.2	Blisters with epidermal loss due to burn (second degree) of multiple specified sites **210**
946.3	Full-thickness skin loss due to burn (third degree NOS) of multiple specified sites **206, 207, 208, 209**
946.4	Deep necrosis of underlying tissues due to burn (deep third degree) of multiple specified sites, without mention of loss of a body part **206, 207, 208, 209**
946.5	Deep necrosis of underlying tissues due to burn (deep third degree) of multiple specified sites, with loss of a body part **206, 207, 208, 209**
947.0	Burn of mouth and pharynx **4, 48**
947.1	Burn of larynx, trachea, and lung **54, 207**
947.2	Burn of esophagus **75**
947.3	Burn of gastrointestinal tract **79**
947.4	Burn of vagina and uterus **128, 131**
947.8	Burn of other specified sites of internal organs **210**
947.9	Burn of internal organs, unspecified site **210**
948.00	Burn (any degree) involving less than 10% of body surface with third degree burn of less than 10% or unspecified amount **210**
948.10	Burn (any degree) involving 10-19% of body surface with third degree burn of less than 10% or unspecified amount **210**
948.11	Burn (any degree) involving 10-19% of body surface with third degree burn of 10-19% **206, 207, 208, 209**
948.20	Burn (any degree) involving 20-29% of body surface with third degree burn of less than 10% or unspecified amount **210**
948.21	Burn (any degree) involving 20-29% of body surface with third degree burn of 10-19% **206, 208**
948.22	Burn (any degree) involving 20-29% of body surface with third degree burn of 20-29% **206, 208**
948.30	Burn (any degree) involving 30-39% of body surface with third degree burn of less than 10% or unspecified amount **210**
948.31	Burn (any degree) involving 30-39% of body surface with third degree burn of 10-19% **206, 208**
948.32	Burn (any degree) involving 30-39% of body surface with third degree burn of 20-29% **206, 208**

948.33	Burn (any degree) involving 30-39% of body surface with third degree burn of 30-39% **206, 208**		948.86	Burn (any degree) involving 80-89% of body surface with third degree burn of 60-69% **207, 209**
948.40	Burn (any degree) involving 40-49% of body surface with third degree burn of less than 10% or unspecified amount **210**		948.87	Burn (any degree) involving 80-89% of body surface with third degree burn of 70-79% **207, 209**
948.41	Burn (any degree) involving 40-49% of body surface with third degree burn of 10-19% **206, 208**		948.88	Burn (any degree) involving 80-89% of body surface with third degree burn of 80-89% **207, 209**
948.42	Burn (any degree) involving 40-49% of body surface with third degree burn of 20-29% **206, 208**		948.90	Burn (any degree) involving 90% or more of body surface with third degree burn of less than 10% or unspecified amount **210**
948.43	Burn (any degree) involving 40-49% of body surface with third degree burn of 30-39% **206, 208**		948.91	Burn (any degree) involving 90% or more of body surface with third degree burn of 10-19% **207, 209**
948.44	Burn (any degree) involving 40-49% of body surface with third degree burn of 40-49% **206, 208**		948.92	Burn (any degree) involving 90% or more of body surface with third degree burn of 20-29% **207, 209**
948.50	Burn (any degree) involving 50-59% of body surface with third degree burn of less than 10% or unspecified amount **210**		948.93	Burn (any degree) involving 90% or more of body surface with third degree burn of 30-39% **207, 209**
948.51	Burn (any degree) involving 50-59% of body surface with third degree burn of 10-19% **206, 208**		948.94	Burn (any degree) involving 90% or more of body surface with third degree burn of 40-49% **207, 209**
948.52	Burn (any degree) involving 50-59% of body surface with third degree burn of 20-29% **206, 208**		948.95	Burn (any degree) involving 90% or more of body surface with third degree burn of 50-59% **207, 209**
948.53	Burn (any degree) involving 50-59% of body surface with third degree burn of 30-39% **206, 208**		948.96	Burn (any degree) involving 90% or more of body surface with third degree burn of 60-69% **207, 209**
948.54	Burn (any degree) involving 50-59% of body surface with third degree burn of 40-49% **206, 208**		948.97	Burn (any degree) involving 90% or more of body surface with third degree burn of 70-79% **207, 209**
948.55	Burn (any degree) involving 50-59% of body surface with third degree burn of 50-59% **206, 208**		948.98	Burn (any degree) involving 90% or more of body surface with third degree burn of 80-89% **207, 209**
948.60	Burn (any degree) involving 60-69% of body surface with third degree burn of less than 10% or unspecified amount **210**		948.99	Burn (any degree) involving 90% or more of body surface with third degree burn of 90% or more of body surface **207, 209**
948.61	Burn (any degree) involving 60-69% of body surface with third degree burn of 10-19% **206, 208**		949.0	Burn of unspecified site, unspecified degree **210**
948.62	Burn (any degree) involving 60-69% of body surface with third degree burn of 20-29% **206, 208**		949.1	Erythema due to burn (first degree), unspecified site **210**
948.63	Burn (any degree) involving 60-69% of body surface with third degree burn of 30-39% **206, 208**		949.2	Blisters with epidermal loss due to burn (second degree), unspecified site **210**
948.64	Burn (any degree) involving 60-69% of body surface with third degree burn of 40-49% **206, 208**		949.3	Full-thickness skin loss due to burn (third degree NOS), unspecified site **206, 207, 208, 209**
948.65	Burn (any degree) involving 60-69% of body surface with third degree burn of 50-59% **206, 208**		949.4	Deep necrosis of underlying tissue due to burn (deep third degree), unspecified site without mention of loss of body part **206, 207, 208, 209**
948.66	Burn (any degree) involving 60-69% of body surface with third degree burn of 60-69% **206, 208**		949.5	Deep necrosis of underlying tissues due to burn (deep third degree, unspecified site with loss of body part **206, 207, 208, 209**
948.70	Burn (any degree) involving 70-79% of body surface with third degree burn of less than 10% or unspecified amount **210**		950.0	Optic nerve injury **40**
948.71	Burn (any degree) involving 70-79% of body surface with third degree burn of 10-19% **206, 208**		950.1	Injury to optic chiasm **33**
			950.2	Injury to optic pathways **33**
948.72	Burn (any degree) involving 70-79% of body surface with third degree burn of 20-29% **206, 208**		950.3	Injury to visual cortex **33**
948.73	Burn (any degree) involving 70-79% of body surface with third degree burn of 30-39% **206, 208**		950.9	Injury to unspecified optic nerve and pathways **33**
948.74	Burn (any degree) involving 70-79% of body surface with third degree burn of 40-49% **206, 208**		950*	Injury to optic nerve and pathways **223**
			951.0	Injury to oculomotor nerve **21**
948.75	Burn (any degree) involving 70-79% of body surface with third degree burn of 50-59% **206, 208**		951.1	Injury to trochlear nerve **21**
			951.2	Injury to trigeminal nerve **21**
948.76	Burn (any degree) involving 70-79% of body surface with third degree burn of 60-69% **206, 208**		951.3	Injury to abducens nerve **21**
			951.4	Injury to facial nerve **21**
948.77	Burn (any degree) involving 70-79% of body surface with third degree burn of 70-79% **206, 208**		951.5	Injury to acoustic nerve **48**
			951.6	Injury to accessory nerve **21**
948.80	Burn (any degree) involving 80-89% of body surface with third degree burn of less than 10% or unspecified amount **210**		951.7	Injury to hypoglossal nerve **21**
			951.8	Injury to other specified cranial nerves **21**
948.81	Burn (any degree) involving 80-89% of body surface with third degree burn of 10-19% **206, 208**		951.9	Injury to unspecified cranial nerve **21**
			951*	Injury to other cranial nerve(s) **223**
948.82	Burn (any degree) involving 80-89% of body surface with third degree burn of 20-29% **207, 208**		952*	Spinal cord injury without evidence of spinal bone injury **19, 223, 227**
948.83	Burn (any degree) involving 80-89% of body surface with third degree burn of 30-39% **207, 208**		953.1	Injury to dorsal nerve root **223**
948.84	Burn (any degree) involving 80-89% of body surface with third degree burn of 40-49% **207, 209**		953.2	Injury to lumbar nerve root **223**
			953.3	Injury to sacral nerve root **223**
948.85	Burn (any degree) involving 80-89% of body surface with third degree burn of 50-59% **207, 209**		953.4	Injury to brachial plexus **166, 170, 223, 227**
			953.5	Injury to lumbosacral plexus **223, 227**
			953.8	Injury to multiple sites of nerve roots and spinal plexus **223, 227**

*Code Range

953.9	Injury to unspecified site of nerve roots and spinal plexus **223**	
953*	Injury to nerve roots and spinal plexus **21, 223**	
954.0	Injury to cervical sympathetic nerve, excluding shoulder and pelvic girdles **223**	
954.1	Injury to other sympathetic nerve, excluding shoulder and pelvic girdles **223**	
954.8	Injury to other specified nerve(s) of trunk, excluding shoulder and pelvic girdles **223, 227**	
954.9	Injury to unspecified nerve of trunk, excluding shoulder and pelvic girdles **223, 227**	
954*	Injury to other nerve(s) of trunk, excluding shoulder and pelvic girdles **21**	
955.0	Injury to axillary nerve **223, 227**	
955.1	Injury to median nerve **223, 227**	
955.2	Injury to ulnar nerve **223, 227**	
955.3	Injury to radial nerve **223, 227**	
955.4	Injury to musculocutaneous nerve **223**	
955.5	Injury to cutaneous sensory nerve, upper limb **223**	
955.6	Injury to digital nerve, upper limb **223**	
955.7	Injury to other specified nerve(s) of shoulder girdle and upper limb **223**	
955.8	Injury to multiple nerves of shoulder girdle and upper limb **224, 227**	
955.9	Injury to unspecified nerve of shoulder girdle and upper limb **224**	
955*	Injury to peripheral nerve(s) of shoulder girdle and upper limb **21**	
956.0	Injury to sciatic nerve **224, 227**	
956.1	Injury to femoral nerve **224, 227**	
956.2	Injury to posterior tibial nerve **224, 228**	
956.3	Injury to peroneal nerve **224, 228**	
956.4	Injury to cutaneous sensory nerve, lower limb **224**	
956.5	Injury to other specified nerve(s) of pelvic girdle and lower limb **224**	
956.8	Injury to multiple nerves of pelvic girdle and lower limb **224, 228**	
956.9	Injury to unspecified nerve of pelvic girdle and lower limb **224, 228**	
956*	Injury to peripheral nerve(s) of pelvic girdle and lower limb **21**	
957*	Injury to other and unspecified nerves **21, 224**	
958.0	Air embolism as an early complication of trauma **51, 166, 170, 224, 226**	
958.1	Fat embolism as an early complication of trauma **51, 166, 170, 224, 227**	
958.2	Secondary and recurrent hemorrhage as an early complication of trauma **166, 171, 204, 224**	
958.3	Posttraumatic wound infection not elsewhere classified **166, 171, 184, 224**	
958.4	Traumatic shock **166, 171, 204, 224**	
958.5	Traumatic anuria **118, 119, 166, 171, 224**	
958.6	Volkmann's ischemic contracture **101, 224, 227**	
958.7	Traumatic subcutaneous emphysema **53, 166, 171, 224**	
958.8	Other early complications of trauma **204, 224**	
958.9*	Traumatic compartment syndrome **204**	
958.90	Compartment syndrome, unspecified **224**	
958.91	Traumatic compartment syndrome of upper extremity **224, 227**	
958.92	Traumatic compartment syndrome of lower extremity **224, 228**	
958.93	Traumatic compartment syndrome of abdomen **224, 227**	
958.99	Traumatic compartment syndrome of other sites **224**	
959.0*	Injury, other and unspecified, head, face, and neck **4, 224**	
959.1*	Injury, other and unspecified, trunk **224**	
959.2	Injury, other and unspecified, shoulder and upper arm **224**	
959.3	Injury, other and unspecified, elbow, forearm, and wrist **224**	
959.4	Injury, other and unspecified, hand, except finger **224**	
959.5	Injury, other and unspecified, finger **224**	

959.6	Injury, other and unspecified, hip and thigh **224**
959.7	Injury, other and unspecified, knee, leg, ankle, and foot **224**
959.8	Injury, other and unspecified, other specified sites, including multiple **224**
959.9	Injury, other and unspecified, unspecified site **224**
959*	Injury, other and unspecified **203**
960*	Poisoning by antibiotics **203**
961*	Poisoning by other anti-infectives **203**
962*	Poisoning by hormones and synthetic substitutes **203**
963*	Poisoning by primarily systemic agents **203**
964*	Poisoning by agents primarily affecting blood constituents **203**
965*	Poisoning by analgesics, antipyretics, and antirheumatics **203**
966*	Poisoning by anticonvulsants and anti-Parkinsonism drugs **203**
967*	Poisoning by sedatives and hypnotics **203**
968*	Poisoning by other central nervous system depressants and anesthetics **203**
969*	Poisoning by psychotropic agents **203**
970*	Poisoning by central nervous system stimulants **203**
971*	Poisoning by drugs primarily affecting the autonomic nervous system **203**
972*	Poisoning by agents primarily affecting the cardiovascular system **203**
973*	Poisoning by agents primarily affecting the gastrointestinal system **203**
974*	Poisoning by water, mineral, and uric acid metabolism drugs **203**
975*	Poisoning by agents primarily acting on the smooth and skeletal muscles and respiratory system **203**
976.0	Poisoning by local anti-infectives and anti-inflammatory drugs **203**
976.1	Poisoning by antipruritics **203**
976.2	Poisoning by local astringents and local detergents **203**
976.3	Poisoning by emollients, demulcents, and protectants **203**
976.4	Poisoning by keratolytics, keratoplastics, other hair treatment drugs and preparations **203**
976.5	Poisoning by eye anti-infectives and other eye drugs **40**
976.6	Poisoning by anti-infectives and other drugs and preparations for ear, nose, and throat **203**
976.7	Poisoning by dental drugs topically applied **203**
976.8	Poisoning by other agents primarily affecting skin and mucous membrane **203**
976.9	Poisoning by unspecified agent primarily affecting skin and mucous membrane **203**
977*	Poisoning by other and unspecified drugs and medicinal substances **203**
978*	Poisoning by bacterial vaccines **203**
979*	Poisoning by other vaccines and biological substances **203**
980*	Toxic effect of alcohol **203**
981	Toxic effect of petroleum products **203**
982*	Toxic effect of solvents other than petroleum-based **203**
983*	Toxic effect of corrosive aromatics, acids, and caustic alkalis **203**
984*	Toxic effect of lead and its compounds (including fumes) **203**
985*	Toxic effect of other metals **203**
986	Toxic effect of carbon monoxide **203**
987.9	Toxic effect of unspecified gas, fume, or vapor **207**
987*	Toxic effect of other gases, fumes, or vapors **203**
988*	Toxic effect of noxious substances eaten as food **203**
989*	Toxic effect of other substances, chiefly nonmedicinal as to source **203**
990	Effects of radiation, unspecified **204**
991*	Effects of reduced temperature **204**
992*	Effects of heat and light **204**
993.0	Barotrauma, otitic **46**

993.1	Barotrauma, sinus **46**	
993.2	Other and unspecified effects of high altitude **204**	
993.3	Caisson disease **204**	
993.4	Effects of air pressure caused by explosion **204**	
993.8	Other specified effects of air pressure **204**	
993.9	Unspecified effect of air pressure **204**	
994.0	Effects of lightning **204**	
994.1	Drowning and nonfatal submersion **204**	
994.2	Effects of hunger **204**	
994.3	Effects of thirst **204**	
994.4	Exhaustion due to exposure **204**	
994.5	Exhaustion due to excessive exertion **204**	
994.6	Motion sickness **46**	
994.7	Asphyxiation and strangulation **204**	
994.8	Electrocution and nonfatal effects of electric current **204**	
994.9	Other effects of external causes **204**	
995.0	Other anaphylactic reaction **203**	
995.1	Angioneurotic edema not elsewhere classified **203**	
995.2*	Other and unspecified adverse effect of drug, medicinal and biological substance **203**	
995.20	Unspecified adverse effect of unspecified drug, medicinal and biological substance **166, 171**	
995.21	Arthus phenomenon **166, 171**	
995.22	Unspecified adverse effect of anesthesia **166, 171**	
995.23	Unspecified adverse effect of insulin **166, 171**	
995.27	Other drug allergy **166, 171**	
995.29	Unspecified adverse effect of other drug, medicinal and biological substance **166, 171**	
995.3	Allergy, unspecified not elsewhere classified **203**	
995.4	Shock due to anesthesia not elsewhere classified **166, 171, 204**	
995.5*	Child maltreatment syndrome **204**	
995.6*	Anaphylactic reaction due to food **203**	
995.7	Other adverse food reactions, not elsewhere classified **204**	
995.8*	Other specified adverse effects, not elsewhere classified **204**	
995.9*	Systemic inflammatory response syndrome (SIRS) **186**	
996.00	Mechanical complication of unspecified cardiac device, implant, and graft **69**	
996.01	Mechanical complication due to cardiac pacemaker (electrode) **68**	
996.02	Mechanical complication due to heart valve prosthesis **68**	
996.03	Mechanical complication due to coronary bypass graft **69**	
996.04	Mechanical complication due to automatic implantable cardiac defibrillator **68**	
996.09	Mechanical complication of cardiac device, implant, and graft, other **69**	
996.1	Mechanical complication of other vascular device, implant, and graft **69**	
996.2	Mechanical complication of nervous system device, implant, and graft **33**	
996.30	Mechanical complication of unspecified genitourinary device, implant, and graft **120**	
996.31	Mechanical complication due to urethral (indwelling) catheter **120**	
996.32	Mechanical complication due to intrauterine contraceptive device **128, 131**	
996.39	Mechanical complication of genitourinary device, implant, and graft, other **120**	
996.4*	Mechanical complication of internal orthopedic device, implant, and graft **99**	
996.51	Mechanical complication due to corneal graft **40**	
996.52	Mechanical complication due to other tissue graft, not elsewhere classified **203**	

996.53	Mechanical complication due to ocular lens prosthesis **40**
996.54	Mechanical complication due to breast prosthesis **106**
996.55	Mechanical complications due to artificial skin graft and decellularized allodermis **203**
996.56	Mechanical complications due to peritoneal dialysis catheter **203**
996.57	Mechanical complication due to insulin pump **203**
996.59	Mechanical complication due to other implant and internal device, not elsewhere classified **203**
996.60	Infection and inflammatory reaction due to unspecified device, implant, and graft **203**
996.61	Infection and inflammatory reaction due to cardiac device, implant, and graft **69**
996.62	Infection and inflammatory reaction due to other vascular device, implant, and graft **69**
996.63	Infection and inflammatory reaction due to nervous system device, implant, and graft **33**
996.64	Infection and inflammatory reaction due to indwelling urinary catheter **120**
996.65	Infection and inflammatory reaction due to other genitourinary device, implant, and graft **120**
996.66	Infection and inflammatory reaction due to internal joint prosthesis **90, 99**
996.67	Infection and inflammatory reaction due to other internal orthopedic device, implant, and graft **90, 99**
996.68	Infection and inflammatory reaction due to peritoneal dialysis catheter **203**
996.69	Infection and inflammatory reaction due to other internal prosthetic device, implant, and graft **203**
996.70	Other complications due to unspecified device, implant, and graft **203**
996.71	Other complications due to heart valve prosthesis **69**
996.72	Other complications due to other cardiac device, implant, and graft **69**
996.73	Other complications due to renal dialysis device, implant, and graft **69**
996.74	Other complications due to other vascular device, implant, and graft **69**
996.75	Other complications due to nervous system device, implant, and graft **33**
996.76	Other complications due to genitourinary device, implant, and graft **120**
996.77	Other complications due to internal joint prosthesis **99**
996.78	Other complications due to other internal orthopedic device, implant, and graft **99**
996.79	Other complications due to other internal prosthetic device, implant, and graft **203**
996.80	Complications of transplanted organ, unspecified site **204**
996.81	Complications of transplanted kidney **120**
996.82	Complications of transplanted liver **83**
996.83	Complications of transplanted heart **69**
996.84	Complications of transplanted lung **54**
996.85	Complications of bone marrow transplant **175**
996.86	Complications of transplanted pancreas **83**
996.87	Complications of transplanted organ, intestine **204**
996.88	Complications of transplanted organ, stem cell **204**
996.89	Complications of other transplanted organ **204**
996.9*	Complications of reattached extremity or body part **99**
997.0*	Nervous system complications **33, 167, 171**
997.1	Cardiac complications **69, 167, 171**
997.2	Peripheral vascular complications **67, 167, 171**
997.3*	Respiratory complications **54, 167, 171**
997.4*	Digestive system complications, not elsewhere classified **79, 167, 171**

997.5	Urinary complications **120**, **167**, **171**
997.6★	Amputation stump complication **101**
997.71	Vascular complications of mesenteric artery **79**, **167**, **171**
997.72	Vascular complications of renal artery **120**, **167**, **171**
997.79	Vascular complications of other vessels **67**, **167**, **171**
997.9★	Complications affecting other specified body systems, not elsewhere classified **204**
998.0★	Postoperative shock **167**, **171**, **204**
998.1★	Hemorrhage or hematoma or seroma complicating procedure, not elsewhere classified **204**
998.11	Hemorrhage complicating a procedure **167**, **171**
998.12	Hematoma complicating a procedure **167**, **171**
998.13	Seroma complicating a procedure **167**, **171**
998.2	Accidental puncture or laceration during procedure **167**, **171**, **204**
998.3★	Disruption of wound **204**
998.4	Foreign body accidentally left during procedure, not elsewhere classified **167**, **171**, **204**
998.5★	Postoperative infection, not elsewhere classified **184**
998.51	Infected postoperative seroma **167**, **171**, **184**
998.59	Other postoperative infection **167**, **171**, **184**
998.6	Persistent postoperative fistula, not elsewhere classified **167**, **171**, **204**
998.7	Acute reaction to foreign substance accidentally left during procedure, not elsewhere classified **167**, **171**, **204**
998.81	Emphysema (subcutaneous) (surgical) resulting from a procedure **204**
998.82	Cataract fragments in eye following surgery **40**
998.83	Non-healing surgical wound **204**
998.89	Other specified complications **204**
998.9	Unspecified complication of procedure, not elsewhere classified **167**, **171**, **204**
999.0	Generalized vaccinia as complication of medical care, not elsewhere classified **185**
999.1	Air embolism as complication of medical care, not elsewhere classified **51**, **167**, **171**
999.2	Other vascular complications of medical care, not elsewhere classified **69**, **167**, **171**
999.31	Other and unspecified infection due to central venous catheter **69**
999.32	Bloodstream infection due to central venous catheter **69**
999.33	Local infection due to central venous catheter **69**
999.34	Acute infection following transfusion, infusion, or injection of blood and blood products **167**, **171**, **184**, **186**
999.39	Complications of medical care, NEC, infection following other infusion, injection, transfusion, or vaccination **167**, **171**, **184**, **186**
999.4★	Anaphylactic reaction due to serum **167**, **171**, **203**
999.5★	Other serum reaction, not elsewhere classified **167**, **171**, **203**
999.6★	ABO incompatibility reaction due to transfusion of blood or blood products **167**, **171**, **176**
999.7★	Rh and other non-ABO incompatibility reaction due to transfusion of blood or blood products **167**, **171**, **176**
999.8★	Other and unspecified infusion and transfusion reaction **167**, **171**
999.80	Transfusion reaction, unspecified **176**
999.81	Extravasation of vesicant chemotherapy **69**
999.82	Extravasation of other vesicant agent **69**
999.83	Hemolytic transfusion reaction, incompatibility unspecified **176**
999.84	Acute hemolytic transfusion reaction, incompatibility unspecified **176**
999.85	Delayed hemolytic transfusion reaction, incompatibility unspecified **176**
999.88	Other infusion reaction **69**
999.89	Other transfusion reaction **176**
999.9	Other and unspecified complications of medical care, not elsewhere classified **204**
V01.81	Contact with or exposure to anthrax **172**
V01.89	Contact or exposure to other communicable diseases **172**
V01★	Contact with or exposure to communicable diseases **213**
V02.0	Carrier or suspected carrier of cholera **213**
V02.1	Carrier or suspected carrier of typhoid **213**
V02.2	Carrier or suspected carrier of amebiasis **213**
V02.3	Carrier or suspected carrier of other gastrointestinal pathogens **213**
V02.4	Carrier or suspected carrier of diphtheria **213**
V02.5★	Carrier or suspected carrier of other specified bacterial diseases **213**
V02.6★	Carrier or suspected carrier of viral hepatitis **83**
V02.7	Carrier or suspected carrier of gonorrhea **213**
V02.8	Carrier or suspected carrier of other venereal diseases **213**
V02.9	Carrier or suspected carrier of other specified infectious organism **213**
V03★	Need for prophylactic vaccination and inoculation against bacterial diseases **213**
V04★	Need for prophylactic vaccination and inoculation against certain viral diseases **213**
V05.3	Need for prophylactic vaccination and inoculation against viral hepatitis **172**
V05.4	Need for prophylactic vaccination and inoculation against varicella **172**
V05.8	Need for prophylactic vaccination and inoculation against other specified disease **172**
V05★	Need for other prophylactic vaccination and inoculation against single diseases **213**
V06★	Need for prophylactic vaccination and inoculation against combinations of diseases **213**
V07★	Need for isolation and other prophylactic or treatment measures **214**
V08	Asymptomatic human immunodeficiency virus (HIV) infection status **185**
V09★	Infection with drug-resistant microorganisms **186**
V10.01	Personal history of malignant neoplasm of tongue **4**
V10.02	Personal history of malignant neoplasm of other and unspecified parts of oral cavity and pharynx **4**
V10.21	Personal history of malignant neoplasm of larynx **4**
V10★	Personal history of malignant neoplasm **180**, **182**
V11★	Personal history of mental disorder **214**
V12★	Personal history of certain other diseases **214**
V13.0★	Personal history of disorders of urinary system **214**
V13.1	Personal history of trophoblastic disease **214**
V13.21	Personal history of pre-term labor **214**
V13.22	Personal history of cervical dysplasia **180**, **182**
V13.23	Personal history of vaginal dysplasia **214**
V13.24	Personal history of vulvar dysplasia **214**
V13.29	Personal history of other genital system and obstetric disorders **214**
V13.3	Personal history of diseases of skin and subcutaneous tissue **214**
V13.4	Personal history of arthritis **214**
V13.5★	Personal history of other musculoskeletal disorders **214**
V13.6★	Personal history of congenital (corrected) malformations **214**
V13.7	Personal history of perinatal problems **214**
V13.8★	Personal history of other specified diseases **214**
V13.9	Personal history of unspecified disease **214**
V14★	Personal history of allergy to medicinal agents **214**
V15★	Other personal history presenting hazards to health **214**
V16★	Family history of malignant neoplasm **214**

V39.1	Liveborn, unspecified whether single, twin or multiple, born before admission to hospital **172**	
V39.2	Liveborn, unspecified whether single, twin or multiple, born outside hospital and not hospitalized **173**	
V40*	Mental and behavioral problems **214**	
V41*	Problems with special senses and other special functions **214**	
V42.0	Kidney replaced by transplant **2**, **120**	
V42.1	Heart replaced by transplant **69**	
V42.2	Heart valve replaced by transplant **69**	
V42.3	Skin replaced by transplant **109**	
V42.4	Bone replaced by transplant **101**	
V42.5	Cornea replaced by transplant **40**	
V42.6	Lung replaced by transplant **54**	
V42.7	Liver replaced by transplant **83**	
V42.81	Bone marrow replaced by transplant **176**	
V42.82	Peripheral stem cells replaced by transplant **176**	
V42.83	Pancreas replaced by transplant **83**	
V42.84	Organ or tissue replaced by transplant, intestines **214**	
V42.89	Other organ or tissue replaced by transplant **214**	
V42.9	Unspecified organ or tissue replaced by transplant **214**	
V43.0	Eye globe replaced by other means **40**	
V43.1	Lens replaced by other means **40**	
V43.2*	Heart replaced by other means **69**	
V43.3	Heart valve replaced by other means **69**	
V43.4	Blood vessel replaced by other means **69**	
V43.5	Bladder replaced by other means **120**	
V43.6*	Joint replaced by other means **101**	
V43.7	Limb replaced by other means **101**	
V43.8*	Other organ or tissue replaced by other means **214**	
V43.89	Other organ or tissue replaced by other means **2**	
V44*	Artificial opening status **214**	
V45.0*	Postsurgical cardiac pacemaker in situ **214**	
V45.1*	Renal dialysis status **214**	
V45.2	Presence of cerebrospinal fluid drainage device **214**	
V45.3	Intestinal bypass or anastomosis status **214**	
V45.4	Arthrodesis status **214**	
V45.5*	Presence of contraceptive device **214**	
V45.61	Cataract extraction status **214**	
V45.69	Other states following surgery of eye and adnexa **214**	
V45.71	Acquired absence of breast and nipple **214**	
V45.72	Acquired absence of intestine (large) (small) **214**	
V45.73	Acquired absence of kidney **214**	
V45.74	Acquired absence of organ, other parts of urinary tract **120**	
V45.75	Acquired absence of organ, stomach **214**	
V45.76	Acquired absence of organ, lung **54**	
V45.77	Acquired absence of organ, genital organs **124**, **128**, **131**	
V45.78	Acquired absence of organ, eye **40**	
V45.79	Other acquired absence of organ **214**	
V45.8*	Other postprocedural status **214**	
V45.88	Status post administration of tPA (rtPA) in a different facility within the last 24 hours prior to admission to current facility **20**	
V46*	Other dependence on machines and devices **214**	
V47*	Other problems with internal organs **214**	
V48*	Problems with head, neck, and trunk **214**	
V49*	Problems with limbs and other problems **214**	
V50.0	Elective hair transplant for purposes other than remedying health states **109**	
V50.1	Other plastic surgery for unacceptable cosmetic appearance **109**	
V50.2	Routine or ritual circumcision **124**, **173**	
V50.3	Ear piercing **214**	

V50.41	Prophylactic breast removal **106**
V50.42	Prophylactic ovary removal **128**, **131**
V50.49	Other prophylactic organ removal **214**
V50.8	Other elective surgery for purposes other than remedying health states **214**
V50.9	Unspecified elective surgery for purposes other than remedying health states **214**
V51*	Aftercare involving the use of plastic surgery **109**
V52.0	Fitting and adjustment of artificial arm (complete) (partial) **99**
V52.1	Fitting and adjustment of artificial leg (complete) (partial) **99**
V52.2	Fitting and adjustment of artificial eye **214**
V52.3	Fitting and adjustment of dental prosthetic device **214**
V52.4	Fitting and adjustment of breast prosthesis and implant **214**
V52.8	Fitting and adjustment of other specified prosthetic device **213**
V52.9	Fitting and adjustment of unspecified prosthetic device **213**
V53.0*	Fitting and adjustment of devices related to nervous system and special senses **33**
V53.1	Fitting and adjustment of spectacles and contact lenses **214**
V53.2	Fitting and adjustment of hearing aid **214**
V53.3*	Fitting and adjustment of cardiac device **69**
V53.4	Fitting and adjustment of orthodontic devices **214**
V53.5*	Fitting and adjustment of other gastrointestinal appliance and device **79**
V53.6	Fitting and adjustment of urinary device **120**
V53.7	Fitting and adjustment of orthopedic device **99**
V53.8	Fitting and adjustment of wheelchair **214**
V53.9*	Fitting and adjustment of other and unspecified device **214**
V54.0*	Aftercare involving internal fixation device **99**
V54.1*	Aftercare for healing traumatic fracture **99**
V54.2*	Aftercare for healing pathologic fracture **99**
V54.8*	Other orthopedic aftercare **99**
V54.9	Unspecified orthopedic aftercare **99**
V55.0	Attention to tracheostomy **54**
V55.1	Attention to gastrostomy **79**
V55.2	Attention to ileostomy **79**
V55.3	Attention to colostomy **79**
V55.4	Attention to other artificial opening of digestive tract **79**
V55.5	Attention to cystostomy **120**
V55.6	Attention to other artificial opening of urinary tract **120**
V55.7	Attention to artificial vagina **128**, **131**
V55.8	Attention to other specified artificial opening **214**
V55.9	Attention to unspecified artificial opening **214**
V56*	Encounter for dialysis and dialysis catheter care **119**
V57.0	Care involving breathing exercises **214**
V57.1	Other physical therapy **213**
V57.2*	Occupational therapy and vocational rehabilitation **213**
V57.3	Care involving use of rehabilitation speech-language therapy **213**
V57.4	Orthoptic training **214**
V57.81	Orthotic training **214**
V57.89	Other specified rehabilitation procedure **213**
V57.9	Unspecified rehabilitation procedure **213**
V58.0	Radiotherapy **180**, **182**
V58.1*	Encounter for antineoplastic chemotherapy and immunotherapy **180**, **181**, **182**
V58.2	Blood transfusion, without reported diagnosis **214**
V58.3*	Attention to dressings and sutures **214**
V58.4*	Other aftercare following surgery **213**
V58.5	Orthodontics aftercare **213**
V58.6*	Long-term (current) drug use **213**

Numeric Index to Diseases

V58.7*	Aftercare following surgery to specified body systems, not elsewhere classified **213**	
V58.8*	Other specified aftercare **213**	
V58.9	Unspecified aftercare **213**	
V59.0*	Blood donor **214**	
V59.1	Skin donor **109**	
V59.2	Bone donor **101**	
V59.3	Bone marrow donor **214**	
V59.4	Kidney donor **120**	
V59.5	Cornea donor **214**	
V59.6	Liver donor **83**	
V59.7*	Egg (oocyte) (ovum) Donor **214**	
V59.8	Donor of other specified organ or tissue **214**	
V59.9	Donor of unspecified organ or tissue **214**	
V60*	Housing, household, and economic circumstances **214**	
V61.0*	Family disruption **214**	
V61.10	Counseling for marital and partner problems, unspecified **214**	
V61.11	Counseling for victim of spousal and partner abuse **214**	
V61.12	Counseling for perpetrator of spousal and partner abuse **214**	
V61.2*	Parent-child problems **214**	
V61.3	Problems with aged parents or in-laws **214**	
V61.4*	Health problems within family **214**	
V61.5	Multiparity **128, 131**	
V61.6	Illegitimacy or illegitimate pregnancy **156, 159**	
V61.7	Other unwanted pregnancy **153**	
V61.8	Other specified family circumstance **214**	
V61.9	Unspecified family circumstance **214**	
V62.0	Unemployment **214**	
V62.1	Adverse effects of work environment **214**	
V62.2*	Other occupational circumstances or maladjustment **214**	
V62.3	Educational circumstance **214**	
V62.4	Social maladjustment **214**	
V62.5	Legal circumstance **214**	
V62.6	Refusal of treatment for reasons of religion or conscience **214**	
V62.81	Interpersonal problem, not elsewhere classified **214**	
V62.82	Bereavement, uncomplicated **214**	
V62.83	Counseling for perpetrator of physical/sexual abuse **214**	
V62.84	Suicidal ideation **188**	
V62.85	Homicidal ideation **214**	
V62.89	Other psychological or physical stress, not elsewhere classified **214**	
V62.9	Unspecified psychosocial circumstance **214**	
V63*	Unavailability of other medical facilities for care **214**	
V64.0*	Vaccination not carried out **173**	
V64.1	Surgical or other procedure not carried out because of contraindication **173**	
V64.2	Surgical or other procedure not carried out because of patient's decision **173**	
V64.3	Procedure not carried out for other reasons **173**	
V64*	Persons encountering health services for specific procedures, not carried out **214**	
V65*	Other persons seeking consultation **214**	
V66*	Convalescence and palliative care **214**	
V67.0*	Surgery follow-up examination **213**	
V67.1	Radiotherapy follow-up examination **180, 182**	
V67.2	Chemotherapy follow-up examination **180, 181, 182**	
V67.3	Psychotherapy and other treatment for mental disorder follow-up examination **214**	
V67.4	Treatment of healed fracture follow-up examination **213**	
V67.5*	Other follow-up examination **214**	

V67.6	Combined treatment follow-up examination **214**	
V67.9	Unspecified follow-up examination **215**	
V68*	Encounters for administrative purposes **215**	
V69*	Problems related to lifestyle **215**	
V70.3	Other general medical exami for administrative purposes **173**	
V70*	General medical examination **215**	
V71.01	Observation of adult antisocial behavior **188**	
V71.02	Observation of childhood or adolescent antisocial behavior **188**	
V71.09	Observation of other suspected mental condition **189**	
V71.1	Observation for suspected malignant neoplasm **180, 182**	
V71.2	Observation for suspected tuberculosis **51**	
V71.3	Observation following accident at work **204**	
V71.4	Observation following other accident **204**	
V71.5	Observation following alleged rape or seduction **215**	
V71.6	Observation following other inflicted injury **204**	
V71.7	Observation for suspected cardiovascular disease **68**	
V71.8*	Observation and evaluation for other specified suspected conditions **215**	
V71.9	Observation for unspecified suspected condition **215**	
V72.1*	Examination of ears and hearing **173**	
V72*	Special investigations and examinations **215**	
V73*	Special screening examination for viral and chlamydial diseases **215**	
V74*	Special screening examination for bacterial and spirochetal diseases **215**	
V75*	Special screening examination for other infectious diseases **215**	
V76*	Special screening for malignant neoplasms **215**	
V77.3	Screening for phenylketonuria (PKU) **173**	
V77*	Special screening for endocrine, nutritional, metabolic, and immunity disorders **215**	
V78*	Special screening for disorders of blood and blood-forming organs **215**	
V79*	Special screening for mental disorders and developmental handicaps **215**	
V80*	Special screening for neurological, eye, and ear diseases **215**	
V81*	Special screening for cardiovascular, respiratory, and genitourinary diseases **215**	
V82*	Special screening for other condition **215**	
V83.01	Asymptomatic hemophilia A carrier **215**	
V83.02	Symptomatic hemophilia A carrier **215**	
V83.8*	Other genetic carrier status **215**	
V84.0*	Genetic susceptibility to malignant neoplasm **215**	
V84.8*	Genetic susceptibility to other disease **215**	
V85.0	Body Mass Index less than 19, adult **215**	
V85.1	Body Mass Index between 19-24, adult **215**	
V85.2*	Body Mass Index between 25-29, adult **215**	
V85.3*	Body Mass Index between 30-39, adult **215**	
V85.4*	Body Mass Index 40 and over, adult **113**	
V85.5*	Body Mass Index, pediatric **215**	
V86*	Estrogen receptor status **215**	
V87.0*	Contact with and (suspected) exposure to hazardous metals **215**	
V87.1*	Contact with and (suspected) exposure to hazardous aromatic compounds **215**	
V87.2	Contact with and (suspected) exposure to other potentially hazardous chemicals **215**	
V87.3*	Contact with and (suspected) exposure to other potentially hazardous substances **215**	
V87.4*	Personal history of drug therapy **213**	
V88.0*	Acquired absence of cervix and uterus **128, 131**	
V88.1*	Acquired absence of pancreas **215**	
V88.2*	Acquired absence of joint **215**	

*Code Range

Numeric Index to Diseases

Alphabetic Index to Procedure

*Code Range

80.03	Arthrotomy for removal of prosthesis without replacement, wrist **92, 193**
69.52	Aspiration curettage following delivery or abortion **139, 140, 234**
69.51	Aspiration curettage of uterus for termination of pregnancy **140, 234**
17.56	Atherectomy of other non-coronary vessel(s) **13, 50, 63, 74, 82, 95, 103, 112, 117, 195**
81.01	Atlas-axis spinal fusion **12, 13, 89, 200**
86.73	Attachment of pedicle or flap graft to hand **94, 194**
27.57	Attachment of pedicle or flap graft to lip and mouth **45, 103, 195, 233**
86.74	Attachment of pedicle or flap graft to other sites **14, 17, 45, 65, 75, 88, 111, 193**
85.50	Augmentation mammoplasty, not otherwise specified **105, 201, 235**
21.85	Augmentation rhinoplasty **44, 95, 103, 195, 233**
41.09	Autologous bone marrow transplant with purging **4**
41.01	Autologous bone marrow transplant without purging **4**
41.07	Autologous hematopoietic stem cell transplant with purging **4**
41.04	Autologous hematopoietic stem cell transplant without purging **4**
52.84	Autotransplantation of cells of islets of Langerhans **118**
50.51	Auxiliary liver transplant **1**
07.3	Bilateral adrenalectomy **103, 111**
85.54	Bilateral breast implant **105, 201, 235**
66.2*	Bilateral endoscopic destruction or occlusion of fallopian tubes **128, 139, 234**
65.5*	Bilateral oophorectomy **104**
62.4*	Bilateral orchiectomy **122, 197**
66.63	Bilateral partial salpingectomy, not otherwise specified **128, 139**
85.32	Bilateral reduction mammoplasty **111**
53.3*	Bilateral repair of femoral hernia **74, 234**
71.62	Bilateral vulvectomy **104**
54.22	Biopsy of abdominal wall or umbilicus **75, 104, 179, 197, 234**
38.21	Biopsy of blood vessel **14, 16, 37, 44, 50, 63, 95, 112, 117, 233**
77.4*	Biopsy of bone **104, 112, 118, 123, 234**
77.40	Biopsy of bone, unspecified site **45, 89**
27.21	Biopsy of bony palate **45, 233**
77.44	Biopsy of carpals and metacarpals **94, 193**
11.22	Biopsy of cornea **194**
70.23	Biopsy of cul-de-sac **128, 140, 234**
34.27	Biopsy of diaphragm **50**
16.23	Biopsy of eyeball and orbit **37, 233**
08.11	Biopsy of eyelid **37, 194, 232**
76.11	Biopsy of facial bone **45, 234**
77.45	Biopsy of femur **89**
77.42	Biopsy of humerus **89**
12.22	Biopsy of iris **37**
09.11	Biopsy of lacrimal gland **194**
09.12	Biopsy of lacrimal sac **44**
40.11	Biopsy of lymphatic structure **14, 16, 44, 50, 82, 118, 129**
20.32	Biopsy of middle and inner ear **44, 233**
77.49	Biopsy of other bone, except facial bones **45, 51, 89, 175**
06.13	Biopsy of parathyroid gland **95, 111**
77.46	Biopsy of patella **89**
64.11	Biopsy of penis **104, 122, 234**
37.24	Biopsy of pericardium **50, 59, 178**
60.15	Biopsy of periprostatic tissue **123, 232**
54.23	Biopsy of peritoneum **75, 82, 129, 175**
07.17	Biopsy of pineal gland **8, 10, 11, 111**
07.13	Biopsy of pituitary gland, transfrontal approach **8, 10, 11, 111**

07.14	Biopsy of pituitary gland, transsphenoidal approach **8, 10, 11, 111**
07.15	Biopsy of pituitary gland, unspecified approach **8, 10, 11, 111**
77.43	Biopsy of radius and ulna **89**
77.41	Biopsy of scapula, clavicle, and thorax (ribs and sternum) **51, 89**
01.15	Biopsy of skull **8, 9, 11, 89, 112**
03.32	Biopsy of spinal cord or spinal meninges **12, 13, 90, 91, 178**
77.48	Biopsy of tarsals and metatarsals **89**
07.16	Biopsy of thymus **50, 112, 175, 178**
77.47	Biopsy of tibia and fibula **89**
28.11	Biopsy of tonsils and adenoids **44, 233**
27.22	Biopsy of uvula and soft palate **45, 233**
78.04	Bone graft of carpals and metacarpals **94, 193**
78.05	Bone graft of femur **89, 198, 219**
78.02	Bone graft of humerus **91, 198**
78.09	Bone graft of other bone, except facial bones **95, 198**
78.06	Bone graft of patella **90, 198**
78.03	Bone graft of radius and ulna **94, 198, 234**
78.01	Bone graft of scapula, clavicle, and thorax (ribs and sternum) **51, 95, 198**
78.08	Bone graft of tarsals and metatarsals **93, 198**
78.07	Bone graft of tibia and fibula **91, 198**
76.91	Bone graft to facial bone **37, 43, 95, 198**
02.04	Bone graft to skull **11, 43, 219**
78.00	Bone graft, unspecified site **95, 198**
41.00	Bone marrow transplant, not otherwise specified **4**
32.27	Bronchoscopic bronchial thermoplasty, ablation of airway smooth muscle **50**
83.5	Bursectomy **92, 200, 235**
82.03	Bursotomy of hand **94, 193**
66.97	Burying of fimbriae in uterine wall **126, 128, 139**
36.1*	Bypass anastomosis for heart revascularization **58, 59**
52.92	Cannulation of pancreatic duct **75, 81, 179, 197**
37.27	Cardiac mapping **62, 63**
37.11	Cardiotomy **58, 195**
81.25	Carporadial fusion **94, 193**
37.26	Catheter based invasive electrophysiologic testing **56, 62, 63**
39.21	Caval-pulmonary artery anastomosis **59**
42.11	Cervical esophagostomy **44**
05.22	Cervical sympathectomy **43**
74.4	Cesarean section of other specified type **139**
51.22	Cholecystectomy **74, 81**
51.2*	Cholecystectomy **81, 179, 197**
51.36	Choledochoenterostomy **75**
03.2*	Chordotomy **12, 13, 82, 178, 194**
02.14	Choroid plexectomy **219**
74.0	Classical cesarean section **139**
39.51	Clipping of aneurysm **8, 10, 11, 63**
57.33	Closed (transurethral) biopsy of bladder **117, 123, 129, 234**
68.15	Closed biopsy of uterine ligaments **128, 234**
68.16	Closed biopsy of uterus **128, 234**
33.27	Closed endoscopic biopsy of lung **50, 64, 233**
35.0*	Closed heart valvotomy or transcatheter replacement of heart valve **59**
79.13	Closed reduction of fracture of carpals and metacarpals with internal fixation **94, 193**
79.15	Closed reduction of fracture of femur with internal fixation **90, 199, 219**
79.11	Closed reduction of fracture of humerus with internal fixation **91, 199**

*Code Range

79.19	Closed reduction of fracture of other specified bone, except facial bones, with internal fixation **95, 199**
79.18	Closed reduction of fracture of phalanges of foot with internal fixation **93, 199**
79.14	Closed reduction of fracture of phalanges of hand with internal fixation **94, 193**
79.12	Closed reduction of fracture of radius and ulna with internal fixation **94, 199, 234**
79.17	Closed reduction of fracture of tarsals and metatarsals with internal fixation **93, 199**
79.16	Closed reduction of fracture of tibia and fibula with internal fixation **91, 199**
79.10	Closed reduction of fracture with internal fixation, unspecified site **95, 199**
79.45	Closed reduction of separated epiphysis of femur **90, 199, 219**
79.41	Closed reduction of separated epiphysis of humerus **91, 199**
79.49	Closed reduction of separated epiphysis of other specified bone **96, 199**
79.42	Closed reduction of separated epiphysis of radius and ulna **94, 199**
79.46	Closed reduction of separated epiphysis of tibia and fibula **91, 199**
79.40	Closed reduction of separated epiphysis, unspecified site **96, 199**
49.73	Closure of anal fistula **74, 104, 196**
47.92	Closure of appendiceal fistula **72, 196**
29.52	Closure of branchial cleft fistula **44, 103**
51.92	Closure of cholecystostomy **81, 197**
57.82	Closure of cystostomy **116, 123, 129, 179, 197, 234**
42.83	Closure of esophagostomy **45, 72, 178, 196**
31.72	Closure of external fistula of trachea **44, 50, 64, 103**
34.83	Closure of fistula of diaphragm **195**
46.72	Closure of fistula of duodenum **72**
46.76	Closure of fistula of large intestine **72**
27.53	Closure of fistula of mouth **45, 195, 233**
46.74	Closure of fistula of small intestine, except duodenum **72**
69.42	Closure of fistula of uterus **73**
46.5*	Closure of intestinal stoma **73, 196**
50.61	Closure of laceration of liver **81**
21.82	Closure of nasal fistula **44, 233**
55.82	Closure of nephrostomy and pyelostomy **197**
51.93	Closure of other biliary fistula **81, 179, 197**
55.83	Closure of other fistula of kidney **197**
29.53	Closure of other fistula of pharynx **44, 195**
34.73	Closure of other fistula of thorax **50, 195**
31.73	Closure of other fistula of trachea **44, 50, 72**
56.84	Closure of other fistula of ureter **73, 123, 129, 179, 197**
58.43	Closure of other fistula of urethra **122, 129, 179, 197**
44.63	Closure of other gastric fistula **72, 82, 179, 196**
48.73	Closure of other rectal fistula **74, 104, 128**
48.72	Closure of proctostomy **72**
46.52	Closure of stoma of large intestine **234**
56.83	Closure of ureterostomy **123, 129, 179, 197**
58.42	Closure of urethrostomy **197**
46.10	Colostomy, not otherwise specified **72, 179, 196**
94.67	Combined alcohol and drug rehabilitation **191**
94.69	Combined alcohol and drug rehabilitation and detoxification **191**
33.6	Combined heart-lung transplantation **1**
88.54	Combined right and left heart angiocardiography **56, 57, 59, 65**
37.23	Combined right and left heart cardiac catheterization **56, 57, 58, 65**
51.42	Common duct exploration for relief of other obstruction **81, 179, 197**
51.41	Common duct exploration for removal of calculus **81**
25.3	Complete glossectomy **43**
30.3	Complete laryngectomy **2**
55.5*	Complete nephrectomy **116, 197**
06.4	Complete thyroidectomy **111**
67.2	Conization of cervix **128, 139, 234**
10.4*	Conjunctivoplasty **194, 232**
18.71	Construction of auricle of ear **103, 233**
64.43	Construction of penis **197**
46.22	Continent ileostomy **72, 179, 196**
96.72	Continuous invasive mechanical ventilation for 96 consecutive hours or more **1, 54, 186, 206, 208**
96.71	Continuous invasive mechanical ventilation for less than 96 consecutive hours **54**
96.70	Continuous invasive mechanical ventilation of unspecified duration **54**
49.95	Control of (postoperative) hemorrhage of anus **196**
57.93	Control of (postoperative) hemorrhage of bladder **116, 197**
60.94	Control of (postoperative) hemorrhage of prostate **123, 197, 232**
21.05	Control of epistaxis by (transantral) ligation of the maxillary artery **44, 64, 195**
21.07	Control of epistaxis by excision of nasal mucosa and skin grafting of septum and lateral nasal wall **44, 64, 195**
21.04	Control of epistaxis by ligation of ethmoidal arteries **44, 64, 195**
21.06	Control of epistaxis by ligation of the external carotid artery **44, 64, 195**
21.09	Control of epistaxis by other means **44, 64, 195, 233**
28.7	Control of hemorrhage after tonsillectomy and adenoidectomy **44, 195**
39.41	Control of hemorrhage following vascular surgery **63, 112**
39.98	Control of hemorrhage, not otherwise specified **44, 50, 64, 74, 82, 95, 104, 112, 118, 123, 129, 139, 178, 196**
41.06	Cord blood stem cell transplant **4**
12.35	Coreoplasty **37**
11.6*	Corneal transplant **194, 232**
11.60	Corneal transplant, not otherwise specified **37**
88.55	Coronary arteriography using single catheter **56, 57, 59, 65**
88.56	Coronary arteriography using two catheters **56, 57, 59, 65**
27.62	Correction of cleft palate **14, 16, 44**
75.36	Correction of fetal defect **140**
08.38	Correction of lid retraction **103, 112**
86.85	Correction of syndactyly **94, 194**
55.87	Correction of ureteropelvic junction **197**
01.20	Cranial implantation or replacement of neurostimulator pulse generator **9, 11, 14, 16**
04.5	Cranial or peripheral nerve graft **14, 16, 194**
02.0*	Cranioplasty **8, 10, 95, 194**
35.94	Creation of conduit between atrium and pulmonary artery **58**
35.93	Creation of conduit between left ventricle and aorta **58**
35.92	Creation of conduit between right ventricle and pulmonary artery **58**
54.93	Creation of cutaneoperitoneal fistula **64, 75, 82, 118, 179, 197**
54.94	Creation of peritoneovascular shunt **75, 81, 179**
35.42	Creation of septal defect in heart **58**
29.31	Cricopharyngeal myotomy **44**
11.43	Cryotherapy of corneal lesion **194**
70.12	Culdotomy **129, 140**
56.5*	Cutaneous uretero-ileostomy **116, 123, 129, 179, 197**

Alphabetic Index to Procedures

*Code Range © 2013 OptumInsight, Inc.

38.16	Endarterectomy of abdominal arteries **59, 74, 117, 196**	77.72	Excision of humerus for graft **92, 198**
38.14	Endarterectomy of aorta **59, 74, 196**	61.2	Excision of hydrocele (of tunica vaginalis) **122, 234**
38.11	Endarterectomy of intracranial vessels **8, 10, 11**	40.24	Excision of inguinal lymph node **50, 64, 74, 95, 118, 123, 129, 139, 233**
38.18	Endarterectomy of lower limb arteries **63, 112, 196**		
38.15	Endarterectomy of other thoracic vessels **50, 59, 196**	40.22	Excision of internal mammary lymph node **50**
38.12	Endarterectomy of other vessels of head and neck **13, 44, 63, 112, 196**	80.51	Excision of intervertebral disc **12, 13, 91, 200**
		09.6	Excision of lacrimal sac and passage **194, 232**
38.13	Endarterectomy of upper limb vessels **63, 112, 196**	12.44	Excision of lesion of ciliary body **37**
38.10	Endarterectomy, unspecified site **13, 63, 196**	16.93	Excision of lesion of eye, unspecified structure **37, 103, 195, 233**
68.23	Endometrial ablation **126, 128**	12.42	Excision of lesion of iris **37**
39.72	Endovascular (total) embolization or occlusion of head and neck vessels **8, 10, 11, 59, 60, 117, 196**	09.21	Excision of lesion of lacrimal gland **194**
		22.62	Excision of lesion of maxillary sinus with other approach **95**
39.75	Endovascular embolization or occlusion of vessel(s) of head or neck using bare coils **8, 10, 11, 59, 60, 117, 196**	20.51	Excision of lesion of middle ear **233**
		83.32	Excision of lesion of muscle **104, 235**
39.76	Endovascular embolization or occlusion of vessel(s) of head or neck using bioactive coils **8, 10, 11, 59, 60, 118, 196**	82.2*	Excision of lesion of muscle, tendon, and fascia of hand **94, 193**
		83.3*	Excision of lesion of muscle, tendon, fascia, and bursa **92, 200**
39.78	Endovascular implantation of branching or fenestrated graft(s) in aorta **59, 60**	16.92	Excision of lesion of orbit **37, 43, 195, 233**
		83.39	Excision of lesion of other soft tissue **45, 104, 113, 235**
39.73	Endovascular implantation of graft in thoracic aorta **56, 117, 196**	26.2*	Excision of lesion of salivary gland **46, 233**
39.71	Endovascular implantation of other graft in abdominal aorta **59, 60, 117, 196**	01.6	Excision of lesion of skull **8, 10, 11, 43, 92, 178, 219**
		83.31	Excision of lesion of tendon sheath **113**
39.74	Endovascular removal of obstruction from head and neck vessel(s) **8, 10, 11, 196**	82.21	Excision of lesion of tendon sheath of hand **104, 113, 235**
		28.92	Excision of lesion of tonsil and adenoid **44**
35.05	Endovascular replacement of aortic valve **56**	61.92	Excision of lesion of tunica vaginalis other than hydrocele **122**
35.07	Endovascular replacement of pulmonary valve **56**	27.3*	Excision of lesion or tissue of bony palate **233**
35.09	Endovascular replacement of unspecified heart valve **56**	01.51	Excision of lesion or tissue of cerebral meninges **8, 10, 11, 219**
45.0*	Enterotomy **196**	34.81	Excision of lesion or tissue of diaphragm **95**
16.4*	Enucleation of eyeball **37, 195, 233**	09.2*	Excision of lesion or tissue of lacrimal gland **232**
63.4	Epididymectomy **122**	45.41	Excision of lesion or tissue of large intestine **74, 112, 179, 234**
63.92	Epididymotomy **122**	41.42	Excision of lesion or tissue of spleen **196**
63.83	Epididymovasostomy **122**	06.6	Excision of lingual thyroid **44, 111**
30.21	Epiglottidectomy **44**	28.5	Excision of lingual tonsil **44**
11.76	Epikeratophakia **37**	08.24	Excision of major lesion of eyelid, full-thickness **103**
42.40	Esophagectomy, not otherwise specified **44**	08.23	Excision of major lesion of eyelid, partial-thickness **103**
44.65	Esophagogastroplasty **72, 196**	83.43	Excision of muscle or fascia for graft **14, 17**
42.7	Esophagomyotomy **45, 72, 178, 196**	85.25	Excision of nipple **105**
42.1*	Esophagostomy **72, 178, 196**	51.69	Excision of other bile duct **75, 81**
42.10	Esophagostomy, not otherwise specified **44**	77.79	Excision of other bone for graft, except facial bones **45, 92, 198**
22.63	Ethmoidectomy **233**	82.29	Excision of other lesion of soft tissue of hand **104, 235**
16.3*	Evisceration of eyeball **37, 195, 233**	63.3	Excision of other lesion or tissue of spermatic cord and epididymis **122, 234**
76.4*	Excision and reconstruction of facial bones **95, 198**		
77.5*	Excision and repair of bunion and other toe deformities **93, 234**	08.22	Excision of other minor lesion of eyelid **103**
41.93	Excision of accessory spleen **175, 178, 196**	77.76	Excision of patella for graft **92, 198**
04.01	Excision of acoustic neuroma **8, 10, 11, 43**	59.91	Excision of perirenal or perivesical tissue **117, 123, 179**
51.62	Excision of ampulla of Vater (with reimplantation of common duct) **75, 81**	58.92	Excision of periurethral tissue **117**
		86.21	Excision of pilonidal cyst or sinus **104, 201, 235**
37.32	Excision of aneurysm of heart **58**	18.21	Excision of preauricular sinus **44, 103, 233**
49.6	Excision of anus **74, 234**	11.3*	Excision of pterygium **37, 232**
40.23	Excision of axillary lymph node **44, 50, 64, 74, 95, 233**	11.32	Excision of pterygium with corneal graft **194**
77.70	Excision of bone for graft, unspecified site **92, 198**	77.73	Excision of radius and ulna for graft **92, 198**
29.2	Excision of branchial cleft cyst or vestige **44, 103**	77.71	Excision of scapula, clavicle, and thorax (ribs and sternum) for graft **51, 92, 198**
77.74	Excision of carpals and metacarpals for graft **94, 193**		
63.2	Excision of cyst of epididymis **122, 234**	80.6	Excision of semilunar cartilage of knee **90, 113, 200, 235**
51.61	Excision of cystic duct remnant **81, 197**	60.73	Excision of seminal vesicle **123**
40.21	Excision of deep cervical lymph node **44, 50, 64, 74, 95, 112, 233**	86.91	Excision of skin for graft **14, 17, 45, 65, 103, 111, 201**
24.4	Excision of dental lesion of jaw **45, 233**	77.78	Excision of tarsals and metatarsals for graft **93, 198**
85.24	Excision of ectopic breast tissue **105**	83.41	Excision of tendon for graft **14, 17**
42.4*	Excision of esophagus **72, 178, 196**	06.7	Excision of thyroglossal duct or tract **44, 111**
77.75	Excision of femur for graft **92, 198**	77.77	Excision of tibia and fibula for graft **92, 198**
49.46	Excision of hemorrhoids **74, 139, 234**		

28.4	Excision of tonsil tag **44**
63.1	Excision of varicocele and hydrocele of spermatic cord **122, 234**
85.2*	Excision or destruction of breast tissue **201**
85.20	Excision or destruction of breast tissue, not otherwise specified **105, 235**
80.50	Excision or destruction of intervertebral disc, unspecified **12, 13, 91, 200**
34.4	Excision or destruction of lesion of chest wall **50, 92, 103, 112, 178, 233**
70.32	Excision or destruction of lesion of cul-de-sac **140**
66.61	Excision or destruction of lesion of fallopian tube **126, 128**
12.4*	Excision or destruction of lesion of iris and ciliary body **194, 232**
12.84	Excision or destruction of lesion of sclera **37**
03.4	Excision or destruction of lesion of spinal cord or spinal meninges **12, 13, 90, 91, 178**
70.33	Excision or destruction of lesion of vagina **104, 147**
54.3	Excision or destruction of lesion or tissue of abdominal wall or umbilicus **75, 92, 104, 112, 179, 234**
10.3*	Excision or destruction of lesion or tissue of conjunctiva **194, 232**
08.2*	Excision or destruction of lesion or tissue of eyelid **37, 194, 232**
30.0*	Excision or destruction of lesion or tissue of larynx **44**
34.3	Excision or destruction of lesion or tissue of mediastinum **50, 112, 178, 233**
29.3*	Excision or destruction of lesion or tissue of pharynx **72**
41.4*	Excision or destruction of lesion or tissue of spleen **175, 178**
25.1	Excision or destruction of lesion or tissue of tongue **45, 64, 233**
37.34	Excision or destruction of other lesion or tissue of heart, endovascular approach **62, 63**
37.33	Excision or destruction of other lesion or tissue of heart, open approach **58**
37.37	Excision or destruction of other lesion or tissue of heart, thoracoscopic approach **58**
54.4	Excision or destruction of peritoneal tissue **75, 82, 112, 129, 179, 234**
62.2	Excision or destruction of testicular lesion **122**
11.4*	Excision or destruction of tissue or other lesion of cornea **37, 232**
71.24	Excision or other destruction of Bartholin's gland (cyst) **104, 128, 140, 234**
86.22	Excisional debridement of wound, infection, or burn **14, 17, 37, 45, 51, 64, 75, 82, 88, 103, 111, 118, 123, 129, 175, 193**
16.51	Exenteration of orbit with removal of adjacent structures **43, 95**
16.52	Exenteration of orbit with therapeutic removal of orbital bone **43**
16.5*	Exenteration of orbital contents **37, 195, 233**
03.0*	Exploration and decompression of spinal canal structures **12, 13, 194**
07.0*	Exploration of adrenal field **111**
51.51	Exploration of common bile duct **81**
82.01	Exploration of tendon sheath of hand **94, 193, 235**
07.91	Exploration of thymus field **194**
54.11	Exploratory laparotomy **50, 64, 82, 104, 112, 122, 139, 175, 179**
34.02	Exploratory thoracotomy **50, 64, 117, 178, 195**
42.12	Exteriorization of esophageal pouch **44**
46.0*	Exteriorization of intestine **72, 179, 196**
46.03	Exteriorization of large intestine **64**
22.3*	External maxillary antrotomy **45**
13.4*	Extracapsular extraction of lens by fragmentation and aspiration technique **233**
13.2	Extracapsular extraction of lens by linear extraction technique **233**
13.3	Extracapsular extraction of lens by simple aspiration (and irrigation) technique **233**
39.65	Extracorporeal membrane oxygenation (ECMO) **1**
98.51	Extracorporeal shockwave lithotripsy (ESWL) of the kidney, ureter and/or bladder **119**
02.3*	Extracranial ventricular shunt **13, 178, 194**
39.28	Extracranial-intracranial (EC-IC) vascular bypass **8, 10, 11, 196**
86.90	Extraction of fat for graft or banking **104**
74.2	Extraperitoneal cesarean section **139**
95.04	Eye examination under anesthesia **37, 235**
86.82	Facial rhytidectomy **45, 201, 235**
12.5*	Facilitation of intraocular circulation **194, 232**
83.14	Fasciotomy **14, 17, 92, 104**
86.87	Fat graft of skin and subcutaneous tissue **45, 111, 201**
85.55	Fat graft to breast **105**
20.6*	Fenestration of inner ear **44**
84.22	Finger reattachment **94, 193**
09.8*	Fistulization of lacrimal tract to nasal cavity **194, 232**
81.42	Five-in-one repair of knee **90**
46.6*	Fixation of intestine **73**
84.26	Foot reattachment **89, 201, 219**
84.23	Forearm, wrist, or hand reattachment **90, 201, 219**
02.03	Formation of cranial bone flap **11, 43, 219**
21.62	Fracture of the turbinates **195, 233**
86.60	Free skin graft, not otherwise specified **14, 17, 64, 75, 88, 103, 111, 193, 206, 207, 235**
39.91	Freeing of vessel **63, 74, 112, 196**
22.4*	Frontal sinusotomy and sinusectomy **45**
85.83	Full-thickness graft to breast **103, 193, 206, 207**
86.61	Full-thickness skin graft to hand **14, 17, 64, 94, 103, 194, 206, 207**
27.55	Full-thickness skin graft to lip and mouth **45, 103, 195, 233**
86.63	Full-thickness skin graft to other sites **14, 17, 45, 64, 75, 88, 103, 111, 193, 206, 207**
81.64	Fusion or refusion of 9 or more vertebrae **87, 88**
04.05	Gasserian ganglionectomy **14, 16, 43, 194**
44.3*	Gastroenterostomy without gastrectomy **72, 111, 179**
44.64	Gastropexy **72, 196**
43.0	Gastrotomy **72, 82, 112, 179, 196**
24.2	Gingivoplasty **45, 195**
12.51	Goniopuncture without goniotomy **37**
12.53	Goniotomy with goniopuncture **37**
12.52	Goniotomy without goniopuncture **37**
49.74	Gracilis muscle transplant for anal incontinence **74**
83.82	Graft of muscle or fascia **14, 17, 93, 104**
36.2	Heart revascularization by arterial implant **58**
37.51	Heart transplantation **1**
30.1	Hemilaryngectomy **43, 50, 195**
01.52	Hemispherectomy **8, 10, 11, 194, 219**
50.0	Hepatotomy **81, 196**
86.65	Heterograft to skin **14, 17, 64, 75, 88, 103, 193, 206, 207, 235**
52.83	Heterotransplant of pancreas **81, 112**
00.15	High-dose infusion interleukin-2 [IL-2] **181**
86.66	Homograft to skin **14, 17, 45, 65, 75, 88, 103, 193, 206, 207**
52.82	Homotransplant of pancreas **2, 81, 112**
70.31	Hymenectomy **147**
70.76	Hymenorrhaphy **128, 234**
04.71	Hypoglossal-facial anastomosis **43**
07.6*	Hypophysectomy **8, 10, 11, 111**
68.0	Hysterotomy **126, 128, 139, 198**
74.91	Hysterotomy to terminate pregnancy **140**
46.20	Ileostomy, not otherwise specified **72, 179, 196**

*Code Range

© 2013 OptumInsight, Inc.

37.61	Implant of pulsation balloon **59**
37.65	Implant of single ventricular (extracorporeal) external heart assist system **1, 56**
58.93	Implantation of artificial urinary sphincter (AUS) **117, 197**
37.95	Implantation of automatic cardioverter/defibrillator leads(s) only **57, 58, 65**
37.96	Implantation of automatic cardioverter/defibrillator pulse generator only **57, 58, 62**
00.51	Implantation of cardiac resynchronization defibrillator, total system (CRT-D) **57**
00.50	Implantation of cardiac resynchronization pacemaker without mention of defibrillation, total system (CRT-P) **60**
37.67	Implantation of cardiomyostimulation system **59**
00.10	Implantation of chemotherapeutic agent **9**
34.85	Implantation of diaphragmatic pacemaker **195**
20.95	Implantation of electromagnetic hearing device **44**
57.96	Implantation of electronic bladder stimulator **117**
56.92	Implantation of electronic ureteral stimulator **116**
14.8*	Implantation of epiretinal visual prosthesis **38, 195**
84.44	Implantation of prosthetic device of arm **94, 201**
84.48	Implantation of prosthetic device of leg **92, 201**
17.51	Implantation of rechargeable cardiac contractility modulation [CCM], total system **57**
37.52	Implantation of total internal biventricular heart replacement system **1**
84.40	Implantation or fitting of prosthetic limb device, not otherwise specified **96, 201**
37.60	Implantation or insertion of biventricular external heart assist system **1, 56**
92.27	Implantation or insertion of radioactive elements **15, 17, 45, 51, 62, 65, 75, 104, 113, 118, 123, 128, 201, 235**
37.94	Implantation or replacement of automatic cardioverter/defibrillator, total system (AICD) **57**
17.52	Implantation or replacement of cardiac contractility modulation [CCM] rechargeable pulse generator only **62**
00.54	Implantation or replacement of cardiac resynchronization defibrillator pulse generator device only (CRT-D) **57, 58, 62**
00.53	Implantation or replacement of cardiac resynchronization pacemaker pulse generator only (CRT-P) **60, 61, 63**
20.98	Implantation or replacement of cochlear prosthetic device, multiple channel **43**
20.96	Implantation or replacement of cochlear prosthetic device, not otherwise specified **43**
20.97	Implantation or replacement of cochlear prosthetic device, single channel **43**
02.93	Implantation or replacement of intracranial neurostimulator lead(s) **8, 9, 10, 11, 178, 194**
55.97	Implantation or replacement of mechanical kidney **116, 197**
04.92	Implantation or replacement of peripheral neurostimulator lead(s) **14, 16, 18, 43, 63, 95, 117, 123, 129**
66.93	Implantation or replacement of prosthesis of fallopian tube **126, 128**
03.93	Implantation or replacement of spinal neurostimulator lead(s) **12, 13, 90, 91, 117, 122, 129, 178, 194**
00.57	Implantation or replacement of subcutaneous device for intracardiac or great vessel hemodynamic monitoring **63, 65**
00.52	Implantation or replacement of transvenous lead (electrode) into left ventricular coronary venous system **57, 60, 65**
49.75	Implantation or revision of artificial anal sphincter **73, 104, 196**
47.1*	Incidental appendectomy **129, 196**
01.21	Incision and drainage of cranial sinus **8, 9, 11, 219**
28.0	Incision and drainage of tonsil and peritonsillar structures **44**
38.06	Incision of abdominal arteries **59, 74, 117**
38.07	Incision of abdominal veins **59, 74, 117**

54.0	Incision of abdominal wall **64, 75, 82, 104, 118, 179, 197**
38.04	Incision of aorta **59, 74**
71.22	Incision of Bartholin's gland (cyst) **128, 140, 234**
01.3*	Incision of brain and cerebral meninges **194**
33.0	Incision of bronchus **50, 195**
01.31	Incision of cerebral meninges **8, 9, 11, 178, 219**
69.95	Incision of cervix **128, 139, 234**
11.1	Incision of cornea **37, 194, 232**
45.01	Incision of duodenum **72, 82**
42.01	Incision of esophageal web **44, 72**
76.0*	Incision of facial bone without division **198**
37.10	Incision of heart, not otherwise specified **58**
45.00	Incision of intestine, not otherwise specified **73**
38.01	Incision of intracranial vessels **8, 10, 11**
09.52	Incision of lacrimal canaliculi **194**
09.0	Incision of lacrimal gland **232**
09.5*	Incision of lacrimal sac and passages **232**
45.03	Incision of large intestine **73, 179**
38.08	Incision of lower limb arteries **63, 112, 178**
38.09	Incision of lower limb veins **64, 233**
33.1	Incision of lung **50, 195**
40.0	Incision of lymphatic structures **104, 175, 233**
20.21	Incision of mastoid **45**
20.2*	Incision of mastoid and middle ear **233**
34.1	Incision of mediastinum **50, 64, 195**
20.23	Incision of middle ear **44**
27.92	Incision of mouth, unspecified structure **45, 103, 195, 233**
83.0*	Incision of muscle, tendon, fascia, and bursa **92, 200, 235**
51.59	Incision of other bile duct **75, 81, 179, 197**
51.49	Incision of other bile ducts for relief of obstruction **81, 179**
38.05	Incision of other thoracic vessels **50, 59, 72**
38.02	Incision of other vessels of head and neck **14, 16, 44, 63, 112**
27.1	Incision of palate **45**
64.92	Incision of penis **122, 234**
49.01	Incision of perianal abscess **74, 104**
54.95	Incision of peritoneum **14, 16, 64, 75, 82, 118, 179, 197**
58.91	Incision of periurethral tissue **117**
59.1*	Incision of perivesical tissue **117, 123, 129, 179, 197**
20.22	Incision of petrous pyramid air cells **45**
07.72	Incision of pituitary gland **103**
60.0	Incision of prostate **123, 232**
48.91	Incision of rectal stricture **196**
60.72	Incision of seminal vesicle **123**
63.93	Incision of spermatic cord **122**
62.0	Incision of testis **122, 197**
38.03	Incision of upper limb vessels **63, 112**
38.0*	Incision of vessel **195**
38.00	Incision of vessel, unspecified site **44, 63, 112, 233**
71.0*	Incision of vulva and perineum **128, 147**
49.1*	Incision or excision of anal fistula **74, 196, 234**
68.22	Incision or excision of congenital septum of uterus **128**
60.8*	Incision or excision of periprostatic tissue **123, 232**
48.8*	Incision or excision of perirectal tissue or lesion **74, 104, 196, 234**
20.7*	Incision, excision, and destruction of inner ear **44**
53.51	Incisional hernia repair **234**
35.34	Infundibulectomy **58**
37.83	Initial insertion of dual-chamber device **15, 16, 17, 18, 61, 201, 202**

37.70	Initial insertion of lead (electrode), not otherwise specified **15, 17, 60, 201**
37.81	Initial insertion of single-chamber device, not specified as rate responsive **15, 17, 18, 60, 61, 201, 202**
37.82	Initial insertion of single-chamber device, rate responsive **15, 16, 17, 18, 60, 61, 201, 202**
37.73	Initial insertion of transvenous lead (electrode) into atrium **15, 17, 18, 61, 201, 202**
37.71	Initial insertion of transvenous lead (electrode) into ventricle **15, 17, 60, 201**
37.72	Initial insertion of transvenous leads (electrodes) into atrium and ventricle **15, 17, 60, 61, 201**
12.92	Injection into anterior chamber **37, 194**
39.92	Injection of sclerosing agent into vein **13, 64**
99.10	Injection or infusion of thrombolytic agent **20**
78.94	Insertion of bone growth stimulator into carpals and metacarpals **94, 193**
78.95	Insertion of bone growth stimulator into femur **90, 199, 219**
78.92	Insertion of bone growth stimulator into humerus **91, 199**
78.99	Insertion of bone growth stimulator into other bone **95, 199**
78.96	Insertion of bone growth stimulator into patella **90, 199**
78.93	Insertion of bone growth stimulator into radius and ulna **94, 199**
78.91	Insertion of bone growth stimulator into scapula, clavicle and thorax (ribs and sternum) **51, 95, 199**
78.98	Insertion of bone growth stimulator into tarsals and metatarsals **93, 199**
78.97	Insertion of bone growth stimulator into tibia and fibula **91, 199**
78.90	Insertion of bone growth stimulator, unspecified site **95, 199**
85.95	Insertion of breast tissue expander **105, 201, 235**
51.43	Insertion of choledochohepatic tube for decompression **81, 179, 197**
36.07	Insertion of drug-eluting coronary artery stent(s) **62**
00.48	Insertion of four or more vascular stents **62**
37.66	Insertion of implantable heart assist system **1**
38.26	Insertion of implantable pressure sensor without lead for intracardiac or great vessel hemodynamic monitoring **64**
13.71	Insertion of intraocular lens prosthesis at time of cataract extraction, one-stage **233**
37.90	Insertion of left atrial appendage device **63**
36.06	Insertion of non-drug-eluting coronary artery stent(s) **62**
84.59	Insertion of other spinal devices **12, 13, 91, 201**
84.61	Insertion of partial spinal disc prosthesis, cervical **91**
84.64	Insertion of partial spinal disc prosthesis, lumbosacral **91**
37.68	Insertion of percutaneous external heart assist device **56**
37.80	Insertion of permanent pacemaker, initial or replacement, type of device not specified **14, 15, 16, 17, 18, 60, 61, 63, 195, 201, 202**
13.70	Insertion of pseudophakos, not otherwise specified **233**
02.05	Insertion of skull plate **11, 43, 219**
84.60	Insertion of spinal disc prosthesis, not otherwise specified **91**
84.63	Insertion of spinal disc prosthesis, thoracic **91**
84.94	Insertion of sternal fixation device with rigid plates **51, 64, 96, 201**
76.92	Insertion of synthetic implant in facial bone **37, 43, 95, 198**
37.62	Insertion of temporary non-implantable extracorporeal circulatory assist device **56**
62.7	Insertion of testicular prosthesis **112, 122**
86.93	Insertion of tissue expander **14, 17, 45, 65, 75, 88, 103, 111, 193, 206, 207**
86.06	Insertion of totally implantable infusion pump **14, 17, 51, 64, 75, 82, 96, 104, 113, 118, 123, 129, 175, 201**
86.07	Insertion of totally implantable vascular access device (VAD) **104, 118**
63.95	Insertion of valve in vas deferens **122**

39.93	Insertion of vessel-to-vessel cannula **64, 112, 118, 196**
37.74	Insertion or replacement of epicardial lead (electrode) into epicardium **14, 15, 16, 18, 57, 58, 61, 64, 195, 202**
84.84	Insertion or replacement of facet replacement device(s) **12, 13, 91**
00.56	Insertion or replacement of implantable pressure sensor with lead for intracardiac or great vessel hemodynamic monitoring **64, 65**
64.97	Insertion or replacement of inflatable penile prosthesis **118, 122, 234**
84.80	Insertion or replacement of interspinous process device(s) **12, 13, 91**
86.98	Insertion or replacement of multiple array (two or more) rechargeable neurostimulator pulse generator **9, 11, 13, 15, 17, 18, 91**
86.95	Insertion or replacement of multiple array neurostimulator pulse generator, not specified as rechargeable **9, 11, 12, 15, 17, 18, 91**
64.95	Insertion or replacement of non-inflatable penile prosthesis **118, 122, 234**
86.96	Insertion or replacement of other neurostimulator pulse generator **15, 17, 63**
84.82	Insertion or replacement of pedicle-based dynamic stabilization device(s) **12, 13, 91**
86.94	Insertion or replacement of single array neurostimulator pulse generator, not specified as rechargeable **12, 15, 17, 18, 91**
86.97	Insertion or replacement of single array rechargeable neurostimulator pulse generator **13, 15, 17, 18, 91**
83.92	Insertion or replacement of skeletal muscle stimulator **14, 17, 93, 200**
02.94	Insertion or replacement of skull tongs or halo traction device **8, 10, 11, 95, 194, 219**
84.8*	Insertion, replacement and revision of posterior spinal motion preservation device(s) **201**
66.95	Insufflation of therapeutic agent into fallopian tubes **129**
35.91	Interatrial transposition of venous return **58**
52.4	Internal drainage of pancreatic cyst **81**
78.50	Internal fixation of bone without fracture reduction, unspecified site **95, 199**
78.54	Internal fixation of carpals and metacarpals without fracture reduction **94, 193**
78.55	Internal fixation of femur without fracture reduction **90, 199, 219**
78.52	Internal fixation of humerus without fracture reduction **91, 199**
78.59	Internal fixation of other bone, except facial bones, without fracture reduction **95, 199**
78.56	Internal fixation of patella without fracture reduction **90, 199**
78.53	Internal fixation of radius and ulna without fracture reduction **94, 199**
78.51	Internal fixation of scapula, clavicle, and thorax (ribs and sternum) without fracture reduction **51, 95, 199**
78.58	Internal fixation of tarsals and metatarsals without fracture reduction **93, 199**
78.57	Internal fixation of tibia and fibula without fracture reduction **91, 199**
81.28	Interphalangeal fusion **94, 193**
38.7	Interruption of the vena cava **14, 16, 50, 63, 74, 82, 95, 112, 117, 123, 129, 139, 175, 196**
84.09	Interthoracoscapular amputation **89, 201**
45.9*	Intestinal anastomosis **72, 196**
45.90	Intestinal anastomosis, not otherwise specified **111, 179**
46.80	Intra-abdominal manipulation of intestine, not otherwise specified **72, 82, 179, 196**
46.82	Intra-abdominal manipulation of large intestine **72, 82, 179, 196**
46.81	Intra-abdominal manipulation of small intestine **72, 82, 179, 196**
39.1	Intra-abdominal venous shunt **59, 72, 81**
13.1*	Intracapsular extraction of lens **112, 233**
87.53	Intraoperative cholangiogram **82, 235**

*Code Range

© 2013 OptumInsight, Inc.

44.92	Intraoperative manipulation of stomach **72, 82, 112, 196**
42.5*	Intrathoracic anastomosis of esophagus **72, 178, 196**
42.55	Intrathoracic esophageal anastomosis with interposition of colon **44**
42.53	Intrathoracic esophageal anastomosis with interposition of small bowel **44**
42.58	Intrathoracic esophageal anastomosis with other interposition **44**
42.51	Intrathoracic esophagoesophagostomy **44**
42.52	Intrathoracic esophagogastrostomy **44**
09.44	Intubation of nasolacrimal duct **44, 194**
12.63	Iridencleisis and iridotasis **232**
12.3*	Iridoplasty and coreoplasty **194, 232**
12.1*	Iridotomy and simple iridectomy **37, 194, 232**
45.5*	Isolation of intestinal segment **72**
45.50	Isolation of intestinal segment, not otherwise specified **179**
81.5*	Joint replacement of lower extremity **200**
11.71	Keratomileusis **37**
11.72	Keratophakia **37**
11.73	Keratoprosthesis **37**
11.61	Lamellar keratoplasty with autograft **37**
50.25	Laparoscopic ablation of liver lesion or tissue **74, 81**
44.98	(Laparoscopic) adjustment of size of adjustable gastric restrictive device **111, 234**
17.2*	Laparoscopic bilateral repair of inguinal hernia **74**
17.32	Laparoscopic cecectomy **64**
51.23	Laparoscopic cholecystectomy **74, 82, 234**
44.95	Laparoscopic gastric restrictive procedure **111, 234**
44.38	Laparoscopic gastroenterostomy **64, 82**
44.68	Laparoscopic gastroplasty **72, 111, 196, 234**
53.62	Laparoscopic incisional hernia repair with graft or prosthesis **197**
17.35	Laparoscopic left hemicolectomy **64, 112, 178**
50.14	Laparoscopic liver biopsy **74, 82, 104, 118, 175, 179, 196**
59.03	Laparoscopic lysis of perirenal or periureteral adhesions **116, 123, 129, 179, 197**
17.31	Laparoscopic multiple segmental resection of large intestine **178**
51.24	Laparoscopic partial cholecystectomy **82**
17.3*	Laparoscopic partial excision of large intestine **72, 195**
44.67	Laparoscopic procedures for creation of esophagogastric sphincteric competence **72, 196, 234**
48.42	Laparoscopic pull-through resection of rectum **196**
68.61	Laparoscopic radical abdominal hysterectomy **126, 139**
68.71	Laparoscopic radical vaginal hysterectomy [LRVH] **126, 139**
65.63	Laparoscopic removal of both ovaries and tubes at same operative episode **104**
44.97	Laparoscopic removal of gastric restrictive device(s) **111, 234**
17.34	Laparoscopic resection of transverse colon **64, 178**
44.96	Laparoscopic revision of gastric restrictive procedure **111, 234**
17.33	Laparoscopic right hemicolectomy **64, 178**
17.36	Laparoscopic sigmoidectomy **178**
68.41	Laparoscopic total abdominal hysterectomy **126, 128, 139**
17.1*	Laparoscopic unilateral repair of inguinal hernia **74**
43.82	Laparoscopic vertical (sleeve) gastrectomy **64, 111**
65.24	Laparoscopic wedge resection of ovary **112**
54.21	Laparoscopy **75, 82, 104, 118, 128, 139, 175, 197, 234**
54.1*	Laparotomy **75, 118, 129, 197**
45.94	Large-to-large intestinal anastomosis **112, 179**
17.61	Laser interstitial thermal therapy [LITT] of lesion or tissue of brain under guidance **8, 10, 11**
17.62	Laser interstitial thermal therapy [LITT] of lesion or tissue of head and neck under guidance **112, 178**

17.63	Laser interstitial thermal therapy [LITT] of lesion or tissue of liver under guidance **74, 81**
17.69	Laser interstitial thermal therapy [LITT] of lesion or tissue of other and unspecified site under guidance **50, 105, 123, 178**
37.22	Left heart cardiac catheterization **56, 57, 58, 65**
59.71	Levator muscle operation for urethrovesical suspension **117, 128**
38.57	Ligation and stripping of abdominal varicose veins **63, 74**
38.59	Ligation and stripping of lower limb varicose veins **64, 233**
38.51	Ligation and stripping of varicose veins of intracranial vessels **8, 10, 11**
38.55	Ligation and stripping of varicose veins of other thoracic vessel **50, 59, 112**
38.52	Ligation and stripping of varicose veins of other vessels of head and neck **63**
38.53	Ligation and stripping of varicose veins of upper limb vessels **64**
38.50	Ligation and stripping of varicose veins, unspecified site **64**
07.43	Ligation of adrenal vessels **194**
33.92	Ligation of bronchus **50, 195**
42.91	Ligation of esophageal varices **72, 82**
44.91	Ligation of gastric varices **72, 82**
49.45	Ligation of hemorrhoids **74, 234**
02.13	Ligation of meningeal vessel **8, 194, 219**
06.92	Ligation of thyroid vessels **112, 194**
56.95	Ligation of ureter **116, 197**
78.34	Limb lengthening procedures, carpals and metacarpals **94, 193**
78.35	Limb lengthening procedures, femur **89, 199, 219**
78.32	Limb lengthening procedures, humerus **91, 199**
78.33	Limb lengthening procedures, radius and ulna **94, 199**
78.38	Limb lengthening procedures, tarsals and metatarsals **93, 199**
78.37	Limb lengthening procedures, tibia and fibula **91, 199**
78.30	Limb lengthening procedures, unspecified site **95, 199**
78.24	Limb shortening procedures, carpals and metacarpals **94, 193**
78.25	Limb shortening procedures, femur **89, 199, 219**
78.22	Limb shortening procedures, humerus **91, 199**
78.29	Limb shortening procedures, other **95, 199**
78.23	Limb shortening procedures, radius and ulna **94, 199**
78.28	Limb shortening procedures, tarsals and metatarsals **93, 199**
78.27	Limb shortening procedures, tibia and fibula **91, 199**
78.20	Limb shortening procedures, unspecified site **95, 198**
21.86	Limited rhinoplasty **44, 95, 103, 195, 233**
01.53	Lobectomy of brain **8, 10, 11, 194, 219**
50.3	Lobectomy of liver **81, 197**
32.4*	Lobectomy of lung **50, 195**
01.32	Lobotomy and tractotomy **8, 9, 11, 178, 219**
42.31	Local excision of esophageal diverticulum **44, 72**
85.21	Local excision of lesion of breast **105, 113, 235**
60.61	Local excision of lesion of prostate **123, 232**
77.6*	Local excision of lesion or tissue of bone **234**
77.60	Local excision of lesion or tissue of bone, unspecified site **92, 198**
77.64	Local excision of lesion or tissue of carpals and metacarpals **94, 193**
77.65	Local excision of lesion or tissue of femur **92, 198**
77.62	Local excision of lesion or tissue of humerus **92, 198**
77.69	Local excision of lesion or tissue of other bone, except facial bones **45, 92, 112, 198**
77.66	Local excision of lesion or tissue of patella **92, 198**
77.63	Local excision of lesion or tissue of radius and ulna **92, 198**
77.61	Local excision of lesion or tissue of scapula, clavicle, and thorax (ribs and sternum) **51, 92, 112, 198**
45.33	Local excision of lesion or tissue of small intestine, except duodenum **74, 179, 234**

*Code Range

© 2013 OptumInsight, Inc.

49.59	Other anal sphincterotomy **147**
57.88	Other anastomosis of bladder **116, 123, 179**
04.74	Other anastomosis of cranial or peripheral nerve **43**
56.7*	Other anastomosis or bypass of ureter **116, 197**
53.69	Other and open repair of other hernia of anterior abdominal wall with graft or prosthesis **234**
53.41	Other and open repair of umbilical hernia with graft or prosthesis **234**
50.26	Other and unspecified ablation of liver lesion or tissue **74, 81**
32.26	Other and unspecified ablation of lung lesion or tissue **50**
88.57	Other and unspecified coronary arteriography **56, 57, 59, 65**
68.9	Other and unspecified hysterectomy **126, 128, 139**
45.79	Other and unspecified partial excision of large intestine **64, 179**
68.69	Other and unspecified radical abdominal hysterectomy **126, 139**
68.79	Other and unspecified radical vaginal hysterectomy **126, 139**
35.7*	Other and unspecified repair of atrial and ventricular septa **58**
80.54	Other and unspecified repair of the anulus fibrosus **12, 13, 91, 179, 200**
07.98	Other and unspecified thoracoscopic operations on thymus **14, 16, 194**
68.49	Other and unspecified total abdominal hysterectomy **126, 128, 139**
48.63	Other anterior resection of rectum **64**
42.69	Other antesternal anastomosis of esophagus **45**
42.68	Other antesternal esophageal anastomosis with interposition **45**
42.66	Other antesternal esophagocolostomy **45**
42.64	Other antesternal esophagoenterostomy **45**
47.09	Other appendectomy **64**
80.17	Other arthrotomy of ankle **91, 200**
80.12	Other arthrotomy of elbow **93, 113, 200**
80.18	Other arthrotomy of foot and toe **93, 200, 235**
80.14	Other arthrotomy of hand and finger **93, 193**
80.15	Other arthrotomy of hip **90, 200, 219**
80.16	Other arthrotomy of knee **90, 113, 200, 235**
80.19	Other arthrotomy of other specified site **96, 200**
80.11	Other arthrotomy of shoulder **93, 200**
80.13	Other arthrotomy of wrist **93, 193**
80.10	Other arthrotomy, unspecified site **96, 112, 200**
66.3*	Other bilateral destruction or occlusion of fallopian tubes **128, 139, 234**
53.1*	Other bilateral repair of inguinal hernia **74, 234**
13.6*	Other cataract extraction **233**
81.02	Other cervical fusion of the anterior column, anterior technique **12, 13, 87, 89, 200**
81.03	Other cervical fusion of the posterior column, posterior technique **12, 13, 87, 89, 200**
74.99	Other cesarean section of unspecified type **139**
83.85	Other change in muscle or tendon length **14, 17, 93**
51.03	Other cholecystostomy **74, 81**
51.04	Other cholecystotomy **81**
11.69	Other corneal transplant **37**
04.42	Other cranial nerve decompression **14, 16, 43, 194**
04.06	Other cranial or peripheral ganglionectomy **14, 16, 43, 95, 194**
04.7*	Other cranial or peripheral neuroplasty **14, 16, 194**
02.06	Other cranial osteoplasty **11, 43, 219**
01.25	Other craniectomy **8, 9, 11, 43, 95, 178, 194, 219**
01.24	Other craniotomy **8, 9, 11, 43, 178, 194, 219**
57.19	Other cystotomy **116, 197**
14.29	Other destruction of chorioretinal lesion **37, 233**
80.59	Other destruction of intervertebral disc **12, 13, 91, 200**

45.32	Other destruction of lesion of duodenum **72, 82, 179, 234**
45.49	Other destruction of lesion of large intestine **73, 179, 234**
50.29	Other destruction of lesion of liver **74, 81**
45.34	Other destruction of lesion of small intestine, except duodenum **73, 179, 234**
42.39	Other destruction of lesion or tissue of esophagus **44, 72, 178**
43.49	Other destruction of lesion or tissue of stomach **72, 233**
54.29	Other diagnostic procedures on abdominal region **75, 82, 129, 175, 179, 197, 234**
07.19	Other diagnostic procedures on adrenal glands, pituitary gland, pineal gland, and thymus **14, 16, 111**
51.19	Other diagnostic procedures on biliary tract **74, 82**
57.39	Other diagnostic procedures on bladder **116, 123, 179, 197, 234**
38.29	Other diagnostic procedures on blood vessels **63, 112**
01.18	Other diagnostic procedures on brain and cerebral meninges **8, 9, 11, 178, 194**
34.28	Other diagnostic procedures on chest wall, pleura, and diaphragm **50**
04.19	Other diagnostic procedures on cranial and peripheral nerves and ganglia **14, 16, 43, 95, 194**
76.19	Other diagnostic procedures on facial bones and joints **43**
12.29	Other diagnostic procedures on iris, ciliary body, sclera, and anterior chamber **37**
81.98	Other diagnostic procedures on joint structures **89, 200**
55.29	Other diagnostic procedures on kidney **116, 175, 179, 197**
09.19	Other diagnostic procedures on lacrimal system **44, 194**
50.19	Other diagnostic procedures on liver **74, 82, 104, 118, 175, 179, 197**
33.29	Other diagnostic procedures on lung or bronchus **50**
40.19	Other diagnostic procedures on lymphatic structures **44, 50, 118**
34.29	Other diagnostic procedures on mediastinum **50, 64**
20.39	Other diagnostic procedures on middle and inner ear **44, 233**
83.29	Other diagnostic procedures on muscle, tendon, fascia, and bursa, including that of hand **200**
16.29	Other diagnostic procedures on orbit and eyeball **37, 233**
52.19	Other diagnostic procedures on pancreas **75, 82, 112, 179, 197**
60.18	Other diagnostic procedures on prostate and periprostatic tissue **123, 232**
60.19	Other diagnostic procedures on seminal vesicles **123**
01.19	Other diagnostic procedures on skull **8, 9, 11, 89, 194**
63.09	Other diagnostic procedures on spermatic cord, epididymis, and vas deferens **122, 234**
03.39	Other diagnostic procedures on spinal cord and spinal canal structures **12, 13, 90, 91, 178**
62.19	Other diagnostic procedures on testes **122**
06.19	Other diagnostic procedures on thyroid and parathyroid glands **95, 111**
28.19	Other diagnostic procedures on tonsils and adenoids **44**
56.39	Other diagnostic procedures on ureter **116, 234**
68.19	Other diagnostic procedures on uterus and supporting structures **126, 128**
70.29	Other diagnostic procedures on vagina and cul-de-sac **128, 140, 234**
69.09	Other dilation and curettage of uterus **128, 139, 234**
77.30	Other division of bone, unspecified site **45, 95, 198**
77.34	Other division of carpals and metacarpals **94, 193**
77.35	Other division of femur **89, 198, 219**
77.32	Other division of humerus **91, 198**
77.39	Other division of other bone, except facial bones **95, 198**
77.36	Other division of patella **90, 198**
77.33	Other division of radius and ulna **94, 198**

*Code Range

© 2013 OptumInsight, Inc.

77.31	Other division of scapula, clavicle, and thorax (ribs and sternum) **51, 95, 198**
83.19	Other division of soft tissue **14, 17, 92, 235**
77.38	Other division of tarsals and metatarsals **93, 112, 198, 234**
77.37	Other division of tibia and fibula **91, 198**
39.79	Other endovascular procedures on other vessels **8, 10, 11, 59, 60, 118, 196**
38.64	Other excision of abdominal aorta **59, 74**
38.66	Other excision of abdominal arteries **59, 74, 117**
38.67	Other excision of abdominal veins **59, 74, 117**
80.97	Other excision of ankle joint **92, 200**
32.1	Other excision of bronchus **50, 195**
51.63	Other excision of common duct **75, 81**
80.92	Other excision of elbow joint **94, 200**
18.39	Other excision of external ear **195, 233**
18.3*	Other excision of external ear **44, 103**
80.95	Other excision of hip joint **90, 200, 219**
38.61	Other excision of intracranial vessels **8, 10, 11**
80.98	Other excision of joint of foot and toe **93, 113, 200, 235**
80.94	Other excision of joint of hand and finger **94, 193**
80.99	Other excision of joint of other specified site **92, 200**
80.90	Other excision of joint, unspecified site **96, 200**
80.96	Other excision of knee joint **90, 200**
27.43	Other excision of lesion or tissue of lip **45, 103, 233**
38.68	Other excision of lower limb arteries **63, 112**
38.69	Other excision of lower limb veins **64**
32.9	Other excision of lung **50, 195**
20.5*	Other excision of middle ear **44**
27.49	Other excision of mouth **45, 195, 233**
83.4*	Other excision of muscle, tendon, and fascia **92, 200**
38.65	Other excision of other thoracic vessel **50, 59, 72**
38.62	Other excision of other vessels of head and neck **13, 44, 63**
49.04	Other excision of perianal tissue **74, 104**
80.91	Other excision of shoulder joint **94, 200**
45.6*	Other excision of small intestine **72, 196**
83.49	Other excision of soft tissue **14, 17, 45, 104**
82.39	Other excision of soft tissue of hand **104**
82.3*	Other excision of soft tissue of hand **94, 193**
38.63	Other excision of upper limb vessels **63, 112**
38.6*	Other excision of vessels **196**
38.60	Other excision of vessels, unspecified site **63, 112**
80.93	Other excision of wrist joint **94, 193**
04.07	Other excision or avulsion of cranial and peripheral nerves **14, 16, 43, 95, 194, 232**
57.5*	Other excision or destruction of bladder tissue **116, 123, 129**
01.5*	Other excision or destruction of brain and meninges **178**
68.29	Other excision or destruction of lesion of uterus **126, 128, 234**
01.59	Other excision or destruction of lesion or tissue of brain **8, 10, 11, 194, 219**
67.39	Other excision or destruction of lesion or tissue of cervix **104**
67.3*	Other excision or destruction of lesion or tissue of cervix **128, 139, 234**
30.09	Other excision or destruction of lesion or tissue of larynx **50, 233**
52.22	Other excision or destruction of lesion or tissue of pancreas or pancreatic duct **81, 112**
29.39	Other excision or destruction of lesion or tissue of pharynx **44**
69.19	Other excision or destruction of uterus and supporting structures **126, 128**
77.58	Other excision, fusion, and repair of toes **198**
16.59	Other exenteration of orbit **43, 95**

03.09	Other exploration and decompression of spinal canal **90, 91, 178**
42.19	Other external fistulization of esophagus **44**
56.6*	Other external urinary diversion **116, 123, 129, 179, 197**
13.59	Other extracapsular extraction of lens **112**
13.5*	Other extracapsular extraction of lens **233**
76.6*	Other facial bone repair and orthognathic surgery **43, 95, 198**
12.59	Other facilitation of intraocular circulation **37**
83.44	Other fasciectomy **104**
81.17	Other fusion of foot **93**
44.39	Other gastroenterostomy without gastrectomy **64, 82**
12.79	Other glaucoma procedures **112**
25.94	Other glossotomy **45**
42.87	Other graft of esophagus **45, 72, 179, 196**
36.3*	Other heart revascularization **58**
53.9	Other hernia repair **74**
77.10	Other incision of bone without division, unspecified site **92, 198**
01.39	Other incision of brain **8, 9, 11, 178, 219**
77.14	Other incision of carpals and metacarpals without division **94, 193**
10.1	Other incision of conjunctiva **232**
04.04	Other incision of cranial and peripheral nerves **14, 16, 43, 95, 194**
42.09	Other incision of esophagus **44, 72, 196**
76.09	Other incision of facial bone **45, 92**
77.15	Other incision of femur without division **92, 198**
77.12	Other incision of humerus without division **92, 198**
31.3	Other incision of larynx or trachea **44, 50**
77.19	Other incision of other bone, except facial bones, without division **45, 92, 198**
77.16	Other incision of patella without division **92, 198**
49.02	Other incision of perianal tissue **74, 104**
59.09	Other incision of perirenal or periureteral tissue **116, 123, 129, 179, 197**
77.13	Other incision of radius and ulna without division **92, 198**
77.11	Other incision of scapula, clavicle, and thorax (ribs and sternum) without division **51, 92, 198**
86.09	Other incision of skin and subcutaneous tissue **104**
45.02	Other incision of small intestine **73, 179**
83.09	Other incision of soft tissue **104**
82.09	Other incision of soft tissue of hand **94, 104, 193, 235**
77.18	Other incision of tarsals and metatarsals without division **93, 198**
07.92	Other incision of thymus **194**
06.09	Other incision of thyroid field **43, 103, 111, 194**
77.17	Other incision of tibia and fibula without division **92, 198**
71.09	Other incision of vulva and perineum **104, 234**
39.26	Other intra-abdominal vascular shunt or bypass **59, 74, 82, 116, 196**
42.59	Other intrathoracic anastomosis of esophagus **44**
42.56	Other intrathoracic esophagocolostomy **44**
42.54	Other intrathoracic esophagoenterostomy **44**
39.23	Other intrathoracic vascular shunt or bypass **59, 196**
12.39	Other iridoplasty **37**
55.69	Other kidney transplantation **2, 116**
00.8*	Other knee and hip procedures **194**
11.62	Other lamellar keratoplasty **37**
17.39	Other laparoscopic partial excision of large intestine **64, 178**
53.43	Other laparoscopic umbilical herniorrhaphy **197**
54.19	Other laparotomy **64, 82, 175, 179**
78.39	Other limb lengthening procedures **95, 199**
45.31	Other local excision of lesion of duodenum **72, 82, 179, 234**
80.87	Other local excision or destruction of lesion of ankle joint **91, 200**

© 2013 OptumInsight, Inc.

*Code Range

80.82	Other local excision or destruction of lesion of elbow joint **92, 113, 200**	18.9	Other operations on external ear **44, 103, 195, 233**
80.85	Other local excision or destruction of lesion of hip joint **92, 200**	15.9	Other operations on extraocular muscles and tendons **195, 233**
80.88	Other local excision or destruction of lesion of joint of foot and toe **93, 113, 200, 235**	16.99	Other operations on eyeball **37, 112, 195, 233**
		08.99	Other operations on eyelids **103**
80.84	Other local excision or destruction of lesion of joint of hand and finger **94, 193**	08.9*	Other operations on eyelids **37, 194, 232**
		76.99	Other operations on facial bones and joints **43, 95, 198**
80.89	Other local excision or destruction of lesion of joint of other specified site **92, 200**	66.99	Other operations on fallopian tubes **126, 128**
		71.9	Other operations on female genital organs **129**
80.80	Other local excision or destruction of lesion of joint, unspecified site **92, 200**	37.99	Other operations on heart and pericardium **59**
		07.79	Other operations on hypophysis **103**
80.86	Other local excision or destruction of lesion of knee joint **92, 200, 235**	07.7*	Other operations on hypophysis **8, 10, 11, 111**
		46.99	Other operations on intestines **72, 82, 179, 196**
80.81	Other local excision or destruction of lesion of shoulder joint **92, 200**	12.97	Other operations on iris **37, 194**
		12.9*	Other operations on iris, ciliary body, and anterior chamber **232**
80.83	Other local excision or destruction of lesion of wrist joint **94, 104, 193**	81.99	Other operations on joint structures **96, 200**
		55.99	Other operations on kidney **116, 197**
49.39	Other local excision or destruction of lesion or tissue of anus **74, 104, 234**	09.3	Other operations on lacrimal gland **194, 232**
		09.9*	Other operations on lacrimal system **194, 232**
32.09	Other local excision or destruction of lesion or tissue of bronchus **50**	09.99	Other operations on lacrimal system **44**
		31.98	Other operations on larynx **44, 50, 233**
32.29	Other local excision or destruction of lesion or tissue of lung **50, 178**	13.9*	Other operations on lens **195, 233**
		33.99	Other operations on lung **50, 195**
86.3	Other local excision or destruction of lesion or tissue of skin and subcutaneous tissue **104**	40.9	Other operations on lymphatic structures **44, 74, 104, 118, 123, 175, 178, 196**
71.3	Other local excision or destruction of vulva and perineum **104, 128, 147, 234**	64.99	Other operations on male genital organs **122, 234**
		20.99	Other operations on middle and inner ear **44**
59.02	Other lysis of perirenal or periureteral adhesions **116, 123, 129, 179, 197**	82.99	Other operations on muscle, tendon, and fascia of hand **94, 193**
		83.99	Other operations on muscle, tendon, fascia, and bursa **93, 200**
54.59	Other lysis of peritoneal adhesions **112**	84.99	Other operations on musculoskeletal system **96, 201**
85.89	Other mammoplasty **105, 201**	22.9	Other operations on nasal sinuses **45**
14.74	Other mechanical vitrectomy **112**	05.9	Other operations on nervous system **14, 16, 194**
83.79	Other muscle transposition **113**	21.99	Other operations on nose **44, 103, 195, 233**
83.45	Other myectomy **14, 17, 104**	15.2*	Other operations on one extraocular muscle **233**
22.6*	Other nasal sinusectomy **45**	27.99	Other operations on oral cavity **45, 195, 233**
22.5*	Other nasal sinusotomy **45**	16.98	Other operations on orbit **37, 43, 195, 233**
75.99	Other obstetric operations **140**	52.99	Other operations on pancreas **75, 81, 197**
53.61	Other open incisional hernia repair with graft or prosthesis **197, 234**	06.99	Other operations on parathyroid glands **112**
		64.98	Other operations on penis **122, 234**
76.79	Other open reduction of facial fracture **37, 43, 95, 198**	59.92	Other operations on perirenal or perivesical tissue **117, 123, 179**
53.49	Other open umbilical herniorrhaphy **197, 234**	29.99	Other operations on pharynx **44, 195**
07.4*	Other operations on adrenal glands, nerves, and vessels **111**	60.99	Other operations on prostate **123, 232**
07.49	Other operations on adrenal glands, nerves, and vessels **194**	48.9*	Other operations on rectum and perirectal tissue **74**
12.99	Other operations on anterior chamber **37, 195**	14.9	Other operations on retina, choroid, and posterior chamber **38, 195, 233**
49.99	Other operations on anus **196**		
49.9*	Other operations on anus **74**	26.99	Other operations on salivary gland or duct **46**
47.99	Other operations on appendix **73**	12.89	Other operations on sclera **37**
71.29	Other operations on Bartholin's gland **128, 140, 234**	61.99	Other operations on scrotum and tunica vaginalis **122, 197**
51.99	Other operations on biliary tract **81, 179, 197, 234**	60.79	Other operations on seminal vesicles **123**
57.99	Other operations on bladder **117, 197**	35.98	Other operations on septa of heart **58**
33.98	Other operations on bronchus **50, 195**	02.99	Other operations on skull, brain, and cerebral meninges **8, 10, 11, 43, 95, 178, 194, 219**
69.99	Other operations on cervix and uterus **129**		
12.98	Other operations on ciliary body **37, 195**	63.99	Other operations on spermatic card, epididymis, and vas deferens **122, 197**
10.9*	Other operations on conjunctiva **232**		
11.9*	Other operations on cornea **194, 232**	51.89	Other operations on sphincter of Oddi **81, 197**
11.99	Other operations on cornea **37**	03.99	Other operations on spinal cord and spinal canal structures **12, 13, 91, 178, 194**
04.99	Other operations on cranial and peripheral nerves **14, 16, 43, 95, 232**		
		41.99	Other operations on spleen **175, 178, 196**
04.9*	Other operations on cranial and peripheral nerves **194**	44.99	Other operations on stomach **72, 111, 196**
70.92	Other operations on cul-de-sac **128**	69.98	Other operations on supporting structures of uterus **128**
70.93	Other operations on cul-de-sac with graft or prosthesis **128**	05.8*	Other operations on sympathetic nerves or ganglia **14, 16**
34.89	Other operations on diaphragm **195**		

*Code Range

05.89	Other operations on sympathetic nerves or ganglia **64**	
62.99	Other operations on testes **122, 197**	
85.99	Other operations on the breast **105, 201, 235**	
34.99	Other operations on thorax **50, 195**	
07.9*	Other operations on thymus **50, 112, 175, 178**	
06.98	Other operations on thyroid glands **112**	
25.99	Other operations on tongue **45**	
28.99	Other operations on tonsils and adenoids **44**	
31.99	Other operations on trachea **44, 50, 195**	
15.4	Other operations on two or more extraocular muscles, one or both eyes **233**	
56.99	Other operations on ureter **116, 197**	
58.99	Other operations on urethra and periurethral tissue **117, 123, 129, 234**	
70.91	Other operations on vagina **128**	
35.99	Other operations on valves of heart **58**	
39.99	Other operations on vessels **44, 50, 63, 74, 139, 178, 196**	
36.9*	Other operations on vessels of heart **58**	
71.8	Other operations on vulva **128**	
73.99	Other operations to assist delivery **147**	
16.09	Other orbitotomy **43**	
51.21	Other partial cholecystectomy **81**	
09.22	Other partial dacryoadenectomy **194**	
43.8*	Other partial gastrectomy **72, 179, 196**	
30.29	Other partial laryngectomy **43**	
30.2*	Other partial laryngectomy **50, 195**	
77.84	Other partial ostectomy of carpals and metacarpals **94, 193**	
77.85	Other partial ostectomy of femur **89, 198, 219**	
77.82	Other partial ostectomy of humerus **91, 198**	
77.89	Other partial ostectomy of other bone, except facial bones **45, 95, 112, 198**	
77.86	Other partial ostectomy of patella **90, 198**	
77.83	Other partial ostectomy of radius and ulna **94, 198**	
77.81	Other partial ostectomy of scapula, clavicle, and thorax (ribs and sternum) **12, 13, 51, 95, 198**	
77.88	Other partial ostectomy of tarsals and metatarsals **93, 112, 198, 234**	
77.87	Other partial ostectomy of tibia and fibula **91, 198**	
77.80	Other partial ostectomy, unspecified site **95, 198**	
45.62	Other partial resection of small intestine **64, 112, 179**	
66.69	Other partial salpingectomy **126, 128, 139**	
06.3*	Other partial thyroidectomy **111**	
11.64	Other penetrating keratoplasty **37**	
04.49	Other peripheral nerve or ganglion decompression or lysis of adhesions **14, 16, 43, 95, 194**	
46.23	Other permanent ileostomy **72, 179, 196**	
31.29	Other permanent tracheostomy **1, 4**	
83.89	Other plastic operations on fascia **14, 17, 93, 104**	
82.89	Other plastic operations on hand **104**	
82.8*	Other plastic operations on hand **14, 17, 94, 193**	
83.87	Other plastic operations on muscle **14, 17, 93, 104**	
83.8*	Other plastic operations on muscle, tendon, and fascia **200**	
83.88	Other plastic operations on tendon **14, 17, 93, 104**	
18.79	Other plastic repair of external ear **103, 233**	
18.7*	Other plastic repair of external ear **44, 195**	
27.59	Other plastic repair of mouth **45, 103, 195, 233**	
27.69	Other plastic repair of palate **14, 16, 44, 103**	
44.66	Other procedures for creation of esophagogastric sphincteric competence **72, 196**	

12.7*	Other procedures for relief of elevated intraocular pressure **37, 232**	
49.49	Other procedures on hemorrhoids **74, 234**	
48.76	Other proctopexy **72**	
60.69	Other prostatectomy **117, 122, 232**	
48.49	Other pull-through resection of rectum **196**	
44.29	Other pyloroplasty **72**	
84.29	Other reattachment of extremity **96, 201**	
08.7*	Other reconstruction of eyelid **37, 103, 194, 232**	
76.43	Other reconstruction of mandible **43, 104**	
76.46	Other reconstruction of other facial bone **37, 43**	
58.46	Other reconstruction of urethra **122, 197**	
11.7*	Other reconstructive and refractive surgery on cornea **194, 232**	
11.79	Other reconstructive surgery on cornea **37**	
65.61	Other removal of both ovaries and tubes at same operative episode **104, 234**	
36.09	Other removal of coronary artery obstruction **62, 63**	
14.72	Other removal of vitreous **112**	
11.49	Other removal or destruction of corneal lesion **194**	
21.89	Other repair and plastic operations on nose **44, 95, 103, 195, 233**	
03.59	Other repair and plastic operations on spinal cord structures **90, 91, 178, 194**	
25.59	Other repair and plastic operations on tongue **45, 195**	
31.79	Other repair and plastic operations on trachea **44, 50**	
86.8*	Other repair and reconstruction of skin and subcutaneous tissue **104**	
86.89	Other repair and reconstruction of skin and subcutaneous tissue **45, 111, 201, 235**	
54.72	Other repair of abdominal wall **74, 82, 104, 179**	
54.7*	Other repair of abdominal wall and peritoneum **197**	
49.79	Other repair of anal sphincter **74, 104, 196, 234**	
39.52	Other repair of aneurysm **8, 10, 11, 59, 117, 196**	
81.49	Other repair of ankle **92**	
57.89	Other repair of bladder **116, 129, 197**	
02.12	Other repair of cerebral meninges **194, 219**	
67.59	Other repair of cervical os **128, 147**	
67.6*	Other repair of cervix **128, 198**	
67.69	Other repair of cervix **147**	
34.79	Other repair of chest wall **50, 95, 103, 195**	
34.84	Other repair of diaphragm **195**	
81.85	Other repair of elbow **93**	
42.89	Other repair of esophagus **45, 72, 179, 196**	
66.79	Other repair of fallopian tube **197**	
81.79	Other repair of hand, fingers, and wrist **14, 16, 93, 193**	
37.49	Other repair of heart and pericardium **195**	
16.89	Other repair of injury of eyeball or orbit **43**	
46.7*	Other repair of intestine **196**	
46.79	Other repair of intestine **72**	
81.96	Other repair of joint **96, 200**	
81.4*	Other repair of joint of lower extremity **200**	
55.8*	Other repair of kidney **116**	
55.89	Other repair of kidney **197**	
81.47	Other repair of knee **90**	
31.69	Other repair of larynx **195**	
50.69	Other repair of liver **81**	
54.75	Other repair of mesentery **75, 82, 179**	
19.9	Other repair of middle ear **233**	
54.74	Other repair of omentum **75, 82, 179**	
52.95	Other repair of pancreas **81, 197**	
64.49	Other repair of penis **104, 197, 234**	

86.70	Pedicle or flap graft, not otherwise specified **14, 17, 45, 65, 75, 88, 111, 193**	
68.8	Pelvic evisceration **73, 126**	
11.63	Penetrating keratoplasty with autograft **37**	
44.32	Percutaneous [endoscopic] gastrojejunostomy **82**	
50.24	Percutaneous ablation of liver lesion or tissue **74, 81**	
32.24	Percutaneous ablation of lung lesion or tissue **50**	
00.61	Percutaneous angioplasty of extracranial vessel(s) **13, 63, 194**	
00.62	Percutaneous angioplasty of intracranial vessel(s) **8, 9, 11, 63, 194**	
17.53	Percutaneous atherectomy of extracranial vessel(s) **13, 63, 195**	
17.54	Percutaneous atherectomy of intracranial vessel(s) **8, 10, 11, 63, 195**	
35.96	Percutaneous balloon valvuloplasty **58, 62, 63**	
00.63	Percutaneous insertion of carotid artery stent(s) **13**	
35.97	Percutaneous mitral valve repair with implant **58, 62, 63**	
00.66	Percutaneous transluminal coronary angioplasty [PTCA] **58, 62, 63**	
81.66	Percutaneous vertebral augmentation **96, 200**	
81.65	Percutaneous vertebroplasty **96, 200**	
37.31	Pericardiectomy **50, 59, 178, 195**	
37.12	Pericardiotomy **50, 59, 178, 195**	
60.62	Perineal prostatectomy **117, 122**	
46.13	Permanent colostomy **64, 72, 179, 196**	
29.32	Pharyngeal diverticulectomy **44**	
29.33	Pharyngectomy (partial) **44**	
29.0	Pharyngotomy **44, 195**	
01.28	Placement of intracerebral catheter(s) via burr hole(s) **8, 9, 11, 178, 194, 219**	
82.72	Plastic operation on hand with graft of muscle or fascia **104**	
82.7*	Plastic operation on hand with graft or implant **14, 17, 94, 193**	
82.79	Plastic operation on hand with other graft or implant **104**	
29.4	Plastic operation on pharynx **14, 16, 44, 195, 233**	
03.5*	Plastic operations on spinal cord structures **12, 13**	
34.5*	Pleurectomy **50, 195**	
32.21	Plication of emphysematous bleb **50**	
59.3	Plication of urethrovesical junction **117**	
32.5*	Pneumonectomy **50, 195**	
12.66	Postoperative revision of scleral fistulization procedure **232**	
05.24	Presacral sympathectomy **129**	
09.43	Probing of nasolacrimal duct **44**	
00.43	Procedure on four or more vessels **62**	
48.1	Proctostomy **72, 196**	
48.0	Proctotomy **73, 196**	
42.86	Production of subcutaneous tunnel without esophageal anastomosis **45, 72, 179, 196**	
73.94	Pubiotomy to assist delivery **140**	
48.4*	Pull-through resection of rectum **73, 179**	
48.40	Pull-through resection of rectum, not otherwise specified **196**	
33.93	Puncture of lung **50**	
55.12	Pyelostomy **234**	
55.1*	Pyelotomy and pyelostomy **116, 197**	
43.3	Pyloromyotomy **72**	
83.86	Quadricepsplasty **93**	
11.75	Radial keratotomy **37**	
32.6	Radical dissection of thoracic structures **50**	
40.51	Radical excision of axillary lymph nodes **95**	
40.4*	Radical excision of cervical lymph nodes **50, 104, 112, 175, 178**	
40.53	Radical excision of iliac lymph nodes **95, 112, 116, 122, 126**	
18.31	Radical excision of lesion of external ear **233**	

40.50	Radical excision of lymph nodes, not otherwise specified **43, 50, 118, 123, 126**
40.59	Radical excision of other lymph nodes **43, 50, 95, 116, 122, 126**
40.5*	Radical excision of other lymph nodes **74, 104, 175, 178**
40.52	Radical excision of periaortic lymph nodes **50, 95, 112, 116, 122, 126**
86.4	Radical excision of skin lesion **14, 17, 37, 45, 64, 93, 103, 201, 235**
25.4	Radical glossectomy **43**
40.54	Radical groin dissection **95, 116, 122, 126**
30.4	Radical laryngectomy **2**
40.42	Radical neck dissection, bilateral **43**
40.40	Radical neck dissection, not otherwise specified **43**
40.41	Radical neck dissection, unilateral **43**
52.7	Radical pancreaticoduodenectomy **72, 81, 197**
60.5	Radical prostatectomy **117, 122**
71.5	Radical vulvectomy **126**
39.54	Re-entry operation (aorta) **50, 59**
58.44	Reanastomosis of urethra **197**
18.72	Reattachment of amputated ear **233**
54.61	Reclosure of postoperative disruption of abdominal wall **82, 129**
18.6	Reconstruction of external auditory canal **44, 103, 195, 233**
08.6*	Reconstruction of eyelid with flaps or grafts **37, 103, 194, 232**
08.70	Reconstruction of eyelid, not otherwise specified **112**
83.7*	Reconstruction of muscle and tendon **14, 17, 93, 200**
64.44	Reconstruction of penis **197**
63.82	Reconstruction of surgically divided vas deferens **122, 197**
82.6*	Reconstruction of thumb **14, 16, 93, 193**
31.75	Reconstruction of trachea and construction of artificial larynx **44, 50**
57.87	Reconstruction of urinary bladder **116, 197**
19*	Reconstructive operations on middle ear **44**
48.74	Rectorectostomy **72**
85.3*	Reduction mammoplasty and subcutaneous mammectomy **104, 105, 201**
76.70	Reduction of facial fracture, not otherwise specified **43, 95, 198**
55.84	Reduction of torsion of renal pedicle **197**
81.31	Refusion of Atlas-axis spine **89**
81.34	Refusion of dorsal and dorsolumbar spine, anterior column, anterior technique **87, 88**
81.35	Refusion of dorsal and dorsolumbar spine, posterior column, posterior technique **87, 88**
81.36	Refusion of lumbar and lumbosacral spine, anterior column, anterior technique **87, 88**
81.38	Refusion of lumbar and lumbosacral spine, anterior column, posterior technique **87, 88**
81.37	Refusion of lumbar and lumbosacral spine, posterior column, posterior technique **87, 88**
81.32	Refusion of other cervical spine, anterior column, anterior technique **87, 89**
81.33	Refusion of other cervical spine, posterior column, posterior technique **87, 89**
81.3*	Refusion of spine **12, 13, 200**
81.39	Refusion of spine, not elsewhere classified **87, 88**
81.30	Refusion of spine, not otherwise specified **87, 88**
40.3	Regional lymph node excision **44, 50, 64, 74, 95, 104, 112, 118, 123, 129, 139, 175, 178, 233**
39.55	Reimplantation of aberrant renal vessel **63, 116**
07.45	Reimplantation of adrenal tissue **194**
52.81	Reimplantation of pancreatic tissue **81**
86.84	Relaxation of scar or web contracture of skin **45, 201, 235**
04.43	Release of carpal tunnel **14, 16, 94, 193**

83.84	Release of clubfoot, not elsewhere classified **93**
04.44	Release of tarsal tunnel **14, 16, 93, 194**
58.5	Release of urethral stricture **117, 122, 129, 197, 234**
39.43	Removal of arteriovenous shunt for renal dialysis **64, 117**
49.76	Removal of artificial anal sphincter **73, 104, 196**
11.92	Removal of artificial implant from cornea **37**
62.41	Removal of both testes at same operative episode **95**
85.96	Removal of breast tissue expander (s) **105, 201, 235**
01.29	Removal of cranial neurostimulator pulse generator **14, 16**
57.98	Removal of electronic bladder stimulator **117, 234**
56.94	Removal of electronic ureteral stimulator **116**
10.0	Removal of embedded foreign body from conjunctiva by incision **194, 232**
37.64	Removal of external heart assist system(s) or device(s) **1, 59**
74.3	Removal of extratubal ectopic pregnancy **140**
13.0*	Removal of foreign body from lens **195, 233**
54.92	Removal of foreign body from peritoneal cavity **75, 118, 197**
14.0*	Removal of foreign body from posterior segment of eye **37, 195, 233**
28.91	Removal of foreign body from tonsil and adenoid by incision **44, 195**
85.94	Removal of implant of breast **105, 201, 235**
78.6*	Removal of implanted device from bone **234**
78.64	Removal of implanted device from carpals and metacarpals **92, 193**
78.65	Removal of implanted device from femur **92, 112, 199**
78.62	Removal of implanted device from humerus **92, 199**
78.69	Removal of implanted device from other bone **92, 199**
78.66	Removal of implanted device from patella **92, 199**
78.63	Removal of implanted device from radius and ulna **92, 199**
78.61	Removal of implanted device from scapula, clavicle, and thorax (ribs and sternum) **51, 92, 199**
78.68	Removal of implanted device from tarsal and metatarsals **92, 199**
78.67	Removal of implanted device from tibia and fibula **92, 199**
78.60	Removal of implanted device, unspecified site **92, 199**
13.8	Removal of implanted lens **195, 233**
37.55	Removal of internal biventricular heart replacement system **59**
76.97	Removal of internal fixation device from facial bone **43, 92, 198**
64.96	Removal of internal prosthesis of penis **118, 122, 234**
01.22	Removal of intracranial neurostimulator lead(s) **8, 9, 11, 178**
12.0*	Removal of intraocular foreign body from anterior segment of eye **37, 194, 232**
37.77	Removal of lead(s) (electrodes) without replacement **14, 16, 64, 195**
12.40	Removal of lesion of anterior segment of eye, not otherwise specified **37**
08.20	Removal of lesion of eyelid, not otherwise specified **103, 112**
56.86	Removal of ligature from ureter **197**
55.98	Removal of mechanical kidney **116, 197**
16.7*	Removal of ocular or orbital implant **37, 195, 233**
69.97	Removal of other penetrating foreign body from cervix **128, 198**
16.1	Removal of penetrating foreign body from eye, not otherwise specified **38, 195, 233**
04.93	Removal of peripheral neurostimulator lead(s) **14, 16, 43, 95, 123, 129**
66.94	Removal of prosthesis of fallopian tube **126, 128**
51.95	Removal of prosthetic device from bile duct **81, 179, 197**
83.93	Removal of skeletal muscle stimulator **14, 17, 93, 200**
02.07	Removal of skull plate **11, 43**
03.94	Removal of spinal neurostimulator lead(s) **12, 13, 90, 91, 117, 122, 129, 194**

03.98	Removal of spinal thecal shunt **12, 13, 91, 194**
14.6	Removal of surgically implanted material from posterior segment of eye **37, 112, 195, 233**
63.85	Removal of valve from vas deferens **122**
02.43	Removal of ventricular shunt **13, 194**
12.93	Removal or destruction of epithelial downgrowth from anterior chamber **37**
55.61	Renal autotransplantation **116, 197**
01.23	Reopening of craniotomy site **8, 9, 11, 43, 178, 194, 219**
03.02	Reopening of laminectomy site **90, 91, 178**
54.12	Reopening of recent laparotomy site **82, 179**
34.03	Reopening of recent thoracotomy site **50, 64, 195**
06.02	Reopening of wound of thyroid field **111, 194, 232**
33.4*	Repair and plastic operation on lung and bronchus **50, 195**
64.4*	Repair and plastic operation on penis **122**
41.95	Repair and plastic operations on spleen **175, 178, 196**
31.7*	Repair and plastic operations on trachea **195**
86.81	Repair for facial weakness **14, 17, 45, 93, 201**
07.44	Repair of adrenal gland **194**
39.53	Repair of arteriovenous fistula **8, 10, 11, 63**
35.6*	Repair of atrial and ventricular septa with tissue graft **58**
35.52	Repair of atrial septal defect with prosthesis, closed technique **63**
35.51	Repair of atrial septal defect with prosthesis, open technique **58**
51.7*	Repair of bile ducts **81, 197**
57.86	Repair of bladder exstrophy **116**
08.3*	Repair of blepharoptosis and lid retraction **37, 194, 232**
39.57	Repair of blood vessel with synthetic patch graft **13, 63, 112, 117, 196**
39.56	Repair of blood vessel with tissue patch graft **13, 63, 112, 117, 196**
39.58	Repair of blood vessel with unspecified type of patch graft **13, 63, 112, 117, 196**
02.92	Repair of brain **8, 10, 11, 194, 219**
09.73	Repair of canaliculus **103**
09.7*	Repair of canaliculus and punctum **194, 232**
02.1*	Repair of cerebral meninges **8, 10, 11**
27.54	Repair of cleft lip **44, 103, 195, 233**
70.72	Repair of colovaginal fistula **72, 128, 179, 198**
11.5*	Repair of cornea **37, 194, 232**
75.61	Repair of current obstetric laceration of bladder and urethra **147**
75.51	Repair of current obstetric laceration of cervix **147**
75.52	Repair of current obstetric laceration of corpus uteri **140**
75.50	Repair of current obstetric laceration of uterus, not otherwise specified **147**
70.51	Repair of cystocele **117**
70.5*	Repair of cystocele and rectocele **129**
70.50	Repair of cystocele and rectocele **75, 117**
70.53	Repair of cystocele and rectocele with graft or prosthesis **72, 116**
70.54	Repair of cystocele with graft or prosthesis **117**
53.7*	Repair of diaphragmatic hernia, abdominal approach **50, 72, 197**
53.8*	Repair of diaphragmatic hernia, thoracic approach **50, 72, 197**
35.54	Repair of endocardial cushion defect with prosthesis **58**
08.4*	Repair of entropion or ectropion **37, 194, 232**
08.44	Repair of entropion or ectropion with lid reconstruction **103**
42.84	Repair of esophageal fistula, not elsewhere classified **45, 72, 178, 196**
42.85	Repair of esophageal stricture **72, 179, 196**
66.7*	Repair of fallopian tube **126, 128**
57.83	Repair of fistula involving bladder and intestine **73, 116, 123, 129, 179, 197**

67.62	Repair of fistula of cervix **139**
71.72	Repair of fistula of vulva or perineum **73**
54.71	Repair of gastroschisis **74**
37.4*	Repair of heart and pericardium **59**
37.63	Repair of heart assist system **1, 56**
81.40	Repair of hip, not elsewhere classified **90, 219**
58.45	Repair of hypospadias or epispadias **122**
15.7	Repair of injury of extraocular muscle **195, 233**
16.8*	Repair of injury of eyeball and orbit **37, 195, 233**
67.5*	Repair of internal cervical os **198**
10.6	Repair of laceration of conjunctiva **194, 232**
51.91	Repair of laceration of gallbladder **81, 197**
31.64	Repair of laryngeal fracture **195**
31.6*	Repair of larynx **44, 50**
50.6*	Repair of liver **197**
22.7*	Repair of nasal sinus **45**
04.76	Repair of old traumatic injury of cranial and peripheral nerves **43**
57.84	Repair of other fistula of bladder **116, 123, 129, 179, 197**
70.75	Repair of other fistula of vagina **73, 128, 179, 198**
53.5*	Repair of other hernia of anterior abdominal wall (without graft or prosthesis) **74**
53.6*	Repair of other hernia of anterior abdominal wall with graft or prosthesis **74**
70.74	Repair of other vaginoenteric fistula **72, 128, 179, 198**
20.93	Repair of oval and round windows **44**
65.7*	Repair of ovary **197**
34.74	Repair of pectus deformity **50, 95**
34.93	Repair of pleura **50, 195**
60.93	Repair of prostate **123, 197, 232**
70.52	Repair of rectocele **72**
70.55	Repair of rectocele with graft or prosthesis **72**
70.73	Repair of rectovaginal fistula **72, 128, 179, 198**
48.7*	Repair of rectum **196**
81.82	Repair of recurrent dislocation of shoulder **94**
14.54	Repair of retinal detachment with laser photocoagulation **112**
14.4*	Repair of retinal detachment with scleral buckling and implant **37, 195, 233**
14.32	Repair of retinal tear by cryotherapy **37, 233**
14.31	Repair of retinal tear by diathermy **37, 195, 233**
26.4*	Repair of salivary gland or duct **46, 195**
12.82	Repair of scleral fistula **37**
12.85	Repair of scleral staphyloma with graft **37**
61.42	Repair of scrotal fistula **122, 197**
62.6*	Repair of testes **122, 197**
80.53	Repair of the anulus fibrosus with graft or prosthesis **12, 13, 91, 179, 200**
07.93	Repair of thymus **194**
53.4*	Repair of umbilical hernia **74**
35.50	Repair of unspecified septal defect of heart with prosthesis **58**
56.8*	Repair of ureter **116**
58.4*	Repair of urethra **117**
69.2*	Repair of uterine supporting structures **128**
35.55	Repair of ventricular septal defect with prosthesis, closed technique **58**
35.53	Repair of ventricular septal defect with prosthesis, open technique **58**
03.53	Repair of vertebral fracture **90, 91, 178, 194**
71.7*	Repair of vulva and perineum **128, 198**
37.87	Replacement of any type of pacemaker device with dual-chamber device **14, 15, 16, 17, 18, 60, 61, 64, 195, 201, 202**

37.85	Replacement of any type of pacemaker device with single-chamber device, not specified as rate responsive **14, 15, 16, 17, 18, 60, 61, 63, 195, 201, 202**
37.86	Replacement of any type of pacemaker device with single-chamber device, rate responsive **14, 15, 16, 17, 18, 60, 61, 63, 195, 201, 202**
37.97	Replacement of automatic cardioverter/defibrillator leads(s) only **57, 58, 65**
37.98	Replacement of automatic cardioverter/defibrillator pulse generator only **57, 58, 62**
57.97	Replacement of electronic bladder stimulator **117, 234**
56.93	Replacement of electronic ureteral stimulator **116**
81.57	Replacement of joint of foot and toe **93, 235**
84.6*	Replacement of spinal disc **12, 13, 91, 201**
37.76	Replacement of transvenous atrial and/or ventricular lead(s) (electrode(s)) **14, 16, 18, 61, 64, 195, 202**
02.42	Replacement of ventricular shunt **13, 178, 194**
39.94	Replacement of vessel-to-vessel cannula **63, 118, 233**
37.54	Replacement or repair of other implantable component of (total) replacement heart system **56**
37.53	Replacement or repair of thoracic unit of (total) replacement heart system **56**
64.45	Replantation of penis **197**
38.44	Resection of abdominal aorta with replacement **59**
38.36	Resection of abdominal arteries with anastomosis **59, 74, 117**
38.46	Resection of abdominal arteries with replacement **59, 74, 117**
38.37	Resection of abdominal veins with anastomosis **59, 74, 117**
38.47	Resection of abdominal veins with replacement **59, 74, 117**
38.34	Resection of aorta with anastomosis **59, 74**
38.31	Resection of intracranial vessels with anastomosis **8, 10, 11**
38.41	Resection of intracranial vessels with replacement **8, 10, 11**
38.38	Resection of lower limb arteries with anastomosis **63, 112**
38.48	Resection of lower limb arteries with replacement **63, 112**
38.39	Resection of lower limb veins with anastomosis **64**
38.49	Resection of lower limb veins with replacement **64**
21.4	Resection of nose **43, 103, 195**
38.35	Resection of other thoracic vessels with anastomosis **50, 59, 72**
38.45	Resection of other thoracic vessels with replacement **50, 56, 72**
38.32	Resection of other vessels of head and neck with anastomosis **13, 44, 63**
38.42	Resection of other vessels of head and neck with replacement **14, 16, 44, 63**
85.22	Resection of quadrant of breast **104, 105**
38.33	Resection of upper limb vessels with anastomosis **63, 112**
38.43	Resection of upper limb vessels with replacement **63, 112**
38.3*	Resection of vessel with anastomosis **196**
38.30	Resection of vessel with anastomosis, unspecified site **63, 112**
38.4*	Resection of vessel with replacement **196**
38.40	Resection of vessel with replacement, unspecified site **63**
00.87	Resurfacing hip, partial, acetabulum **88, 112, 219**
00.86	Resurfacing hip, partial, femoral head **88, 112, 219**
00.85	Resurfacing hip, total, acetabulum and femoral head **88, 219**
59.00	Retroperitoneal dissection, not otherwise specified **95, 104, 116, 122, 129, 179**
60.4	Retropubic prostatectomy **117, 122**
59.5	Retropubic urethral suspension **117, 128**
81.88	Reverse total shoulder replacement **90**
84.3	Revision of amputation stump **63, 89, 104, 111, 201**
51.94	Revision of anastomosis of biliary tract **81, 179, 197**
46.94	Revision of anastomosis of large intestine **72, 196**
46.93	Revision of anastomosis of small intestine **72, 196**

     *Code Range

39.42	Revision of arteriovenous shunt for renal dialysis **64, 112, 117**
27.63	Revision of cleft palate repair **44, 103**
35.95	Revision of corrective procedure on heart **58**
56.52	Revision of cutaneous uretero-ileostomy **234**
16.63	Revision of enucleation socket with graft **43**
15.6	Revision of extraocular muscle surgery **233**
84.85	Revision of facet replacement device(s) **96**
44.5	Revision of gastric anastomosis **72, 111, 196**
00.71	Revision of hip replacement, acetabular component **88, 112, 194, 219**
00.73	Revision of hip replacement, acetabular liner and/or femoral head only **88, 112, 194, 219**
00.70	Revision of hip replacement, both acetabular and femoral components **88, 112, 194, 219**
00.72	Revision of hip replacement, femoral component **88, 112, 194, 219**
81.53	Revision of hip replacement, not otherwise specified **88, 113, 219**
85.93	Revision of implant of breast **105, 201, 235**
84.81	Revision of interspinous process device(s) **96**
46.4*	Revision of intestinal stoma **74, 196**
46.40	Revision of intestinal stoma, not otherwise specified **179**
81.59	Revision of joint replacement of lower extremity, not elsewhere classified **96**
81.97	Revision of joint replacement of upper extremity **96, 200**
00.82	Revision of knee replacement, femoral component **88**
81.55	Revision of knee replacement, not otherwise specified **88**
00.83	Revision of knee replacement, patellar component **90**
00.81	Revision of knee replacement, tibial component **88**
00.80	Revision of knee replacement, total (all components) **88**
37.75	Revision of lead (electrode) **14, 16, 64, 195**
20.92	Revision of mastoidectomy **45**
12.83	Revision of operative wound of anterior segment, not elsewhere classified **37**
86.75	Revision of pedicle or flap graft **14, 17, 45, 65, 75, 88, 111, 193**
84.83	Revision of pedicle-based dynamic stabilization device(s) **96**
04.75	Revision of previous repair of cranial and peripheral nerves **43**
03.97	Revision of spinal thecal shunt **12, 13, 90, 91, 178, 194**
46.41	Revision of stoma of small intestine **179, 234**
00.84	Revision of total knee replacement, tibial insert (liner) **90**
31.74	Revision of tracheostomy **44, 50, 64, 103**
56.72	Revision of ureterointestinal anastomosis **123, 129, 179**
39.4*	Revision of vascular procedure **196**
57.22	Revision or closure of vesicostomy **129, 179, 234**
37.79	Revision or relocation of cardiac device pocket **14, 16, 64, 103, 195**
37.89	Revision or removal of pacemaker device **14, 16, 64, 195, 233**
84.66	Revision or replacement of artificial spinal disc prosthesis, cervical **91**
84.68	Revision or replacement of artificial spinal disc prosthesis, lumbosacral **91**
84.69	Revision or replacement of artificial spinal disc prosthesis, not otherwise specified **91**
84.67	Revision or replacement of artificial spinal disc prosthesis, thoracic **91**
21.84	Revision rhinoplasty **44, 95, 103, 195, 233**
37.21	Right heart cardiac catheterization **56, 57, 58, 65**
83.63	Rotator cuff repair **94**
66.62	Salpingectomy with removal of tubal pregnancy **126, 128, 139**
66.0*	Salpingotomy **126, 128**
34.6	Scarification of pleura **50, 178, 195**
12.6*	Scleral fistulization **37, 194**

12.87	Scleral reinforcement with graft **37**
16.65	Secondary graft to exenteration cavity **44**
13.72	Secondary insertion of intraocular lens prosthesis **195, 233**
16.6*	Secondary procedures after removal of eyeball **37, 195, 233**
32.3*	Segmental resection of lung **50, 178, 195**
84.92	Separation of equal conjoined twins **96**
84.93	Separation of unequal conjoined twins **96**
77.04	Sequestrectomy of carpals and metacarpals **94, 193**
76.01	Sequestrectomy of facial bone **43, 95**
77.05	Sequestrectomy of femur **89, 198, 219**
77.02	Sequestrectomy of humerus **91, 198**
77.09	Sequestrectomy of other bone, except facial bones **95, 198**
77.06	Sequestrectomy of patella **90, 198**
77.03	Sequestrectomy of radius and ulna **94, 198**
77.01	Sequestrectomy of scapula, clavicle, and thorax (ribs and sternum) **50, 95, 198**
77.08	Sequestrectomy of tarsals and metatarsals **93, 198**
77.07	Sequestrectomy of tibia and fibula **91, 198**
77.00	Sequestrectomy, unspecified site **95, 198**
03.7*	Shunt of spinal theca **12, 13, 178**
26.3*	Sialoadenectomy **46, 233**
26.30	Sialoadenectomy, not otherwise specified **175**
40.2*	Simple excision of lymphatic structure **104, 175**
40.29	Simple excision of other lymphatic structure **44, 50, 64, 74, 95, 112, 118, 123, 129, 196, 233**
02.11	Simple suture of dura mater of brain **194, 219**
66.71	Simple suture of fallopian tube **197**
86.83	Size reduction plastic operation **111, 201, 235**
45.91	Small-to-small intestinal anastomosis **111, 179**
05.21	Sphenopalatine ganglionectomy **43**
57.91	Sphincterotomy of bladder **116, 234**
81.00	Spinal fusion, not otherwise specified **12, 13, 87, 88, 200**
41.2	Splenotomy **175, 178, 196**
85.82	Split-thickness graft to breast **103, 193, 206, 207**
19.1*	Stapedectomy **233**
92.3*	Stereotactic radiosurgery **16, 18, 113, 180**
21.5	Submucous resection of nasal septum **44, 195, 233**
06.5*	Substernal thyroidectomy **111**
81.13	Subtalar fusion **93**
81.18	Subtalar joint arthroereisis **96**
68.3*	Subtotal abdominal hysterectomy **126, 128, 139**
85.23	Subtotal mastectomy **104, 105, 235**
60.3	Suprapubic prostatectomy **117, 122**
59.4	Suprapubic sling operation **117, 128**
75.93	Surgical correction of inverted uterus **140**
18.5	Surgical correction of prominent ear **44, 103, 233**
54.6*	Suture of abdominal wall and peritoneum **75, 197**
39.31	Suture of artery **50, 63, 104, 112**
81.94	Suture of capsule or ligament of ankle and foot **93, 200**
81.95	Suture of capsule or ligament of other lower extremity **92, 200**
81.93	Suture of capsule or ligament of upper extremity **94, 200**
04.3	Suture of cranial and peripheral nerves **14, 16, 194**
44.42	Suture of duodenal ulcer site **72**
44.41	Suture of gastric ulcer site **72**
49.71	Suture of laceration of anus **74, 104, 196**
57.81	Suture of laceration of bladder **116, 197**
67.61	Suture of laceration of cervix **147**
34.82	Suture of laceration of diaphragm **195**
46.71	Suture of laceration of duodenum **72**

*Code Range

42.82	Suture of laceration of esophagus **45, 72, 178, 196**
55.81	Suture of laceration of kidney **197**
46.75	Suture of laceration of large intestine **72**
31.61	Suture of laceration of larynx **195**
27.61	Suture of laceration of palate **45, 195**
64.41	Suture of laceration of penis **197**
29.51	Suture of laceration of pharynx **44, 195**
48.71	Suture of laceration of rectum **72, 147**
12.81	Suture of laceration of sclera **37**
46.73	Suture of laceration of small intestine, except duodenum **72**
63.51	Suture of laceration of spermatic cord and epididymis **122, 197**
44.61	Suture of laceration of stomach **72, 196**
31.71	Suture of laceration of trachea **44, 50**
56.82	Suture of laceration of ureter **197**
58.41	Suture of laceration of urethra **197**
69.41	Suture of laceration of uterus **139**
70.71	Suture of laceration of vagina **104, 128, 147, 198**
63.81	Suture of laceration of vas deferens and epididymis **122, 197**
71.71	Suture of laceration of vulva or perineum **104, 147, 234**
82.46	Suture of muscle or fascia of hand **235**
83.6*	Suture of muscle, tendon, and fascia **200, 235**
82.4*	Suture of muscle, tendon, and fascia of hand **94, 193**
44.40	Suture of peptic ulcer, not otherwise specified **72**
54.64	Suture of peritoneum **82, 179, 234**
83.61	Suture of tendon sheath **92**
82.41	Suture of tendon sheath of hand **235**
06.93	Suture of thyroid gland **112, 194**
39.30	Suture of unspecified blood vessel **63**
39.32	Suture of vein **64**
39.3*	Suture of vessel **13, 196**
05.2*	Sympathectomy **14, 16, 64**
80.7*	Synovectomy **235**
80.77	Synovectomy of ankle **91, 200**
80.72	Synovectomy of elbow **94, 200**
80.78	Synovectomy of foot and toe **93, 200**
80.74	Synovectomy of hand and finger **94, 193**
80.75	Synovectomy of hip **90, 200**
80.76	Synovectomy of knee **90, 200**
80.79	Synovectomy of other specified site **92, 200**
80.71	Synovectomy of shoulder **94, 200**
80.73	Synovectomy of wrist **94, 193**
80.70	Synovectomy, unspecified site **92, 200**
39.0	Systemic to pulmonary artery shunt **59**
81.15	Tarsometatarsal fusion **93**
11.91	Tattooing of cornea **37**
39.77	Temporary (partial) therapeutic endovascular occlusion of vessel **13, 63, 196**
46.11	Temporary colostomy **72, 179, 196**
46.21	Temporary ileostomy **72, 179, 196**
31.1	Temporary tracheostomy **1, 4**
76.5	Temporomandibular arthroplasty **45, 95, 198**
83.81	Tendon graft **14, 17, 93**
83.83	Tendon pulley reconstruction on muscle, tendon, and fascia **14, 17, 93**
83.75	Tendon transfer or transplantation **113**
82.11	Tenotomy of hand **235**
12.91	Therapeutic evacuation of anterior chamber **37, 194**
11.42	Thermocauterization of corneal lesion **194**
12.62	Thermocauterization of sclera with iridectomy **232**

11.74	Thermokeratoplasty **37**
84.28	Thigh reattachment **89, 201, 219**
33.34	Thoracoplasty **50**
32.25	Thoracoscopic ablation of lung lesion or tissue **50, 178**
34.52	Thoracoscopic decortication of lung **178**
34.06	Thoracoscopic drainage of pleural cavity **50**
32.20	Thoracoscopic excision of lesion or tissue of lung **50, 178, 195**
07.95	Thoracoscopic incision of thymus **14, 16, 194**
33.20	Thoracoscopic lung biopsy **50, 64, 95, 117**
34.20	Thoracoscopic pleural biopsy **50**
84.21	Thumb reattachment **94, 193**
07.8*	Thymectomy **14, 16, 50, 112, 175, 178, 194**
06.94	Thyroid tissue reimplantation **112**
84.25	Toe reattachment **93, 201**
28.3	Tonsillectomy with adenoidectomy **44**
28.2	Tonsillectomy without adenoidectomy **44, 233**
81.56	Total ankle replacement **88, 89**
66.5*	Total bilateral salpingectomy **126, 128, 139**
57.7*	Total cystectomy **116, 122, 129, 179**
09.23	Total dacryoadenectomy **194**
81.84	Total elbow replacement **90**
42.42	Total esophagectomy **44**
07.68	Total excision of pituitary gland, other specified approach **103**
07.64	Total excision of pituitary gland, transfrontal approach **103**
07.65	Total excision of pituitary gland, transsphenoidal approach **103**
07.69	Total excision of pituitary gland, unspecified approach **103**
43.9*	Total gastrectomy **72, 179, 196**
50.4	Total hepatectomy **81, 197**
81.51	Total hip replacement **88, 89, 219**
45.8*	Total intra-abdominal colectomy **64, 72, 179, 196**
81.54	Total knee replacement **88, 89**
76.41	Total mandibulectomy with synchronous reconstruction **43**
21.83	Total nasal reconstruction **44, 95, 103, 195, 233**
77.94	Total ostectomy of carpals and metacarpals **94, 193**
77.95	Total ostectomy of femur **89, 198, 219**
77.92	Total ostectomy of humerus **91, 198**
77.99	Total ostectomy of other bone, except facial bones **45, 95, 198**
76.44	Total ostectomy of other facial bone with synchronous reconstruction **43**
77.96	Total ostectomy of patella **90, 198**
77.93	Total ostectomy of radius and ulna **94, 198**
77.91	Total ostectomy of scapula, clavicle, and thorax (ribs and sternum) **12, 13, 51, 95, 198**
77.98	Total ostectomy of tarsals and metatarsals **93, 198, 234**
77.97	Total ostectomy of tibia and fibula **91, 198**
77.90	Total ostectomy, unspecified site **95, 198**
52.6	Total pancreatectomy **81, 197**
85.7*	Total reconstruction of breast **104, 105, 201**
45.63	Total removal of small intestine **179**
35.8*	Total repair of certain congenital cardiac anomalies **58**
41.5	Total splenectomy **64, 74, 95, 175, 178, 196**
66.4	Total unilateral salpingectomy **126, 128, 139**
81.73	Total wrist replacement **90, 200**
12.64	Trabeculectomy ab externo **112, 232**
12.54	Trabeculotomy ab externo **37**
67.51	Transabdominal cerclage of cervix **128, 147**
45.21	Transabdominal endoscopy of large intestine **73, 196, 234**
45.11	Transabdominal endoscopy of small intestine **73, 179, 196, 234**
44.11	Transabdominal gastroscopy **72, 82, 179, 196**

Numeric Index to Procedures

Code	Description
03.93	Implantation or replacement of spinal neurostimulator lead(s) **12, 13, 90, 91, 117, 122, 129, 178, 194**
03.94	Removal of spinal neurostimulator lead(s) **12, 13, 90, 91, 117, 122, 129, 194**
03.97	Revision of spinal thecal shunt **12, 13, 90, 91, 178, 194**
03.98	Removal of spinal thecal shunt **12, 13, 91, 194**
03.99	Other operations on spinal cord and spinal canal structures **12, 13, 91, 178, 194**
04.01	Excision of acoustic neuroma **8, 10, 11, 43**
04.02	Division of trigeminal nerve **14, 16, 43, 194**
04.03	Division or crushing of other cranial and peripheral nerves **14, 16, 43, 95, 194**
04.04	Other incision of cranial and peripheral nerves **14, 16, 43, 95, 194**
04.05	Gasserian ganglionectomy **14, 16, 43, 194**
04.06	Other cranial or peripheral ganglionectomy **14, 16, 43, 95, 194**
04.07	Other excision or avulsion of cranial and peripheral nerves **14, 16, 43, 95, 194, 232**
04.12	Open biopsy of cranial or peripheral nerve or ganglion **14, 16, 43, 95, 194**
04.19	Other diagnostic procedures on cranial and peripheral nerves and ganglia **14, 16, 43, 95, 194**
04.3	Suture of cranial and peripheral nerves **14, 16, 194**
04.4*	Lysis of adhesions and decompression of cranial and peripheral nerves **232**
04.41	Decompression of trigeminal nerve root **8, 10, 11, 43, 194, 219**
04.42	Other cranial nerve decompression **14, 16, 43, 194**
04.43	Release of carpal tunnel **14, 16, 94, 193**
04.44	Release of tarsal tunnel **14, 16, 93, 194**
04.49	Other peripheral nerve or ganglion decompression or lysis of adhesions **14, 16, 43, 95, 194**
04.5	Cranial or peripheral nerve graft **14, 16, 194**
04.6	Transposition of cranial and peripheral nerves **14, 16, 194**
04.7*	Other cranial or peripheral neuroplasty **14, 16, 194**
04.71	Hypoglossal-facial anastomosis **43**
04.72	Accessory-facial anastomosis **43**
04.73	Accessory-hypoglossal anastomosis **43**
04.74	Other anastomosis of cranial or peripheral nerve **43**
04.75	Revision of previous repair of cranial and peripheral nerves **43**
04.76	Repair of old traumatic injury of cranial and peripheral nerves **43**
04.9*	Other operations on cranial and peripheral nerves **194**
04.91	Neurectasis **14, 16**
04.92	Implantation or replacement of peripheral neurostimulator lead(s) **14, 16, 18, 43, 63, 95, 117, 123, 129**
04.93	Removal of peripheral neurostimulator lead(s) **14, 16, 43, 95, 123, 129**
04.99	Other operations on cranial and peripheral nerves **14, 16, 43, 95, 232**
05.0	Division of sympathetic nerve or ganglion **14, 16, 64**
05.1*	Diagnostic procedures on sympathetic nerves or ganglia **14, 16**
05.2*	Sympathectomy **14, 16, 64**
05.21	Sphenopalatine ganglionectomy **43**
05.22	Cervical sympathectomy **43**
05.23	Lumbar sympathectomy **232**
05.24	Presacral sympathectomy **129**
05.8*	Other operations on sympathetic nerves or ganglia **14, 16**
05.89	Other operations on sympathetic nerves or ganglia **64**
05.9	Other operations on nervous system **14, 16, 194**
06.02	Reopening of wound of thyroid field **111, 194, 232**
06.09	Other incision of thyroid field **43, 103, 111, 194**
06.12	Open biopsy of thyroid gland **111**
06.13	Biopsy of parathyroid gland **95, 111**
06.19	Other diagnostic procedures on thyroid and parathyroid glands **95, 111**
06.2	Unilateral thyroid lobectomy **111**
06.3*	Other partial thyroidectomy **111**
06.4	Complete thyroidectomy **111**
06.5*	Substernal thyroidectomy **111**
06.6	Excision of lingual thyroid **44, 111**
06.7	Excision of thyroglossal duct or tract **44, 111**
06.8*	Parathyroidectomy **111, 117**
06.91	Division of thyroid isthmus **111**
06.92	Ligation of thyroid vessels **112, 194**
06.93	Suture of thyroid gland **112, 194**
06.94	Thyroid tissue reimplantation **112**
06.95	Parathyroid tissue reimplantation **112**
06.98	Other operations on thyroid glands **112**
06.99	Other operations on parathyroid glands **112**
07.0*	Exploration of adrenal field **111**
07.12	Open biopsy of adrenal gland **111**
07.13	Biopsy of pituitary gland, transfrontal approach **8, 10, 11, 111**
07.14	Biopsy of pituitary gland, transsphenoidal approach **8, 10, 11, 111**
07.15	Biopsy of pituitary gland, unspecified approach **8, 10, 11, 111**
07.16	Biopsy of thymus **50, 112, 175, 178**
07.17	Biopsy of pineal gland **8, 10, 11, 111**
07.19	Other diagnostic procedures on adrenal glands, pituitary gland, pineal gland, and thymus **14, 16, 111**
07.2*	Partial adrenalectomy **111**
07.22	Unilateral adrenalectomy **103**
07.3	Bilateral adrenalectomy **103, 111**
07.4*	Other operations on adrenal glands, nerves, and vessels **111**
07.43	Ligation of adrenal vessels **194**
07.44	Repair of adrenal gland **194**
07.45	Reimplantation of adrenal tissue **194**
07.49	Other operations on adrenal glands, nerves, and vessels **194**
07.5*	Operations on pineal gland **8, 10, 11, 111**
07.6*	Hypophysectomy **8, 10, 11, 111**
07.63	Partial excision of pituitary gland, unspecified approach **103**
07.64	Total excision of pituitary gland, transfrontal approach **103**
07.65	Total excision of pituitary gland, transsphenoidal approach **103**
07.68	Total excision of pituitary gland, other specified approach **103**
07.69	Total excision of pituitary gland, unspecified approach **103**
07.7*	Other operations on hypophysis **8, 10, 11, 111**
07.72	Incision of pituitary gland **103**
07.79	Other operations on hypophysis **103**
07.8*	Thymectomy **14, 16, 50, 112, 175, 178, 194**
07.9*	Other operations on thymus **50, 112, 175, 178**
07.91	Exploration of thymus field **194**
07.92	Other incision of thymus **194**
07.93	Repair of thymus **194**
07.95	Thoracoscopic incision of thymus **14, 16, 194**
07.98	Other and unspecified thoracoscopic operations on thymus **14, 16, 194**
08.11	Biopsy of eyelid **37, 194, 232**
08.2*	Excision or destruction of lesion or tissue of eyelid **37, 194, 232**
08.20	Removal of lesion of eyelid, not otherwise specified **103, 112**
08.22	Excision of other minor lesion of eyelid **103**
08.23	Excision of major lesion of eyelid, partial-thickness **103**
08.24	Excision of major lesion of eyelid, full-thickness **103**
08.25	Destruction of lesion of eyelid **103**
08.3*	Repair of blepharoptosis and lid retraction **37, 194, 232**

*Code Range

© 2013 OptumInsight, Inc.

08.38	Correction of lid retraction **103, 112**	
08.4*	Repair of entropion or ectropion **37, 194, 232**	
08.44	Repair of entropion or ectropion with lid reconstruction **103**	
08.5*	Other adjustment of lid position **14, 16, 37, 103, 194, 232**	
08.6*	Reconstruction of eyelid with flaps or grafts **37, 103, 194, 232**	
08.7*	Other reconstruction of eyelid **37, 103, 194, 232**	
08.70	Reconstruction of eyelid, not otherwise specified **112**	
08.9*	Other operations on eyelids **37, 194, 232**	
08.99	Other operations on eyelids **103**	
09.0	Incision of lacrimal gland **232**	
09.1*	Diagnostic procedures on lacrimal system **232**	
09.11	Biopsy of lacrimal gland **194**	
09.12	Biopsy of lacrimal sac **44**	
09.19	Other diagnostic procedures on lacrimal system **44, 194**	
09.2*	Excision of lesion or tissue of lacrimal gland **232**	
09.21	Excision of lesion of lacrimal gland **194**	
09.22	Other partial dacryoadenectomy **194**	
09.23	Total dacryoadenectomy **194**	
09.3	Other operations on lacrimal gland **194, 232**	
09.4*	Manipulation of lacrimal passage **232**	
09.43	Probing of nasolacrimal duct **44**	
09.44	Intubation of nasolacrimal duct **44, 194**	
09.5*	Incision of lacrimal sac and passages **232**	
09.52	Incision of lacrimal canaliculi **194**	
09.6	Excision of lacrimal sac and passage **194, 232**	
09.7*	Repair of canaliculus and punctum **194, 232**	
09.73	Repair of canaliculus **103**	
09.8*	Fistulization of lacrimal tract to nasal cavity **194, 232**	
09.81	Dacryocystorhinostomy (DCR) **44**	
09.9*	Other operations on lacrimal system **194, 232**	
09.99	Other operations on lacrimal system **44**	
09*	Operations on lacrimal system **37**	
10.0	Removal of embedded foreign body from conjunctiva by incision **194, 232**	
10.1	Other incision of conjunctiva **232**	
10.2*	Diagnostic procedures on conjunctiva **232**	
10.3*	Excision or destruction of lesion or tissue of conjunctiva **194, 232**	
10.4*	Conjunctivoplasty **194, 232**	
10.5	Lysis of adhesions of conjunctiva and eyelid **232**	
10.6	Repair of laceration of conjunctiva **194, 232**	
10.9*	Other operations on conjunctiva **232**	
10*	Operations on conjunctiva **37**	
11.0	Magnetic removal of embedded foreign body from cornea **37, 194, 232**	
11.1	Incision of cornea **37, 194, 232**	
11.2*	Diagnostic procedures on cornea **37, 232**	
11.22	Biopsy of cornea **194**	
11.3*	Excision of pterygium **37, 232**	
11.32	Excision of pterygium with corneal graft **194**	
11.4*	Excision or destruction of tissue or other lesion of cornea **37, 232**	
11.42	Thermocauterization of corneal lesion **194**	
11.43	Cryotherapy of corneal lesion **194**	
11.49	Other removal or destruction of corneal lesion **194**	
11.5*	Repair of cornea **37, 194, 232**	
11.6*	Corneal transplant **194, 232**	
11.60	Corneal transplant, not otherwise specified **37**	
11.61	Lamellar keratoplasty with autograft **37**	
11.62	Other lamellar keratoplasty **37**	
11.63	Penetrating keratoplasty with autograft **37**	

11.64	Other penetrating keratoplasty **37**	
11.69	Other corneal transplant **37**	
11.7*	Other reconstructive and refractive surgery on cornea **194, 232**	
11.71	Keratomileusis **37**	
11.72	Keratophakia **37**	
11.73	Keratoprosthesis **37**	
11.74	Thermokeratoplasty **37**	
11.75	Radial keratotomy **37**	
11.76	Epikeratophakia **37**	
11.79	Other reconstructive surgery on cornea **37**	
11.9*	Other operations on cornea **194, 232**	
11.91	Tattooing of cornea **37**	
11.92	Removal of artificial implant from cornea **37**	
11.99	Other operations on cornea **37**	
12.0*	Removal of intraocular foreign body from anterior segment of eye **37, 194, 232**	
12.1*	Iridotomy and simple iridectomy **37, 194, 232**	
12.2*	Diagnostic procedures on iris, ciliary body, sclera, and anterior chamber **194, 232**	
12.21	Diagnostic aspiration of anterior chamber of eye **37**	
12.22	Biopsy of iris **37**	
12.29	Other diagnostic procedures on iris, ciliary body, sclera, and anterior chamber **37**	
12.3*	Iridoplasty and coreoplasty **194, 232**	
12.31	Lysis of goniosynechiae **37**	
12.32	Lysis of other anterior synechiae **37**	
12.33	Lysis of posterior synechiae **37**	
12.34	Lysis of corneovitreal adhesions **37**	
12.35	Coreoplasty **37**	
12.39	Other iridoplasty **37**	
12.4*	Excision or destruction of lesion of iris and ciliary body **194, 232**	
12.40	Removal of lesion of anterior segment of eye, not otherwise specified **37**	
12.41	Destruction of lesion of iris, nonexcisional **37**	
12.42	Excision of lesion of iris **37**	
12.43	Destruction of lesion of ciliary body, nonexcisional **37**	
12.44	Excision of lesion of ciliary body **37**	
12.5*	Facilitation of intraocular circulation **194, 232**	
12.51	Goniopuncture without goniotomy **37**	
12.52	Goniotomy without goniopuncture **37**	
12.53	Goniotomy with goniopuncture **37**	
12.54	Trabeculotomy ab externo **37**	
12.55	Cyclodialysis **37**	
12.59	Other facilitation of intraocular circulation **37**	
12.6*	Scleral fistulization **37, 194**	
12.61	Trephination of sclera with iridectomy **232**	
12.62	Thermocauterization of sclera with iridectomy **232**	
12.63	Iridencleisis and iridotasis **232**	
12.64	Trabeculectomy ab externo **112, 232**	
12.65	Other scleral fistulization with iridectomy **232**	
12.66	Postoperative revision of scleral fistulization procedure **232**	
12.69	Other scleral fistulizing procedure **232**	
12.7*	Other procedures for relief of elevated intraocular pressure **37, 232**	
12.72	Cyclocryotherapy **112**	
12.79	Other glaucoma procedures **112**	
12.8*	Operations on sclera **194, 232**	
12.81	Suture of laceration of sclera **37**	
12.82	Repair of scleral fistula **37**	

Numeric Index to Procedures

*Code Range

17.62	Laser interstitial thermal therapy [LITT] of lesion or tissue of head and neck under guidance **112, 178**
17.63	Laser interstitial thermal therapy [LITT] of lesion or tissue of liver under guidance **74, 81**
17.69	Laser interstitial thermal therapy [LITT] of lesion or tissue of other and unspecified site under guidance **50, 105, 123, 178**
18.21	Excision of preauricular sinus **44, 103, 233**
18.3*	Other excision of external ear **44, 103**
18.31	Radical excision of lesion of external ear **233**
18.39	Other excision of external ear **195, 233**
18.5	Surgical correction of prominent ear **44, 103, 233**
18.6	Reconstruction of external auditory canal **44, 103, 195, 233**
18.7*	Other plastic repair of external ear **44, 195**
18.71	Construction of auricle of ear **103, 233**
18.72	Reattachment of amputated ear **233**
18.79	Other plastic repair of external ear **103, 233**
18.9	Other operations on external ear **44, 103, 195, 233**
19.1*	Stapedectomy **233**
19.4	Myringoplasty **233**
19.9	Other repair of middle ear **233**
19*	Reconstructive operations on middle ear **44**
20.01	Myringotomy with insertion of tube **44, 233**
20.2*	Incision of mastoid and middle ear **233**
20.21	Incision of mastoid **45**
20.22	Incision of petrous pyramid air cells **45**
20.23	Incision of middle ear **44**
20.32	Biopsy of middle and inner ear **44, 233**
20.39	Other diagnostic procedures on middle and inner ear **44, 233**
20.4*	Mastoidectomy **45**
20.5*	Other excision of middle ear **44**
20.51	Excision of lesion of middle ear **233**
20.6*	Fenestration of inner ear **44**
20.7*	Incision, excision, and destruction of inner ear **44**
20.91	Tympanosympathectomy **44**
20.92	Revision of mastoidectomy **45**
20.93	Repair of oval and round windows **44**
20.95	Implantation of electromagnetic hearing device **44**
20.96	Implantation or replacement of cochlear prosthetic device, not otherwise specified **43**
20.97	Implantation or replacement of cochlear prosthetic device, single channel **43**
20.98	Implantation or replacement of cochlear prosthetic device, multiple channel **43**
20.99	Other operations on middle and inner ear **44**
21.04	Control of epistaxis by ligation of ethmoidal arteries **44, 64, 195**
21.05	Control of epistaxis by (transantral) ligation of the maxillary artery **44, 64, 195**
21.06	Control of epistaxis by ligation of the external carotid artery **44, 64, 195**
21.07	Control of epistaxis by excision of nasal mucosa and skin grafting of septum and lateral nasal wall **44, 64, 195**
21.09	Control of epistaxis by other means **44, 64, 195, 233**
21.4	Resection of nose **43, 103, 195**
21.5	Submucous resection of nasal septum **44, 195, 233**
21.6*	Turbinectomy **44**
21.62	Fracture of the turbinates **195, 233**
21.69	Other turbinectomy **195, 233**
21.72	Open reduction of nasal fracture **43, 95, 103, 195, 233**
21.82	Closure of nasal fistula **44, 233**
21.83	Total nasal reconstruction **44, 95, 103, 195, 233**
21.84	Revision rhinoplasty **44, 95, 103, 195, 233**
21.85	Augmentation rhinoplasty **44, 95, 103, 195, 233**
21.86	Limited rhinoplasty **44, 95, 103, 195, 233**
21.87	Other rhinoplasty **44, 95, 103, 195, 233**
21.88	Other septoplasty **44, 95, 103, 195, 233**
21.89	Other repair and plastic operations on nose **44, 95, 103, 195, 233**
21.99	Other operations on nose **44, 103, 195, 233**
22.12	Open biopsy of nasal sinus **45**
22.3*	External maxillary antrotomy **45**
22.4*	Frontal sinusotomy and sinusectomy **45**
22.5*	Other nasal sinusotomy **45**
22.6*	Other nasal sinusectomy **45**
22.62	Excision of lesion of maxillary sinus with other approach **95**
22.63	Ethmoidectomy **233**
22.7*	Repair of nasal sinus **45**
22.9	Other operations on nasal sinuses **45**
24.2	Gingivoplasty **45, 195**
24.4	Excision of dental lesion of jaw **45, 233**
24.5	Alveoloplasty **45, 195, 233**
25.02	Open biopsy of tongue **45**
25.1	Excision or destruction of lesion or tissue of tongue **45, 64, 233**
25.2	Partial glossectomy **45**
25.3	Complete glossectomy **43**
25.4	Radical glossectomy **43**
25.59	Other repair and plastic operations on tongue **45, 195**
25.94	Other glossotomy **45**
25.99	Other operations on tongue **45**
26.12	Open biopsy of salivary gland or duct **46, 233**
26.2*	Excision of lesion of salivary gland **46, 233**
26.3*	Sialoadenectomy **45, 233**
26.30	Sialoadenectomy, not otherwise specified **175**
26.4*	Repair of salivary gland or duct **46, 195**
26.99	Other operations on salivary gland or duct **46**
27.0	Drainage of face and floor of mouth **45, 103, 195**
27.1	Incision of palate **45**
27.21	Biopsy of bony palate **45, 233**
27.22	Biopsy of uvula and soft palate **45, 233**
27.3*	Excision of lesion or tissue of bony palate **233**
27.31	Local excision or destruction of lesion or tissue of bony palate **45**
27.32	Wide excision or destruction of lesion or tissue of bony palate **43**
27.42	Wide excision of lesion of lip **45, 103, 233**
27.43	Other excision of lesion or tissue of lip **45, 103, 233**
27.49	Other excision of mouth **45, 195, 233**
27.53	Closure of fistula of mouth **45, 195, 233**
27.54	Repair of cleft lip **44, 103, 195, 233**
27.55	Full-thickness skin graft to lip and mouth **45, 103, 195, 233**
27.56	Other skin graft to lip and mouth **45, 103, 195, 233**
27.57	Attachment of pedicle or flap graft to lip and mouth **45, 103, 195, 233**
27.59	Other plastic repair of mouth **45, 103, 195, 233**
27.61	Suture of laceration of palate **45, 195**
27.62	Correction of cleft palate **14, 16, 44**
27.63	Revision of cleft palate repair **44, 103**
27.69	Other plastic repair of palate **14, 16, 44, 103**
27.7*	Operations on uvula **45, 233**
27.92	Incision of mouth, unspecified structure **45, 103, 195, 233**
27.99	Other operations on oral cavity **45, 195, 233**
28.0	Incision and drainage of tonsil and peritonsillar structures **44**
28.11	Biopsy of tonsils and adenoids **44, 233**
28.19	Other diagnostic procedures on tonsils and adenoids **44**

*Code Range

37.89	Revision or removal of pacemaker device **14, 16, 64, 195, 233**
37.90	Insertion of left atrial appendage device **63**
37.91	Open chest cardiac massage **50, 59, 178, 195**
37.94	Implantation or replacement of automatic cardioverter/defibrillator, total system (AICD) **57**
37.95	Implantation of automatic cardioverter/defibrillator leads(s) only **57, 58, 65**
37.96	Implantation of automatic cardioverter/defibrillator pulse generator only **57, 58, 62**
37.97	Replacement of automatic cardioverter/defibrillator leads(s) only **57, 58, 65**
37.98	Replacement of automatic cardioverter/defibrillator pulse generator only **57, 58, 62**
37.99	Other operations on heart and pericardium **59**
38.0*	Incision of vessel **195**
38.00	Incision of vessel, unspecified site **44, 63, 112, 233**
38.01	Incision of intracranial vessels **8, 10, 11**
38.02	Incision of other vessels of head and neck **14, 16, 44, 63, 112**
38.03	Incision of upper limb vessels **63, 112**
38.04	Incision of aorta **59, 74**
38.05	Incision of other thoracic vessels **50, 59, 72**
38.06	Incision of abdominal arteries **59, 74, 117**
38.07	Incision of abdominal veins **59, 74, 117**
38.08	Incision of lower limb arteries **63, 112, 178**
38.09	Incision of lower limb veins **64, 233**
38.10	Endarterectomy, unspecified site **13, 63, 196**
38.11	Endarterectomy of intracranial vessels **8, 10, 11**
38.12	Endarterectomy of other vessels of head and neck **13, 44, 63, 112, 196**
38.13	Endarterectomy of upper limb vessels **63, 112, 196**
38.14	Endarterectomy of aorta **59, 74, 196**
38.15	Endarterectomy of other thoracic vessels **50, 59, 196**
38.16	Endarterectomy of abdominal arteries **59, 74, 117, 196**
38.18	Endarterectomy of lower limb arteries **63, 112, 196**
38.21	Biopsy of blood vessel **14, 16, 37, 44, 50, 63, 95, 112, 117, 233**
38.26	Insertion of implantable pressure sensor without lead for intracardiac or great vessel hemodynamic monitoring **64**
38.29	Other diagnostic procedures on blood vessels **63, 112**
38.3*	Resection of vessel with anastomosis **196**
38.30	Resection of vessel with anastomosis, unspecified site **63, 112**
38.31	Resection of intracranial vessels with anastomosis **8, 10, 11**
38.32	Resection of other vessels of head and neck with anastomosis **13, 44, 63**
38.33	Resection of upper limb vessels with anastomosis **63, 112**
38.34	Resection of aorta with anastomosis **59, 74**
38.35	Resection of other thoracic vessels with anastomosis **50, 59, 72**
38.36	Resection of abdominal arteries with anastomosis **59, 74, 117**
38.37	Resection of abdominal veins with anastomosis **59, 74, 117**
38.38	Resection of lower limb arteries with anastomosis **63, 112**
38.39	Resection of lower limb veins with anastomosis **64**
38.4*	Resection of vessel with replacement **196**
38.40	Resection of vessel with replacement, unspecified site **63**
38.41	Resection of intracranial vessels with replacement **8, 10, 11**
38.42	Resection of other vessels of head and neck with replacement **14, 16, 44, 63**
38.43	Resection of upper limb vessels with replacement **63, 112**
38.44	Resection of abdominal aorta with replacement **59**
38.45	Resection of other thoracic vessels with replacement **50, 56, 72**
38.46	Resection of abdominal arteries with replacement **59, 74, 117**
38.47	Resection of abdominal veins with replacement **59, 74, 117**
38.48	Resection of lower limb arteries with replacement **63, 112**

38.49	Resection of lower limb veins with replacement **64**
38.50	Ligation and stripping of varicose veins, unspecified site **64**
38.51	Ligation and stripping of varicose veins of intracranial vessels **8, 10, 11**
38.52	Ligation and stripping of varicose veins of other vessels of head and neck **63**
38.53	Ligation and stripping of varicose veins of upper limb vessels **64**
38.55	Ligation and stripping of varicose veins of other thoracic vessel **50, 59, 112**
38.57	Ligation and stripping of abdominal varicose veins **63, 74**
38.59	Ligation and stripping of lower limb varicose veins **64, 233**
38.6*	Other excision of vessels **196**
38.60	Other excision of vessels, unspecified site **63, 112**
38.61	Other excision of intracranial vessels **8, 10, 11**
38.62	Other excision of other vessels of head and neck **13, 44, 63**
38.63	Other excision of upper limb vessels **63, 112**
38.64	Other excision of abdominal aorta **59, 74**
38.65	Other excision of other thoracic vessel **50, 59, 72**
38.66	Other excision of abdominal arteries **59, 74, 117**
38.67	Other excision of abdominal veins **59, 74, 117**
38.68	Other excision of lower limb arteries **63, 112**
38.69	Other excision of lower limb veins **64**
38.7	Interruption of the vena cava **14, 16, 50, 63, 74, 82, 95, 112, 117, 123, 129, 139, 175, 196**
38.8*	Other surgical occlusion of vessels **196**
38.80	Other surgical occlusion of vessels, unspecified site **63**
38.81	Other surgical occlusion of intracranial vessels **8, 10, 11, 219**
38.82	Other surgical occlusion of other vessels of head and neck **14, 16, 44, 63**
38.83	Other surgical occlusion of upper limb vessels **63, 112**
38.84	Other surgical occlusion of abdominal aorta **59, 74**
38.85	Other surgical occlusion of other thoracic vessel **50, 59, 72**
38.86	Other surgical occlusion of abdominal arteries **59, 74, 117, 233**
38.87	Other surgical occlusion of abdominal veins **59, 74, 117**
38.88	Other surgical occlusion of lower limb arteries **63, 112**
38.89	Other surgical occlusion of lower limb veins **64**
39.0	Systemic to pulmonary artery shunt **59**
39.1	Intra-abdominal venous shunt **59, 72, 81**
39.21	Caval-pulmonary artery anastomosis **59**
39.22	Aorta-subclavian-carotid bypass **13, 59, 196**
39.23	Other intrathoracic vascular shunt or bypass **59, 196**
39.24	Aorta-renal bypass **59, 116, 196**
39.25	Aorta-iliac-femoral bypass **59, 104, 112, 196**
39.26	Other intra-abdominal vascular shunt or bypass **59, 74, 82, 116, 196**
39.27	Arteriovenostomy for renal dialysis **64, 74, 112, 117, 196**
39.28	Extracranial-intracranial (EC-IC) vascular bypass **8, 10, 11, 196**
39.29	Other (peripheral) vascular shunt or bypass **13, 50, 63, 82, 104, 112, 196**
39.3*	Suture of vessel **13, 196**
39.30	Suture of unspecified blood vessel **63**
39.31	Suture of artery **50, 63, 104, 112**
39.32	Suture of vein **64**
39.4*	Revision of vascular procedure **196**
39.41	Control of hemorrhage following vascular surgery **63, 112**
39.42	Revision of arteriovenous shunt for renal dialysis **64, 112, 117**
39.43	Removal of arteriovenous shunt for renal dialysis **64, 117**
39.49	Other revision of vascular procedure **63, 74, 82, 112, 117**
39.50	Angioplasty of other non-coronary vessel(s) **13, 50, 63, 74, 82, 95, 104, 112, 117, 196**

*Code Range

39.51	Clipping of aneurysm **8, 10, 11, 63**	
39.52	Other repair of aneurysm **8, 10, 11, 59, 117, 196**	
39.53	Repair of arteriovenous fistula **8, 10, 11, 63**	
39.54	Re-entry operation (aorta) **50, 59**	
39.55	Reimplantation of aberrant renal vessel **63, 116**	
39.56	Repair of blood vessel with tissue patch graft **13, 63, 112, 117, 196**	
39.57	Repair of blood vessel with synthetic patch graft **13, 63, 112, 117, 196**	
39.58	Repair of blood vessel with unspecified type of patch graft **13, 63, 112, 117, 196**	
39.59	Other repair of vessel **13, 63, 104, 112, 117, 196**	
39.65	Extracorporeal membrane oxygenation (ECMO) **1**	
39.71	Endovascular implantation of other graft in abdominal aorta **59, 60, 117, 196**	
39.72	Endovascular (total) embolization or occlusion of head and neck vessels **8, 10, 11, 59, 60, 117, 196**	
39.73	Endovascular implantation of graft in thoracic aorta **56, 117, 196**	
39.74	Endovascular removal of obstruction from head and neck vessel(s) **8, 10, 11, 196**	
39.75	Endovascular embolization or occlusion of vessel(s) of head or neck using bare coils **8, 10, 11, 59, 60, 117, 196**	
39.76	Endovascular embolization or occlusion of vessel(s) of head or neck using bioactive coils **8, 10, 11, 59, 60, 118, 196**	
39.77	Temporary (partial) therapeutic endovascular occlusion of vessel **13, 63, 196**	
39.78	Endovascular implantation of branching or fenestrated graft(s) in aorta **59, 60**	
39.79	Other endovascular procedures on other vessels **8, 10, 11, 59, 60, 118, 196**	
39.8*	Operations on carotid body, carotid sinus and other vascular bodies **63**	
39.91	Freeing of vessel **63, 74, 112, 196**	
39.92	Injection of sclerosing agent into vein **13, 64**	
39.93	Insertion of vessel-to-vessel cannula **64, 112, 118, 196**	
39.94	Replacement of vessel-to-vessel cannula **63, 118, 233**	
39.98	Control of hemorrhage, not otherwise specified **44, 50, 64, 74, 82, 95, 104, 112, 118, 123, 129, 139, 178, 196**	
39.99	Other operations on vessels **44, 50, 63, 74, 139, 178, 196**	
40.0	Incision of lymphatic structures **104, 175, 233**	
40.1*	Diagnostic procedures on lymphatic structures **64, 74, 95, 104, 112, 123, 175, 233**	
40.11	Biopsy of lymphatic structure **14, 16, 44, 50, 82, 118, 129**	
40.19	Other diagnostic procedures on lymphatic structures **44, 50, 118**	
40.2*	Simple excision of lymphatic structure **104, 175**	
40.21	Excision of deep cervical lymph node **44, 50, 64, 74, 95, 112, 233**	
40.22	Excision of internal mammary lymph node **50**	
40.23	Excision of axillary lymph node **44, 50, 64, 74, 95, 233**	
40.24	Excision of inguinal lymph node **50, 64, 74, 95, 118, 123, 129, 139, 233**	
40.29	Simple excision of other lymphatic structure **44, 50, 64, 74, 95, 112, 118, 123, 129, 196, 233**	
40.3	Regional lymph node excision **44, 50, 64, 74, 95, 104, 112, 118, 123, 129, 139, 175, 178, 233**	
40.4*	Radical excision of cervical lymph nodes **50, 104, 112, 175, 178**	
40.40	Radical neck dissection, not otherwise specified **43**	
40.41	Radical neck dissection, unilateral **43**	
40.42	Radical neck dissection, bilateral **43**	
40.5*	Radical excision of other lymph nodes **74, 104, 175, 178**	
40.50	Radical excision of lymph nodes, not otherwise specified **43, 50, 118, 123, 126**	
40.51	Radical excision of axillary lymph nodes **95**	

40.52	Radical excision of periaortic lymph nodes **50, 95, 112, 116, 122, 126**
40.53	Radical excision of iliac lymph nodes **95, 112, 116, 122, 126**
40.54	Radical groin dissection **95, 116, 122, 126**
40.59	Radical excision of other lymph nodes **43, 50, 95, 116, 122, 126**
40.6*	Operations on thoracic duct **50, 196**
40.9	Other operations on lymphatic structures **44, 74, 104, 118, 123, 175, 178, 196**
41.00	Bone marrow transplant, not otherwise specified **4**
41.01	Autologous bone marrow transplant without purging **4**
41.02	Allogeneic bone marrow transplant with purging **4**
41.03	Allogeneic bone marrow transplant without purging **4**
41.04	Autologous hematopoietic stem cell transplant without purging **4**
41.05	Allogeneic hematopoietic stem cell transplant without purging **4**
41.06	Cord blood stem cell transplant **4**
41.07	Autologous hematopoietic stem cell transplant with purging **4**
41.08	Allogeneic hematopoietic stem cell transplant with purging **4**
41.09	Autologous bone marrow transplant with purging **4**
41.2	Splenotomy **175, 178, 196**
41.33	Open biopsy of spleen **175, 178**
41.4*	Excision or destruction of lesion or tissue of spleen **175, 178**
41.42	Excision of lesion or tissue of spleen **196**
41.43	Partial splenectomy **95, 196**
41.5	Total splenectomy **64, 74, 95, 175, 178, 196**
41.93	Excision of accessory spleen **175, 178, 196**
41.94	Transplantation of spleen **175, 178**
41.95	Repair and plastic operations on spleen **175, 178, 196**
41.99	Other operations on spleen **175, 178, 196**
42.01	Incision of esophageal web **44, 72**
42.09	Other incision of esophagus **44, 72, 196**
42.1*	Esophagostomy **72, 178, 196**
42.10	Esophagostomy, not otherwise specified **44**
42.11	Cervical esophagostomy **44**
42.12	Exteriorization of esophageal pouch **44**
42.19	Other external fistulization of esophagus **44**
42.21	Operative esophagoscopy by incision **44, 72, 178, 196**
42.25	Open biopsy of esophagus **44, 72, 178**
42.31	Local excision of esophageal diverticulum **44, 72**
42.32	Local excision of other lesion or tissue of esophagus **44, 72, 178**
42.39	Other destruction of lesion or tissue of esophagus **44, 72, 178**
42.4*	Excision of esophagus **72, 178, 196**
42.40	Esophagectomy, not otherwise specified **44**
42.41	Partial esophagectomy **44**
42.42	Total esophagectomy **44**
42.5*	Intrathoracic anastomosis of esophagus **72, 178, 196**
42.51	Intrathoracic esophagoesophagostomy **44**
42.52	Intrathoracic esophagogastrostomy **44**
42.53	Intrathoracic esophageal anastomosis with interposition of small bowel **44**
42.54	Other intrathoracic esophagoenterostomy **44**
42.55	Intrathoracic esophageal anastomosis with interposition of colon **44**
42.56	Other intrathoracic esophagocolostomy **44**
42.58	Intrathoracic esophageal anastomosis with other interposition **44**
42.59	Other intrathoracic anastomosis of esophagus **44**
42.6*	Antesternal anastomosis of esophagus **72, 178, 196**
42.61	Antesternal esophagoesophagostomy **45**
42.62	Antesternal esophagogastrostomy **45**
42.63	Antesternal esophageal anastomosis with interposition of small bowel **45**

42.64	Other antesternal esophagoenterostomy **45**	
42.65	Antesternal esophageal anastomosis with interposition of colon **45**	
42.66	Other antesternal esophagocolostomy **45**	
42.68	Other antesternal esophageal anastomosis with interposition **45**	
42.69	Other antesternal anastomosis of esophagus **45**	
42.7	Esophagomyotomy **45, 72, 178, 196**	
42.82	Suture of laceration of esophagus **45, 72, 178, 196**	
42.83	Closure of esophagostomy **45, 72, 178, 196**	
42.84	Repair of esophageal fistula, not elsewhere classified **45, 72, 178, 196**	
42.85	Repair of esophageal stricture **72, 179, 196**	
42.86	Production of subcutaneous tunnel without esophageal anastomosis **45, 72, 179, 196**	
42.87	Other graft of esophagus **45, 72, 179, 196**	
42.89	Other repair of esophagus **45, 72, 179, 196**	
42.91	Ligation of esophageal varices **72, 82**	
43.0	Gastrotomy **72, 82, 112, 179, 196**	
43.3	Pyloromyotomy **72**	
43.42	Local excision of other lesion or tissue of stomach **72, 82, 112**	
43.49	Other destruction of lesion or tissue of stomach **72, 233**	
43.5	Partial gastrectomy with anastomosis to esophagus **72, 179, 196**	
43.6	Partial gastrectomy with anastomosis to duodenum **64, 72, 179, 196**	
43.7	Partial gastrectomy with anastomosis to jejunum **64, 72, 112, 179, 196**	
43.8*	Other partial gastrectomy **72, 179, 196**	
43.82	Laparoscopic vertical (sleeve) gastrectomy **64, 111**	
43.89	Open and other partial gastrectomy **64, 111**	
43.9*	Total gastrectomy **72, 179, 196**	
43.99	Other total gastrectomy **64**	
44.0*	Vagotomy **72**	
44.00	Vagotomy, not otherwise specified **14, 16**	
44.11	Transabdominal gastroscopy **72, 82, 179, 196**	
44.15	Open biopsy of stomach **72, 233**	
44.21	Dilation of pylorus by incision **72**	
44.29	Other pyloroplasty **72**	
44.3*	Gastroenterostomy without gastrectomy **72, 111, 179**	
44.32	Percutaneous [endoscopic] gastrojejunostomy **82**	
44.38	Laparoscopic gastroenterostomy **64, 82**	
44.39	Other gastroenterostomy without gastrectomy **64, 82**	
44.40	Suture of peptic ulcer, not otherwise specified **72**	
44.41	Suture of gastric ulcer site **72**	
44.42	Suture of duodenal ulcer site **72**	
44.5	Revision of gastric anastomosis **72, 111, 196**	
44.61	Suture of laceration of stomach **72, 196**	
44.63	Closure of other gastric fistula **72, 82, 179, 196**	
44.64	Gastropexy **72, 196**	
44.65	Esophagogastroplasty **72, 196**	
44.66	Other procedures for creation of esophagogastric sphincteric competence **72, 196**	
44.67	Laparoscopic procedures for creation of esophagogastric sphincteric competence **72, 196, 234**	
44.68	Laparoscopic gastroplasty **72, 111, 196, 234**	
44.69	Other repair of stomach **72, 111, 196**	
44.91	Ligation of gastric varices **72, 82**	
44.92	Intraoperative manipulation of stomach **72, 82, 112, 196**	
44.95	Laparoscopic gastric restrictive procedure **111, 234**	
44.96	Laparoscopic revision of gastric restrictive procedure **111, 234**	
44.97	Laparoscopic removal of gastric restrictive device(s) **111, 234**	

44.98	(Laparoscopic) adjustment of size of adjustable gastric restrictive device **111, 234**	
44.99	Other operations on stomach **72, 111, 196**	
45.0*	Enterotomy **196**	
45.00	Incision of intestine, not otherwise specified **73**	
45.01	Incision of duodenum **72, 82**	
45.02	Other incision of small intestine **73, 179**	
45.03	Incision of large intestine **73, 179**	
45.11	Transabdominal endoscopy of small intestine **73, 179, 196, 234**	
45.15	Open biopsy of small intestine **73**	
45.21	Transabdominal endoscopy of large intestine **73, 196, 234**	
45.26	Open biopsy of large intestine **73, 234**	
45.31	Other local excision of lesion of duodenum **72, 82, 179, 234**	
45.32	Other destruction of lesion of duodenum **72, 82, 179, 234**	
45.33	Local excision of lesion or tissue of small intestine, except duodenum **74, 179, 234**	
45.34	Other destruction of lesion of small intestine, except duodenum **73, 179, 234**	
45.41	Excision of lesion or tissue of large intestine **74, 112, 179, 234**	
45.49	Other destruction of lesion of large intestine **73, 179, 234**	
45.5*	Isolation of intestinal segment **72**	
45.50	Isolation of intestinal segment, not otherwise specified **179**	
45.6*	Other excision of small intestine **72, 196**	
45.61	Multiple segmental resection of small intestine **64, 179**	
45.62	Other partial resection of small intestine **64, 112, 179**	
45.63	Total removal of small intestine **179**	
45.7*	Open and other partial excision of large intestine **72, 196**	
45.71	Open and other multiple segmental resection of large intestine **179**	
45.72	Open and other cecectomy **64**	
45.73	Open and other right hemicolectomy **64, 179**	
45.74	Open and other resection of transverse colon **64, 179**	
45.75	Open and other left hemicolectomy **64, 112, 179**	
45.76	Open and other sigmoidectomy **179**	
45.79	Other and unspecified partial excision of large intestine **64, 179**	
45.8*	Total intra-abdominal colectomy **64, 72, 179, 196**	
45.9*	Intestinal anastomosis **72, 196**	
45.90	Intestinal anastomosis, not otherwise specified **111, 179**	
45.91	Small-to-small intestinal anastomosis **111, 179**	
45.92	Anastomosis of small intestine to rectal stump **179**	
45.93	Other small-to-large intestinal anastomosis **64, 112, 179**	
45.94	Large-to-large intestinal anastomosis **112, 179**	
45.95	Anastomosis to anus **179**	
46.0*	Exteriorization of intestine **72, 179, 196**	
46.03	Exteriorization of large intestine **64**	
46.10	Colostomy, not otherwise specified **72, 179, 196**	
46.11	Temporary colostomy **72, 179, 196**	
46.13	Permanent colostomy **64, 72, 179, 196**	
46.20	Ileostomy, not otherwise specified **72, 179, 196**	
46.21	Temporary ileostomy **72, 179, 196**	
46.22	Continent ileostomy **72, 179, 196**	
46.23	Other permanent ileostomy **72, 179, 196**	
46.4*	Revision of intestinal stoma **74, 196**	
46.40	Revision of intestinal stoma, not otherwise specified **179**	
46.41	Revision of stoma of small intestine **179, 234**	
46.43	Other revision of stoma of large intestine **234**	
46.5*	Closure of intestinal stoma **73, 196**	
46.52	Closure of stoma of large intestine **234**	
46.6*	Fixation of intestine **73**	
46.7*	Other repair of intestine **196**	

*Code Range

© 2013 OptumInsight, Inc.

46.71	Suture of laceration of duodenum **72**	49.45	Ligation of hemorrhoids **74, 234**
46.72	Closure of fistula of duodenum **72**	49.46	Excision of hemorrhoids **74, 139, 234**
46.73	Suture of laceration of small intestine, except duodenum **72**	49.49	Other procedures on hemorrhoids **74, 234**
46.74	Closure of fistula of small intestine, except duodenum **72**	49.5*	Division of anal sphincter **74, 234**
46.75	Suture of laceration of large intestine **72**	49.59	Other anal sphincterotomy **147**
46.76	Closure of fistula of large intestine **72**	49.6	Excision of anus **74, 234**
46.79	Other repair of intestine **72**	49.71	Suture of laceration of anus **74, 104, 196**
46.80	Intra-abdominal manipulation of intestine, not otherwise specified **72, 82, 179, 196**	49.72	Anal cerclage **74, 104**
46.81	Intra-abdominal manipulation of small intestine **72, 82, 179, 196**	49.73	Closure of anal fistula **74, 104, 196**
46.82	Intra-abdominal manipulation of large intestine **72, 82, 179, 196**	49.74	Gracilis muscle transplant for anal incontinence **74**
46.91	Myotomy of sigmoid colon **72**	49.75	Implantation or revision of artificial anal sphincter **73, 104, 196**
46.92	Myotomy of other parts of colon **72**	49.76	Removal of artificial anal sphincter **73, 104, 196**
46.93	Revision of anastomosis of small intestine **72, 196**	49.79	Other repair of anal sphincter **74, 104, 196, 234**
46.94	Revision of anastomosis of large intestine **72, 196**	49.9*	Other operations on anus **74**
46.97	Transplant of intestine **1**	49.95	Control of (postoperative) hemorrhage of anus **196**
46.99	Other operations on intestines **72, 82, 179, 196**	49.99	Other operations on anus **196**
47.0*	Appendectomy **73**	50.0	Hepatotomy **81, 196**
47.09	Other appendectomy **64**	50.12	Open biopsy of liver **45, 50, 64, 74, 82, 95, 104, 112, 118, 123, 129, 175, 179, 196**
47.1*	Incidental appendectomy **129, 196**	50.14	Laparoscopic liver biopsy **74, 82, 104, 118, 175, 179, 196**
47.2	Drainage of appendiceal abscess **73**	50.19	Other diagnostic procedures on liver **74, 82, 104, 118, 175, 179, 197**
47.91	Appendicostomy **73**	50.21	Marsupialization of lesion of liver **81**
47.92	Closure of appendiceal fistula **72, 196**	50.22	Partial hepatectomy **81, 197**
47.99	Other operations on appendix **73**	50.23	Open ablation of liver lesion or tissue **74, 81**
48.0	Proctotomy **73, 196**	50.24	Percutaneous ablation of liver lesion or tissue **74, 81**
48.1	Proctostomy **72, 196**	50.25	Laparoscopic ablation of liver lesion or tissue **74, 81**
48.21	Transabdominal proctosigmoidoscopy **73, 196**	50.26	Other and unspecified ablation of liver lesion or tissue **74, 81**
48.25	Open biopsy of rectum **64, 73, 234**	50.29	Other destruction of lesion of liver **74, 81**
48.35	Local excision of rectal lesion or tissue **64, 74, 104, 234**	50.3	Lobectomy of liver **81, 197**
48.4*	Pull-through resection of rectum **73, 179**	50.4	Total hepatectomy **81, 197**
48.40	Pull-through resection of rectum, not otherwise specified **196**	50.51	Auxiliary liver transplant **1**
48.42	Laparoscopic pull-through resection of rectum **196**	50.59	Other transplant of liver **1**
48.43	Open pull-through resection of rectum **196**	50.6*	Repair of liver **197**
48.49	Other pull-through resection of rectum **196**	50.61	Closure of laceration of liver **81**
48.5*	Abdominoperineal resection of rectum **73, 179, 196**	50.69	Other repair of liver **81**
48.6*	Other resection of rectum **73, 179, 196**	51.02	Trocar cholecystostomy **81**
48.62	Anterior resection of rectum with synchronous colostomy **64**	51.03	Other cholecystostomy **74, 81**
48.63	Other anterior resection of rectum **64**	51.04	Other cholecystotomy **81**
48.69	Other resection of rectum **64, 122**	51.13	Open biopsy of gallbladder or bile ducts **74, 82**
48.7*	Repair of rectum **196**	51.19	Other diagnostic procedures on biliary tract **74, 82**
48.71	Suture of laceration of rectum **72, 147**	51.2*	Cholecystectomy **81, 179, 197**
48.72	Closure of proctostomy **72**	51.21	Other partial cholecystectomy **81**
48.73	Closure of other rectal fistula **74, 104, 128**	51.22	Cholecystectomy **74, 81**
48.74	Rectorectostomy **72**	51.23	Laparoscopic cholecystectomy **74, 82, 234**
48.75	Abdominal proctopexy **72**	51.24	Laparoscopic partial cholecystectomy **82**
48.76	Other proctopexy **72**	51.3*	Anastomosis of gallbladder or bile duct **81, 179, 197**
48.79	Other repair of rectum **74, 139**	51.32	Anastomosis of gallbladder to intestine **75**
48.8*	Incision or excision of perirectal tissue or lesion **74, 104, 196, 234**	51.36	Choledochoenterostomy **75**
48.9*	Other operations on rectum and perirectal tissue **74**	51.37	Anastomosis of hepatic duct to gastrointestinal tract **75**
48.91	Incision of rectal stricture **196**	51.41	Common duct exploration for removal of calculus **81**
49.01	Incision of perianal abscess **74, 104**	51.42	Common duct exploration for relief of other obstruction **81, 179, 197**
49.02	Other incision of perianal tissue **74, 104**	51.43	Insertion of choledochohepatic tube for decompression **81, 179, 197**
49.04	Other excision of perianal tissue **74, 104**		
49.1*	Incision or excision of anal fistula **74, 196, 234**	51.49	Incision of other bile ducts for relief of obstruction **81, 179**
49.11	Anal fistulotomy **104**	51.51	Exploration of common bile duct **81**
49.12	Anal fistulectomy **104**	51.59	Incision of other bile duct **75, 81, 179, 197**
49.39	Other local excision or destruction of lesion or tissue of anus **74, 104, 234**	51.61	Excision of cystic duct remnant **81, 197**
49.44	Destruction of hemorrhoids by cryotherapy **74, 234**		

Numeric Index to Procedures

56.4*	Ureterectomy **116, 197**	
56.41	Partial ureterectomy **123, 129**	
56.5*	Cutaneous uretero-ileostomy **116, 123, 129, 179, 197**	
56.52	Revision of cutaneous uretero-ileostomy **234**	
56.6*	Other external urinary diversion **116, 123, 129, 179, 197**	
56.7*	Other anastomosis or bypass of ureter **116, 197**	
56.71	Urinary diversion to intestine **123, 129, 179**	
56.72	Revision of ureterointestinal anastomosis **123, 129, 179**	
56.73	Nephrocystanastomosis, not otherwise specified **123, 129, 179**	
56.75	Transureteroureterostomy **123, 129, 179**	
56.8*	Repair of ureter **116**	
56.81	Lysis of intraluminal adhesions of ureter **197**	
56.82	Suture of laceration of ureter **197**	
56.83	Closure of ureterostomy **123, 129, 179, 197**	
56.84	Closure of other fistula of ureter **73, 123, 129, 179, 197**	
56.86	Removal of ligature from ureter **197**	
56.89	Other repair of ureter **197**	
56.92	Implantation of electronic ureteral stimulator **116**	
56.93	Replacement of electronic ureteral stimulator **116**	
56.94	Removal of electronic ureteral stimulator **116**	
56.95	Ligation of ureter **116, 197**	
56.99	Other operations on ureter **116, 197**	
57.12	Lysis of intraluminal adhesions with incision into bladder **116, 197**	
57.18	Other suprapubic cystostomy **116, 123, 128, 179, 197**	
57.19	Other cystotomy **116, 197**	
57.2*	Vesicostomy **116, 123, 197**	
57.21	Vesicostomy **128, 179**	
57.22	Revision or closure of vesicostomy **129, 179, 234**	
57.33	Closed (transurethral) biopsy of bladder **117, 123, 129, 234**	
57.34	Open biopsy of bladder **116, 123, 129, 179**	
57.39	Other diagnostic procedures on bladder **116, 123, 179, 197, 234**	
57.4*	Transurethral excision or destruction of bladder tissue **117**	
57.49	Other transurethral excision or destruction of lesion or tissue of bladder **123, 234**	
57.5*	Other excision or destruction of bladder tissue **116, 123, 129**	
57.59	Open excision or destruction of other lesion or tissue of bladder **179, 234**	
57.6	Partial cystectomy **116, 122, 129, 179, 197**	
57.7*	Total cystectomy **116, 122, 129, 179**	
57.79	Other total cystectomy **197**	
57.81	Suture of laceration of bladder **116, 197**	
57.82	Closure of cystostomy **116, 123, 129, 179, 197, 234**	
57.83	Repair of fistula involving bladder and intestine **73, 116, 123, 129, 179, 197**	
57.84	Repair of other fistula of bladder **116, 123, 129, 179, 197**	
57.85	Cystourethroplasty and plastic repair of bladder neck **116, 128**	
57.86	Repair of bladder exstrophy **116**	
57.87	Reconstruction of urinary bladder **116, 197**	
57.88	Other anastomosis of bladder **116, 123, 179**	
57.89	Other repair of bladder **116, 129, 197**	
57.91	Sphincterotomy of bladder **116, 234**	
57.93	Control of (postoperative) hemorrhage of bladder **116, 197**	
57.96	Implantation of electronic bladder stimulator **117**	
57.97	Replacement of electronic bladder stimulator **117, 234**	
57.98	Removal of electronic bladder stimulator **117, 234**	
57.99	Other operations on bladder **117, 197**	
58.0	Urethrotomy **117, 129, 197, 234**	
58.1	Urethral meatotomy **117, 123, 197, 234**	
58.4*	Repair of urethra **117**	
58.41	Suture of laceration of urethra **197**	
58.42	Closure of urethrostomy **197**	
58.43	Closure of other fistula of urethra **122, 129, 179, 197**	
58.44	Reanastomosis of urethra **197**	
58.45	Repair of hypospadias or epispadias **122**	
58.46	Other reconstruction of urethra **122, 197**	
58.47	Urethral meatoplasty **123**	
58.49	Other repair of urethra **122, 129, 197**	
58.5	Release of urethral stricture **117, 122, 129, 197, 234**	
58.91	Incision of periurethral tissue **117**	
58.92	Excision of periurethral tissue **117**	
58.93	Implantation of artificial urinary sphincter (AUS) **117, 197**	
58.99	Other operations on urethra and periurethral tissue **117, 123, 129, 234**	
59.00	Retroperitoneal dissection, not otherwise specified **95, 104, 116, 122, 129, 179**	
59.02	Other lysis of perirenal or periureteral adhesions **116, 123, 129, 179, 197**	
59.03	Laparoscopic lysis of perirenal or periureteral adhesions **116, 123, 129, 179, 197**	
59.09	Other incision of perirenal or periureteral tissue **116, 123, 129, 179, 197**	
59.1*	Incision of perivesical tissue **117, 123, 129, 179, 197**	
59.2*	Diagnostic procedures on perirenal and perivesical tissue **117, 123, 179, 197**	
59.3	Plication of urethrovesical junction **117**	
59.4	Suprapubic sling operation **117, 128**	
59.5	Retropubic urethral suspension **117, 128**	
59.6	Paraurethral suspension **117, 128**	
59.71	Levator muscle operation for urethrovesical suspension **117, 128**	
59.79	Other repair of urinary stress incontinence **117, 128, 234**	
59.91	Excision of perirenal or perivesical tissue **117, 123, 179**	
59.92	Other operations on perirenal or perivesical tissue **117, 123, 179**	
60.0	Incision of prostate **123, 232**	
60.12	Open biopsy of prostate **117, 123, 232**	
60.14	Open biopsy of seminal vesicles **123**	
60.15	Biopsy of periprostatic tissue **123, 232**	
60.18	Other diagnostic procedures on prostate and periprostatic tissue **123, 232**	
60.19	Other diagnostic procedures on seminal vesicles **123**	
60.2*	Transurethral prostatectomy **117, 122, 232**	
60.3	Suprapubic prostatectomy **117, 122**	
60.4	Retropubic prostatectomy **117, 122**	
60.5	Radical prostatectomy **117, 122**	
60.61	Local excision of lesion of prostate **123, 232**	
60.62	Perineal prostatectomy **117, 122**	
60.69	Other prostatectomy **117, 122, 232**	
60.72	Incision of seminal vesicle **123**	
60.73	Excision of seminal vesicle **123**	
60.79	Other operations on seminal vesicles **123**	
60.8*	Incision or excision of periprostatic tissue **123, 232**	
60.93	Repair of prostate **123, 197, 232**	
60.94	Control of (postoperative) hemorrhage of prostate **123, 197, 232**	
60.95	Transurethral balloon dilation of the prostatic urethra **117, 123, 232**	
60.96	Transurethral destruction of prostate tissue by microwave thermotherapy **117, 122, 232**	
60.97	Other transurethral destruction of prostate tissue by other thermotherapy **117, 122, 232**	
60.99	Other operations on prostate **123, 232**	
61.2	Excision of hydrocele (of tunica vaginalis) **122, 234**	

61.42	Repair of scrotal fistula **122**, **197**
61.49	Other repair of scrotum and tunica vaginalis **122**, **197**
61.92	Excision of lesion of tunica vaginalis other than hydrocele **122**
61.99	Other operations on scrotum and tunica vaginalis **122**, **197**
62.0	Incision of testis **122**, **197**
62.12	Open biopsy of testis **122**
62.19	Other diagnostic procedures on testes **122**
62.2	Excision or destruction of testicular lesion **122**
62.3	Unilateral orchiectomy **122**, **197**
62.4*	Bilateral orchiectomy **122**, **197**
62.41	Removal of both testes at same operative episode **95**
62.5	Orchiopexy **122**
62.6*	Repair of testes **122**, **197**
62.7	Insertion of testicular prosthesis **112**, **122**
62.99	Other operations on testes **122**, **197**
63.09	Other diagnostic procedures on spermatic cord, epididymis, and vas deferens **122**, **234**
63.1	Excision of varicocele and hydrocele of spermatic cord **122**, **234**
63.2	Excision of cyst of epididymis **122**, **234**
63.3	Excision of other lesion or tissue of spermatic cord and epididymis **122**, **234**
63.4	Epididymectomy **122**
63.51	Suture of laceration of spermatic cord and epididymis **122**, **197**
63.53	Transplantation of spermatic cord **122**, **197**
63.59	Other repair of spermatic cord and epididymis **122**, **197**
63.81	Suture of laceration of vas deferens and epididymis **122**, **197**
63.82	Reconstruction of surgically divided vas deferens **122**, **197**
63.83	Epididymovasostomy **122**
63.85	Removal of valve from vas deferens **122**
63.89	Other repair of vas deferens and epididymis **122**, **197**
63.92	Epididymotomy **122**
63.93	Incision of spermatic cord **122**
63.94	Lysis of adhesions of spermatic cord **122**, **197**
63.95	Insertion of valve in vas deferens **122**
63.99	Other operations on spermatic card, epididymis, and vas deferens **122**, **197**
64.11	Biopsy of penis **104**, **122**, **234**
64.2	Local excision or destruction of lesion of penis **104**, **122**, **234**
64.3	Amputation of penis **122**
64.4*	Repair and plastic operation on penis **122**
64.41	Suture of laceration of penis **197**
64.43	Construction of penis **197**
64.44	Reconstruction of penis **197**
64.45	Replantation of penis **197**
64.49	Other repair of penis **104**, **197**, **234**
64.5	Operations for sex transformation, not elsewhere classified **122**, **128**
64.92	Incision of penis **122**, **234**
64.93	Division of penile adhesions **122**, **234**
64.95	Insertion or replacement of non-inflatable penile prosthesis **118**, **122**, **234**
64.96	Removal of internal prosthesis of penis **118**, **122**, **234**
64.97	Insertion or replacement of inflatable penile prosthesis **118**, **122**, **234**
64.98	Other operations on penis **122**, **234**
64.99	Other operations on male genital organs **122**, **234**
65.22	Wedge resection of ovary **112**
65.24	Laparoscopic wedge resection of ovary **112**
65.5*	Bilateral oophorectomy **104**

65.61	Other removal of both ovaries and tubes at same operative episode **104**, **234**
65.63	Laparoscopic removal of both ovaries and tubes at same operative episode **104**
65.7*	Repair of ovary **197**
65.8*	Lysis of adhesions of ovary and fallopian tube **197**
65*	Operations on ovary **126**, **128**
66.0*	Salpingotomy **126**, **128**
66.1*	Diagnostic procedures on fallopian tubes **126**, **128**
66.2*	Bilateral endoscopic destruction or occlusion of fallopian tubes **128**, **139**, **234**
66.3*	Other bilateral destruction or occlusion of fallopian tubes **128**, **139**, **234**
66.4	Total unilateral salpingectomy **126**, **128**, **139**
66.5*	Total bilateral salpingectomy **126**, **128**, **139**
66.61	Excision or destruction of lesion of fallopian tube **126**, **128**
66.62	Salpingectomy with removal of tubal pregnancy **126**, **128**, **139**
66.63	Bilateral partial salpingectomy, not otherwise specified **128**, **139**
66.69	Other partial salpingectomy **126**, **128**, **139**
66.7*	Repair of fallopian tube **126**, **128**
66.71	Simple suture of fallopian tube **197**
66.79	Other repair of fallopian tube **197**
66.92	Unilateral destruction or occlusion of fallopian tube **126**, **128**, **139**, **234**
66.93	Implantation or replacement of prosthesis of fallopian tube **126**, **128**
66.94	Removal of prosthesis of fallopian tube **126**, **128**
66.95	Insufflation of therapeutic agent into fallopian tubes **129**
66.96	Dilation of fallopian tube **126**, **128**
66.97	Burying of fimbriae in uterine wall **126**, **128**, **139**
66.99	Other operations on fallopian tubes **126**, **128**
67.1*	Diagnostic procedures on cervix **104**, **128**, **139**, **234**
67.2	Conization of cervix **128**, **139**, **234**
67.3*	Other excision or destruction of lesion or tissue of cervix **128**, **139**, **234**
67.39	Other excision or destruction of lesion or tissue of cervix **104**
67.4	Amputation of cervix **128**
67.5*	Repair of internal cervical os **198**
67.51	Transabdominal cerclage of cervix **128**, **147**
67.59	Other repair of cervical os **128**, **147**
67.6*	Other repair of cervix **128**, **198**
67.61	Suture of laceration of cervix **147**
67.62	Repair of fistula of cervix **139**
67.69	Other repair of cervix **147**
68.0	Hysterotomy **126**, **128**, **139**, **198**
68.13	Open biopsy of uterus **126**, **128**
68.14	Open biopsy of uterine ligaments **126**, **128**
68.15	Closed biopsy of uterine ligaments **128**, **234**
68.16	Closed biopsy of uterus **128**, **234**
68.19	Other diagnostic procedures on uterus and supporting structures **126**, **128**
68.21	Division of endometrial synechiae **128**
68.22	Incision or excision of congenital septum of uterus **128**
68.23	Endometrial ablation **126**, **128**
68.24	Uterine artery embolization [UAE] with coils **129**
68.25	Uterine artery embolization [UAE] without coils **129**
68.29	Other excision or destruction of lesion of uterus **126**, **128**, **234**
68.3*	Subtotal abdominal hysterectomy **126**, **128**, **139**
68.41	Laparoscopic total abdominal hysterectomy **126**, **128**, **139**
68.49	Other and unspecified total abdominal hysterectomy **126**, **128**, **139**

*Code Range

68.5*	Vaginal hysterectomy **126, 128, 139, 234**	
68.61	Laparoscopic radical abdominal hysterectomy **126, 139**	
68.69	Other and unspecified radical abdominal hysterectomy **126, 139**	
68.71	Laparoscopic radical vaginal hysterectomy [LRVH] **126, 139**	
68.79	Other and unspecified radical vaginal hysterectomy **126, 139**	
68.8	Pelvic evisceration **73, 126**	
68.9	Other and unspecified hysterectomy **126, 128, 139**	
69.0*	Dilation and curettage of uterus **140**	
69.01	Dilation and curettage for termination of pregnancy **234**	
69.02	Dilation and curettage following delivery or abortion **139**	
69.09	Other dilation and curettage of uterus **128, 139, 234**	
69.19	Other excision or destruction of uterus and supporting structures **126, 128**	
69.2*	Repair of uterine supporting structures **128**	
69.23	Vaginal repair of chronic inversion of uterus **198**	
69.29	Other repair of uterus and supporting structures **198**	
69.3	Paracervical uterine denervation **126, 128**	
69.4*	Uterine repair **126, 128, 198**	
69.41	Suture of laceration of uterus **139**	
69.42	Closure of fistula of uterus **73**	
69.49	Other repair of uterus **139**	
69.51	Aspiration curettage of uterus for termination of pregnancy **140, 234**	
69.52	Aspiration curettage following delivery or abortion **139, 140, 234**	
69.95	Incision of cervix **128, 139, 234**	
69.97	Removal of other penetrating foreign body from cervix **128, 198**	
69.98	Other operations on supporting structures of uterus **128**	
69.99	Other operations on cervix and uterus **129**	
70.12	Culdotomy **129, 140**	
70.13	Lysis of intraluminal adhesions of vagina **128, 147, 198**	
70.14	Other vaginotomy **128, 147, 234**	
70.23	Biopsy of cul-de-sac **128, 140, 234**	
70.24	Vaginal biopsy **104, 128, 147, 234**	
70.29	Other diagnostic procedures on vagina and cul-de-sac **128, 140, 234**	
70.3*	Local excision or destruction of vagina and cul-de-sac **128, 234**	
70.31	Hymenectomy **147**	
70.32	Excision or destruction of lesion of cul-de-sac **140**	
70.33	Excision or destruction of lesion of vagina **104, 147**	
70.4	Obliteration and total excision of vagina **128**	
70.5*	Repair of cystocele and rectocele **129**	
70.50	Repair of cystocele and rectocele **75, 117**	
70.51	Repair of cystocele **117**	
70.52	Repair of rectocele **72**	
70.53	Repair of cystocele and rectocele with graft or prosthesis **72, 116**	
70.54	Repair of cystocele with graft or prosthesis **117**	
70.55	Repair of rectocele with graft or prosthesis **72**	
70.6*	Vaginal construction and reconstruction **129**	
70.62	Vaginal reconstruction **198**	
70.64	Vaginal reconstruction with graft or prosthesis **198**	
70.71	Suture of laceration of vagina **104, 128, 147, 198**	
70.72	Repair of colovaginal fistula **72, 128, 179, 198**	
70.73	Repair of rectovaginal fistula **72, 128, 179, 198**	
70.74	Repair of other vaginoenteric fistula **72, 128, 179, 198**	
70.75	Repair of other fistula of vagina **73, 128, 179, 198**	
70.76	Hymenorrhaphy **128, 234**	
70.77	Vaginal suspension and fixation **117, 129**	
70.78	Vaginal suspension and fixation with graft or prosthesis **117, 129**	
70.79	Other repair of vagina **128, 147, 198**	

70.8	Obliteration of vaginal vault **129**
70.91	Other operations on vagina **128**
70.92	Other operations on cul-de-sac **128**
70.93	Other operations on cul-de-sac with graft or prosthesis **128**
71.0*	Incision of vulva and perineum **128, 147**
71.01	Lysis of vulvar adhesions **198**
71.09	Other incision of vulva and perineum **104, 234**
71.1*	Diagnostic procedures on vulva **104, 128, 147, 234**
71.22	Incision of Bartholin's gland (cyst) **128, 140, 234**
71.23	Marsupialization of Bartholin's gland (cyst) **128, 140, 234**
71.24	Excision or other destruction of Bartholin's gland (cyst) **104, 128, 140, 234**
71.29	Other operations on Bartholin's gland **128, 140, 234**
71.3	Other local excision or destruction of vulva and perineum **104, 128, 147, 234**
71.4	Operations on clitoris **128, 234**
71.5	Radical vulvectomy **126**
71.6*	Other vulvectomy **128**
71.62	Bilateral vulvectomy **104**
71.7*	Repair of vulva and perineum **128, 198**
71.71	Suture of laceration of vulva or perineum **104, 147, 234**
71.72	Repair of fistula of vulva or perineum **73**
71.79	Other repair of vulva and perineum **147, 234**
71.8	Other operations on vulva **128**
71.9	Other operations on female genital organs **129**
73.94	Pubiotomy to assist delivery **140**
73.99	Other operations to assist delivery **147**
74.0	Classical cesarean section **139**
74.1	Low cervical cesarean section **139**
74.2	Extraperitoneal cesarean section **139**
74.3	Removal of extratubal ectopic pregnancy **140**
74.4	Cesarean section of other specified type **139**
74.91	Hysterotomy to terminate pregnancy **140**
74.99	Other cesarean section of unspecified type **139**
75.36	Correction of fetal defect **140**
75.50	Repair of current obstetric laceration of uterus, not otherwise specified **147**
75.51	Repair of current obstetric laceration of cervix **147**
75.52	Repair of current obstetric laceration of corpus uteri **140**
75.61	Repair of current obstetric laceration of bladder and urethra **147**
75.93	Surgical correction of inverted uterus **140**
75.99	Other obstetric operations **140**
76.0*	Incision of facial bone without division **198**
76.01	Sequestrectomy of facial bone **43, 95**
76.09	Other incision of facial bone **45, 92**
76.1*	Diagnostic procedures on facial bones and joints **89, 198**
76.11	Biopsy of facial bone **45, 234**
76.19	Other diagnostic procedures on facial bones and joints **43**
76.2	Local excision or destruction of lesion of facial bone **43, 92, 198, 234**
76.3*	Partial ostectomy of facial bone **198**
76.31	Partial mandibulectomy **43, 95**
76.39	Partial ostectomy of other facial bone **43, 95**
76.4*	Excision and reconstruction of facial bones **95, 198**
76.41	Total mandibulectomy with synchronous reconstruction **43**
76.42	Other total mandibulectomy **43**
76.43	Other reconstruction of mandible **43, 104**
76.44	Total ostectomy of other facial bone with synchronous reconstruction **43**
76.45	Other total ostectomy of other facial bone **43**

76.46	Other reconstruction of other facial bone **37, 43**	77.4*	Biopsy of bone **104, 112, 118, 123, 234**
76.5	Temporomandibular arthroplasty **45, 95, 198**	77.40	Biopsy of bone, unspecified site **45, 89**
76.6*	Other facial bone repair and orthognathic surgery **43, 95, 198**	77.41	Biopsy of scapula, clavicle, and thorax (ribs and sternum) **51, 89**
76.70	Reduction of facial fracture, not otherwise specified **43, 95, 198**	77.42	Biopsy of humerus **89**
76.72	Open reduction of malar and zygomatic fracture **43, 95, 198**	77.43	Biopsy of radius and ulna **89**
76.74	Open reduction of maxillary fracture **43, 95, 198**	77.44	Biopsy of carpals and metacarpals **94, 193**
76.76	Open reduction of mandibular fracture **43, 95, 198**	77.45	Biopsy of femur **89**
76.77	Open reduction of alveolar fracture **43, 95, 198**	77.46	Biopsy of patella **89**
76.79	Other open reduction of facial fracture **37, 43, 95, 198**	77.47	Biopsy of tibia and fibula **89**
76.91	Bone graft to facial bone **37, 43, 95, 198**	77.48	Biopsy of tarsals and metatarsals **89**
76.92	Insertion of synthetic implant in facial bone **37, 43, 95, 198**	77.49	Biopsy of other bone, except facial bones **45, 51, 89, 175**
76.94	Open reduction of temporomandibular dislocation **43, 95, 198**	77.5*	Excision and repair of bunion and other toe deformities **93, 234**
76.97	Removal of internal fixation device from facial bone **43, 92, 198**	77.58	Other excision, fusion, and repair of toes **198**
76.99	Other operations on facial bones and joints **43, 95, 198**	77.6*	Local excision of lesion or tissue of bone **234**
77.00	Sequestrectomy, unspecified site **95, 198**	77.60	Local excision of lesion or tissue of bone, unspecified site **92, 198**
77.01	Sequestrectomy of scapula, clavicle, and thorax (ribs and sternum) **50, 95, 198**	77.61	Local excision of lesion or tissue of scapula, clavicle, and thorax (ribs and sternum) **51, 92, 112, 198**
77.02	Sequestrectomy of humerus **91, 198**	77.62	Local excision of lesion or tissue of humerus **92, 198**
77.03	Sequestrectomy of radius and ulna **94, 198**	77.63	Local excision of lesion or tissue of radius and ulna **92, 198**
77.04	Sequestrectomy of carpals and metacarpals **94, 193**	77.64	Local excision of lesion or tissue of carpals and metacarpals **94, 193**
77.05	Sequestrectomy of femur **89, 198, 219**	77.65	Local excision of lesion or tissue of femur **92, 198**
77.06	Sequestrectomy of patella **90, 198**	77.66	Local excision of lesion or tissue of patella **92, 198**
77.07	Sequestrectomy of tibia and fibula **91, 198**	77.67	Local excision of lesion or tissue of tibia and fibula **92, 198**
77.08	Sequestrectomy of tarsals and metatarsals **93, 198**	77.68	Local excision of lesion or tissue of tarsals and metatarsals **93, 112, 198**
77.09	Sequestrectomy of other bone, except facial bones **95, 198**	77.69	Local excision of lesion or tissue of other bone, except facial bones **45, 92, 112, 198**
77.10	Other incision of bone without division, unspecified site **92, 198**	77.70	Excision of bone for graft, unspecified site **92, 198**
77.11	Other incision of scapula, clavicle, and thorax (ribs and sternum) without division **51, 92, 198**	77.71	Excision of scapula, clavicle, and thorax (ribs and sternum) for graft **51, 92, 198**
77.12	Other incision of humerus without division **92, 198**	77.72	Excision of humerus for graft **92, 198**
77.13	Other incision of radius and ulna without division **92, 198**	77.73	Excision of radius and ulna for graft **92, 198**
77.14	Other incision of carpals and metacarpals without division **94, 193**	77.74	Excision of carpals and metacarpals for graft **94, 193**
77.15	Other incision of femur without division **92, 198**	77.75	Excision of femur for graft **92, 198**
77.16	Other incision of patella without division **92, 198**	77.76	Excision of patella for graft **92, 198**
77.17	Other incision of tibia and fibula without division **92, 198**	77.77	Excision of tibia and fibula for graft **92, 198**
77.18	Other incision of tarsals and metatarsals without division **93, 198**	77.78	Excision of tarsals and metatarsals for graft **93, 198**
77.19	Other incision of other bone, except facial bones, without division **45, 92, 198**	77.79	Excision of other bone for graft, except facial bones **45, 92, 198**
77.20	Wedge osteotomy, unspecified site **95, 198**	77.80	Other partial ostectomy, unspecified site **95, 198**
77.21	Wedge osteotomy of scapula, clavicle, and thorax (ribs and sternum) **51, 95, 198**	77.81	Other partial ostectomy of scapula, clavicle, and thorax (ribs and sternum) **12, 13, 51, 95, 198**
77.22	Wedge osteotomy of humerus **91, 198**	77.82	Other partial ostectomy of humerus **91, 198**
77.23	Wedge osteotomy of radius and ulna **94, 198**	77.83	Other partial ostectomy of radius and ulna **94, 198**
77.24	Wedge osteotomy of carpals and metacarpals **94, 193**	77.84	Other partial ostectomy of carpals and metacarpals **94, 193**
77.25	Wedge osteotomy of femur **89, 198, 219**	77.85	Other partial ostectomy of femur **89, 198, 219**
77.26	Wedge osteotomy of patella **90, 198**	77.86	Other partial ostectomy of patella **90, 198**
77.27	Wedge osteotomy of tibia and fibula **91, 112, 198**	77.87	Other partial ostectomy of tibia and fibula **91, 198**
77.28	Wedge osteotomy of tarsals and metatarsals **93, 104, 198**	77.88	Other partial ostectomy of tarsals and metatarsals **93, 112, 198, 234**
77.29	Wedge osteotomy of other bone, except facial bones **95, 198**	77.89	Other partial ostectomy of other bone, except facial bones **45, 95, 112, 198**
77.30	Other division of bone, unspecified site **45, 95, 198**	77.90	Total ostectomy, unspecified site **95, 198**
77.31	Other division of scapula, clavicle, and thorax (ribs and sternum) **51, 95, 198**	77.91	Total ostectomy of scapula, clavicle, and thorax (ribs and sternum) **12, 13, 51, 95, 198**
77.32	Other division of humerus **91, 198**	77.92	Total ostectomy of humerus **91, 198**
77.33	Other division of radius and ulna **94, 198**	77.93	Total ostectomy of radius and ulna **94, 198**
77.34	Other division of carpals and metacarpals **94, 193**	77.94	Total ostectomy of carpals and metacarpals **94, 193**
77.35	Other division of femur **89, 198, 219**	77.95	Total ostectomy of femur **89, 198, 219**
77.36	Other division of patella **90, 198**	77.96	Total ostectomy of patella **90, 198**
77.37	Other division of tibia and fibula **91, 198**	77.97	Total ostectomy of tibia and fibula **91, 198**
77.38	Other division of tarsals and metatarsals **93, 112, 198, 234**		
77.39	Other division of other bone, except facial bones **95, 198**		

*Code Range

77.98	Total ostectomy of tarsals and metatarsals **93**, **198**, **234**	
77.99	Total ostectomy of other bone, except facial bones **45**, **95**, **198**	
78.00	Bone graft, unspecified site **95**, **198**	
78.01	Bone graft of scapula, clavicle, and thorax (ribs and sternum) **51**, **95**, **198**	
78.02	Bone graft of humerus **91**, **198**	
78.03	Bone graft of radius and ulna **94**, **198**, **234**	
78.04	Bone graft of carpals and metacarpals **94**, **193**	
78.05	Bone graft of femur **89**, **198**, **219**	
78.06	Bone graft of patella **90**, **198**	
78.07	Bone graft of tibia and fibula **91**, **198**	
78.08	Bone graft of tarsals and metatarsals **93**, **198**	
78.09	Bone graft of other bone, except facial bones **95**, **198**	
78.10	Application of external fixator device, unspecified site **95**, **198**	
78.11	Application of external fixator device, scapula, clavicle, and thorax [ribs and sternum] **51**, **95**, **198**	
78.12	Application of external fixator device, humerus **91**, **198**	
78.13	Application of external fixator device, radius and ulna **94**, **198**	
78.14	Application of external fixator device, carpals and metacarpals **94**, **193**	
78.15	Application of external fixator device, femur **89**, **198**, **219**	
78.16	Application of external fixator device, patella **90**, **198**	
78.17	Application of external fixator device, tibia and fibula **91**, **198**	
78.18	Application of external fixator device, tarsals and metatarsals **93**, **198**	
78.19	Application of external fixator device, other **95**, **198**	
78.20	Limb shortening procedures, unspecified site **95**, **198**	
78.22	Limb shortening procedures, humerus **91**, **199**	
78.23	Limb shortening procedures, radius and ulna **94**, **199**	
78.24	Limb shortening procedures, carpals and metacarpals **94**, **193**	
78.25	Limb shortening procedures, femur **89**, **199**, **219**	
78.27	Limb shortening procedures, tibia and fibula **91**, **199**	
78.28	Limb shortening procedures, tarsals and metatarsals **93**, **199**	
78.29	Limb shortening procedures, other **95**, **199**	
78.30	Limb lengthening procedures, unspecified site **95**, **199**	
78.32	Limb lengthening procedures, humerus **91**, **199**	
78.33	Limb lengthening procedures, radius and ulna **94**, **199**	
78.34	Limb lengthening procedures, carpals and metacarpals **94**, **193**	
78.35	Limb lengthening procedures, femur **89**, **199**, **219**	
78.37	Limb lengthening procedures, tibia and fibula **91**, **199**	
78.38	Limb lengthening procedures, tarsals and metatarsals **93**, **199**	
78.39	Other limb lengthening procedures **95**, **199**	
78.40	Other repair or plastic operations on bone, unspecified site **95**, **199**	
78.41	Other repair or plastic operations on scapula, clavicle, and thorax (ribs and sternum) **51**, **95**, **199**	
78.42	Other repair or plastic operation on humerus **91**, **199**	
78.43	Other repair or plastic operations on radius and ulna **94**, **199**	
78.44	Other repair or plastic operations on carpals and metacarpals **94**, **193**	
78.45	Other repair or plastic operations on femur **90**, **199**, **219**	
78.46	Other repair or plastic operations on patella **90**, **199**	
78.47	Other repair or plastic operations on tibia and fibula **91**, **199**	
78.48	Other repair or plastic operations on tarsals and metatarsals **93**, **199**	
78.49	Other repair or plastic operations on other bone, except facial bones **95**, **199**	
78.50	Internal fixation of bone without fracture reduction, unspecified site **95**, **199**	
78.51	Internal fixation of scapula, clavicle, and thorax (ribs and sternum) without fracture reduction **51**, **95**, **199**	

78.52	Internal fixation of humerus without fracture reduction **91**, **199**
78.53	Internal fixation of radius and ulna without fracture reduction **94**, **199**
78.54	Internal fixation of carpals and metacarpals without fracture reduction **94**, **193**
78.55	Internal fixation of femur without fracture reduction **90**, **199**, **219**
78.56	Internal fixation of patella without fracture reduction **90**, **199**
78.57	Internal fixation of tibia and fibula without fracture reduction **91**, **199**
78.58	Internal fixation of tarsals and metatarsals without fracture reduction **93**, **199**
78.59	Internal fixation of other bone, except facial bones, without fracture reduction **95**, **199**
78.6*	Removal of implanted device from bone **234**
78.60	Removal of implanted device, unspecified site **92**, **199**
78.61	Removal of implanted device from scapula, clavicle, and thorax (ribs and sternum) **51**, **92**, **199**
78.62	Removal of implanted device from humerus **92**, **199**
78.63	Removal of implanted device from radius and ulna **92**, **199**
78.64	Removal of implanted device from carpals and metacarpals **92**, **193**
78.65	Removal of implanted device from femur **92**, **112**, **199**
78.66	Removal of implanted device from patella **92**, **199**
78.67	Removal of implanted device from tibia and fibula **92**, **199**
78.68	Removal of implanted device from tarsal and metatarsals **92**, **199**
78.69	Removal of implanted device from other bone **92**, **199**
78.70	Osteoclasis, unspecified site **95**, **199**
78.71	Osteoclasis of scapula, clavicle, and thorax (ribs and sternum) **51**, **95**, **199**
78.72	Osteoclasis of humerus **91**, **199**
78.73	Osteoclasis of radius and ulna **94**, **199**
78.74	Osteoclasis of carpals and metacarpals **94**, **193**
78.75	Osteoclasis of femur **90**, **199**, **219**
78.76	Osteoclasis of patella **90**, **199**
78.77	Osteoclasis of tibia and fibula **91**, **199**
78.78	Osteoclasis of tarsals and metatarsals **93**, **199**
78.79	Osteoclasis of other bone, except facial bones **95**, **199**
78.80	Diagnostic procedures on bone, not elsewhere classified, unspecified site **89**
78.81	Diagnostic procedures on scapula, clavicle, and thorax (ribs and sternum) not elsewhere classified **51**, **89**
78.82	Diagnostic procedures on humerus, not elsewhere classified **89**
78.83	Diagnostic procedures on radius and ulna, not elsewhere classified **89**
78.84	Diagnostic procedures on carpals and metacarpals, not elsewhere classified **94**, **193**
78.85	Diagnostic procedures on femur, not elsewhere classified **89**
78.86	Diagnostic procedures on patella, not elsewhere classified **89**
78.87	Diagnostic procedures on tibia and fibula, not elsewhere classified **89**
78.88	Diagnostic procedures on tarsals and metatarsals, not elsewhere classified **93**
78.89	Diagnostic procedures on other bone, except facial bones, not elsewhere classified **89**
78.90	Insertion of bone growth stimulator, unspecified site **95**, **199**
78.91	Insertion of bone growth stimulator into scapula, clavicle and thorax (ribs and sternum) **51**, **95**, **199**
78.92	Insertion of bone growth stimulator into humerus **91**, **199**
78.93	Insertion of bone growth stimulator into radius and ulna **94**, **199**
78.94	Insertion of bone growth stimulator into carpals and metacarpals **94**, **193**
78.95	Insertion of bone growth stimulator into femur **90**, **199**, **219**

*Code Range

Numeric Index to Procedures

78.96	Insertion of bone growth stimulator into patella **90**, **199**
78.97	Insertion of bone growth stimulator into tibia and fibula **91**, **199**
78.98	Insertion of bone growth stimulator into tarsals and metatarsals **93**, **199**
78.99	Insertion of bone growth stimulator into other bone **95**, **199**
79.10	Closed reduction of fracture with internal fixation, unspecified site **95**, **199**
79.11	Closed reduction of fracture of humerus with internal fixation **91**, **199**
79.12	Closed reduction of fracture of radius and ulna with internal fixation **94**, **199**, **234**
79.13	Closed reduction of fracture of carpals and metacarpals with internal fixation **94**, **193**
79.14	Closed reduction of fracture of phalanges of hand with internal fixation **94**, **193**
79.15	Closed reduction of fracture of femur with internal fixation **90**, **199**, **219**
79.16	Closed reduction of fracture of tibia and fibula with internal fixation **91**, **199**
79.17	Closed reduction of fracture of tarsals and metatarsals with internal fixation **93**, **199**
79.18	Closed reduction of fracture of phalanges of foot with internal fixation **93**, **199**
79.19	Closed reduction of fracture of other specified bone, except facial bones, with internal fixation **95**, **199**
79.20	Open reduction of fracture without internal fixation, unspecified site **96**, **199**
79.21	Open reduction of fracture of humerus without internal fixation **91**, **199**
79.22	Open reduction of fracture of radius and ulna without internal fixation **94**, **199**
79.23	Open reduction of fracture of carpals and metacarpals without internal fixation **94**, **193**
79.24	Open reduction of fracture of phalanges of hand without internal fixation **94**, **193**
79.25	Open reduction of fracture of femur without internal fixation **90**, **199**, **219**
79.26	Open reduction of fracture of tibia and fibula without internal fixation **91**, **199**
79.27	Open reduction of fracture of tarsals and metatarsals without internal fixation **93**, **199**
79.28	Open reduction of fracture of phalanges of foot without internal fixation **93**, **199**
79.29	Open reduction of fracture of other specified bone, except facial bones, without internal fixation **45**, **96**, **199**
79.30	Open reduction of fracture with internal fixation, unspecified site **96**, **199**
79.31	Open reduction of fracture of humerus with internal fixation **91**, **199**
79.32	Open reduction of fracture of radius and ulna with internal fixation **94**, **199**
79.33	Open reduction of fracture of carpals and metacarpals with internal fixation **94**, **193**
79.34	Open reduction of fracture of phalanges of hand with internal fixation **94**, **193**
79.35	Open reduction of fracture of femur with internal fixation **90**, **112**, **199**, **219**
79.36	Open reduction of fracture of tibia and fibula with internal fixation **91**, **199**
79.37	Open reduction of fracture of tarsals and metatarsals with internal fixation **93**, **199**
79.38	Open reduction of fracture of phalanges of foot with internal fixation **93**, **199**
79.39	Open reduction of fracture of other specified bone, except facial bones, with internal fixation **45**, **96**, **199**

79.40	Closed reduction of separated epiphysis, unspecified site **96**, **199**
79.41	Closed reduction of separated epiphysis of humerus **91**, **199**
79.42	Closed reduction of separated epiphysis of radius and ulna **94**, **199**
79.45	Closed reduction of separated epiphysis of femur **90**, **199**, **219**
79.46	Closed reduction of separated epiphysis of tibia and fibula **91**, **199**
79.49	Closed reduction of separated epiphysis of other specified bone **96**, **199**
79.50	Open reduction of separated epiphysis, unspecified site **96**, **199**
79.51	Open reduction of separated epiphysis of humerus **91**, **199**
79.52	Open reduction of separated epiphysis of radius and ulna **94**, **199**
79.55	Open reduction of separated epiphysis of femur **90**, **199**, **219**
79.56	Open reduction of separated epiphysis of tibia and fibula **91**, **199**
79.59	Open reduction of separated epiphysis of other specified bone **96**, **199**
79.60	Debridement of open fracture, unspecified site **96**, **199**
79.61	Debridement of open fracture of humerus **91**, **199**
79.62	Debridement of open fracture of radius and ulna **94**, **199**
79.63	Debridement of open fracture of carpals and metacarpals **94**, **193**
79.64	Debridement of open fracture of phalanges of hand **94**, **193**
79.65	Debridement of open fracture of femur **90**, **199**, **219**
79.66	Debridement of open fracture of tibia and fibula **91**, **199**
79.67	Debridement of open fracture of tarsals and metatarsals **93**, **199**
79.68	Debridement of open fracture of phalanges of foot **93**, **199**
79.69	Debridement of open fracture of other specified bone, except facial bones **45**, **96**, **199**
79.80	Open reduction of dislocation of unspecified site **96**, **199**
79.81	Open reduction of dislocation of shoulder **94**, **199**
79.82	Open reduction of dislocation of elbow **94**, **199**
79.83	Open reduction of dislocation of wrist **94**, **193**
79.84	Open reduction of dislocation of hand and finger **94**, **193**
79.85	Open reduction of dislocation of hip **90**, **200**, **219**
79.86	Open reduction of dislocation of knee **90**, **200**
79.87	Open reduction of dislocation of ankle **91**, **200**
79.88	Open reduction of dislocation of foot and toe **93**, **200**
79.89	Open reduction of dislocation of other specified site, except temporomandibular **96**, **200**
79.90	Unspecified operation on bone injury, unspecified site **96**, **200**
79.91	Unspecified operation on bone injury of humerus **91**, **200**
79.92	Unspecified operation on bone injury of radius and ulna **94**, **200**
79.93	Unspecified operation on bone injury of carpals and metacarpals **94**, **193**
79.94	Unspecified operation on bone injury of phalanges of hand **94**, **193**
79.95	Unspecified operation on bone injury of femur **90**, **200**, **219**
79.96	Unspecified operation on bone injury of tibia and fibula **91**, **200**
79.97	Unspecified operation on bone injury of tarsals and metatarsals **91**, **200**
79.98	Unspecified operation on bone injury of phalanges of foot **93**, **200**
79.99	Unspecified operation on bone injury of other specified bone **96**, **200**
80.00	Arthrotomy for removal of prosthesis without replacement, unspecified site **92**, **200**
80.01	Arthrotomy for removal of prosthesis without replacement, shoulder **92**, **200**
80.02	Arthrotomy for removal of prosthesis without replacement, elbow **92**, **200**
80.03	Arthrotomy for removal of prosthesis without replacement, wrist **92**, **193**
80.04	Arthrotomy for removal of prosthesis without replacement, hand and finger **92**, **193**

*Code Range

80.05	Arthrotomy for removal of prosthesis without replacement, hip **88, 200, 219**
80.06	Arthrotomy for removal of prosthesis without replacement, knee **88, 200**
80.07	Arthrotomy for removal of prosthesis without replacement, ankle **92, 200**
80.08	Arthrotomy for removal of prosthesis without replacement, foot and toe **92, 200**
80.09	Arthrotomy for removal of prosthesis without replacement, other specified site **92, 200**
80.10	Other arthrotomy, unspecified site **96, 112, 200**
80.11	Other arthrotomy of shoulder **93, 200**
80.12	Other arthrotomy of elbow **93, 113, 200**
80.13	Other arthrotomy of wrist **93, 193**
80.14	Other arthrotomy of hand and finger **93, 193**
80.15	Other arthrotomy of hip **90, 200, 219**
80.16	Other arthrotomy of knee **90, 113, 200, 235**
80.17	Other arthrotomy of ankle **91, 200**
80.18	Other arthrotomy of foot and toe **93, 200, 235**
80.19	Other arthrotomy of other specified site **96, 200**
80.2*	Arthroscopy **93, 200**
80.26	Arthroscopy of knee **113, 235**
80.40	Division of joint capsule, ligament, or cartilage, unspecified site **96, 200**
80.41	Division of joint capsule, ligament, or cartilage of shoulder **94, 200**
80.42	Division of joint capsule, ligament, or cartilage of elbow **94, 200**
80.43	Division of joint capsule, ligament, or cartilage of wrist **94, 193**
80.44	Division of joint capsule, ligament, or cartilage of hand and finger **94, 193**
80.45	Division of joint capsule, ligament, or cartilage of hip **90, 200, 219**
80.46	Division of joint capsule, ligament, or cartilage of knee **90, 200, 235**
80.47	Division of joint capsule, ligament, or cartilage of ankle **91, 200**
80.48	Division of joint capsule, ligament, or cartilage of foot and toe **93, 200**
80.49	Division of joint capsule, ligament, or cartilage of other specified site **96, 200**
80.50	Excision or destruction of intervertebral disc, unspecified **12, 13, 91, 200**
80.51	Excision of intervertebral disc **12, 13, 91, 200**
80.53	Repair of the anulus fibrosus with graft or prosthesis **12, 13, 91, 179, 200**
80.54	Other and unspecified repair of the anulus fibrosus **12, 13, 91, 179, 200**
80.59	Other destruction of intervertebral disc **12, 13, 91, 200**
80.6	Excision of semilunar cartilage of knee **90, 113, 200, 235**
80.7*	Synovectomy **235**
80.70	Synovectomy, unspecified site **92, 200**
80.71	Synovectomy of shoulder **94, 200**
80.72	Synovectomy of elbow **94, 200**
80.73	Synovectomy of wrist **94, 193**
80.74	Synovectomy of hand and finger **94, 193**
80.75	Synovectomy of hip **90, 200**
80.76	Synovectomy of knee **90, 200**
80.77	Synovectomy of ankle **91, 200**
80.78	Synovectomy of foot and toe **93, 200**
80.79	Synovectomy of other specified site **92, 200**
80.80	Other local excision or destruction of lesion of joint, unspecified site **92, 200**
80.81	Other local excision or destruction of lesion of shoulder joint **92, 200**

80.82	Other local excision or destruction of lesion of elbow joint **92, 113, 200**
80.83	Other local excision or destruction of lesion of wrist joint **94, 104, 193**
80.84	Other local excision or destruction of lesion of joint of hand and finger **94, 193**
80.85	Other local excision or destruction of lesion of hip joint **92, 200**
80.86	Other local excision or destruction of lesion of knee joint **92, 200, 235**
80.87	Other local excision or destruction of lesion of ankle joint **91, 200**
80.88	Other local excision or destruction of lesion of joint of foot and toe **93, 113, 200, 235**
80.89	Other local excision or destruction of lesion of joint of other specified site **92, 200**
80.90	Other excision of joint, unspecified site **96, 200**
80.91	Other excision of shoulder joint **94, 200**
80.92	Other excision of elbow joint **94, 200**
80.93	Other excision of wrist joint **94, 193**
80.94	Other excision of joint of hand and finger **94, 193**
80.95	Other excision of hip joint **90, 200, 219**
80.96	Other excision of knee joint **90, 200**
80.97	Other excision of ankle joint **92, 200**
80.98	Other excision of joint of foot and toe **93, 113, 200, 235**
80.99	Other excision of joint of other specified site **92, 200**
81.00	Spinal fusion, not otherwise specified **12, 13, 87, 88, 200**
81.01	Atlas-axis spinal fusion **12, 13, 89, 200**
81.02	Other cervical fusion of the anterior column, anterior technique **12, 13, 87, 89, 200**
81.03	Other cervical fusion of the posterior column, posterior technique **12, 13, 87, 89, 200**
81.04	Dorsal and dorsolumbar fusion of the anterior column, anterior technique **12, 13, 87, 88, 200**
81.05	Dorsal and dorsolumbar fusion of the posterior column, posterior technique **12, 13, 87, 88, 200**
81.06	Lumbar and lumbosacral fusion of the anterior column, anterior technique **12, 13, 87, 88, 200**
81.07	Lumbar and lumbosacral fusion of the posterior column, posterior technique **12, 13, 87, 88, 200**
81.08	Lumbar and lumbosacral fusion of the anterior column, posterior technique **12, 13, 87, 88, 200**
81.1*	Arthrodesis and arthroereisis of foot and ankle **200**
81.11	Ankle fusion **92, 113**
81.12	Triple arthrodesis **92**
81.13	Subtalar fusion **93**
81.14	Midtarsal fusion **93**
81.15	Tarsometatarsal fusion **93**
81.16	Metatarsophalangeal fusion **93**
81.17	Other fusion of foot **93**
81.18	Subtalar joint arthroereisis **96**
81.20	Arthrodesis of unspecified joint **96, 200**
81.21	Arthrodesis of hip **90, 200, 219**
81.22	Arthrodesis of knee **90, 200**
81.23	Arthrodesis of shoulder **93, 113, 200**
81.24	Arthrodesis of elbow **93, 200**
81.25	Carporadial fusion **94, 193**
81.26	Metacarpocarpal fusion **94, 193**
81.27	Metacarpophalangeal fusion **94, 193**
81.28	Interphalangeal fusion **94, 193**
81.29	Arthrodesis of other specified joint **96, 200**
81.3*	Refusion of spine **12, 13, 200**
81.30	Refusion of spine, not otherwise specified **87, 88**
81.31	Refusion of Atlas-axis spine **89**

81.32	Refusion of other cervical spine, anterior column, anterior technique **87**, **89**	
81.33	Refusion of other cervical spine, posterior column, posterior technique **87**, **89**	
81.34	Refusion of dorsal and dorsolumbar spine, anterior column, anterior technique **87**, **88**	
81.35	Refusion of dorsal and dorsolumbar spine, posterior column, posterior technique **87**, **88**	
81.36	Refusion of lumbar and lumbosacral spine, anterior column, anterior technique **87**, **88**	
81.37	Refusion of lumbar and lumbosacral spine, posterior column, posterior technique **87**, **88**	
81.38	Refusion of lumbar and lumbosacral spine, anterior column, posterior technique **87**, **88**	
81.39	Refusion of spine, not elsewhere classified **87**, **88**	
81.4*	Other repair of joint of lower extremity **200**	
81.40	Repair of hip, not elsewhere classified **90**, **219**	
81.42	Five-in-one repair of knee **90**	
81.43	Triad knee repair **90**	
81.44	Patellar stabilization **90**	
81.45	Other repair of the cruciate ligaments **90**	
81.46	Other repair of the collateral ligaments **90**	
81.47	Other repair of knee **90**	
81.49	Other repair of ankle **92**	
81.5*	Joint replacement of lower extremity **200**	
81.51	Total hip replacement **88**, **89**, **219**	
81.52	Partial hip replacement **88**, **89**, **113**, **219**	
81.53	Revision of hip replacement, not otherwise specified **88**, **113**, **219**	
81.54	Total knee replacement **88**, **89**	
81.55	Revision of knee replacement, not otherwise specified **88**	
81.56	Total ankle replacement **88**, **89**	
81.57	Replacement of joint of foot and toe **93**, **235**	
81.59	Revision of joint replacement of lower extremity, not elsewhere classified **96**	
81.64	Fusion or refusion of 9 or more vertebrae **87**, **88**	
81.65	Percutaneous vertebroplasty **96**, **200**	
81.66	Percutaneous vertebral augmentation **96**, **200**	
81.71	Arthroplasty of metacarpophalangeal and interphalangeal joint with implant **14**, **16**, **93**, **193**	
81.72	Arthroplasty of metacarpophalangeal and interphalangeal joint without implant **14**, **16**, **93**, **193**	
81.73	Total wrist replacement **90**, **200**	
81.74	Arthroplasty of carpocarpal or carpometacarpal joint with implant **14**, **16**, **93**, **193**	
81.75	Arthroplasty of carpocarpal or carpometacarpal joint without implant **14**, **16**, **93**, **193**	
81.79	Other repair of hand, fingers, and wrist **14**, **16**, **93**, **193**	
81.8*	Arthroplasty and repair of shoulder and elbow **200**	
81.80	Other total shoulder replacement **90**	
81.81	Partial shoulder replacement **90**	
81.82	Repair of recurrent dislocation of shoulder **94**	
81.83	Other repair of shoulder **93**, **235**	
81.84	Total elbow replacement **90**	
81.85	Other repair of elbow **93**	
81.88	Reverse total shoulder replacement **90**	
81.93	Suture of capsule or ligament of upper extremity **94**, **200**	
81.94	Suture of capsule or ligament of ankle and foot **93**, **200**	
81.95	Suture of capsule or ligament of other lower extremity **92**, **200**	
81.96	Other repair of joint **96**, **200**	
81.97	Revision of joint replacement of upper extremity **96**, **200**	
81.98	Other diagnostic procedures on joint structures **89**, **200**	

81.99	Other operations on joint structures **96**, **200**
82.01	Exploration of tendon sheath of hand **94**, **193**, **235**
82.02	Myotomy of hand **94**, **193**
82.03	Bursotomy of hand **94**, **193**
82.09	Other incision of soft tissue of hand **94**, **104**, **193**, **235**
82.1*	Division of muscle, tendon, and fascia of hand **94**, **193**
82.11	Tenotomy of hand **235**
82.2*	Excision of lesion of muscle, tendon, and fascia of hand **94**, **193**
82.21	Excision of lesion of tendon sheath of hand **104**, **113**, **235**
82.29	Excision of other lesion of soft tissue of hand **104**, **235**
82.3*	Other excision of soft tissue of hand **94**, **193**
82.33	Other tenonectomy of hand **113**
82.39	Other excision of soft tissue of hand **104**
82.4*	Suture of muscle, tendon, and fascia of hand **94**, **193**
82.41	Suture of tendon sheath of hand **235**
82.45	Other suture of other tendon of hand **104**, **235**
82.46	Suture of muscle or fascia of hand **235**
82.5*	Transplantation of muscle and tendon of hand **14**, **16**, **94**, **193**
82.6*	Reconstruction of thumb **14**, **16**, **93**, **193**
82.7*	Plastic operation on hand with graft or implant **14**, **17**, **94**, **193**
82.72	Plastic operation on hand with graft of muscle or fascia **104**
82.79	Plastic operation on hand with other graft or implant **104**
82.8*	Other plastic operations on hand **14**, **17**, **94**, **193**
82.89	Other plastic operations on hand **104**
82.91	Lysis of adhesions of hand **94**, **104**, **193**
82.99	Other operations on muscle, tendon, and fascia of hand **94**, **193**
83.0*	Incision of muscle, tendon, fascia, and bursa **92**, **200**, **235**
83.02	Myotomy **45**, **104**
83.09	Other incision of soft tissue **104**
83.1*	Division of muscle, tendon, and fascia **200**
83.11	Achillotenotomy **93**
83.12	Adductor tenotomy of hip **90**, **219**
83.13	Other tenotomy **14**, **17**, **92**, **113**, **235**
83.14	Fasciotomy **14**, **17**, **92**, **104**
83.19	Other division of soft tissue **14**, **17**, **92**, **235**
83.2*	Diagnostic procedures on muscle, tendon, fascia, and bursa, including that of hand **92**
83.21	Open biopsy of soft tissue **14**, **17**, **51**, **104**, **175**, **235**
83.29	Other diagnostic procedures on muscle, tendon, fascia, and bursa, including that of hand **200**
83.3*	Excision of lesion of muscle, tendon, fascia, and bursa **92**, **200**
83.31	Excision of lesion of tendon sheath **113**
83.32	Excision of lesion of muscle **104**, **235**
83.39	Excision of lesion of other soft tissue **45**, **104**, **113**, **235**
83.4*	Other excision of muscle, tendon, and fascia **92**, **200**
83.41	Excision of tendon for graft **14**, **17**
83.43	Excision of muscle or fascia for graft **14**, **17**
83.44	Other fasciectomy **104**
83.45	Other myectomy **14**, **17**, **104**
83.49	Other excision of soft tissue **14**, **17**, **45**, **104**
83.5	Bursectomy **92**, **200**, **235**
83.6*	Suture of muscle, tendon, and fascia **200**, **235**
83.61	Suture of tendon sheath **92**
83.62	Delayed suture of tendon **92**
83.63	Rotator cuff repair **94**
83.64	Other suture of tendon **93**
83.65	Other suture of muscle or fascia **93**, **104**, **113**
83.7*	Reconstruction of muscle and tendon **14**, **17**, **93**, **200**
83.71	Advancement of tendon **104**

*Code Range

83.75	Tendon transfer or transplantation **113**	
83.79	Other muscle transposition **113**	
83.8*	Other plastic operations on muscle, tendon, and fascia **200**	
83.81	Tendon graft **14, 17, 93**	
83.82	Graft of muscle or fascia **14, 17, 93, 104**	
83.83	Tendon pulley reconstruction on muscle, tendon, and fascia **14, 17, 93**	
83.84	Release of clubfoot, not elsewhere classified **93**	
83.85	Other change in muscle or tendon length **14, 17, 93**	
83.86	Quadricepsplasty **93**	
83.87	Other plastic operations on muscle **14, 17, 93, 104**	
83.88	Other plastic operations on tendon **14, 17, 93, 104**	
83.89	Other plastic operations on fascia **14, 17, 93, 104**	
83.91	Lysis of adhesions of muscle, tendon, fascia, and bursa **93, 200**	
83.92	Insertion or replacement of skeletal muscle stimulator **14, 17, 93, 200**	
83.93	Removal of skeletal muscle stimulator **14, 17, 93, 200**	
83.99	Other operations on muscle, tendon, fascia, and bursa **93, 200**	
84.0*	Amputation of upper limb **63, 104**	
84.00	Upper limb amputation, not otherwise specified **89, 200**	
84.01	Amputation and disarticulation of finger **94, 193, 235**	
84.02	Amputation and disarticulation of thumb **94, 193**	
84.03	Amputation through hand **89, 200**	
84.04	Disarticulation of wrist **89, 200**	
84.05	Amputation through forearm **89, 200**	
84.06	Disarticulation of elbow **89, 201**	
84.07	Amputation through humerus **89, 201**	
84.08	Disarticulation of shoulder **89, 201**	
84.09	Interthoracoscapular amputation **89, 201**	
84.1*	Amputation of lower limb **104, 201**	
84.10	Lower limb amputation, not otherwise specified **60, 89, 111**	
84.11	Amputation of toe **14, 17, 63, 93, 111**	
84.12	Amputation through foot **14, 17, 60, 89, 111**	
84.13	Disarticulation of ankle **14, 17, 60, 89, 111**	
84.14	Amputation of ankle through malleoli of tibia and fibula **14, 17, 60, 89, 111**	
84.15	Other amputation below knee **14, 17, 60, 89, 111**	
84.16	Disarticulation of knee **14, 17, 60, 89, 111**	
84.17	Amputation above knee **14, 17, 60, 89, 111**	
84.18	Disarticulation of hip **60, 89**	
84.19	Abdominopelvic amputation **60, 89**	
84.21	Thumb reattachment **94, 193**	
84.22	Finger reattachment **94, 193**	
84.23	Forearm, wrist, or hand reattachment **90, 201, 219**	
84.24	Upper arm reattachment **90, 201, 219**	
84.25	Toe reattachment **93, 201**	
84.26	Foot reattachment **89, 201, 219**	
84.27	Lower leg or ankle reattachment **89, 201, 219**	
84.28	Thigh reattachment **89, 201, 219**	
84.29	Other reattachment of extremity **96, 201**	
84.3	Revision of amputation stump **63, 89, 104, 111, 201**	
84.40	Implantation or fitting of prosthetic limb device, not otherwise specified **96, 201**	
84.44	Implantation of prosthetic device of arm **94, 201**	
84.48	Implantation of prosthetic device of leg **92, 201**	
84.59	Insertion of other spinal devices **12, 13, 91, 201**	
84.6*	Replacement of spinal disc **12, 13, 91, 201**	
84.60	Insertion of spinal disc prosthesis, not otherwise specified **91**	
84.61	Insertion of partial spinal disc prosthesis, cervical **91**	
84.63	Insertion of spinal disc prosthesis, thoracic **91**	

84.64	Insertion of partial spinal disc prosthesis, lumbosacral **91**	
84.66	Revision or replacement of artificial spinal disc prosthesis, cervical **91**	
84.67	Revision or replacement of artificial spinal disc prosthesis, thoracic **91**	
84.68	Revision or replacement of artificial spinal disc prosthesis, lumbosacral **91**	
84.69	Revision or replacement of artificial spinal disc prosthesis, not otherwise specified **91**	
84.8*	Insertion, replacement and revision of posterior spinal motion preservation device(s) **201**	
84.80	Insertion or replacement of interspinous process device(s) **12, 13, 91**	
84.81	Revision of interspinous process device(s) **96**	
84.82	Insertion or replacement of pedicle-based dynamic stabilization device(s) **12, 13, 91**	
84.83	Revision of pedicle-based dynamic stabilization device(s) **96**	
84.84	Insertion or replacement of facet replacement device(s) **12, 13, 91**	
84.85	Revision of facet replacement device(s) **96**	
84.91	Amputation, not otherwise specified **60, 89, 104, 201**	
84.92	Separation of equal conjoined twins **96**	
84.93	Separation of unequal conjoined twins **96**	
84.94	Insertion of sternal fixation device with rigid plates **51, 64, 96, 201**	
84.99	Other operations on musculoskeletal system **96, 201**	
85.12	Open biopsy of breast **105, 113, 201, 235**	
85.2*	Excision or destruction of breast tissue **201**	
85.20	Excision or destruction of breast tissue, not otherwise specified **105, 235**	
85.21	Local excision of lesion of breast **105, 113, 235**	
85.22	Resection of quadrant of breast **104, 105**	
85.23	Subtotal mastectomy **104, 105, 235**	
85.24	Excision of ectopic breast tissue **105**	
85.25	Excision of nipple **105**	
85.3*	Reduction mammoplasty and subcutaneous mammectomy **104, 105, 201**	
85.31	Unilateral reduction mammoplasty **111**	
85.32	Bilateral reduction mammoplasty **111**	
85.4*	Mastectomy **104, 105, 201**	
85.50	Augmentation mammoplasty, not otherwise specified **105, 201, 235**	
85.53	Unilateral breast implant **105, 201, 235**	
85.54	Bilateral breast implant **105, 201, 235**	
85.55	Fat graft to breast **105**	
85.6	Mastopexy **105, 201**	
85.7*	Total reconstruction of breast **104, 105, 201**	
85.82	Split-thickness graft to breast **103, 193, 206, 207**	
85.83	Full-thickness graft to breast **103, 193, 206, 207**	
85.84	Pedicle graft to breast **103, 193, 206, 207**	
85.85	Muscle flap graft to breast **103, 201**	
85.86	Transposition of nipple **105, 201**	
85.87	Other repair or reconstruction of nipple **105, 201**	
85.89	Other mammoplasty **105, 201**	
85.93	Revision of implant of breast **105, 201, 235**	
85.94	Removal of implant of breast **105, 201, 235**	
85.95	Insertion of breast tissue expander **105, 201, 235**	
85.96	Removal of breast tissue expander (s) **105, 201, 235**	
85.99	Other operations on the breast **105, 201, 235**	
86.06	Insertion of totally implantable infusion pump **14, 17, 51, 64, 75, 82, 96, 104, 113, 118, 123, 129, 175, 201**	
86.07	Insertion of totally implantable vascular access device (VAD) **104, 118**	

Numeric Index to Procedures

86.09	Other incision of skin and subcutaneous tissue **104**	
86.21	Excision of pilonidal cyst or sinus **104, 201, 235**	
86.22	Excisional debridement of wound, infection, or burn **14, 17, 37, 45, 51, 64, 75, 82, 88, 103, 111, 118, 123, 129, 175, 193**	
86.25	Dermabrasion **104, 235**	
86.3	Other local excision or destruction of lesion or tissue of skin and subcutaneous tissue **104**	
86.4	Radical excision of skin lesion **14, 17, 37, 45, 64, 93, 103, 201, 235**	
86.60	Free skin graft, not otherwise specified **14, 17, 64, 75, 88, 103, 111, 193, 206, 207, 235**	
86.61	Full-thickness skin graft to hand **14, 17, 64, 94, 103, 194, 206, 207**	
86.62	Other skin graft to hand **14, 17, 64, 94, 103, 194, 206, 207, 235**	
86.63	Full-thickness skin graft to other sites **14, 17, 45, 64, 75, 88, 103, 111, 193, 206, 207**	
86.65	Heterograft to skin **14, 17, 64, 75, 88, 103, 193, 206, 207, 235**	
86.66	Homograft to skin **14, 17, 45, 65, 75, 88, 103, 193, 206, 207**	
86.67	Dermal regenerative graft **14, 17, 45, 65, 75, 88, 103, 111, 193, 206, 207**	
86.69	Other skin graft to other sites **14, 17, 45, 51, 65, 75, 88, 103, 111, 193, 206, 207**	
86.7*	Pedicle grafts or flaps **103, 206, 207**	
86.70	Pedicle or flap graft, not otherwise specified **14, 17, 45, 65, 75, 88, 111, 193**	
86.71	Cutting and preparation of pedicle grafts or flaps **14, 17, 45, 65, 75, 88, 111, 193**	
86.72	Advancement of pedicle graft **14, 17, 45, 65, 75, 88, 111, 193**	
86.73	Attachment of pedicle or flap graft to hand **94, 194**	
86.74	Attachment of pedicle or flap graft to other sites **14, 17, 45, 65, 75, 88, 111, 193**	
86.75	Revision of pedicle or flap graft **14, 17, 45, 65, 75, 88, 111, 193**	
86.8*	Other repair and reconstruction of skin and subcutaneous tissue **104**	
86.81	Repair for facial weakness **14, 17, 45, 93, 201**	
86.82	Facial rhytidectomy **45, 201, 235**	
86.83	Size reduction plastic operation **111, 201, 235**	
86.84	Relaxation of scar or web contracture of skin **45, 201, 235**	
86.85	Correction of syndactyly **94, 194**	
86.86	Onychoplasty **201**	
86.87	Fat graft of skin and subcutaneous tissue **45, 111, 201**	
86.89	Other repair and reconstruction of skin and subcutaneous tissue **45, 111, 201, 235**	

86.90	Extraction of fat for graft or banking **104**
86.91	Excision of skin for graft **14, 17, 45, 65, 103, 111, 201**
86.93	Insertion of tissue expander **14, 17, 45, 65, 75, 88, 103, 111, 193, 206, 207**
86.94	Insertion or replacement of single array neurostimulator pulse generator, not specified as rechargeable **12, 15, 17, 18, 91**
86.95	Insertion or replacement of multiple array neurostimulator pulse generator, not specified as rechargeable **9, 11, 12, 15, 17, 18, 91**
86.96	Insertion or replacement of other neurostimulator pulse generator **15, 17, 63**
86.97	Insertion or replacement of single array rechargeable neurostimulator pulse generator **13, 15, 17, 18, 91**
86.98	Insertion or replacement of multiple array (two or more) rechargeable neurostimulator pulse generator **9, 11, 13, 15, 17, 18, 91**
87.53	Intraoperative cholangiogram **82, 235**
88.52	Angiocardiography of right heart structures **56, 57, 59, 65**
88.53	Angiocardiography of left heart structures **56, 57, 59, 65**
88.54	Combined right and left heart angiocardiography **56, 57, 59, 65**
88.55	Coronary arteriography using single catheter **56, 57, 59, 65**
88.56	Coronary arteriography using two catheters **56, 57, 59, 65**
88.57	Other and unspecified coronary arteriography **56, 57, 59, 65**
88.58	Negative-contrast cardiac roentgenography **56, 57, 59, 65**
92.27	Implantation or insertion of radioactive elements **15, 17, 45, 51, 62, 65, 75, 104, 113, 118, 123, 128, 201, 235**
92.3*	Stereotactic radiosurgery **16, 18, 113, 180**
94.61	Alcohol rehabilitation **191**
94.63	Alcohol rehabilitation and detoxification **191**
94.64	Drug rehabilitation **191**
94.66	Drug rehabilitation and detoxification **191**
94.67	Combined alcohol and drug rehabilitation **191**
94.69	Combined alcohol and drug rehabilitation and detoxification **191**
95.04	Eye examination under anesthesia **37, 235**
96.70	Continuous invasive mechanical ventilation of unspecified duration **54**
96.71	Continuous invasive mechanical ventilation for less than 96 consecutive hours **54**
96.72	Continuous invasive mechanical ventilation for 96 consecutive hours or more **1, 54, 186, 206, 208**
98.51	Extracorporeal shockwave lithotripsy (ESWL) of the kidney, ureter and/or bladder **119**
99.10	Injection or infusion of thrombolytic agent **20**

*Code Range

© 2013 OptumInsight, Inc.

Appendix A — Lists of CCs and MCCs

Numeric CC List

001.0	Cholera due to vibrio cholerae
001.1	Cholera due to vibrio cholerae el tor
001.9	Cholera, unspecified
002.0	Typhoid fever
002.1	Paratyphoid fever A
002.2	Paratyphoid fever B
002.3	Paratyphoid fever C
002.9	Paratyphoid fever, unspecified
003.0	Salmonella gastroenteritis
003.23	Salmonella arthritis
003.24	Salmonella osteomyelitis
003.29	Other localized salmonella infections
003.8	Other specified salmonella infections
003.9	Salmonella infection, unspecified
004.0	Shigella dysenteriae
005.0	Staphylococcal food poisoning
005.1	Botulism food poisoning
005.2	Food poisoning due to Clostridium perfringens (C. welchii)
005.3	Food poisoning due to other Clostridia
005.4	Food poisoning due to Vibrio parahaemolyticus
005.81	Food poisoning due to Vibrio vulnificus
005.89	Other bacterial food poisoning
006.0	Acute amebic dysentery without mention of abscess
006.1	Chronic intestinal amebiasis without mention of abscess
006.2	Amebic nondysenteric colitis
006.8	Amebic infection of other sites
007.1	Giardiasis
007.2	Coccidiosis
007.4	Cryptosporidiosis
007.5	Cyclosporiasis
007.8	Other specified protozoal intestinal diseases
007.9	Unspecified protozoal intestinal disease
008.00	Intestinal infection due to E. coli, unspecified
008.01	Intestinal infection due to enteropathogenic E. coli
008.02	Intestinal infection due to enterotoxigenic E. coli
008.03	Intestinal infection due to enteroinvasive E. coli
008.04	Intestinal infection due to enterohemorrhagic E. coli
008.09	Intestinal infection due to other intestinal E. coli infections
008.1	Intestinal infection due to arizona group of paracolon bacilli
008.2	Intestinal infection due to aerobacter aerogenes
008.3	Intestinal infection due to proteus (mirabilis) (morganii)
008.41	Intestinal infection due to staphylococcus
008.42	Intestinal infection due to pseudomonas
008.43	Intestinal infection due to campylobacter
008.44	Intestinal infection due to yersinia enterocolitica
008.45	Intestinal infection due to Clostridium difficile
008.46	Intestinal infection due to other anaerobes
008.47	Intestinal infection due to other gram-negative bacteria
008.49	Intestinal infection due to other organisms
008.5	Bacterial enteritis, unspecified
008.61	Enteritis due to rotavirus
008.62	Enteritis due to adenovirus
008.63	Enteritis due to norwalk virus

008.64	Enteritis due to other small round viruses [SRV's]
008.65	Enteritis due to calicivirus
008.66	Enteritis due to astrovirus
008.67	Enteritis due to enterovirus nec
008.69	Enteritis due to other viral enteritis
009.0	Infectious colitis, enteritis, and gastroenteritis
009.1	Colitis, enteritis, and gastroenteritis of presumed infectious origin
009.2	Infectious diarrhea
009.3	Diarrhea of presumed infectious origin
010.00	Primary tuberculous infection, unspecified
010.01	Primary tuberculous infection, bacteriological or histological examination not done
010.02	Primary tuberculous infection, bacteriological or histological examination unknown (at present)
010.03	Primary tuberculous infection, tubercle bacilli found (in sputum) by microscopy
010.04	Primary tuberculous infection, tubercle bacilli not found (in sputum) by microscopy, but found by bacterial culture
010.05	Primary tuberculous infection, tubercle bacilli not found by bacteriological examination, but tuberculosis confirmed histologically
010.06	Primary tuberculous infection, tubercle bacilli not found by bacteriological or histological examination, but tuberculosis confirmed by other methods [inoculation of animals]
010.10	Tuberculous pleurisy in primary progressive tuberculosis, unspecified
010.11	Tuberculous pleurisy in primary progressive tuberculosis, bacteriological or histological examination not done
010.12	Tuberculous pleurisy in primary progressive tuberculosis, bacteriological or histological examination unknown (at present)
010.13	Tuberculous pleurisy in primary progressive tuberculosis, tubercle bacilli found (in sputum) by microscopy
010.14	Tuberculous pleurisy in primary progressive tuberculosis, tubercle bacilli not found (in sputum) by microscopy, but found by bacterial culture
010.15	Tuberculous pleurisy in primary progressive tuberculosis, tubercle bacilli not found by bacteriological examination, but tuberculosis confirmed histologically
010.16	Tuberculous pleurisy in primary progressive tuberculosis, tubercle bacilli not found by bacteriological or histological examination, but tuberculosis confirmed by other methods [inoculation of animals]
010.80	Other primary progressive tuberculosis, unspecified
010.81	Other primary progressive tuberculosis, bacteriological or histological examination not done
010.82	Other primary progressive tuberculosis, bacteriological or histological examination unknown (at present)
010.83	Other primary progressive tuberculosis, tubercle bacilli found (in sputum) by microscopy
010.84	Other primary progressive tuberculosis, tubercle bacilli not found (in sputum) by microscopy, but found by bacterial culture
010.85	Other primary progressive tuberculosis, tubercle bacilli not found by bacteriological examination, but tuberculosis confirmed histologically
010.86	Other primary progressive tuberculosis, tubercle bacilli not found by bacteriological or histological examination, but tuberculosis confirmed by other methods [inoculation of animals]
010.90	Primary tuberculous infection, unspecified, unspecified
010.91	Primary tuberculous infection, unspecified, bacteriological or histological examination not done
010.92	Primary tuberculous infection, unspecified, bacteriological or histological examination unknown (at present)

010.93 Primary tuberculous infection, unspecified, tubercle bacilli found (in sputum) by microscopy

010.94 Primary tuberculous infection, unspecified, tubercle bacilli not found (in sputum) by microscopy, but found by bacterial culture

010.95 Primary tuberculous infection, unspecified, tubercle bacilli not found by bacteriological examination, but tuberculosis confirmed histologically

010.96 Primary tuberculous infection, unspecified, tubercle bacilli not found by bacteriological or histological examination, but tuberculosis confirmed by other methods [inoculation of animals]

011.00 Tuberculosis of lung, infiltrative, unspecified

011.01 Tuberculosis of lung, infiltrative, bacteriological or histological examination not done

011.02 Tuberculosis of lung, infiltrative, bacteriological or histological examination unknown (at present)

011.03 Tuberculosis of lung, infiltrative, tubercle bacilli found (in sputum) by microscopy

011.04 Tuberculosis of lung, infiltrative, tubercle bacilli not found (in sputum) by microscopy, but found by bacterial culture

011.05 Tuberculosis of lung, infiltrative, tubercle bacilli not found by bacteriological examination, but tuberculosis confirmed histologically

011.06 Tuberculosis of lung, infiltrative, tubercle bacilli not found bacteriological or histological examination, but tuberculosis confirmed by other methods [inoculation of animals]

011.10 Tuberculosis of lung, nodular, unspecified

011.11 Tuberculosis of lung, nodular, bacteriological or histological examination not done

011.12 Tuberculosis of lung, nodular, bacteriological or histological examination unknown (at present)

011.13 Tuberculosis of lung, nodular, tubercle bacilli found (in sputum) by microscopy

011.14 Tuberculosis of lung, nodular, tubercle bacilli not found (in sputum) by microscopy, but found by bacterial culture

011.15 Tuberculosis of lung, nodular, tubercle bacilli not found by bacteriological examination, but tuberculosis confirmed histologically

011.16 Tuberculosis of lung, nodular, tubercle bacilli not found by bacteriological or histological examination, but tuberculosis confirmed by other methods [inoculation of animals]

011.20 Tuberculosis of lung with cavitation, unspecified

011.21 Tuberculosis of lung with cavitation, bacteriological or histological examination not done

011.22 Tuberculosis of lung with cavitation, bacteriological or histological examination unknown (at present)

011.23 Tuberculosis of lung with cavitation, tubercle bacilli found (in sputum) by microscopy

011.24 Tuberculosis of lung with cavitation, tubercle bacilli not found (in sputum) by microscopy, but found by bacterial culture

011.25 Tuberculosis of lung with cavitation, tubercle bacilli not found by bacteriological examination, but tuberculosis confirmed histologically

011.26 Tuberculosis of lung with cavitation, tubercle bacilli not found by bacteriological or histological examination, but tuberculosis confirmed by other methods [inoculation of animals]

011.30 Tuberculosis of bronchus, unspecified

011.31 Tuberculosis of bronchus, bacteriological or histological examination not done

011.32 Tuberculosis of bronchus, bacteriological or histological examination unknown (at present)

011.33 Tuberculosis of bronchus, tubercle bacilli found (in sputum) by microscopy

011.34 Tuberculosis of bronchus, tubercle bacilli not found (in sputum) by microscopy, but found in bacterial culture

011.35 Tuberculosis of bronchus, tubercle bacilli not found by bacteriological examination, but tuberculosis confirmed histologically

011.36 Tuberculosis of bronchus, tubercle bacilli not found by bacteriological or histological examination, but tuberculosis confirmed by other methods [inoculation of animals]

011.40 Tuberculous fibrosis of lung, unspecified

011.41 Tuberculous fibrosis of lung, bacteriological or histological examination not done

011.42 Tuberculous fibrosis of lung, bacteriological or histological examination unknown (at present)

011.43 Tuberculous fibrosis of lung, tubercle bacilli found (in sputum) by microscopy

011.44 Tuberculous fibrosis of lung, tubercle bacilli not found (in sputum) by microscopy, but found by bacterial culture

011.45 Tuberculous fibrosis of lung, tubercle bacilli not found by bacteriological examination, but tuberculosis confirmed histologically

011.46 Tuberculous fibrosis of lung, tubercle bacilli not found by bacteriological or histological examination, but tuberculosis confirmed by other methods [inoculation of animals]

011.50 Tuberculous bronchiectasis, unspecified

011.51 Tuberculous bronchiectasis, bacteriological or histological examination not done

011.52 Tuberculous bronchiectasis, bacteriological or histological examination unknown (at present)

011.53 Tuberculous bronchiectasis, tubercle bacilli found (in sputum) by microscopy

011.54 Tuberculous bronchiectasis, tubercle bacilli not found (in sputum) by microscopy, but found by bacterial culture

011.55 Tuberculous bronchiectasis, tubercle bacilli not found by bacteriological examination, but tuberculosis confirmed histologically

011.56 Tuberculous bronchiectasis, tubercle bacilli not found by bacteriological or histological examination, but tuberculosis confirmed by other methods [inoculation of animals]

011.70 Tuberculous pneumothorax, unspecified

011.71 Tuberculous pneumothorax, bacteriological or histological examination not done

011.72 Tuberculous pneumothorax, bacteriological or histological examination unknown (at present)

011.73 Tuberculous pneumothorax, tubercle bacilli found (in sputum) by microscopy

011.74 Tuberculous pneumothorax, tubercle bacilli not found (in sputum) by microscopy, but found by bacterial culture

011.75 Tuberculous pneumothorax, tubercle bacilli not found by bacteriological examination, but tuberculosis confirmed histologically

011.76 Tuberculous pneumothorax, tubercle bacilli not found by bacteriological or histological examination, but tuberculosis confirmed by other methods [inoculation of animals]

011.80 Other specified pulmonary tuberculosis, unspecified

011.81 Other specified pulmonary tuberculosis, bacteriological or histological examination not done

011.82 Other specified pulmonary tuberculosis, bacteriological or histological examination unknown (at present)

011.83 Other specified pulmonary tuberculosis, tubercle bacilli found (in sputum) by microscopy

011.84 Other specified pulmonary tuberculosis, tubercle bacilli not found (in sputum) by microscopy, but found by bacterial culture

011.85 Other specified pulmonary tuberculosis, tubercle bacilli not found by bacteriological examination, but tuberculosis confirmed histologically

011.86 Other specified pulmonary tuberculosis, tubercle bacilli not found by bacteriological or histological examination, but tuberculosis confirmed by other methods [inoculation of animals]

011.90 Pulmonary tuberculosis, unspecified, unspecified

011.91 Pulmonary tuberculosis, unspecified, bacteriological or histological examination not done

011.92   Pulmonary tuberculosis, unspecified, bacteriological or histological examination unknown (at present)

011.93   Pulmonary tuberculosis, unspecified, tubercle bacilli found (in sputum) by microscopy

011.94   Pulmonary tuberculosis, unspecified, tubercle bacilli not found (in sputum) by microscopy, but found by bacterial culture

011.95   Pulmonary tuberculosis, unspecified, tubercle bacilli not found by bacteriological examination, but tuberculosis confirmed histologically

011.96   Pulmonary tuberculosis, unspecified, tubercle bacilli not found by bacteriological or histological examination, but tuberculosis confirmed by other methods [inoculation of animals]

012.00   Tuberculous pleurisy, unspecified

012.01   Tuberculous pleurisy, bacteriological or histological examination not done

012.02   Tuberculous pleurisy, bacteriological or histological examination unknown (at present)

012.03   Tuberculous pleurisy, tubercle bacilli found (in sputum) by microscopy

012.04   Tuberculous pleurisy, tubercle bacilli not found (in sputum) by microscopy, but found by bacterial culture

012.05   Tuberculous pleurisy, tubercle bacilli not found by bacteriological examination, but tuberculosis confirmed histologically

012.06   Tuberculous pleurisy, tubercle bacilli not found by bacteriological or histological examination, but tuberculosis confirmed by other methods [inoculation of animals]

012.10   Tuberculosis of intrathoracic lymph nodes, unspecified

012.11   Tuberculosis of intrathoracic lymph nodes, bacteriological or histological examination not done

012.12   Tuberculosis of intrathoracic lymph nodes, bacteriological or histological examination unknown (at present)

012.13   Tuberculosis of intrathoracic lymph nodes, tubercle bacilli found (in sputum) by microscopy

012.14   Tuberculosis of intrathoracic lymph nodes, tubercle bacilli not found (in sputum) by microscopy, but found by bacterial culture

012.15   Tuberculosis of intrathoracic lymph nodes, tubercle bacilli not found by bacteriological examination, but tuberculosis confirmed histologically

012.16   Tuberculosis of intrathoracic lymph nodes, tubercle bacilli not found by bacteriological or histological examination, but tuberculosis confirmed by other methods [inoculation of animals]

012.20   Isolated tracheal or bronchial tuberculosis, unspecified

012.21   Isolated tracheal or bronchial tuberculosis, bacteriological or histological examination not done

012.22   Isolated tracheal or bronchial tuberculosis, bacteriological or histological examination unknown (at present)

012.23   Isolated tracheal or bronchial tuberculosis, tubercle bacilli found (in sputum) by microscopy

012.24   Isolated tracheal or bronchial tuberculosis, tubercle bacilli not found (in sputum) by microscopy, but found by bacterial culture

012.25   Isolated tracheal or bronchial tuberculosis, tubercle bacilli not found by bacteriological examination, but tuberculosis confirmed histologically

012.26   Isolated tracheal or bronchial tuberculosis, tubercle bacilli not found by bacteriological or histological examination, but tuberculosis confirmed by other methods [inoculation of animals]

012.30   Tuberculous laryngitis, unspecified

012.31   Tuberculous laryngitis, bacteriological or histological examination not done

012.32   Tuberculous laryngitis, bacteriological or histological examination unknown (at present)

012.33   Tuberculous laryngitis, tubercle bacilli found (in sputum) by microscopy

012.34   Tuberculous laryngitis, tubercle bacilli not found (in sputum) by microscopy, but found by bacterial culture

012.35   Tuberculous laryngitis, tubercle bacilli not found by bacteriological examination, but tuberculosis confirmed histologically

012.36   Tuberculous laryngitis, tubercle bacilli not found by bacteriological or histological examination, but tuberculosis confirmed by other methods [inoculation of animals]

012.80   Other specified respiratory tuberculosis, unspecified

012.81   Other specified respiratory tuberculosis, bacteriological or histological examination not done

012.82   Other specified respiratory tuberculosis, bacteriological or histological examination unknown (at present)

012.83   Other specified respiratory tuberculosis, tubercle bacilli found (in sputum) by microscopy

012.84   Other specified respiratory tuberculosis, tubercle bacilli not found (in sputum) by microscopy, but found by bacterial culture

012.85   Other specified respiratory tuberculosis, tubercle bacilli not found by bacteriological examination, but tuberculosis confirmed histologically

012.86   Other specified respiratory tuberculosis, tubercle bacilli not found by bacteriological or histological examination, but tuberculosis confirmed by other methods [inoculation of animals]

014.80   Other tuberculosis of intestines, peritoneum, and mesenteric glands, unspecified

014.81   Other tuberculosis of intestines, peritoneum, and mesenteric glands, bacteriological or histological examination not done

014.82   Other tuberculosis of intestines, peritoneum, and mesenteric glands, bacteriological or histological examination unknown (at present)

014.83   Other tuberculosis of intestines, peritoneum, and mesenteric glands, tubercle bacilli found (in sputum) by microscopy

014.84   Other tuberculosis of intestines, peritoneum, and mesenteric glands, tubercle bacilli not found (in sputum) by microscopy, but found by bacterial culture

014.85   Other tuberculosis of intestines, peritoneum, and mesenteric glands, tubercle bacilli not found by bacteriological examination, but tuberculosis confirmed histologically

014.86   Other tuberculosis of intestines, peritoneum, and mesenteric glands, tubercle bacilli not found by bacteriological or histological examination, but tuberculosis confirmed by other methods [inoculation of animals]

015.00   Tuberculosis of vertebral column, unspecified

015.01   Tuberculosis of vertebral column, bacteriological or histological examination not done

015.02   Tuberculosis of vertebral column, bacteriological or histological examination unknown (at present)

015.03   Tuberculosis of vertebral column, tubercle bacilli found (in sputum) by microscopy

015.04   Tuberculosis of vertebral column, tubercle bacilli not found (in sputum) by microscopy, but found by bacterial culture

015.05   Tuberculosis of vertebral column, tubercle bacilli not found by bacteriological examination, but tuberculosis confirmed histologically

015.06   Tuberculosis of vertebral column, tubercle bacilli not found by bacteriological or histological examination, but tuberculosis confirmed by other methods [inoculation of animals]

015.10   Tuberculosis of hip, unspecified

015.11   Tuberculosis of hip, bacteriological or histological examination not done

015.12   Tuberculosis of hip, bacteriological or histological examination unknown (at present)

015.13   Tuberculosis of hip, tubercle bacilli found (in sputum) by microscopy

015.14   Tuberculosis of hip, tubercle bacilli not found (in sputum) by microscopy, but found by bacterial culture

015.15   Tuberculosis of hip, tubercle bacilli not found by bacteriological examination, but tuberculosis confirmed histologically

015.16 Tuberculosis of hip, tubercle bacilli not found by bacteriological or histological examination, but tuberculosis confirmed by other methods [inoculation of animals]

015.20 Tuberculosis of knee, unspecified

015.21 Tuberculosis of knee, bacteriological or histological examination not done

015.22 Tuberculosis of knee, bacteriological or histological examination unknown (at present)

015.23 Tuberculosis of knee, tubercle bacilli found (in sputum) by microscopy

015.24 Tuberculosis of knee, tubercle bacilli not found (in sputum) by microscopy, but found by bacterial culture

015.25 Tuberculosis of knee, tubercle bacilli not found by bacteriological examination, but tuberculosis confirmed histologically

015.26 Tuberculosis of knee, tubercle bacilli not found by bacteriological or histological examination, but tuberculosis confirmed by other methods [inoculation of animals]

015.50 Tuberculosis of limb bones, unspecified

015.51 Tuberculosis of limb bones, bacteriological or histological examination not done

015.52 Tuberculosis of limb bones, bacteriological or histological examination unknown (at present)

015.53 Tuberculosis of limb bones, tubercle bacilli found (in sputum) by microscopy

015.54 Tuberculosis of limb bones, tubercle bacilli not found (in sputum) by microscopy, but found by bacterial culture

015.55 Tuberculosis of limb bones, tubercle bacilli not found by bacteriological examination, but tuberculosis confirmed histologically

015.56 Tuberculosis of limb bones, tubercle bacilli not found by bacteriological or histological examination, but tuberculosis confirmed by other methods [inoculation of animals]

015.60 Tuberculosis of mastoid, unspecified

015.61 Tuberculosis of mastoid, bacteriological or histological examination not done

015.62 Tuberculosis of mastoid, bacteriological or histological examination unknown (at present)

015.63 Tuberculosis of mastoid, tubercle bacilli found (in sputum) by microscopy

015.64 Tuberculosis of mastoid, tubercle bacilli not found (in sputum) by microscopy, but found by bacterial culture

015.65 Tuberculosis of mastoid, tubercle bacilli not found by bacteriological examination, but tuberculosis confirmed histologically

015.66 Tuberculosis of mastoid, tubercle bacilli not found by bacteriological or histological examination, but tuberculosis confirmed by other methods [inoculation of animals]

015.70 Tuberculosis of other specified bone, unspecified

015.71 Tuberculosis of other specified bone, bacteriological or histological examination not done

015.72 Tuberculosis of other specified bone, bacteriological or histological examination unknown (at present)

015.73 Tuberculosis of other specified bone, tubercle bacilli found (in sputum) by microscopy

015.74 Tuberculosis of other specified bone, tubercle bacilli not found (in sputum) by microscopy, but found by bacterial culture

015.75 Tuberculosis of other specified bone, tubercle bacilli not found by bacteriological examination, but tuberculosis confirmed histologically

015.76 Tuberculosis of other specified bone, tubercle bacilli not found by bacteriological or histological examination, but tuberculosis confirmed by other methods [inoculation of animals]

015.80 Tuberculosis of other specified joint, unspecified

015.81 Tuberculosis of other specified joint, bacteriological or histological examination not done

015.82 Tuberculosis of other specified joint, bacteriological or histological examination unknown (at present)

015.83 Tuberculosis of other specified joint, tubercle bacilli found (in sputum) by microscopy

015.84 Tuberculosis of other specified joint, tubercle bacilli not found (in sputum) by microscopy, but found by bacterial culture

015.85 Tuberculosis of other specified joint, tubercle bacilli not found by bacteriological examination, but tuberculosis confirmed histologically

015.86 Tuberculosis of other specified joint, tubercle bacilli not found by bacteriological or histological examination, but tuberculosis confirmed by other methods [inoculation of animals]

015.90 Tuberculosis of unspecified bones and joints, unspecified

015.91 Tuberculosis of unspecified bones and joints, bacteriological or histological examination not done

015.92 Tuberculosis of unspecified bones and joints, bacteriological or histological examination unknown (at present)

015.93 Tuberculosis of unspecified bones and joints, tubercle bacilli found (in sputum) by microscopy

015.94 Tuberculosis of unspecified bones and joints, tubercle bacilli not found (in sputum) by microscopy, but found by bacterial culture

015.95 Tuberculosis of unspecified bones and joints, tubercle bacilli not found by bacteriological examination, but tuberculosis confirmed histologically

015.96 Tuberculosis of unspecified bones and joints, tubercle bacilli not found by bacteriological or histological examination, but tuberculosis confirmed by other methods [inoculation of animals]

016.00 Tuberculosis of kidney, unspecified

016.01 Tuberculosis of kidney, bacteriological or histological examination not done

016.02 Tuberculosis of kidney, bacteriological or histological examination unknown (at present)

016.03 Tuberculosis of kidney, tubercle bacilli found (in sputum) by microscopy

016.04 Tuberculosis of kidney, tubercle bacilli not found (in sputum) by microscopy, but found by bacterial culture

016.05 Tuberculosis of kidney, tubercle bacilli not found by bacteriological examination, but tuberculosis confirmed histologically

016.06 Tuberculosis of kidney, tubercle bacilli not found by bacteriological or histological examination, but tuberculosis confirmed by other methods [inoculation of animals]

016.10 Tuberculosis of bladder, unspecified

016.11 Tuberculosis of bladder, bacteriological or histological examination not done

016.12 Tuberculosis of bladder, bacteriological or histological examination unknown (at present)

016.13 Tuberculosis of bladder, tubercle bacilli found (in sputum) by microscopy

016.14 Tuberculosis of bladder, tubercle bacilli not found (in sputum) by microscopy, but found by bacterial culture

016.15 Tuberculosis of bladder, tubercle bacilli not found by bacteriological examination, but tuberculosis confirmed histologically

016.16 Tuberculosis of bladder, tubercle bacilli not found by bacteriological or histological examination, but tuberculosis confirmed by other methods [inoculation of animals]

016.20 Tuberculosis of ureter, unspecified

016.21 Tuberculosis of ureter, bacteriological or histological examination not done

016.22 Tuberculosis of ureter, bacteriological or histological examination unknown (at present)

016.23 Tuberculosis of ureter, tubercle bacilli found (in sputum) by microscopy

016.24 Tuberculosis of ureter, tubercle bacilli not found (in sputum) by microscopy, but found by bacterial culture

016.25 Tuberculosis of ureter, tubercle bacilli not found by bacteriological examination, but tuberculosis confirmed histologically

016.26 Tuberculosis of ureter, tubercle bacilli not found by bacteriological or histological examination, but tuberculosis confirmed by other methods [inoculation of animals]

016.30 Tuberculosis of other urinary organs, unspecified

016.31 Tuberculosis of other urinary organs, bacteriological or histological examination not done

016.32 Tuberculosis of other urinary organs, bacteriological or histological examination unknown (at present)

016.33 Tuberculosis of other urinary organs, tubercle bacilli found (in sputum) by microscopy

016.34 Tuberculosis of other urinary organs, tubercle bacilli not found (in sputum) by microscopy, but found by bacterial culture

016.35 Tuberculosis of other urinary organs, tubercle bacilli not found by bacteriological examination, but tuberculosis confirmed histologically

016.36 Tuberculosis of other urinary organs, tubercle bacilli not found by bacteriological or histological examination, but tuberculosis confirmed by other methods [inoculation of animals]

016.40 Tuberculosis of epididymis, unspecified

016.41 Tuberculosis of epididymis, bacteriological or histological examination not done

016.42 Tuberculosis of epididymis, bacteriological or histological examination unknown (at present)

016.43 Tuberculosis of epididymis, tubercle bacilli found (in sputum) by microscopy

016.44 Tuberculosis of epididymis, tubercle bacilli not found (in sputum) by microscopy, but found by bacterial culture

016.45 Tuberculosis of epididymis, tubercle bacilli not found by bacteriological examination, but tuberculosis confirmed histologically

016.46 Tuberculosis of epididymis, tubercle bacilli not found by bacteriological or histological examination, but tuberculosis confirmed by other methods [inoculation of animals]

016.50 Tuberculosis of other male genital organs, unspecified

016.51 Tuberculosis of other male genital organs, bacteriological or histological examination not done

016.52 Tuberculosis of other male genital organs, bacteriological or histological examination unknown (at present)

016.53 Tuberculosis of other male genital organs, tubercle bacilli found (in sputum) by microscopy

016.54 Tuberculosis of other male genital organs, tubercle bacilli not found (in sputum) by microscopy, but found by bacterial culture

016.55 Tuberculosis of other male genital organs, tubercle bacilli not found by bacteriological examination, but tuberculosis confirmed histologically

016.56 Tuberculosis of other male genital organs, tubercle bacilli not found by bacteriological or histological examination, but tuberculosis confirmed by other methods [inoculation of animals]

016.60 Tuberculous oophoritis and salpingitis, unspecified

016.61 Tuberculous oophoritis and salpingitis, bacteriological or histological examination not done

016.62 Tuberculous oophoritis and salpingitis, bacteriological or histological examination unknown (at present)

016.63 Tuberculous oophoritis and salpingitis, tubercle bacilli found (in sputum) by microscopy

016.64 Tuberculous oophoritis and salpingitis, tubercle bacilli not found (in sputum) by microscopy, but found by bacterial culture

016.65 Tuberculous oophoritis and salpingitis, tubercle bacilli not found by bacteriological examination, but tuberculosis confirmed histologically

016.66 Tuberculous oophoritis and salpingitis, tubercle bacilli not found by bacteriological or histological examination, but tuberculosis confirmed by other methods [inoculation of animals]

016.70 Tuberculosis of other female genital organs, unspecified

016.71 Tuberculosis of other female genital organs, bacteriological or histological examination not done

016.72 Tuberculosis of other female genital organs, bacteriological or histological examination unknown (at present)

016.73 Tuberculosis of other female genital organs, tubercle bacilli found (in sputum) by microscopy

016.74 Tuberculosis of other female genital organs, tubercle bacilli not found (in sputum) by microscopy, but found by bacterial culture

016.75 Tuberculosis of other female genital organs, tubercle bacilli not found by bacteriological examination, but tuberculosis confirmed histologically

016.76 Tuberculosis of other female genital organs, tubercle bacilli not found by bacteriological or histological examination, but tuberculosis confirmed by other methods [inoculation of animals]

016.90 Genitourinary tuberculosis, unspecified, unspecified

016.91 Genitourinary tuberculosis, unspecified, bacteriological or histological examination not done

016.92 Genitourinary tuberculosis, unspecified, bacteriological or histological examination unknown (at present)

016.93 Genitourinary tuberculosis, unspecified, tubercle bacilli found (in sputum) by microscopy

016.94 Genitourinary tuberculosis, unspecified, tubercle bacilli not found (in sputum) by microscopy, but found by bacterial culture

016.95 Genitourinary tuberculosis, unspecified, tubercle bacilli not found by bacteriological examination, but tuberculosis confirmed histologically

016.96 Genitourinary tuberculosis, unspecified, tubercle bacilli not found by bacteriological or histological examination, but tuberculosis confirmed by other methods [inoculation of animals]

017.00 Tuberculosis of skin and subcutaneous cellular tissue, unspecified

017.01 Tuberculosis of skin and subcutaneous cellular tissue, bacteriological or histological examination not done

017.02 Tuberculosis of skin and subcutaneous cellular tissue, bacteriological or histological examination unknown (at present)

017.03 Tuberculosis of skin and subcutaneous cellular tissue, tubercle bacilli found (in sputum) by microscopy

017.04 Tuberculosis of skin and subcutaneous cellular tissue, tubercle bacilli not found (in sputum) by microscopy, but found by bacterial culture

017.05 Tuberculosis of skin and subcutaneous cellular tissue, tubercle bacilli not found by bacteriological examination, but tuberculosis confirmed histologically

017.06 Tuberculosis of skin and subcutaneous cellular tissue, tubercle bacilli not found by bacteriological or histological examination, but tuberculosis confirmed by other methods [inoculation of animals]

017.20 Tuberculosis of peripheral lymph nodes, unspecified

017.21 Tuberculosis of peripheral lymph nodes, bacteriological or histological examination not done

017.22 Tuberculosis of peripheral lymph nodes, bacteriological or histological examination unknown (at present)

017.23 Tuberculosis of peripheral lymph nodes, tubercle bacilli found (in sputum) by microscopy

017.24 Tuberculosis of peripheral lymph nodes, tubercle bacilli not found (in sputum) by microscopy, but found by bacterial culture

017.25 Tuberculosis of peripheral lymph nodes, tubercle bacilli not found by bacteriological examination, but tuberculosis confirmed histologically

017.26 Tuberculosis of peripheral lymph nodes, tubercle bacilli not found by bacteriological or histological examination, but tuberculosis confirmed by other methods [inoculation of animals]

017.30 Tuberculosis of eye, unspecified

017.31 Tuberculosis of eye, bacteriological or histological examination not done

017.32 Tuberculosis of eye, bacteriological or histological examination unknown (at present)

017.33 Tuberculosis of eye, tubercle bacilli found (in sputum) by microscopy

017.34 Tuberculosis of eye, tubercle bacilli not found (in sputum) by microscopy, but found by bacterial culture

017.35 Tuberculosis of eye, tubercle bacilli not found by bacteriological examination, but tuberculosis confirmed histologically

017.36 Tuberculosis of eye, tubercle bacilli not found by bacteriological or histological examination, but tuberculosis confirmed by other methods [inoculation of animals]

017.40 Tuberculosis of ear, unspecified

017.41 Tuberculosis of ear, bacteriological or histological examination not done

017.42 Tuberculosis of ear, bacteriological or histological examination unknown (at present)

017.43 Tuberculosis of ear, tubercle bacilli found (in sputum) by microscopy

017.44 Tuberculosis of ear, tubercle bacilli not found (in sputum) by microscopy, but found by bacterial culture

017.45 Tuberculosis of ear, tubercle bacilli not found by bacteriological examination, but tuberculosis confirmed histologically

017.46 Tuberculosis of ear, tubercle bacilli not found by bacteriological or histological examination, but tuberculosis confirmed by other methods [inoculation of animals]

017.50 Tuberculosis of thyroid gland, unspecified

017.51 Tuberculosis of thyroid gland, bacteriological or histological examination not done

017.52 Tuberculosis of thyroid gland, bacteriological or histological examination unknown (at present)

017.53 Tuberculosis of thyroid gland, tubercle bacilli found (in sputum) by microscopy

017.54 Tuberculosis of thyroid gland, tubercle bacilli not found (in sputum) by microscopy, but found by bacterial culture

017.55 Tuberculosis of thyroid gland, tubercle bacilli not found by bacteriological examination, but tuberculosis confirmed histologically

017.56 Tuberculosis of thyroid gland, tubercle bacilli not found by bacteriological or histological examination, but tuberculosis confirmed by other methods [inoculation of animals]

017.60 Tuberculosis of adrenal glands, unspecified

017.61 Tuberculosis of adrenal glands, bacteriological or histological examination not done

017.62 Tuberculosis of adrenal glands, bacteriological or histological examination unknown (at present)

017.63 Tuberculosis of adrenal glands, tubercle bacilli found (in sputum) by microscopy

017.64 Tuberculosis of adrenal glands, tubercle bacilli not found (in sputum) by microscopy, but found by bacterial culture

017.65 Tuberculosis of adrenal glands, tubercle bacilli not found by bacteriological examination, but tuberculosis confirmed histologically

017.66 Tuberculosis of adrenal glands, tubercle bacilli not found by bacteriological or histological examination, but tuberculosis confirmed by other methods [inoculation of animals]

017.70 Tuberculosis of spleen, unspecified

017.71 Tuberculosis of spleen, bacteriological or histological examination not done

017.72 Tuberculosis of spleen, bacteriological or histological examination unknown (at present)

017.73 Tuberculosis of spleen, tubercle bacilli found (in sputum) by microscopy

017.74 Tuberculosis of spleen, tubercle bacilli not found (in sputum) by microscopy, but found by bacterial culture

017.75 Tuberculosis of spleen, tubercle bacilli not found by bacteriological examination, but tuberculosis confirmed histologically

017.76 Tuberculosis of spleen, tubercle bacilli not found by bacteriological or histological examination, but tuberculosis confirmed by other methods [inoculation of animals]

017.80 Tuberculosis of esophagus, unspecified

017.81 Tuberculosis of esophagus, bacteriological or histological examination not done

017.82 Tuberculosis of esophagus, bacteriological or histological examination unknown (at present)

017.83 Tuberculosis of esophagus, tubercle bacilli found (in sputum) by microscopy

017.84 Tuberculosis of esophagus, tubercle bacilli not found (in sputum) by microscopy, but found by bacterial culture

017.85 Tuberculosis of esophagus, tubercle bacilli not found by bacteriological examination, but tuberculosis confirmed histologically

017.86 Tuberculosis of esophagus, tubercle bacilli not found by bacteriological or histological examination, but tuberculosis confirmed by other methods [inoculation of animals]

017.90 Tuberculosis of other specified organs, unspecified

017.91 Tuberculosis of other specified organs, bacteriological or histological examination not done

017.92 Tuberculosis of other specified organs, bacteriological or histological examination unknown (at present)

017.93 Tuberculosis of other specified organs, tubercle bacilli found (in sputum) by microscopy

017.94 Tuberculosis of other specified organs, tubercle bacilli not found (in sputum) by microscopy, but found by bacterial culture

017.95 Tuberculosis of other specified organs, tubercle bacilli not found by bacteriological examination, but tuberculosis confirmed histologically

017.96 Tuberculosis of other specified organs, tubercle bacilli not found by bacteriological or histological examination, but tuberculosis confirmed by other methods [inoculation of animals]

021.0 Ulceroglandular tularemia

021.1 Enteric tularemia

021.2 Pulmonary tularemia

021.3 Oculoglandular tularemia

021.8 Other specified tularemia

021.9 Unspecified tularemia

022.0 Cutaneous anthrax

022.2 Gastrointestinal anthrax

022.8 Other specified manifestations of anthrax

022.9 Anthrax, unspecified

023.8 Other brucellosis

023.9 Brucellosis, unspecified

024 Glanders

025 Melioidosis

026.0 Spirillary fever

026.1 Streptobacillary fever

026.9 Unspecified rat-bite fever

027.0 Listeriosis

027.2 Pasteurellosis

027.8 Other specified zoonotic bacterial diseases

027.9 Unspecified zoonotic bacterial disease

030.0 Lepromatous leprosy [type L]

030.1 Tuberculoid leprosy [type T]

030.2 Indeterminate leprosy [group I]

030.3 Borderline leprosy [group B]

030.8 Other specified leprosy

030.9 Leprosy, unspecified

031.0 Pulmonary diseases due to other mycobacteria

031.1 Cutaneous diseases due to other mycobacteria

031.2 Disseminated due to other mycobacteria

031.8	Other specified mycobacterial diseases	052.7	Chickenpox with other specified complications
031.9	Unspecified diseases due to mycobacteria	052.8	Chickenpox with unspecified complication
032.0	Faucial diphtheria	052.9	Varicella without mention of complication
032.1	Nasopharyngeal diphtheria	053.10	Herpes zoster with unspecified nervous system complication
032.2	Anterior nasal diphtheria	053.11	Geniculate herpes zoster
032.3	Laryngeal diphtheria	053.12	Postherpetic trigeminal neuralgia
032.81	Conjunctival diphtheria	053.13	Postherpetic polyneuropathy
032.82	Diphtheritic myocarditis	053.19	Herpes zoster with other nervous system complications
032.83	Diphtheritic peritonitis	053.20	Herpes zoster dermatitis of eyelid
032.84	Diphtheritic cystitis	053.21	Herpes zoster keratoconjunctivitis
032.85	Cutaneous diphtheria	053.22	Herpes zoster iridocyclitis
032.89	Other specified diphtheria	053.29	Herpes zoster with other ophthalmic complications
032.9	Diphtheria, unspecified	053.71	Otitis externa due to herpes zoster
033.0	Whooping cough due to bordetella pertussis [B. pertussis]	053.79	Herpes zoster with other specified complications
033.1	Whooping cough due to bordetella parapertussis [B. parapertussis]	053.8	Herpes zoster with unspecified complication
033.8	Whooping cough due to other specified organism	054.2	Herpetic gingivostomatitis
033.9	Whooping cough, unspecified organism	054.40	Herpes simplex with unspecified ophthalmic complication
034.1	Scarlet fever	054.41	Herpes simplex dermatitis of eyelid
036.81	Meningococcal optic neuritis	054.42	Dendritic keratitis
036.82	Meningococcal arthropathy	054.43	Herpes simplex disciform keratitis
036.89	Other specified meningococcal infections	054.44	Herpes simplex iridocyclitis
036.9	Meningococcal infection, unspecified	054.49	Herpes simplex with other ophthalmic complications
039.0	Cutaneous actinomycotic infection	054.71	Visceral herpes simplex
039.1	Pulmonary actinomycotic infection	054.79	Herpes simplex with other specified complications
039.2	Abdominal actinomycotic infection	055.71	Measles keratoconjunctivitis
039.3	Cervicofacial actinomycotic infection	055.79	Measles with other specified complications
039.4	Madura foot	056.00	Rubella with unspecified neurological complication
039.8	Actinomycotic infection of other specified sites	056.09	Rubella with other neurological complications
039.9	Actinomycotic infection of unspecified site	056.71	Arthritis due to rubella
040.2	Whipple's disease	056.79	Rubella with other specified complications
040.3	Necrobacillosis	057.0	Erythema infectiosum (fifth disease)
040.41	Infant botulism	059.01	Monkeypox
040.42	Wound botulism	059.21	Tanapox
040.81	Tropical pyomyositis	060.0	Sylvatic yellow fever
046.0	Kuru	060.1	Urban yellow fever
046.11	Variant Creutzfeldt-Jakob disease	060.9	Yellow fever, unspecified
046.19	Other and unspecified Creutzfeldt-Jakob disease	061	Dengue
046.2	Subacute sclerosing panencephalitis	065.0	Crimean hemorrhagic fever [CHF Congo virus]
046.3	Progressive multifocal leukoencephalopathy	065.1	Omsk hemorrhagic fever
046.71	Gerstmann-Sträussler-Scheinker syndrome	065.2	Kyasanur forest disease
046.72	Fatal familial insomnia	065.3	Other tick-borne hemorrhagic fever
046.79	Other and unspecified prion disease of central nervous system	065.4	Mosquito-borne hemorrhagic fever
046.8	Other specified slow virus infection of central nervous system	065.8	Other specified arthropod-borne hemorrhagic fever
046.9	Unspecified slow virus infection of central nervous system	065.9	Arthropod-borne hemorrhagic fever, unspecified
047.0	Meningitis due to coxsackie virus	066.0	Phlebotomus fever
047.1	Meningitis due to echo virus	066.1	Tick-borne fever
047.8	Other specified viral meningitis	066.2	Venezuelan equine fever
047.9	Unspecified viral meningitis	066.3	Other mosquito-borne fever
048	Other enterovirus diseases of central nervous system	066.8	Other specified arthropod-borne viral diseases
049.0	Lymphocytic choriomeningitis	066.9	Arthropod-borne viral disease, unspecified
049.1	Meningitis due to adenovirus	070.1	Viral hepatitis A without mention of hepatic coma
049.8	Other specified non-arthropod-borne viral diseases of central nervous system	070.30	Viral hepatitis B without mention of hepatic coma, acute or unspecified, without mention of hepatitis delta
049.9	Unspecified non-arthropod-borne viral diseases of central nervous system	070.31	Viral hepatitis B without mention of hepatic coma, acute or unspecified, with hepatitis delta
050.0	Variola major	070.32	Chronic viral hepatitis B without mention of hepatic coma without mention of hepatitis delta
050.1	Alastrim	070.33	Chronic viral hepatitis B without mention of hepatic coma with hepatitis delta
050.2	Modified smallpox		
050.9	Smallpox, unspecified	070.51	Acute hepatitis C without mention of hepatic coma

070.52	Hepatitis delta without mention of active hepatitis B disease or hepatic coma
070.53	Hepatitis E without mention of hepatic coma
070.59	Other specified viral hepatitis without mention of hepatic coma
070.9	Unspecified viral hepatitis without mention of hepatic coma
071	Rabies
072.0	Mumps orchitis
072.3	Mumps pancreatitis
072.71	Mumps hepatitis
072.72	Mumps polyneuropathy
072.79	Other mumps with other specified complications
072.8	Mumps with unspecified complication
073.7	Ornithosis with other specified complications
073.8	Ornithosis with unspecified complication
073.9	Ornithosis, unspecified
074.20	Coxsackie carditis, unspecified
074.21	Coxsackie pericarditis
074.22	Coxsackie endocarditis
074.23	Coxsackie myocarditis
078.3	Cat-scratch disease
078.5	Cytomegaloviral disease
078.6	Hemorrhagic nephrosonephritis
078.7	Arenaviral hemorrhagic fever
079.51	Human T-cell lymphotrophic virus, type I [HTLV-I]
079.52	Human T-cell lymphotrophic virus, type II [HTLV-II]
079.53	Human immunodeficiency virus, type 2 [HIV-2]
079.81	Hantavirus infection
079.82	SARS-associated coronavirus
079.83	Parvovirus B19
080	Louse-borne (epidemic) typhus
081.0	Murine (endemic) typhus
081.1	Brill's disease
081.2	Scrub typhus
081.9	Typhus, unspecified
082.0	Spotted fevers
082.1	Boutonneuse fever
082.2	North Asian tick fever
082.3	Queensland tick typhus
082.40	Ehrlichiosis, unspecified
082.41	Ehrlichiosis chafeensis [E. chafeensis]
082.49	Other ehrlichiosis
082.8	Other specified tick-borne rickettsioses
082.9	Tick-borne rickettsiosis, unspecified
083.0	Q fever
083.1	Trench fever
083.2	Rickettsialpox
083.8	Other specified rickettsioses
083.9	Rickettsiosis, unspecified
084.1	Vivax malaria [benign tertian]
084.2	Quartan malaria
084.3	Ovale malaria
084.4	Other malaria
084.5	Mixed malaria
084.6	Malaria, unspecified
084.7	Induced malaria
084.8	Blackwater fever
084.9	Other pernicious complications of malaria
085.0	Visceral [kala-azar] leishmaniasis
085.1	Cutaneous leishmaniasis, urban
085.2	Cutaneous leishmaniasis, Asian desert
085.3	Cutaneous leishmaniasis, Ethiopian
085.4	Cutaneous leishmaniasis, American
085.5	Mucocutaneous leishmaniasis, (American)
085.9	Leishmaniasis, unspecified
086.0	Chagas' disease with heart involvement
086.1	Chagas' disease with other organ involvement
086.2	Chagas' disease without mention of organ involvement
086.3	Gambian trypanosomiasis
086.4	Rhodesian trypanosomiasis
086.5	African trypanosomiasis, unspecified
086.9	Trypanosomiasis, unspecified
087.0	Relapsing fever, louse-borne
087.1	Relapsing fever, tick-borne
087.9	Relapsing fever, unspecified
088.0	Bartonellosis
088.81	Lyme Disease
088.82	Babesiosis
090.0	Early congenital syphilis, symptomatic
090.2	Early congenital syphilis, unspecified
090.3	Syphilitic interstitial keratitis
090.40	Juvenile neurosyphilis, unspecified
090.49	Other juvenile neurosyphilis
090.5	Other late congenital syphilis, symptomatic
091.3	Secondary syphilis of skin or mucous membranes
091.4	Adenopathy due to secondary syphilis
091.50	Syphilitic uveitis, unspecified
091.51	Syphilitic chorioretinitis (secondary)
091.52	Syphilitic iridocyclitis (secondary)
091.61	Secondary syphilitic periostitis
091.62	Secondary syphilitic hepatitis
091.69	Secondary syphilis of other viscera
091.7	Secondary syphilis, relapse
091.82	Syphilitic alopecia
091.89	Other forms of secondary syphilis
091.9	Unspecified secondary syphilis
093.0	Aneurysm of aorta, specified as syphilitic
093.1	Syphilitic aortitis
093.20	Syphilitic endocarditis of valve, unspecified
093.21	Syphilitic endocarditis of mitral valve
093.22	Syphilitic endocarditis of aortic valve
093.23	Syphilitic endocarditis of tricuspid valve
093.24	Syphilitic endocarditis of pulmonary valve
093.81	Syphilitic pericarditis
093.82	Syphilitic myocarditis
093.89	Other specified cardiovascular syphilis
093.9	Cardiovascular syphilis, unspecified
094.0	Tabes dorsalis
094.1	General paresis
094.3	Asymptomatic neurosyphilis
094.82	Syphilitic parkinsonism
094.83	Syphilitic disseminated retinochoroiditis
094.84	Syphilitic optic atrophy
094.85	Syphilitic retrobulbar neuritis
094.86	Syphilitic acoustic neuritis
094.89	Other specified neurosyphilis
094.9	Neurosyphilis, unspecified
095.0	Syphilitic episcleritis
095.1	Syphilis of lung

095.2	Syphilitic peritonitis		117.5	Cryptococcosis
095.3	Syphilis of liver		117.6	Allescheriosis [Petriellidosis]
095.4	Syphilis of kidney		117.8	Infection by dematiacious fungi [Phaehyphomycosis]
095.5	Syphilis of bone		117.9	Other and unspecified mycoses
095.6	Syphilis of muscle		118	Opportunistic mycoses
095.7	Syphilis of synovium, tendon, and bursa		120.0	Schistosomiasis due to schistosoma haematobium
095.8	Other specified forms of late symptomatic syphilis		120.1	Schistosomiasis due to schistosoma mansoni
095.9	Late symptomatic syphilis, unspecified		120.2	Schistosomiasis due to schistosoma japonicum
098.0	Gonococcal infection (acute) of lower genitourinary tract		120.3	Cutaneous schistosomiasis
098.10	Gonococcal infection (acute) of upper genitourinary tract, site unspecified		120.8	Other specified schistosomiasis
			120.9	Schistosomiasis, unspecified
098.11	Gonococcal cystitis (acute)		121.0	Opisthorchiasis
098.12	Gonococcal prostatitis (acute)		121.1	Clonorchiasis
098.13	Gonococcal epididymo-orchitis (acute)		121.2	Paragonimiasis
098.14	Gonococcal seminal vesiculitis (acute)		121.3	Fascioliasis
098.15	Gonococcal cervicitis (acute)		121.4	Fasciolopsiasis
098.16	Gonococcal endometritis (acute)		121.5	Metagonimiasis
098.17	Gonococcal salpingitis, specified as acute		121.6	Heterophyiasis
098.19	Other gonococcal infection (acute) of upper genitourinary tract		121.8	Other specified trematode infections
098.40	Gonococcal conjunctivitis (neonatorum)		122.0	Echinococcus granulosus infection of liver
098.41	Gonococcal iridocyclitis		122.1	Echinococcus granulosus infection of lung
098.42	Gonococcal endophthalmia		122.2	Echinococcus granulosus infection of thyroid
098.43	Gonococcal keratitis		122.3	Echinococcus granulosus infection, other
098.49	Other gonococcal infection of eye		122.4	Echinococcus granulosus infection, unspecified
098.50	Gonococcal arthritis		122.5	Echinococcus multilocularis infection of liver
098.51	Gonococcal synovitis and tenosynovitis		122.6	Echinococcus multilocularis infection, other
098.52	Gonococcal bursitis		122.7	Echinococcus multilocularis infection, unspecified
098.53	Gonococcal spondylitis		122.8	Echinococcosis, unspecified, of liver
098.59	Other gonococcal infection of joint		122.9	Echinococcosis, other and unspecified
098.81	Gonococcal keratosis (blennorrhagica)		123.0	Taenia solium infection, intestinal form
098.85	Other gonococcal heart disease		123.1	Cysticercosis
098.86	Gonococcal peritonitis		123.2	Taenia saginata infection
098.89	Gonococcal infection of other specified sites		123.3	Taeniasis, unspecified
099.56	Other venereal diseases due to chlamydia trachomatis, peritoneum		123.4	Diphyllobothriasis, intestinal
			123.5	Sparganosis [larval diphyllobothriasis]
100.0	Leptospirosis icterohemorrhagica		123.6	Hymenolepiasis
100.89	Other specified leptospiral infections		123.8	Other specified cestode infection
100.9	Leptospirosis, unspecified		124	Trichinosis
101	Vincent's angina		125.0	Bancroftian filariasis
112.0	Candidiasis of mouth		125.1	Malayan filariasis
112.2	Candidiasis of other urogenital sites		125.2	Loiasis
112.82	Candidal otitis externa		125.3	Onchocerciasis
112.84	Candidal esophagitis		125.4	Dipetalonemiasis
112.85	Candidal enteritis		125.5	Mansonella ozzardi infection
112.89	Other candidiasis of other specified sites		125.6	Other specified filariasis
114.0	Primary coccidioidomycosis (pulmonary)		125.7	Dracontiasis
114.1	Primary extrapulmonary coccidioidomycosis		125.9	Unspecified filariasis
114.3	Other forms of progressive coccidioidomycosis		126.0	Ancylostomiasis due to ancylostoma duodenale
114.4	Chronic pulmonary coccidioidomycosis		126.1	Necatoriasis due to necator americanus
114.5	Pulmonary coccidioidomycosis, unspecified		126.2	Ancylostomiasis due to ancylostoma braziliense
114.9	Coccidioidomycosis, unspecified		126.3	Ancylostomiasis due to ancylostoma ceylanicum
115.02	Infection by Histoplasma capsulatum, retinitis		126.8	Other specified ancylostoma
115.09	Infection by Histoplasma capsulatum, other		126.9	Ancylostomiasis and necatoriasis, unspecified
115.12	Infection by Histoplasma duboisii, retinitis		127.0	Ascariasis
115.19	Infection by Histoplasma duboisii, other		127.1	Anisakiasis
115.92	Histoplasmosis, unspecified, retinitis		127.2	Strongyloidiasis
116.0	Blastomycosis		127.3	Trichuriasis
116.1	Paracoccidioidomycosis		127.4	Enterobiasis
117.3	Aspergillosis		127.5	Capillariasis
117.4	Mycotic mycetomas			

Appendix A — Numeric CC List

127.6	Trichostrongyliasis
127.7	Other specified intestinal helminthiasis
127.8	Mixed intestinal helminthiasis
127.9	Intestinal helminthiasis, unspecified
130.1	Conjunctivitis due to toxoplasmosis
130.2	Chorioretinitis due to toxoplasmosis
130.5	Hepatitis due to toxoplasmosis
130.7	Toxoplasmosis of other specified sites
130.9	Toxoplasmosis, unspecified
136.29	Other specific infections by free-living amebae
136.4	Psorospermiasis
136.5	Sarcosporidiosis
150.0	Malignant neoplasm of cervical esophagus
150.1	Malignant neoplasm of thoracic esophagus
150.2	Malignant neoplasm of abdominal esophagus
150.3	Malignant neoplasm of upper third of esophagus
150.4	Malignant neoplasm of middle third of esophagus
150.5	Malignant neoplasm of lower third of esophagus
150.8	Malignant neoplasm of other specified part of esophagus
150.9	Malignant neoplasm of esophagus, unspecified site
151.0	Malignant neoplasm of cardia
151.1	Malignant neoplasm of pylorus
151.2	Malignant neoplasm of pyloric antrum
151.3	Malignant neoplasm of fundus of stomach
151.4	Malignant neoplasm of body of stomach
151.5	Malignant neoplasm of lesser curvature of stomach, unspecified
151.6	Malignant neoplasm of greater curvature of stomach, unspecified
151.8	Malignant neoplasm of other specified sites of stomach
151.9	Malignant neoplasm of stomach, unspecified site
152.0	Malignant neoplasm of duodenum
152.1	Malignant neoplasm of jejunum
152.2	Malignant neoplasm of ileum
152.3	Malignant neoplasm of Meckel's diverticulum
152.8	Malignant neoplasm of other specified sites of small intestine
152.9	Malignant neoplasm of small intestine, unspecified site
153.0	Malignant neoplasm of hepatic flexure
153.1	Malignant neoplasm of transverse colon
153.2	Malignant neoplasm of descending colon
153.3	Malignant neoplasm of sigmoid colon
153.4	Malignant neoplasm of cecum
153.5	Malignant neoplasm of appendix vermiformis
153.6	Malignant neoplasm of ascending colon
153.7	Malignant neoplasm of splenic flexure
153.8	Malignant neoplasm of other specified sites of large intestine
153.9	Malignant neoplasm of colon, unspecified site
154.0	Malignant neoplasm of rectosigmoid junction
154.1	Malignant neoplasm of rectum
154.2	Malignant neoplasm of anal canal
154.3	Malignant neoplasm of anus, unspecified site
154.8	Malignant neoplasm of other sites of rectum, rectosigmoid junction, and anus
155.0	Malignant neoplasm of liver, primary
155.1	Malignant neoplasm of intrahepatic bile ducts
155.2	Malignant neoplasm of liver, not specified as primary or secondary
156.0	Malignant neoplasm of gallbladder
156.1	Malignant neoplasm of extrahepatic bile ducts
156.2	Malignant neoplasm of ampulla of vater
156.8	Malignant neoplasm of other specified sites of gallbladder and extrahepatic bile ducts
156.9	Malignant neoplasm of biliary tract, part unspecified site
157.0	Malignant neoplasm of head of pancreas
157.1	Malignant neoplasm of body of pancreas
157.2	Malignant neoplasm of tail of pancreas
157.3	Malignant neoplasm of pancreatic duct
157.4	Malignant neoplasm of islets of langerhans
157.8	Malignant neoplasm of other specified sites of pancreas
157.9	Malignant neoplasm of pancreas, part unspecified
158.0	Malignant neoplasm of retroperitoneum
158.8	Malignant neoplasm of specified parts of peritoneum
158.9	Malignant neoplasm of peritoneum, unspecified
162.0	Malignant neoplasm of trachea
162.2	Malignant neoplasm of main bronchus
162.3	Malignant neoplasm of upper lobe, bronchus or lung
162.4	Malignant neoplasm of middle lobe, bronchus or lung
162.5	Malignant neoplasm of lower lobe, bronchus or lung
162.8	Malignant neoplasm of other parts of bronchus or lung
162.9	Malignant neoplasm of bronchus and lung, unspecified
163.0	Malignant neoplasm of parietal pleura
163.1	Malignant neoplasm of visceral pleura
163.8	Malignant neoplasm of other specified sites of pleura
163.9	Malignant neoplasm of pleura, unspecified
164.0	Malignant neoplasm of thymus
164.1	Malignant neoplasm of heart
164.2	Malignant neoplasm of anterior mediastinum
164.3	Malignant neoplasm of posterior mediastinum
164.8	Malignant neoplasm of other parts of mediastinum
164.9	Malignant neoplasm of mediastinum, part unspecified
170.0	Malignant neoplasm of bones of skull and face, except mandible
170.1	Malignant neoplasm of mandible
170.2	Malignant neoplasm of vertebral column, excluding sacrum and coccyx
170.3	Malignant neoplasm of ribs, sternum, and clavicle
170.4	Malignant neoplasm of scapula and long bones of upper limb
170.5	Malignant neoplasm of short bones of upper limb
170.6	Malignant neoplasm of pelvic bones, sacrum, and coccyx
170.7	Malignant neoplasm of long bones of lower limb
170.8	Malignant neoplasm of short bones of lower limb
170.9	Malignant neoplasm of bone and articular cartilage, site unspecified
171.0	Malignant neoplasm of connective and other soft tissue of head, face, and neck
171.2	Malignant neoplasm of connective and other soft tissue of upper limb, including shoulder
171.3	Malignant neoplasm of connective and other soft tissue of lower limb, including hip
171.4	Malignant neoplasm of connective and other soft tissue of thorax
171.5	Malignant neoplasm of connective and other soft tissue of abdomen
171.6	Malignant neoplasm of connective and other soft tissue of pelvis
171.7	Malignant neoplasm of connective and other soft tissue of trunk, unspecified
171.8	Malignant neoplasm of other specified sites of connective and other soft tissue
171.9	Malignant neoplasm of connective and other soft tissue, site unspecified
176.0	Kaposi's sarcoma, skin
176.1	Kaposi's sarcoma, soft tissue
176.2	Kaposi's sarcoma, palate
176.3	Kaposi's sarcoma, gastrointestinal sites
176.4	Kaposi's sarcoma, lung

Appendix A — Numeric CC List

176.5	Kaposi's sarcoma, lymph nodes
176.8	Kaposi's sarcoma, other specified sites
176.9	Kaposi's sarcoma, unspecified site
183.0	Malignant neoplasm of ovary
189.0	Malignant neoplasm of kidney, except pelvis
189.1	Malignant neoplasm of renal pelvis
189.2	Malignant neoplasm of ureter
189.3	Malignant neoplasm of urethra
189.4	Malignant neoplasm of paraurethral glands
189.8	Malignant neoplasm of other specified sites of urinary organs
189.9	Malignant neoplasm of urinary organ, site unspecified
191.0	Malignant neoplasm of cerebrum, except lobes and ventricles
191.1	Malignant neoplasm of frontal lobe
191.2	Malignant neoplasm of temporal lobe
191.3	Malignant neoplasm of parietal lobe
191.4	Malignant neoplasm of occipital lobe
191.5	Malignant neoplasm of ventricles
191.6	Malignant neoplasm of cerebellum nos
191.7	Malignant neoplasm of brain stem
191.8	Malignant neoplasm of other parts of brain
191.9	Malignant neoplasm of brain, unspecified
192.0	Malignant neoplasm of cranial nerves
192.1	Malignant neoplasm of cerebral meninges
192.2	Malignant neoplasm of spinal cord
192.3	Malignant neoplasm of spinal meninges
192.8	Malignant neoplasm of other specified sites of nervous system
192.9	Malignant neoplasm of nervous system, part unspecified
194.0	Malignant neoplasm of adrenal gland
194.1	Malignant neoplasm of parathyroid gland
194.3	Malignant neoplasm of pituitary gland and craniopharyngeal duct
194.4	Malignant neoplasm of pineal gland
194.5	Malignant neoplasm of carotid body
194.6	Malignant neoplasm of aortic body and other paraganglia
194.8	Malignant neoplasm of other endocrine glands and related structures
194.9	Malignant neoplasm of endocrine gland, site unspecified
196.0	Secondary and unspecified malignant neoplasm of lymph nodes of head, face, and neck
196.1	Secondary and unspecified malignant neoplasm of intrathoracic lymph nodes
196.2	Secondary and unspecified malignant neoplasm of intra-abdominal lymph nodes
196.3	Secondary and unspecified malignant neoplasm of lymph nodes of axilla and upper limb
196.5	Secondary and unspecified malignant neoplasm of lymph nodes of inguinal region and lower limb
196.6	Secondary and unspecified malignant neoplasm of intrapelvic lymph nodes
196.8	Secondary and unspecified malignant neoplasm of lymph nodes of multiple sites
196.9	Secondary and unspecified malignant neoplasm of lymph nodes, site unspecified
197.0	Secondary malignant neoplasm of lung
197.1	Secondary malignant neoplasm of mediastinum
197.2	Secondary malignant neoplasm of pleura
197.3	Secondary malignant neoplasm of other respiratory organs
197.4	Secondary malignant neoplasm of small intestine including duodenum
197.5	Secondary malignant neoplasm of large intestine and rectum
197.6	Secondary malignant neoplasm of retroperitoneum and peritoneum
197.7	Malignant neoplasm of liver, secondary
197.8	Secondary malignant neoplasm of other digestive organs and spleen
198.0	Secondary malignant neoplasm of kidney
198.1	Secondary malignant neoplasm of other urinary organs
198.2	Secondary malignant neoplasm of skin
198.3	Secondary malignant neoplasm of brain and spinal cord
198.4	Secondary malignant neoplasm of other parts of nervous system
198.5	Secondary malignant neoplasm of bone and bone marrow
198.6	Secondary malignant neoplasm of ovary
198.7	Secondary malignant neoplasm of adrenal gland
198.81	Secondary malignant neoplasm of breast
198.82	Secondary malignant neoplasm of genital organs
198.89	Secondary malignant neoplasm of other specified sites
199.0	Disseminated malignant neoplasm without specification of site
199.2	Malignant neoplasm associated with transplant organ
200.00	Reticulosarcoma, unspecified site, extranodal and solid organ sites
200.01	Reticulosarcoma, lymph nodes of head, face, and neck
200.02	Reticulosarcoma, intrathoracic lymph nodes
200.03	Reticulosarcoma, intra-abdominal lymph nodes
200.04	Reticulosarcoma, lymph nodes of axilla and upper limb
200.05	Reticulosarcoma, lymph nodes of inguinal region and lower limb
200.06	Reticulosarcoma, intrapelvic lymph nodes
200.07	Reticulosarcoma, spleen
200.08	Reticulosarcoma, lymph nodes of multiple sites
200.10	Lymphosarcoma, unspecified site, extranodal and solid organ sites
200.11	Lymphosarcoma, lymph nodes of head, face, and neck
200.12	Lymphosarcoma, intrathoracic lymph nodes
200.13	Lymphosarcoma, intra-abdominal lymph nodes
200.14	Lymphosarcoma, lymph nodes of axilla and upper limb
200.15	Lymphosarcoma, lymph nodes of inguinal region and lower limb
200.16	Lymphosarcoma, intrapelvic lymph nodes
200.17	Lymphosarcoma, spleen
200.18	Lymphosarcoma, lymph nodes of multiple sites
200.20	Burkitt's tumor or lymphoma, unspecified site, extranodal and solid organ sites
200.21	Burkitt's tumor or lymphoma, lymph nodes of head, face, and neck
200.22	Burkitt's tumor or lymphoma, intrathoracic lymph nodes
200.23	Burkitt's tumor or lymphoma, intra-abdominal lymph nodes
200.24	Burkitt's tumor or lymphoma, lymph nodes of axilla and upper limb
200.25	Burkitt's tumor or lymphoma, lymph nodes of inguinal region and lower limb
200.26	Burkitt's tumor or lymphoma, intrapelvic lymph nodes
200.27	Burkitt's tumor or lymphoma, spleen
200.28	Burkitt's tumor or lymphoma, lymph nodes of multiple sites
200.30	Marginal zone lymphoma, unspecified site, extranodal and solid organ sites
200.31	Marginal zone lymphoma, lymph nodes of head, face, and neck
200.32	Marginal zone lymphoma, intrathoracic lymph nodes
200.33	Marginal zone lymphoma, intraabdominal lymph nodes
200.34	Marginal zone lymphoma, lymph nodes of axilla and upper limb
200.35	Marginal zone lymphoma, lymph nodes of inguinal region and lower limb
200.36	Marginal zone lymphoma, intrapelvic lymph nodes
200.37	Marginal zone lymphoma, spleen
200.38	Marginal zone lymphoma, lymph nodes of multiple sites
200.40	Mantle cell lymphoma, unspecified site, extranodal and solid organ sites
200.41	Mantle cell lymphoma, lymph nodes of head, face, and neck

200.42	Mantle cell lymphoma, intrathoracic lymph nodes
200.43	Mantle cell lymphoma, intra-abdominal lymph nodes
200.44	Mantle cell lymphoma, lymph nodes of axilla and upper limb
200.45	Mantle cell lymphoma, lymph nodes of inguinal region and lower limb
200.46	Mantle cell lymphoma, intrapelvic lymph nodes
200.47	Mantle cell lymphoma, spleen
200.48	Mantle cell lymphoma, lymph nodes of multiple sites
200.50	Primary central nervous system lymphoma, unspecified site, extranodal and solid organ sites
200.51	Primary central nervous system lymphoma, lymph nodes of head, face, and neck
200.52	Primary central nervous system lymphoma, intrathoracic lymph nodes
200.53	Primary central nervous system lymphoma, intra-abdominal lymph nodes
200.54	Primary central nervous system lymphoma, lymph nodes of axilla and upper limb
200.55	Primary central nervous system lymphoma, lymph nodes of inguinal region and lower limb
200.56	Primary central nervous system lymphoma, intrapelvic lymph nodes
200.57	Primary central nervous system lymphoma, spleen
200.58	Primary central nervous system lymphoma, lymph nodes of multiple sites
200.60	Anaplastic large cell lymphoma, unspecified site, extranodal and solid organ sites
200.61	Anaplastic large cell lymphoma, lymph nodes of head, face, and neck
200.62	Anaplastic large cell lymphoma, intrathoracic lymph nodes
200.63	Anaplastic large cell lymphoma, intra-abdominal lymph nodes
200.64	Anaplastic large cell lymphoma, lymph nodes of axilla and upper limb
200.65	Anaplastic large cell lymphoma, lymph nodes of inguinal region and lower limb
200.66	Anaplastic large cell lymphoma, intrapelvic lymph nodes
200.67	Anaplastic large cell lymphoma, spleen
200.68	Anaplastic large cell lymphoma, lymph nodes of multiple sites
200.70	Large cell lymphoma, unspecified site, extranodal and solid organ sites
200.71	Large cell lymphoma, lymph nodes of head, face, and neck
200.72	Large cell lymphoma, intrathoracic lymph nodes
200.73	Large cell lymphoma, intra-abdominal lymph nodes
200.74	Large cell lymphoma, lymph nodes of axilla and upper limb
200.75	Large cell lymphoma, lymph nodes of inguinal region and lower limb
200.76	Large cell lymphoma, intrapelvic lymph nodes
200.77	Large cell lymphoma, spleen
200.78	Large cell lymphoma, lymph nodes of multiple sites
200.80	Other named variants of lymphosarcoma and reticulosarcoma, unspecified site, extranodal and solid organ sites
200.81	Other named variants of lymphosarcoma and reticulosarcoma, lymph nodes of head, face, and neck
200.82	Other named variants of lymphosarcoma and reticulosarcoma,intrathoracic lymph nodes
200.83	Other named variants of lymphosarcoma and reticulosarcoma, intra-abdominal lymph nodes
200.84	Other named variants of lymphosarcoma and reticulosarcoma, lymph nodes of axilla and upper limb
200.85	Other named variants of lymphosarcoma and reticulosarcoma, lymph nodes of inguinal region and lower limb
200.86	Other named variants of lymphosarcoma and reticulosarcoma, intrapelvic lymph nodes
200.87	Other named variants of lymphosarcoma and reticulosarcoma, spleen
200.88	Other named variants of lymphosarcoma and reticulosarcoma, lymph nodes of multiple sites
201.00	Hodgkin's paragranuloma, unspecified site, extranodal and solid organ sites
201.01	Hodgkin's paragranuloma, lymph nodes of head, face, and neck
201.02	Hodgkin's paragranuloma, intrathoracic lymph nodes
201.03	Hodgkin's paragranuloma, intra-abdominal lymph nodes
201.04	Hodgkin's paragranuloma, lymph nodes of axilla and upper limb
201.05	Hodgkin's paragranuloma, lymph nodes of inguinal region and lower limb
201.06	Hodgkin's paragranuloma, intrapelvic lymph nodes
201.07	Hodgkin's paragranuloma, spleen
201.08	Hodgkin's paragranuloma, lymph nodes of multiple sites
201.10	Hodgkin's granuloma, unspecified site, extranodal and solid organ sites
201.11	Hodgkin's granuloma, lymph nodes of head, face, and neck
201.12	Hodgkin's granuloma, intrathoracic lymph nodes
201.13	Hodgkin's granuloma, intra-abdominal lymph nodes
201.14	Hodgkin's granuloma, lymph nodes of axilla and upper limb
201.15	Hodgkin's granuloma, lymph nodes of inguinal region and lower limb
201.16	Hodgkin's granuloma, intrapelvic lymph nodes
201.17	Hodgkin's granuloma, spleen
201.18	Hodgkin's granuloma, lymph nodes of multiple sites
201.20	Hodgkin's sarcoma, unspecified site, extranodal and solid organ sites
201.21	Hodgkin's sarcoma, lymph nodes of head, face, and neck
201.22	Hodgkin's sarcoma, intrathoracic lymph nodes
201.23	Hodgkin's sarcoma, intra-abdominal lymph nodes
201.24	Hodgkin's sarcoma, lymph nodes of axilla and upper limb
201.25	Hodgkin's sarcoma, lymph nodes of inguinal region and lower limb
201.26	Hodgkin's sarcoma, intrapelvic lymph nodes
201.27	Hodgkin's sarcoma, spleen
201.28	Hodgkin's sarcoma, lymph nodes of multiple sites
201.40	Hodgkin's disease, lymphocytic-histiocytic predominance, unspecified site, extranodal and solid organ sites
201.41	Hodgkin's disease, lymphocytic-histiocytic predominance, lymph nodes of head, face, and neck
201.42	Hodgkin's disease, lymphocytic-histiocytic predominance, intrathoracic lymph nodes
201.43	Hodgkin's disease, lymphocytic-histiocytic predominance, intra-abdominal lymph nodes
201.44	Hodgkin's disease, lymphocytic-histiocytic predominance, lymph nodes of axilla and upper limb
201.45	Hodgkin's disease, lymphocytic-histiocytic predominance, lymph nodes of inguinal region and lower limb
201.46	Hodgkin's disease, lymphocytic-histiocytic predominance, intrapelvic lymph nodes
201.47	Hodgkin's disease, lymphocytic-histiocytic predominance, spleen
201.48	Hodgkin's disease, lymphocytic-histiocytic predominance, lymph nodes of multiple sites
201.50	Hodgkin's disease, nodular sclerosis, unspecified site, extranodal and solid organ sites
201.51	Hodgkin's disease, nodular sclerosis, lymph nodes of head, face, and neck
201.52	Hodgkin's disease, nodular sclerosis, intrathoracic lymph nodes
201.53	Hodgkin's disease, nodular sclerosis, intra-abdominal lymph nodes
201.54	Hodgkin's disease, nodular sclerosis, lymph nodes of axilla and upper limb
201.55	Hodgkin's disease, nodular sclerosis, lymph nodes of inguinal region and lower limb

201.56	Hodgkin's disease, nodular sclerosis, intrapelvic lymph nodes
201.57	Hodgkin's disease, nodular sclerosis, spleen
201.58	Hodgkin's disease, nodular sclerosis, lymph nodes of multiple sites
201.60	Hodgkin's disease, mixed cellularity, unspecified site, extranodal and solid organ sites
201.61	Hodgkin's disease, mixed cellularity, lymph nodes of head, face, and neck
201.62	Hodgkin's disease, mixed cellularity, intrathoracic lymph nodes
201.63	Hodgkin's disease, mixed cellularity, intra-abdominal lymph nodes
201.64	Hodgkin's disease, mixed cellularity, lymph nodes of axilla and upper limb
201.65	Hodgkin's disease, mixed cellularity, lymph nodes of inguinal region and lower limb
201.66	Hodgkin's disease, mixed cellularity, intrapelvic lymph nodes
201.67	Hodgkin's disease, mixed cellularity, spleen
201.68	Hodgkin's disease, mixed cellularity, lymph nodes of multiple sites
201.70	Hodgkin's disease, lymphocytic depletion, unspecified site, extranodal and solid organ sites
201.71	Hodgkin's disease, lymphocytic depletion, lymph nodes of head, face, and neck
201.72	Hodgkin's disease, lymphocytic depletion, intrathoracic lymph nodes
201.73	Hodgkin's disease, lymphocytic depletion, intra-abdominal lymph nodes
201.74	Hodgkin's disease, lymphocytic depletion, lymph nodes of axilla and upper limb
201.75	Hodgkin's disease, lymphocytic depletion, lymph nodes of inguinal region and lower limb
201.76	Hodgkin's disease, lymphocytic depletion, intrapelvic lymph nodes
201.77	Hodgkin's disease, lymphocytic depletion, spleen
201.78	Hodgkin's disease, lymphocytic depletion, lymph nodes of multiple sites
201.90	Hodgkin's disease, unspecified type, unspecified site, extranodal and solid organ sites
201.91	Hodgkin's disease, unspecified type, lymph nodes of head, face, and neck
201.92	Hodgkin's disease, unspecified type, intrathoracic lymph nodes
201.93	Hodgkin's disease, unspecified type, intra-abdominal lymph nodes
201.94	Hodgkin's disease, unspecified type, lymph nodes of axilla and upper limb
201.95	Hodgkin's disease, unspecified type, lymph nodes of inguinal region and lower limb
201.96	Hodgkin's disease, unspecified type, intrapelvic lymph nodes
201.97	Hodgkin's disease, unspecified type, spleen
201.98	Hodgkin's disease, unspecified type, lymph nodes of multiple sites
202.00	Nodular lymphoma, unspecified site, extranodal and solid organ sites
202.01	Nodular lymphoma, lymph nodes of head, face, and neck
202.02	Nodular lymphoma, intrathoracic lymph nodes
202.03	Nodular lymphoma, intra-abdominal lymph nodes
202.04	Nodular lymphoma, lymph nodes of axilla and upper limb
202.05	Nodular lymphoma, lymph nodes of inguinal region and lower limb
202.06	Nodular lymphoma, intrapelvic lymph nodes
202.07	Nodular lymphoma, spleen
202.08	Nodular lymphoma, lymph nodes of multiple sites
202.10	Mycosis fungoides, unspecified site, extranodal and solid organ sites
202.11	Mycosis fungoides, lymph nodes of head, face, and neck
202.12	Mycosis fungoides, intrathoracic lymph nodes
202.13	Mycosis fungoides, intra-abdominal lymph nodes
202.14	Mycosis fungoides, lymph nodes of axilla and upper limb
202.15	Mycosis fungoides, lymph nodes of inguinal region and lower limb

202.16	Mycosis fungoides, intrapelvic lymph nodes
202.17	Mycosis fungoides, spleen
202.18	Mycosis fungoides, lymph nodes of multiple sites
202.20	Sezary's disease, unspecified site, extranodal and solid organ sites
202.21	Sezary's disease, lymph nodes of head, face, and neck
202.22	Sezary's disease, intrathoracic lymph nodes
202.23	Sezary's disease, intra-abdominal lymph nodes
202.24	Sezary's disease, lymph nodes of axilla and upper limb
202.25	Sezary's disease, lymph nodes of inguinal region and lower limb
202.26	Sezary's disease, intrapelvic lymph nodes
202.27	Sezary's disease, spleen
202.28	Sezary's disease, lymph nodes of multiple sites
202.30	Malignant histiocytosis, unspecified site, extranodal and solid organ sites
202.31	Malignant histiocytosis, lymph nodes of head, face, and neck
202.32	Malignant histiocytosis, intrathoracic lymph nodes
202.33	Malignant histiocytosis, intra-abdominal lymph nodes
202.34	Malignant histiocytosis, lymph nodes of axilla and upper limb
202.35	Malignant histiocytosis, lymph nodes of inguinal region and lower limb
202.36	Malignant histiocytosis, intrapelvic lymph nodes
202.37	Malignant histiocytosis, spleen
202.38	Malignant histiocytosis, lymph nodes of multiple sites
202.40	Leukemic reticuloendotheliosis, unspecified site, extranodal and solid organ sites
202.41	Leukemic reticuloendotheliosis, lymph nodes of head, face, and neck
202.42	Leukemic reticuloendotheliosis, intrathoracic lymph nodes
202.43	Leukemic reticuloendotheliosis, intra-abdominal lymph nodes
202.44	Leukemic reticuloendotheliosis, lymph nodes of axilla and upper arm
202.45	Leukemic reticuloendotheliosis, lymph nodes of inguinal region and lower limb
202.46	Leukemic reticuloendotheliosis, intrapelvic lymph nodes
202.47	Leukemic reticuloendotheliosis, spleen
202.48	Leukemic reticuloendotheliosis, lymph nodes of multiple sites
202.50	Letterer-siwe disease, unspecified site, extranodal and solid organ sites
202.51	Letterer-siwe disease, lymph nodes of head, face, and neck
202.52	Letterer-siwe disease, intrathoracic lymph nodes
202.53	Letterer-siwe disease, intra-abdominal lymph nodes
202.54	Letterer-siwe disease, lymph nodes of axilla and upper limb
202.55	Letterer-siwe disease, lymph nodes of inguinal region and lower limb
202.56	Letterer-siwe disease, intrapelvic lymph nodes
202.57	Letterer-siwe disease, spleen
202.58	Letterer-siwe disease, lymph nodes of multiple sites
202.60	Malignant mast cell tumors, unspecified site, extranodal and solid organ sites
202.61	Malignant mast cell tumors, lymph nodes of head, face, and neck
202.62	Malignant mast cell tumors, intrathoracic lymph nodes
202.63	Malignant mast cell tumors, intra-abdominal lymph nodes
202.64	Malignant mast cell tumors, lymph nodes of axilla and upper limb
202.65	Malignant mast cell tumors, lymph nodes of inguinal region and lower limb
202.66	Malignant mast cell tumors, intrapelvic lymph nodes
202.67	Malignant mast cell tumors, spleen
202.68	Malignant mast cell tumors, lymph nodes of multiple sites
202.70	Peripheral T cell lymphoma, unspecified site, extranodal and solid organ sites
202.71	Peripheral T cell lymphoma, lymph nodes of head, face, and neck

202.72	Peripheral T cell lymphoma, intrathoracic lymph nodes
202.73	Peripheral T cell lymphoma, intra-abdominal lymph nodes
202.74	Peripheral T cell lymphoma, lymph nodes of axilla and upper limb
202.75	Peripheral T cell lymphoma, lymph nodes of inguinal region and lower limb
202.76	Peripheral T cell lymphoma, intrapelvic lymph nodes
202.77	Peripheral T cell lymphoma, spleen
202.78	Peripheral T cell lymphoma, lymph nodes of multiple sites
202.80	Other malignant lymphomas, unspecified site, extranodal and solid organ sites
202.81	Other malignant lymphomas, lymph nodes of head, face, and neck
202.82	Other malignant lymphomas, intrathoracic lymph nodes
202.83	Other malignant lymphomas, intra-abdominal lymph nodes
202.84	Other malignant lymphomas, lymph nodes of axilla and upper limb
202.85	Other malignant lymphomas, lymph nodes of inguinal region and lower limb
202.86	Other malignant lymphomas, intrapelvic lymph nodes
202.87	Other malignant lymphomas, spleen
202.88	Other malignant lymphomas, lymph nodes of multiple sites
202.90	Other and unspecified malignant neoplasms of lymphoid and histiocytic tissue, unspecified site, extranodal and solid organ sites
202.91	Other and unspecified malignant neoplasms of lymphoid and histiocytic tissue, lymph nodes of head, face, and neck
202.92	Other and unspecified malignant neoplasms of lymphoid and histiocytic tissue, intrathoracic lymph nodes
202.93	Other and unspecified malignant neoplasms of lymphoid and histiocytic tissue, intra-abdominal lymph nodes
202.94	Other and unspecified malignant neoplasms of lymphoid and histiocytic tissue, lymph nodes of axilla and upper limb
202.95	Other and unspecified malignant neoplasms of lymphoid and histiocytic tissue, lymph nodes of inguinal region and lower limb
202.96	Other and unspecified malignant neoplasms of lymphoid and histiocytic tissue, intrapelvic lymph nodes
202.97	Other and unspecified malignant neoplasms of lymphoid and histiocytic tissue, spleen
202.98	Other and unspecified malignant neoplasms of lymphoid and histiocytic tissue, lymph nodes of multiple sites
203.00	Multiple myeloma, without mention of having achieved remission
203.01	Multiple myeloma, in remission
203.02	Multiple myeloma, in relapse
203.10	Plasma cell leukemia, without mention of having achieved remission
203.11	Plasma cell leukemia, in remission
203.12	Plasma cell leukemia, in relapse
203.80	Other immunoproliferative neoplasms, without mention of having achieved remission
203.81	Other immunoproliferative neoplasms, in remission
203.82	Other immunoproliferative neoplasms, in relapse
204.00	Acute lymphoid leukemia, without mention of having achieved remission
204.01	Acute lymphoid leukemia, in remission
204.02	Acute lymphoid leukemia, in relapse
204.10	Chronic lymphoid leukemia, without mention of having achieved remission
204.11	Chronic lymphoid leukemia, in remission
204.12	Chronic lymphoid leukemia, in relapse
204.20	Subacute lymphoid leukemia, without mention of having achieved remission
204.21	Subacute lymphoid leukemia, in remission
204.22	Subacute lymphoid leukemia, in relapse
204.80	Other lymphoid leukemia, without mention of having achieved remission
204.81	Other lymphoid leukemia, in remission
204.82	Other lymphoid leukemia, in relapse
204.90	Unspecified lymphoid leukemia, without mention of having achieved remission
204.91	Unspecified lymphoid leukemia, in remission
204.92	Unspecified lymphoid leukemia, in relapse
205.00	Acute myeloid leukemia, without mention of having achieved remission
205.01	Acute myeloid leukemia, in remission
205.02	Acute myeloid leukemia, in relapse
205.10	Chronic myeloid leukemia, without mention of having achieved remission
205.11	Chronic myeloid leukemia, in remission
205.12	Chronic myeloid leukemia, in relapse
205.20	Subacute myeloid leukemia, without mention of having achieved remission
205.21	Subacute myeloid leukemia, in remission
205.22	Subacute myeloid leukemia, in relapse
205.30	Myeloid sarcoma, without mention of having achieved remission
205.31	Myeloid sarcoma, in remission
205.32	Myeloid sarcoma, in relapse
205.80	Other myeloid leukemia, without mention of having achieved remission
205.81	Other myeloid leukemia, in remission
205.82	Other myeloid leukemia, in relapse
205.90	Unspecified myeloid leukemia, without mention of having achieved remission
205.91	Unspecified myeloid leukemia, in remission
205.92	Unspecified myeloid leukemia, in relapse
206.00	Acute monocytic leukemia, without mention of having achieved remission
206.01	Acute monocytic leukemia, in remission
206.02	Acute monocytic leukemia, in relapse
206.10	Chronic monocytic leukemia, without mention of having achieved remission
206.11	Chronic monocytic leukemia, in remission
206.12	Chronic monocytic leukemia, in relapse
206.20	Subacute monocytic leukemia, without mention of having achieved remission
206.21	Subacute monocytic leukemia, in remission
206.22	Subacute monocytic leukemia, in relapse
206.80	Other monocytic leukemia, without mention of having achieved remission
206.81	Other monocytic leukemia, in remission
206.82	Other monocytic leukemia, in relapse
206.90	Unspecified monocytic leukemia, without mention of having achieved remission
206.91	Unspecified monocytic leukemia, in remission
206.92	Unspecified monocytic leukemia, in relapse
207.00	Acute erythremia and erythroleukemia, without mention of having achieved remission
207.01	Acute erythremia and erythroleukemia, in remission
207.02	Acute erythremia and erythroleukemia, in relapse
207.10	Chronic erythremia, without mention of having achieved remission
207.11	Chronic erythremia, in remission
207.12	Chronic erythremia, in relapse
207.20	Megakaryocytic leukemia, without mention of having achieved remission
207.21	Megakaryocytic leukemia, in remission
207.22	Megakaryocytic leukemia, in relapse
207.80	Other specified leukemia, without mention of having achieved remission

207.81	Other specified leukemia, in remission
207.82	Other specified leukemia, in relapse
208.00	Acute leukemia of unspecified cell type, without mention of having achieved remission
208.01	Acute leukemia of unspecified cell type, in remission
208.02	Acute leukemia of unspecified cell type, in relapse
208.10	Chronic leukemia of unspecified cell type, without mention of having achieved remission
208.11	Chronic leukemia of unspecified cell type, in remission
208.12	Chronic leukemia of unspecified cell type, in relapse
208.20	Subacute leukemia of unspecified cell type, without mention of having achieved remission
208.21	Subacute leukemia of unspecified cell type, in remission
208.22	Subacute leukemia of unspecified cell type, in relapse
208.80	Other leukemia of unspecified cell type, without mention of having achieved remission
208.81	Other leukemia of unspecified cell type, in remission
208.82	Other leukemia of unspecified cell type, in relapse
208.90	Unspecified leukemia, without mention of having achieved remission
208.91	Unspecified leukemia, in remission
208.92	Unspecified leukemia, in relapse
209.00	Malignant carcinoid tumor of the small intestine, unspecified portion
209.01	Malignant carcinoid tumor of the duodenum
209.02	Malignant carcinoid tumor of the jejunum
209.03	Malignant carcinoid tumor of the ileum
209.10	Malignant carcinoid tumor of the large intestine, unspecified portion
209.11	Malignant carcinoid tumor of the appendix
209.12	Malignant carcinoid tumor of the cecum
209.13	Malignant carcinoid tumor of the ascending colon
209.14	Malignant carcinoid tumor of the transverse colon
209.15	Malignant carcinoid tumor of the descending colon
209.16	Malignant carcinoid tumor of the sigmoid colon
209.17	Malignant carcinoid tumor of the rectum
209.20	Malignant carcinoid tumor of unknown primary site
209.21	Malignant carcinoid tumor of the bronchus and lung
209.22	Malignant carcinoid tumor of the thymus
209.23	Malignant carcinoid tumor of the stomach
209.24	Malignant carcinoid tumor of the kidney
209.25	Malignant carcinoid tumor of foregut, not otherwise specified
209.26	Malignant carcinoid tumor of midgut, not otherwise specified
209.27	Malignant carcinoid tumor of hindgut, not otherwise specified
209.29	Malignant carcinoid tumor of other sites
209.30	Malignant poorly differentiated neuroendocrine carcinoma, any site
209.71	Secondary neuroendocrine tumor of distant lymph nodes
209.72	Secondary neuroendocrine tumor of liver
209.73	Secondary neuroendocrine tumor of bone
209.74	Secondary neuroendocrine tumor of peritoneum
209.79	Secondary neuroendocrine tumor of other sites
238.5	Neoplasm of uncertain behavior of histiocytic and mast cells
238.6	Neoplasm of uncertain behavior of plasma cells
238.73	High grade myelodysplastic syndrome lesions
238.74	Myelodysplastic syndrome with 5q deletion
238.76	Myelofibrosis with myeloid metaplasia
238.77	Post-transplant lymphoproliferative disorder (PTLD)
238.79	Other lymphatic and hematopoietic tissues
245.0	Acute thyroiditis

246.3	Hemorrhage and infarction of thyroid
251.0	Hypoglycemic coma
251.3	Postsurgical hypoinsulinemia
253.1	Other and unspecified anterior pituitary hyperfunction
253.2	Panhypopituitarism
253.5	Diabetes insipidus
253.6	Other disorders of neurohypophysis
254.1	Abscess of thymus
255.0	Cushing's syndrome
255.3	Other corticoadrenal overactivity
255.41	Glucocorticoid deficiency
255.42	Mineralocorticoid deficiency
255.5	Other adrenal hypofunction
255.6	Medulloadrenal hyperfunction
259.2	Carcinoid syndrome
263.0	Malnutrition of moderate degree
263.1	Malnutrition of mild degree
263.2	Arrested development following protein-calorie malnutrition
263.8	Other protein-calorie malnutrition
263.9	Unspecified protein-calorie malnutrition
265.0	Beriberi
265.1	Other and unspecified manifestations of thiamine deficiency
266.0	Ariboflavinosis
268.0	Rickets, active
270.0	Disturbances of amino-acid transport
270.1	Phenylketonuria [PKU]
270.2	Other disturbances of aromatic amino-acid metabolism
270.3	Disturbances of branched-chain amino-acid metabolism
270.4	Disturbances of sulphur-bearing amino-acid metabolism
270.5	Disturbances of histidine metabolism
270.6	Disorders of urea cycle metabolism
270.7	Other disturbances of straight-chain amino-acid metabolism
270.8	Other specified disorders of amino-acid metabolism
270.9	Unspecified disorder of amino-acid metabolism
271.0	Glycogenosis
271.1	Galactosemia
271.8	Other specified disorders of carbohydrate transport and metabolism
274.11	Uric acid nephrolithiasis
276.0	Hyperosmolality and/or hypernatremia
276.1	Hyposmolality and/or hyponatremia
276.2	Acidosis
276.3	Alkalosis
276.4	Mixed acid-base balance disorder
277.00	Cystic fibrosis without mention of meconium ileus
277.03	Cystic fibrosis with gastrointestinal manifestations
277.09	Cystic fibrosis with other manifestations
277.1	Disorders of porphyrin metabolism
277.2	Other disorders of purine and pyrimidine metabolism
277.30	Amyloidosis, unspecified
277.31	Familial Mediterranean fever
277.39	Other amyloidosis
277.5	Mucopolysaccharidosis
277.85	Disorders of fatty acid oxidation
277.86	Peroxisomal disorders
277.87	Disorders of mitochondrial metabolism
277.89	Other specified disorders of metabolism
278.03	Obesity hypoventilation syndrome
279.00	Hypogammaglobulinemia, unspecified

279.01	Selective IgA immunodeficiency
279.02	Selective IgM immunodeficiency
279.03	Other selective immunoglobulin deficiencies
279.04	Congenital hypogammaglobulinemia
279.05	Immunodeficiency with increased IgM
279.06	Common variable immunodeficiency
279.09	Other deficiency of humoral immunity
279.10	Immunodeficiency with predominant T-cell defect, unspecified
279.11	Digeorge's syndrome
279.12	Wiskott-aldrich syndrome
279.13	Nezelof's syndrome
279.19	Other deficiency of cell-mediated immunity
279.2	Combined immunity deficiency
279.3	Unspecified immunity deficiency
279.50	Graft-versus-host disease, unspecified
279.51	Acute graft-versus-host disease
279.52	Chronic graft-versus-host disease
279.53	Acute on chronic graft-versus-host disease
282.8	Other specified hereditary hemolytic anemias
282.9	Hereditary hemolytic anemia, unspecified
283.0	Autoimmune hemolytic anemias
283.10	Non-autoimmune hemolytic anemia, unspecified
283.19	Other non-autoimmune hemolytic anemias
283.9	Acquired hemolytic anemia, unspecified
284.01	Constitutional red blood cell aplasia
284.09	Other constitutional aplastic anemia
284.19	Other pancytopenia
284.2	Myelophthisis
284.9	Aplastic anemia, unspecified
285.1	Acute posthemorrhagic anemia
286.2	Congenital factor XI deficiency
286.3	Congenital deficiency of other clotting factors
286.4	Von Willebrand's disease
286.52	Acquired hemophilia
286.53	Antiphospholipid antibody with hemorrhagic disorder
286.59	Other hemorrhagic disorder due to intrinsic circulating anticoagulants, antibodies, or inhibitors
286.7	Acquired coagulation factor deficiency
286.9	Other and unspecified coagulation defects
287.0	Allergic purpura
287.31	Immune thrombocytopenic purpura
287.32	Evans' syndrome
287.33	Congenital and hereditary thrombocytopenic purpura
288.4	Hemophagocytic syndromes
289.7	Methemoglobinemia
289.81	Primary hypercoagulable state
289.82	Secondary hypercoagulable state
289.83	Myelofibrosis
290.11	Presenile dementia with delirium
290.12	Presenile dementia with delusional features
290.13	Presenile dementia with depressive features
290.20	Senile dementia with delusional features
290.21	Senile dementia with depressive features
290.3	Senile dementia with delirium
290.41	Vascular dementia, with delirium
290.42	Vascular dementia, with delusions
290.43	Vascular dementia, with depressed mood
290.8	Other specified senile psychotic conditions
290.9	Unspecified senile psychotic condition
291.0	Alcohol withdrawal delirium
291.2	Alcohol-induced persisting dementia
291.3	Alcohol-induced psychotic disorder with hallucinations
291.81	Alcohol withdrawal
291.89	Other alcohol-induced mental disorders
291.9	Unspecified alcohol-induced mental disorders
292.0	Drug withdrawal
292.11	Drug-induced psychotic disorder with delusions
292.12	Drug-induced psychotic disorder with hallucinations
292.81	Drug-induced delirium
292.82	Drug-induced persisting dementia
293.0	Delirium due to conditions classified elsewhere
293.1	Subacute delirium
293.81	Psychotic disorder with delusions in conditions classified elsewhere
293.82	Psychotic disorder with hallucinations in conditions classified elsewhere
293.9	Unspecified transient mental disorder in conditions classified elsewhere
294.11	Dementia in conditions classified elsewhere with behavioral disturbance
294.21	Dementia, unspecified, with behavioral disturbance
295.00	Simple type schizophrenia, unspecified
295.01	Simple type schizophrenia, subchronic
295.02	Simple type schizophrenia, chronic
295.03	Simple type schizophrenia, subchronic with acute exacerbation
295.04	Simple type schizophrenia, chronic with acute exacerbation
295.10	Disorganized type schizophrenia, unspecified
295.11	Disorganized type schizophrenia, subchronic
295.12	Disorganized type schizophrenia, chronic
295.13	Disorganized type schizophrenia, subchronic with acute exacerbation
295.14	Disorganized type schizophrenia, chronic with acute exacerbation
295.20	Catatonic type schizophrenia, unspecified
295.21	Catatonic type schizophrenia, subchronic
295.22	Catatonic type schizophrenia, chronic
295.23	Catatonic type schizophrenia, subchronic with acute exacerbation
295.24	Catatonic type schizophrenia, chronic with acute exacerbation
295.30	Paranoid type schizophrenia, unspecified
295.31	Paranoid type schizophrenia, subchronic
295.32	Paranoid type schizophrenia, chronic
295.33	Paranoid type schizophrenia, subchronic with acute exacerbation
295.34	Paranoid type schizophrenia, chronic with acute exacerbation
295.40	Schizophreniform disorder, unspecified
295.41	Schizophreniform disorder, subchronic
295.42	Schizophreniform disorder, chronic
295.43	Schizophreniform disorder, subchronic with acute exacerbation
295.44	Schizophreniform disorder, chronic with acute exacerbation
295.53	Latent schizophrenia, subchronic with acute exacerbation
295.54	Latent schizophrenia, chronic with acute exacerbation
295.60	Schizophrenic disorders, residual type, unspecified
295.61	Schizophrenic disorders, residual type, subchronic
295.62	Schizophrenic disorders, residual type, chronic
295.63	Schizophrenic disorders, residual type, subchronic with acute exacerbation
295.64	Schizophrenic disorders, residual type, chronic with acute exacerbation
295.71	Schizoaffective disorder, subchronic
295.72	Schizoaffective disorder, chronic
295.73	Schizoaffective disorder, subchronic with acute exacerbation

295.74	Schizoaffective disorder, chronic with acute exacerbation
295.80	Other specified types of schizophrenia, unspecified
295.81	Other specified types of schizophrenia, subchronic
295.82	Other specified types of schizophrenia, chronic
295.83	Other specified types of schizophrenia, subchronic with acute exacerbation
295.84	Other specified types of schizophrenia, chronic with acute exacerbation
295.91	Unspecified schizophrenia, subchronic
295.92	Unspecified schizophrenia, chronic
295.93	Unspecified schizophrenia, subchronic with acute exacerbation
295.94	Unspecified schizophrenia, chronic with acute exacerbation
296.00	Bipolar I disorder, single manic episode, unspecified
296.01	Bipolar I disorder, single manic episode, mild
296.02	Bipolar I disorder, single manic episode, moderate
296.03	Bipolar I disorder, single manic episode, severe, without mention of psychotic behavior
296.04	Bipolar I disorder, single manic episode, severe, specified as with psychotic behavior
296.10	Manic affective disorder, recurrent episode, unspecified
296.11	Manic affective disorder, recurrent episode, mild
296.12	Manic affective disorder, recurrent episode, moderate
296.13	Manic affective disorder, recurrent episode, severe, without mention of psychotic behavior
296.14	Manic affective disorder, recurrent episode, severe, specified as with psychotic behavior
296.20	Major depressive affective disorder, single episode, unspecified
296.21	Major depressive affective disorder, single episode, mild
296.22	Major depressive affective disorder, single episode, moderate
296.23	Major depressive affective disorder, single episode, severe, without mention of psychotic behavior
296.24	Major depressive affective disorder, single episode, severe, specified as with psychotic behavior
296.30	Major depressive affective disorder, recurrent episode, unspecified
296.31	Major depressive affective disorder, recurrent episode, mild
296.32	Major depressive affective disorder, recurrent episode, moderate
296.33	Major depressive affective disorder, recurrent episode, severe, without mention of psychotic behavior
296.34	Major depressive affective disorder, recurrent episode, severe, specified as with psychotic behavior
296.40	Bipolar I disorder, most recent episode (or current) manic, unspecified
296.41	Bipolar I disorder, most recent episode (or current) manic, mild
296.42	Bipolar I disorder, most recent episode (or current) manic, moderate
296.43	Bipolar I disorder, most recent episode (or current) manic, severe, without mention of psychotic behavior
296.44	Bipolar I disorder, most recent episode (or current) manic, severe, specified as with psychotic behavior
296.50	Bipolar I disorder, most recent episode (or current) depressed, unspecified
296.51	Bipolar I disorder, most recent episode (or current) depressed, mild
296.52	Bipolar I disorder, most recent episode (or current) depressed, moderate
296.53	Bipolar I disorder, most recent episode (or current) depressed, severe, without mention of psychotic behavior
296.54	Bipolar I disorder, most recent episode (or current) depressed, severe, specified as with psychotic behavior
296.60	Bipolar I disorder, most recent episode (or current) mixed, unspecified
296.61	Bipolar I disorder, most recent episode (or current) mixed, mild
296.62	Bipolar I disorder, most recent episode (or current) mixed, moderate

296.63	Bipolar I disorder, most recent episode (or current) mixed, severe, without mention of psychotic behavior
296.64	Bipolar I disorder, most recent episode (or current) mixed, severe, specified as with psychotic behavior
296.89	Other bipolar disorders
296.99	Other specified episodic mood disorder
298.0	Depressive type psychosis
298.1	Excitative type psychosis
298.3	Acute paranoid reaction
298.4	Psychogenic paranoid psychosis
299.00	Autistic disorder, current or active state
299.01	Autistic disorder, residual state
299.10	Childhood disintegrative disorder, current or active state
299.11	Childhood disintegrative disorder, residual state
299.80	Other specified pervasive developmental disorders, current or active state
299.81	Other specified pervasive developmental disorders, residual state
299.90	Unspecified pervasive developmental disorder, current or active state
299.91	Unspecified pervasive developmental disorder, residual state
301.51	Chronic factitious illness with physical symptoms
304.01	Opioid type dependence, continuous
304.11	Sedative, hypnotic or anxiolytic dependence, continuous
304.21	Cocaine dependence, continuous
304.41	Amphetamine and other psychostimulant dependence, continuous
304.51	Hallucinogen dependence, continuous
304.61	Other specified drug dependence, continuous
304.71	Combinations of opioid type drug with any other drug dependence, continuous
304.81	Combinations of drug dependence excluding opioid type drug, continuous
304.91	Unspecified drug dependence, continuous
307.1	Anorexia nervosa
307.51	Bulimia nervosa
318.1	Severe intellectual disabilities
318.2	Profound intellectual disabilities
322.2	Chronic meningitis
330.0	Leukodystrophy
330.1	Cerebral lipidoses
330.2	Cerebral degeneration in generalized lipidoses
330.3	Cerebral degeneration of childhood in other diseases classified elsewhere
330.8	Other specified cerebral degenerations in childhood
330.9	Unspecified cerebral degeneration in childhood
331.3	Communicating hydrocephalus
331.4	Obstructive hydrocephalus
331.5	Idiopathic normal pressure hydrocephalus (INPH)
332.1	Secondary parkinsonism
333.0	Other degenerative diseases of the basal ganglia
333.4	Huntington's chorea
333.71	Athetoid cerebral palsy
333.72	Acute dystonia due to drugs
333.79	Other acquired torsion dystonia
333.90	Unspecified extrapyramidal disease and abnormal movement disorder
333.91	Stiff-man syndrome
334.0	Friedreich's ataxia
334.1	Hereditary spastic paraplegia
334.2	Primary cerebellar degeneration
334.3	Other cerebellar ataxia

334.4	Cerebellar ataxia in diseases classified elsewhere
334.8	Other spinocerebellar diseases
334.9	Spinocerebellar disease, unspecified
335.0	Werdnig-Hoffmann disease
335.10	Spinal muscular atrophy, unspecified
335.11	Kugelberg-Welander disease
335.19	Other spinal muscular atrophy
335.20	Amyotrophic lateral sclerosis
335.21	Progressive muscular atrophy
335.22	Progressive bulbar palsy
335.23	Pseudobulbar palsy
335.24	Primary lateral sclerosis
335.29	Other motor neuron disease
335.8	Other anterior horn cell diseases
335.9	Anterior horn cell disease, unspecified
336.0	Syringomyelia and syringobulbia
336.2	Subacute combined degeneration of spinal cord in diseases classified elsewhere
336.3	Myelopathy in other diseases classified elsewhere
336.8	Other myelopathy
336.9	Unspecified disease of spinal cord
337.1	Peripheral autonomic neuropathy in disorders classified elsewhere
337.20	Reflex sympathetic dystrophy, unspecified
337.21	Reflex sympathetic dystrophy of the upper limb
337.22	Reflex sympathetic dystrophy of the lower limb
337.29	Reflex sympathetic dystrophy of other specified site
341.0	Neuromyelitis optica
341.1	Schilder's disease
341.20	Acute (transverse) myelitis NOS
341.21	Acute (transverse) myelitis in conditions classified elsewhere
341.22	Idiopathic transverse myelitis
341.8	Other demyelinating diseases of central nervous system
341.9	Demyelinating disease of central nervous system, unspecified
342.00	Flaccid hemiplegia and hemiparesis affecting unspecified side
342.01	Flaccid hemiplegia and hemiparesis affecting dominant side
342.02	Flaccid hemiplegia and hemiparesis affecting nondominant side
342.10	Spastic hemiplegia and hemiparesis affecting unspecified side
342.11	Spastic hemiplegia and hemiparesis affecting dominant side
342.12	Spastic hemiplegia and hemiparesis affecting nondominant side
342.80	Other specified hemiplegia and hemiparesis affecting unspecified side
342.81	Other specified hemiplegia and hemiparesis affecting dominant side
342.82	Other specified hemiplegia and hemiparesis affecting nondominant side
342.90	Hemiplegia, unspecified, affecting unspecified side
342.91	Hemiplegia, unspecified, affecting dominant side
342.92	Hemiplegia, unspecified, affecting nondominant side
343.0	Congenital diplegia
343.1	Congenital hemiplegia
343.4	Infantile hemiplegia
344.1	Paraplegia
344.2	Diplegia of upper limbs
344.60	Cauda equina syndrome without mention of neurogenic bladder
344.61	Cauda equina syndrome with neurogenic bladder
345.01	Generalized nonconvulsive epilepsy, with intractable epilepsy
345.11	Generalized convulsive epilepsy, with intractable epilepsy
345.40	Localization-related (focal) (partial) epilepsy and epileptic syndromes with complex partial seizures, without mention of intractable epilepsy
345.41	Localization-related (focal) (partial) epilepsy and epileptic syndromes with complex partial seizures, with intractable epilepsy
345.50	Localization-related (focal) (partial) epilepsy and epileptic syndromes with simple partial seizures, without mention of intractable epilepsy
345.51	Localization-related (focal) (partial) epilepsy and epileptic syndromes with simple partial seizures, with intractable epilepsy
345.60	Infantile spasms, without mention of intractable epilepsy
345.61	Infantile spasms, with intractable epilepsy
345.70	Epilepsia partialis continua, without mention of intractable epilepsy
345.80	Other forms of epilepsy and recurrent seizures, without mention of intractable epilepsy
345.81	Other forms of epilepsy and recurrent seizures, with intractable epilepsy
345.91	Epilepsy, unspecified, with intractable epilepsy
346.60	Persistent migraine aura with cerebral infarction, without mention of intractable migraine without mention of status migrainosus
346.61	Persistent migraine aura with cerebral infarction, with intractable migraine, so stated, without mention of status migrainosus
346.62	Persistent migraine aura with cerebral infarction, without mention of intractable migraine with status migrainosus
346.63	Persistent migraine aura with cerebral infarction, with intractable migraine, so stated, with status migrainosus
348.1	Anoxic brain damage
349.1	Nervous system complications from surgically implanted device
349.31	Accidental puncture or laceration of dura during a procedure
349.39	Other dural tear
349.81	Cerebrospinal fluid rhinorrhea
356.3	Refsum's disease
357.0	Acute infective polyneuritis
357.81	Chronic inflammatory demyelinating polyneuritis
357.82	Critical illness polyneuropathy
358.1	Myasthenic syndromes in diseases classified elsewhere
358.30	Lambert-Eaton syndrome, unspecified
358.31	Lambert-Eaton syndrome in neoplastic disease
358.39	Lambert-Eaton syndrome in other diseases classified elsewhere
359.0	Congenital hereditary muscular dystrophy
359.1	Hereditary progressive muscular dystrophy
359.4	Toxic myopathy
359.6	Symptomatic inflammatory myopathy in diseases classified elsewhere
359.81	Critical illness myopathy
360.00	Purulent endophthalmitis, unspecified
360.01	Acute endophthalmitis
360.02	Panophthalmitis
360.04	Vitreous abscess
360.11	Sympathetic uveitis
360.12	Panuveitis
360.13	Parasitic endophthalmitis NOS
360.19	Other endophthalmitis
361.2	Serous retinal detachment
361.81	Traction detachment of retina
361.89	Other forms of retinal detachment
361.9	Unspecified retinal detachment
362.30	Retinal vascular occlusion, unspecified
362.31	Central retinal artery occlusion
362.32	Retinal arterial branch occlusion
362.33	Partial retinal arterial occlusion
362.34	Transient retinal arterial occlusion
362.35	Central retinal vein occlusion

362.40	Retinal layer separation, unspecified
362.42	Serous detachment of retinal pigment epithelium
362.43	Hemorrhagic detachment of retinal pigment epithelium
362.84	Retinal ischemia
363.10	Disseminated chorioretinitis, unspecified
363.11	Disseminated choroiditis and chorioretinitis, posterior pole
363.12	Disseminated choroiditis and chorioretinitis, peripheral
363.13	Disseminated choroiditis and chorioretinitis, generalized
363.14	Disseminated retinitis and retinochoroiditis, metastatic
363.15	Disseminated retinitis and retinochoroiditis, pigment epitheliopathy
363.20	Chorioretinitis, unspecified
363.63	Choroidal rupture
363.70	Choroidal detachment, unspecified
363.71	Serous choroidal detachment
363.72	Hemorrhagic choroidal detachment
364.00	Acute and subacute iridocyclitis, unspecified
364.01	Primary iridocyclitis
364.02	Recurrent iridocyclitis
364.03	Secondary iridocyclitis, infectious
364.22	Glaucomatocyclitic crises
364.3	Unspecified iridocyclitis
365.22	Acute angle-closure glaucoma
368.11	Sudden visual loss
368.12	Transient visual loss
376.01	Orbital cellulitis
376.02	Orbital periostitis
376.03	Orbital osteomyelitis
377.00	Papilledema, unspecified
377.01	Papilledema associated with increased intracranial pressure
377.30	Optic neuritis, unspecified
377.31	Optic papillitis
377.32	Retrobulbar neuritis (acute)
377.39	Other optic neuritis
377.51	Disorders of optic chiasm associated with pituitary neoplasms and disorders
377.52	Disorders of optic chiasm associated with other neoplasms
377.53	Disorders of optic chiasm associated with vascular disorders
377.54	Disorders of optic chiasm associated with inflammatory disorders
377.61	Disorders of other visual pathways associated with neoplasms
377.62	Disorders of other visual pathways associated with vascular disorders
377.63	Disorders of other visual pathways associated with inflammatory disorders
377.71	Disorders of visual cortex associated with neoplasms
377.72	Disorders of visual cortex associated with vascular disorders
377.73	Disorders of visual cortex associated with inflammatory disorders
380.14	Malignant otitis externa
383.00	Acute mastoiditis without complications
383.01	Subperiosteal abscess of mastoid
383.02	Acute mastoiditis with other complications
388.61	Cerebrospinal fluid otorrhea
391.0	Acute rheumatic pericarditis
391.1	Acute rheumatic endocarditis
391.2	Acute rheumatic myocarditis
391.8	Other acute rheumatic heart disease
391.9	Acute rheumatic heart disease, unspecified
392.0	Rheumatic chorea with heart involvement
392.9	Rheumatic chorea without mention of heart involvement
393	Chronic rheumatic pericarditis
398.0	Rheumatic myocarditis
398.91	Rheumatic heart failure (congestive)
401.0	Malignant essential hypertension
402.00	Malignant hypertensive heart disease without heart failure
402.01	Malignant hypertensive heart disease with heart failure
403.00	Hypertensive chronic kidney disease, malignant, with chronic kidney disease stage I through stage IV, or unspecified
403.01	Hypertensive chronic kidney disease, malignant, with chronic kidney disease stage V or end stage renal disease
403.11	Hypertensive chronic kidney disease, benign, with chronic kidney disease stage V or end stage renal disease
403.91	Hypertensive chronic kidney disease, unspecified, with chronic kidney disease stage V or end stage renal disease
404.00	Hypertensive heart and chronic kidney disease, malignant, without heart failure and with chronic kidney disease stage I through stage IV, or unspecified
404.01	Hypertensive heart and chronic kidney disease, malignant, with heart failure and with chronic kidney disease stage I through stage IV, or unspecified
404.02	Hypertensive heart and chronic kidney disease, malignant, without heart failure and with chronic kidney disease stage V or end stage renal disease
404.03	Hypertensive heart and chronic kidney disease, malignant, with heart failure and with chronic kidney disease stage V or end stage renal disease
404.11	Hypertensive heart and chronic kidney disease, benign, with heart failure and with chronic kidney disease stage I through stage IV, or unspecified
404.12	Hypertensive heart and chronic kidney disease, benign, without heart failure and with chronic kidney disease stage V or end stage renal disease
404.13	Hypertensive heart and chronic kidney disease, benign, with heart failure and chronic kidney disease stage V or end stage renal disease
404.91	Hypertensive heart and chronic kidney disease, unspecified, with heart failure and with chronic kidney disease stage I through stage IV, or unspecified
404.92	Hypertensive heart and chronic kidney disease, unspecified, without heart failure and with chronic kidney disease stage V or end stage renal disease
404.93	Hypertensive heart and chronic kidney disease, unspecified, with heart failure and chronic kidney disease stage V or end stage renal disease
405.01	Malignant renovascular hypertension
405.09	Other malignant secondary hypertension
411.0	Postmyocardial infarction syndrome
411.1	Intermediate coronary syndrome
411.81	Acute coronary occlusion without myocardial infarction
411.89	Other acute and subacute forms of ischemic heart disease, other
413.0	Angina decubitus
413.1	Prinzmetal angina
414.02	Coronary atherosclerosis of autologous vein bypass graft
414.03	Coronary atherosclerosis of nonautologous biological bypass graft
414.04	Coronary atherosclerosis of artery bypass graft
414.06	Coronary atherosclerosis of native coronary artery of transplanted heart
414.07	Coronary atherosclerosis of bypass graft (artery) (vein) of transplanted heart
414.10	Aneurysm of heart (wall)
414.19	Other aneurysm of heart
416.0	Primary pulmonary hypertension
416.1	Kyphoscoliotic heart disease
416.2	Chronic pulmonary embolism
417.0	Arteriovenous fistula of pulmonary vessels

417.1	Aneurysm of pulmonary artery
420.0	Acute pericarditis in diseases classified elsewhere
420.90	Acute pericarditis, unspecified
420.91	Acute idiopathic pericarditis
420.99	Other acute pericarditis
423.0	Hemopericardium
423.1	Adhesive pericarditis
423.2	Constrictive pericarditis
423.3	Cardiac tamponade
423.8	Other specified diseases of pericardium
423.9	Unspecified disease of pericardium
424.90	Endocarditis, valve unspecified, unspecified cause
424.91	Endocarditis in diseases classified elsewhere
424.99	Other endocarditis, valve unspecified
425.0	Endomyocardial fibrosis
425.11	Hypertrophic obstructive cardiomyopathy
425.18	Other hypertrophic cardiomyopathy
425.2	Obscure cardiomyopathy of Africa
425.3	Endocardial fibroelastosis
425.4	Other primary cardiomyopathies
425.5	Alcoholic cardiomyopathy
425.7	Nutritional and metabolic cardiomyopathy
425.8	Cardiomyopathy in other diseases classified elsewhere
425.9	Secondary cardiomyopathy, unspecified
426.0	Atrioventricular block, complete
426.12	Mobitz (type) II atrioventricular block
426.53	Other bilateral bundle branch block
426.54	Trifascicular block
426.89	Other specified conduction disorders
427.0	Paroxysmal supraventricular tachycardia
427.1	Paroxysmal ventricular tachycardia
427.32	Atrial flutter
428.1	Left heart failure
428.20	Systolic heart failure, unspecified
428.22	Chronic systolic heart failure
428.30	Diastolic heart failure, unspecified
428.32	Chronic diastolic heart failure
428.40	Combined systolic and diastolic heart failure, unspecified
428.42	Chronic combined systolic and diastolic heart failure
429.71	Acquired cardiac septal defect
429.79	Certain sequelae of myocardial infarction, not elsewhere classified, other
429.81	Other disorders of papillary muscle
429.82	Hyperkinetic heart disease
429.83	Takotsubo syndrome
432.9	Unspecified intracranial hemorrhage
435.0	Basilar artery syndrome
435.1	Vertebral artery syndrome
435.2	Subclavian steal syndrome
435.3	Vertebrobasilar artery syndrome
435.8	Other specified transient cerebral ischemias
435.9	Unspecified transient cerebral ischemia
436	Acute, but ill-defined, cerebrovascular disease
437.1	Other generalized ischemic cerebrovascular disease
437.2	Hypertensive encephalopathy
437.4	Cerebral arteritis
437.5	Moyamoya disease
437.6	Nonpyogenic thrombosis of intracranial venous sinus

438.20	Late effects of cerebrovascular disease, hemiplegia affecting unspecified side
438.21	Late effects of cerebrovascular disease, hemiplegia affecting dominant side
438.22	Late effects of cerebrovascular disease, hemiplegia affecting nondominant side
440.24	Atherosclerosis of native arteries of the extremities with gangrene
440.4	Chronic total occlusion of artery of the extremities
444.09	Other arterial embolism and thrombosis of abdominal aorta
444.1	Embolism and thrombosis of thoracic aorta
444.21	Arterial embolism and thrombosis of upper extremity
444.22	Arterial embolism and thrombosis of lower extremity
444.81	Embolism and thrombosis of iliac artery
444.89	Embolism and thrombosis of other specified artery
444.9	Embolism and thrombosis of unspecified artery
445.01	Atheroembolism of upper extremity
445.02	Atheroembolism of lower extremity
445.81	Atheroembolism of kidney
445.89	Atheroembolism of other site
446.0	Polyarteritis nodosa
446.1	Acute febrile mucocutaneous lymph node syndrome [MCLS]
446.20	Hypersensitivity angiitis, unspecified
446.21	Goodpasture's syndrome
446.29	Other specified hypersensitivity angiitis
446.3	Lethal midline granuloma
446.4	Wegener's granulomatosis
446.7	Takayasu's disease
447.2	Rupture of artery
447.4	Celiac artery compression syndrome
447.5	Necrosis of artery
449	Septic arterial embolism
451.11	Phlebitis and thrombophlebitis of femoral vein (deep) (superficial)
451.19	Phlebitis and thrombophlebitis of deep veins of lower extremities, other
451.81	Phlebitis and thrombophlebitis of iliac vein
451.83	Phlebitis and thrombophlebitis of deep veins of upper extremities
451.89	Phlebitis and thrombophlebitis of other sites
453.1	Thrombophlebitis migrans
453.3	Other venous embolism and thrombosis of renal vein
453.40	Acute venous embolism and thrombosis of unspecified deep vessels of lower extremity
453.41	Acute venous embolism and thrombosis of deep vessels of proximal lower extremity
453.42	Acute venous embolism and thrombosis of deep vessels of distal lower extremity
453.50	Chronic venous embolism and thrombosis of unspecified deep vessels of lower extremity
453.51	Chronic venous embolism and thrombosis of deep vessels of proximal lower extremity
453.52	Chronic venous embolism and thrombosis of deep vessels of distal lower extremity
453.6	Venous embolism and thrombosis of superficial vessels of lower extremity
453.71	Chronic venous embolism and thrombosis of superficial veins of upper extremity
453.72	Chronic venous embolism and thrombosis of deep veins of upper extremity
453.73	Chronic venous embolism and thrombosis of upper extremity, unspecified
453.74	Chronic venous embolism and thrombosis of axillary veins
453.75	Chronic venous embolism and thrombosis of subclavian veins
453.76	Chronic venous embolism and thrombosis of internal jugular veins

453.77	Chronic venous embolism and thrombosis of other thoracic veins
453.79	Chronic venous embolism and thrombosis of other specified veins
453.81	Acute venous embolism and thrombosis of superficial veins of upper extremity
453.82	Acute venous embolism and thrombosis of deep veins of upper extremity
453.83	Acute venous embolism and thrombosis of upper extremity, unspecified
453.84	Acute venous embolism and thrombosis of axillary veins
453.85	Acute venous embolism and thrombosis of subclavian veins
453.86	Acute venous embolism and thrombosis of internal jugular veins
453.87	Acute venous embolism and thrombosis of other thoracic veins
453.89	Acute venous embolism and thrombosis of other specified veins
453.9	Other venous embolism and thrombosis of unspecified site
454.2	Varicose veins of lower extremities with ulcer and inflammation
456.1	Esophageal varices without mention of bleeding
456.21	Esophageal varices in diseases classified elsewhere, without mention of bleeding
459.11	Postphlebetic syndrome with ulcer
459.13	Postphlebetic syndrome with ulcer and inflammation
459.2	Compression of vein
459.31	Chronic venous hypertension with ulcer
459.33	Chronic venous hypertension with ulcer and inflammation
464.30	Acute epiglottitis without mention of obstruction
466.11	Acute bronchiolitis due to respiratory syncytial virus (RSV)
466.19	Acute bronchiolitis due to other infectious organisms
475	Peritonsillar abscess
478.21	Cellulitis of pharynx or nasopharynx
478.22	Parapharyngeal abscess
478.24	Retropharyngeal abscess
478.34	Bilateral paralysis of vocal cords or larynx, complete
478.71	Cellulitis and perichondritis of larynx
488.02	Influenza due to identified avian influenza virus with other respiratory manifestations
488.09	Influenza due to identified avian influenza virus with other manifestations
491.21	Obstructive chronic bronchitis with (acute) exacerbation
491.22	Obstructive chronic bronchitis with acute bronchitis
493.01	Extrinsic asthma with status asthmaticus
493.02	Extrinsic asthma with (acute) exacerbation
493.11	Intrinsic asthma with status asthmaticus
493.12	Intrinsic asthma with (acute) exacerbation
493.21	Chronic obstructive asthma with status asthmaticus
493.22	Chronic obstructive asthma with (acute) exacerbation
493.91	Asthma, unspecified type, with status asthmaticus
493.92	Asthma, unspecified type, with (acute) exacerbation
494.1	Bronchiectasis with acute exacerbation
495.7	"Ventilation" pneumonitis
495.8	Other specified allergic alveolitis and pneumonitis
495.9	Unspecified allergic alveolitis and pneumonitis
506.0	Bronchitis and pneumonitis due to fumes and vapors
508.0	Acute pulmonary manifestations due to radiation
508.1	Chronic and other pulmonary manifestations due to radiation
511.81	Malignant pleural effusion
511.89	Other specified forms of effusion, except tuberculous
511.9	Unspecified pleural effusion
512.1	Iatrogenic pneumothorax
512.2	Postoperative air leak
512.81	Primary spontaneous pneumothorax
512.82	Secondary spontaneous pneumothorax

512.83	Chronic pneumothorax
512.84	Other air leak
512.89	Other pneumothorax
514	Pulmonary congestion and hypostasis
516.0	Pulmonary alveolar proteinosis
516.1	Idiopathic pulmonary hemosiderosis
516.2	Pulmonary alveolar microlithiasis
516.33	Acute interstitial pneumonitis
516.35	Idiopathic lymphoid interstitial pneumonia
516.36	Cryptogenic organizing pneumonia
516.37	Desquamative interstitial pneumonia
516.5	Adult pulmonary Langerhans cell histiocytosis
516.8	Other specified alveolar and parietoalveolar pneumonopathies
516.9	Unspecified alveolar and parietoalveolar pneumonopathy
517.1	Rheumatic pneumonia
517.2	Lung involvement in systemic sclerosis
517.3	Acute chest syndrome
518.0	Pulmonary collapse
518.3	Pulmonary eosinophilia
518.6	Allergic bronchopulmonary aspergillosis
518.7	Transfusion related acute lung injury (TRALI)
518.82	Other pulmonary insufficiency, not elsewhere classified
518.83	Chronic respiratory failure
519.00	Tracheostomy complication, unspecified
519.01	Infection of tracheostomy
519.02	Mechanical complication of tracheostomy
519.09	Other tracheostomy complications
522.0	Pulpitis
522.4	Acute apical periodontitis of pulpal origin
527.3	Abscess of salivary gland
527.4	Fistula of salivary gland
528.3	Cellulitis and abscess of oral soft tissues
530.12	Acute esophagitis
530.20	Ulcer of esophagus without bleeding
530.86	Infection of esophagostomy
530.87	Mechanical complication of esophagostomy
531.30	Acute gastric ulcer without mention of hemorrhage or perforation, without mention of obstruction
532.30	Acute duodenal ulcer without mention of hemorrhage or perforation, without mention of obstruction
533.30	Acute peptic ulcer of unspecified site without mention of hemorrhage and perforation, without mention of obstruction
534.30	Acute gastrojejunal ulcer without mention of hemorrhage or perforation, without mention of obstruction
536.1	Acute dilatation of stomach
536.41	Infection of gastrostomy
536.42	Mechanical complication of gastrostomy
537.0	Acquired hypertrophic pyloric stenosis
537.3	Other obstruction of duodenum
537.4	Fistula of stomach or duodenum
538	Gastrointestinal mucositis (ulcerative)
539.01	Infection due to gastric band procedure
539.09	Other complications of gastric band procedure
539.81	Infection due to other bariatric procedure
539.89	Other complications of other bariatric procedure
540.9	Acute appendicitis without mention of peritonitis
550.10	Inguinal hernia, with obstruction, without mention of gangrene, unilateral or unspecified (not specified as recurrent)
550.11	Inguinal hernia, with obstruction, without mention of gangrene, unilateral or unspecified, recurrent

550.12	Inguinal hernia, with obstruction, without mention of gangrene, bilateral (not specified as recurrent)
550.13	Inguinal hernia, with obstruction, without mention of gangrene, bilateral, recurrent
552.00	Femoral hernia with obstruction, unilateral or unspecified (not specified as recurrent)
552.01	Femoral hernia with obstruction, unilateral or unspecified, recurrent
552.02	Femoral hernia with obstruction, bilateral (not specified as recurrent)
552.03	Femoral hernia with obstruction, bilateral, recurrent
552.1	Umbilical hernia with obstruction
552.20	Ventral, unspecified, hernia with obstruction
552.21	Incisional ventral hernia with obstruction
552.29	Other ventral hernia with obstruction
552.3	Diaphragmatic hernia with obstruction
552.8	Hernia of other specified sites, with obstruction
552.9	Hernia of unspecified site, with obstruction
555.0	Regional enteritis of small intestine
555.1	Regional enteritis of large intestine
555.2	Regional enteritis of small intestine with large intestine
555.9	Regional enteritis of unspecified site
556.0	Ulcerative (chronic) enterocolitis
556.1	Ulcerative (chronic) ileocolitis
556.2	Ulcerative (chronic) proctitis
556.3	Ulcerative (chronic) proctosigmoiditis
556.4	Pseudopolyposis of colon
556.5	Left-sided ulcerative (chronic) colitis
556.6	Universal ulcerative (chronic) colitis
556.8	Other ulcerative colitis
556.9	Ulcerative colitis, unspecified
557.1	Chronic vascular insufficiency of intestine
557.9	Unspecified vascular insufficiency of intestine
558.1	Gastroenteritis and colitis due to radiation
558.2	Toxic gastroenteritis and colitis
560.0	Intussusception
560.1	Paralytic ileus
560.30	Impaction of intestine, unspecified
560.31	Gallstone ileus
560.39	Other impaction of intestine
560.81	Intestinal or peritoneal adhesions with obstruction (postoperative) (postinfection)
560.89	Other specified intestinal obstruction
560.9	Unspecified intestinal obstruction
562.01	Diverticulitis of small intestine (without mention of hemorrhage)
562.11	Diverticulitis of colon (without mention of hemorrhage)
564.7	Megacolon, other than Hirschsprung's
564.81	Neurogenic bowel
566	Abscess of anal and rectal regions
567.82	Sclerosing mesenteritis
568.82	Peritoneal effusion (chronic)
569.3	Hemorrhage of rectum and anus
569.41	Ulcer of anus and rectum
569.5	Abscess of intestine
569.61	Infection of colostomy or enterostomy
569.62	Mechanical complication of colostomy and enterostomy
569.69	Other colostomy and enterostomy complication
569.71	Pouchitis
569.79	Other complications of intestinal pouch
569.81	Fistula of intestine, excluding rectum and anus
569.82	Ulceration of intestine
572.3	Portal hypertension
573.1	Hepatitis in viral diseases classified elsewhere
573.2	Hepatitis in other infectious diseases classified elsewhere
574.00	Calculus of gallbladder with acute cholecystitis, without mention of obstruction
574.01	Calculus of gallbladder with acute cholecystitis, with obstruction
574.10	Calculus of gallbladder with other cholecystitis, without mention of obstruction
574.11	Calculus of gallbladder with other cholecystitis, with obstruction
574.21	Calculus of gallbladder without mention of cholecystitis, with obstruction
574.30	Calculus of bile duct with acute cholecystitis, without mention of obstruction
574.31	Calculus of bile duct with acute cholecystitis, with obstruction
574.40	Calculus of bile duct with other cholecystitis, without mention of obstruction
574.41	Calculus of bile duct with other cholecystitis, with obstruction
574.51	Calculus of bile duct without mention of cholecystitis, with obstruction
574.60	Calculus of gallbladder and bile duct with acute cholecystitis, without mention of obstruction
574.61	Calculus of gallbladder and bile duct with acute cholecystitis, with obstruction
574.70	Calculus of gallbladder and bile duct with other cholecystitis, without mention of obstruction
574.71	Calculus of gallbladder and bile duct with other cholecystitis, with obstruction
574.80	Calculus of gallbladder and bile duct with acute and chronic cholecystitis, without mention of obstruction
574.91	Calculus of gallbladder and bile duct without cholecystitis, with obstruction
575.0	Acute cholecystitis
575.12	Acute and chronic cholecystitis
575.2	Obstruction of gallbladder
575.3	Hydrops of gallbladder
575.5	Fistula of gallbladder
576.1	Cholangitis
576.4	Fistula of bile duct
577.1	Chronic pancreatitis
577.2	Cyst and pseudocyst of pancreas
578.0	Hematemesis
578.1	Blood in stool
578.9	Hemorrhage of gastrointestinal tract, unspecified
579.1	Tropical sprue
579.2	Blind loop syndrome
579.3	Other and unspecified postsurgical nonabsorption
579.4	Pancreatic steatorrhea
579.8	Other specified intestinal malabsorption
579.9	Unspecified intestinal malabsorption
581.0	Nephrotic syndrome with lesion of proliferative glomerulonephritis
581.1	Nephrotic syndrome with lesion of membranous glomerulonephritis
581.2	Nephrotic syndrome with lesion of membranoproliferative glomerulonephritis
581.3	Nephrotic syndrome with lesion of minimal change glomerulonephritis
581.81	Nephrotic syndrome in diseases classified elsewhere
581.89	Nephrotic syndrome with other specified pathological lesion in kidney
581.9	Nephrotic syndrome with unspecified pathological lesion in kidney

582.0	Chronic glomerulonephritis with lesion of proliferative glomerulonephritis
582.1	Chronic glomerulonephritis with lesion of membranous glomerulonephritis
582.2	Chronic glomerulonephritis with lesion of membranoproliferative glomerulonephritis
582.4	Chronic glomerulonephritis with lesion of rapidly progressive glomerulonephritis
582.81	Chronic glomerulonephritis in diseases classified elsewhere
582.89	Chronic glomerulonephritis with other specified pathological lesion in kidney
582.9	Chronic glomerulonephritis with unspecified pathological lesion in kidney
583.0	Nephritis and nephropathy, not specified as acute or chronic, with lesion of proliferative glomerulonephritis
583.1	Nephritis and nephropathy, not specified as acute or chronic, with lesion of membranous glomerulonephritis
583.2	Nephritis and nephropathy, not specified as acute or chronic, with lesion of membranoproliferative glomerulonephritis
583.7	Nephritis and nephropathy, not specified as acute or chronic, with lesion of renal medullary necrosis
584.8	Acute kidney failure with other specified pathological lesion in kidney
584.9	Acute kidney failure, unspecified
585.4	Chronic kidney disease, Stage IV (severe)
585.5	Chronic kidney disease, Stage V
588.1	Nephrogenic diabetes insipidus
588.81	Secondary hyperparathyroidism (of renal origin)
590.01	Chronic pyelonephritis with lesion of renal medullary necrosis
590.10	Acute pyelonephritis without lesion of renal medullary necrosis
590.3	Pyeloureteritis cystica
590.80	Pyelonephritis, unspecified
590.81	Pyelitis or pyelonephritis in diseases classified elsewhere
591	Hydronephrosis
592.1	Calculus of ureter
593.4	Other ureteric obstruction
593.5	Hydroureter
593.81	Vascular disorders of kidney
593.82	Ureteral fistula
595.0	Acute cystitis
595.82	Irradiation cystitis
596.1	Intestinovesical fistula
596.2	Vesical fistula, not elsewhere classified
596.7	Hemorrhage into bladder wall
596.81	Infection of cystostomy
596.82	Mechanical complication of cystostomy
596.83	Other complication of cystostomy
597.0	Urethral abscess
599.0	Urinary tract infection, site not specified
599.1	Urethral fistula
601.0	Acute prostatitis
601.2	Abscess of prostate
603.1	Infected hydrocele
604.0	Orchitis, epididymitis, and epididymo-orchitis, with abscess
607.3	Priapism
607.82	Vascular disorders of penis
608.20	Torsion of testis, unspecified
608.21	Extravaginal torsion of spermatic cord
608.22	Intravaginal torsion of spermatic cord
608.23	Torsion of appendix testis
608.24	Torsion of appendix epididymis

614.0	Acute salpingitis and oophoritis
614.3	Acute parametritis and pelvic cellulitis
614.7	Other chronic pelvic peritonitis, female
615.0	Acute inflammatory diseases of uterus, except cervix
616.3	Abscess of Bartholin's gland
616.4	Other abscess of vulva
616.81	Mucositis (ulcerative) of cervix, vagina, and vulva
619.0	Urinary-genital tract fistula, female
619.1	Digestive-genital tract fistula, female
619.2	Genital tract-skin fistula, female
619.8	Other specified fistulas involving female genital tract
619.9	Unspecified fistula involving female genital tract
620.5	Torsion of ovary, ovarian pedicle, or fallopian tube
633.00	Abdominal pregnancy without intrauterine pregnancy
633.01	Abdominal pregnancy with intrauterine pregnancy
633.10	Tubal pregnancy without intrauterine pregnancy
633.11	Tubal pregnancy with intrauterine pregnancy
633.20	Ovarian pregnancy without intrauterine pregnancy
633.21	Ovarian pregnancy with intrauterine pregnancy
633.80	Other ectopic pregnancy without intrauterine pregnancy
633.81	Other ectopic pregnancy with intrauterine pregnancy
633.90	Unspecified ectopic pregnancy without intrauterine pregnancy
633.91	Unspecified ectopic pregnancy with intrauterine pregnancy
634.00	Spontaneous abortion, complicated by genital tract and pelvic infection, unspecified
634.01	Spontaneous abortion, complicated by genital tract and pelvic infection, incomplete
634.02	Spontaneous abortion, complicated by genital tract and pelvic infection, complete
634.20	Spontaneous abortion, complicated by damage to pelvic organs or tissues, unspecified
634.21	Spontaneous abortion, complicated by damage to pelvic organs or tissues, incomplete
634.22	Spontaneous abortion, complicated by damage to pelvic organs or tissues, complete
634.40	Spontaneous abortion, complicated by metabolic disorder, unspecified
634.41	Spontaneous abortion, complicated by metabolic disorder, incomplete
634.42	Spontaneous abortion, complicated by metabolic disorder, complete
634.60	Spontaneous abortion, complicated by embolism, unspecified
634.70	Spontaneous abortion, with other specified complications, unspecified
634.71	Spontaneous abortion, with other specified complications, incomplete
634.72	Spontaneous abortion, with other specified complications, complete
634.80	Spontaneous abortion, with unspecified complication, unspecified
634.81	Spontaneous abortion, with unspecified complication, incomplete
634.82	Spontaneous abortion, with unspecified complication, complete
635.00	Legally induced abortion, complicated by genital tract and pelvic infection, unspecified
635.01	Legally induced abortion, complicated by genital tract and pelvic infection, incomplete
635.02	Legally induced abortion, complicated by genital tract and pelvic infection, complete
635.20	Legally induced abortion, complicated by damage to pelvic organs or tissues, unspecified
635.21	Legally induced abortion, complicated by damage to pelvic organs or tissues, incomplete
635.22	Legally induced abortion, complicated by damage to pelvic organs or tissues, complete

635.40	Legally induced abortion, complicated by metabolic disorder, unspecified
635.41	Legally induced abortion, complicated by metabolic disorder, incomplete
635.42	Legally induced abortion, complicated by metabolic disorder, complete
635.70	Legally induced abortion, with other specified complications, unspecified
635.71	Legally induced abortion, with other specified complications, incomplete
635.72	Legally induced abortion, with other specified complications, complete
635.80	Legally induced abortion, with unspecified complication, unspecified
635.81	Legally induced abortion, with unspecified complication, incomplete
635.82	Legally induced abortion, with unspecified complication, complete
636.00	Illegally induced abortion, complicated by genital tract and pelvic infection, unspecified
636.01	Illegally induced abortion, complicated by genital tract and pelvic infection, incomplete
636.02	Illegally induced abortion, complicated by genital tract and pelvic infection, complete
636.20	Illegally induced abortion, complicated by damage to pelvic organs or tissues, unspecified
636.21	Illegally induced abortion, complicated by damage to pelvic organs or tissues, incomplete
636.22	Illegally induced abortion, complicated by damage to pelvic organs or tissues, complete
636.40	Illegally induced abortion, complicated by metabolic disorder, unspecified
636.41	Illegally induced abortion, complicated by metabolic disorder, incomplete
636.42	Illegally induced abortion, complicated by metabolic disorder, complete
636.70	Illegally induced abortion, with other specified complications, unspecified
636.71	Illegally induced abortion, with other specified complications, incomplete
636.72	Illegally induced abortion, with other specified complications, complete
636.80	Illegally induced abortion, with unspecified complication, unspecified
636.81	Illegally induced abortion, with unspecified complication, incomplete
636.82	Illegally induced abortion, with unspecified complication, complete
637.00	Unspecified abortion, complicated by genital tract and pelvic infection, unspecified
637.01	Unspecified abortion, complicated by genital tract and pelvic infection, incomplete
637.02	Unspecified abortion, complicated by genital tract and pelvic infection, complete
637.20	Unspecified abortion, complicated by damage to pelvic organs or tissues, unspecified
637.21	Unspecified abortion, complicated by damage to pelvic organs or tissues, incomplete
637.22	Unspecified abortion, complicated by damage to pelvic organs or tissues, complete
637.40	Unspecified abortion, complicated by metabolic disorder, unspecified
637.41	Unspecified abortion, complicated by metabolic disorder, incomplete
637.42	Unspecified abortion, complicated by metabolic disorder, complete

637.70	Unspecified abortion, with other specified complications, unspecified
637.71	Unspecified abortion, with other specified complications, incomplete
637.72	Unspecified abortion, with other specified complications, complete
637.80	Unspecified abortion, with unspecified complication, unspecified
637.81	Unspecified abortion, with unspecified complication, incomplete
637.82	Unspecified abortion, with unspecified complication, complete
638.0	Failed attempted abortion complicated by genital tract and pelvic infection
638.1	Failed attempted abortion complicated by delayed or excessive hemorrhage
638.2	Failed attempted abortion complicated by damage to pelvic organs or tissues
638.4	Failed attempted abortion complicated by metabolic disorder
638.7	Failed attempted abortion with other specified complications
638.8	Failed attempted abortion with unspecified complication
639.0	Genital tract and pelvic infection following abortion or ectopic and molar pregnancies
639.1	Delayed or excessive hemorrhage following abortion or ectopic and molar pregnancies
639.2	Damage to pelvic organs and tissues following abortion or ectopic and molar pregnancies
639.4	Metabolic disorders following abortion or ectopic and molar pregnancies
639.8	Other specified complications following abortion or ectopic and molar pregnancy
639.9	Unspecified complication following abortion or ectopic and molar pregnancy
640.01	Threatened abortion, delivered, with or without mention of antepartum condition
640.03	Threatened abortion, antepartum condition or complication
640.93	Unspecified hemorrhage in early pregnancy, antepartum condition or complication
641.01	Placenta previa without hemorrhage, delivered, with or without mention of antepartum condition
641.03	Placenta previa without hemorrhage, antepartum condition or complication
641.23	Premature separation of placenta, antepartum condition or complication
642.01	Benign essential hypertension complicating pregnancy, childbirth, and the puerperium, delivered, with or without mention of antepartum condition
642.02	Benign essential hypertension, complicating pregnancy, childbirth, and the puerperium, delivered, with mention of postpartum complication
642.03	Benign essential hypertension complicating pregnancy, childbirth, and the puerperium, antepartum condition or complication
642.13	Hypertension secondary to renal disease, complicating pregnancy, childbirth, and the puerperium, antepartum condition or complication
642.14	Hypertension secondary to renal disease, complicating pregnancy, childbirth, and the puerperium, postpartum condition or complication
642.31	Transient hypertension of pregnancy, delivered , with or without mention of antepartum condition
642.32	Transient hypertension of pregnancy, delivered, with mention of postpartum complication
642.41	Mild or unspecified pre-eclampsia, delivered, with or without mention of antepartum condition
642.43	Mild or unspecified pre-eclampsia, antepartum condition or complication
642.44	Mild or unspecified pre-eclampsia, postpartum condition or complication

642.91 Unspecified hypertension complicating pregnancy, childbirth, or the puerperium, delivered, with or without mention of antepartum condition

642.92 Unspecified hypertension complicating pregnancy, childbirth, or the puerperium, delivered, with mention of postpartum complication

642.93 Unspecified hypertension complicating pregnancy, childbirth, or the puerperium, antepartum condition or complication

642.94 Unspecified hypertension complicating pregnancy, childbirth, or the puerperium, postpartum condition or complication

644.13 Other threatened labor, antepartum condition or complication

644.20 Early onset of delivery, unspecified as to episode of care or not applicable

646.21 Unspecified renal disease in pregnancy, without mention of hypertension, delivered, with or without mention of antepartum condition

646.22 Unspecified renal disease in pregnancy, without mention of hypertension, delivered, with mention of postpartum complication

646.23 Unspecified renal disease in pregnancy, without mention of hypertension, antepartum condition or complication

646.24 Unspecified renal disease in pregnancy, without mention of hypertension, postpartum condition or complication

646.31 Recurrent pregnancy loss, delivered, with or without mention of antepartum condition

646.61 Infections of genitourinary tract in pregnancy, delivered, with or without mention of antepartum condition

646.62 Infections of genitourinary tract in pregnancy, delivered, with mention of postpartum complication

646.63 Infections of genitourinary tract in pregnancy, antepartum condition or complication

646.64 Infections of genitourinary tract in pregnancy, postpartum condition or complication

646.71 Liver and biliary tract disorders in pregnancy, delivered, with or without mention of antepartum condition

646.73 Liver and biliary tract disorders in pregnancy, antepartum condition or complication

647.01 Syphilis of mother, complicating pregnancy, childbirth, or the puerperium, delivered, with or without mention of antepartum condition

647.02 Syphilis of mother, complicating pregnancy, childbirth, or the puerperium, delivered, with mention of postpartum complication

647.03 Syphilis of mother, complicating pregnancy, childbirth, or the puerperium, antepartum condition or complication

647.04 Syphilis of mother, complicating pregnancy, childbirth, or the puerperium, postpartum condition or complication

647.11 Gonorrhea of mother, complicating pregnancy, childbirth, or the puerperium, delivered, with or without mention of antepartum condition

647.12 Gonorrhea of mother, complicating pregnancy, childbirth, or the puerperium, delivered, with mention of postpartum complication

647.13 Gonorrhea of mother, complicating pregnancy, childbirth, or the puerperium, antepartum condition or complication

647.14 Gonorrhea of mother, complicating pregnancy, childbirth, or the puerperium, postpartum condition or complication

647.21 Other venereal diseases of mother, complicating pregnancy, childbirth, or the puerperium, delivered, with or without mention of antepartum condition

647.22 Other venereal diseases of mother, complicating pregnancy, childbirth, or the puerperium, delivered, with mention of postpartum complication

647.23 Other venereal diseases of mother, complicating pregnancy, childbirth, or the puerperium, antepartum condition or complication

647.24 Other venereal diseases of mother, complicating pregnancy, childbirth, or the puerperium, postpartum condition or complication

647.31 Tuberculosis of mother, complicating pregnancy, childbirth, or the puerperium, delivered, with or without mention of antepartum condition

647.32 Tuberculosis of mother, complicating pregnancy, childbirth, or the puerperium, delivered, with mention of postpartum complication

647.33 Tuberculosis of mother, complicating pregnancy, childbirth, or the puerperium, antepartum condition or complication

647.34 Tuberculosis of mother, complicating pregnancy, childbirth, or the puerperium, postpartum condition or complication

647.41 Malaria in the mother, delivered, with or without mention of antepartum condition

647.42 Malaria in the mother, delivered, with mention of postpartum complication

647.43 Malaria in the mother, antepartum condition or complication

647.44 Malaria in the mother, postpartum condition or complication

647.51 Rubella in the mother, delivered, with or without mention of antepartum condition

647.52 Rubella in the mother, delivered, with mention of postpartum complication

647.53 Rubella in the mother, antepartum condition or complication

647.54 Rubella in the mother, postpartum condition or complication

647.61 Other viral diseases in the mother, delivered, with or without mention of antepartum condition

647.62 Other viral diseases in the mother, delivered, with mention of postpartum complication

647.63 Other viral diseases in the mother, antepartum condition or complication

647.64 Other viral diseases in the mother, postpartum condition or complication

647.81 Other specified infectious and parasitic diseases of mother, delivered, with or without mention of antepartum condition

647.82 Other specified infectious and parasitic diseases of mother, delivered, with mention of postpartum complication

647.83 Other specified infectious and parasitic diseases of mother, antepartum condition or complication

647.84 Other specified infectious and parasitic diseases of mother, postpartum condition or complication

647.91 Unspecified infection or infestation of mother, delivered, with or without mention of antepartum condition

647.92 Unspecified infection or infestation of mother, delivered, with mention of postpartum complication

647.93 Unspecified infection or infestation of mother, antepartum condition or complication

647.94 Unspecified infection or infestation of mother, postpartum condition or complication

648.00 Diabetes mellitus of mother, complicating pregnancy, childbirth, or the puerperium, unspecified as to episode of care or not applicable

648.03 Diabetes mellitus of mother, complicating pregnancy, childbirth, or the puerperium, antepartum condition or complication

648.04 Diabetes mellitus of mother, complicating pregnancy, childbirth, or the puerperium, postpartum condition or complication

648.31 Drug dependence of mother, delivered, with or without mention of antepartum condition

648.32 Drug dependence of mother, delivered, with mention of postpartum complication

648.33 Drug dependence of mother, antepartum condition or complication

648.34 Drug dependence of mother, postpartum condition or complication

648.51 Congenital cardiovascular disorders of mother, delivered, with or without mention of antepartum condition

648.52 Congenital cardiovascular disorders of mother, delivered, with mention of postpartum complication

648.53 Congenital cardiovascular disorders of mother, antepartum condition or complication

648.54	Congenital cardiovascular disorders of mother, postpartum condition or complication
648.61	Other cardiovascular diseases of mother, delivered, with or without mention of antepartum condition
648.62	Other cardiovascular diseases of mother, delivered, with mention of postpartum complication
648.63	Other cardiovascular diseases of mother, antepartum condition or complication
648.64	Other cardiovascular diseases of mother, postpartum condition or complication
648.71	Bone and joint disorders of back, pelvis, and lower limbs of mother, delivered, with or without mention of antepartum condition
648.72	Bone and joint disorders of back, pelvis, and lower limbs of mother, delivered, with mention of postpartum complication
648.73	Bone and joint disorders of back, pelvis, and lower limbs of mother, antepartum condition or complication
648.74	Bone and joint disorders of back, pelvis, and lower limbs of mother, postpartum condition or complication
649.30	Coagulation defects complicating pregnancy, childbirth, or the puerperium, unspecified as to episode of care or not applicable
649.31	Coagulation defects complicating pregnancy, childbirth, or the puerperium, delivered, with or without mention of antepartum condition
649.32	Coagulation defects complicating pregnancy, childbirth, or the puerperium, delivered, with mention of postpartum complication
649.33	Coagulation defects complicating pregnancy, childbirth, or the puerperium, antepartum condition or complication
649.34	Coagulation defects complicating pregnancy, childbirth, or the puerperium, postpartum condition or complication
649.41	Epilepsy complicating pregnancy, childbirth, or the puerperium, delivered, with or without mention of antepartum condition
649.42	Epilepsy complicating pregnancy, childbirth, or the puerperium, delivered, with mention of postpartum complication
649.43	Epilepsy complicating pregnancy, childbirth, or the puerperium, antepartum condition or complication
649.44	Epilepsy complicating pregnancy, childbirth, or the puerperium, postpartum condition or complication
649.70	Cervical shortening, unspecified as to episode of care or not applicable
649.71	Cervical shortening, delivered, with or without mention of antepartum condition
649.73	Cervical shortening, antepartum condition or complication
651.01	Twin pregnancy, delivered, with or without mention of antepartum condition
651.11	Triplet pregnancy, delivered, with or without mention of antepartum condition
651.13	Triplet pregnancy, antepartum condition or complication
651.21	Quadruplet pregnancy, delivered, with or without mention of antepartum condition
651.23	Quadruplet pregnancy, antepartum condition or complication
651.41	Triplet pregnancy with fetal loss and retention of one or more fetus(es), delivered, with or without mention of antepartum condition
651.43	Triplet pregnancy with fetal loss and retention of one or more fetus(es), antepartum condition or complication
651.51	Quadruplet pregnancy with fetal loss and retention of one or more fetus(es), delivered, with or without mention of antepartum condition
651.53	Quadruplet pregnancy with fetal loss and retention of one or more fetus(es), antepartum condition or complication
651.81	Other specified multiple gestation, delivered, with or without mention of antepartum condition
651.83	Other specified multiple gestation, antepartum condition or complication
656.13	Rhesus isoimmunization, antepartum condition or complication

656.31	Fetal distress, affecting management of mother, delivered, with or without mention of antepartum condition
656.41	Intrauterine death, affecting management of mother, delivered, with or without mention of antepartum condition
656.43	Intrauterine death, affecting management of mother, antepartum condition or complication
656.51	Poor fetal growth, affecting management of mother, delivered, with or without mention of antepartum condition
657.01	Polyhydramnios, delivered, with or without mention of antepartum condition
658.01	Oligohydramnios, delivered, with or without mention of antepartum condition
658.03	Oligohydramnios, antepartum condition or complication
658.81	Other problems associated with amniotic cavity and membranes, delivered, with or without mention of antepartum condition
659.21	Maternal pyrexia during labor, unspecified, delivered, with or without mention of antepartum condition
660.03	Obstruction caused by malposition of fetus at onset of labor, antepartum condition or complication
662.11	Unspecified prolonged labor, delivered, with or without mention of antepartum condition
664.21	Third-degree perineal laceration, delivered, with or without mention of antepartum condition
664.31	Fourth-degree perineal laceration, delivered, with or without mention of antepartum condition
664.61	Anal sphincter tear complicating delivery, not associated with third-degree perineal laceration, delivered, with or without mention of antepartum condition
664.64	Anal sphincter tear complicating delivery, not associated with third-degree perineal laceration, postpartum condition or complication
665.22	Inversion of uterus, delivered, with mention of postpartum complication
665.31	Laceration of cervix, delivered, with or without mention of antepartum condition
665.41	High vaginal laceration, delivered, with or without mention of antepartum condition
665.51	Other injury to pelvic organs, delivered, with or without mention of antepartum condition
665.61	Damage to pelvic joints and ligaments, delivered, with or without mention of antepartum condition
665.71	Pelvic hematoma, delivered, with or without mention of antepartum condition
665.72	Pelvic hematoma, delivered with mention of postpartum complication
666.02	Third-stage postpartum hemorrhage, delivered, with mention of postpartum complication
666.04	Third-stage postpartum hemorrhage, postpartum condition or complication
666.12	Other immediate postpartum hemorrhage, delivered, with mention of postpartum complication
666.14	Other immediate postpartum hemorrhage, postpartum condition or complication
666.22	Delayed and secondary postpartum hemorrhage, delivered, with mention of postpartum complication
666.24	Delayed and secondary postpartum hemorrhage, postpartum condition or complication
666.32	Postpartum coagulation defects, delivered, with mention of postpartum complication
669.24	Maternal hypotension syndrome, postpartum condition or complication
670.10	Puerperal endometritis, unspecified as to episode of care or not applicable
670.12	Puerperal endometritis, delivered, with mention of postpartum complication
670.14	Puerperal endometritis, postpartum condition or complication

670.20	Puerperal sepsis, unspecified as to episode of care or not applicable
670.30	Puerperal septic thrombophlebitis, unspecified as to episode of care or not applicable
671.20	Superficial thrombophlebitis complicating pregnancy and the puerperium, unspecified as to episode of care or not applicable
671.21	Superficial thrombophlebitis complicating pregnancy and the puerperium, delivered, with or without mention of antepartum condition
671.22	Superficial thrombophlebitis complicating pregnancy and the puerperium, delivered, with mention of postpartum complication
671.23	Superficial thrombophlebitis complicating pregnancy and the puerperium, antepartum condition or complication
671.24	Superficial thrombophlebitis complicating pregnancy and the puerperium, postpartum condition or complication
671.30	Deep phlebothrombosis, antepartum, unspecified as to episode of care or not applicable
671.40	Deep phlebothrombosis, postpartum, unspecified as to episode of care or not applicable
671.50	Other phlebitis and thrombosis complicating pregnancy and the puerperium, unspecified as to episode of care or not applicable
671.51	Other phlebitis and thrombosis complicating pregnancy and the puerperium, delivered, with or without mention of antepartum condition
671.52	Other phlebitis and thrombosis complicating pregnancy and the puerperium, delivered, with mention of postpartum complication
671.53	Other phlebitis and thrombosis complicating pregnancy and the puerperium, antepartum condition or complication
671.54	Other phlebitis and thrombosis complicating pregnancy and the puerperium, postpartum condition or complication
671.80	Other venous complications of pregnancy and the puerperium, unspecified as to episode of care or not applicable
671.81	Other venous complications of pregnancy and the puerperium, delivered, with or without mention of antepartum condition
671.82	Other venous complications of pregnancy and the puerperium, delivered, with mention of postpartum complication
671.83	Other venous complications of pregnancy and the puerperium, antepartum condition or complication
671.84	Other venous complications of pregnancy and the puerperium, postpartum condition or complication
671.90	Unspecified venous complication of pregnancy and the puerperium, unspecified as to episode of care or not applicable
671.91	Unspecified venous complication of pregnancy and the puerperium, delivered, with or without mention of antepartum condition
671.92	Unspecified venous complication of pregnancy and the puerperium, delivered, with mention of postpartum complication
672.02	Pyrexia of unknown origin during the puerperium, delivered, with mention of postpartum complication
672.04	Pyrexia of unknown origin during the puerperium, postpartum condition or complication
673.30	Obstetrical pyemic and septic embolism, unspecified as to episode of care or not applicable
674.02	Cerebrovascular disorders in the puerperium, delivered, with mention of postpartum complication
674.03	Cerebrovascular disorders in the puerperium, antepartum condition or complication
674.04	Cerebrovascular disorders in the puerperium, postpartum condition or complication
675.11	Abscess of breast associated with childbirth, delivered, with or without mention of antepartum condition
675.12	Abscess of breast associated with childbirth, delivered, with mention of postpartum complication
682.0	Cellulitis and abscess of face
682.1	Cellulitis and abscess of neck
682.2	Cellulitis and abscess of trunk
682.3	Cellulitis and abscess of upper arm and forearm

682.4	Cellulitis and abscess of hand, except fingers and thumb
682.5	Cellulitis and abscess of buttock
682.6	Cellulitis and abscess of leg, except foot
682.7	Cellulitis and abscess of foot, except toes
682.8	Cellulitis and abscess of other specified sites
682.9	Cellulitis and abscess of unspecified sites
685.0	Pilonidal cyst with abscess
686.01	Pyoderma gangrenosum
694.4	Pemphigus
694.5	Pemphigoid
695.0	Toxic erythema
695.12	Erythema multiforme major
695.13	Stevens-Johnson syndrome
695.14	Stevens-Johnson syndrome-toxic epidermal necrolysis overlap syndrome
695.15	Toxic epidermal necrolysis
695.53	Exfoliation due to erythematous condition involving 30-39 percent of body surface
695.54	Exfoliation due to erythematous condition involving 40-49 percent of body surface
695.55	Exfoliation due to erythematous condition involving 50-59 percent of body surface
695.56	Exfoliation due to erythematous condition involving 60-69 percent of body surface
695.57	Exfoliation due to erythematous condition involving 70-79 percent of body surface
695.58	Exfoliation due to erythematous condition involving 80-89 percent of body surface
695.59	Exfoliation due to erythematous condition involving 90 percent or more of body surface
707.10	Ulcer of lower limb, unspecified
707.11	Ulcer of thigh
707.12	Ulcer of calf
707.13	Ulcer of ankle
707.14	Ulcer of heel and midfoot
707.19	Ulcer of other part of lower limb
710.3	Dermatomyositis
710.4	Polymyositis
710.5	Eosinophilia myalgia syndrome
710.8	Other specified diffuse diseases of connective tissue
711.00	Pyogenic arthritis, site unspecified
711.01	Pyogenic arthritis, shoulder region
711.02	Pyogenic arthritis, upper arm
711.03	Pyogenic arthritis, forearm
711.04	Pyogenic arthritis, hand
711.05	Pyogenic arthritis, pelvic region and thigh
711.06	Pyogenic arthritis, lower leg
711.07	Pyogenic arthritis, ankle and foot
711.08	Pyogenic arthritis, other specified sites
711.09	Pyogenic arthritis, multiple sites
711.10	Arthropathy associated with Reiter's disease and nonspecific urethritis, site unspecified
711.11	Arthropathy associated with Reiter's disease and nonspecific urethritis, shoulder region
711.12	Arthropathy associated with Reiter's disease and nonspecific urethritis, upper arm
711.13	Arthropathy associated with Reiter's disease and nonspecific urethritis, forearm
711.14	Arthropathy associated with Reiter's disease and nonspecific urethritis, hand
711.15	Arthropathy associated with Reiter's disease and nonspecific urethritis, pelvic region and thigh

711.16 Arthropathy associated with Reiter's disease and nonspecific urethritis, lower leg

711.17 Arthropathy associated with Reiter's disease and nonspecific urethritis, ankle and foot

711.18 Arthropathy associated with Reiter's disease and nonspecific urethritis, other specified sites

711.19 Arthropathy associated with Reiter's disease and nonspecific urethritis, multiple sites

711.20 Arthropathy in Behcet's syndrome, site unspecified

711.21 Arthropathy in Behcet's syndrome, shoulder region

711.22 Arthropathy in Behcet's syndrome, upper arm

711.23 Arthropathy in Behcet's syndrome, forearm

711.24 Arthropathy in Behcet's syndrome, hand

711.25 Arthropathy in Behcet's syndrome, pelvic region and thigh

711.26 Arthropathy in Behcet's syndrome, lower leg

711.27 Arthropathy in Behcet's syndrome, ankle and foot

711.28 Arthropathy in Behcet's syndrome, other specified sites

711.29 Arthropathy in Behcet's syndrome, multiple sites

711.30 Postdysenteric arthropathy, site unspecified

711.31 Postdysenteric arthropathy, shoulder region

711.32 Postdysenteric arthropathy, upper arm

711.33 Postdysenteric arthropathy, forearm

711.34 Postdysenteric arthropathy, hand

711.35 Postdysenteric arthropathy, pelvic region and thigh

711.36 Postdysenteric arthropathy, lower leg

711.37 Postdysenteric arthropathy, ankle and foot

711.38 Postdysenteric arthropathy, other specified sites

711.39 Postdysenteric arthropathy, multiple sites

711.40 Arthropathy associated with other bacterial diseases, site unspecified

711.41 Arthropathy associated with other bacterial diseases, shoulder region

711.42 Arthropathy associated with other bacterial diseases, upper arm

711.43 Arthropathy associated with other bacterial diseases, forearm

711.44 Arthropathy associated with other bacterial diseases, hand

711.45 Arthropathy associated with other bacterial diseases, pelvic region and thigh

711.46 Arthropathy associated with other bacterial diseases, lower leg

711.47 Arthropathy associated with other bacterial diseases, ankle and foot

711.48 Arthropathy associated with other bacterial diseases, other specified sites

711.49 Arthropathy associated with other bacterial diseases, multiple sites

711.50 Arthropathy associated with other viral diseases, site unspecified

711.51 Arthropathy associated with other viral diseases, shoulder region

711.52 Arthropathy associated with other viral diseases, upper arm

711.53 Arthropathy associated with other viral diseases, forearm

711.54 Arthropathy associated with other viral diseases, hand

711.55 Arthropathy associated with other viral diseases, pelvic region and thigh

711.56 Arthropathy associated with other viral diseases, lower leg

711.57 Arthropathy associated with other viral diseases, ankle and foot

711.58 Arthropathy associated with other viral diseases, other specified sites

711.59 Arthropathy associated with other viral diseases, multiple sites

711.60 Arthropathy associated with mycoses, site unspecified

711.61 Arthropathy associated with mycoses, shoulder region

711.62 Arthropathy associated with mycoses, upper arm

711.63 Arthropathy associated with mycoses, forearm

711.64 Arthropathy associated with mycoses, hand

711.65 Arthropathy associated with mycoses, pelvic region and thigh

711.66 Arthropathy associated with mycoses, lower leg

711.67 Arthropathy associated with mycoses, ankle and foot

711.68 Arthropathy associated with mycoses, other specified sites

711.69 Arthropathy associated with mycoses, involving multiple sites

711.70 Arthropathy associated with helminthiasis, site unspecified

711.71 Arthropathy associated with helminthiasis, shoulder region

711.72 Arthropathy associated with helminthiasis, upper arm

711.73 Arthropathy associated with helminthiasis, forearm

711.74 Arthropathy associated with helminthiasis, hand

711.75 Arthropathy associated with helminthiasis, pelvic region and thigh

711.76 Arthropathy associated with helminthiasis, lower leg

711.77 Arthropathy associated with helminthiasis, ankle and foot

711.78 Arthropathy associated with helminthiasis, other specified sites

711.79 Arthropathy associated with helminthiasis, multiple sites

711.80 Arthropathy associated with other infectious and parasitic diseases, site unspecified

711.81 Arthropathy associated with other infectious and parasitic diseases, shoulder region

711.82 Arthropathy associated with other infectious and parasitic diseases, upper arm

711.83 Arthropathy associated with other infectious and parasitic diseases, forearm

711.84 Arthropathy associated with other infectious and parasitic diseases, hand

711.85 Arthropathy associated with other infectious and parasitic diseases, pelvic region and thigh

711.86 Arthropathy associated with other infectious and parasitic diseases, lower leg

711.87 Arthropathy associated with other infectious and parasitic diseases, ankle and foot

711.88 Arthropathy associated with other infectious and parasitic diseases, other specified sites

711.89 Arthropathy associated with other infectious and parasitic diseases, multiple sites

711.90 Unspecified infective arthritis, site unspecified

711.91 Unspecified infective arthritis, shoulder region

711.92 Unspecified infective arthritis, upper arm

711.93 Unspecified infective arthritis, forearm

711.94 Unspecified infective arthritis, hand

711.95 Unspecified infective arthritis, pelvic region and thigh

711.96 Unspecified infective arthritis, lower leg

711.97 Unspecified infective arthritis, ankle and foot

711.98 Unspecified infective arthritis, other specified sites

711.99 Unspecified infective arthritis, multiple sites

714.31 Polyarticular juvenile rheumatoid arthritis, acute

719.10 Hemarthrosis, site unspecified

719.11 Hemarthrosis, shoulder region

719.12 Hemarthrosis, upper arm

719.13 Hemarthrosis, forearm

719.14 Hemarthrosis, hand

719.15 Hemarthrosis, pelvic region and thigh

719.16 Hemarthrosis, lower leg

719.17 Hemarthrosis, ankle and foot

719.18 Hemarthrosis, other specified sites

719.19 Hemarthrosis, multiple sites

721.1 Cervical spondylosis with myelopathy

721.41 Spondylosis with myelopathy, thoracic region

721.42 Spondylosis with myelopathy, lumbar region

721.7 Traumatic spondylopathy

721.91 Spondylosis of unspecified site, with myelopathy

722.71 Intervertebral disc disorder with myelopathy, cervical region

722.72	Intervertebral disc disorder with myelopathy, thoracic region
722.73	Intervertebral disc disorder with myelopathy, lumbar region
728.0	Infective myositis
728.88	Rhabdomyolysis
729.71	Nontraumatic compartment syndrome of upper extremity
729.72	Nontraumatic compartment syndrome of lower extremity
729.73	Nontraumatic compartment syndrome of abdomen
729.79	Nontraumatic compartment syndrome of other sites
730.00	Acute osteomyelitis, site unspecified
730.01	Acute osteomyelitis, shoulder region
730.02	Acute osteomyelitis, upper arm
730.03	Acute osteomyelitis, forearm
730.04	Acute osteomyelitis, hand
730.05	Acute osteomyelitis, pelvic region and thigh
730.06	Acute osteomyelitis, lower leg
730.07	Acute osteomyelitis, ankle and foot
730.08	Acute osteomyelitis, other specified sites
730.09	Acute osteomyelitis, multiple sites
730.10	Chronic osteomyelitis, site unspecified
730.11	Chronic osteomyelitis, shoulder region
730.12	Chronic osteomyelitis, upper arm
730.13	Chronic osteomyelitis, forearm
730.14	Chronic osteomyelitis, hand
730.15	Chronic osteomyelitis, pelvic region and thigh
730.16	Chronic osteomyelitis, lower leg
730.17	Chronic osteomyelitis, ankle and foot
730.18	Chronic osteomyelitis, other specified sites
730.19	Chronic osteomyelitis, multiple sites
730.20	Unspecified osteomyelitis, site unspecified
730.21	Unspecified osteomyelitis, shoulder region
730.22	Unspecified osteomyelitis, upper arm
730.23	Unspecified osteomyelitis, forearm
730.24	Unspecified osteomyelitis, hand
730.25	Unspecified osteomyelitis, pelvic region and thigh
730.26	Unspecified osteomyelitis, lower leg
730.27	Unspecified osteomyelitis, ankle and foot
730.28	Unspecified osteomyelitis, other specified sites
730.29	Unspecified osteomyelitis, multiple sites
730.80	Other infections involving bone in diseases classified elsewhere, site unspecified
730.81	Other infections involving bone in diseases classified elsewhere, shoulder region
730.82	Other infections involving bone in diseases classified elsewhere, upper arm
730.83	Other infections involving bone in diseases classified elsewhere, forearm
730.84	Other infections involving bone in diseases classified elsewhere, hand
730.85	Other infections involving bone in diseases classified elsewhere, pelvic region and thigh
730.86	Other infections involving bone in diseases classified elsewhere, lower leg
730.87	Other infections involving bone in diseases classified elsewhere, ankle and foot
730.88	Other infections involving bone in diseases classified elsewhere, other specified sites
730.89	Other infections involving bone in diseases classified elsewhere, multiple sites
730.90	Unspecified infection of bone, site unspecified
730.91	Unspecified infection of bone, shoulder region
730.92	Unspecified infection of bone, upper arm
730.93	Unspecified infection of bone, forearm
730.94	Unspecified infection of bone, hand
730.95	Unspecified infection of bone, pelvic region and thigh
730.96	Unspecified infection of bone, lower leg
730.97	Unspecified infection of bone, ankle and foot
730.98	Unspecified infection of bone, other specified sites
730.99	Unspecified infection of bone, multiple sites
733.10	Pathologic fracture, unspecified site
733.11	Pathologic fracture of humerus
733.12	Pathologic fracture of distal radius and ulna
733.13	Pathologic fracture of vertebrae
733.14	Pathologic fracture of neck of femur
733.15	Pathologic fracture of other specified part of femur
733.16	Pathologic fracture of tibia or fibula
733.19	Pathologic fracture of other specified site
733.40	Aseptic necrosis of bone, site unspecified
733.41	Aseptic necrosis of head of humerus
733.42	Aseptic necrosis of head and neck of femur
733.43	Aseptic necrosis of medial femoral condyle
733.44	Aseptic necrosis of talus
733.45	Aseptic necrosis of bone, jaw
733.49	Aseptic necrosis of bone, other
733.81	Malunion of fracture
733.82	Nonunion of fracture
741.00	Spina bifida with hydrocephalus, unspecified region
741.01	Spina bifida with hydrocephalus, cervical region
741.02	Spina bifida with hydrocephalus, dorsal (thoracic) region
741.03	Spina bifida with hydrocephalus, lumbar region
742.0	Encephalocele
742.4	Other specified congenital anomalies of brain
745.12	Corrected transposition of great vessels
745.4	Ventricular septal defect
745.5	Ostium secundum type atrial septal defect
745.60	Endocardial cushion defect, unspecified type
745.61	Ostium primum defect
745.69	Other endocardial cushion defects
746.00	Congenital pulmonary valve anomaly, unspecified
746.02	Stenosis of pulmonary valve, congenital
746.09	Other congenital anomalies of pulmonary valve
746.3	Congenital stenosis of aortic valve
746.4	Congenital insufficiency of aortic valve
746.5	Congenital mitral stenosis
746.6	Congenital mitral insufficiency
746.83	Infundibular pulmonic stenosis
746.85	Coronary artery anomaly
746.87	Malposition of heart and cardiac apex
747.0	Patent ductus arteriosus
747.10	Coarctation of aorta (preductal) (postductal)
747.20	Anomaly of aorta, unspecified
747.21	Anomalies of aortic arch
747.22	Atresia and stenosis of aorta
747.29	Other anomalies of aorta
747.40	Anomaly of great veins, unspecified
747.41	Total anomalous pulmonary venous connection
747.42	Partial anomalous pulmonary venous connection
747.49	Other anomalies of great veins
747.82	Spinal vessel anomaly
747.89	Other specified anomalies of circulatory system
747.9	Unspecified anomaly of circulatory system

748.3	Other anomalies of larynx, trachea, and bronchus
748.4	Congenital cystic lung
748.61	Congenital bronchiectasis
750.4	Other specified anomalies of esophagus
751.1	Atresia and stenosis of small intestine
751.2	Atresia and stenosis of large intestine, rectum, and anal canal
751.3	Hirschsprung's disease and other congenital functional disorders of colon
751.4	Anomalies of intestinal fixation
751.5	Other anomalies of intestine
751.60	Unspecified anomaly of gallbladder, bile ducts, and liver
751.62	Congenital cystic disease of liver
751.69	Other anomalies of gallbladder, bile ducts, and liver
751.7	Anomalies of pancreas
753.0	Renal agenesis and dysgenesis
753.10	Cystic kidney disease, unspecified
753.11	Congenital single renal cyst
753.12	Polycystic kidney, unspecified type
753.13	Polycystic kidney, autosomal dominant
753.14	Polycystic kidney, autosomal recessive
753.15	Renal dysplasia
753.16	Medullary cystic kidney
753.17	Medullary sponge kidney
753.19	Other specified cystic kidney disease
753.20	Unspecified obstructive defect of renal pelvis and ureter
753.21	Congenital obstruction of ureteropelvic junction
753.22	Congenital obstruction of ureterovesical junction
753.23	Congenital ureterocele
753.29	Other obstructive defects of renal pelvis and ureter
753.5	Exstrophy of urinary bladder
753.6	Atresia and stenosis of urethra and bladder neck
754.2	Congenital musculoskeletal deformities of spine
754.89	Other specified nonteratogenic anomalies
756.13	Absence of vertebra, congenital
756.3	Other anomalies of ribs and sternum
756.51	Osteogenesis imperfecta
756.52	Osteopetrosis
756.83	Ehlers-Danlos syndrome
758.1	Patau's syndrome
758.2	Edwards' syndrome
758.31	Cri-du-chat syndrome
758.33	Other microdeletions
758.39	Other autosomal deletions
759.0	Anomalies of spleen
759.3	Situs inversus
759.5	Tuberous sclerosis
759.6	Other hamartoses, not elsewhere classified
759.7	Multiple congenital anomalies, so described
759.81	Prader-Willi syndrome
759.82	Marfan syndrome
759.89	Other specified congenital anomalies
767.11	Epicranial subaponeurotic hemorrhage (massive)
768.70	Hypoxic-ischemic encephalopathy, unspecified
768.71	Mild hypoxic-ischemic encephalopathy
768.72	Moderate hypoxic-ischemic encephalopathy
770.4	Primary atelectasis
770.5	Other and unspecified atelectasis
770.81	Primary apnea of newborn
770.82	Other apnea of newborn
770.83	Cyanotic attacks of newborn
771.0	Congenital rubella
771.4	Omphalitis of the newborn
771.5	Neonatal infective mastitis
771.82	Urinary tract infection of newborn
771.83	Bacteremia of newborn
771.89	Other infections specific to the perinatal period
772.10	Intraventricular hemorrhage unspecified grade
772.11	Intraventricular hemorrhage, grade I
772.12	Intraventricular hemorrhage, grade II
772.5	Adrenal hemorrhage of fetus or newborn
775.1	Neonatal diabetes mellitus
775.2	Neonatal myasthenia gravis
775.3	Neonatal thyrotoxicosis
775.4	Hypocalcemia and hypomagnesemia of newborn
775.81	Other acidosis of newborn
775.89	Other neonatal endocrine and metabolic disturbances
776.0	Hemorrhagic disease of newborn
776.3	Other transient neonatal disorders of coagulation
776.5	Congenital anemia
776.6	Anemia of prematurity
777.4	Transitory ileus of newborn
778.1	Sclerema neonatorum
778.5	Other and unspecified edema of newborn
779.4	Drug reactions and intoxications specific to newborn
779.5	Drug withdrawal syndrome in newborn
780.03	Persistent vegetative state
780.1	Hallucinations
780.31	Febrile convulsions (simple), unspecified
780.32	Complex febrile convulsions
780.33	Post traumatic seizures
781.4	Transient paralysis of limb
781.6	Meningismus
781.7	Tetany
781.8	Neurologic neglect syndrome
782.4	Jaundice, unspecified, not of newborn
784.3	Aphasia
785.4	Gangrene
785.50	Shock, unspecified
786.04	Cheyne-Stokes respiration
786.30	Hemoptysis, unspecified
786.31	Acute idiopathic pulmonary hemorrhage in infants [AIPHI]
786.39	Other hemoptysis
788.8	Extravasation of urine
789.51	Malignant ascites
789.59	Other ascites
790.01	Precipitous drop in hematocrit
790.7	Bacteremia
791.1	Chyluria
791.3	Myoglobinuria
799.01	Asphyxia
799.4	Cachexia
800.00	Closed fracture of vault of skull without mention of intracranial injury, unspecified state of consciousness
800.01	Closed fracture of vault of skull without mention of intracranial injury, with no loss of consciousness
800.02	Closed fracture of vault of skull without mention of intracranial injury, with brief [less than one hour] loss of consciousness
800.06	Closed fracture of vault of skull without mention of intracranial injury, with loss of consciousness of unspecified duration

800.09	Closed fracture of vault of skull without mention of intracranial injury, with concussion, unspecified
800.40	Closed fracture of vault of skull with intracranial injury of other and unspecified nature, unspecified state of consciousness
800.41	Closed fracture of vault of skull with intracranial injury of other and unspecified nature, with no loss of consciousness
800.42	Closed fracture of vault of skull with intracranial injury of other and unspecified nature, with brief [less than one hour] loss of consciousness
800.46	Closed fracture of vault of skull with intracranial injury of other and unspecified nature, with loss of consciousness of unspecified duration
800.49	Closed fracture of vault of skull with intracranial injury of other and unspecified nature, with concussion, unspecified
801.00	Closed fracture of base of skull without mention of intra cranial injury, unspecified state of consciousness
801.01	Closed fracture of base of skull without mention of intra cranial injury, with no loss of consciousness
801.02	Closed fracture of base of skull without mention of intra cranial injury, with brief [less than one hour] loss of consciousness
801.06	Closed fracture of base of skull without mention of intra cranial injury, with loss of consciousness of unspecified duration
801.09	Closed fracture of base of skull without mention of intra cranial injury, with concussion, unspecified
801.40	Closed fracture of base of skull with intracranial injury of other and unspecified nature, unspecified state of consciousness
801.41	Closed fracture of base of skull with intracranial injury of other and unspecified nature, with no loss of consciousness
801.42	Closed fracture of base of skull with intracranial injury of other and unspecified nature, with brief [less than one hour] loss of consciousness
801.46	Closed fracture of base of skull with intracranial injury of other and unspecified nature, with loss of consciousness of unspecified duration
801.49	Closed fracture of base of skull with intracranial injury of other and unspecified nature, with concussion, unspecified
802.1	Open fracture of nasal bones
802.20	Closed fracture of mandible, unspecified site
802.21	Closed fracture of mandible, condylar process
802.22	Closed fracture of mandible, subcondylar
802.23	Closed fracture of mandible, coronoid process
802.24	Closed fracture of mandible, ramus, unspecified
802.25	Closed fracture of mandible, angle of jaw
802.26	Closed fracture of mandible, symphysis of body
802.27	Closed fracture of mandible, alveolar border of body
802.28	Closed fracture of mandible, body, other and unspecified
802.29	Closed fracture of mandible, multiple sites
802.30	Open fracture of mandible, unspecified site
802.31	Open fracture of mandible, condylar process
802.32	Open fracture of mandible, subcondylar
802.33	Open fracture of mandible, coronoid process
802.34	Open fracture of mandible, ramus, unspecified
802.35	Open fracture of mandible, angle of jaw
802.36	Open fracture of mandible, symphysis of body
802.37	Open fracture of mandible, alveolar border of body
802.38	Open fracture of mandible, body, other and unspecified
802.39	Open fracture of mandible, multiple sites
802.4	Closed fracture of malar and maxillary bones
802.5	Open fracture of malar and maxillary bones
802.6	Closed fracture of orbital floor (blow-out)
802.7	Open fracture of orbital floor (blow-out)
802.8	Closed fracture of other facial bones
802.9	Open fracture of other facial bones

803.00	Other closed skull fracture without mention of intracranial injury, unspecified state of consciousness
803.01	Other closed skull fracture without mention of intracranial injury, with no loss of consciousness
803.02	Other closed skull fracture without mention of intracranial injury, with brief [less than one hour] loss of consciousness
803.06	Other closed skull fracture without mention of intracranial injury, with loss of consciousness of unspecified duration
803.09	Other closed skull fracture without mention of intracranial injury, with concussion, unspecified
803.40	Other closed skull fracture with intracranial injury of other and unspecified nature, unspecified state of consciousness
803.41	Other closed skull fracture with intracranial injury of other and unspecified nature, with no loss of consciousness
803.42	Other closed skull fracture with intracranial injury of other and unspecified nature, with brief [less than one hour] loss of consciousness
803.46	Other closed skull fracture with intracranial injury of other and unspecified nature, with loss of consciousness of unspecified duration
803.49	Other closed skull fracture with intracranial injury of other and unspecified nature, with concussion, unspecified
804.00	Closed fractures involving skull or face with other bones, without mention of intracranial injury, unspecified state of consciousness
804.01	Closed fractures involving skull or face with other bones, without mention of intracranial injury, with no loss of consciousness
804.02	Closed fractures involving skull or face with other bones, without mention of intracranial injury, with brief [less than one hour] loss of consciousness
804.06	Closed fractures involving skull of face with other bones, without mention of intracranial injury, with loss of consciousness of unspecified duration
804.09	Closed fractures involving skull of face with other bones, without mention of intracranial injury, with concussion, unspecified
804.40	Closed fractures involving skull or face with other bones, with intracranial injury of other and unspecified nature, unspecified state of consciousness
804.41	Closed fractures involving skull or face with other bones, with intracranial injury of other and unspecified nature, with no loss of consciousness
804.42	Closed fractures involving skull or face with other bones, with intracranial injury of other and unspecified nature, with brief [less than one hour] loss of consciousness
804.46	Closed fractures involving skull or face with other bones, with intracranial injury of other and unspecified nature, with loss of consciousness of unspecified duration
804.49	Closed fractures involving skull or face with other bones, with intracranial injury of other and unspecified nature, with concussion, unspecified
804.50	Open fractures involving skull or face with other bones, without mention of intracranial injury, unspecified state of consciousness
804.51	Open fractures involving skull or face with other bones, without mention of intracranial injury, with no loss of consciousness
804.52	Open fractures involving skull or face with other bones, without mention of intracranial injury, with brief [less than one hour] loss of consciousness
804.56	Open fractures involving skull or face with other bones, without mention of intracranial injury, with loss of consciousness of unspecified duration
804.59	Open fractures involving skull or face with other bones, without mention of intracranial injury, with concussion, unspecified
804.90	Open fractures involving skull or face with other bones, with intracranial injury of other and unspecified nature, unspecified state of consciousness
804.91	Open fractures involving skull or face with other bones, with intracranial injury of other and unspecified nature, with no loss of consciousness

804.92	Open fractures involving skull or face with other bones, with intracranial injury of other and unspecified nature, with brief [less than one hour] loss of consciousness
804.96	Open fractures involving skull or face with other bones, with intracranial injury of other and unspecified nature, with loss of consciousness of unspecified duration
804.99	Open fractures involving skull or face with other bones, with intracranial injury of other and unspecified nature, with concussion, unspecified
805.00	Closed fracture of cervical vertebra, unspecified level
805.01	Closed fracture of first cervical vertebra
805.02	Closed fracture of second cervical vertebra
805.03	Closed fracture of third cervical vertebra
805.04	Closed fracture of fourth cervical vertebra
805.05	Closed fracture of fifth cervical vertebra
805.06	Closed fracture of sixth cervical vertebra
805.07	Closed fracture of seventh cervical vertebra
805.08	Closed fracture of multiple cervical vertebrae
805.2	Closed fracture of dorsal [thoracic] vertebra without mention of spinal cord injury
805.4	Closed fracture of lumbar vertebra without mention of spinal cord injury
805.6	Closed fracture of sacrum and coccyx without mention of spinal cord injury
805.8	Closed fracture of unspecified vertebral column without mention of spinal cord injury
807.00	Closed fracture of rib(s), unspecified
807.01	Closed fracture of one rib
807.02	Closed fracture of two ribs
807.03	Closed fracture of three ribs
807.04	Closed fracture of four ribs
807.05	Closed fracture of five ribs
807.06	Closed fracture of six ribs
807.07	Closed fracture of seven ribs
807.08	Closed fracture of eight or more ribs
807.09	Closed fracture of multiple ribs, unspecified
807.2	Closed fracture of sternum
808.2	Closed fracture of pubis
808.41	Closed fracture of ilium
808.42	Closed fracture of ischium
808.43	Multiple closed pelvic fractures with disruption of pelvic circle
808.44	Multiple closed pelvic fractures without disruption of pelvic circle
808.49	Closed fracture of other specified part of pelvis
808.8	Closed unspecified fracture of pelvis
809.0	Fracture of bones of trunk, closed
810.10	Open fracture of clavicle, unspecified part
810.11	Open fracture of sternal end of clavicle
810.12	Open fracture of shaft of clavicle
810.13	Open fracture of acromial end of clavicle
811.10	Open fracture of scapula, unspecified part
811.11	Open fracture of acromial process of scapula
811.12	Open fracture of coracoid process
811.13	Open fracture of glenoid cavity and neck of scapula
811.19	Open fracture of scapula, other
812.00	Closed fracture of unspecified part of upper end of humerus
812.01	Closed fracture of surgical neck of humerus
812.02	Closed fracture of anatomical neck of humerus
812.03	Closed fracture of greater tuberosity of humerus
812.09	Other closed fracture of upper end of humerus
812.20	Closed fracture of unspecified part of humerus
812.21	Closed fracture of shaft of humerus

812.40	Closed fracture of unspecified part of lower end of humerus
812.41	Closed supracondylar fracture of humerus
812.42	Closed fracture of lateral condyle of humerus
812.43	Closed fracture of medial condyle of humerus
812.44	Closed fracture of unspecified condyle(s) of humerus
812.49	Other closed fracture of lower end of humerus
813.20	Closed fracture of shaft of radius or ulna, unspecified
813.21	Closed fracture of shaft of radius (alone)
813.22	Closed fracture of shaft of ulna (alone)
813.23	Closed fracture of shaft of radius with ulna
813.40	Closed fracture of lower end of forearm, unspecified
813.41	Closed Colles' fracture
813.42	Other closed fractures of distal end of radius (alone)
813.43	Closed fracture of distal end of ulna (alone)
813.44	Closed fracture of lower end of radius with ulna
813.45	Torus fracture of radius (alone)
813.46	Torus fracture of ulna (alone)
813.47	Torus fracture of radius and ulna
813.80	Closed fracture of unspecified part of forearm
813.82	Closed fracture of unspecified part of ulna (alone)
813.83	Closed fracture of unspecified part of radius with ulna
814.10	Open fracture of carpal bone, unspecified
814.11	Open fracture of navicular [scaphoid] bone of wrist
814.12	Open fracture of lunate [semilunar] bone of wrist
814.13	Open fracture of triquetral [cuneiform] bone of wrist
814.14	Open fracture of pisiform bone of wrist
814.15	Open fracture of trapezium bone [larger multangular] of wrist
814.16	Open fracture of trapezoid bone [smaller multangular] of wrist
814.17	Open fracture of capitate bone [os magnum] of wrist
814.18	Open fracture of hamate [unciform] bone of wrist
814.19	Open fracture of other bone of wrist
815.10	Open fracture of metacarpal bone(s), site unspecified
815.11	Open fracture of base of thumb [first] metacarpal
815.12	Open fracture of base of other metacarpal bone(s)
815.13	Open fracture of shaft of metacarpal bone(s)
815.14	Open fracture of neck of metacarpal bone(s)
815.19	Open fracture of multiple sites of metacarpus
816.10	Open fracture of phalanx or phalanges of hand, unspecified
816.11	Open fracture of middle or proximal phalanx or phalanges of hand
816.12	Open fracture of distal phalanx or phalanges of hand
816.13	Open fracture of multiple sites of phalanx or phalanges of hand
817.1	Multiple open fractures of hand bones
818.1	Ill-defined open fractures of upper limb
819.0	Multiple closed fractures involving both upper limbs, and upper limb with rib(s) and sternum
819.1	Multiple open fractures involving both upper limbs, and upper limb with rib(s) and sternum
821.20	Closed fracture of lower end of femur, unspecified part
821.21	Closed fracture of condyle, femoral
821.22	Closed fracture of epiphysis, lower (separation) of femur
821.23	Closed supracondylar fracture of femur
821.29	Other closed fracture of lower end of femur
822.0	Closed fracture of patella
822.1	Open fracture of patella
823.00	Closed fracture of upper end of tibia alone
823.02	Closed fracture of upper end of fibula with tibia
823.20	Closed fracture of shaft of tibia alone
823.22	Closed fracture of shaft of fibula with tibia
823.40	Torus fracture, tibia alone

823.42	Torus fracture, fibula with tibia
823.80	Closed fracture of unspecified part of tibia alone
823.82	Closed fracture of unspecified part of fibula with tibia
824.1	Fracture of medial malleolus, open
824.3	Fracture of lateral malleolus, open
824.5	Bimalleolar fracture, open
824.7	Trimalleolar fracture, open
824.9	Unspecified fracture of ankle, open
825.1	Fracture of calcaneus, open
825.30	Open fracture of unspecified bone(s) of foot [except toes]
825.31	Open fracture of astragalus
825.32	Open fracture of navicular [scaphoid], foot
825.33	Open fracture of cuboid
825.34	Open fracture of cuneiform, foot
825.35	Open fracture of metatarsal bone(s)
825.39	Other open fracture of tarsal and metatarsal bones
827.1	Other, multiple and ill-defined fractures of lower limb, open
830.1	Open dislocation of jaw
831.10	Open dislocation of shoulder, unspecified
831.11	Open anterior dislocation of humerus
831.12	Open posterior dislocation of humerus
831.13	Open inferior dislocation of humerus
831.14	Open dislocation of acromioclavicular (joint)
831.19	Open dislocation of shoulder, other
832.10	Open dislocation of elbow, unspecified
832.11	Open anterior dislocation of elbow
832.12	Open posterior dislocation of elbow
832.13	Open medial dislocation of elbow
832.14	Open lateral dislocation of elbow
832.19	Open dislocation of elbow, other
833.10	Open dislocation of wrist, unspecified part
833.11	Open dislocation of radioulnar (joint), distal
833.12	Open dislocation of radiocarpal (joint)
833.13	Open dislocation of midcarpal (joint)
833.14	Open dislocation of carpometacarpal (joint)
833.15	Open dislocation of metacarpal (bone), proximal end
833.19	Open dislocation of wrist, other
835.00	Closed dislocation of hip, unspecified site
835.01	Closed posterior dislocation of hip
835.02	Closed obturator dislocation of hip
835.03	Other closed anterior dislocation of hip
836.4	Dislocation of patella, open
836.60	Dislocation of knee, unspecified, open
836.61	Anterior dislocation of tibia, proximal end, open
836.62	Posterior dislocation of tibia, proximal end, open
836.63	Medial dislocation of tibia, proximal end, open
836.64	Lateral dislocation of tibia, proximal end, open
836.69	Other dislocation of knee, open
837.1	Open dislocation of ankle
839.00	Closed dislocation, cervical vertebra, unspecified
839.01	Closed dislocation, first cervical vertebra
839.02	Closed dislocation, second cervical vertebra
839.03	Closed dislocation, third cervical vertebra
839.04	Closed dislocation, fourth cervical vertebra
839.05	Closed dislocation, fifth cervical vertebra
839.06	Closed dislocation, sixth cervical vertebra
839.07	Closed dislocation, seventh cervical vertebra
839.08	Closed dislocation, multiple cervical vertebrae
839.51	Open dislocation, coccyx

839.52	Open dislocation, sacrum
839.61	Closed dislocation, sternum
839.79	Open dislocation, other location
839.9	Open dislocation, multiple and ill-defined sites
850.11	Concussion, with loss of consciousness of 30 minutes or less
850.12	Concussion, with loss of consciousness from 31 to 59 minutes
850.2	Concussion with moderate loss of consciousness
850.3	Concussion with prolonged loss of consciousness and return to pre-existing conscious level
850.5	Concussion with loss of consciousness of unspecified duration
851.02	Cortex (cerebral) contusion without mention of open intracranial wound, with brief [less than one hour] loss of consciousness
851.03	Cortex (cerebral) contusion without mention of open intracranial wound, with moderate [1-24 hours] loss of consciousness
851.04	Cortex (cerebral) contusion without mention of open intracranial wound, with prolonged [more than 24 hours] loss of consciousness and return to pre-existing conscious level
851.06	Cortex (cerebral) contusion without mention of open intracranial wound, with loss of consciousness of unspecified duration
851.42	Cerebellar or brain stem contusion without mention of open intracranial wound, with brief [less than one hour] loss of consciousness
851.43	Cerebellar or brain stem contusion without mention of open intracranial wound, with moderate [1-24 hours] loss of consciousness
851.44	Cerebellar or brain stem contusion without mention of open intracranial wound, with prolonged [more than 24 hours] loss consciousness and return to pre-existing conscious level
851.46	Cerebellar or brain stem contusion without mention of open intracranial wound, with loss of consciousness of unspecified duration
854.02	Intracranial injury of other and unspecified nature without mention of open intracranial wound, with brief [less than one hour] loss of consciousness
854.03	Intracranial injury of other and unspecified nature without mention of open intracranial wound, with moderate [1-24 hours] loss of consciousness
854.04	Intracranial injury of other and unspecified nature without mention of open intracranial wound, with prolonged [more than 24 hours] loss of consciousness and return to pre-existing conscious level
854.06	Intracranial injury of other and unspecified nature without mention of open intracranial wound, with loss of consciousness of unspecified duration
860.0	Traumatic pneumothorax without mention of open wound into thorax
861.00	Unspecified injury of heart without mention of open wound into thorax
861.01	Contusion of heart without mention of open wound into thorax
861.20	Unspecified injury of lung without mention of open wound into thorax
861.21	Contusion of lung without mention of open wound into thorax
862.0	Injury to diaphragm, without mention of open wound into cavity
862.29	Injury to other specified intrathoracic organs without mention of open wound into cavity
862.8	Injury to multiple and unspecified intrathoracic organs, without mention of open wound into cavity
863.0	Injury to stomach, without mention of open wound into cavity
863.20	Injury to small intestine, unspecified site, without open wound into cavity
863.21	Injury to duodenum, without open wound into cavity
863.29	Other injury to small intestine, without mention of open wound into cavity
863.40	Injury to colon, unspecified site, without mention of open wound into cavity

863.41 Injury to ascending [right] colon, without mention of open wound into cavity

863.42 Injury to transverse colon, without mention of open wound into cavity

863.43 Injury to descending [left] colon, without mention of open wound into cavity

863.44 Injury to sigmoid colon, without mention of open wound into cavity

863.45 Injury to rectum, without mention of open wound into cavity

863.46 Injury to multiple sites in colon and rectum, without mention of open wound into cavity

863.49 Other injury to colon or rectum, without mention of open wound into cavity

863.80 Injury to gastrointestinal tract, unspecified site, without mention of open wound into cavity

863.81 Injury to pancreas, head, without mention of open wound into cavity

863.82 Injury to pancreas, body, without mention of open wound into cavity

863.83 Injury to pancreas, tail, without mention of open wound into cavity

863.84 Injury to pancreas, multiple and unspecified sites, without mention of open wound into cavity

863.85 Injury to appendix, without mention of open wound into cavity

863.89 Injury to other gastrointestinal sites, without mention of open wound into cavity

864.00 Injury to liver without mention of open wound into cavity, unspecified injury

864.01 Injury to liver without mention of open wound into cavity, hematoma and contusion

864.02 Injury to liver without mention of open wound into cavity, laceration, minor

864.05 Injury to liver without mention of open wound into cavity laceration, unspecified

864.09 Other injury to liver without mention of open wound into cavity

865.00 Injury to spleen without mention of open wound into cavity, unspecified injury

865.01 Injury to spleen without mention of open wound into cavity, hematoma without rupture of capsule

865.02 Injury to spleen without mention of open wound into cavity, capsular tears, without major disruption of parenchyma

865.09 Other injury into spleen without mention of open wound into cavity

866.00 Injury to kidney without mention of open wound into cavity, unspecified injury

866.01 Injury to kidney without mention of open wound into cavity, hematoma without rupture of capsule

866.02 Injury to kidney without mention of open wound into cavity, laceration

867.0 Injury to bladder and urethra, without mention of open wound into cavity

867.2 Injury to ureter, without mention of open wound into cavity

867.4 Injury to uterus, without mention of open wound into cavity

867.6 Injury to other specified pelvic organs, without mention of open wound into cavity

867.8 Injury to unspecified pelvic organ, without mention of open wound into cavity

868.00 Injury to other intra-abdominal organs without mention of open wound into cavity, unspecified intra-abdominal organ

868.01 Injury to other intra-abdominal organs without mention of open wound into cavity, adrenal gland

868.02 Injury to other intra-abdominal organs without mention of open wound into cavity, bile duct and gallbladder

868.03 Injury to other intra-abdominal organs without mention of open wound into cavity, peritoneum

868.04 Injury to other intra-abdominal organs without mention of open wound into cavity, retroperitoneum

868.09 Injury to other and multiple intra-abdominal organs without mention of open wound into cavity

869.0 Internal injury to unspecified or ill-defined organs without mention of open wound into cavity

870.2 Laceration of eyelid involving lacrimal passages

870.3 Penetrating wound of orbit, without mention of foreign body

870.4 Penetrating wound of orbit with foreign body

870.8 Other specified open wounds of ocular adnexa

870.9 Unspecified open wound of ocular adnexa

871.0 Ocular laceration without prolapse of intraocular tissue

871.1 Ocular laceration with prolapse or exposure of intraocular tissue

871.2 Rupture of eye with partial loss of intraocular tissue

871.3 Avulsion of eye

871.5 Penetration of eyeball with magnetic foreign body

871.6 Penetration of eyeball with (nonmagnetic) foreign body

871.9 Unspecified open wound of eyeball

872.12 Open wound of auditory canal, complicated

872.61 Open wound of ear drum, without mention of complication

872.62 Open wound of ossicles, without mention of complication

872.63 Open wound of eustachian tube, without mention of complication

872.64 Open wound of cochlea, without mention of complication

872.69 Open wound of other and multiple sites of ear, without mention of complication

872.71 Open wound of ear drum, complicated

872.72 Open wound of ossicles, complicated

872.73 Open wound of eustachian tube, complicated

872.74 Open wound of cochlea, complicated

872.79 Open wound of other and multiple sites of ear, complicated

873.23 Open wound of nasal sinus, without mention of complication

873.33 Open wound of nasal sinus, complicated

874.2 Open wound of thyroid gland, without mention of complication

874.3 Open wound of thyroid gland, complicated

874.4 Open wound of pharynx, without mention of complication

874.5 Open wound of pharynx, complicated

875.0 Open wound of chest (wall), without mention of complication

875.1 Open wound of chest (wall), complicated

880.20 Open wound of shoulder region, with tendon involvement

880.21 Open wound of scapular region, with tendon involvement

880.22 Open wound of axillary region, with tendon involvement

880.23 Open wound of upper arm, with tendon involvement

880.29 Open wound of multiple sites of shoulder and upper arm, with tendon involvement

881.20 Open wound of forearm, with tendon involvement

881.21 Open wound of elbow, with tendon involvement

881.22 Open wound of wrist, with tendon involvement

882.2 Open wound of hand except finger(s) alone, with tendon involvement

883.2 Open wound of finger(s), with tendon involvement

884.2 Multiple and unspecified open wound of upper limb, with tendon involvement

887.0 Traumatic amputation of arm and hand (complete) (partial), unilateral, below elbow, without mention of complication

887.1 Traumatic amputation of arm and hand (complete) (partial), unilateral, below elbow, complicated

887.2 Traumatic amputation of arm and hand (complete) (partial), unilateral, at or above elbow, without mention of complication

887.3 Traumatic amputation of arm and hand (complete) (partial), unilateral, at or above elbow, complicated

887.4	Traumatic amputation of arm and hand (complete) (partial), unilateral, level not specified, without mention of complication
887.5	Traumatic amputation of arm and hand (complete) (partial), unilateral, level not specified, complicated
890.2	Open wound of hip and thigh, with tendon involvement
891.2	Open wound of knee, leg [except thigh], and ankle, with tendon involvement
892.2	Open wound of foot except toe(s) alone, with tendon involvement
893.2	Open wound of toe(s), with tendon involvement
894.2	Multiple and unspecified open wound of lower limb, with tendon involvement
896.0	Traumatic amputation of foot (complete) (partial), unilateral, without mention of complication
896.1	Traumatic amputation of foot (complete) (partial), unilateral, complicated
897.0	Traumatic amputation of leg(s) (complete) (partial), unilateral, below knee, without mention of complication
897.1	Traumatic amputation of leg(s) (complete) (partial), unilateral, below knee, complicated
897.2	Traumatic amputation of leg(s) (complete) (partial), unilateral, at or above knee, without mention of complication
897.3	Traumatic amputation of leg(s) (complete) (partial), unilateral, at or above knee, complicated
897.4	Traumatic amputation of leg(s) (complete) (partial), unilateral, level not specified, without mention of complication
897.5	Traumatic amputation of leg(s) (complete) (partial), unilateral, level not specified, complicated
900.00	Injury to carotid artery, unspecified
900.01	Injury to common carotid artery
900.02	Injury to external carotid artery
900.03	Injury to internal carotid artery
900.1	Injury to internal jugular vein
900.81	Injury to external jugular vein
900.82	Injury to multiple blood vessels of head and neck
900.89	Injury to other specified blood vessels of head and neck
900.9	Injury to unspecified blood vessel of head and neck
901.81	Injury to intercostal artery or vein
901.82	Injury to internal mammary artery or vein
901.89	Injury to other specified blood vessels of thorax
901.9	Injury to unspecified blood vessel of thorax
902.55	Injury to uterine artery
902.56	Injury to uterine vein
902.81	Injury to ovarian artery
902.82	Injury to ovarian vein
902.89	Injury to other specified blood vessels of abdomen and pelvis
902.9	Injury to unspecified blood vessel of abdomen and pelvis
903.1	Injury to brachial blood vessels
903.2	Injury to radial blood vessels
903.3	Injury to ulnar blood vessels
903.4	Injury to palmar artery
903.5	Injury to digital blood vessels
903.8	Injury to other specified blood vessels of upper extremity
903.9	Injury to unspecified blood vessel of upper extremity
904.3	Injury to saphenous veins
904.50	Injury to tibial vessel(s), unspecified
904.51	Injury to anterior tibial artery
904.52	Injury to anterior tibial vein
904.53	Injury to posterior tibial artery
904.54	Injury to posterior tibial vein
904.6	Injury to deep plantar blood vessels
904.7	Injury to other specified blood vessels of lower extremity

904.8	Injury to unspecified blood vessel of lower extremity
904.9	Injury to blood vessels of unspecified site
925.1	Crushing injury of face and scalp
925.2	Crushing injury of neck
928.00	Crushing injury of thigh
928.01	Crushing injury of hip
934.0	Foreign body in trachea
934.1	Foreign body in main bronchus
934.8	Foreign body in other specified parts bronchus and lung
940.5	Burn with resulting rupture and destruction of eyeball
941.30	Full-thickness skin loss [third degree, not otherwise specified] of face and head, unspecified site
941.31	Full-thickness skin loss [third degree, not otherwise specified] of ear [any part]
941.32	Full-thickness skin loss [third degree, not otherwise specified] of eye (with other parts of face, head, and neck)
941.33	Full-thickness skin loss [third degree, not otherwise specified] of lip(s)
941.34	Full-thickness skin loss [third degree, not otherwise specified] of chin
941.35	Full-thickness skin loss [third degree, not otherwise specified] of nose (septum)
941.36	Full-thickness skin loss [third degree, not otherwise specified] of scalp [any part]
941.37	Full-thickness skin loss [third degree, not otherwise specified] of forehead and cheek
941.38	Full-thickness skin loss [third degree, not otherwise specified] of neck
941.39	Full-thickness skin loss [third degree, not otherwise specified] of multiple sites [except with eye] of face, head, and neck
941.40	Deep necrosis of underlying tissues [deep third degree] without mention of loss of a body part, face and head, unspecified site
941.41	Deep necrosis of underlying tissues [deep third degree]) without mention of loss of a body part, ear [any part]
941.42	Deep necrosis of underlying tissues [deep third degree] without mention of loss of a body part, of eye (with other parts of face, head, and neck)
941.43	Deep necrosis of underlying tissues [deep third degree] without mention of loss of a body part, of lip(s)
941.44	Deep necrosis of underlying tissues [deep third degree] without mention of loss of a body part, of chin
941.45	Deep necrosis of underlying tissues [deep third degree] without mention of loss of a body part, of nose (septum)
941.46	Deep necrosis of underlying tissues [deep third degree] without mention of loss of a body part of scalp [any part]
941.47	Deep necrosis of underlying tissues [deep third degree] without mention of loss of a body part, of forehead and cheek
941.48	Deep necrosis of underlying tissues [deep third degree] without mention of loss of a body part, of neck
941.49	Deep necrosis of underlying tissues [deep third degree] without mention of loss of a body part, of multiple sites [except with eye] of face, head, and neck
941.50	Deep necrosis of underlying tissues [deep third degree] with loss of a body part, of face and head, unspecified site
941.51	Deep necrosis of underlying tissues [deep third degree] with loss of a body part, of ear [any part]
941.52	Deep necrosis of underlying tissues [deep third degree] with loss of a body part, of eye (with other parts of face, head, and neck)
941.53	Deep necrosis of underlying tissues [deep third degree] with loss of a body part, of lip(s)
941.54	Deep necrosis of underlying tissues [deep third degree] with loss of a body part, of chin
941.55	Deep necrosis of underlying tissues [deep third degree] with loss of a body part, of nose (septum)

941.56 Deep necrosis of underlying tissues [deep third degree] with loss of a body part, of scalp [any part]

941.57 Deep necrosis of underlying tissues [deep third degree] with loss of a body part, of forehead and cheek

941.58 Deep necrosis of underlying tissues [deep third degree] with loss of a body part, of neck

941.59 Deep necrosis of underlying tissues [deep third degree] with loss of a body part, of multiple sites [except with eye] of face, head, and neck

942.30 Full-thickness skin loss [third degree, not otherwise specified] of trunk, unspecified site

942.31 Full-thickness skin loss [third degree,not otherwise specified] of breast

942.32 Full-thickness skin loss [third degree, not otherwise specified] of chest wall, excluding breast and nipple

942.33 Full-thickness skin loss [third degree, not otherwise specified] of abdominal wall

942.34 Full-thickness skin loss [third degree,not otherwise specified] of back [any part]

942.35 Full-thickness skin loss [third degree, not otherwise specified] of genitalia

942.39 Full-thickness skin loss [third degree, not otherwise specified] of other and multiple sites of trunk

942.40 Deep necrosis of underlying tissues [deep third degree]) without mention of loss of a body part, of trunk, unspecified site

942.41 Deep necrosis of underlying tissues [deep third degree]) without mention of loss of a body part, of breast

942.42 Deep necrosis of underlying tissues [deep third degree] without mention of loss of a body part, of chest wall, excluding breast and nipple

942.43 Deep necrosis of underlying tissues [deep third degree] without mention of loss of a body part, of abdominal wall

942.44 Deep necrosis of underlying tissues [deep third degree] without mention of loss of a body part, of back [any part]

942.45 Deep necrosis of underlying tissues [deep third degree] without mention of loss of a body part, of genitalia

942.49 Deep necrosis of underlying tissues [deep third degree] without mention of loss of a body part, of other and multiple sites of trunk

942.50 Deep necrosis of underlying tissues [deep third degree] with loss of a body part, trunk, unspecified site

942.51 Deep necrosis of underlying tissues [deep third degree] with loss of a body part, of breast

942.52 Deep necrosis of underlying tissues [deep third degree] with loss of a body part, of chest wall, excluding breast and nipple

942.53 Deep necrosis of underlying tissues [deep third degree] with loss of a body part, of abdominal wall

942.54 Deep necrosis of underlying tissues [deep third degree] with loss of a body part, of back [any part]

942.55 Deep necrosis of underlying tissues [deep third degree] with loss of a body part, of genitalia

942.59 Deep necrosis of underlying tissues [deep third degree] with loss of a body part, of other and multiple sites of trunk,

943.30 Full-thickness skin [third degree, not otherwise specified] of upper limb, unspecified site

943.31 Full-thickness skin loss [third degree, not otherwise specified] of forearm

943.32 Full-thickness skin loss [third degree, not otherwise specified] of elbow

943.33 Full-thickness skin loss [third degree, not otherwise specified] of upper arm

943.34 Full-thickness skin loss [third degree, not otherwise specified] of axilla

943.35 Full-thickness skin loss [third degree, not otherwise specified] of shoulder

943.36 Full-thickness skin loss [third degree, not otherwise specified] of scapular region

943.39 Full-thickness skin loss [third degree, not otherwise specified] of multiple sites of upper limb, except wrist and hand

943.40 Deep necrosis of underlying tissues [deep third degree] without mention of loss of a body part, of upper limb,unspecified site

943.41 Deep necrosis of underlying tissues [deep third degree] without mention of loss of a body part, of forearm

943.42 Deep necrosis of underlying tissues [deep third degree] without mention of loss of a body part, of elbow

943.43 Deep necrosis of underlying tissues [deep third degree] without mention of loss of a body part, of upper arm

943.44 Deep necrosis of underlying tissues [deep third degree] without mention of loss of a body part, of axilla

943.45 Deep necrosis of underlying tissues [deep third degree] without mention of loss of a body part, of shoulder

943.46 Deep necrosis of underlying tissues [deep third degree] without mention of loss of a body part, of scapular region

943.49 Deep necrosis of underlying tissues [deep third degree] without mention of loss of a body part, of multiple sites of upper limb, except wrist and hand

943.50 Deep necrosis of underlying tissues [deep third degree] with loss of a body part, of upper limb, unspecified site

943.51 Deep necrosis of underlying tissues [deep third degree] with loss of a body part, of forearm

943.52 Deep necrosis of underlying tissues [deep third degree] with loss of a body part, of elbow

943.53 Deep necrosis of underlying tissues [deep third degree] with loss of a body part, of upper arm

943.54 Deep necrosis of underlying tissues [deep third degree] with loss of a body part, of axilla

943.55 Deep necrosis of underlying tissues [deep third degree] with loss of a body part, of shoulder

943.56 Deep necrosis of underlying tissues [deep third degree] with loss of a body part, of scapular region

943.59 Deep necrosis of underlying tissues [deep third degree] with loss of a body part, of multiple sites of upper limb, except wrist and hand

944.30 Full-thickness skin loss [third degree, not otherwise specified] of hand, unspecified site

944.31 Full-thickness skin loss [third degree, not otherwise specified] of single digit [finger (nail)] other than thumb

944.32 Full-thickness skin loss [third degree, not otherwise specified] of thumb (nail)

944.33 Full-thickness skin loss [third degree, not otherwise specified]of two or more digits of hand, not including thumb

944.34 Full-thickness skin loss [third degree, not otherwise specified] of two or more digits of hand including thumb

944.35 Full-thickness skin loss [third degree, not otherwise specified] of palm of hand

944.36 Full-thickness skin loss [third degree, not otherwise specified] of back of hand

944.37 Full-thickness skin loss [third degree, not otherwise specified] of wrist

944.38 Full-thickness skin loss [third degree, not otherwise specified] of multiple sites of wrist(s) and hand(s)

944.40 Deep necrosis of underlying tissues [deep third degree] without mention of loss of a body part, hand, unspecified site

944.41 Deep necrosis of underlying tissues [deep third degree] without mention of loss of a body part, single digit [finger (nail)] other than thumb

944.42 Deep necrosis of underlying tissues [deep third degree] without mention of loss of a body part, thumb (nail)

944.43 Deep necrosis of underlying tissues [deep third degree] without mention of loss of a body part, two or more digits of hand, not including thumb

944.44 Deep necrosis of underlying tissues [deep third degree] without mention of loss of a body part, two or more digits of hand including thumb

944.45   Deep necrosis of underlying tissues [deep third degree] without mention of loss of a body part, of palm of hand

944.46   Deep necrosis of underlying tissues [deep third degree] without mention of loss of a body part, of back of hand

944.47   Deep necrosis of underlying tissues [deep third degree] without mention of loss of a body part, of wrist

944.48   Deep necrosis of underlying tissues [deep third degree] without mention of loss of a body part, of multiple sites of wrist(s) and hand(s)

944.50   Deep necrosis of underlying tissues [deep third degree] with loss of a body part, of hand, unspecified site

944.51   Deep necrosis of underlying tissues [deep third degree] with loss of a body part, of single digit [finger (nail)] other than thumb

944.52   Deep necrosis of underlying tissues [deep third degree] with loss of a body part, of thumb (nail)

944.53   Deep necrosis of underlying tissues [deep third degree] with loss of a body part, of two or more digits of hand, not including thumb

944.54   Deep necrosis of underlying tissues [deep third degree] with loss of a body part, of two or more digits of hand including thumb

944.55   Deep necrosis of underlying tissues [deep third degree] with loss of a body part, of palm of hand

944.56   Deep necrosis of underlying tissues [deep third degree] with loss of a body part, of back of hand

944.57   Deep necrosis of underlying tissues [deep third degree] with loss of a body part, of wrist

944.58   Deep necrosis of underlying tissues [deep third degree] with loss of a body part, of multiple sites of wrist(s) and hand(s)

945.30   Full-thickness skin loss [third degree NOS] of lower limb [leg] unspecified site

945.31   Full-thickness skin loss [third degree NOS] of toe(s) (nail)

945.32   Full-thickness skin loss [third degree NOS] of foot

945.33   Full-thickness skin loss [third degree NOS] of ankle

945.34   Full-thickness skin loss [third degree nos] of lower leg

945.35   Full-thickness skin loss [third degree NOS] of knee

945.36   Full-thickness skin loss [third degree NOS] of thigh [any part]

945.39   Full-thickness skin loss [third degree NOS] of multiple sites of lower limb(s)

945.40   Deep necrosis of underlying tissues [deep third degree] without mention of loss of a body part, lower limb [leg], unspecified site

945.41   Deep necrosis of underlying tissues [deep third degree] without mention of loss of a body part, of toe(s)(nail)

945.42   Deep necrosis of underlying tissues [deep third degree] without mention of loss of a body part, of foot

945.43   Deep necrosis of underlying tissues [deep third degree] without mention of loss of a body part, of ankle

945.44   Deep necrosis of underlying tissues [deep third degree] without mention of loss of a body part, of lower leg

945.45   Deep necrosis of underlying tissues [deep third degree] without mention of loss of a body part, of knee

945.46   Deep necrosis of underlying tissues [deep third degree] without mention of loss of a body part, of thigh [any part]

945.49   Deep necrosis of underlying tissues [deep third degree] without mention of loss of a body part, of multiple sites of lower limb(s)

945.50   Deep necrosis of underlying tissues [deep third degree] with loss of a body part, of lower limb [leg], unspecified site

945.51   Deep necrosis of underlying tissues [deep third degree] with loss of a body part, of toe(s) (nail)

945.52   Deep necrosis of underlying tissues [deep third degree] with loss of a body part, of foot

945.53   Deep necrosis of underlying tissues [deep third degree] with loss of a body part, of ankle

945.54   Deep necrosis of underlying tissues [deep third degree] with loss of a body part, of lower leg

945.55   Deep necrosis of underlying tissues [deep third degree] with loss of a body part, of knee

945.56   Deep necrosis of underlying tissues [deep third degree] with loss of a body part, of thigh [any part]

945.59   Deep necrosis of underlying tissues [deep third degree] with loss of a body part, of multiple sites of lower limb(s)

946.3   Full-thickness skin loss [third degree NOS] of multiple specified sites

946.4   Deep necrosis of underlying tissues [deep third degree] without mention of loss of a body part, of multiple specified sites

946.5   Deep necrosis of underlying tissues [deep third degree] with loss of a body part, of multiple specified sites

947.1   Burn of larynx, trachea, and lung

947.2   Burn of esophagus

947.3   Burn of gastrointestinal tract

947.4   Burn of vagina and uterus

948.10   Burn [any degree] involving 10-19 percent of body surface with third degree burn, less than 10 percent or unspecified

948.11   Burn [any degree] involving 10-19 percent of body surface with third degree burn, 10-19%

948.20   Burn [any degree] involving 20-29 percent of body surface with third degree burn, less than 10 percent or unspecified

948.30   Burn [any degree] involving 30-39 percent of body surface with third degree burn, less than 10 percent or unspecified

948.40   Burn [any degree] involving 40-49 percent of body surface with third degree burn, less than 10 percent or unspecified

948.50   Burn [any degree] involving 50-59 percent of body surface with third degree burn, less than 10 percent or unspecified

948.60   Burn [any degree] involving 60-69 percent of body surface with third degree burn, less than 10 percent or unspecified

948.70   Burn [any degree] involving 70-79 percent of body surface with third degree burn, less than 10 percent or unspecified

948.80   Burn [any degree] involving 80-89 percent of body surface with third degree burn, less than 10 percent or unspecified

948.90   Burn [any degree] involving 90 percent or more of body surface with third degree burn, less than 10 percent or unspecified

949.3   Full-thickness skin loss [third degree nos]

949.4   Deep necrosis of underlying tissue [deep third degree] without mention of loss of a body part, unspecified

949.5   Deep necrosis of underlying tissues [deep third degree] with loss of a body part, unspecified

950.0   Optic nerve injury

950.1   Injury to optic chiasm

950.2   Injury to optic pathways

950.3   Injury to visual cortex

950.9   Injury to unspecified optic nerve and pathways

951.0   Injury to oculomotor nerve

951.1   Injury to trochlear nerve

951.2   Injury to trigeminal nerve

951.3   Injury to abducens nerve

951.4   Injury to facial nerve

951.5   Injury to acoustic nerve

951.6   Injury to accessory nerve

951.7   Injury to hypoglossal nerve

951.8   Injury to other specified cranial nerves

951.9   Injury to unspecified cranial nerve

958.2   Secondary and recurrent hemorrhage

958.3   Posttraumatic wound infection not elsewhere classified

958.7   Traumatic subcutaneous emphysema

958.90   Compartment syndrome, unspecified

958.91   Traumatic compartment syndrome of upper extremity

958.92   Traumatic compartment syndrome of lower extremity

958.93   Traumatic compartment syndrome of abdomen

958.99   Traumatic compartment syndrome of other sites

991.0	Frostbite of face
991.1	Frostbite of hand
991.2	Frostbite of foot
991.3	Frostbite of other and unspecified sites
991.4	Immersion foot
992.0	Heat stroke and sunstroke
993.3	Caisson disease
994.1	Drowning and nonfatal submersion
994.7	Asphyxiation and strangulation
995.0	Other anaphylactic reaction
995.4	Shock due to anesthesia, not elsewhere classified
995.50	Child abuse, unspecified
995.51	Child emotional/psychological abuse
995.52	Child neglect (nutritional)
995.53	Child sexual abuse
995.54	Child physical abuse
995.55	Shaken baby syndrome
995.59	Other child abuse and neglect
995.60	Anaphylactic reaction due to unspecified food
995.61	Anaphylactic reaction due to peanuts
995.62	Anaphylactic reaction due to crustaceans
995.63	Anaphylactic reaction due to fruits and vegetables
995.64	Anaphylactic reaction due to tree nuts and seeds
995.65	Anaphylactic reaction due to fish
995.66	Anaphylactic reaction due to food additives
995.67	Anaphylactic reaction due to milk products
995.68	Anaphylactic reaction due to eggs
995.69	Anaphylactic reaction due to other specified food
995.80	Adult maltreatment, unspecified
995.81	Adult physical abuse
995.83	Adult sexual abuse
995.84	Adult neglect (nutritional)
995.85	Other adult abuse and neglect
995.86	Malignant hyperthermia
995.90	Systemic inflammatory response syndrome, unspecified
995.93	Systemic inflammatory response syndrome due to noninfectious process without acute organ dysfunction
996.00	Mechanical complication of unspecified cardiac device, implant, and graft
996.01	Mechanical complication due to cardiac pacemaker (electrode)
996.02	Mechanical complication due to heart valve prosthesis
996.03	Mechanical complication due to coronary bypass graft
996.04	Mechanical complication of automatic implantable cardiac defibrillator
996.09	Other mechanical complication of cardiac device, implant, and graft
996.1	Mechanical complication of other vascular device, implant, and graft
996.2	Mechanical complication of nervous system device, implant, and graft
996.30	Mechanical complication of unspecified genitourinary device, implant, and graft
996.39	Other mechanical complication of genitourinary device, implant, and graft
996.40	Unspecified mechanical complication of internal orthopedic device, implant, and graft
996.41	Mechanical loosening of prosthetic joint
996.42	Dislocation of prosthetic joint
996.43	Broken prosthetic joint implant
996.44	Peri-prosthetic fracture around prosthetic joint
996.45	Peri-prosthetic osteolysis
996.46	Articular bearing surface wear of prosthetic joint
996.47	Other mechanical complication of prosthetic joint implant
996.49	Other mechanical complication of other internal orthopedic device, implant, and graft
996.51	Mechanical complication due to corneal graft
996.52	Mechanical complication due to graft of other tissue, not elsewhere classified
996.53	Mechanical complication due to ocular lens prosthesis
996.54	Mechanical complication due to breast prosthesis
996.55	Mechanical complication due to artificial skin graft and decellularized allodermis
996.56	Mechanical complication due to peritoneal dialysis catheter
996.57	Mechanical complication due to insulin pump
996.59	Mechanical complication due to other implant and internal device, not elsewhere classified
996.60	Infection and inflammatory reaction due to unspecified device, implant, and graft
996.61	Infection and inflammatory reaction due to cardiac device, implant, and graft
996.62	Infection and inflammatory reaction due to other vascular device, implant, and graft
996.63	Infection and inflammatory reaction due to nervous system device, implant, and graft
996.64	Infection and inflammatory reaction due to indwelling urinary catheter
996.65	Infection and inflammatory reaction due to other genitourinary device, implant, and graft
996.66	Infection and inflammatory reaction due to internal joint prosthesis
996.67	Infection and inflammatory reaction due to other internal orthopedic device, implant, and graft
996.68	Infection and inflammatory reaction due to peritoneal dialysis catheter
996.69	Infection and inflammatory reaction due to other internal prosthetic device, implant, and graft
996.71	Other complications due to heart valve prosthesis
996.72	Other complications due to other cardiac device, implant, and graft
996.73	Other complications due to renal dialysis device, implant, and graft
996.74	Other complications due to other vascular device, implant, and graft
996.75	Other complications due to nervous system device, implant, and graft
996.76	Other complications due to genitourinary device, implant, and graft
996.77	Other complications due to internal joint prosthesis
996.78	Other complications due to other internal orthopedic device, implant, and graft
996.79	Other complications due to other internal prosthetic device, implant, and graft
996.80	Complications of transplanted organ, unspecified
996.81	Complications of transplanted kidney
996.82	Complications of transplanted liver
996.83	Complications of transplanted heart
996.84	Complications of transplanted lung
996.85	Complications of transplanted bone marrow
996.86	Complications of transplanted pancreas
996.87	Complications of transplanted intestine
996.88	Complications of transplanted organ, stem cell
996.89	Complications of other specified transplanted organ
996.90	Complications of unspecified reattached extremity
996.91	Complications of reattached forearm
996.92	Complications of reattached hand
996.93	Complications of reattached finger(s)

996.94	Complications of reattached upper extremity, other and unspecified
996.95	Complication of reattached foot and toe(s)
996.96	Complication of reattached lower extremity, other and unspecified
996.99	Complication of other specified reattached body part
997.01	Central nervous system complication
997.02	Iatrogenic cerebrovascular infarction or hemorrhage
997.09	Other nervous system complications
997.1	Cardiac complications, not elsewhere classified
997.2	Peripheral vascular complications, not elsewhere classified
997.31	Ventilator associated pneumonia
997.32	Postprocedural aspiration pneumonia
997.39	Other respiratory complications
997.41	Retained cholelithiasis following cholecystectomy
997.49	Other digestive system complications
997.62	Infection (chronic) of amputation stump
997.71	Vascular complications of mesenteric artery
997.72	Vascular complications of renal artery
997.79	Vascular complications of other vessels
997.99	Complications affecting other specified body systems, not elsewhere classified
998.00	Postoperative shock, unspecified
998.11	Hemorrhage complicating a procedure
998.12	Hematoma complicating a procedure
998.13	Seroma complicating a procedure
998.2	Accidental puncture or laceration during a procedure, not elsewhere classified
998.30	Disruption of wound, unspecified
998.31	Disruption of internal operation (surgical) wound
998.32	Disruption of external operation (surgical) wound
998.33	Disruption of traumatic injury wound repair
998.4	Foreign body accidentally left during a procedure
998.51	Infected postoperative seroma
998.59	Other postoperative infection
998.6	Persistent postoperative fistula
998.7	Acute reaction to foreign substance accidentally left during a procedure
998.83	Non-healing surgical wound
999.0	Generalized vaccinia as a complication of medical care, not elsewhere classified
999.2	Other vascular complications of medical care, not elsewhere classified
999.31	Other and unspecified infection due to central venous catheter
999.32	Bloodstream infection due to central venous catheter
999.33	Local infection due to central venous catheter
999.34	Acute infection following transfusion, infusion, or injection of blood and blood products
999.39	Infection following other infusion, injection, transfusion, or vaccination
999.41	Anaphylactic reaction due to administration of blood and blood products
999.42	Anaphylactic reaction due to vaccination
999.49	Anaphylactic reaction due to other serum
999.51	Other serum reaction due to administration of blood and blood products
999.52	Other serum reaction due to vaccination
999.59	Other serum reaction
999.60	ABO incompatibility reaction, unspecified
999.61	ABO incompatibility with hemolytic transfusion reaction not specified as acute or delayed
999.62	ABO incompatibility with acute hemolytic transfusion reaction

999.63	ABO incompatibility with delayed hemolytic transfusion reaction
999.69	Other ABO incompatibility reaction
999.70	Rh incompatibility reaction, unspecified
999.71	Rh incompatibility with hemolytic transfusion reaction not specified as acute or delayed
999.72	Rh incompatibility with acute hemolytic transfusion reaction
999.73	Rh incompatibility with delayed hemolytic transfusion reaction
999.74	Other Rh incompatibility reaction
999.75	Non-ABO incompatibility reaction, unspecified
999.76	Non-ABO incompatibility with hemolytic transfusion reaction not specified as acute or delayed
999.77	Non-ABO incompatibility with acute hemolytic transfusion reaction
999.78	Non-ABO incompatibility with delayed hemolytic transfusion reaction
999.79	Other non-ABO incompatibility reaction
999.81	Extravasation of vesicant chemotherapy
999.82	Extravasation of other vesicant agent
999.83	Hemolytic transfusion reaction, incompatibility unspecified
999.84	Acute hemolytic transfusion reaction, incompatibility unspecified
999.85	Delayed hemolytic transfusion reaction, incompatibility unspecified
V42.0	Kidney replaced by transplant
V42.1	Heart replaced by transplant
V42.6	Lung replaced by transplant
V42.7	Liver replaced by transplant
V42.81	Bone marrow replaced by transplant
V42.82	Peripheral stem cells replaced by transplant
V42.83	Pancreas replaced by transplant
V42.84	Organ or tissue replaced by transplant, intestines
V43.21	Organ or tissue replaced by other means, heart assist device
V43.22	Organ or tissue replaced by other means, fully implantable artificial heart
V46.11	Dependence on respirator, status
V46.12	Encounter for respirator dependence during power failure
V46.13	Encounter for weaning from respirator [ventilator]
V46.14	Mechanical complication of respirator [ventilator]
V55.1	Attention to gastrostomy
V62.84	Suicidal ideation
V85.0	Body Mass Index less than 19, adult
V85.41	Body Mass Index 40.0-44.9, adult
V85.42	Body Mass Index 45.0-49.9, adult
V85.43	Body Mass Index 50.0-59.9, adult
V85.44	Body Mass Index 60.0-69.9, adult
V85.45	Body Mass Index 70 and over, adult

Appendix A — Numeric CC List

Alphabetic CC List

039.2	Abdominal actinomycotic infection
633.01	Abdominal pregnancy with intrauterine pregnancy
633.00	Abdominal pregnancy without intrauterine pregnancy
999.60	ABO incompatibility reaction, unspecified
999.62	ABO incompatibility with acute hemolytic transfusion reaction
999.63	ABO incompatibility with delayed hemolytic transfusion reaction
999.61	ABO incompatibility with hemolytic transfusion reaction not specified as acute or delayed
566	Abscess of anal and rectal regions
616.3	Abscess of Bartholin's gland
675.12	Abscess of breast associated with childbirth, delivered, with mention of postpartum complication
675.11	Abscess of breast associated with childbirth, delivered, with or without mention of antepartum condition
569.5	Abscess of intestine
601.2	Abscess of prostate
527.3	Abscess of salivary gland
254.1	Abscess of thymus
756.13	Absence of vertebra, congenital
998.2	Accidental puncture or laceration during a procedure, not elsewhere classified
349.31	Accidental puncture or laceration of dura during a procedure
276.2	Acidosis
429.71	Acquired cardiac septal defect
286.7	Acquired coagulation factor deficiency
283.9	Acquired hemolytic anemia, unspecified
286.52	Acquired hemophilia
537.0	Acquired hypertrophic pyloric stenosis
039.8	Actinomycotic infection of other specified sites
039.9	Actinomycotic infection of unspecified site
341.21	Acute (transverse) myelitis in conditions classified elsewhere
341.20	Acute (transverse) myelitis NOS
006.0	Acute amebic dysentery without mention of abscess
575.12	Acute and chronic cholecystitis
364.00	Acute and subacute iridocyclitis, unspecified
365.22	Acute angle-closure glaucoma
522.4	Acute apical periodontitis of pulpal origin
540.9	Acute appendicitis without mention of peritonitis
466.19	Acute bronchiolitis due to other infectious organisms
466.11	Acute bronchiolitis due to respiratory syncytial virus (RSV)
517.3	Acute chest syndrome
575.0	Acute cholecystitis
411.81	Acute coronary occlusion without myocardial infarction
595.0	Acute cystitis
536.1	Acute dilatation of stomach
532.30	Acute duodenal ulcer without mention of hemorrhage or perforation, without mention of obstruction
333.72	Acute dystonia due to drugs
360.01	Acute endophthalmitis
464.30	Acute epiglottitis without mention of obstruction
207.02	Acute erythremia and erythroleukemia, in relapse
207.01	Acute erythremia and erythroleukemia, in remission
207.00	Acute erythremia and erythroleukemia, without mention of having achieved remission
530.12	Acute esophagitis
446.1	Acute febrile mucocutaneous lymph node syndrome [MCLS]
531.30	Acute gastric ulcer without mention of hemorrhage or perforation, without mention of obstruction
534.30	Acute gastrojejunal ulcer without mention of hemorrhage or perforation, without mention of obstruction
279.51	Acute graft-versus-host disease
999.84	Acute hemolytic transfusion reaction, incompatibility unspecified
070.51	Acute hepatitis C without mention of hepatic coma
420.91	Acute idiopathic pericarditis
786.31	Acute idiopathic pulmonary hemorrhage in infants [AIPHI]
999.34	Acute infection following transfusion, infusion, or injection of blood and blood products
357.0	Acute infective polyneuritis
615.0	Acute inflammatory diseases of uterus, except cervix
516.33	Acute interstitial pneumonitis
584.8	Acute kidney failure with other specified pathological lesion in kidney
584.9	Acute kidney failure, unspecified
208.02	Acute leukemia of unspecified cell type, in relapse
208.01	Acute leukemia of unspecified cell type, in remission
208.00	Acute leukemia of unspecified cell type, without mention of having achieved remission
204.02	Acute lymphoid leukemia, in relapse
204.01	Acute lymphoid leukemia, in remission
204.00	Acute lymphoid leukemia, without mention of having achieved remission
383.02	Acute mastoiditis with other complications
383.00	Acute mastoiditis without complications
206.02	Acute monocytic leukemia, in relapse
206.00	Acute monocytic leukemia, without mention of having achieved remission
206.01	Acute monocytic leukemia, in remission
205.02	Acute myeloid leukemia, in relapse
205.01	Acute myeloid leukemia, in remission
205.00	Acute myeloid leukemia, without mention of having achieved remission
279.53	Acute on chronic graft-versus-host disease
730.07	Acute osteomyelitis, ankle and foot
730.03	Acute osteomyelitis, forearm
730.04	Acute osteomyelitis, hand
730.06	Acute osteomyelitis, lower leg
730.09	Acute osteomyelitis, multiple sites
730.08	Acute osteomyelitis, other specified sites
730.05	Acute osteomyelitis, pelvic region and thigh
730.01	Acute osteomyelitis, shoulder region
730.00	Acute osteomyelitis, site unspecified
730.02	Acute osteomyelitis, upper arm
614.3	Acute parametritis and pelvic cellulitis
298.3	Acute paranoid reaction
533.30	Acute peptic ulcer of unspecified site without mention of hemorrhage and perforation, without mention of obstruction
420.0	Acute pericarditis in diseases classified elsewhere
420.90	Acute pericarditis, unspecified
285.1	Acute posthemorrhagic anemia
601.0	Acute prostatitis
508.0	Acute pulmonary manifestations due to radiation
590.10	Acute pyelonephritis without lesion of renal medullary necrosis
998.7	Acute reaction to foreign substance accidentally left during a procedure
391.1	Acute rheumatic endocarditis
391.9	Acute rheumatic heart disease, unspecified
391.2	Acute rheumatic myocarditis
391.0	Acute rheumatic pericarditis
614.0	Acute salpingitis and oophoritis

245.0	Acute thyroiditis
453.84	Acute venous embolism and thrombosis of axillary veins
453.82	Acute venous embolism and thrombosis of deep veins of upper extremity
453.42	Acute venous embolism and thrombosis of deep vessels of distal lower extremity
453.41	Acute venous embolism and thrombosis of deep vessels of proximal lower extremity
453.86	Acute venous embolism and thrombosis of internal jugular veins
453.89	Acute venous embolism and thrombosis of other specified veins
453.87	Acute venous embolism and thrombosis of other thoracic veins
453.85	Acute venous embolism and thrombosis of subclavian veins
453.81	Acute venous embolism and thrombosis of superficial veins of upper extremity
453.40	Acute venous embolism and thrombosis of unspecified deep vessels of lower extremity
453.83	Acute venous embolism and thrombosis of upper extremity, unspecified
436	Acute, but ill-defined, cerebrovascular disease
091.4	Adenopathy due to secondary syphilis
423.1	Adhesive pericarditis
772.5	Adrenal hemorrhage of fetus or newborn
995.80	Adult maltreatment, unspecified
995.84	Adult neglect (nutritional)
995.81	Adult physical abuse
516.5	Adult pulmonary Langerhans cell histiocytosis
995.83	Adult sexual abuse
086.5	African trypanosomiasis, unspecified
050.1	Alastrim
291.81	Alcohol withdrawal
291.0	Alcohol withdrawal delirium
291.2	Alcohol-induced persisting dementia
291.3	Alcohol-induced psychotic disorder with hallucinations
425.5	Alcoholic cardiomyopathy
276.3	Alkalosis
518.6	Allergic bronchopulmonary aspergillosis
287.0	Allergic purpura
117.6	Allescheriosis [Petriellidosis]
006.8	Amebic infection of other sites
006.2	Amebic nondysenteric colitis
304.41	Amphetamine and other psychostimulant dependence, continuous
277.30	Amyloidosis, unspecified
335.20	Amyotrophic lateral sclerosis
664.61	Anal sphincter tear complicating delivery, not associated with third-degree perineal laceration, delivered, with or without mention of antepartum condition
664.64	Anal sphincter tear complicating delivery, not associated with third-degree perineal laceration, postpartum condition or complication
999.41	Anaphylactic reaction due to administration of blood and blood products
995.62	Anaphylactic reaction due to crustaceans
995.68	Anaphylactic reaction due to eggs
995.65	Anaphylactic reaction due to fish
995.66	Anaphylactic reaction due to food additives
995.63	Anaphylactic reaction due to fruits and vegetables
995.67	Anaphylactic reaction due to milk products
999.49	Anaphylactic reaction due to other serum
995.69	Anaphylactic reaction due to other specified food
995.61	Anaphylactic reaction due to peanuts
995.64	Anaphylactic reaction due to tree nuts and seeds
995.60	Anaphylactic reaction due to unspecified food
999.42	Anaphylactic reaction due to vaccination
200.63	Anaplastic large cell lymphoma, intra-abdominal lymph nodes
200.66	Anaplastic large cell lymphoma, intrapelvic lymph nodes
200.62	Anaplastic large cell lymphoma, intrathoracic lymph nodes
200.64	Anaplastic large cell lymphoma, lymph nodes of axilla and upper limb
200.61	Anaplastic large cell lymphoma, lymph nodes of head, face, and neck
200.65	Anaplastic large cell lymphoma, lymph nodes of inguinal region and lower limb
200.68	Anaplastic large cell lymphoma, lymph nodes of multiple sites
200.67	Anaplastic large cell lymphoma, spleen
200.60	Anaplastic large cell lymphoma, unspecified site, extranodal and solid organ sites
126.9	Ancylostomiasis and necatoriasis, unspecified
126.2	Ancylostomiasis due to ancylostoma braziliense
126.3	Ancylostomiasis due to ancylostoma ceylanicum
126.0	Ancylostomiasis due to ancylostoma duodenale
776.6	Anemia of prematurity
093.0	Aneurysm of aorta, specified as syphilitic
414.10	Aneurysm of heart (wall)
417.1	Aneurysm of pulmonary artery
413.0	Angina decubitus
127.1	Anisakiasis
747.21	Anomalies of aortic arch
751.4	Anomalies of intestinal fixation
751.7	Anomalies of pancreas
759.0	Anomalies of spleen
747.20	Anomaly of aorta, unspecified
747.40	Anomaly of great veins, unspecified
307.1	Anorexia nervosa
348.1	Anoxic brain damage
836.61	Anterior dislocation of tibia, proximal end, open
335.9	Anterior horn cell disease, unspecified
032.2	Anterior nasal diphtheria
022.9	Anthrax, unspecified
286.53	Antiphospholipid antibody with hemorrhagic disorder
784.3	Aphasia
284.9	Aplastic anemia, unspecified
078.7	Arenaviral hemorrhagic fever
266.0	Ariboflavinosis
263.2	Arrested development following protein-calorie malnutrition
444.22	Arterial embolism and thrombosis of lower extremity
444.21	Arterial embolism and thrombosis of upper extremity
417.0	Arteriovenous fistula of pulmonary vessels
056.71	Arthritis due to rubella
711.77	Arthropathy associated with helminthiasis, ankle and foot
711.73	Arthropathy associated with helminthiasis, forearm
711.74	Arthropathy associated with helminthiasis, hand
711.76	Arthropathy associated with helminthiasis, lower leg
711.79	Arthropathy associated with helminthiasis, multiple sites
711.78	Arthropathy associated with helminthiasis, other specified sites
711.75	Arthropathy associated with helminthiasis, pelvic region and thigh
711.71	Arthropathy associated with helminthiasis, shoulder region
711.70	Arthropathy associated with helminthiasis, site unspecified
711.72	Arthropathy associated with helminthiasis, upper arm
711.67	Arthropathy associated with mycoses, ankle and foot
711.63	Arthropathy associated with mycoses, forearm

Appendix A — Alphabetic CC List

711.64	Arthropathy associated with mycoses, hand
711.69	Arthropathy associated with mycoses, involving multiple sites
711.66	Arthropathy associated with mycoses, lower leg
711.68	Arthropathy associated with mycoses, other specified sites
711.65	Arthropathy associated with mycoses, pelvic region and thigh
711.61	Arthropathy associated with mycoses, shoulder region
711.60	Arthropathy associated with mycoses, site unspecified
711.62	Arthropathy associated with mycoses, upper arm
711.47	Arthropathy associated with other bacterial diseases, ankle and foot
711.43	Arthropathy associated with other bacterial diseases, forearm
711.44	Arthropathy associated with other bacterial diseases, hand
711.46	Arthropathy associated with other bacterial diseases, lower leg
711.49	Arthropathy associated with other bacterial diseases, multiple sites
711.48	Arthropathy associated with other bacterial diseases, other specified sites
711.45	Arthropathy associated with other bacterial diseases, pelvic region and thigh
711.41	Arthropathy associated with other bacterial diseases, shoulder region
711.40	Arthropathy associated with other bacterial diseases, site unspecified
711.42	Arthropathy associated with other bacterial diseases, upper arm
711.87	Arthropathy associated with other infectious and parasitic diseases, ankle and foot
711.83	Arthropathy associated with other infectious and parasitic diseases, forearm
711.84	Arthropathy associated with other infectious and parasitic diseases, hand
711.86	Arthropathy associated with other infectious and parasitic diseases, lower leg
711.89	Arthropathy associated with other infectious and parasitic diseases, multiple sites
711.88	Arthropathy associated with other infectious and parasitic diseases, other specified sites
711.85	Arthropathy associated with other infectious and parasitic diseases, pelvic region and thigh
711.81	Arthropathy associated with other infectious and parasitic diseases, shoulder region
711.80	Arthropathy associated with other infectious and parasitic diseases, site unspecified
711.82	Arthropathy associated with other infectious and parasitic diseases, upper arm
711.57	Arthropathy associated with other viral diseases, ankle and foot
711.53	Arthropathy associated with other viral diseases, forearm
711.54	Arthropathy associated with other viral diseases, hand
711.56	Arthropathy associated with other viral diseases, lower leg
711.59	Arthropathy associated with other viral diseases, multiple sites
711.58	Arthropathy associated with other viral diseases, other specified sites
711.55	Arthropathy associated with other viral diseases, pelvic region and thigh
711.51	Arthropathy associated with other viral diseases, shoulder region
711.50	Arthropathy associated with other viral diseases, site unspecified
711.52	Arthropathy associated with other viral diseases, upper arm
711.17	Arthropathy associated with Reiter's disease and nonspecific urethritis, ankle and foot
711.13	Arthropathy associated with Reiter's disease and nonspecific urethritis, forearm
711.14	Arthropathy associated with Reiter's disease and nonspecific urethritis, hand
711.16	Arthropathy associated with Reiter's disease and nonspecific urethritis, lower leg

711.19	Arthropathy associated with Reiter's disease and nonspecific urethritis, multiple sites
711.18	Arthropathy associated with Reiter's disease and nonspecific urethritis, other specified sites
711.15	Arthropathy associated with Reiter's disease and nonspecific urethritis, pelvic region and thigh
711.11	Arthropathy associated with Reiter's disease and nonspecific urethritis, shoulder region
711.10	Arthropathy associated with Reiter's disease and nonspecific urethritis, site unspecified
711.12	Arthropathy associated with Reiter's disease and nonspecific urethritis, upper arm
711.27	Arthropathy in Behcet's syndrome, ankle and foot
711.23	Arthropathy in Behcet's syndrome, forearm
711.24	Arthropathy in Behcet's syndrome, hand
711.26	Arthropathy in Behcet's syndrome, lower leg
711.29	Arthropathy in Behcet's syndrome, multiple sites
711.28	Arthropathy in Behcet's syndrome, other specified sites
711.25	Arthropathy in Behcet's syndrome, pelvic region and thigh
711.21	Arthropathy in Behcet's syndrome, shoulder region
711.20	Arthropathy in Behcet's syndrome, site unspecified
711.22	Arthropathy in Behcet's syndrome, upper arm
065.9	Arthropod-borne hemorrhagic fever, unspecified
066.9	Arthropod-borne viral disease, unspecified
996.46	Articular bearing surface wear of prosthetic joint
127.0	Ascariasis
733.45	Aseptic necrosis of bone, jaw
733.49	Aseptic necrosis of bone, other
733.40	Aseptic necrosis of bone, site unspecified
733.42	Aseptic necrosis of head and neck of femur
733.41	Aseptic necrosis of head of humerus
733.43	Aseptic necrosis of medial femoral condyle
733.44	Aseptic necrosis of talus
117.3	Aspergillosis
799.01	Asphyxia
994.7	Asphyxiation and strangulation
493.92	Asthma, unspecified type, with (acute) exacerbation
493.91	Asthma, unspecified type, with status asthmaticus
094.3	Asymptomatic neurosyphilis
445.81	Atheroembolism of kidney
445.02	Atheroembolism of lower extremity
445.89	Atheroembolism of other site
445.01	Atheroembolism of upper extremity
440.24	Atherosclerosis of native arteries of the extremities with gangrene
333.71	Athetoid cerebral palsy
747.22	Atresia and stenosis of aorta
751.2	Atresia and stenosis of large intestine, rectum, and anal canal
751.1	Atresia and stenosis of small intestine
753.6	Atresia and stenosis of urethra and bladder neck
427.32	Atrial flutter
426.0	Atrioventricular block, complete
V55.1	Attention to gastrostomy
299.00	Autistic disorder, current or active state
299.01	Autistic disorder, residual state
283.0	Autoimmune hemolytic anemias
871.3	Avulsion of eye
088.82	Babesiosis
790.7	Bacteremia
771.83	Bacteremia of newborn
008.5	Bacterial enteritis, unspecified

125.0	Bancroftian filariasis
088.0	Bartonellosis
435.0	Basilar artery syndrome
642.03	Benign essential hypertension complicating pregnancy, childbirth, and the puerperium, antepartum condition or complication
642.01	Benign essential hypertension complicating pregnancy, childbirth, and the puerperium, delivered, with or without mention of antepartum condition
642.02	Benign essential hypertension, complicating pregnancy, childbirth, and the puerperium, delivered, with mention of postpartum complication
265.0	Beriberi
478.34	Bilateral paralysis of vocal cords or larynx, complete
824.5	Bimalleolar fracture, open
296.51	Bipolar I disorder, most recent episode (or current) depressed, mild
296.52	Bipolar I disorder, most recent episode (or current) depressed, moderate
296.54	Bipolar I disorder, most recent episode (or current) depressed, severe, specified as with psychotic behavior
296.53	Bipolar I disorder, most recent episode (or current) depressed, severe, without mention of psychotic behavior
296.50	Bipolar I disorder, most recent episode (or current) depressed, unspecified
296.41	Bipolar I disorder, most recent episode (or current) manic, mild
296.42	Bipolar I disorder, most recent episode (or current) manic, moderate
296.44	Bipolar I disorder, most recent episode (or current) manic, severe, specified as with psychotic behavior
296.43	Bipolar I disorder, most recent episode (or current) manic, severe, without mention of psychotic behavior
296.40	Bipolar I disorder, most recent episode (or current) manic, unspecified
296.61	Bipolar I disorder, most recent episode (or current) mixed, mild
296.62	Bipolar I disorder, most recent episode (or current) mixed, moderate
296.64	Bipolar I disorder, most recent episode (or current) mixed, severe, specified as with psychotic behavior
296.63	Bipolar I disorder, most recent episode (or current) mixed, severe, without mention of psychotic behavior
296.60	Bipolar I disorder, most recent episode (or current) mixed, unspecified
296.01	Bipolar I disorder, single manic episode, mild
296.02	Bipolar I disorder, single manic episode, moderate
296.04	Bipolar I disorder, single manic episode, severe, specified as with psychotic behavior
296.03	Bipolar I disorder, single manic episode, severe, without mention of psychotic behavior
296.00	Bipolar I disorder, single manic episode, unspecified
084.8	Blackwater fever
116.0	Blastomycosis
579.2	Blind loop syndrome
578.1	Blood in stool
999.32	Bloodstream infection due to central venous catheter
V85.41	Body Mass Index 40.0-44.9, adult
V85.42	Body Mass Index 45.0-49.9, adult
V85.43	Body Mass Index 50.0-59.9, adult
V85.44	Body Mass Index 60.0-69.9, adult
V85.45	Body Mass Index 70 and over, adult
V85.0	Body Mass Index less than 19, adult
648.73	Bone and joint disorders of back, pelvis, and lower limbs of mother, antepartum condition or complication
648.72	Bone and joint disorders of back, pelvis, and lower limbs of mother, delivered, with mention of postpartum complication

648.71	Bone and joint disorders of back, pelvis, and lower limbs of mother, delivered, with or without mention of antepartum condition
648.74	Bone and joint disorders of back, pelvis, and lower limbs of mother, postpartum condition or complication
V42.81	Bone marrow replaced by transplant
030.3	Borderline leprosy [group B]
005.1	Botulism food poisoning
082.1	Boutonneuse fever
081.1	Brill's disease
996.43	Broken prosthetic joint implant
494.1	Bronchiectasis with acute exacerbation
506.0	Bronchitis and pneumonitis due to fumes and vapors
023.9	Brucellosis, unspecified
307.51	Bulimia nervosa
200.23	Burkitt's tumor or lymphoma, intra-abdominal lymph nodes
200.26	Burkitt's tumor or lymphoma, intrapelvic lymph nodes
200.22	Burkitt's tumor or lymphoma, intrathoracic lymph nodes
200.24	Burkitt's tumor or lymphoma, lymph nodes of axilla and upper limb
200.21	Burkitt's tumor or lymphoma, lymph nodes of head, face, and neck
200.25	Burkitt's tumor or lymphoma, lymph nodes of inguinal region and lower limb
200.28	Burkitt's tumor or lymphoma, lymph nodes of multiple sites
200.27	Burkitt's tumor or lymphoma, spleen
200.20	Burkitt's tumor or lymphoma, unspecified site, extranodal and solid organ sites
948.11	Burn [any degree] involving 10-19 percent of body surface with third degree burn, 10-19%
948.10	Burn [any degree] involving 10-19 percent of body surface with third degree burn, less than 10 percent or unspecified
948.20	Burn [any degree] involving 20-29 percent of body surface with third degree burn, less than 10 percent or unspecified
948.30	Burn [any degree] involving 30-39 percent of body surface with third degree burn, less than 10 percent or unspecified
948.40	Burn [any degree] involving 40-49 percent of body surface with third degree burn, less than 10 percent or unspecified
948.50	Burn [any degree] involving 50-59 percent of body surface with third degree burn, less than 10 percent or unspecified
948.60	Burn [any degree] involving 60-69 percent of body surface with third degree burn, less than 10 percent or unspecified
948.70	Burn [any degree] involving 70-79 percent of body surface with third degree burn, less than 10 percent or unspecified
948.80	Burn [any degree] involving 80-89 percent of body surface with third degree burn, less than 10 percent or unspecified
948.90	Burn [any degree] involving 90 percent or more of body surface with third degree burn, less than 10 percent or unspecified
947.2	Burn of esophagus
947.3	Burn of gastrointestinal tract
947.1	Burn of larynx, trachea, and lung
947.4	Burn of vagina and uterus
940.5	Burn with resulting rupture and destruction of eyeball
799.4	Cachexia
993.3	Caisson disease
574.31	Calculus of bile duct with acute cholecystitis, with obstruction
574.30	Calculus of bile duct with acute cholecystitis, without mention of obstruction
574.41	Calculus of bile duct with other cholecystitis, with obstruction
574.40	Calculus of bile duct with other cholecystitis, without mention of obstruction
574.51	Calculus of bile duct without mention of cholecystitis, with obstruction
574.80	Calculus of gallbladder and bile duct with acute and chronic cholecystitis, without mention of obstruction

574.61	Calculus of gallbladder and bile duct with acute cholecystitis, with obstruction
574.60	Calculus of gallbladder and bile duct with acute cholecystitis, without mention of obstruction
574.71	Calculus of gallbladder and bile duct with other cholecystitis, with obstruction
574.70	Calculus of gallbladder and bile duct with other cholecystitis, without mention of obstruction
574.91	Calculus of gallbladder and bile duct without cholecystitis, with obstruction
574.01	Calculus of gallbladder with acute cholecystitis, with obstruction
574.00	Calculus of gallbladder with acute cholecystitis, without mention of obstruction
574.11	Calculus of gallbladder with other cholecystitis, with obstruction
574.10	Calculus of gallbladder with other cholecystitis, without mention of obstruction
574.21	Calculus of gallbladder without mention of cholecystitis, with obstruction
592.1	Calculus of ureter
112.85	Candidal enteritis
112.84	Candidal esophagitis
112.82	Candidal otitis externa
112.0	Candidiasis of mouth
112.2	Candidiasis of other urogenital sites
127.5	Capillariasis
259.2	Carcinoid syndrome
997.1	Cardiac complications, not elsewhere classified
423.3	Cardiac tamponade
425.8	Cardiomyopathy in other diseases classified elsewhere
093.9	Cardiovascular syphilis, unspecified
078.3	Cat-scratch disease
295.22	Catatonic type schizophrenia, chronic
295.24	Catatonic type schizophrenia, chronic with acute exacerbation
295.21	Catatonic type schizophrenia, subchronic
295.23	Catatonic type schizophrenia, subchronic with acute exacerbation
295.20	Catatonic type schizophrenia, unspecified
344.61	Cauda equina syndrome with neurogenic bladder
344.60	Cauda equina syndrome without mention of neurogenic bladder
447.4	Celiac artery compression syndrome
682.5	Cellulitis and abscess of buttock
682.0	Cellulitis and abscess of face
682.7	Cellulitis and abscess of foot, except toes
682.4	Cellulitis and abscess of hand, except fingers and thumb
682.6	Cellulitis and abscess of leg, except foot
682.1	Cellulitis and abscess of neck
528.3	Cellulitis and abscess of oral soft tissues
682.8	Cellulitis and abscess of other specified sites
682.2	Cellulitis and abscess of trunk
682.9	Cellulitis and abscess of unspecified sites
682.3	Cellulitis and abscess of upper arm and forearm
478.71	Cellulitis and perichondritis of larynx
478.21	Cellulitis of pharynx or nasopharynx
997.01	Central nervous system complication
362.31	Central retinal artery occlusion
362.35	Central retinal vein occlusion
334.4	Cerebellar ataxia in diseases classified elsewhere
851.42	Cerebellar or brain stem contusion without mention of open intracranial wound, with brief [less than one hour] loss of consciousness
851.46	Cerebellar or brain stem contusion without mention of open intracranial wound, with loss of consciousness of unspecified duration
851.43	Cerebellar or brain stem contusion without mention of open intracranial wound, with moderate [1-24 hours] loss of consciousness
851.44	Cerebellar or brain stem contusion without mention of open intracranial wound, with prolonged [more than 24 hours] loss consciousness and return to pre-existing conscious level
437.4	Cerebral arteritis
330.2	Cerebral degeneration in generalized lipidoses
330.3	Cerebral degeneration of childhood in other diseases classified elsewhere
330.1	Cerebral lipidoses
388.61	Cerebrospinal fluid otorrhea
349.81	Cerebrospinal fluid rhinorrhea
674.03	Cerebrovascular disorders in the puerperium, antepartum condition or complication
674.02	Cerebrovascular disorders in the puerperium, delivered, with mention of postpartum complication
674.04	Cerebrovascular disorders in the puerperium, postpartum condition or complication
429.79	Certain sequelae of myocardial infarction, not elsewhere classified, other
649.73	Cervical shortening, antepartum condition or complication
649.71	Cervical shortening, delivered, with or without mention of antepartum condition
649.70	Cervical shortening, unspecified as to episode of care or not applicable
721.1	Cervical spondylosis with myelopathy
039.3	Cervicofacial actinomycotic infection
086.0	Chagas' disease with heart involvement
086.1	Chagas' disease with other organ involvement
086.2	Chagas' disease without mention of organ involvement
786.04	Cheyne-Stokes respiration
052.7	Chickenpox with other specified complications
052.8	Chickenpox with unspecified complication
995.50	Child abuse, unspecified
995.51	Child emotional/psychological abuse
995.52	Child neglect (nutritional)
995.54	Child physical abuse
995.53	Child sexual abuse
299.10	Childhood disintegrative disorder, current or active state
299.11	Childhood disintegrative disorder, residual state
576.1	Cholangitis
001.0	Cholera due to vibrio cholerae
001.1	Cholera due to vibrio cholerae el tor
001.9	Cholera, unspecified
130.2	Chorioretinitis due to toxoplasmosis
363.20	Chorioretinitis, unspecified
363.70	Choroidal detachment, unspecified
363.63	Choroidal rupture
508.1	Chronic and other pulmonary manifestations due to radiation
428.42	Chronic combined systolic and diastolic heart failure
428.32	Chronic diastolic heart failure
207.12	Chronic erythremia, in relapse
207.11	Chronic erythremia, in remission
207.10	Chronic erythremia, without mention of having achieved remission
301.51	Chronic factitious illness with physical symptoms
582.81	Chronic glomerulonephritis in diseases classified elsewhere
582.2	Chronic glomerulonephritis with lesion of membranoproliferative glomerulonephritis

582.1	Chronic glomerulonephritis with lesion of membranous glomerulonephritis
582.0	Chronic glomerulonephritis with lesion of proliferative glomerulonephritis
582.4	Chronic glomerulonephritis with lesion of rapidly progressive glomerulonephritis
582.89	Chronic glomerulonephritis with other specified pathological lesion in kidney
582.9	Chronic glomerulonephritis with unspecified pathological lesion in kidney
279.52	Chronic graft-versus-host disease
357.81	Chronic inflammatory demyelinating polyneuritis
006.1	Chronic intestinal amebiasis without mention of abscess
585.4	Chronic kidney disease, Stage IV (severe)
585.5	Chronic kidney disease, Stage V
208.12	Chronic leukemia of unspecified cell type, in relapse
208.11	Chronic leukemia of unspecified cell type, in remission
208.10	Chronic leukemia of unspecified cell type, without mention of having achieved remission
204.12	Chronic lymphoid leukemia, in relapse
204.11	Chronic lymphoid leukemia, in remission
204.10	Chronic lymphoid leukemia, without mention of having achieved remission
322.2	Chronic meningitis
206.12	Chronic monocytic leukemia, in relapse
206.11	Chronic monocytic leukemia, in remission
206.10	Chronic monocytic leukemia, without mention of having achieved remission
205.12	Chronic myeloid leukemia, in relapse
205.11	Chronic myeloid leukemia, in remission
205.10	Chronic myeloid leukemia, without mention of having achieved remission
493.22	Chronic obstructive asthma with (acute) exacerbation
493.21	Chronic obstructive asthma with status asthmaticus
730.17	Chronic osteomyelitis, ankle and foot
730.13	Chronic osteomyelitis, forearm
730.14	Chronic osteomyelitis, hand
730.16	Chronic osteomyelitis, lower leg
730.19	Chronic osteomyelitis, multiple sites
730.18	Chronic osteomyelitis, other specified sites
730.15	Chronic osteomyelitis, pelvic region and thigh
730.11	Chronic osteomyelitis, shoulder region
730.10	Chronic osteomyelitis, site unspecified
730.12	Chronic osteomyelitis, upper arm
577.1	Chronic pancreatitis
512.83	Chronic pneumothorax
114.4	Chronic pulmonary coccidioidomycosis
416.2	Chronic pulmonary embolism
590.01	Chronic pyelonephritis with lesion of renal medullary necrosis
518.83	Chronic respiratory failure
393	Chronic rheumatic pericarditis
428.22	Chronic systolic heart failure
440.4	Chronic total occlusion of artery of the extremities
557.1	Chronic vascular insufficiency of intestine
453.74	Chronic venous embolism and thrombosis of axillary veins
453.72	Chronic venous embolism and thrombosis of deep veins of upper extremity
453.52	Chronic venous embolism and thrombosis of deep vessels of distal lower extremity
453.51	Chronic venous embolism and thrombosis of deep vessels of proximal lower extremity

453.76	Chronic venous embolism and thrombosis of internal jugular veins
453.79	Chronic venous embolism and thrombosis of other specified veins
453.77	Chronic venous embolism and thrombosis of other thoracic veins
453.75	Chronic venous embolism and thrombosis of subclavian veins
453.71	Chronic venous embolism and thrombosis of superficial veins of upper extremity
453.50	Chronic venous embolism and thrombosis of unspecified deep vessels of lower extremity
453.73	Chronic venous embolism and thrombosis of upper extremity, unspecified
459.31	Chronic venous hypertension with ulcer
459.33	Chronic venous hypertension with ulcer and inflammation
070.33	Chronic viral hepatitis B without mention of hepatic coma with hepatitis delta
070.32	Chronic viral hepatitis B without mention of hepatic coma without mention of hepatitis delta
791.1	Chyluria
121.1	Clonorchiasis
813.41	Closed Colles' fracture
835.00	Closed dislocation of hip, unspecified site
839.00	Closed dislocation, cervical vertebra, unspecified
839.05	Closed dislocation, fifth cervical vertebra
839.01	Closed dislocation, first cervical vertebra
839.04	Closed dislocation, fourth cervical vertebra
839.08	Closed dislocation, multiple cervical vertebrae
839.02	Closed dislocation, second cervical vertebra
839.07	Closed dislocation, seventh cervical vertebra
839.06	Closed dislocation, sixth cervical vertebra
839.61	Closed dislocation, sternum
839.03	Closed dislocation, third cervical vertebra
812.02	Closed fracture of anatomical neck of humerus
801.40	Closed fracture of base of skull with intracranial injury of other and unspecified nature, unspecified state of consciousness
801.42	Closed fracture of base of skull with intracranial injury of other and unspecified nature, with brief [less than one hour] loss of consciousness
801.49	Closed fracture of base of skull with intracranial injury of other and unspecified nature, with concussion, unspecified
801.46	Closed fracture of base of skull with intracranial injury of other and unspecified nature, with loss of consciousness of unspecified duration
801.41	Closed fracture of base of skull with intracranial injury of other and unspecified nature, with no loss of consciousness
801.00	Closed fracture of base of skull without mention of intra cranial injury, unspecified state of consciousness
801.02	Closed fracture of base of skull without mention of intra cranial injury, with brief [less than one hour] loss of consciousness
801.09	Closed fracture of base of skull without mention of intra cranial injury, with concussion, unspecified
801.06	Closed fracture of base of skull without mention of intra cranial injury, with loss of consciousness of unspecified duration
801.01	Closed fracture of base of skull without mention of intra cranial injury, with no loss of consciousness
805.00	Closed fracture of cervical vertebra, unspecified level
821.21	Closed fracture of condyle, femoral
813.43	Closed fracture of distal end of ulna (alone)
805.2	Closed fracture of dorsal [thoracic] vertebra without mention of spinal cord injury
807.08	Closed fracture of eight or more ribs
821.22	Closed fracture of epiphysis, lower (separation) of femur
805.05	Closed fracture of fifth cervical vertebra
805.01	Closed fracture of first cervical vertebra
807.05	Closed fracture of five ribs

807.04	Closed fracture of four ribs
805.04	Closed fracture of fourth cervical vertebra
812.03	Closed fracture of greater tuberosity of humerus
808.41	Closed fracture of ilium
808.42	Closed fracture of ischium
812.42	Closed fracture of lateral condyle of humerus
821.20	Closed fracture of lower end of femur, unspecified part
813.40	Closed fracture of lower end of forearm, unspecified
813.44	Closed fracture of lower end of radius with ulna
805.4	Closed fracture of lumbar vertebra without mention of spinal cord injury
802.4	Closed fracture of malar and maxillary bones
802.27	Closed fracture of mandible, alveolar border of body
802.25	Closed fracture of mandible, angle of jaw
802.28	Closed fracture of mandible, body, other and unspecified
802.21	Closed fracture of mandible, condylar process
802.23	Closed fracture of mandible, coronoid process
802.29	Closed fracture of mandible, multiple sites
802.24	Closed fracture of mandible, ramus, unspecified
802.22	Closed fracture of mandible, subcondylar
802.26	Closed fracture of mandible, symphysis of body
802.20	Closed fracture of mandible, unspecified site
812.43	Closed fracture of medial condyle of humerus
805.08	Closed fracture of multiple cervical vertebrae
807.09	Closed fracture of multiple ribs, unspecified
807.01	Closed fracture of one rib
802.6	Closed fracture of orbital floor (blow-out)
802.8	Closed fracture of other facial bones
808.49	Closed fracture of other specified part of pelvis
822.0	Closed fracture of patella
808.2	Closed fracture of pubis
807.00	Closed fracture of rib(s), unspecified
805.6	Closed fracture of sacrum and coccyx without mention of spinal cord injury
805.02	Closed fracture of second cervical vertebra
807.07	Closed fracture of seven ribs
805.07	Closed fracture of seventh cervical vertebra
823.22	Closed fracture of shaft of fibula with tibia
812.21	Closed fracture of shaft of humerus
813.21	Closed fracture of shaft of radius (alone)
813.20	Closed fracture of shaft of radius or ulna, unspecified
813.23	Closed fracture of shaft of radius with ulna
823.20	Closed fracture of shaft of tibia alone
813.22	Closed fracture of shaft of ulna (alone)
807.06	Closed fracture of six ribs
805.06	Closed fracture of sixth cervical vertebra
807.2	Closed fracture of sternum
812.01	Closed fracture of surgical neck of humerus
805.03	Closed fracture of third cervical vertebra
807.03	Closed fracture of three ribs
807.02	Closed fracture of two ribs
812.44	Closed fracture of unspecified condyle(s) of humerus
823.82	Closed fracture of unspecified part of fibula with tibia
813.80	Closed fracture of unspecified part of forearm
812.20	Closed fracture of unspecified part of humerus
812.40	Closed fracture of unspecified part of lower end of humerus
813.83	Closed fracture of unspecified part of radius with ulna
823.80	Closed fracture of unspecified part of tibia alone
813.82	Closed fracture of unspecified part of ulna (alone)

812.00	Closed fracture of unspecified part of upper end of humerus
805.8	Closed fracture of unspecified vertebral column without mention of spinal cord injury
823.02	Closed fracture of upper end of fibula with tibia
823.00	Closed fracture of upper end of tibia alone
800.40	Closed fracture of vault of skull with intracranial injury of other and unspecified nature, unspecified state of consciousness
800.42	Closed fracture of vault of skull with intracranial injury of other and unspecified nature, with brief [less than one hour] loss of consciousness
800.49	Closed fracture of vault of skull with intracranial injury of other and unspecified nature, with concussion, unspecified
800.46	Closed fracture of vault of skull with intracranial injury of other and unspecified nature, with loss of consciousness of unspecified duration
800.41	Closed fracture of vault of skull with intracranial injury of other and unspecified nature, with no loss of consciousness
800.00	Closed fracture of vault of skull without mention of intracranial injury, unspecified state of consciousness
800.02	Closed fracture of vault of skull without mention of intracranial injury, with brief [less than one hour] loss of consciousness
800.09	Closed fracture of vault of skull without mention of intracranial injury, with concussion, unspecified
800.06	Closed fracture of vault of skull without mention of intracranial injury, with loss of consciousness of unspecified duration
800.01	Closed fracture of vault of skull without mention of intracranial injury, with no loss of consciousness
804.09	Closed fractures involving skull of face with other bones, without mention of intracranial injury, with concussion, unspecified
804.06	Closed fractures involving skull of face with other bones, without mention of intracranial injury, with loss of consciousness of unspecified duration
804.40	Closed fractures involving skull or face with other bones, with intracranial injury of other and unspecified nature, unspecified state of consciousness
804.42	Closed fractures involving skull or face with other bones, with intracranial injury of other and unspecified nature, with brief [less than one hour] loss of consciousness
804.49	Closed fractures involving skull or face with other bones, with intracranial injury of other and unspecified nature, with concussion, unspecified
804.46	Closed fractures involving skull or face with other bones, with intracranial injury of other and unspecified nature, with loss of consciousness of unspecified duration
804.41	Closed fractures involving skull or face with other bones, with intracranial injury of other and unspecified nature, with no loss of consciousness
804.00	Closed fractures involving skull or face with other bones, without mention of intracranial injury, unspecified state of consciousness
804.02	Closed fractures involving skull or face with other bones, without mention of intracranial injury, with brief [less than one hour] loss of consciousness
804.01	Closed fractures involving skull or face with other bones, without mention of intracranial injury, with no loss of consciousness
835.02	Closed obturator dislocation of hip
835.01	Closed posterior dislocation of hip
821.23	Closed supracondylar fracture of femur
812.41	Closed supracondylar fracture of humerus
808.8	Closed unspecified fracture of pelvis
649.33	Coagulation defects complicating pregnancy, childbirth, or the puerperium, antepartum condition or complication
649.32	Coagulation defects complicating pregnancy, childbirth, or the puerperium, delivered, with mention of postpartum complication
649.31	Coagulation defects complicating pregnancy, childbirth, or the puerperium, delivered, with or without mention of antepartum condition

Appendix A — Alphabetic CC List

649.34	Coagulation defects complicating pregnancy, childbirth, or the puerperium, postpartum condition or complication
649.30	Coagulation defects complicating pregnancy, childbirth, or the puerperium, unspecified as to episode of care or not applicable
747.10	Coarctation of aorta (preductal) (postductal)
304.21	Cocaine dependence, continuous
114.9	Coccidioidomycosis, unspecified
007.2	Coccidiosis
009.1	Colitis, enteritis, and gastroenteritis of presumed infectious origin
304.81	Combinations of drug dependence excluding opioid type drug, continuous
304.71	Combinations of opioid type drug with any other drug dependence, continuous
279.2	Combined immunity deficiency
428.40	Combined systolic and diastolic heart failure, unspecified
279.06	Common variable immunodeficiency
331.3	Communicating hydrocephalus
958.90	Compartment syndrome, unspecified
780.32	Complex febrile convulsions
996.99	Complication of other specified reattached body part
996.95	Complication of reattached foot and toe(s)
996.96	Complication of reattached lower extremity, other and unspecified
997.99	Complications affecting other specified body systems, not elsewhere classified
996.89	Complications of other specified transplanted organ
996.93	Complications of reattached finger(s)
996.91	Complications of reattached forearm
996.92	Complications of reattached hand
996.94	Complications of reattached upper extremity, other and unspecified
996.85	Complications of transplanted bone marrow
996.83	Complications of transplanted heart
996.87	Complications of transplanted intestine
996.81	Complications of transplanted kidney
996.82	Complications of transplanted liver
996.84	Complications of transplanted lung
996.88	Complications of transplanted organ, stem cell
996.80	Complications of transplanted organ, unspecified
996.86	Complications of transplanted pancreas
996.90	Complications of unspecified reattached extremity
459.2	Compression of vein
850.5	Concussion with loss of consciousness of unspecified duration
850.2	Concussion with moderate loss of consciousness
850.3	Concussion with prolonged loss of consciousness and return to pre-existing conscious level
850.12	Concussion, with loss of consciousness from 31 to 59 minutes
850.11	Concussion, with loss of consciousness of 30 minutes or less
287.33	Congenital and hereditary thrombocytopenic purpura
776.5	Congenital anemia
748.61	Congenital bronchiectasis
648.53	Congenital cardiovascular disorders of mother, antepartum condition or complication
648.52	Congenital cardiovascular disorders of mother, delivered, with mention of postpartum complication
648.51	Congenital cardiovascular disorders of mother, delivered, with or without mention of antepartum condition
648.54	Congenital cardiovascular disorders of mother, postpartum condition or complication
751.62	Congenital cystic disease of liver
748.4	Congenital cystic lung
286.3	Congenital deficiency of other clotting factors

343.0	Congenital diplegia
286.2	Congenital factor XI deficiency
343.1	Congenital hemiplegia
359.0	Congenital hereditary muscular dystrophy
279.04	Congenital hypogammaglobulinemia
746.4	Congenital insufficiency of aortic valve
746.6	Congenital mitral insufficiency
746.5	Congenital mitral stenosis
754.2	Congenital musculoskeletal deformities of spine
753.21	Congenital obstruction of ureteropelvic junction
753.22	Congenital obstruction of ureterovesical junction
746.00	Congenital pulmonary valve anomaly, unspecified
771.0	Congenital rubella
753.11	Congenital single renal cyst
746.3	Congenital stenosis of aortic valve
753.23	Congenital ureterocele
032.81	Conjunctival diphtheria
130.1	Conjunctivitis due to toxoplasmosis
284.01	Constitutional red blood cell aplasia
423.2	Constrictive pericarditis
861.01	Contusion of heart without mention of open wound into thorax
861.21	Contusion of lung without mention of open wound into thorax
746.85	Coronary artery anomaly
414.04	Coronary atherosclerosis of artery bypass graft
414.02	Coronary atherosclerosis of autologous vein bypass graft
414.07	Coronary atherosclerosis of bypass graft (artery) (vein) of transplanted heart
414.06	Coronary atherosclerosis of native coronary artery of transplanted heart
414.03	Coronary atherosclerosis of nonautologous biological bypass graft
745.12	Corrected transposition of great vessels
851.02	Cortex (cerebral) contusion without mention of open intracranial wound, with brief [less than one hour] loss of consciousness
851.06	Cortex (cerebral) contusion without mention of open intracranial wound, with loss of consciousness of unspecified duration
851.03	Cortex (cerebral) contusion without mention of open intracranial wound, with moderate [1-24 hours] loss of consciousness
851.04	Cortex (cerebral) contusion without mention of open intracranial wound, with prolonged [more than 24 hours] loss of consciousness and return to pre-existing conscious level
074.20	Coxsackie carditis, unspecified
074.22	Coxsackie endocarditis
074.23	Coxsackie myocarditis
074.21	Coxsackie pericarditis
758.31	Cri-du-chat syndrome
065.0	Crimean hemorrhagic fever [CHF Congo virus]
359.81	Critical illness myopathy
357.82	Critical illness polyneuropathy
925.1	Crushing injury of face and scalp
928.01	Crushing injury of hip
925.2	Crushing injury of neck
928.00	Crushing injury of thigh
117.5	Cryptococcosis
516.36	Cryptogenic organizing pneumonia
007.4	Cryptosporidiosis
255.0	Cushing's syndrome
039.0	Cutaneous actinomycotic infection
022.0	Cutaneous anthrax
032.85	Cutaneous diphtheria
031.1	Cutaneous diseases due to other mycobacteria

085.4	Cutaneous leishmaniasis, American
085.2	Cutaneous leishmaniasis, Asian desert
085.3	Cutaneous leishmaniasis, Ethiopian
085.1	Cutaneous leishmaniasis, urban
120.3	Cutaneous schistosomiasis
770.83	Cyanotic attacks of newborn
007.5	Cyclosporiasis
577.2	Cyst and pseudocyst of pancreas
277.03	Cystic fibrosis with gastrointestinal manifestations
277.09	Cystic fibrosis with other manifestations
277.00	Cystic fibrosis without mention of meconium ileus
753.10	Cystic kidney disease, unspecified
123.1	Cysticercosis
078.5	Cytomegaloviral disease
665.61	Damage to pelvic joints and ligaments, delivered, with or without mention of antepartum condition
639.2	Damage to pelvic organs and tissues following abortion or ectopic and molar pregnancies
949.4	Deep necrosis of underlying tissue [deep third degree] without mention of loss of a body part, unspecified
943.51	Deep necrosis of underlying tissues [deep third degree) with loss of a body part, of forearm
942.40	Deep necrosis of underlying tissues [deep third degree]) without mention of loss of a body part, of trunk, unspecified site
942.53	Deep necrosis of underlying tissues [deep third degree] with loss of a body part, of abdominal wall
945.53	Deep necrosis of underlying tissues [deep third degree] with loss of a body part, of ankle
943.54	Deep necrosis of underlying tissues [deep third degree] with loss of a body part, of axilla
942.54	Deep necrosis of underlying tissues [deep third degree] with loss of a body part, of back [any part]
944.56	Deep necrosis of underlying tissues [deep third degree] with loss of a body part, of back of hand
942.51	Deep necrosis of underlying tissues [deep third degree] with loss of a body part, of breast
942.52	Deep necrosis of underlying tissues [deep third degree] with loss of a body part, of chest wall, excluding breast and nipple
941.54	Deep necrosis of underlying tissues [deep third degree] with loss of a body part, of chin
941.51	Deep necrosis of underlying tissues [deep third degree] with loss of a body part, of ear [any part]
943.52	Deep necrosis of underlying tissues [deep third degree] with loss of a body part, of elbow
941.52	Deep necrosis of underlying tissues [deep third degree] with loss of a body part, of eye (with other parts of face, head, and neck)
941.50	Deep necrosis of underlying tissues [deep third degree] with loss of a body part, of face and head, unspecified site
945.52	Deep necrosis of underlying tissues [deep third degree] with loss of a body part, of foot
941.57	Deep necrosis of underlying tissues [deep third degree] with loss of a body part, of forehead and cheek
942.55	Deep necrosis of underlying tissues [deep third degree] with loss of a body part, of genitalia
944.50	Deep necrosis of underlying tissues [deep third degree] with loss of a body part, of hand, unspecified site
945.55	Deep necrosis of underlying tissues [deep third degree] with loss of a body part, of knee
941.53	Deep necrosis of underlying tissues [deep third degree] with loss of a body part, of lip(s)
945.54	Deep necrosis of underlying tissues [deep third degree] with loss of a body part, of lower leg
945.50	Deep necrosis of underlying tissues [deep third degree] with loss of a body part, of lower limb [leg], unspecified site
941.59	Deep necrosis of underlying tissues [deep third degree] with loss of a body part, of multiple sites [except with eye] of face, head, and neck
945.59	Deep necrosis of underlying tissues [deep third degree] with loss of a body part, of multiple sites of lower limb(s)
943.59	Deep necrosis of underlying tissues [deep third degree] with loss of a body part, of multiple sites of upper limb, except wrist and hand
944.58	Deep necrosis of underlying tissues [deep third degree] with loss of a body part, of multiple sites of wrist(s) and hand(s)
946.5	Deep necrosis of underlying tissues [deep third degree] with loss of a body part, of multiple specified sites
941.58	Deep necrosis of underlying tissues [deep third degree] with loss of a body part, of neck
941.55	Deep necrosis of underlying tissues [deep third degree] with loss of a body part, of nose (septum)
942.59	Deep necrosis of underlying tissues [deep third degree] with loss of a body part, of other and multiple sites of trunk,
944.55	Deep necrosis of underlying tissues [deep third degree] with loss of a body part, of palm of hand
941.56	Deep necrosis of underlying tissues [deep third degree] with loss of a body part, of scalp [any part]
943.56	Deep necrosis of underlying tissues [deep third degree] with loss of a body part, of scapular region
943.55	Deep necrosis of underlying tissues [deep third degree] with loss of a body part, of shoulder
944.51	Deep necrosis of underlying tissues [deep third degree] with loss of a body part, of single digit [finger (nail)] other than thumb
945.56	Deep necrosis of underlying tissues [deep third degree] with loss of a body part, of thigh [any part]
944.52	Deep necrosis of underlying tissues [deep third degree] with loss of a body part, of thumb (nail)
945.51	Deep necrosis of underlying tissues [deep third degree] with loss of a body part, of toe(s) (nail)
944.54	Deep necrosis of underlying tissues [deep third degree] with loss of a body part, of two or more digits of hand including thumb
944.53	Deep necrosis of underlying tissues [deep third degree] with loss of a body part, of two or more digits of hand, not including thumb
943.53	Deep necrosis of underlying tissues [deep third degree] with loss of a body part, of upper arm
943.50	Deep necrosis of underlying tissues [deep third degree] with loss of a body part, of upper limb, unspecified site
944.57	Deep necrosis of underlying tissues [deep third degree] with loss of a body part, of wrist
942.50	Deep necrosis of underlying tissues [deep third degree] with loss of a body part, trunk, unspecified site
949.5	Deep necrosis of underlying tissues [deep third degree] with loss of a body part, unspecified
941.46	Deep necrosis of underlying tissues [deep third degree] without mention of loss of a body part of scalp [any part]
941.40	Deep necrosis of underlying tissues [deep third degree] without mention of loss of a body part, face and head, unspecified site
944.40	Deep necrosis of underlying tissues [deep third degree] without mention of loss of a body part, hand, unspecified site
945.40	Deep necrosis of underlying tissues [deep third degree] without mention of loss of a body part, lower limb [leg], unspecified site
942.43	Deep necrosis of underlying tissues [deep third degree] without mention of loss of a body part, of abdominal wall
945.43	Deep necrosis of underlying tissues [deep third degree] without mention of loss of a body part, of ankle
943.44	Deep necrosis of underlying tissues [deep third degree] without mention of loss of a body part, of axilla
942.44	Deep necrosis of underlying tissues [deep third degree] without mention of loss of a body part, of back [any part]
944.46	Deep necrosis of underlying tissues [deep third degree] without mention of loss of a body part, of back of hand

Appendix A — Alphabetic CC List

942.42	Deep necrosis of underlying tissues [deep third degree] without mention of loss of a body part, of chest wall, excluding breast and nipple
941.44	Deep necrosis of underlying tissues [deep third degree] without mention of loss of a body part, of chin
943.42	Deep necrosis of underlying tissues [deep third degree] without mention of loss of a body part, of elbow
941.42	Deep necrosis of underlying tissues [deep third degree] without mention of loss of a body part, of eye (with other parts of face, head, and neck)
945.42	Deep necrosis of underlying tissues [deep third degree] without mention of loss of a body part, of foot
943.41	Deep necrosis of underlying tissues [deep third degree] without mention of loss of a body part, of forearm
941.47	Deep necrosis of underlying tissues [deep third degree] without mention of loss of a body part, of forehead and cheek
942.45	Deep necrosis of underlying tissues [deep third degree] without mention of loss of a body part, of genitalia
945.45	Deep necrosis of underlying tissues [deep third degree] without mention of loss of a body part, of knee
941.43	Deep necrosis of underlying tissues [deep third degree] without mention of loss of a body part, of lip(s)
945.44	Deep necrosis of underlying tissues [deep third degree] without mention of loss of a body part, of lower leg
941.49	Deep necrosis of underlying tissues [deep third degree] without mention of loss of a body part, of multiple sites [except with eye] of face, head, and neck
945.49	Deep necrosis of underlying tissues [deep third degree] without mention of loss of a body part, of multiple sites of lower limb(s)
943.49	Deep necrosis of underlying tissues [deep third degree] without mention of loss of a body part, of multiple sites of upper limb, except wrist and hand
944.48	Deep necrosis of underlying tissues [deep third degree] without mention of loss of a body part, of multiple sites of wrist(s) and hand(s)
946.4	Deep necrosis of underlying tissues [deep third degree] without mention of loss of a body part, of multiple specified sites
941.48	Deep necrosis of underlying tissues [deep third degree] without mention of loss of a body part, of neck
941.45	Deep necrosis of underlying tissues [deep third degree] without mention of loss of a body part, of nose (septum)
942.49	Deep necrosis of underlying tissues [deep third degree] without mention of loss of a body part, of other and multiple sites of trunk
944.45	Deep necrosis of underlying tissues [deep third degree] without mention of loss of a body part, of palm of hand
943.46	Deep necrosis of underlying tissues [deep third degree] without mention of loss of a body part, of scapular region
943.45	Deep necrosis of underlying tissues [deep third degree] without mention of loss of a body part, of shoulder
945.46	Deep necrosis of underlying tissues [deep third degree] without mention of loss of a body part, of thigh [any part]
945.41	Deep necrosis of underlying tissues [deep third degree] without mention of loss of a body part, of toe(s)(nail)
943.43	Deep necrosis of underlying tissues [deep third degree] without mention of loss of a body part, of upper arm
943.40	Deep necrosis of underlying tissues [deep third degree] without mention of loss of a body part, of upper limb,unspecified site
944.47	Deep necrosis of underlying tissues [deep third degree] without mention of loss of a body part, of wrist
944.41	Deep necrosis of underlying tissues [deep third degree] without mention of loss of a body part, single digit [finger (nail)] other than thumb
944.42	Deep necrosis of underlying tissues [deep third degree] without mention of loss of a body part, thumb (nail)
944.44	Deep necrosis of underlying tissues [deep third degree] without mention of loss of a body part, two or more digits of hand including thumb

944.43	Deep necrosis of underlying tissues [deep third degree] without mention of loss of a body part, two or more digits of hand, not including thumb
941.41	Deep necrosis of underlying tissues [deep third degree]) without mention of loss of a body part, ear [any part]
942.41	Deep necrosis of underlying tissues [deep third degree]) without mention of loss of a body part, of breast
671.30	Deep phlebothrombosis, antepartum, unspecified as to episode of care or not applicable
671.40	Deep phlebothrombosis, postpartum, unspecified as to episode of care or not applicable
666.22	Delayed and secondary postpartum hemorrhage, delivered, with mention of postpartum complication
666.24	Delayed and secondary postpartum hemorrhage, postpartum condition or complication
999.85	Delayed hemolytic transfusion reaction, incompatibility unspecified
639.1	Delayed or excessive hemorrhage following abortion or ectopic and molar pregnancies
293.0	Delirium due to conditions classified elsewhere
294.11	Dementia in conditions classified elsewhere with behavioral disturbance
294.21	Dementia, unspecified, with behavioral disturbance
341.9	Demyelinating disease of central nervous system, unspecified
054.42	Dendritic keratitis
061	Dengue
V46.11	Dependence on respirator, status
298.0	Depressive type psychosis
710.3	Dermatomyositis
516.37	Desquamative interstitial pneumonia
253.5	Diabetes insipidus
648.03	Diabetes mellitus of mother, complicating pregnancy, childbirth, or the puerperium, antepartum condition or complication
648.04	Diabetes mellitus of mother, complicating pregnancy, childbirth, or the puerperium, postpartum condition or complication
648.00	Diabetes mellitus of mother, complicating pregnancy, childbirth, or the puerperium, unspecified as to episode of care or not applicable
552.3	Diaphragmatic hernia with obstruction
009.3	Diarrhea of presumed infectious origin
428.30	Diastolic heart failure, unspecified
279.11	Digeorge's syndrome
619.1	Digestive-genital tract fistula, female
125.4	Dipetalonemiasis
032.9	Diphtheria, unspecified
032.84	Diphtheritic cystitis
032.82	Diphtheritic myocarditis
032.83	Diphtheritic peritonitis
123.4	Diphyllobothriasis, intestinal
344.2	Diplegia of upper limbs
836.60	Dislocation of knee, unspecified, open
836.4	Dislocation of patella, open
996.42	Dislocation of prosthetic joint
277.85	Disorders of fatty acid oxidation
277.87	Disorders of mitochondrial metabolism
377.54	Disorders of optic chiasm associated with inflammatory disorders
377.52	Disorders of optic chiasm associated with other neoplasms
377.51	Disorders of optic chiasm associated with pituitary neoplasms and disorders
377.53	Disorders of optic chiasm associated with vascular disorders
377.63	Disorders of other visual pathways associated with inflammatory disorders
377.61	Disorders of other visual pathways associated with neoplasms

377.62	Disorders of other visual pathways associated with vascular disorders
277.1	Disorders of porphyrin metabolism
270.6	Disorders of urea cycle metabolism
377.73	Disorders of visual cortex associated with inflammatory disorders
377.71	Disorders of visual cortex associated with neoplasms
377.72	Disorders of visual cortex associated with vascular disorders
295.12	Disorganized type schizophrenia, chronic
295.14	Disorganized type schizophrenia, chronic with acute exacerbation
295.11	Disorganized type schizophrenia, subchronic
295.13	Disorganized type schizophrenia, subchronic with acute exacerbation
295.10	Disorganized type schizophrenia, unspecified
998.32	Disruption of external operation (surgical) wound
998.31	Disruption of internal operation (surgical) wound
998.33	Disruption of traumatic injury wound repair
998.30	Disruption of wound, unspecified
363.10	Disseminated chorioretinitis, unspecified
363.13	Disseminated choroiditis and chorioretinitis, generalized
363.12	Disseminated choroiditis and chorioretinitis, peripheral
363.11	Disseminated choroiditis and chorioretinitis, posterior pole
031.2	Disseminated due to other mycobacteria
199.0	Disseminated malignant neoplasm without specification of site
363.14	Disseminated retinitis and retinochoroiditis, metastatic
363.15	Disseminated retinitis and retinochoroiditis, pigment epitheliopathy
270.0	Disturbances of amino-acid transport
270.3	Disturbances of branched-chain amino-acid metabolism
270.5	Disturbances of histidine metabolism
270.4	Disturbances of sulphur-bearing amino-acid metabolism
562.11	Diverticulitis of colon (without mention of hemorrhage)
562.01	Diverticulitis of small intestine (without mention of hemorrhage)
125.7	Dracontiasis
994.1	Drowning and nonfatal submersion
648.33	Drug dependence of mother, antepartum condition or complication
648.32	Drug dependence of mother, delivered, with mention of postpartum complication
648.31	Drug dependence of mother, delivered, with or without mention of antepartum condition
648.34	Drug dependence of mother, postpartum condition or complication
779.4	Drug reactions and intoxications specific to newborn
292.0	Drug withdrawal
779.5	Drug withdrawal syndrome in newborn
292.81	Drug-induced delirium
292.82	Drug-induced persisting dementia
292.11	Drug-induced psychotic disorder with delusions
292.12	Drug-induced psychotic disorder with hallucinations
090.0	Early congenital syphilis, symptomatic
090.2	Early congenital syphilis, unspecified
644.20	Early onset of delivery, unspecified as to episode of care or not applicable
122.9	Echinococcosis, other and unspecified
122.8	Echinococcosis, unspecified, of liver
122.0	Echinococcus granulosus infection of liver
122.1	Echinococcus granulosus infection of lung
122.2	Echinococcus granulosus infection of thyroid
122.3	Echinococcus granulosus infection, other
122.4	Echinococcus granulosus infection, unspecified
122.5	Echinococcus multilocularis infection of liver
122.6	Echinococcus multilocularis infection, other
122.7	Echinococcus multilocularis infection, unspecified
758.2	Edwards' syndrome
756.83	Ehlers-Danlos syndrome
082.41	Ehrlichiosis chafeensis [E. chafeensis]
082.40	Ehrlichiosis, unspecified
444.81	Embolism and thrombosis of iliac artery
444.89	Embolism and thrombosis of other specified artery
444.1	Embolism and thrombosis of thoracic aorta
444.9	Embolism and thrombosis of unspecified artery
742.0	Encephalocele
V46.12	Encounter for respirator dependence during power failure
V46.13	Encounter for weaning from respirator [ventilator]
745.60	Endocardial cushion defect, unspecified type
425.3	Endocardial fibroelastosis
424.91	Endocarditis in diseases classified elsewhere
424.90	Endocarditis, valve unspecified, unspecified cause
425.0	Endomyocardial fibrosis
021.1	Enteric tularemia
008.62	Enteritis due to adenovirus
008.66	Enteritis due to astrovirus
008.65	Enteritis due to calicivirus
008.67	Enteritis due to enterovirus nec
008.63	Enteritis due to norwalk virus
008.64	Enteritis due to other small round viruses [SRV's]
008.69	Enteritis due to other viral enteritis
008.61	Enteritis due to rotavirus
127.4	Enterobiasis
710.5	Eosinophilia myalgia syndrome
767.11	Epicranial subaponeurotic hemorrhage (massive)
345.70	Epilepsia partialis continua, without mention of intractable epilepsy
649.43	Epilepsy complicating pregnancy, childbirth, or the puerperium, antepartum condition or complication
649.42	Epilepsy complicating pregnancy, childbirth, or the puerperium, delivered, with mention of postpartum complication
649.41	Epilepsy complicating pregnancy, childbirth, or the puerperium, delivered, with or without mention of antepartum condition
649.44	Epilepsy complicating pregnancy, childbirth, or the puerperium, postpartum condition or complication
345.91	Epilepsy, unspecified, with intractable epilepsy
057.0	Erythema infectiosum (fifth disease)
695.12	Erythema multiforme major
456.21	Esophageal varices in diseases classified elsewhere, without mention of bleeding
456.1	Esophageal varices without mention of bleeding
287.32	Evans' syndrome
298.1	Excitative type psychosis
695.53	Exfoliation due to erythematous condition involving 30-39 percent of body surface
695.54	Exfoliation due to erythematous condition involving 40-49 percent of body surface
695.55	Exfoliation due to erythematous condition involving 50-59 percent of body surface
695.56	Exfoliation due to erythematous condition involving 60-69 percent of body surface
695.57	Exfoliation due to erythematous condition involving 70-79 percent of body surface
695.58	Exfoliation due to erythematous condition involving 80-89 percent of body surface

695.59	Exfoliation due to erythematous condition involving 90 percent or more of body surface
753.5	Exstrophy of urinary bladder
608.21	Extravaginal torsion of spermatic cord
999.82	Extravasation of other vesicant agent
788.8	Extravasation of urine
999.81	Extravasation of vesicant chemotherapy
493.02	Extrinsic asthma with (acute) exacerbation
493.01	Extrinsic asthma with status asthmaticus
638.2	Failed attempted abortion complicated by damage to pelvic organs or tissues
638.1	Failed attempted abortion complicated by delayed or excessive hemorrhage
638.0	Failed attempted abortion complicated by genital tract and pelvic infection
638.4	Failed attempted abortion complicated by metabolic disorder
638.7	Failed attempted abortion with other specified complications
638.8	Failed attempted abortion with unspecified complication
277.31	Familial Mediterranean fever
121.3	Fascioliasis
121.4	Fasciolopsiasis
046.72	Fatal familial insomnia
032.0	Faucial diphtheria
780.31	Febrile convulsions (simple), unspecified
552.02	Femoral hernia with obstruction, bilateral (not specified as recurrent)
552.03	Femoral hernia with obstruction, bilateral, recurrent
552.00	Femoral hernia with obstruction, unilateral or unspecified (not specified as recurrent)
552.01	Femoral hernia with obstruction, unilateral or unspecified, recurrent
656.31	Fetal distress, affecting management of mother, delivered, with or without mention of antepartum condition
576.4	Fistula of bile duct
575.5	Fistula of gallbladder
569.81	Fistula of intestine, excluding rectum and anus
527.4	Fistula of salivary gland
537.4	Fistula of stomach or duodenum
342.01	Flaccid hemiplegia and hemiparesis affecting dominant side
342.02	Flaccid hemiplegia and hemiparesis affecting nondominant side
342.00	Flaccid hemiplegia and hemiparesis affecting unspecified side
005.2	Food poisoning due to Clostridium perfringens (C. welchii)
005.3	Food poisoning due to other Clostridia
005.4	Food poisoning due to Vibrio parahaemolyticus
005.81	Food poisoning due to Vibrio vulnificus
998.4	Foreign body accidentally left during a procedure
934.1	Foreign body in main bronchus
934.8	Foreign body in other specified parts bronchus and lung
934.0	Foreign body in trachea
664.31	Fourth-degree perineal laceration, delivered, with or without mention of antepartum condition
809.0	Fracture of bones of trunk, closed
825.1	Fracture of calcaneus, open
824.3	Fracture of lateral malleolus, open
824.1	Fracture of medial malleolus, open
334.0	Friedreich's ataxia
991.0	Frostbite of face
991.2	Frostbite of foot
991.1	Frostbite of hand
991.3	Frostbite of other and unspecified sites

943.30	Full-thickness skin [third degree, not otherwise specified] of upper limb, unspecified site
949.3	Full-thickness skin loss [third degree nos]
945.33	Full-thickness skin loss [third degree NOS] of ankle
945.32	Full-thickness skin loss [third degree NOS] of foot
945.35	Full-thickness skin loss [third degree NOS] of knee
945.34	Full-thickness skin loss [third degree nos] of lower leg
945.30	Full-thickness skin loss [third degree NOS] of lower limb [leg] unspecified site
945.39	Full-thickness skin loss [third degree NOS] of multiple sites of lower limb(s)
946.3	Full-thickness skin loss [third degree NOS] of multiple specified sites
945.36	Full-thickness skin loss [third degree NOS] of thigh [any part]
945.31	Full-thickness skin loss [third degree NOS] of toe(s) (nail)
942.33	Full-thickness skin loss [third degree, not otherwise specified] of abdominal wall
943.34	Full-thickness skin loss [third degree, not otherwise specified] of axilla
944.36	Full-thickness skin loss [third degree, not otherwise specified] of back of hand
942.32	Full-thickness skin loss [third degree, not otherwise specified] of chest wall, excluding breast and nipple
941.34	Full-thickness skin loss [third degree, not otherwise specified] of chin
941.31	Full-thickness skin loss [third degree, not otherwise specified] of ear [any part]
943.32	Full-thickness skin loss [third degree, not otherwise specified] of elbow
941.32	Full-thickness skin loss [third degree, not otherwise specified] of eye (with other parts of face, head, and neck)
941.30	Full-thickness skin loss [third degree, not otherwise specified] of face and head, unspecified site
943.31	Full-thickness skin loss [third degree, not otherwise specified] of forearm
941.37	Full-thickness skin loss [third degree, not otherwise specified] of forehead and cheek
942.35	Full-thickness skin loss [third degree, not otherwise specified] of genitalia
944.30	Full-thickness skin loss [third degree, not otherwise specified] of hand, unspecified site
941.33	Full-thickness skin loss [third degree, not otherwise specified] of lip(s)
941.39	Full-thickness skin loss [third degree, not otherwise specified] of multiple sites [except with eye] of face, head, and neck
943.39	Full-thickness skin loss [third degree, not otherwise specified] of multiple sites of upper limb, except wrist and hand
944.38	Full-thickness skin loss [third degree, not otherwise specified] of multiple sites of wrist(s) and hand(s)
941.38	Full-thickness skin loss [third degree, not otherwise specified] of neck
941.35	Full-thickness skin loss [third degree, not otherwise specified] of nose (septum)
942.39	Full-thickness skin loss [third degree, not otherwise specified] of other and multiple sites of trunk
944.35	Full-thickness skin loss [third degree, not otherwise specified] of palm of hand
941.36	Full-thickness skin loss [third degree, not otherwise specified] of scalp [any part]
943.36	Full-thickness skin loss [third degree, not otherwise specified] of scapular region
943.35	Full-thickness skin loss [third degree, not otherwise specified] of shoulder
944.31	Full-thickness skin loss [third degree, not otherwise specified] of single digit [finger (nail)] other than thumb

944.32	Full-thickness skin loss [third degree, not otherwise specified] of thumb (nail)
942.30	Full-thickness skin loss [third degree, not otherwise specified] of trunk, unspecified site
944.34	Full-thickness skin loss [third degree, not otherwise specified] of two or more digits of hand including thumb
943.33	Full-thickness skin loss [third degree, not otherwise specified] of upper arm
944.37	Full-thickness skin loss [third degree, not otherwise specified] of wrist
944.33	Full-thickness skin loss [third degree, not otherwise specified]of two or more digits of hand, not including thumb
942.34	Full-thickness skin loss [third degree,not otherwise specified] of back [any part]
942.31	Full-thickness skin loss [third degree,not otherwise specified] of breast
271.1	Galactosemia
560.31	Gallstone ileus
086.3	Gambian trypanosomiasis
785.4	Gangrene
558.1	Gastroenteritis and colitis due to radiation
022.2	Gastrointestinal anthrax
538	Gastrointestinal mucositis (ulcerative)
094.1	General paresis
345.11	Generalized convulsive epilepsy, with intractable epilepsy
345.01	Generalized nonconvulsive epilepsy, with intractable epilepsy
999.0	Generalized vaccinia as a complication of medical care, not elsewhere classified
053.11	Geniculate herpes zoster
639.0	Genital tract and pelvic infection following abortion or ectopic and molar pregnancies
619.2	Genital tract-skin fistula, female
016.91	Genitourinary tuberculosis, unspecified, bacteriological or histological examination not done
016.92	Genitourinary tuberculosis, unspecified, bacteriological or histological examination unknown (at present)
016.93	Genitourinary tuberculosis, unspecified, tubercle bacilli found (in sputum) by microscopy
016.94	Genitourinary tuberculosis, unspecified, tubercle bacilli not found (in sputum) by microscopy, but found by bacterial culture
016.95	Genitourinary tuberculosis, unspecified, tubercle bacilli not found by bacteriological examination, but tuberculosis confirmed histologically
016.96	Genitourinary tuberculosis, unspecified, tubercle bacilli not found by bacteriological or histological examination, but tuberculosis confirmed by other methods [inoculation of animals]
016.90	Genitourinary tuberculosis, unspecified, unspecified
046.71	Gerstmann-Sträussler-Scheinker syndrome
007.1	Giardiasis
024	Glanders
364.22	Glaucomatocyclitic crises
255.41	Glucocorticoid deficiency
271.0	Glycogenosis
098.50	Gonococcal arthritis
098.52	Gonococcal bursitis
098.15	Gonococcal cervicitis (acute)
098.40	Gonococcal conjunctivitis (neonatorum)
098.11	Gonococcal cystitis (acute)
098.16	Gonococcal endometritis (acute)
098.42	Gonococcal endophthalmia
098.13	Gonococcal epididymo-orchitis (acute)
098.0	Gonococcal infection (acute) of lower genitourinary tract

098.10	Gonococcal infection (acute) of upper genitourinary tract, site unspecified
098.89	Gonococcal infection of other specified sites
098.41	Gonococcal iridocyclitis
098.43	Gonococcal keratitis
098.81	Gonococcal keratosis (blennorrhagica)
098.86	Gonococcal peritonitis
098.12	Gonococcal prostatitis (acute)
098.17	Gonococcal salpingitis, specified as acute
098.14	Gonococcal seminal vesiculitis (acute)
098.53	Gonococcal spondylitis
098.51	Gonococcal synovitis and tenosynovitis
647.13	Gonorrhea of mother, complicating pregnancy, childbirth, or the puerperium, antepartum condition or complication
647.12	Gonorrhea of mother, complicating pregnancy, childbirth, or the puerperium, delivered, with mention of postpartum complication
647.11	Gonorrhea of mother, complicating pregnancy, childbirth, or the puerperium, delivered, with or without mention of antepartum condition
647.14	Gonorrhea of mother, complicating pregnancy, childbirth, or the puerperium, postpartum condition or complication
446.21	Goodpasture's syndrome
279.50	Graft-versus-host disease, unspecified
780.1	Hallucinations
304.51	Hallucinogen dependence, continuous
079.81	Hantavirus infection
V42.1	Heart replaced by transplant
992.0	Heat stroke and sunstroke
719.17	Hemarthrosis, ankle and foot
719.13	Hemarthrosis, forearm
719.14	Hemarthrosis, hand
719.16	Hemarthrosis, lower leg
719.19	Hemarthrosis, multiple sites
719.18	Hemarthrosis, other specified sites
719.15	Hemarthrosis, pelvic region and thigh
719.11	Hemarthrosis, shoulder region
719.10	Hemarthrosis, site unspecified
719.12	Hemarthrosis, upper arm
578.0	Hematemesis
998.12	Hematoma complicating a procedure
342.91	Hemiplegia, unspecified, affecting dominant side
342.92	Hemiplegia, unspecified, affecting nondominant side
342.90	Hemiplegia, unspecified, affecting unspecified side
999.83	Hemolytic transfusion reaction, incompatibility unspecified
423.0	Hemopericardium
288.4	Hemophagocytic syndromes
786.30	Hemoptysis, unspecified
246.3	Hemorrhage and infarction of thyroid
998.11	Hemorrhage complicating a procedure
596.7	Hemorrhage into bladder wall
578.9	Hemorrhage of gastrointestinal tract, unspecified
569.3	Hemorrhage of rectum and anus
363.72	Hemorrhagic choroidal detachment
362.43	Hemorrhagic detachment of retinal pigment epithelium
776.0	Hemorrhagic disease of newborn
078.6	Hemorrhagic nephrosonephritis
070.52	Hepatitis delta without mention of active hepatitis B disease or hepatic coma
130.5	Hepatitis due to toxoplasmosis
070.53	Hepatitis E without mention of hepatic coma

573.2	Hepatitis in other infectious diseases classified elsewhere
573.1	Hepatitis in viral diseases classified elsewhere
282.9	Hereditary hemolytic anemia, unspecified
359.1	Hereditary progressive muscular dystrophy
334.1	Hereditary spastic paraplegia
552.8	Hernia of other specified sites, with obstruction
552.9	Hernia of unspecified site, with obstruction
054.41	Herpes simplex dermatitis of eyelid
054.43	Herpes simplex disciform keratitis
054.44	Herpes simplex iridocyclitis
054.49	Herpes simplex with other ophthalmic complications
054.79	Herpes simplex with other specified complications
054.40	Herpes simplex with unspecified ophthalmic complication
053.20	Herpes zoster dermatitis of eyelid
053.22	Herpes zoster iridocyclitis
053.21	Herpes zoster keratoconjunctivitis
053.19	Herpes zoster with other nervous system complications
053.29	Herpes zoster with other ophthalmic complications
053.79	Herpes zoster with other specified complications
053.8	Herpes zoster with unspecified complication
053.10	Herpes zoster with unspecified nervous system complication
054.2	Herpetic gingivostomatitis
121.6	Heterophyiasis
238.73	High grade myelodysplastic syndrome lesions
665.41	High vaginal laceration, delivered, with or without mention of antepartum condition
751.3	Hirschsprung's disease and other congenital functional disorders of colon
115.92	Histoplasmosis, unspecified, retinitis
201.73	Hodgkin's disease, lymphocytic depletion, intra-abdominal lymph nodes
201.76	Hodgkin's disease, lymphocytic depletion, intrapelvic lymph nodes
201.72	Hodgkin's disease, lymphocytic depletion, intrathoracic lymph nodes
201.74	Hodgkin's disease, lymphocytic depletion, lymph nodes of axilla and upper limb
201.71	Hodgkin's disease, lymphocytic depletion, lymph nodes of head, face, and neck
201.75	Hodgkin's disease, lymphocytic depletion, lymph nodes of inguinal region and lower limb
201.78	Hodgkin's disease, lymphocytic depletion, lymph nodes of multiple sites
201.77	Hodgkin's disease, lymphocytic depletion, spleen
201.70	Hodgkin's disease, lymphocytic depletion, unspecified site, extranodal and solid organ sites
201.43	Hodgkin's disease, lymphocytic-histiocytic predominance, intra-abdominal lymph nodes
201.46	Hodgkin's disease, lymphocytic-histiocytic predominance, intrapelvic lymph nodes
201.42	Hodgkin's disease, lymphocytic-histiocytic predominance, intrathoracic lymph nodes
201.44	Hodgkin's disease, lymphocytic-histiocytic predominance, lymph nodes of axilla and upper limb
201.41	Hodgkin's disease, lymphocytic-histiocytic predominance, lymph nodes of head, face, and neck
201.45	Hodgkin's disease, lymphocytic-histiocytic predominance, lymph nodes of inguinal region and lower limb
201.48	Hodgkin's disease, lymphocytic-histiocytic predominance, lymph nodes of multiple sites
201.47	Hodgkin's disease, lymphocytic-histiocytic predominance, spleen
201.40	Hodgkin's disease, lymphocytic-histiocytic predominance, unspecified site, extranodal and solid organ sites
201.63	Hodgkin's disease, mixed cellularity, intra-abdominal lymph nodes
201.66	Hodgkin's disease, mixed cellularity, intrapelvic lymph nodes
201.62	Hodgkin's disease, mixed cellularity, intrathoracic lymph nodes
201.64	Hodgkin's disease, mixed cellularity, lymph nodes of axilla and upper limb
201.61	Hodgkin's disease, mixed cellularity, lymph nodes of head, face, and neck
201.65	Hodgkin's disease, mixed cellularity, lymph nodes of inguinal region and lower limb
201.68	Hodgkin's disease, mixed cellularity, lymph nodes of multiple sites
201.67	Hodgkin's disease, mixed cellularity, spleen
201.60	Hodgkin's disease, mixed cellularity, unspecified site, extranodal and solid organ sites
201.53	Hodgkin's disease, nodular sclerosis, intra-abdominal lymph nodes
201.56	Hodgkin's disease, nodular sclerosis, intrapelvic lymph nodes
201.52	Hodgkin's disease, nodular sclerosis, intrathoracic lymph nodes
201.54	Hodgkin's disease, nodular sclerosis, lymph nodes of axilla and upper limb
201.51	Hodgkin's disease, nodular sclerosis, lymph nodes of head, face, and neck
201.55	Hodgkin's disease, nodular sclerosis, lymph nodes of inguinal region and lower limb
201.58	Hodgkin's disease, nodular sclerosis, lymph nodes of multiple sites
201.57	Hodgkin's disease, nodular sclerosis, spleen
201.50	Hodgkin's disease, nodular sclerosis, unspecified site, extranodal and solid organ sites
201.93	Hodgkin's disease, unspecified type, intra-abdominal lymph nodes
201.96	Hodgkin's disease, unspecified type, intrapelvic lymph nodes
201.92	Hodgkin's disease, unspecified type, intrathoracic lymph nodes
201.94	Hodgkin's disease, unspecified type, lymph nodes of axilla and upper limb
201.91	Hodgkin's disease, unspecified type, lymph nodes of head, face, and neck
201.95	Hodgkin's disease, unspecified type, lymph nodes of inguinal region and lower limb
201.98	Hodgkin's disease, unspecified type, lymph nodes of multiple sites
201.97	Hodgkin's disease, unspecified type, spleen
201.90	Hodgkin's disease, unspecified type, unspecified site, extranodal and solid organ sites
201.13	Hodgkin's granuloma, intra-abdominal lymph nodes
201.16	Hodgkin's granuloma, intrapelvic lymph nodes
201.12	Hodgkin's granuloma, intrathoracic lymph nodes
201.14	Hodgkin's granuloma, lymph nodes of axilla and upper limb
201.11	Hodgkin's granuloma, lymph nodes of head, face, and neck
201.15	Hodgkin's granuloma, lymph nodes of inguinal region and lower limb
201.18	Hodgkin's granuloma, lymph nodes of multiple sites
201.17	Hodgkin's granuloma, spleen
201.10	Hodgkin's granuloma, unspecified site, extranodal and solid organ sites
201.03	Hodgkin's paragranuloma, intra-abdominal lymph nodes
201.06	Hodgkin's paragranuloma, intrapelvic lymph nodes
201.02	Hodgkin's paragranuloma, intrathoracic lymph nodes
201.04	Hodgkin's paragranuloma, lymph nodes of axilla and upper limb
201.01	Hodgkin's paragranuloma, lymph nodes of head, face, and neck
201.05	Hodgkin's paragranuloma, lymph nodes of inguinal region and lower limb
201.08	Hodgkin's paragranuloma, lymph nodes of multiple sites
201.07	Hodgkin's paragranuloma, spleen
201.00	Hodgkin's paragranuloma, unspecified site, extranodal and solid organ sites
201.23	Hodgkin's sarcoma, intra-abdominal lymph nodes

201.26	Hodgkin's sarcoma, intrapelvic lymph nodes
201.22	Hodgkin's sarcoma, intrathoracic lymph nodes
201.24	Hodgkin's sarcoma, lymph nodes of axilla and upper limb
201.21	Hodgkin's sarcoma, lymph nodes of head, face, and neck
201.25	Hodgkin's sarcoma, lymph nodes of inguinal region and lower limb
201.28	Hodgkin's sarcoma, lymph nodes of multiple sites
201.27	Hodgkin's sarcoma, spleen
201.20	Hodgkin's sarcoma, unspecified site, extranodal and solid organ sites
079.53	Human immunodeficiency virus, type 2 [HIV-2]
079.51	Human T-cell lymphotrophic virus, type I [HTLV-I]
079.52	Human T-cell lymphotrophic virus, type II [HTLV-II]
333.4	Huntington's chorea
591	Hydronephrosis
575.3	Hydrops of gallbladder
593.5	Hydroureter
123.6	Hymenolepiasis
429.82	Hyperkinetic heart disease
276.0	Hyperosmolality and/or hypernatremia
446.20	Hypersensitivity angiitis, unspecified
642.13	Hypertension secondary to renal disease, complicating pregnancy, childbirth, and the puerperium, antepartum condition or complication
642.14	Hypertension secondary to renal disease, complicating pregnancy, childbirth, and the puerperium, postpartum condition or complication
403.11	Hypertensive chronic kidney disease, benign, with chronic kidney disease stage V or end stage renal disease
403.00	Hypertensive chronic kidney disease, malignant, with chronic kidney disease stage I through stage IV, or unspecified
403.01	Hypertensive chronic kidney disease, malignant, with chronic kidney disease stage V or end stage renal disease
403.91	Hypertensive chronic kidney disease, unspecified, with chronic kidney disease stage V or end stage renal disease
437.2	Hypertensive encephalopathy
404.13	Hypertensive heart and chronic kidney disease, benign, with heart failure and chronic kidney disease stage V or end stage renal disease
404.11	Hypertensive heart and chronic kidney disease, benign, with heart failure and with chronic kidney disease stage I through stage IV, or unspecified
404.12	Hypertensive heart and chronic kidney disease, benign, without heart failure and with chronic kidney disease stage V or end stage renal disease
404.01	Hypertensive heart and chronic kidney disease, malignant, with heart failure and with chronic kidney disease stage I through stage IV, or unspecified
404.03	Hypertensive heart and chronic kidney disease, malignant, with heart failure and with chronic kidney disease stage V or end stage renal disease
404.00	Hypertensive heart and chronic kidney disease, malignant, without heart failure and with chronic kidney disease stage I through stage IV, or unspecified
404.02	Hypertensive heart and chronic kidney disease, malignant, without heart failure and with chronic kidney disease stage V or end stage renal disease
404.93	Hypertensive heart and chronic kidney disease, unspecified, with heart failure and chronic kidney disease stage V or end stage renal disease
404.91	Hypertensive heart and chronic kidney disease, unspecified, with heart failure and with chronic kidney disease stage I through stage IV, or unspecified
404.92	Hypertensive heart and chronic kidney disease, unspecified, without heart failure and with chronic kidney disease stage V or end stage renal disease
425.11	Hypertrophic obstructive cardiomyopathy
775.4	Hypocalcemia and hypomagnesemia of newborn
279.00	Hypogammaglobulinemia, unspecified
251.0	Hypoglycemic coma
276.1	Hyposmolality and/or hyponatremia
768.70	Hypoxic-ischemic encephalopathy, unspecified
997.02	Iatrogenic cerebrovascular infarction or hemorrhage
512.1	Iatrogenic pneumothorax
516.35	Idiopathic lymphoid interstitial pneumonia
331.5	Idiopathic normal pressure hydrocephalus (INPH)
516.1	Idiopathic pulmonary hemosiderosis
341.22	Idiopathic transverse myelitis
818.1	Ill-defined open fractures of upper limb
636.22	Illegally induced abortion, complicated by damage to pelvic organs or tissues, complete
636.21	Illegally induced abortion, complicated by damage to pelvic organs or tissues, incomplete
636.20	Illegally induced abortion, complicated by damage to pelvic organs or tissues, unspecified
636.02	Illegally induced abortion, complicated by genital tract and pelvic infection, complete
636.01	Illegally induced abortion, complicated by genital tract and pelvic infection, incomplete
636.00	Illegally induced abortion, complicated by genital tract and pelvic infection, unspecified
636.42	Illegally induced abortion, complicated by metabolic disorder, complete
636.41	Illegally induced abortion, complicated by metabolic disorder, incomplete
636.40	Illegally induced abortion, complicated by metabolic disorder, unspecified
636.72	Illegally induced abortion, with other specified complications, complete
636.71	Illegally induced abortion, with other specified complications, incomplete
636.70	Illegally induced abortion, with other specified complications, unspecified
636.82	Illegally induced abortion, with unspecified complication, complete
636.81	Illegally induced abortion, with unspecified complication, incomplete
636.80	Illegally induced abortion, with unspecified complication, unspecified
991.4	Immersion foot
287.31	Immune thrombocytopenic purpura
279.05	Immunodeficiency with increased IgM
279.10	Immunodeficiency with predominant T-cell defect, unspecified
560.30	Impaction of intestine, unspecified
552.21	Incisional ventral hernia with obstruction
030.2	Indeterminate leprosy [group I]
084.7	Induced malaria
040.41	Infant botulism
343.4	Infantile hemiplegia
345.61	Infantile spasms, with intractable epilepsy
345.60	Infantile spasms, without mention of intractable epilepsy
603.1	Infected hydrocele
998.51	Infected postoperative seroma
997.62	Infection (chronic) of amputation stump
996.61	Infection and inflammatory reaction due to cardiac device, implant, and graft
996.64	Infection and inflammatory reaction due to indwelling urinary catheter

996.66	Infection and inflammatory reaction due to internal joint prosthesis
996.63	Infection and inflammatory reaction due to nervous system device, implant, and graft
996.65	Infection and inflammatory reaction due to other genitourinary device, implant, and graft
996.67	Infection and inflammatory reaction due to other internal orthopedic device, implant, and graft
996.69	Infection and inflammatory reaction due to other internal prosthetic device, implant, and graft
996.62	Infection and inflammatory reaction due to other vascular device, implant, and graft
996.68	Infection and inflammatory reaction due to peritoneal dialysis catheter
996.60	Infection and inflammatory reaction due to unspecified device, implant, and graft
117.8	Infection by dematiacious fungi [Phaehyphomycosis]
115.09	Infection by Histoplasma capsulatum, other
115.02	Infection by Histoplasma capsulatum, retinitis
115.19	Infection by Histoplasma duboisii, other
115.12	Infection by Histoplasma duboisii, retinitis
539.01	Infection due to gastric band procedure
539.81	Infection due to other bariatric procedure
999.39	Infection following other infusion, injection, transfusion, or vaccination
569.61	Infection of colostomy or enterostomy
596.81	Infection of cystostomy
530.86	Infection of esophagostomy
536.41	Infection of gastrostomy
519.01	Infection of tracheostomy
646.63	Infections of genitourinary tract in pregnancy, antepartum condition or complication
646.62	Infections of genitourinary tract in pregnancy, delivered, with mention of postpartum complication
646.61	Infections of genitourinary tract in pregnancy, delivered, with or without mention of antepartum condition
646.64	Infections of genitourinary tract in pregnancy, postpartum condition or complication
009.0	Infectious colitis, enteritis, and gastroenteritis
009.2	Infectious diarrhea
728.0	Infective myositis
488.09	Influenza due to identified avian influenza virus with other manifestations
488.02	Influenza due to identified avian influenza virus with other respiratory manifestations
746.83	Infundibular pulmonic stenosis
550.12	Inguinal hernia, with obstruction, without mention of gangrene, bilateral (not specified as recurrent)
550.13	Inguinal hernia, with obstruction, without mention of gangrene, bilateral, recurrent
550.10	Inguinal hernia, with obstruction, without mention of gangrene, unilateral or unspecified (not specified as recurrent)
550.11	Inguinal hernia, with obstruction, without mention of gangrene, unilateral or unspecified,recurrent
951.3	Injury to abducens nerve
951.6	Injury to accessory nerve
951.5	Injury to acoustic nerve
904.51	Injury to anterior tibial artery
904.52	Injury to anterior tibial vein
863.85	Injury to appendix, without mention of open wound into cavity
863.41	Injury to ascending [right] colon, without mention of open wound into cavity

867.0	Injury to bladder and urethra, without mention of open wound into cavity
904.9	Injury to blood vessels of unspecified site
903.1	Injury to brachial blood vessels
900.00	Injury to carotid artery, unspecified
863.40	Injury to colon, unspecified site, without mention of open wound into cavity
900.01	Injury to common carotid artery
904.6	Injury to deep plantar blood vessels
863.43	Injury to descending [left] colon, without mention of open wound into cavity
862.0	Injury to diaphragm, without mention of open wound into cavity
903.5	Injury to digital blood vessels
863.21	Injury to duodenum, without open wound into cavity
900.02	Injury to external carotid artery
900.81	Injury to external jugular vein
951.4	Injury to facial nerve
863.80	Injury to gastrointestinal tract, unspecified site, without mention of open wound into cavity
951.7	Injury to hypoglossal nerve
901.81	Injury to intercostal artery or vein
900.03	Injury to internal carotid artery
900.1	Injury to internal jugular vein
901.82	Injury to internal mammary artery or vein
866.01	Injury to kidney without mention of open wound into cavity, hematoma without rupture of capsule
866.02	Injury to kidney without mention of open wound into cavity, laceration
866.00	Injury to kidney without mention of open wound into cavity, unspecified injury
864.05	Injury to liver without mention of open wound into cavity laceration, unspecified
864.01	Injury to liver without mention of open wound into cavity, hematoma and contusion
864.02	Injury to liver without mention of open wound into cavity, laceration, minor
864.00	Injury to liver without mention of open wound into cavity, unspecified injury
862.8	Injury to multiple and unspecified intrathoracic organs, without mention of open wound into cavity
900.82	Injury to multiple blood vessels of head and neck
863.46	Injury to multiple sites in colon and rectum, without mention of open wound into cavity
951.0	Injury to oculomotor nerve
950.1	Injury to optic chiasm
950.2	Injury to optic pathways
868.09	Injury to other and multiple intra-abdominal organs without mention of open wound into cavity
863.89	Injury to other gastrointestinal sites, without mention of open wound into cavity
868.01	Injury to other intra-abdominal organs without mention of open wound into cavity, adrenal gland
868.02	Injury to other intra-abdominal organs without mention of open wound into cavity, bile duct and gallbladder
868.03	Injury to other intra-abdominal organs without mention of open wound into cavity, peritoneum
868.04	Injury to other intra-abdominal organs without mention of open wound into cavity, retroperitoneum
868.00	Injury to other intra-abdominal organs without mention of open wound into cavity, unspecified intra-abdominal organ
902.89	Injury to other specified blood vessels of abdomen and pelvis
900.89	Injury to other specified blood vessels of head and neck
904.7	Injury to other specified blood vessels of lower extremity

901.89	Injury to other specified blood vessels of thorax
903.8	Injury to other specified blood vessels of upper extremity
951.8	Injury to other specified cranial nerves
862.29	Injury to other specified intrathoracic organs without mention of open wound into cavity
867.6	Injury to other specified pelvic organs, without mention of open wound into cavity
902.81	Injury to ovarian artery
902.82	Injury to ovarian vein
903.4	Injury to palmar artery
863.82	Injury to pancreas, body, without mention of open wound into cavity
863.81	Injury to pancreas, head, without mention of open wound into cavity
863.84	Injury to pancreas, multiple and unspecified sites, without mention of open wound into cavity
863.83	Injury to pancreas, tail, without mention of open wound into cavity
904.53	Injury to posterior tibial artery
904.54	Injury to posterior tibial vein
903.2	Injury to radial blood vessels
863.45	Injury to rectum, without mention of open wound into cavity
904.3	Injury to saphenous veins
863.44	Injury to sigmoid colon, without mention of open wound into cavity
863.20	Injury to small intestine, unspecified site, without open wound into cavity
865.02	Injury to spleen without mention of open wound into cavity, capsular tears, without major disruption of parenchyma
865.01	Injury to spleen without mention of open wound into cavity, hematoma without rupture of capsule
865.00	Injury to spleen without mention of open wound into cavity, unspecified injury
863.0	Injury to stomach, without mention of open wound into cavity
904.50	Injury to tibial vessel(s), unspecified
863.42	Injury to transverse colon, without mention of open wound into cavity
951.2	Injury to trigeminal nerve
951.1	Injury to trochlear nerve
903.3	Injury to ulnar blood vessels
902.9	Injury to unspecified blood vessel of abdomen and pelvis
900.9	Injury to unspecified blood vessel of head and neck
904.8	Injury to unspecified blood vessel of lower extremity
901.9	Injury to unspecified blood vessel of thorax
903.9	Injury to unspecified blood vessel of upper extremity
951.9	Injury to unspecified cranial nerve
950.9	Injury to unspecified optic nerve and pathways
867.8	Injury to unspecified pelvic organ, without mention of open wound into cavity
867.2	Injury to ureter, without mention of open wound into cavity
902.55	Injury to uterine artery
902.56	Injury to uterine vein
867.4	Injury to uterus, without mention of open wound into cavity
950.3	Injury to visual cortex
411.1	Intermediate coronary syndrome
869.0	Internal injury to unspecified or ill-defined organs without mention of open wound into cavity
722.71	Intervertebral disc disorder with myelopathy, cervical region
722.73	Intervertebral disc disorder with myelopathy, lumbar region
722.72	Intervertebral disc disorder with myelopathy, thoracic region
127.9	Intestinal helminthiasis, unspecified
008.2	Intestinal infection due to aerobacter aerogenes
008.1	Intestinal infection due to arizona group of paracolon bacilli

008.43	Intestinal infection due to campylobacter
008.45	Intestinal infection due to Clostridium difficile
008.00	Intestinal infection due to E. coli, unspecified
008.04	Intestinal infection due to enterohemorrhagic E. coli
008.03	Intestinal infection due to enteroinvasive E. coli
008.01	Intestinal infection due to enteropathogenic E. coli
008.02	Intestinal infection due to enterotoxigenic E. coli
008.46	Intestinal infection due to other anaerobes
008.47	Intestinal infection due to other gram-negative bacteria
008.09	Intestinal infection due to other intestinal E. coli infections
008.49	Intestinal infection due to other organisms
008.3	Intestinal infection due to proteus (mirabilis) (morganii)
008.42	Intestinal infection due to pseudomonas
008.41	Intestinal infection due to staphylococcus
008.44	Intestinal infection due to yersinia enterocolitica
560.81	Intestinal or peritoneal adhesions with obstruction (postoperative) (postinfection)
596.1	Intestinovesical fistula
854.02	Intracranial injury of other and unspecified nature without mention of open intracranial wound, with brief [less than one hour] loss of consciousness
854.06	Intracranial injury of other and unspecified nature without mention of open intracranial wound, with loss of consciousness of unspecified duration
854.03	Intracranial injury of other and unspecified nature without mention of open intracranial wound, with moderate [1-24 hours] loss of consciousness
854.04	Intracranial injury of other and unspecified nature without mention of open intracranial wound, with prolonged [more than 24 hours] loss of consciousness and return to pre-existing conscious level
656.43	Intrauterine death, affecting management of mother, antepartum condition or complication
656.41	Intrauterine death, affecting management of mother, delivered, with or without mention of antepartum condition
608.22	Intravaginal torsion of spermatic cord
772.10	Intraventricular hemorrhage unspecified grade
772.11	Intraventricular hemorrhage, grade I
772.12	Intraventricular hemorrhage, grade II
493.12	Intrinsic asthma with (acute) exacerbation
493.11	Intrinsic asthma with status asthmaticus
560.0	Intussusception
665.22	Inversion of uterus, delivered, with mention of postpartum complication
595.82	Irradiation cystitis
012.21	Isolated tracheal or bronchial tuberculosis, bacteriological or histological examination not done
012.22	Isolated tracheal or bronchial tuberculosis, bacteriological or histological examination unknown (at present)
012.23	Isolated tracheal or bronchial tuberculosis, tubercle bacilli found (in sputum) by microscopy
012.24	Isolated tracheal or bronchial tuberculosis, tubercle bacilli not found (in sputum) by microscopy, but found by bacterial culture
012.25	Isolated tracheal or bronchial tuberculosis, tubercle bacilli not found by bacteriological examination, but tuberculosis confirmed histologically
012.26	Isolated tracheal or bronchial tuberculosis, tubercle bacilli not found by bacteriological or histological examination, but tuberculosis confirmed by other methods [inoculation of animals]
012.20	Isolated tracheal or bronchial tuberculosis, unspecified
782.4	Jaundice, unspecified, not of newborn
090.40	Juvenile neurosyphilis, unspecified
176.3	Kaposi's sarcoma, gastrointestinal sites

176.4	Kaposi's sarcoma, lung
176.5	Kaposi's sarcoma, lymph nodes
176.8	Kaposi's sarcoma, other specified sites
176.2	Kaposi's sarcoma, palate
176.0	Kaposi's sarcoma, skin
176.1	Kaposi's sarcoma, soft tissue
176.9	Kaposi's sarcoma, unspecified site
V42.0	Kidney replaced by transplant
335.11	Kugelberg-Welander disease
046.0	Kuru
065.2	Kyasanur forest disease
416.1	Kyphoscoliotic heart disease
665.31	Laceration of cervix, delivered, with or without mention of antepartum condition
870.2	Laceration of eyelid involving lacrimal passages
358.31	Lambert-Eaton syndrome in neoplastic disease
358.39	Lambert-Eaton syndrome in other diseases classified elsewhere
358.30	Lambert-Eaton syndrome, unspecified
200.73	Large cell lymphoma, intra-abdominal lymph nodes
200.76	Large cell lymphoma, intrapelvic lymph nodes
200.72	Large cell lymphoma, intrathoracic lymph nodes
200.74	Large cell lymphoma, lymph nodes of axilla and upper limb
200.71	Large cell lymphoma, lymph nodes of head, face, and neck
200.75	Large cell lymphoma, lymph nodes of inguinal region and lower limb
200.78	Large cell lymphoma, lymph nodes of multiple sites
200.77	Large cell lymphoma, spleen
200.70	Large cell lymphoma, unspecified site, extranodal and solid organ sites
032.3	Laryngeal diphtheria
438.21	Late effects of cerebrovascular disease, hemiplegia affecting dominant side
438.22	Late effects of cerebrovascular disease, hemiplegia affecting nondominant side
438.20	Late effects of cerebrovascular disease, hemiplegia affecting unspecified side
095.9	Late symptomatic syphilis, unspecified
295.54	Latent schizophrenia, chronic with acute exacerbation
295.53	Latent schizophrenia, subchronic with acute exacerbation
836.64	Lateral dislocation of tibia, proximal end, open
428.1	Left heart failure
556.5	Left-sided ulcerative (chronic) colitis
635.22	Legally induced abortion, complicated by damage to pelvic organs or tissues, complete
635.21	Legally induced abortion, complicated by damage to pelvic organs or tissues, incomplete
635.20	Legally induced abortion, complicated by damage to pelvic organs or tissues, unspecified
635.02	Legally induced abortion, complicated by genital tract and pelvic infection, complete
635.01	Legally induced abortion, complicated by genital tract and pelvic infection, incomplete
635.00	Legally induced abortion, complicated by genital tract and pelvic infection, unspecified
635.42	Legally induced abortion, complicated by metabolic disorder, complete
635.41	Legally induced abortion, complicated by metabolic disorder, incomplete
635.40	Legally induced abortion, complicated by metabolic disorder, unspecified
635.72	Legally induced abortion, with other specified complications, complete

635.71	Legally induced abortion, with other specified complications, incomplete
635.70	Legally induced abortion, with other specified complications, unspecified
635.82	Legally induced abortion, with unspecified complication, complete
635.81	Legally induced abortion, with unspecified complication, incomplete
635.80	Legally induced abortion, with unspecified complication, unspecified
085.9	Leishmaniasis, unspecified
030.0	Lepromatous leprosy [type L]
030.9	Leprosy, unspecified
100.0	Leptospirosis icterohemorrhagica
100.9	Leptospirosis, unspecified
446.3	Lethal midline granuloma
202.53	Letterer-siwe disease, intra-abdominal lymph nodes
202.56	Letterer-siwe disease, intrapelvic lymph nodes
202.52	Letterer-siwe disease, intrathoracic lymph nodes
202.54	Letterer-siwe disease, lymph nodes of axilla and upper limb
202.51	Letterer-siwe disease, lymph nodes of head, face, and neck
202.55	Letterer-siwe disease, lymph nodes of inguinal region and lower limb
202.58	Letterer-siwe disease, lymph nodes of multiple sites
202.57	Letterer-siwe disease, spleen
202.50	Letterer-siwe disease, unspecified site, extranodal and solid organ sites
202.43	Leukemic reticuloendotheliosis, intra-abdominal lymph nodes
202.46	Leukemic reticuloendotheliosis, intrapelvic lymph nodes
202.42	Leukemic reticuloendotheliosis, intrathoracic lymph nodes
202.44	Leukemic reticuloendotheliosis, lymph nodes of axilla and upper arm
202.41	Leukemic reticuloendotheliosis, lymph nodes of head, face, and neck
202.45	Leukemic reticuloendotheliosis, lymph nodes of inguinal region and lower limb
202.48	Leukemic reticuloendotheliosis, lymph nodes of multiple sites
202.47	Leukemic reticuloendotheliosis, spleen
202.40	Leukemic reticuloendotheliosis, unspecified site, extranodal and solid organ sites
330.0	Leukodystrophy
027.0	Listeriosis
646.73	Liver and biliary tract disorders in pregnancy, antepartum condition or complication
646.71	Liver and biliary tract disorders in pregnancy, delivered, with or without mention of antepartum condition
V42.7	Liver replaced by transplant
999.33	Local infection due to central venous catheter
345.41	Localization-related (focal) (partial) epilepsy and epileptic syndromes with complex partial seizures, with intractable epilepsy
345.40	Localization-related (focal) (partial) epilepsy and epileptic syndromes with complex partial seizures, without mention of intractable epilepsy
345.51	Localization-related (focal) (partial) epilepsy and epileptic syndromes with simple partial seizures, with intractable epilepsy
345.50	Localization-related (focal) (partial) epilepsy and epileptic syndromes with simple partial seizures, without mention of intractable epilepsy
125.2	Loiasis
080	Louse-borne (epidemic) typhus
517.2	Lung involvement in systemic sclerosis
V42.6	Lung replaced by transplant
088.81	Lyme Disease
049.0	Lymphocytic choriomeningitis

200.13	Lymphosarcoma, intra-abdominal lymph nodes
200.16	Lymphosarcoma, intrapelvic lymph nodes
200.12	Lymphosarcoma, intrathoracic lymph nodes
200.14	Lymphosarcoma, lymph nodes of axilla and upper limb
200.11	Lymphosarcoma, lymph nodes of head, face, and neck
200.15	Lymphosarcoma, lymph nodes of inguinal region and lower limb
200.18	Lymphosarcoma, lymph nodes of multiple sites
200.17	Lymphosarcoma, spleen
200.10	Lymphosarcoma, unspecified site, extranodal and solid organ sites
039.4	Madura foot
296.31	Major depressive affective disorder, recurrent episode, mild
296.32	Major depressive affective disorder, recurrent episode, moderate
296.34	Major depressive affective disorder, recurrent episode, severe, specified as with psychotic behavior
296.33	Major depressive affective disorder, recurrent episode, severe, without mention of psychotic behavior
296.30	Major depressive affective disorder, recurrent episode, unspecified
296.21	Major depressive affective disorder, single episode, mild
296.22	Major depressive affective disorder, single episode, moderate
296.24	Major depressive affective disorder, single episode, severe, specified as with psychotic behavior
296.23	Major depressive affective disorder, single episode, severe, without mention of psychotic behavior
296.20	Major depressive affective disorder, single episode, unspecified
647.43	Malaria in the mother, antepartum condition or complication
647.42	Malaria in the mother, delivered, with mention of postpartum complication
647.41	Malaria in the mother, delivered, with or without mention of antepartum condition
647.44	Malaria in the mother, postpartum condition or complication
084.6	Malaria, unspecified
125.1	Malayan filariasis
789.51	Malignant ascites
209.25	Malignant carcinoid tumor of foregut, not otherwise specified
209.27	Malignant carcinoid tumor of hindgut, not otherwise specified
209.26	Malignant carcinoid tumor of midgut, not otherwise specified
209.29	Malignant carcinoid tumor of other sites
209.11	Malignant carcinoid tumor of the appendix
209.13	Malignant carcinoid tumor of the ascending colon
209.21	Malignant carcinoid tumor of the bronchus and lung
209.12	Malignant carcinoid tumor of the cecum
209.15	Malignant carcinoid tumor of the descending colon
209.01	Malignant carcinoid tumor of the duodenum
209.03	Malignant carcinoid tumor of the ileum
209.02	Malignant carcinoid tumor of the jejunum
209.24	Malignant carcinoid tumor of the kidney
209.10	Malignant carcinoid tumor of the large intestine, unspecified portion
209.17	Malignant carcinoid tumor of the rectum
209.16	Malignant carcinoid tumor of the sigmoid colon
209.00	Malignant carcinoid tumor of the small intestine, unspecified portion
209.23	Malignant carcinoid tumor of the stomach
209.22	Malignant carcinoid tumor of the thymus
209.14	Malignant carcinoid tumor of the transverse colon
209.20	Malignant carcinoid tumor of unknown primary site
401.0	Malignant essential hypertension
202.33	Malignant histiocytosis, intra-abdominal lymph nodes
202.36	Malignant histiocytosis, intrapelvic lymph nodes
202.32	Malignant histiocytosis, intrathoracic lymph nodes

202.34	Malignant histiocytosis, lymph nodes of axilla and upper limb
202.31	Malignant histiocytosis, lymph nodes of head, face, and neck
202.35	Malignant histiocytosis, lymph nodes of inguinal region and lower limb
202.38	Malignant histiocytosis, lymph nodes of multiple sites
202.37	Malignant histiocytosis, spleen
202.30	Malignant histiocytosis, unspecified site, extranodal and solid organ sites
402.01	Malignant hypertensive heart disease with heart failure
402.00	Malignant hypertensive heart disease without heart failure
995.86	Malignant hyperthermia
202.63	Malignant mast cell tumors, intra-abdominal lymph nodes
202.66	Malignant mast cell tumors, intrapelvic lymph nodes
202.62	Malignant mast cell tumors, intrathoracic lymph nodes
202.64	Malignant mast cell tumors, lymph nodes of axilla and upper limb
202.61	Malignant mast cell tumors, lymph nodes of head, face, and neck
202.65	Malignant mast cell tumors, lymph nodes of inguinal region and lower limb
202.68	Malignant mast cell tumors, lymph nodes of multiple sites
202.67	Malignant mast cell tumors, spleen
202.60	Malignant mast cell tumors, unspecified site, extranodal and solid organ sites
199.2	Malignant neoplasm associated with transplant organ
150.2	Malignant neoplasm of abdominal esophagus
194.0	Malignant neoplasm of adrenal gland
156.2	Malignant neoplasm of ampulla of vater
154.2	Malignant neoplasm of anal canal
164.2	Malignant neoplasm of anterior mediastinum
154.3	Malignant neoplasm of anus, unspecified site
194.6	Malignant neoplasm of aortic body and other paraganglia
153.5	Malignant neoplasm of appendix vermiformis
153.6	Malignant neoplasm of ascending colon
156.9	Malignant neoplasm of biliary tract, part unspecified site
157.1	Malignant neoplasm of body of pancreas
151.4	Malignant neoplasm of body of stomach
170.9	Malignant neoplasm of bone and articular cartilage, site unspecified
170.0	Malignant neoplasm of bones of skull and face, except mandible
191.7	Malignant neoplasm of brain stem
191.9	Malignant neoplasm of brain, unspecified
162.9	Malignant neoplasm of bronchus and lung, unspecified
151.0	Malignant neoplasm of cardia
194.5	Malignant neoplasm of carotid body
153.4	Malignant neoplasm of cecum
191.6	Malignant neoplasm of cerebellum nos
192.1	Malignant neoplasm of cerebral meninges
191.0	Malignant neoplasm of cerebrum, except lobes and ventricles
150.0	Malignant neoplasm of cervical esophagus
153.9	Malignant neoplasm of colon, unspecified site
171.5	Malignant neoplasm of connective and other soft tissue of abdomen
171.0	Malignant neoplasm of connective and other soft tissue of head, face, and neck
171.3	Malignant neoplasm of connective and other soft tissue of lower limb, including hip
171.6	Malignant neoplasm of connective and other soft tissue of pelvis
171.4	Malignant neoplasm of connective and other soft tissue of thorax
171.7	Malignant neoplasm of connective and other soft tissue of trunk, unspecified
171.2	Malignant neoplasm of connective and other soft tissue of upper limb, including shoulder

171.9	Malignant neoplasm of connective and other soft tissue, site unspecified
192.0	Malignant neoplasm of cranial nerves
153.2	Malignant neoplasm of descending colon
152.0	Malignant neoplasm of duodenum
194.9	Malignant neoplasm of endocrine gland, site unspecified
150.9	Malignant neoplasm of esophagus, unspecified site
156.1	Malignant neoplasm of extrahepatic bile ducts
191.1	Malignant neoplasm of frontal lobe
151.3	Malignant neoplasm of fundus of stomach
156.0	Malignant neoplasm of gallbladder
151.6	Malignant neoplasm of greater curvature of stomach, unspecified
157.0	Malignant neoplasm of head of pancreas
164.1	Malignant neoplasm of heart
153.0	Malignant neoplasm of hepatic flexure
152.2	Malignant neoplasm of ileum
155.1	Malignant neoplasm of intrahepatic bile ducts
157.4	Malignant neoplasm of islets of langerhans
152.1	Malignant neoplasm of jejunum
189.0	Malignant neoplasm of kidney, except pelvis
151.5	Malignant neoplasm of lesser curvature of stomach, unspecified
155.2	Malignant neoplasm of liver, not specified as primary or secondary
155.0	Malignant neoplasm of liver, primary
197.7	Malignant neoplasm of liver, secondary
170.7	Malignant neoplasm of long bones of lower limb
162.5	Malignant neoplasm of lower lobe, bronchus or lung
150.5	Malignant neoplasm of lower third of esophagus
162.2	Malignant neoplasm of main bronchus
170.1	Malignant neoplasm of mandible
152.3	Malignant neoplasm of Meckel's diverticulum
164.9	Malignant neoplasm of mediastinum, part unspecified
162.4	Malignant neoplasm of middle lobe, bronchus or lung
150.4	Malignant neoplasm of middle third of esophagus
192.9	Malignant neoplasm of nervous system, part unspecified
191.4	Malignant neoplasm of occipital lobe
194.8	Malignant neoplasm of other endocrine glands and related structures
191.8	Malignant neoplasm of other parts of brain
162.8	Malignant neoplasm of other parts of bronchus or lung
164.8	Malignant neoplasm of other parts of mediastinum
154.8	Malignant neoplasm of other sites of rectum, rectosigmoid junction, and anus
150.8	Malignant neoplasm of other specified part of esophagus
171.8	Malignant neoplasm of other specified sites of connective and other soft tissue
156.8	Malignant neoplasm of other specified sites of gallbladder and extrahepatic bile ducts
153.8	Malignant neoplasm of other specified sites of large intestine
192.8	Malignant neoplasm of other specified sites of nervous system
157.8	Malignant neoplasm of other specified sites of pancreas
163.8	Malignant neoplasm of other specified sites of pleura
152.8	Malignant neoplasm of other specified sites of small intestine
151.8	Malignant neoplasm of other specified sites of stomach
189.8	Malignant neoplasm of other specified sites of urinary organs
183.0	Malignant neoplasm of ovary
157.9	Malignant neoplasm of pancreas, part unspecified
157.3	Malignant neoplasm of pancreatic duct
194.1	Malignant neoplasm of parathyroid gland
189.4	Malignant neoplasm of paraurethral glands
191.3	Malignant neoplasm of parietal lobe

163.0	Malignant neoplasm of parietal pleura
170.6	Malignant neoplasm of pelvic bones, sacrum, and coccyx
158.9	Malignant neoplasm of peritoneum, unspecified
194.4	Malignant neoplasm of pineal gland
194.3	Malignant neoplasm of pituitary gland and craniopharyngeal duct
163.9	Malignant neoplasm of pleura, unspecified
164.3	Malignant neoplasm of posterior mediastinum
151.2	Malignant neoplasm of pyloric antrum
151.1	Malignant neoplasm of pylorus
154.0	Malignant neoplasm of rectosigmoid junction
154.1	Malignant neoplasm of rectum
189.1	Malignant neoplasm of renal pelvis
158.0	Malignant neoplasm of retroperitoneum
170.3	Malignant neoplasm of ribs, sternum, and clavicle
170.4	Malignant neoplasm of scapula and long bones of upper limb
170.8	Malignant neoplasm of short bones of lower limb
170.5	Malignant neoplasm of short bones of upper limb
153.3	Malignant neoplasm of sigmoid colon
152.9	Malignant neoplasm of small intestine, unspecified site
158.8	Malignant neoplasm of specified parts of peritoneum
192.2	Malignant neoplasm of spinal cord
192.3	Malignant neoplasm of spinal meninges
153.7	Malignant neoplasm of splenic flexure
151.9	Malignant neoplasm of stomach, unspecified site
157.2	Malignant neoplasm of tail of pancreas
191.2	Malignant neoplasm of temporal lobe
150.1	Malignant neoplasm of thoracic esophagus
164.0	Malignant neoplasm of thymus
162.0	Malignant neoplasm of trachea
153.1	Malignant neoplasm of transverse colon
162.3	Malignant neoplasm of upper lobe, bronchus or lung
150.3	Malignant neoplasm of upper third of esophagus
189.2	Malignant neoplasm of ureter
189.3	Malignant neoplasm of urethra
189.9	Malignant neoplasm of urinary organ, site unspecified
191.5	Malignant neoplasm of ventricles
170.2	Malignant neoplasm of vertebral column, excluding sacrum and coccyx
163.1	Malignant neoplasm of visceral pleura
380.14	Malignant otitis externa
511.81	Malignant pleural effusion
209.30	Malignant poorly differentiated neuroendocrine carcinoma, any site
405.01	Malignant renovascular hypertension
263.1	Malnutrition of mild degree
263.0	Malnutrition of moderate degree
746.87	Malposition of heart and cardiac apex
733.81	Malunion of fracture
296.11	Manic affective disorder, recurrent episode, mild
296.12	Manic affective disorder, recurrent episode, moderate
296.14	Manic affective disorder, recurrent episode, severe, specified as with psychotic behavior
296.13	Manic affective disorder, recurrent episode, severe, without mention of psychotic behavior
296.10	Manic affective disorder, recurrent episode, unspecified
125.5	Mansonella ozzardi infection
200.43	Mantle cell lymphoma, intra-abdominal lymph nodes
200.46	Mantle cell lymphoma, intrapelvic lymph nodes
200.42	Mantle cell lymphoma, intrathoracic lymph nodes
200.44	Mantle cell lymphoma, lymph nodes of axilla and upper limb

Appendix A — Alphabetic CC List

200.41	Mantle cell lymphoma, lymph nodes of head, face, and neck
200.45	Mantle cell lymphoma, lymph nodes of inguinal region and lower limb
200.48	Mantle cell lymphoma, lymph nodes of multiple sites
200.47	Mantle cell lymphoma, spleen
200.40	Mantle cell lymphoma, unspecified site, extranodal and solid organ sites
759.82	Marfan syndrome
200.33	Marginal zone lymphoma, intraabdominal lymph nodes
200.36	Marginal zone lymphoma, intrapelvic lymph nodes
200.32	Marginal zone lymphoma, intrathoracic lymph nodes
200.34	Marginal zone lymphoma, lymph nodes of axilla and upper limb
200.31	Marginal zone lymphoma, lymph nodes of head, face, and neck
200.35	Marginal zone lymphoma, lymph nodes of inguinal region and lower limb
200.38	Marginal zone lymphoma, lymph nodes of multiple sites
200.37	Marginal zone lymphoma, spleen
200.30	Marginal zone lymphoma, unspecified site, extranodal and solid organ sites
669.24	Maternal hypotension syndrome, postpartum condition or complication
659.21	Maternal pyrexia during labor, unspecified, delivered, with or without mention of antepartum condition
055.71	Measles keratoconjunctivitis
055.79	Measles with other specified complications
996.55	Mechanical complication due to artificial skin graft and decellularized allodermis
996.54	Mechanical complication due to breast prosthesis
996.01	Mechanical complication due to cardiac pacemaker (electrode)
996.51	Mechanical complication due to corneal graft
996.03	Mechanical complication due to coronary bypass graft
996.52	Mechanical complication due to graft of other tissue, not elsewhere classified
996.02	Mechanical complication due to heart valve prosthesis
996.57	Mechanical complication due to insulin pump
996.53	Mechanical complication due to ocular lens prosthesis
996.59	Mechanical complication due to other implant and internal device, not elsewhere classified
996.56	Mechanical complication due to peritoneal dialysis catheter
996.04	Mechanical complication of automatic implantable cardiac defibrillator
569.62	Mechanical complication of colostomy and enterostomy
596.82	Mechanical complication of cystostomy
530.87	Mechanical complication of esophagostomy
536.42	Mechanical complication of gastrostomy
996.2	Mechanical complication of nervous system device, implant, and graft
996.1	Mechanical complication of other vascular device, implant, and graft
V46.14	Mechanical complication of respirator [ventilator]
519.02	Mechanical complication of tracheostomy
996.00	Mechanical complication of unspecified cardiac device, implant, and graft
996.30	Mechanical complication of unspecified genitourinary device, implant, and graft
996.41	Mechanical loosening of prosthetic joint
836.63	Medial dislocation of tibia, proximal end, open
753.16	Medullary cystic kidney
753.17	Medullary sponge kidney
255.6	Medulloadrenal hyperfunction
564.7	Megacolon, other than Hirschsprung's
207.22	Megakaryocytic leukemia, in relapse
207.21	Megakaryocytic leukemia, in remission
207.20	Megakaryocytic leukemia, without mention of having achieved remission
025	Melioidosis
781.6	Meningismus
049.1	Meningitis due to adenovirus
047.0	Meningitis due to coxsackie virus
047.1	Meningitis due to echo virus
036.82	Meningococcal arthropathy
036.9	Meningococcal infection, unspecified
036.81	Meningococcal optic neuritis
639.4	Metabolic disorders following abortion or ectopic and molar pregnancies
121.5	Metagonimiasis
289.7	Methemoglobinemia
768.71	Mild hypoxic-ischemic encephalopathy
642.43	Mild or unspecified pre-eclampsia, antepartum condition or complication
642.41	Mild or unspecified pre-eclampsia, delivered, with or without mention of antepartum condition
642.44	Mild or unspecified pre-eclampsia, postpartum condition or complication
255.42	Mineralocorticoid deficiency
276.4	Mixed acid-base balance disorder
127.8	Mixed intestinal helminthiasis
084.5	Mixed malaria
426.12	Mobitz (type) II atrioventricular block
768.72	Moderate hypoxic-ischemic encephalopathy
050.2	Modified smallpox
059.01	Monkeypox
065.4	Mosquito-borne hemorrhagic fever
437.5	Moyamoya disease
085.5	Mucocutaneous leishmaniasis, (American)
277.5	Mucopolysaccharidosis
616.81	Mucositis (ulcerative) of cervix, vagina, and vulva
894.2	Multiple and unspecified open wound of lower limb, with tendon involvement
884.2	Multiple and unspecified open wound of upper limb, with tendon involvement
819.0	Multiple closed fractures involving both upper limbs, and upper limb with rib(s) and sternum
808.43	Multiple closed pelvic fractures with disruption of pelvic circle
808.44	Multiple closed pelvic fractures without disruption of pelvic circle
759.7	Multiple congenital anomalies, so described
203.02	Multiple myeloma, in relapse
203.01	Multiple myeloma, in remission
203.00	Multiple myeloma, without mention of having achieved remission
819.1	Multiple open fractures involving both upper limbs, and upper limb with rib(s) and sternum
817.1	Multiple open fractures of hand bones
072.71	Mumps hepatitis
072.0	Mumps orchitis
072.3	Mumps pancreatitis
072.72	Mumps polyneuropathy
072.8	Mumps with unspecified complication
081.0	Murine (endemic) typhus
358.1	Myasthenic syndromes in diseases classified elsewhere
202.13	Mycosis fungoides, intra-abdominal lymph nodes
202.16	Mycosis fungoides, intrapelvic lymph nodes
202.12	Mycosis fungoides, intrathoracic lymph nodes
202.14	Mycosis fungoides, lymph nodes of axilla and upper limb

202.11	Mycosis fungoides, lymph nodes of head, face, and neck
202.15	Mycosis fungoides, lymph nodes of inguinal region and lower limb
202.18	Mycosis fungoides, lymph nodes of multiple sites
202.17	Mycosis fungoides, spleen
202.10	Mycosis fungoides, unspecified site, extranodal and solid organ sites
117.4	Mycotic mycetomas
238.74	Myelodysplastic syndrome with 5q deletion
289.83	Myelofibrosis
238.76	Myelofibrosis with myeloid metaplasia
205.32	Myeloid sarcoma, in relapse
205.31	Myeloid sarcoma, in remission
205.30	Myeloid sarcoma, without mention of having achieved remission
336.3	Myelopathy in other diseases classified elsewhere
284.2	Myelophthisis
791.3	Myoglobinuria
032.1	Nasopharyngeal diphtheria
126.1	Necatoriasis due to necator americanus
040.3	Necrobacillosis
447.5	Necrosis of artery
775.1	Neonatal diabetes mellitus
771.5	Neonatal infective mastitis
775.2	Neonatal myasthenia gravis
775.3	Neonatal thyrotoxicosis
238.5	Neoplasm of uncertain behavior of histiocytic and mast cells
238.6	Neoplasm of uncertain behavior of plasma cells
583.2	Nephritis and nephropathy, not specified as acute or chronic, with lesion of membranoproliferative glomerulonephritis
583.1	Nephritis and nephropathy, not specified as acute or chronic, with lesion of membranous glomerulonephritis
583.0	Nephritis and nephropathy, not specified as acute or chronic, with lesion of proliferative glomerulonephritis
583.7	Nephritis and nephropathy, not specified as acute or chronic, with lesion of renal medullary necrosis
588.1	Nephrogenic diabetes insipidus
581.81	Nephrotic syndrome in diseases classified elsewhere
581.2	Nephrotic syndrome with lesion of membranoproliferative glomerulonephritis
581.1	Nephrotic syndrome with lesion of membranous glomerulonephritis
581.3	Nephrotic syndrome with lesion of minimal change glomerulonephritis
581.0	Nephrotic syndrome with lesion of proliferative glomerulonephritis
581.89	Nephrotic syndrome with other specified pathological lesion in kidney
581.9	Nephrotic syndrome with unspecified pathological lesion in kidney
349.1	Nervous system complications from surgically implanted device
564.81	Neurogenic bowel
781.8	Neurologic neglect syndrome
341.0	Neuromyelitis optica
094.9	Neurosyphilis, unspecified
279.13	Nezelof's syndrome
202.03	Nodular lymphoma, intra-abdominal lymph nodes
202.06	Nodular lymphoma, intrapelvic lymph nodes
202.02	Nodular lymphoma, intrathoracic lymph nodes
202.04	Nodular lymphoma, lymph nodes of axilla and upper limb
202.01	Nodular lymphoma, lymph nodes of head, face, and neck
202.05	Nodular lymphoma, lymph nodes of inguinal region and lower limb
202.08	Nodular lymphoma, lymph nodes of multiple sites
202.07	Nodular lymphoma, spleen
202.00	Nodular lymphoma, unspecified site, extranodal and solid organ sites
999.75	Non-ABO incompatibility reaction, unspecified
999.77	Non-ABO incompatibility with acute hemolytic transfusion reaction
999.78	Non-ABO incompatibility with delayed hemolytic transfusion reaction
999.76	Non-ABO incompatibility with hemolytic transfusion reaction not specified as acute or delayed
283.10	Non-autoimmune hemolytic anemia, unspecified
998.83	Non-healing surgical wound
437.6	Nonpyogenic thrombosis of intracranial venous sinus
729.73	Nontraumatic compartment syndrome of abdomen
729.72	Nontraumatic compartment syndrome of lower extremity
729.79	Nontraumatic compartment syndrome of other sites
729.71	Nontraumatic compartment syndrome of upper extremity
733.82	Nonunion of fracture
082.2	North Asian tick fever
425.7	Nutritional and metabolic cardiomyopathy
278.03	Obesity hypoventilation syndrome
425.2	Obscure cardiomyopathy of Africa
673.30	Obstetrical pyemic and septic embolism, unspecified as to episode of care or not applicable
660.03	Obstruction caused by malposition of fetus at onset of labor, antepartum condition or complication
575.2	Obstruction of gallbladder
491.21	Obstructive chronic bronchitis with (acute) exacerbation
491.22	Obstructive chronic bronchitis with acute bronchitis
331.4	Obstructive hydrocephalus
871.1	Ocular laceration with prolapse or exposure of intraocular tissue
871.0	Ocular laceration without prolapse of intraocular tissue
021.3	Oculoglandular tularemia
658.03	Oligohydramnios, antepartum condition or complication
658.01	Oligohydramnios, delivered, with or without mention of antepartum condition
771.4	Omphalitis of the newborn
065.1	Omsk hemorrhagic fever
125.3	Onchocerciasis
832.11	Open anterior dislocation of elbow
831.11	Open anterior dislocation of humerus
831.14	Open dislocation of acromioclavicular (joint)
837.1	Open dislocation of ankle
833.14	Open dislocation of carpometacarpal (joint)
832.19	Open dislocation of elbow, other
832.10	Open dislocation of elbow, unspecified
830.1	Open dislocation of jaw
833.15	Open dislocation of metacarpal (bone), proximal end
833.13	Open dislocation of midcarpal (joint)
833.12	Open dislocation of radiocarpal (joint)
833.11	Open dislocation of radioulnar (joint), distal
831.19	Open dislocation of shoulder, other
831.10	Open dislocation of shoulder, unspecified
833.19	Open dislocation of wrist, other
833.10	Open dislocation of wrist, unspecified part
839.51	Open dislocation, coccyx
839.9	Open dislocation, multiple and ill-defined sites
839.79	Open dislocation, other location
839.52	Open dislocation, sacrum
810.13	Open fracture of acromial end of clavicle
811.11	Open fracture of acromial process of scapula

825.31	Open fracture of astragalus
815.12	Open fracture of base of other metacarpal bone(s)
815.11	Open fracture of base of thumb [first] metacarpal
814.17	Open fracture of capitate bone [os magnum] of wrist
814.10	Open fracture of carpal bone, unspecified
810.10	Open fracture of clavicle, unspecified part
811.12	Open fracture of coracoid process
825.33	Open fracture of cuboid
825.34	Open fracture of cuneiform, foot
816.12	Open fracture of distal phalanx or phalanges of hand
811.13	Open fracture of glenoid cavity and neck of scapula
814.18	Open fracture of hamate [unciform] bone of wrist
814.12	Open fracture of lunate [semilunar] bone of wrist
802.5	Open fracture of malar and maxillary bones
802.37	Open fracture of mandible, alveolar border of body
802.35	Open fracture of mandible, angle of jaw
802.38	Open fracture of mandible, body, other and unspecified
802.31	Open fracture of mandible, condylar process
802.33	Open fracture of mandible, coronoid process
802.39	Open fracture of mandible, multiple sites
802.34	Open fracture of mandible, ramus, unspecified
802.32	Open fracture of mandible, subcondylar
802.36	Open fracture of mandible, symphysis of body
802.30	Open fracture of mandible, unspecified site
815.10	Open fracture of metacarpal bone(s), site unspecified
825.35	Open fracture of metatarsal bone(s)
816.11	Open fracture of middle or proximal phalanx or phalanges of hand
815.19	Open fracture of multiple sites of metacarpus
816.13	Open fracture of multiple sites of phalanx or phalanges of hand
802.1	Open fracture of nasal bones
814.11	Open fracture of navicular [scaphoid] bone of wrist
825.32	Open fracture of navicular [scaphoid], foot
815.14	Open fracture of neck of metacarpal bone(s)
802.7	Open fracture of orbital floor (blow-out)
814.19	Open fracture of other bone of wrist
802.9	Open fracture of other facial bones
822.1	Open fracture of patella
816.10	Open fracture of phalanx or phalanges of hand, unspecified
814.14	Open fracture of pisiform bone of wrist
811.19	Open fracture of scapula, other
811.10	Open fracture of scapula, unspecified part
810.12	Open fracture of shaft of clavicle
815.13	Open fracture of shaft of metacarpal bone(s)
810.11	Open fracture of sternal end of clavicle
814.15	Open fracture of trapezium bone [larger multangular] of wrist
814.16	Open fracture of trapezoid bone [smaller multangular] of wrist
814.13	Open fracture of triquetral [cuneiform] bone of wrist
825.30	Open fracture of unspecified bone(s) of foot [except toes]
804.90	Open fractures involving skull or face with other bones, with intracranial injury of other and unspecified nature, unspecified state of consciousness
804.92	Open fractures involving skull or face with other bones, with intracranial injury of other and unspecified nature, with brief [less than one hour] loss of consciousness
804.99	Open fractures involving skull or face with other bones, with intracranial injury of other and unspecified nature, with concussion, unspecified
804.96	Open fractures involving skull or face with other bones, with intracranial injury of other and unspecified nature, with loss of consciousness of unspecified duration
804.91	Open fractures involving skull or face with other bones, with intracranial injury of other and unspecified nature, with no loss of consciousness
804.50	Open fractures involving skull or face with other bones, without mention of intracranial injury, unspecified state of consciousness
804.52	Open fractures involving skull or face with other bones, without mention of intracranial injury, with brief [less than one hour] loss of consciousness
804.59	Open fractures involving skull or face with other bones, without mention of intracranial injury, with concussion, unspecified
804.56	Open fractures involving skull or face with other bones, without mention of intracranial injury, with loss of consciousness of unspecified duration
804.51	Open fractures involving skull or face with other bones, without mention of intracranial injury, with no loss of consciousness
831.13	Open inferior dislocation of humerus
832.14	Open lateral dislocation of elbow
832.13	Open medial dislocation of elbow
832.12	Open posterior dislocation of elbow
831.12	Open posterior dislocation of humerus
872.12	Open wound of auditory canal, complicated
880.22	Open wound of axillary region, with tendon involvement
875.1	Open wound of chest (wall), complicated
875.0	Open wound of chest (wall), without mention of complication
872.74	Open wound of cochlea, complicated
872.64	Open wound of cochlea, without mention of complication
872.71	Open wound of ear drum, complicated
872.61	Open wound of ear drum, without mention of complication
881.21	Open wound of elbow, with tendon involvement
872.73	Open wound of eustachian tube, complicated
872.63	Open wound of eustachian tube, without mention of complication
883.2	Open wound of finger(s), with tendon involvement
892.2	Open wound of foot except toe(s) alone, with tendon involvement
881.20	Open wound of forearm, with tendon involvement
882.2	Open wound of hand except finger(s) alone, with tendon involvement
890.2	Open wound of hip and thigh, with tendon involvement
891.2	Open wound of knee, leg [except thigh], and ankle, with tendon involvement
880.29	Open wound of multiple sites of shoulder and upper arm, with tendon involvement
873.33	Open wound of nasal sinus, complicated
873.23	Open wound of nasal sinus, without mention of complication
872.72	Open wound of ossicles, complicated
872.62	Open wound of ossicles, without mention of complication
872.79	Open wound of other and multiple sites of ear, complicated
872.69	Open wound of other and multiple sites of ear, without mention of complication
874.5	Open wound of pharynx, complicated
874.4	Open wound of pharynx, without mention of complication
880.21	Open wound of scapular region, with tendon involvement
880.20	Open wound of shoulder region, with tendon involvement
874.3	Open wound of thyroid gland, complicated
874.2	Open wound of thyroid gland, without mention of complication
893.2	Open wound of toe(s), with tendon involvement
880.23	Open wound of upper arm, with tendon involvement
881.22	Open wound of wrist, with tendon involvement
304.01	Opioid type dependence, continuous
121.0	Opisthorchiasis
118	Opportunistic mycoses
950.0	Optic nerve injury
377.30	Optic neuritis, unspecified

377.31	Optic papillitis
376.01	Orbital cellulitis
376.03	Orbital osteomyelitis
376.02	Orbital periostitis
604.0	Orchitis, epididymitis, and epididymo-orchitis, with abscess
V43.22	Organ or tissue replaced by other means, fully implantable artificial heart
V43.21	Organ or tissue replaced by other means, heart assist device
V42.84	Organ or tissue replaced by transplant, intestines
073.7	Ornithosis with other specified complications
073.8	Ornithosis with unspecified complication
073.9	Ornithosis, unspecified
756.51	Osteogenesis imperfecta
756.52	Osteopetrosis
745.61	Ostium primum defect
745.5	Ostium secundum type atrial septal defect
999.69	Other ABO incompatibility reaction
616.4	Other abscess of vulva
775.81	Other acidosis of newborn
333.79	Other acquired torsion dystonia
411.89	Other acute and subacute forms of ischemic heart disease, other
420.99	Other acute pericarditis
391.8	Other acute rheumatic heart disease
255.5	Other adrenal hypofunction
995.85	Other adult abuse and neglect
512.84	Other air leak
291.89	Other alcohol-induced mental disorders
277.39	Other amyloidosis
995.0	Other anaphylactic reaction
253.1	Other and unspecified anterior pituitary hyperfunction
770.5	Other and unspecified atelectasis
286.9	Other and unspecified coagulation defects
046.19	Other and unspecified Creutzfeldt-Jakob disease
778.5	Other and unspecified edema of newborn
999.31	Other and unspecified infection due to central venous catheter
202.93	Other and unspecified malignant neoplasms of lymphoid and histiocytic tissue, intra-abdominal lymph nodes
202.96	Other and unspecified malignant neoplasms of lymphoid and histiocytic tissue, intrapelvic lymph nodes
202.92	Other and unspecified malignant neoplasms of lymphoid and histiocytic tissue, intrathoracic lymph nodes
202.94	Other and unspecified malignant neoplasms of lymphoid and histiocytic tissue, lymph nodes of axilla and upper limb
202.91	Other and unspecified malignant neoplasms of lymphoid and histiocytic tissue, lymph nodes of head, face, and neck
202.95	Other and unspecified malignant neoplasms of lymphoid and histiocytic tissue, lymph nodes of inguinal region and lower limb
202.98	Other and unspecified malignant neoplasms of lymphoid and histiocytic tissue, lymph nodes of multiple sites
202.97	Other and unspecified malignant neoplasms of lymphoid and histiocytic tissue, spleen
202.90	Other and unspecified malignant neoplasms of lymphoid and histiocytic tissue, unspecified site, extranodal and solid organ sites
265.1	Other and unspecified manifestations of thiamine deficiency
117.9	Other and unspecified mycoses
579.3	Other and unspecified postsurgical nonabsorption
046.79	Other and unspecified prion disease of central nervous system
414.19	Other aneurysm of heart
747.29	Other anomalies of aorta
751.69	Other anomalies of gallbladder, bile ducts, and liver
747.49	Other anomalies of great veins

751.5	Other anomalies of intestine
748.3	Other anomalies of larynx, trachea, and bronchus
756.3	Other anomalies of ribs and sternum
335.8	Other anterior horn cell diseases
770.82	Other apnea of newborn
444.09	Other arterial embolism and thrombosis of abdominal aorta
789.59	Other ascites
758.39	Other autosomal deletions
005.89	Other bacterial food poisoning
426.53	Other bilateral bundle branch block
296.89	Other bipolar disorders
023.8	Other brucellosis
112.89	Other candidiasis of other specified sites
648.63	Other cardiovascular diseases of mother, antepartum condition or complication
648.62	Other cardiovascular diseases of mother, delivered, with mention of postpartum complication
648.61	Other cardiovascular diseases of mother, delivered, with or without mention of antepartum condition
648.64	Other cardiovascular diseases of mother, postpartum condition or complication
334.3	Other cerebellar ataxia
995.59	Other child abuse and neglect
614.7	Other chronic pelvic peritonitis, female
835.03	Other closed anterior dislocation of hip
821.29	Other closed fracture of lower end of femur
812.49	Other closed fracture of lower end of humerus
812.09	Other closed fracture of upper end of humerus
813.42	Other closed fractures of distal end of radius (alone)
803.40	Other closed skull fracture with intracranial injury of other and unspecified nature, unspecified state of consciousness
803.42	Other closed skull fracture with intracranial injury of other and unspecified nature, with brief [less than one hour] loss of consciousness
803.49	Other closed skull fracture with intracranial injury of other and unspecified nature, with concussion, unspecified
803.46	Other closed skull fracture with intracranial injury of other and unspecified nature, with loss of consciousness of unspecified duration
803.41	Other closed skull fracture with intracranial injury of other and unspecified nature, with no loss of consciousness
803.00	Other closed skull fracture without mention of intracranial injury, unspecified state of consciousness
803.02	Other closed skull fracture without mention of intracranial injury, with brief [less than one hour] loss of consciousness
803.09	Other closed skull fracture without mention of intracranial injury, with concussion, unspecified
803.06	Other closed skull fracture without mention of intracranial injury, with loss of consciousness of unspecified duration
803.01	Other closed skull fracture without mention of intracranial injury, with no loss of consciousness
569.69	Other colostomy and enterostomy complication
596.83	Other complication of cystostomy
996.76	Other complications due to genitourinary device, implant, and graft
996.71	Other complications due to heart valve prosthesis
996.77	Other complications due to internal joint prosthesis
996.75	Other complications due to nervous system device, implant, and graft
996.72	Other complications due to other cardiac device, implant, and graft
996.78	Other complications due to other internal orthopedic device, implant, and graft

996.79	Other complications due to other internal prosthetic device, implant, and graft
996.74	Other complications due to other vascular device, implant, and graft
996.73	Other complications due to renal dialysis device, implant, and graft
539.09	Other complications of gastric band procedure
569.79	Other complications of intestinal pouch
539.89	Other complications of other bariatric procedure
746.09	Other congenital anomalies of pulmonary valve
284.09	Other constitutional aplastic anemia
255.3	Other corticoadrenal overactivity
279.19	Other deficiency of cell-mediated immunity
279.09	Other deficiency of humoral immunity
333.0	Other degenerative diseases of the basal ganglia
341.8	Other demyelinating diseases of central nervous system
997.49	Other digestive system complications
836.69	Other dislocation of knee, open
253.6	Other disorders of neurohypophysis
429.81	Other disorders of papillary muscle
277.2	Other disorders of purine and pyrimidine metabolism
270.2	Other disturbances of aromatic amino-acid metabolism
270.7	Other disturbances of straight-chain amino-acid metabolism
349.39	Other dural tear
633.81	Other ectopic pregnancy with intrauterine pregnancy
633.80	Other ectopic pregnancy without intrauterine pregnancy
082.49	Other ehrlichiosis
745.69	Other endocardial cushion defects
424.99	Other endocarditis, valve unspecified
360.19	Other endophthalmitis
048	Other enterovirus diseases of central nervous system
345.81	Other forms of epilepsy and recurrent seizures, with intractable epilepsy
345.80	Other forms of epilepsy and recurrent seizures, without mention of intractable epilepsy
114.3	Other forms of progressive coccidioidomycosis
361.89	Other forms of retinal detachment
091.89	Other forms of secondary syphilis
437.1	Other generalized ischemic cerebrovascular disease
098.85	Other gonococcal heart disease
098.19	Other gonococcal infection (acute) of upper genitourinary tract
098.49	Other gonococcal infection of eye
098.59	Other gonococcal infection of joint
759.6	Other hamartoses, not elsewhere classified
786.39	Other hemoptysis
286.59	Other hemorrhagic disorder due to intrinsic circulating anticoagulants, antibodies, or inhibitors
425.18	Other hypertrophic cardiomyopathy
666.12	Other immediate postpartum hemorrhage, delivered, with mention of postpartum complication
666.14	Other immediate postpartum hemorrhage, postpartum condition or complication
203.82	Other immunoproliferative neoplasms, in relapse
203.81	Other immunoproliferative neoplasms, in remission
203.80	Other immunoproliferative neoplasms, without mention of having achieved remission
560.39	Other impaction of intestine
730.87	Other infections involving bone in diseases classified elsewhere, ankle and foot
730.83	Other infections involving bone in diseases classified elsewhere, forearm

730.84	Other infections involving bone in diseases classified elsewhere, hand
730.86	Other infections involving bone in diseases classified elsewhere, lower leg
730.89	Other infections involving bone in diseases classified elsewhere, multiple sites
730.88	Other infections involving bone in diseases classified elsewhere, other specified sites
730.85	Other infections involving bone in diseases classified elsewhere, pelvic region and thigh
730.81	Other infections involving bone in diseases classified elsewhere, shoulder region
730.80	Other infections involving bone in diseases classified elsewhere, site unspecified
730.82	Other infections involving bone in diseases classified elsewhere, upper arm
771.89	Other infections specific to the perinatal period
865.09	Other injury into spleen without mention of open wound into cavity
863.49	Other injury to colon or rectum, without mention of open wound into cavity
864.09	Other injury to liver without mention of open wound into cavity
665.51	Other injury to pelvic organs, delivered, with or without mention of antepartum condition
863.29	Other injury to small intestine, without mention of open wound into cavity
090.49	Other juvenile neurosyphilis
090.5	Other late congenital syphilis, symptomatic
208.82	Other leukemia of unspecified cell type, in relapse
208.81	Other leukemia of unspecified cell type, in remission
208.80	Other leukemia of unspecified cell type, without mention of having achieved remission
003.29	Other localized salmonella infections
238.79	Other lymphatic and hematopoietic tissues
204.82	Other lymphoid leukemia, in relapse
204.81	Other lymphoid leukemia, in remission
204.80	Other lymphoid leukemia, without mention of having achieved remission
084.4	Other malaria
202.83	Other malignant lymphomas, intra-abdominal lymph nodes
202.86	Other malignant lymphomas, intrapelvic lymph nodes
202.82	Other malignant lymphomas, intrathoracic lymph nodes
202.84	Other malignant lymphomas, lymph nodes of axilla and upper limb
202.81	Other malignant lymphomas, lymph nodes of head, face, and neck
202.85	Other malignant lymphomas, lymph nodes of inguinal region and lower limb
202.88	Other malignant lymphomas, lymph nodes of multiple sites
202.87	Other malignant lymphomas, spleen
202.80	Other malignant lymphomas, unspecified site, extranodal and solid organ sites
405.09	Other malignant secondary hypertension
996.09	Other mechanical complication of cardiac device, implant, and graft
996.39	Other mechanical complication of genitourinary device, implant, and graft
996.49	Other mechanical complication of other internal orthopedic device, implant, and graft
996.47	Other mechanical complication of prosthetic joint implant
758.33	Other microdeletions
206.82	Other monocytic leukemia, in relapse
206.81	Other monocytic leukemia, in remission

206.80	Other monocytic leukemia, without mention of having achieved remission
066.3	Other mosquito-borne fever
335.29	Other motor neuron disease
072.79	Other mumps with other specified complications
205.82	Other myeloid leukemia, in relapse
205.81	Other myeloid leukemia, in remission
205.80	Other myeloid leukemia, without mention of having achieved remission
336.8	Other myelopathy
200.83	Other named variants of lymphosarcoma and reticulosarcoma, intra-abdominal lymph nodes
200.86	Other named variants of lymphosarcoma and reticulosarcoma, intrapelvic lymph nodes
200.84	Other named variants of lymphosarcoma and reticulosarcoma, lymph nodes of axilla and upper limb
200.81	Other named variants of lymphosarcoma and reticulosarcoma, lymph nodes of head, face, and neck
200.85	Other named variants of lymphosarcoma and reticulosarcoma, lymph nodes of inguinal region and lower limb
200.88	Other named variants of lymphosarcoma and reticulosarcoma, lymph nodes of multiple sites
200.87	Other named variants of lymphosarcoma and reticulosarcoma, spleen
200.80	Other named variants of lymphosarcoma and reticulosarcoma, unspecified site, extranodal and solid organ sites
200.82	Other named variants of lymphosarcoma and reticulosarcoma,intrathoracic lymph nodes
775.89	Other neonatal endocrine and metabolic disturbances
997.09	Other nervous system complications
999.79	Other non-ABO incompatibility reaction
283.19	Other non-autoimmune hemolytic anemias
537.3	Other obstruction of duodenum
753.29	Other obstructive defects of renal pelvis and ureter
825.39	Other open fracture of tarsal and metatarsal bones
377.39	Other optic neuritis
284.19	Other pancytopenia
084.9	Other pernicious complications of malaria
671.53	Other phlebitis and thrombosis complicating pregnancy and the puerperium, antepartum condition or complication
671.52	Other phlebitis and thrombosis complicating pregnancy and the puerperium, delivered, with mention of postpartum complication
671.51	Other phlebitis and thrombosis complicating pregnancy and the puerperium, delivered, with or without mention of antepartum condition
671.54	Other phlebitis and thrombosis complicating pregnancy and the puerperium, postpartum condition or complication
671.50	Other phlebitis and thrombosis complicating pregnancy and the puerperium, unspecified as to episode of care or not applicable
512.89	Other pneumothorax
998.59	Other postoperative infection
425.4	Other primary cardiomyopathies
010.81	Other primary progressive tuberculosis, bacteriological or histological examination not done
010.82	Other primary progressive tuberculosis, bacteriological or histological examination unknown (at present)
010.83	Other primary progressive tuberculosis, tubercle bacilli found (in sputum) by microscopy
010.84	Other primary progressive tuberculosis, tubercle bacilli not found (in sputum) by microscopy, but found by bacterial culture
010.85	Other primary progressive tuberculosis, tubercle bacilli not found by bacteriological examination, but tuberculosis confirmed histologically
010.86	Other primary progressive tuberculosis, tubercle bacilli not found by bacteriological or histological examination, but tuberculosis confirmed by other methods [inoculation of animals]
010.80	Other primary progressive tuberculosis, unspecified
658.81	Other problems associated with amniotic cavity and membranes, delivered, with or without mention of antepartum condition
263.8	Other protein-calorie malnutrition
518.82	Other pulmonary insufficiency, not elsewhere classified
997.39	Other respiratory complications
999.74	Other Rh incompatibility reaction
279.03	Other selective immunoglobulin deficiencies
999.59	Other serum reaction
999.51	Other serum reaction due to administration of blood and blood products
999.52	Other serum reaction due to vaccination
136.29	Other specific infections by free-living amebae
495.8	Other specified allergic alveolitis and pneumonitis
516.8	Other specified alveolar and parietoalveolar pneumonopathies
126.8	Other specified ancylostoma
747.89	Other specified anomalies of circulatory system
750.4	Other specified anomalies of esophagus
065.8	Other specified arthropod-borne hemorrhagic fever
066.8	Other specified arthropod-borne viral diseases
093.89	Other specified cardiovascular syphilis
330.8	Other specified cerebral degenerations in childhood
123.8	Other specified cestode infection
639.8	Other specified complications following abortion or ectopic and molar pregnancy
426.89	Other specified conduction disorders
759.89	Other specified congenital anomalies
742.4	Other specified congenital anomalies of brain
753.19	Other specified cystic kidney disease
710.8	Other specified diffuse diseases of connective tissue
032.89	Other specified diphtheria
423.8	Other specified diseases of pericardium
270.8	Other specified disorders of amino-acid metabolism
271.8	Other specified disorders of carbohydrate transport and metabolism
277.89	Other specified disorders of metabolism
304.61	Other specified drug dependence, continuous
296.99	Other specified episodic mood disorder
125.6	Other specified filariasis
619.8	Other specified fistulas involving female genital tract
511.89	Other specified forms of effusion, except tuberculous
095.8	Other specified forms of late symptomatic syphilis
342.81	Other specified hemiplegia and hemiparesis affecting dominant side
342.82	Other specified hemiplegia and hemiparesis affecting nondominant side
342.80	Other specified hemiplegia and hemiparesis affecting unspecified side
282.8	Other specified hereditary hemolytic anemias
446.29	Other specified hypersensitivity angiitis
647.83	Other specified infectious and parasitic diseases of mother, antepartum condition or complication
647.82	Other specified infectious and parasitic diseases of mother, delivered, with mention of postpartum complication
647.81	Other specified infectious and parasitic diseases of mother, delivered, with or without mention of antepartum condition
647.84	Other specified infectious and parasitic diseases of mother, postpartum condition or complication

127.7	Other specified intestinal helminthiasis
579.8	Other specified intestinal malabsorption
560.89	Other specified intestinal obstruction
030.8	Other specified leprosy
100.89	Other specified leptospiral infections
207.82	Other specified leukemia, in relapse
207.81	Other specified leukemia, in remission
207.80	Other specified leukemia, without mention of having achieved remission
022.8	Other specified manifestations of anthrax
036.89	Other specified meningococcal infections
651.83	Other specified multiple gestation, antepartum condition or complication
651.81	Other specified multiple gestation, delivered, with or without mention of antepartum condition
031.8	Other specified mycobacterial diseases
094.89	Other specified neurosyphilis
049.8	Other specified non-arthropod-borne viral diseases of central nervous system
754.89	Other specified nonteratogenic anomalies
870.8	Other specified open wounds of ocular adnexa
299.80	Other specified pervasive developmental disorders, current or active state
299.81	Other specified pervasive developmental disorders, residual state
007.8	Other specified protozoal intestinal diseases
011.81	Other specified pulmonary tuberculosis, bacteriological or histological examination not done
011.82	Other specified pulmonary tuberculosis, bacteriological or histological examination unknown (at present)
011.83	Other specified pulmonary tuberculosis, tubercle bacilli found (in sputum) by microscopy
011.84	Other specified pulmonary tuberculosis, tubercle bacilli not found (in sputum) by microscopy, but found by bacterial culture
011.85	Other specified pulmonary tuberculosis, tubercle bacilli not found by bacteriological examination, but tuberculosis confirmed histologically
011.86	Other specified pulmonary tuberculosis, tubercle bacilli not found by bacteriological or histological examination, but tuberculosis confirmed by other methods [inoculation of animals]
011.80	Other specified pulmonary tuberculosis, unspecified
012.81	Other specified respiratory tuberculosis, bacteriological or histological examination not done
012.82	Other specified respiratory tuberculosis, bacteriological or histological examination unknown (at present)
012.83	Other specified respiratory tuberculosis, tubercle bacilli found (in sputum) by microscopy
012.84	Other specified respiratory tuberculosis, tubercle bacilli not found (in sputum) by microscopy, but found by bacterial culture
012.85	Other specified respiratory tuberculosis, tubercle bacilli not found by bacteriological examination, but tuberculosis confirmed histologically
012.86	Other specified respiratory tuberculosis, tubercle bacilli not found by bacteriological or histological examination, but tuberculosis confirmed by other methods [inoculation of animals]
012.80	Other specified respiratory tuberculosis, unspecified
083.8	Other specified rickettsioses
003.8	Other specified salmonella infections
120.8	Other specified schistosomiasis
290.8	Other specified senile psychotic conditions
046.8	Other specified slow virus infection of central nervous system
082.8	Other specified tick-borne rickettsioses
435.8	Other specified transient cerebral ischemias
121.8	Other specified trematode infections

021.8	Other specified tularemia
295.82	Other specified types of schizophrenia, chronic
295.84	Other specified types of schizophrenia, chronic with acute exacerbation
295.81	Other specified types of schizophrenia, subchronic
295.83	Other specified types of schizophrenia, subchronic with acute exacerbation
295.80	Other specified types of schizophrenia, unspecified
070.59	Other specified viral hepatitis without mention of hepatic coma
047.8	Other specified viral meningitis
027.8	Other specified zoonotic bacterial diseases
335.19	Other spinal muscular atrophy
334.8	Other spinocerebellar diseases
644.13	Other threatened labor, antepartum condition or complication
065.3	Other tick-borne hemorrhagic fever
519.09	Other tracheostomy complications
776.3	Other transient neonatal disorders of coagulation
014.81	Other tuberculosis of intestines, peritoneum, and mesenteric glands, bacteriological or histological examination not done
014.82	Other tuberculosis of intestines, peritoneum, and mesenteric glands, bacteriological or histological examination unknown (at present)
014.83	Other tuberculosis of intestines, peritoneum, and mesenteric glands, tubercle bacilli found (in sputum) by microscopy
014.84	Other tuberculosis of intestines, peritoneum, and mesenteric glands, tubercle bacilli not found (in sputum) by microscopy, but found by bacterial culture
014.85	Other tuberculosis of intestines, peritoneum, and mesenteric glands, tubercle bacilli not found by bacteriological examination, but tuberculosis confirmed histologically
014.86	Other tuberculosis of intestines, peritoneum, and mesenteric glands, tubercle bacilli not found by bacteriological or histological examination, but tuberculosis confirmed by other methods [inoculation of animals]
014.80	Other tuberculosis of intestines, peritoneum, and mesenteric glands, unspecified
556.8	Other ulcerative colitis
593.4	Other ureteric obstruction
999.2	Other vascular complications of medical care, not elsewhere classified
099.56	Other venereal diseases due to chlamydia trachomatis, peritoneum
647.23	Other venereal diseases of mother, complicating pregnancy, childbirth, or the puerperium, antepartum condition or complication
647.22	Other venereal diseases of mother, complicating pregnancy, childbirth, or the puerperium, delivered, with mention of postpartum complication
647.21	Other venereal diseases of mother, complicating pregnancy, childbirth, or the puerperium, delivered, with or without mention of antepartum condition
647.24	Other venereal diseases of mother, complicating pregnancy, childbirth, or the puerperium, postpartum condition or complication
671.83	Other venous complications of pregnancy and the puerperium, antepartum condition or complication
671.82	Other venous complications of pregnancy and the puerperium, delivered, with mention of postpartum complication
671.81	Other venous complications of pregnancy and the puerperium, delivered, with or without mention of antepartum condition
671.84	Other venous complications of pregnancy and the puerperium, postpartum condition or complication
671.80	Other venous complications of pregnancy and the puerperium, unspecified as to episode of care or not applicable
453.3	Other venous embolism and thrombosis of renal vein
453.9	Other venous embolism and thrombosis of unspecified site

552.29	Other ventral hernia with obstruction
647.63	Other viral diseases in the mother, antepartum condition or complication
647.62	Other viral diseases in the mother, delivered, with mention of postpartum complication
647.61	Other viral diseases in the mother, delivered, with or without mention of antepartum condition
647.64	Other viral diseases in the mother, postpartum condition or complication
827.1	Other, multiple and ill-defined fractures of lower limb, open
053.71	Otitis externa due to herpes zoster
084.3	Ovale malaria
633.21	Ovarian pregnancy with intrauterine pregnancy
633.20	Ovarian pregnancy without intrauterine pregnancy
V42.83	Pancreas replaced by transplant
579.4	Pancreatic steatorrhea
253.2	Panhypopituitarism
360.02	Panophthalmitis
360.12	Panuveitis
377.01	Papilledema associated with increased intracranial pressure
377.00	Papilledema, unspecified
116.1	Paracoccidioidomycosis
121.2	Paragonimiasis
560.1	Paralytic ileus
295.32	Paranoid type schizophrenia, chronic
295.34	Paranoid type schizophrenia, chronic with acute exacerbation
295.31	Paranoid type schizophrenia, subchronic
295.33	Paranoid type schizophrenia, subchronic with acute exacerbation
295.30	Paranoid type schizophrenia, unspecified
478.22	Parapharyngeal abscess
344.1	Paraplegia
360.13	Parasitic endophthalmitis NOS
002.1	Paratyphoid fever A
002.2	Paratyphoid fever B
002.3	Paratyphoid fever C
002.9	Paratyphoid fever, unspecified
427.0	Paroxysmal supraventricular tachycardia
427.1	Paroxysmal ventricular tachycardia
747.42	Partial anomalous pulmonary venous connection
362.33	Partial retinal arterial occlusion
079.83	Parvovirus B19
027.2	Pasteurellosis
758.1	Patau's syndrome
747.0	Patent ductus arteriosus
733.12	Pathologic fracture of distal radius and ulna
733.11	Pathologic fracture of humerus
733.14	Pathologic fracture of neck of femur
733.15	Pathologic fracture of other specified part of femur
733.19	Pathologic fracture of other specified site
733.16	Pathologic fracture of tibia or fibula
733.13	Pathologic fracture of vertebrae
733.10	Pathologic fracture, unspecified site
665.72	Pelvic hematoma, delivered with mention of postpartum complication
665.71	Pelvic hematoma, delivered, with or without mention of antepartum condition
694.5	Pemphigoid
694.4	Pemphigus
870.4	Penetrating wound of orbit with foreign body
870.3	Penetrating wound of orbit, without mention of foreign body

871.6	Penetration of eyeball with (nonmagnetic) foreign body
871.5	Penetration of eyeball with magnetic foreign body
996.44	Peri-prosthetic fracture around prosthetic joint
996.45	Peri-prosthetic osteolysis
337.1	Peripheral autonomic neuropathy in disorders classified elsewhere
V42.82	Peripheral stem cells replaced by transplant
202.73	Peripheral T cell lymphoma, intra-abdominal lymph nodes
202.76	Peripheral T cell lymphoma, intrapelvic lymph nodes
202.72	Peripheral T cell lymphoma, intrathoracic lymph nodes
202.74	Peripheral T cell lymphoma, lymph nodes of axilla and upper limb
202.71	Peripheral T cell lymphoma, lymph nodes of head, face, and neck
202.75	Peripheral T cell lymphoma, lymph nodes of inguinal region and lower limb
202.78	Peripheral T cell lymphoma, lymph nodes of multiple sites
202.77	Peripheral T cell lymphoma, spleen
202.70	Peripheral T cell lymphoma, unspecified site, extranodal and solid organ sites
997.2	Peripheral vascular complications, not elsewhere classified
568.82	Peritoneal effusion (chronic)
475	Peritonsillar abscess
277.86	Peroxisomal disorders
346.63	Persistent migraine aura with cerebral infarction, with intractable migraine, so stated, with status migrainosus
346.61	Persistent migraine aura with cerebral infarction, with intractable migraine, so stated, without mention of status migrainosus
346.62	Persistent migraine aura with cerebral infarction, without mention of intractable migraine with status migrainosus
346.60	Persistent migraine aura with cerebral infarction, without mention of intractable migraine without mention of status migrainosus
998.6	Persistent postoperative fistula
780.03	Persistent vegetative state
270.1	Phenylketonuria [PKU]
451.19	Phlebitis and thrombophlebitis of deep veins of lower extremities, other
451.83	Phlebitis and thrombophlebitis of deep veins of upper extremities
451.11	Phlebitis and thrombophlebitis of femoral vein (deep) (superficial)
451.81	Phlebitis and thrombophlebitis of iliac vein
451.89	Phlebitis and thrombophlebitis of other sites
066.0	Phlebotomus fever
685.0	Pilonidal cyst with abscess
641.03	Placenta previa without hemorrhage, antepartum condition or complication
641.01	Placenta previa without hemorrhage, delivered, with or without mention of antepartum condition
203.12	Plasma cell leukemia, in relapse
203.11	Plasma cell leukemia, in remission
203.10	Plasma cell leukemia, without mention of having achieved remission
446.0	Polyarteritis nodosa
714.31	Polyarticular juvenile rheumatoid arthritis, acute
753.13	Polycystic kidney, autosomal dominant
753.14	Polycystic kidney, autosomal recessive
753.12	Polycystic kidney, unspecified type
657.01	Polyhydramnios, delivered, with or without mention of antepartum condition
710.4	Polymyositis
656.51	Poor fetal growth, affecting management of mother, delivered, with or without mention of antepartum condition
572.3	Portal hypertension
780.33	Post traumatic seizures
238.77	Post-transplant lymphoproliferative disorder (PTLD)

711.37	Postdysenteric arthropathy, ankle and foot
711.33	Postdysenteric arthropathy, forearm
711.34	Postdysenteric arthropathy, hand
711.36	Postdysenteric arthropathy, lower leg
711.39	Postdysenteric arthropathy, multiple sites
711.38	Postdysenteric arthropathy, other specified sites
711.35	Postdysenteric arthropathy, pelvic region and thigh
711.31	Postdysenteric arthropathy, shoulder region
711.30	Postdysenteric arthropathy, site unspecified
711.32	Postdysenteric arthropathy, upper arm
836.62	Posterior dislocation of tibia, proximal end, open
053.13	Postherpetic polyneuropathy
053.12	Postherpetic trigeminal neuralgia
411.0	Postmyocardial infarction syndrome
512.2	Postoperative air leak
998.00	Postoperative shock, unspecified
666.32	Postpartum coagulation defects, delivered, with mention of postpartum complication
459.11	Postphlebetic syndrome with ulcer
459.13	Postphlebetic syndrome with ulcer and inflammation
997.32	Postprocedural aspiration pneumonia
251.3	Postsurgical hypoinsulinemia
958.3	Posttraumatic wound infection not elsewhere classified
569.71	Pouchitis
759.81	Prader-Willi syndrome
790.01	Precipitous drop in hematocrit
641.23	Premature separation of placenta, antepartum condition or complication
290.11	Presenile dementia with delirium
290.12	Presenile dementia with delusional features
290.13	Presenile dementia with depressive features
607.3	Priapism
770.81	Primary apnea of newborn
770.4	Primary atelectasis
200.53	Primary central nervous system lymphoma, intra-abdominal lymph nodes
200.56	Primary central nervous system lymphoma, intrapelvic lymph nodes
200.52	Primary central nervous system lymphoma, intrathoracic lymph nodes
200.54	Primary central nervous system lymphoma, lymph nodes of axilla and upper limb
200.51	Primary central nervous system lymphoma, lymph nodes of head, face, and neck
200.55	Primary central nervous system lymphoma, lymph nodes of inguinal region and lower limb
200.58	Primary central nervous system lymphoma, lymph nodes of multiple sites
200.57	Primary central nervous system lymphoma, spleen
200.50	Primary central nervous system lymphoma, unspecified site, extranodal and solid organ sites
334.2	Primary cerebellar degeneration
114.0	Primary coccidioidomycosis (pulmonary)
114.1	Primary extrapulmonary coccidioidomycosis
289.81	Primary hypercoagulable state
364.01	Primary iridocyclitis
335.24	Primary lateral sclerosis
416.0	Primary pulmonary hypertension
512.81	Primary spontaneous pneumothorax
010.01	Primary tuberculous infection, bacteriological or histological examination not done

010.02	Primary tuberculous infection, bacteriological or histological examination unknown (at present)
010.03	Primary tuberculous infection, tubercle bacilli found (in sputum) by microscopy
010.04	Primary tuberculous infection, tubercle bacilli not found (in sputum) by microscopy, but found by bacterial culture
010.05	Primary tuberculous infection, tubercle bacilli not found by bacteriological examination, but tuberculosis confirmed histologically
010.06	Primary tuberculous infection, tubercle bacilli not found by bacteriological or histological examination, but tuberculosis confirmed by other methods [inoculation of animals]
010.00	Primary tuberculous infection, unspecified
010.91	Primary tuberculous infection, unspecified, bacteriological or histological examination not done
010.92	Primary tuberculous infection, unspecified, bacteriological or histological examination unknown (at present)
010.93	Primary tuberculous infection, unspecified, tubercle bacilli found (in sputum) by microscopy
010.94	Primary tuberculous infection, unspecified, tubercle bacilli not found (in sputum) by microscopy, but found by bacterial culture
010.95	Primary tuberculous infection, unspecified, tubercle bacilli not found by bacteriological examination, but tuberculosis confirmed histologically
010.96	Primary tuberculous infection, unspecified, tubercle bacilli not found by bacteriological or histological examination, but tuberculosis confirmed by other methods [inoculation of animals]
010.90	Primary tuberculous infection, unspecified, unspecified
413.1	Prinzmetal angina
318.2	Profound intellectual disabilities
335.22	Progressive bulbar palsy
046.3	Progressive multifocal leukoencephalopathy
335.21	Progressive muscular atrophy
335.23	Pseudobulbar palsy
556.4	Pseudopolyposis of colon
136.4	Psorospermiasis
298.4	Psychogenic paranoid psychosis
293.81	Psychotic disorder with delusions in conditions classified elsewhere
293.82	Psychotic disorder with hallucinations in conditions classified elsewhere
670.12	Puerperal endometritis, delivered, with mention of postpartum complication
670.14	Puerperal endometritis, postpartum condition or complication
670.10	Puerperal endometritis, unspecified as to episode of care or not applicable
670.20	Puerperal sepsis, unspecified as to episode of care or not applicable
670.30	Puerperal septic thrombophlebitis, unspecified as to episode of care or not applicable
039.1	Pulmonary actinomycotic infection
516.2	Pulmonary alveolar microlithiasis
516.0	Pulmonary alveolar proteinosis
114.5	Pulmonary coccidioidomycosis, unspecified
518.0	Pulmonary collapse
514	Pulmonary congestion and hypostasis
031.0	Pulmonary diseases due to other mycobacteria
518.3	Pulmonary eosinophilia
011.91	Pulmonary tuberculosis, unspecified, bacteriological or histological examination not done
011.92	Pulmonary tuberculosis, unspecified, bacteriological or histological examination unknown (at present)
011.93	Pulmonary tuberculosis, unspecified, tubercle bacilli found (in sputum) by microscopy

011.94	Pulmonary tuberculosis, unspecified, tubercle bacilli not found (in sputum) by microscopy, but found by bacterial culture
011.95	Pulmonary tuberculosis, unspecified, tubercle bacilli not found by bacteriological examination, but tuberculosis confirmed histologically
011.96	Pulmonary tuberculosis, unspecified, tubercle bacilli not found by bacteriological or histological examination, but tuberculosis confirmed by other methods [inoculation of animals]
011.90	Pulmonary tuberculosis, unspecified, unspecified
021.2	Pulmonary tularemia
522.0	Pulpitis
360.00	Purulent endophthalmitis, unspecified
590.81	Pyelitis or pyelonephritis in diseases classified elsewhere
590.80	Pyelonephritis, unspecified
590.3	Pyeloureteritis cystica
686.01	Pyoderma gangrenosum
711.07	Pyogenic arthritis, ankle and foot
711.03	Pyogenic arthritis, forearm
711.04	Pyogenic arthritis, hand
711.06	Pyogenic arthritis, lower leg
711.09	Pyogenic arthritis, multiple sites
711.08	Pyogenic arthritis, other specified sites
711.05	Pyogenic arthritis, pelvic region and thigh
711.01	Pyogenic arthritis, shoulder region
711.00	Pyogenic arthritis, site unspecified
711.02	Pyogenic arthritis, upper arm
672.02	Pyrexia of unknown origin during the puerperium, delivered, with mention of postpartum complication
672.04	Pyrexia of unknown origin during the puerperium, postpartum condition or complication
083.0	Q fever
651.53	Quadruplet pregnancy with fetal loss and retention of one or more fetus(es), antepartum condition or complication
651.51	Quadruplet pregnancy with fetal loss and retention of one or more fetus(es), delivered, with or without mention of antepartum condition
651.23	Quadruplet pregnancy, antepartum condition or complication
651.21	Quadruplet pregnancy, delivered, with or without mention of antepartum condition
084.2	Quartan malaria
082.3	Queensland tick typhus
071	Rabies
364.02	Recurrent iridocyclitis
646.31	Recurrent pregnancy loss, delivered, with or without mention of antepartum condition
337.29	Reflex sympathetic dystrophy of other specified site
337.22	Reflex sympathetic dystrophy of the lower limb
337.21	Reflex sympathetic dystrophy of the upper limb
337.20	Reflex sympathetic dystrophy, unspecified
356.3	Refsum's disease
555.1	Regional enteritis of large intestine
555.0	Regional enteritis of small intestine
555.2	Regional enteritis of small intestine with large intestine
555.9	Regional enteritis of unspecified site
087.0	Relapsing fever, louse-borne
087.1	Relapsing fever, tick-borne
087.9	Relapsing fever, unspecified
753.0	Renal agenesis and dysgenesis
753.15	Renal dysplasia
997.41	Retained cholelithiasis following cholecystectomy
200.03	Reticulosarcoma, intra-abdominal lymph nodes

200.06	Reticulosarcoma, intrapelvic lymph nodes
200.02	Reticulosarcoma, intrathoracic lymph nodes
200.04	Reticulosarcoma, lymph nodes of axilla and upper limb
200.01	Reticulosarcoma, lymph nodes of head, face, and neck
200.05	Reticulosarcoma, lymph nodes of inguinal region and lower limb
200.08	Reticulosarcoma, lymph nodes of multiple sites
200.07	Reticulosarcoma, spleen
200.00	Reticulosarcoma, unspecified site, extranodal and solid organ sites
362.32	Retinal arterial branch occlusion
362.84	Retinal ischemia
362.40	Retinal layer separation, unspecified
362.30	Retinal vascular occlusion, unspecified
377.32	Retrobulbar neuritis (acute)
478.24	Retropharyngeal abscess
999.70	Rh incompatibility reaction, unspecified
999.72	Rh incompatibility with acute hemolytic transfusion reaction
999.73	Rh incompatibility with delayed hemolytic transfusion reaction
999.71	Rh incompatibility with hemolytic transfusion reaction not specified as acute or delayed
728.88	Rhabdomyolysis
656.13	Rhesus isoimmunization, antepartum condition or complication
392.0	Rheumatic chorea with heart involvement
392.9	Rheumatic chorea without mention of heart involvement
398.91	Rheumatic heart failure (congestive)
398.0	Rheumatic myocarditis
517.1	Rheumatic pneumonia
086.4	Rhodesian trypanosomiasis
268.0	Rickets, active
083.2	Rickettsialpox
083.9	Rickettsiosis, unspecified
647.53	Rubella in the mother, antepartum condition or complication
647.52	Rubella in the mother, delivered, with mention of postpartum complication
647.51	Rubella in the mother, delivered, with or without mention of antepartum condition
647.54	Rubella in the mother, postpartum condition or complication
056.09	Rubella with other neurological complications
056.79	Rubella with other specified complications
056.00	Rubella with unspecified neurological complication
447.2	Rupture of artery
871.2	Rupture of eye with partial loss of intraocular tissue
003.23	Salmonella arthritis
003.0	Salmonella gastroenteritis
003.9	Salmonella infection, unspecified
003.24	Salmonella osteomyelitis
136.5	Sarcosporidiosis
079.82	SARS-associated coronavirus
034.1	Scarlet fever
341.1	Schilder's disease
120.0	Schistosomiasis due to schistosoma haematobium
120.2	Schistosomiasis due to schistosoma japonicum
120.1	Schistosomiasis due to schistosoma mansoni
120.9	Schistosomiasis, unspecified
295.72	Schizoaffective disorder, chronic
295.74	Schizoaffective disorder, chronic with acute exacerbation
295.71	Schizoaffective disorder, subchronic
295.73	Schizoaffective disorder, subchronic with acute exacerbation
295.62	Schizophrenic disorders, residual type, chronic
295.64	Schizophrenic disorders, residual type, chronic with acute exacerbation

295.61	Schizophrenic disorders, residual type, subchronic
295.63	Schizophrenic disorders, residual type, subchronic with acute exacerbation
295.60	Schizophrenic disorders, residual type, unspecified
295.42	Schizophreniform disorder, chronic
295.44	Schizophreniform disorder, chronic with acute exacerbation
295.41	Schizophreniform disorder, subchronic
295.43	Schizophreniform disorder, subchronic with acute exacerbation
295.40	Schizophreniform disorder, unspecified
778.1	Sclerema neonatorum
567.82	Sclerosing mesenteritis
081.2	Scrub typhus
958.2	Secondary and recurrent hemorrhage
196.2	Secondary and unspecified malignant neoplasm of intra-abdominal lymph nodes
196.6	Secondary and unspecified malignant neoplasm of intrapelvic lymph nodes
196.1	Secondary and unspecified malignant neoplasm of intrathoracic lymph nodes
196.3	Secondary and unspecified malignant neoplasm of lymph nodes of axilla and upper limb
196.0	Secondary and unspecified malignant neoplasm of lymph nodes of head, face, and neck
196.5	Secondary and unspecified malignant neoplasm of lymph nodes of inguinal region and lower limb
196.8	Secondary and unspecified malignant neoplasm of lymph nodes of multiple sites
196.9	Secondary and unspecified malignant neoplasm of lymph nodes, site unspecified
425.9	Secondary cardiomyopathy, unspecified
289.82	Secondary hypercoagulable state
588.81	Secondary hyperparathyroidism (of renal origin)
364.03	Secondary iridocyclitis, infectious
198.7	Secondary malignant neoplasm of adrenal gland
198.5	Secondary malignant neoplasm of bone and bone marrow
198.3	Secondary malignant neoplasm of brain and spinal cord
198.81	Secondary malignant neoplasm of breast
198.82	Secondary malignant neoplasm of genital organs
198.0	Secondary malignant neoplasm of kidney
197.5	Secondary malignant neoplasm of large intestine and rectum
197.0	Secondary malignant neoplasm of lung
197.1	Secondary malignant neoplasm of mediastinum
197.8	Secondary malignant neoplasm of other digestive organs and spleen
198.4	Secondary malignant neoplasm of other parts of nervous system
197.3	Secondary malignant neoplasm of other respiratory organs
198.89	Secondary malignant neoplasm of other specified sites
198.1	Secondary malignant neoplasm of other urinary organs
198.6	Secondary malignant neoplasm of ovary
197.2	Secondary malignant neoplasm of pleura
197.6	Secondary malignant neoplasm of retroperitoneum and peritoneum
198.2	Secondary malignant neoplasm of skin
197.4	Secondary malignant neoplasm of small intestine including duodenum
209.73	Secondary neuroendocrine tumor of bone
209.71	Secondary neuroendocrine tumor of distant lymph nodes
209.72	Secondary neuroendocrine tumor of liver
209.79	Secondary neuroendocrine tumor of other sites
209.74	Secondary neuroendocrine tumor of peritoneum
332.1	Secondary parkinsonism
512.82	Secondary spontaneous pneumothorax
091.69	Secondary syphilis of other viscera
091.3	Secondary syphilis of skin or mucous membranes
091.7	Secondary syphilis, relapse
091.62	Secondary syphilitic hepatitis
091.61	Secondary syphilitic periostitis
304.11	Sedative, hypnotic or anxiolytic dependence, continuous
279.01	Selective IgA immunodeficiency
279.02	Selective IgM immunodeficiency
290.3	Senile dementia with delirium
290.20	Senile dementia with delusional features
290.21	Senile dementia with depressive features
449	Septic arterial embolism
998.13	Seroma complicating a procedure
363.71	Serous choroidal detachment
362.42	Serous detachment of retinal pigment epithelium
361.2	Serous retinal detachment
318.1	Severe intellectual disabilities
202.23	Sezary's disease, intra-abdominal lymph nodes
202.26	Sezary's disease, intrapelvic lymph nodes
202.22	Sezary's disease, intrathoracic lymph nodes
202.24	Sezary's disease, lymph nodes of axilla and upper limb
202.21	Sezary's disease, lymph nodes of head, face, and neck
202.25	Sezary's disease, lymph nodes of inguinal region and lower limb
202.28	Sezary's disease, lymph nodes of multiple sites
202.27	Sezary's disease, spleen
202.20	Sezary's disease, unspecified site, extranodal and solid organ sites
995.55	Shaken baby syndrome
004.0	Shigella dysenteriae
995.4	Shock due to anesthesia, not elsewhere classified
785.50	Shock, unspecified
295.02	Simple type schizophrenia, chronic
295.04	Simple type schizophrenia, chronic with acute exacerbation
295.01	Simple type schizophrenia, subchronic
295.03	Simple type schizophrenia, subchronic with acute exacerbation
295.00	Simple type schizophrenia, unspecified
759.3	Situs inversus
050.9	Smallpox, unspecified
123.5	Sparganosis [larval diphyllobothriasis]
342.11	Spastic hemiplegia and hemiparesis affecting dominant side
342.12	Spastic hemiplegia and hemiparesis affecting nondominant side
342.10	Spastic hemiplegia and hemiparesis affecting unspecified side
741.01	Spina bifida with hydrocephalus, cervical region
741.02	Spina bifida with hydrocephalus, dorsal (thoracic) region
741.03	Spina bifida with hydrocephalus, lumbar region
741.00	Spina bifida with hydrocephalus, unspecified region
335.10	Spinal muscular atrophy, unspecified
747.82	Spinal vessel anomaly
334.9	Spinocerebellar disease, unspecified
026.0	Spirillary fever
721.91	Spondylosis of unspecified site, with myelopathy
721.42	Spondylosis with myelopathy, lumbar region
721.41	Spondylosis with myelopathy, thoracic region
634.22	Spontaneous abortion, complicated by damage to pelvic organs or tissues, complete
634.21	Spontaneous abortion, complicated by damage to pelvic organs or tissues, incomplete
634.20	Spontaneous abortion, complicated by damage to pelvic organs or tissues, unspecified

634.60	Spontaneous abortion, complicated by embolism, unspecified
634.02	Spontaneous abortion, complicated by genital tract and pelvic infection, complete
634.01	Spontaneous abortion, complicated by genital tract and pelvic infection, incomplete
634.00	Spontaneous abortion, complicated by genital tract and pelvic infection, unspecified
634.42	Spontaneous abortion, complicated by metabolic disorder, complete
634.41	Spontaneous abortion, complicated by metabolic disorder, incomplete
634.40	Spontaneous abortion, complicated by metabolic disorder, unspecified
634.72	Spontaneous abortion, with other specified complications, complete
634.71	Spontaneous abortion, with other specified complications, incomplete
634.70	Spontaneous abortion, with other specified complications, unspecified
634.82	Spontaneous abortion, with unspecified complication, complete
634.81	Spontaneous abortion, with unspecified complication, incomplete
634.80	Spontaneous abortion, with unspecified complication, unspecified
082.0	Spotted fevers
005.0	Staphylococcal food poisoning
746.02	Stenosis of pulmonary valve, congenital
695.13	Stevens-Johnson syndrome
695.14	Stevens-Johnson syndrome-toxic epidermal necrolysis overlap syndrome
333.91	Stiff-man syndrome
026.1	Streptobacillary fever
127.2	Strongyloidiasis
336.2	Subacute combined degeneration of spinal cord in diseases classified elsewhere
293.1	Subacute delirium
208.22	Subacute leukemia of unspecified cell type, in relapse
208.21	Subacute leukemia of unspecified cell type, in remission
208.20	Subacute leukemia of unspecified cell type, without mention of having achieved remission
204.22	Subacute lymphoid leukemia, in relapse
204.21	Subacute lymphoid leukemia, in remission
204.20	Subacute lymphoid leukemia, without mention of having achieved remission
206.22	Subacute monocytic leukemia, in relapse
206.21	Subacute monocytic leukemia, in remission
206.20	Subacute monocytic leukemia, without mention of having achieved remission
205.22	Subacute myeloid leukemia, in relapse
205.20	Subacute myeloid leukemia, without mention of having achieved remission
205.21	Subacute myeloid leukemia, in remission
046.2	Subacute sclerosing panencephalitis
435.2	Subclavian steal syndrome
383.01	Subperiosteal abscess of mastoid
368.11	Sudden visual loss
V62.84	Suicidal ideation
671.23	Superficial thrombophlebitis complicating pregnancy and the puerperium, antepartum condition or complication
671.22	Superficial thrombophlebitis complicating pregnancy and the puerperium, delivered, with mention of postpartum complication
671.21	Superficial thrombophlebitis complicating pregnancy and the puerperium, delivered, with or without mention of antepartum condition

671.24	Superficial thrombophlebitis complicating pregnancy and the puerperium, postpartum condition or complication
671.20	Superficial thrombophlebitis complicating pregnancy and the puerperium, unspecified as to episode of care or not applicable
060.0	Sylvatic yellow fever
360.11	Sympathetic uveitis
359.6	Symptomatic inflammatory myopathy in diseases classified elsewhere
095.5	Syphilis of bone
095.4	Syphilis of kidney
095.3	Syphilis of liver
095.1	Syphilis of lung
647.03	Syphilis of mother, complicating pregnancy, childbirth, or the puerperium, antepartum condition or complication
647.02	Syphilis of mother, complicating pregnancy, childbirth, or the puerperium, delivered, with mention of postpartum complication
647.01	Syphilis of mother, complicating pregnancy, childbirth, or the puerperium, delivered, with or without mention of antepartum condition
647.04	Syphilis of mother, complicating pregnancy, childbirth, or the puerperium, postpartum condition or complication
095.6	Syphilis of muscle
095.7	Syphilis of synovium, tendon, and bursa
094.86	Syphilitic acoustic neuritis
091.82	Syphilitic alopecia
093.1	Syphilitic aortitis
091.51	Syphilitic chorioretinitis (secondary)
094.83	Syphilitic disseminated retinochoroiditis
093.22	Syphilitic endocarditis of aortic valve
093.21	Syphilitic endocarditis of mitral valve
093.24	Syphilitic endocarditis of pulmonary valve
093.23	Syphilitic endocarditis of tricuspid valve
093.20	Syphilitic endocarditis of valve, unspecified
095.0	Syphilitic episcleritis
090.3	Syphilitic interstitial keratitis
091.52	Syphilitic iridocyclitis (secondary)
093.82	Syphilitic myocarditis
094.84	Syphilitic optic atrophy
094.82	Syphilitic parkinsonism
093.81	Syphilitic pericarditis
095.2	Syphilitic peritonitis
094.85	Syphilitic retrobulbar neuritis
091.50	Syphilitic uveitis, unspecified
336.0	Syringomyelia and syringobulbia
995.93	Systemic inflammatory response syndrome due to noninfectious process without acute organ dysfunction
995.90	Systemic inflammatory response syndrome, unspecified
428.20	Systolic heart failure, unspecified
094.0	Tabes dorsalis
123.2	Taenia saginata infection
123.0	Taenia solium infection, intestinal form
123.3	Taeniasis, unspecified
446.7	Takayasu's disease
429.83	Takotsubo syndrome
059.21	Tanapox
781.7	Tetany
664.21	Third-degree perineal laceration, delivered, with or without mention of antepartum condition
666.02	Third-stage postpartum hemorrhage, delivered, with mention of postpartum complication

666.04	Third-stage postpartum hemorrhage, postpartum condition or complication
640.03	Threatened abortion, antepartum condition or complication
640.01	Threatened abortion, delivered, with or without mention of antepartum condition
453.1	Thrombophlebitis migrans
066.1	Tick-borne fever
082.9	Tick-borne rickettsiosis, unspecified
608.24	Torsion of appendix epididymis
608.23	Torsion of appendix testis
620.5	Torsion of ovary, ovarian pedicle, or fallopian tube
608.20	Torsion of testis, unspecified
813.45	Torus fracture of radius (alone)
813.47	Torus fracture of radius and ulna
813.46	Torus fracture of ulna (alone)
823.42	Torus fracture, fibula with tibia
823.40	Torus fracture, tibia alone
747.41	Total anomalous pulmonary venous connection
695.15	Toxic epidermal necrolysis
695.0	Toxic erythema
558.2	Toxic gastroenteritis and colitis
359.4	Toxic myopathy
130.7	Toxoplasmosis of other specified sites
130.9	Toxoplasmosis, unspecified
519.00	Tracheostomy complication, unspecified
361.81	Traction detachment of retina
518.7	Transfusion related acute lung injury (TRALI)
642.31	Transient hypertension of pregnancy, delivered , with or without mention of antepartum condition
642.32	Transient hypertension of pregnancy, delivered, with mention of postpartum complication
781.4	Transient paralysis of limb
362.34	Transient retinal arterial occlusion
368.12	Transient visual loss
777.4	Transitory ileus of newborn
887.3	Traumatic amputation of arm and hand (complete) (partial), unilateral, at or above elbow, complicated
887.2	Traumatic amputation of arm and hand (complete) (partial), unilateral, at or above elbow, without mention of complication
887.1	Traumatic amputation of arm and hand (complete) (partial), unilateral, below elbow, complicated
887.0	Traumatic amputation of arm and hand (complete) (partial), unilateral, below elbow, without mention of complication
887.5	Traumatic amputation of arm and hand (complete) (partial), unilateral, level not specified, complicated
887.4	Traumatic amputation of arm and hand (complete) (partial), unilateral, level not specified, without mention of complication
896.1	Traumatic amputation of foot (complete) (partial), unilateral, complicated
896.0	Traumatic amputation of foot (complete) (partial), unilateral, without mention of complication
897.3	Traumatic amputation of leg(s) (complete) (partial), unilateral, at or above knee, complicated
897.2	Traumatic amputation of leg(s) (complete) (partial), unilateral, at or above knee, without mention of complication
897.1	Traumatic amputation of leg(s) (complete) (partial), unilateral, below knee, complicated
897.0	Traumatic amputation of leg(s) (complete) (partial), unilateral, below knee, without mention of complication
897.5	Traumatic amputation of leg(s) (complete) (partial), unilateral, level not specified, complicated
897.4	Traumatic amputation of leg(s) (complete) (partial), unilateral, level not specified, without mention of complication

958.93	Traumatic compartment syndrome of abdomen
958.92	Traumatic compartment syndrome of lower extremity
958.99	Traumatic compartment syndrome of other sites
958.91	Traumatic compartment syndrome of upper extremity
860.0	Traumatic pneumothorax without mention of open wound into thorax
721.7	Traumatic spondylopathy
958.7	Traumatic subcutaneous emphysema
083.1	Trench fever
124	Trichinosis
127.6	Trichostrongyliasis
127.3	Trichuriasis
426.54	Trifascicular block
824.7	Trimalleolar fracture, open
651.43	Triplet pregnancy with fetal loss and retention of one or more fetus(es), antepartum condition or complication
651.41	Triplet pregnancy with fetal loss and retention of one or more fetus(es), delivered, with or without mention of antepartum condition
651.13	Triplet pregnancy, antepartum condition or complication
651.11	Triplet pregnancy, delivered, with or without mention of antepartum condition
040.81	Tropical pyomyositis
579.1	Tropical sprue
086.9	Trypanosomiasis, unspecified
633.11	Tubal pregnancy with intrauterine pregnancy
633.10	Tubal pregnancy without intrauterine pregnancy
030.1	Tuberculoid leprosy [type T]
017.61	Tuberculosis of adrenal glands, bacteriological or histological examination not done
017.62	Tuberculosis of adrenal glands, bacteriological or histological examination unknown (at present)
017.63	Tuberculosis of adrenal glands, tubercle bacilli found (in sputum) by microscopy
017.64	Tuberculosis of adrenal glands, tubercle bacilli not found (in sputum) by microscopy, but found by bacterial culture
017.65	Tuberculosis of adrenal glands, tubercle bacilli not found by bacteriological examination, but tuberculosis confirmed histologically
017.66	Tuberculosis of adrenal glands, tubercle bacilli not found by bacteriological or histological examination, but tuberculosis confirmed by other methods [inoculation of animals]
017.60	Tuberculosis of adrenal glands, unspecified
016.11	Tuberculosis of bladder, bacteriological or histological examination not done
016.12	Tuberculosis of bladder, bacteriological or histological examination unknown (at present)
016.13	Tuberculosis of bladder, tubercle bacilli found (in sputum) by microscopy
016.14	Tuberculosis of bladder, tubercle bacilli not found (in sputum) by microscopy, but found by bacterial culture
016.15	Tuberculosis of bladder, tubercle bacilli not found by bacteriological examination, but tuberculosis confirmed histologically
016.16	Tuberculosis of bladder, tubercle bacilli not found by bacteriological or histological examination, but tuberculosis confirmed by other methods [inoculation of animals]
016.10	Tuberculosis of bladder, unspecified
011.31	Tuberculosis of bronchus, bacteriological or histological examination not done
011.32	Tuberculosis of bronchus, bacteriological or histological examination unknown (at present)
011.33	Tuberculosis of bronchus, tubercle bacilli found (in sputum) by microscopy

011.34 Tuberculosis of bronchus, tubercle bacilli not found (in sputum) by microscopy, but found in bacterial culture

011.35 Tuberculosis of bronchus, tubercle bacilli not found by bacteriological examination, but tuberculosis confirmed histologically

011.36 Tuberculosis of bronchus, tubercle bacilli not found by bacteriological or histological examination, but tuberculosis confirmed by other methods [inoculation of animals]

011.30 Tuberculosis of bronchus, unspecified

017.41 Tuberculosis of ear, bacteriological or histological examination not done

017.42 Tuberculosis of ear, bacteriological or histological examination unknown (at present)

017.43 Tuberculosis of ear, tubercle bacilli found (in sputum) by microscopy

017.44 Tuberculosis of ear, tubercle bacilli not found (in sputum) by microscopy, but found by bacterial culture

017.45 Tuberculosis of ear, tubercle bacilli not found by bacteriological examination, but tuberculosis confirmed histologically

017.46 Tuberculosis of ear, tubercle bacilli not found by bacteriological or histological examination, but tuberculosis confirmed by other methods [inoculation of animals]

017.40 Tuberculosis of ear, unspecified

016.41 Tuberculosis of epididymis, bacteriological or histological examination not done

016.42 Tuberculosis of epididymis, bacteriological or histological examination unknown (at present)

016.43 Tuberculosis of epididymis, tubercle bacilli found (in sputum) by microscopy

016.44 Tuberculosis of epididymis, tubercle bacilli not found (in sputum) by microscopy, but found by bacterial culture

016.45 Tuberculosis of epididymis, tubercle bacilli not found by bacteriological examination, but tuberculosis confirmed histologically

016.46 Tuberculosis of epididymis, tubercle bacilli not found by bacteriological or histological examination, but tuberculosis confirmed by other methods [inoculation of animals]

016.40 Tuberculosis of epididymis, unspecified

017.81 Tuberculosis of esophagus, bacteriological or histological examination not done

017.82 Tuberculosis of esophagus, bacteriological or histological examination unknown (at present)

017.83 Tuberculosis of esophagus, tubercle bacilli found (in sputum) by microscopy

017.84 Tuberculosis of esophagus, tubercle bacilli not found (in sputum) by microscopy, but found by bacterial culture

017.85 Tuberculosis of esophagus, tubercle bacilli not found by bacteriological examination, but tuberculosis confirmed histologically

017.86 Tuberculosis of esophagus, tubercle bacilli not found by bacteriological or histological examination, but tuberculosis confirmed by other methods [inoculation of animals]

017.80 Tuberculosis of esophagus, unspecified

017.31 Tuberculosis of eye, bacteriological or histological examination not done

017.32 Tuberculosis of eye, bacteriological or histological examination unknown (at present)

017.33 Tuberculosis of eye, tubercle bacilli found (in sputum) by microscopy

017.34 Tuberculosis of eye, tubercle bacilli not found (in sputum) by microscopy, but found by bacterial culture

017.35 Tuberculosis of eye, tubercle bacilli not found by bacteriological examination, but tuberculosis confirmed histologically

017.36 Tuberculosis of eye, tubercle bacilli not found by bacteriological or histological examination, but tuberculosis confirmed by other methods [inoculation of animals]

017.30 Tuberculosis of eye, unspecified

015.11 Tuberculosis of hip, bacteriological or histological examination not done

015.12 Tuberculosis of hip, bacteriological or histological examination unknown (at present)

015.13 Tuberculosis of hip, tubercle bacilli found (in sputum) by microscopy

015.14 Tuberculosis of hip, tubercle bacilli not found (in sputum) by microscopy, but found by bacterial culture

015.15 Tuberculosis of hip, tubercle bacilli not found by bacteriological examination, but tuberculosis confirmed histologically

015.16 Tuberculosis of hip, tubercle bacilli not found by bacteriological or histological examination, but tuberculosis confirmed by other methods [inoculation of animals]

015.10 Tuberculosis of hip, unspecified

012.11 Tuberculosis of intrathoracic lymph nodes, bacteriological or histological examination not done

012.12 Tuberculosis of intrathoracic lymph nodes, bacteriological or histological examination unknown (at present)

012.13 Tuberculosis of intrathoracic lymph nodes, tubercle bacilli found (in sputum) by microscopy

012.14 Tuberculosis of intrathoracic lymph nodes, tubercle bacilli not found (in sputum) by microscopy, but found by bacterial culture

012.15 Tuberculosis of intrathoracic lymph nodes, tubercle bacilli not found by bacteriological examination, but tuberculosis confirmed histologically

012.16 Tuberculosis of intrathoracic lymph nodes, tubercle bacilli not found by bacteriological or histological examination, but tuberculosis confirmed by other methods [inoculation of animals]

012.10 Tuberculosis of intrathoracic lymph nodes, unspecified

016.01 Tuberculosis of kidney, bacteriological or histological examination not done

016.02 Tuberculosis of kidney, bacteriological or histological examination unknown (at present)

016.03 Tuberculosis of kidney, tubercle bacilli found (in sputum) by microscopy

016.04 Tuberculosis of kidney, tubercle bacilli not found (in sputum) by microscopy, but found by bacterial culture

016.05 Tuberculosis of kidney, tubercle bacilli not found by bacteriological examination, but tuberculosis confirmed histologically

016.06 Tuberculosis of kidney, tubercle bacilli not found by bacteriological or histological examination, but tuberculosis confirmed by other methods [inoculation of animals]

016.00 Tuberculosis of kidney, unspecified

015.21 Tuberculosis of knee, bacteriological or histological examination not done

015.22 Tuberculosis of knee, bacteriological or histological examination unknown (at present)

015.23 Tuberculosis of knee, tubercle bacilli found (in sputum) by microscopy

015.24 Tuberculosis of knee, tubercle bacilli not found (in sputum) by microscopy, but found by bacterial culture

015.25 Tuberculosis of knee, tubercle bacilli not found by bacteriological examination, but tuberculosis confirmed histologically

015.26 Tuberculosis of knee, tubercle bacilli not found by bacteriological or histological examination, but tuberculosis confirmed by other methods [inoculation of animals]

015.20 Tuberculosis of knee, unspecified

015.51 Tuberculosis of limb bones, bacteriological or histological examination not done

015.52 Tuberculosis of limb bones, bacteriological or histological examination unknown (at present)

015.53 Tuberculosis of limb bones, tubercle bacilli found (in sputum) by microscopy

015.54 Tuberculosis of limb bones, tubercle bacilli not found (in sputum) by microscopy, but found by bacterial culture

015.55	Tuberculosis of limb bones, tubercle bacilli not found by bacteriological examination, but tuberculosis confirmed histologically
015.56	Tuberculosis of limb bones, tubercle bacilli not found by bacteriological or histological examination, but tuberculosis confirmed by other methods [inoculation of animals]
015.50	Tuberculosis of limb bones, unspecified
011.21	Tuberculosis of lung with cavitation, bacteriological or histological examination not done
011.22	Tuberculosis of lung with cavitation, bacteriological or histological examination unknown (at present)
011.23	Tuberculosis of lung with cavitation, tubercle bacilli found (in sputum) by microscopy
011.24	Tuberculosis of lung with cavitation, tubercle bacilli not found (in sputum) by microscopy, but found by bacterial culture
011.25	Tuberculosis of lung with cavitation, tubercle bacilli not found by bacteriological examination, but tuberculosis confirmed histologically
011.26	Tuberculosis of lung with cavitation, tubercle bacilli not found by bacteriological or histological examination, but tuberculosis confirmed by other methods [inoculation of animals]
011.20	Tuberculosis of lung with cavitation, unspecified
011.01	Tuberculosis of lung, infiltrative, bacteriological or histological examination not done
011.02	Tuberculosis of lung, infiltrative, bacteriological or histological examination unknown (at present)
011.03	Tuberculosis of lung, infiltrative, tubercle bacilli found (in sputum) by microscopy
011.04	Tuberculosis of lung, infiltrative, tubercle bacilli not found (in sputum) by microscopy, but found by bacterial culture
011.06	Tuberculosis of lung, infiltrative, tubercle bacilli not found bacteriological or histological examination, but tuberculosis confirmed by other methods [inoculation of animals]
011.05	Tuberculosis of lung, infiltrative, tubercle bacilli not found by bacteriological examination, but tuberculosis confirmed histologically
011.00	Tuberculosis of lung, infiltrative, unspecified
011.11	Tuberculosis of lung, nodular, bacteriological or histological examination not done
011.12	Tuberculosis of lung, nodular, bacteriological or histological examination unknown (at present)
011.13	Tuberculosis of lung, nodular, tubercle bacilli found (in sputum) by microscopy
011.14	Tuberculosis of lung, nodular, tubercle bacilli not found (in sputum) by microscopy, but found by bacterial culture
011.15	Tuberculosis of lung, nodular, tubercle bacilli not found by bacteriological examination, but tuberculosis confirmed histologically
011.16	Tuberculosis of lung, nodular, tubercle bacilli not found by bacteriological or histological examination, but tuberculosis confirmed by other methods [inoculation of animals]
011.10	Tuberculosis of lung, nodular, unspecified
015.61	Tuberculosis of mastoid, bacteriological or histological examination not done
015.62	Tuberculosis of mastoid, bacteriological or histological examination unknown (at present)
015.63	Tuberculosis of mastoid, tubercle bacilli found (in sputum) by microscopy
015.64	Tuberculosis of mastoid, tubercle bacilli not found (in sputum) by microscopy, but found by bacterial culture
015.65	Tuberculosis of mastoid, tubercle bacilli not found by bacteriological examination, but tuberculosis confirmed histologically
015.66	Tuberculosis of mastoid, tubercle bacilli not found by bacteriological or histological examination, but tuberculosis confirmed by other methods [inoculation of animals]
015.60	Tuberculosis of mastoid, unspecified

647.33	Tuberculosis of mother, complicating pregnancy, childbirth, or the puerperium, antepartum condition or complication
647.32	Tuberculosis of mother, complicating pregnancy, childbirth, or the puerperium, delivered, with mention of postpartum complication
647.31	Tuberculosis of mother, complicating pregnancy, childbirth, or the puerperium, delivered, with or without mention of antepartum condition
647.34	Tuberculosis of mother, complicating pregnancy, childbirth, or the puerperium,postpartum condition or complication
016.71	Tuberculosis of other female genital organs, bacteriological or histological examination not done
016.72	Tuberculosis of other female genital organs, bacteriological or histological examination unknown (at present)
016.73	Tuberculosis of other female genital organs, tubercle bacilli found (in sputum) by microscopy
016.74	Tuberculosis of other female genital organs, tubercle bacilli not found (in sputum) by microscopy, but found by bacterial culture
016.75	Tuberculosis of other female genital organs, tubercle bacilli not found by bacteriological examination, but tuberculosis confirmed histologically
016.76	Tuberculosis of other female genital organs, tubercle bacilli not found by bacteriological or histological examination, but tuberculosis confirmed by other methods [inoculation of animals]
016.70	Tuberculosis of other female genital organs, unspecified
016.51	Tuberculosis of other male genital organs, bacteriological or histological examination not done
016.52	Tuberculosis of other male genital organs, bacteriological or histological examination unknown (at present)
016.53	Tuberculosis of other male genital organs, tubercle bacilli found (in sputum) by microscopy
016.54	Tuberculosis of other male genital organs, tubercle bacilli not found (in sputum) by microscopy, but found by bacterial culture
016.55	Tuberculosis of other male genital organs, tubercle bacilli not found by bacteriological examination, but tuberculosis confirmed histologically
016.56	Tuberculosis of other male genital organs, tubercle bacilli not found by bacteriological or histological examination, but tuberculosis confirmed by other methods [inoculation of animals]
016.50	Tuberculosis of other male genital organs, unspecified
015.71	Tuberculosis of other specified bone, bacteriological or histological examination not done
015.72	Tuberculosis of other specified bone, bacteriological or histological examination unknown (at present)
015.73	Tuberculosis of other specified bone, tubercle bacilli found (in sputum) by microscopy
015.74	Tuberculosis of other specified bone, tubercle bacilli not found (in sputum) by microscopy, but found by bacterial culture
015.75	Tuberculosis of other specified bone, tubercle bacilli not found by bacteriological examination, but tuberculosis confirmed histologically
015.76	Tuberculosis of other specified bone, tubercle bacilli not found by bacteriological or histological examination, but tuberculosis confirmed by other methods [inoculation of animals]
015.70	Tuberculosis of other specified bone, unspecified
015.81	Tuberculosis of other specified joint, bacteriological or histological examination not done
015.82	Tuberculosis of other specified joint, bacteriological or histological examination unknown (at present)
015.83	Tuberculosis of other specified joint, tubercle bacilli found (in sputum) by microscopy
015.84	Tuberculosis of other specified joint, tubercle bacilli not found (in sputum) by microscopy, but found by bacterial culture
015.85	Tuberculosis of other specified joint, tubercle bacilli not found by bacteriological examination, but tuberculosis confirmed histologically

015.86	Tuberculosis of other specified joint, tubercle bacilli not found by bacteriological or histological examination, but tuberculosis confirmed by other methods [inoculation of animals]
015.80	Tuberculosis of other specified joint, unspecified
017.91	Tuberculosis of other specified organs, bacteriological or histological examination not done
017.92	Tuberculosis of other specified organs, bacteriological or histological examination unknown (at present)
017.93	Tuberculosis of other specified organs, tubercle bacilli found (in sputum) by microscopy
017.94	Tuberculosis of other specified organs, tubercle bacilli not found (in sputum) by microscopy, but found by bacterial culture
017.95	Tuberculosis of other specified organs, tubercle bacilli not found by bacteriological examination, but tuberculosis confirmed histologically
017.96	Tuberculosis of other specified organs, tubercle bacilli not found by bacteriological or histological examination, but tuberculosis confirmed by other methods [inoculation of animals]
017.90	Tuberculosis of other specified organs, unspecified
016.31	Tuberculosis of other urinary organs, bacteriological or histological examination not done
016.32	Tuberculosis of other urinary organs, bacteriological or histological examination unknown (at present)
016.33	Tuberculosis of other urinary organs, tubercle bacilli found (in sputum) by microscopy
016.34	Tuberculosis of other urinary organs, tubercle bacilli not found (in sputum) by microscopy, but found by bacterial culture
016.35	Tuberculosis of other urinary organs, tubercle bacilli not found by bacteriological examination, but tuberculosis confirmed histologically
016.36	Tuberculosis of other urinary organs, tubercle bacilli not found by bacteriological or histological examination, but tuberculosis confirmed by other methods [inoculation of animals]
016.30	Tuberculosis of other urinary organs, unspecified
017.21	Tuberculosis of peripheral lymph nodes, bacteriological or histological examination not done
017.22	Tuberculosis of peripheral lymph nodes, bacteriological or histological examination unknown (at present)
017.23	Tuberculosis of peripheral lymph nodes, tubercle bacilli found (in sputum) by microscopy
017.24	Tuberculosis of peripheral lymph nodes, tubercle bacilli not found (in sputum) by microscopy, but found by bacterial culture
017.25	Tuberculosis of peripheral lymph nodes, tubercle bacilli not found by bacteriological examination, but tuberculosis confirmed histologically
017.26	Tuberculosis of peripheral lymph nodes, tubercle bacilli not found by bacteriological or histological examination, but tuberculosis confirmed by other methods [inoculation of animals]
017.20	Tuberculosis of peripheral lymph nodes, unspecified
017.01	Tuberculosis of skin and subcutaneous cellular tissue, bacteriological or histological examination not done
017.02	Tuberculosis of skin and subcutaneous cellular tissue, bacteriological or histological examination unknown (at present)
017.03	Tuberculosis of skin and subcutaneous cellular tissue, tubercle bacilli found (in sputum) by microscopy
017.04	Tuberculosis of skin and subcutaneous cellular tissue, tubercle bacilli not found (in sputum) by microscopy, but found by bacterial culture
017.05	Tuberculosis of skin and subcutaneous cellular tissue, tubercle bacilli not found by bacteriological examination, but tuberculosis confirmed histologically
017.06	Tuberculosis of skin and subcutaneous cellular tissue, tubercle bacilli not found by bacteriological or histological examination, but tuberculosis confirmed by other methods [inoculation of animals]
017.00	Tuberculosis of skin and subcutaneous cellular tissue, unspecified

017.71	Tuberculosis of spleen, bacteriological or histological examination not done
017.72	Tuberculosis of spleen, bacteriological or histological examination unknown (at present)
017.73	Tuberculosis of spleen, tubercle bacilli found (in sputum) by microscopy
017.74	Tuberculosis of spleen, tubercle bacilli not found (in sputum) by microscopy, but found by bacterial culture
017.75	Tuberculosis of spleen, tubercle bacilli not found by bacteriological examination, but tuberculosis confirmed histologically
017.76	Tuberculosis of spleen, tubercle bacilli not found by bacteriological or histological examination, but tuberculosis confirmed by other methods [inoculation of animals]
017.70	Tuberculosis of spleen, unspecified
017.51	Tuberculosis of thyroid gland, bacteriological or histological examination not done
017.52	Tuberculosis of thyroid gland, bacteriological or histological examination unknown (at present)
017.53	Tuberculosis of thyroid gland, tubercle bacilli found (in sputum) by microscopy
017.54	Tuberculosis of thyroid gland, tubercle bacilli not found (in sputum) by microscopy, but found by bacterial culture
017.55	Tuberculosis of thyroid gland, tubercle bacilli not found by bacteriological examination, but tuberculosis confirmed histologically
017.56	Tuberculosis of thyroid gland, tubercle bacilli not found by bacteriological or histological examination, but tuberculosis confirmed by other methods [inoculation of animals]
017.50	Tuberculosis of thyroid gland, unspecified
015.91	Tuberculosis of unspecified bones and joints, bacteriological or histological examination not done
015.92	Tuberculosis of unspecified bones and joints, bacteriological or histological examination unknown (at present)
015.93	Tuberculosis of unspecified bones and joints, tubercle bacilli found (in sputum) by microscopy
015.94	Tuberculosis of unspecified bones and joints, tubercle bacilli not found (in sputum) by microscopy, but found by bacterial culture
015.95	Tuberculosis of unspecified bones and joints, tubercle bacilli not found by bacteriological examination, but tuberculosis confirmed histologically
015.96	Tuberculosis of unspecified bones and joints, tubercle bacilli not found by bacteriological or histological examination, but tuberculosis confirmed by other methods [inoculation of animals]
015.90	Tuberculosis of unspecified bones and joints, unspecified
016.21	Tuberculosis of ureter, bacteriological or histological examination not done
016.22	Tuberculosis of ureter, bacteriological or histological examination unknown (at present)
016.23	Tuberculosis of ureter, tubercle bacilli found (in sputum) by microscopy
016.24	Tuberculosis of ureter, tubercle bacilli not found (in sputum) by microscopy, but found by bacterial culture
016.25	Tuberculosis of ureter, tubercle bacilli not found by bacteriological examination, but tuberculosis confirmed histologically
016.26	Tuberculosis of ureter, tubercle bacilli not found by bacteriological or histological examination, but tuberculosis confirmed by other methods [inoculation of animals]
016.20	Tuberculosis of ureter, unspecified
015.01	Tuberculosis of vertebral column, bacteriological or histological examination not done
015.02	Tuberculosis of vertebral column, bacteriological or histological examination unknown (at present)
015.03	Tuberculosis of vertebral column, tubercle bacilli found (in sputum) by microscopy
015.04	Tuberculosis of vertebral column, tubercle bacilli not found (in sputum) by microscopy, but found by bacterial culture

015.05   Tuberculosis of vertebral column, tubercle bacilli not found by bacteriological examination, but tuberculosis confirmed histologically

015.06   Tuberculosis of vertebral column, tubercle bacilli not found by bacteriological or histological examination, but tuberculosis confirmed by other methods [inoculation of animals]

015.00   Tuberculosis of vertebral column, unspecified

011.51   Tuberculous bronchiectasis, bacteriological or histological examination not done

011.52   Tuberculous bronchiectasis, bacteriological or histological examination unknown (at present)

011.53   Tuberculous bronchiectasis, tubercle bacilli found (in sputum) by microscopy

011.54   Tuberculous bronchiectasis, tubercle bacilli not found (in sputum) by microscopy, but found by bacterial culture

011.55   Tuberculous bronchiectasis, tubercle bacilli not found by bacteriological examination, but tuberculosis confirmed histologically

011.56   Tuberculous bronchiectasis, tubercle bacilli not found by bacteriological or histological examination, but tuberculosis confirmed by other methods [inoculation of animals]

011.50   Tuberculous bronchiectasis, unspecified

011.41   Tuberculous fibrosis of lung, bacteriological or histological examination not done

011.42   Tuberculous fibrosis of lung, bacteriological or histological examination unknown (at present)

011.43   Tuberculous fibrosis of lung, tubercle bacilli found (in sputum) by microscopy

011.44   Tuberculous fibrosis of lung, tubercle bacilli not found (in sputum) by microscopy, but found by bacterial culture

011.45   Tuberculous fibrosis of lung, tubercle bacilli not found by bacteriological examination, but tuberculosis confirmed histologically

011.46   Tuberculous fibrosis of lung, tubercle bacilli not found by bacteriological or histological examination, but tuberculosis confirmed by other methods [inoculation of animals]

011.40   Tuberculous fibrosis of lung, unspecified

012.31   Tuberculous laryngitis, bacteriological or histological examination not done

012.32   Tuberculous laryngitis, bacteriological or histological examination unknown (at present)

012.33   Tuberculous laryngitis, tubercle bacilli found (in sputum) by microscopy

012.34   Tuberculous laryngitis, tubercle bacilli not found (in sputum) by microscopy, but found by bacterial culture

012.35   Tuberculous laryngitis, tubercle bacilli not found by bacteriological examination, but tuberculosis confirmed histologically

012.36   Tuberculous laryngitis, tubercle bacilli not found by bacteriological or histological examination, but tuberculosis confirmed by other methods [inoculation of animals]

012.30   Tuberculous laryngitis, unspecified

016.61   Tuberculous oophoritis and salpingitis, bacteriological or histological examination not done

016.62   Tuberculous oophoritis and salpingitis, bacteriological or histological examination unknown (at present)

016.63   Tuberculous oophoritis and salpingitis, tubercle bacilli found (in sputum) by microscopy

016.64   Tuberculous oophoritis and salpingitis, tubercle bacilli not found (in sputum) by microscopy, but found by bacterial culture

016.65   Tuberculous oophoritis and salpingitis, tubercle bacilli not found by bacteriological examination, but tuberculosis confirmed histologically

016.66   Tuberculous oophoritis and salpingitis, tubercle bacilli not found by bacteriological or histological examination, but tuberculosis confirmed by other methods [inoculation of animals]

016.60   Tuberculous oophoritis and salpingitis, unspecified

010.11   Tuberculous pleurisy in primary progressive tuberculosis, bacteriological or histological examination not done

010.12   Tuberculous pleurisy in primary progressive tuberculosis, bacteriological or histological examination unknown (at present)

010.13   Tuberculous pleurisy in primary progressive tuberculosis, tubercle bacilli found (in sputum) by microscopy

010.14   Tuberculous pleurisy in primary progressive tuberculosis, tubercle bacilli not found (in sputum) by microscopy, but found by bacterial culture

010.15   Tuberculous pleurisy in primary progressive tuberculosis, tubercle bacilli not found by bacteriological examination, but tuberculosis confirmed histologically

010.16   Tuberculous pleurisy in primary progressive tuberculosis, tubercle bacilli not found by bacteriological or histological examination, but tuberculosis confirmed by other methods [inoculation of animals]

010.10   Tuberculous pleurisy in primary progressive tuberculosis, unspecified

012.01   Tuberculous pleurisy, bacteriological or histological examination not done

012.02   Tuberculous pleurisy, bacteriological or histological examination unknown (at present)

012.03   Tuberculous pleurisy, tubercle bacilli found (in sputum) by microscopy

012.04   Tuberculous pleurisy, tubercle bacilli not found (in sputum) by microscopy, but found by bacterial culture

012.05   Tuberculous pleurisy, tubercle bacilli not found by bacteriological examination, but tuberculosis confirmed histologically

012.06   Tuberculous pleurisy, tubercle bacilli not found by bacteriological or histological examination, but tuberculosis confirmed by other methods [inoculation of animals]

012.00   Tuberculous pleurisy, unspecified

011.71   Tuberculous pneumothorax, bacteriological or histological examination not done

011.72   Tuberculous pneumothorax, bacteriological or histological examination unknown (at present)

011.73   Tuberculous pneumothorax, tubercle bacilli found (in sputum) by microscopy

011.74   Tuberculous pneumothorax, tubercle bacilli not found (in sputum) by microscopy, but found by bacterial culture

011.75   Tuberculous pneumothorax, tubercle bacilli not found by bacteriological examination, but tuberculosis confirmed histologically

011.76   Tuberculous pneumothorax, tubercle bacilli not found by bacteriological or histological examination, but tuberculosis confirmed by other methods [inoculation of animals]

011.70   Tuberculous pneumothorax, unspecified

759.5   Tuberous sclerosis

651.01   Twin pregnancy, delivered, with or without mention of antepartum condition

002.0   Typhoid fever

081.9   Typhus, unspecified

707.13   Ulcer of ankle

569.41   Ulcer of anus and rectum

707.12   Ulcer of calf

530.20   Ulcer of esophagus without bleeding

707.14   Ulcer of heel and midfoot

707.10   Ulcer of lower limb, unspecified

707.19   Ulcer of other part of lower limb

707.11   Ulcer of thigh

569.82   Ulceration of intestine

556.0   Ulcerative (chronic) enterocolitis

556.1   Ulcerative (chronic) ileocolitis

556.2   Ulcerative (chronic) proctitis

556.3   Ulcerative (chronic) proctosigmoiditis

556.9	Ulcerative colitis, unspecified
021.0	Ulceroglandular tularemia
552.1	Umbilical hernia with obstruction
556.6	Universal ulcerative (chronic) colitis
637.22	Unspecified abortion, complicated by damage to pelvic organs or tissues, complete
637.21	Unspecified abortion, complicated by damage to pelvic organs or tissues, incomplete
637.20	Unspecified abortion, complicated by damage to pelvic organs or tissues, unspecified
637.02	Unspecified abortion, complicated by genital tract and pelvic infection, complete
637.01	Unspecified abortion, complicated by genital tract and pelvic infection, incomplete
637.00	Unspecified abortion, complicated by genital tract and pelvic infection, unspecified
637.42	Unspecified abortion, complicated by metabolic disorder, complete
637.41	Unspecified abortion, complicated by metabolic disorder, incomplete
637.40	Unspecified abortion, complicated by metabolic disorder, unspecified
637.72	Unspecified abortion, with other specified complications, complete
637.71	Unspecified abortion, with other specified complications, incomplete
637.70	Unspecified abortion, with other specified complications, unspecified
637.82	Unspecified abortion, with unspecified complication, complete
637.81	Unspecified abortion, with unspecified complication, incomplete
637.80	Unspecified abortion, with unspecified complication, unspecified
291.9	Unspecified alcohol-induced mental disorders
495.9	Unspecified allergic alveolitis and pneumonitis
516.9	Unspecified alveolar and parietoalveolar pneumonopathy
747.9	Unspecified anomaly of circulatory system
751.60	Unspecified anomaly of gallbladder, bile ducts, and liver
330.9	Unspecified cerebral degeneration in childhood
639.9	Unspecified complication following abortion or ectopic and molar pregnancy
423.9	Unspecified disease of pericardium
336.9	Unspecified disease of spinal cord
031.9	Unspecified diseases due to mycobacteria
270.9	Unspecified disorder of amino-acid metabolism
304.91	Unspecified drug dependence, continuous
633.91	Unspecified ectopic pregnancy with intrauterine pregnancy
633.90	Unspecified ectopic pregnancy without intrauterine pregnancy
333.90	Unspecified extrapyramidal disease and abnormal movement disorder
125.9	Unspecified filariasis
619.9	Unspecified fistula involving female genital tract
824.9	Unspecified fracture of ankle, open
640.93	Unspecified hemorrhage in early pregnancy, antepartum condition or complication
642.93	Unspecified hypertension complicating pregnancy, childbirth, or the puerperium, antepartum condition or complication
642.92	Unspecified hypertension complicating pregnancy, childbirth, or the puerperium, delivered, with mention of postpartum complication
642.91	Unspecified hypertension complicating pregnancy, childbirth, or the puerperium, delivered, with or without mention of antepartum condition
642.94	Unspecified hypertension complicating pregnancy, childbirth, or the puerperium, postpartum condition or complication

279.3	Unspecified immunity deficiency
730.97	Unspecified infection of bone, ankle and foot
730.93	Unspecified infection of bone, forearm
730.94	Unspecified infection of bone, hand
730.96	Unspecified infection of bone, lower leg
730.99	Unspecified infection of bone, multiple sites
730.98	Unspecified infection of bone, other specified sites
730.95	Unspecified infection of bone, pelvic region and thigh
730.91	Unspecified infection of bone, shoulder region
730.90	Unspecified infection of bone, site unspecified
730.92	Unspecified infection of bone, upper arm
647.93	Unspecified infection or infestation of mother, antepartum condition or complication
647.92	Unspecified infection or infestation of mother, delivered, with mention of postpartum complication
647.91	Unspecified infection or infestation of mother, delivered, with or without mention of antepartum condition
647.94	Unspecified infection or infestation of mother, postpartum condition or complication
711.97	Unspecified infective arthritis, ankle and foot
711.93	Unspecified infective arthritis, forearm
711.94	Unspecified infective arthritis, hand
711.96	Unspecified infective arthritis, lower leg
711.99	Unspecified infective arthritis, multiple sites
711.98	Unspecified infective arthritis, other specified sites
711.95	Unspecified infective arthritis, pelvic region and thigh
711.91	Unspecified infective arthritis, shoulder region
711.90	Unspecified infective arthritis, site unspecified
711.92	Unspecified infective arthritis, upper arm
861.00	Unspecified injury of heart without mention of open wound into thorax
861.20	Unspecified injury of lung without mention of open wound into thorax
579.9	Unspecified intestinal malabsorption
560.9	Unspecified intestinal obstruction
432.9	Unspecified intracranial hemorrhage
364.3	Unspecified iridocyclitis
208.92	Unspecified leukemia, in relapse
208.91	Unspecified leukemia, in remission
208.90	Unspecified leukemia, without mention of having achieved remission
204.92	Unspecified lymphoid leukemia, in relapse
204.91	Unspecified lymphoid leukemia, in remission
204.90	Unspecified lymphoid leukemia, without mention of having achieved remission
996.40	Unspecified mechanical complication of internal orthopedic device, implant, and graft
206.92	Unspecified monocytic leukemia, in relapse
206.91	Unspecified monocytic leukemia, in remission
206.90	Unspecified monocytic leukemia, without mention of having achieved remission
205.92	Unspecified myeloid leukemia, in relapse
205.91	Unspecified myeloid leukemia, in remission
205.90	Unspecified myeloid leukemia, without mention of having achieved remission
049.9	Unspecified non-arthropod-borne viral diseases of central nervous system
753.20	Unspecified obstructive defect of renal pelvis and ureter
871.9	Unspecified open wound of eyeball
870.9	Unspecified open wound of ocular adnexa
730.27	Unspecified osteomyelitis, ankle and foot

730.23	Unspecified osteomyelitis, forearm
730.24	Unspecified osteomyelitis, hand
730.26	Unspecified osteomyelitis, lower leg
730.29	Unspecified osteomyelitis, multiple sites
730.28	Unspecified osteomyelitis, other specified sites
730.25	Unspecified osteomyelitis, pelvic region and thigh
730.21	Unspecified osteomyelitis, shoulder region
730.20	Unspecified osteomyelitis, site unspecified
730.22	Unspecified osteomyelitis, upper arm
299.90	Unspecified pervasive developmental disorder, current or active state
299.91	Unspecified pervasive developmental disorder, residual state
511.9	Unspecified pleural effusion
662.11	Unspecified prolonged labor, delivered, with or without mention of antepartum condition
263.9	Unspecified protein-calorie malnutrition
007.9	Unspecified protozoal intestinal disease
026.9	Unspecified rat-bite fever
646.23	Unspecified renal disease in pregnancy, without mention of hypertension, antepartum condition or complication
646.22	Unspecified renal disease in pregnancy, without mention of hypertension, delivered, with mention of postpartum complication
646.21	Unspecified renal disease in pregnancy, without mention of hypertension, delivered, with or without mention of antepartum condition
646.24	Unspecified renal disease in pregnancy, without mention of hypertension, postpartum condition or complication
361.9	Unspecified retinal detachment
295.92	Unspecified schizophrenia, chronic
295.94	Unspecified schizophrenia, chronic with acute exacerbation
295.91	Unspecified schizophrenia, subchronic
295.93	Unspecified schizophrenia, subchronic with acute exacerbation
091.9	Unspecified secondary syphilis
290.9	Unspecified senile psychotic condition
046.9	Unspecified slow virus infection of central nervous system
435.9	Unspecified transient cerebral ischemia
293.9	Unspecified transient mental disorder in conditions classified elsewhere
021.9	Unspecified tularemia
557.9	Unspecified vascular insufficiency of intestine
671.92	Unspecified venous complication of pregnancy and the puerperium, delivered, with mention of postpartum complication
671.91	Unspecified venous complication of pregnancy and the puerperium, delivered, with or without mention of antepartum condition
671.90	Unspecified venous complication of pregnancy and the puerperium, unspecified as to episode of care or not applicable
070.9	Unspecified viral hepatitis without mention of hepatic coma
047.9	Unspecified viral meningitis
027.9	Unspecified zoonotic bacterial disease
060.1	Urban yellow fever
593.82	Ureteral fistula
597.0	Urethral abscess
599.1	Urethral fistula
274.11	Uric acid nephrolithiasis
771.82	Urinary tract infection of newborn
599.0	Urinary tract infection, site not specified
619.0	Urinary-genital tract fistula, female
046.11	Variant Creutzfeldt-Jakob disease
052.9	Varicella without mention of complication
454.2	Varicose veins of lower extremities with ulcer and inflammation
050.0	Variola major
997.71	Vascular complications of mesenteric artery
997.79	Vascular complications of other vessels
997.72	Vascular complications of renal artery
290.41	Vascular dementia, with delirium
290.42	Vascular dementia, with delusions
290.43	Vascular dementia, with depressed mood
593.81	Vascular disorders of kidney
607.82	Vascular disorders of penis
066.2	Venezuelan equine fever
453.6	Venous embolism and thrombosis of superficial vessels of lower extremity
495.7	"Ventilation" pneumonitis
997.31	Ventilator associated pneumonia
552.20	Ventral, unspecified, hernia with obstruction
745.4	Ventricular septal defect
435.1	Vertebral artery syndrome
435.3	Vertebrobasilar artery syndrome
596.2	Vesical fistula, not elsewhere classified
101	Vincent's angina
070.1	Viral hepatitis A without mention of hepatic coma
070.31	Viral hepatitis B without mention of hepatic coma, acute or unspecified, with hepatitis delta
070.30	Viral hepatitis B without mention of hepatic coma, acute or unspecified, without mention of hepatitis delta
085.0	Visceral [kala-azar] leishmaniasis
054.71	Visceral herpes simplex
360.04	Vitreous abscess
084.1	Vivax malaria [benign tertian]
286.4	Von Willebrand's disease
446.4	Wegener's granulomatosis
335.0	Werdnig-Hoffmann disease
040.2	Whipple's disease
033.1	Whooping cough due to bordetella parapertussis [B. parapertussis]
033.0	Whooping cough due to bordetella pertussis [B. pertussis]
033.8	Whooping cough due to other specified organism
033.9	Whooping cough, unspecified organism
279.12	Wiskott-aldrich syndrome
040.42	Wound botulism
060.9	Yellow fever, unspecified

Numeric MCC List

003.1	Salmonella septicemia
003.21	Salmonella meningitis
003.22	Salmonella pneumonia
006.3	Amebic liver abscess
006.4	Amebic lung abscess
006.5	Amebic brain abscess
011.60	Tuberculous pneumonia [any form], unspecified
011.61	Tuberculous pneumonia [any form], bacteriological or histological examination not done
011.62	Tuberculous pneumonia [any form], bacteriological or histological examination unknown (at present)
011.63	Tuberculous pneumonia [any form], tubercle bacilli found (in sputum) by microscopy
011.64	Tuberculous pneumonia [any form], tubercle bacilli not found (in sputum) by microscopy, but found by bacterial culture
011.65	Tuberculous pneumonia [any form], tubercle bacilli not found by bacteriological examination, but tuberculosis confirmed histologically
011.66	Tuberculous pneumonia [any form], tubercle bacilli not found by bacteriological or histological examination, but tuberculosis confirmed by other methods [inoculation of animals]
013.00	Tuberculous meningitis, unspecified
013.01	Tuberculous meningitis, bacteriological or histological examination not done
013.02	Tuberculous meningitis, bacteriological or histological examination unknown (at present)
013.03	Tuberculous meningitis, tubercle bacilli found (in sputum) by microscopy
013.04	Tuberculous meningitis, tubercle bacilli not found (in sputum) by microscopy, but found by bacterial culture
013.05	Tuberculous meningitis, tubercle bacilli not found by bacteriological examination, but tuberculosis confirmed histologically
013.06	Tuberculous meningitis, tubercle bacilli not found by bacteriological or histological examination, but tuberculosis confirmed by other methods [inoculation of animals]
013.10	Tuberculoma of meninges, unspecified
013.11	Tuberculoma of meninges, bacteriological or histological examination not done
013.12	Tuberculoma of meninges, bacteriological or histological examination unknown (at present)
013.13	Tuberculoma of meninges, tubercle bacilli found (in sputum) by microscopy
013.14	Tuberculoma of meninges, tubercle bacilli not found (in sputum) by microscopy, but found by bacterial culture
013.15	Tuberculoma of meninges, tubercle bacilli not found by bacteriological examination, but tuberculosis confirmed histologically
013.16	Tuberculoma of meninges, tubercle bacilli not found by bacteriological or histological examination, but tuberculosis confirmed by other methods [inoculation of animals]
013.20	Tuberculoma of brain, unspecified
013.21	Tuberculoma of brain, bacteriological or histological examination not done
013.22	Tuberculoma of brain, bacteriological or histological examination unknown (at present)
013.23	Tuberculoma of brain, tubercle bacilli found (in sputum) by microscopy
013.24	Tuberculoma of brain, tubercle bacilli not found (in sputum) by microscopy, but found by bacterial culture
013.25	Tuberculoma of brain, tubercle bacilli not found by bacteriological examination, but tuberculosis confirmed histologically
013.26	Tuberculoma of brain, tubercle bacilli not found by bacteriological or histological examination, but tuberculosis confirmed by other methods [inoculation of animals]
013.30	Tuberculous abscess of brain, unspecified
013.31	Tuberculous abscess of brain, bacteriological or histological examination not done
013.32	Tuberculous abscess of brain, bacteriological or histological examination unknown (at present)
013.33	Tuberculous abscess of brain, tubercle bacilli found (in sputum) by microscopy
013.34	Tuberculous abscess of brain, tubercle bacilli not found (in sputum) by microscopy, but found by bacterial culture
013.35	Tuberculous abscess of brain, tubercle bacilli not found by bacteriological examination, but tuberculosis confirmed histologically
013.36	Tuberculous abscess of brain, tubercle bacilli not found by bacteriological or histological examination, but tuberculosis confirmed by other methods [inoculation of animals]
013.40	Tuberculoma of spinal cord, unspecified
013.41	Tuberculoma of spinal cord, bacteriological or histological examination not done
013.42	Tuberculoma of spinal cord, bacteriological or histological examination unknown (at present)
013.43	Tuberculoma of spinal cord, tubercle bacilli found (in sputum) by microscopy
013.44	Tuberculoma of spinal cord, tubercle bacilli not found (in sputum) by microscopy, but found by bacterial culture
013.45	Tuberculoma of spinal cord, tubercle bacilli not found by bacteriological examination, but tuberculosis confirmed histologically
013.46	Tuberculoma of spinal cord, tubercle bacilli not found by bacteriological or histological examination, but tuberculosis confirmed by other methods [inoculation of animals]
013.50	Tuberculous abscess of spinal cord, unspecified
013.51	Tuberculous abscess of spinal cord, bacteriological or histological examination not done
013.52	Tuberculous abscess of spinal cord, bacteriological or histological examination unknown (at present)
013.53	Tuberculous abscess of spinal cord, tubercle bacilli found (in sputum) by microscopy
013.54	Tuberculous abscess of spinal cord, tubercle bacilli not found (in sputum) by microscopy, but found by bacterial culture
013.55	Tuberculous abscess of spinal cord, tubercle bacilli not found by bacteriological examination, but tuberculosis confirmed histologically
013.56	Tuberculous abscess of spinal cord, tubercle bacilli not found by bacteriological or histological examination, but tuberculosis confirmed by other methods [inoculation of animals]
013.60	Tuberculous encephalitis or myelitis, unspecified
013.61	Tuberculous encephalitis or myelitis, bacteriological or histological examination not done
013.62	Tuberculous encephalitis or myelitis, bacteriological or histological examination unknown (at present)
013.63	Tuberculous encephalitis or myelitis, tubercle bacilli found (in sputum) by microscopy
013.64	Tuberculous encephalitis or myelitis, tubercle bacilli not found (in sputum) by microscopy, but found by bacterial culture
013.65	Tuberculous encephalitis or myelitis, tubercle bacilli not found by bacteriological examination, but tuberculosis confirmed histologically
013.66	Tuberculous encephalitis or myelitis, tubercle bacilli not found by bacteriological or histological examination, but tuberculosis confirmed by other methods [inoculation of animals]
013.80	Other specified tuberculosis of central nervous system, unspecified
013.81	Other specified tuberculosis of central nervous system, bacteriological or histological examination not done

013.82	Other specified tuberculosis of central nervous system, bacteriological or histological examination unknown (at present)
013.83	Other specified tuberculosis of central nervous system, tubercle bacilli found (in sputum) by microscopy
013.84	Other specified tuberculosis of central nervous system, tubercle bacilli not found (in sputum) by microscopy, but found by bacterial culture
013.85	Other specified tuberculosis of central nervous system, tubercle bacilli not found by bacteriological examination, but tuberculosis confirmed histologically
013.86	Other specified tuberculosis of central nervous system, tubercle bacilli not found by bacteriological or histological examination, but tuberculosis confirmed by other methods [inoculation of animals]
013.90	Unspecified tuberculosis of central nervous system, unspecified
013.91	Unspecified tuberculosis of central nervous system, bacteriological or histological examination not done
013.92	Unspecified tuberculosis of central nervous system, bacteriological or histological examination unknown (at present)
013.93	Unspecified tuberculosis of central nervous system, tubercle bacilli found (in sputum) by microscopy
013.94	Unspecified tuberculosis of central nervous system, tubercle bacilli not found (in sputum) by microscopy, but found by bacterial culture
013.95	Unspecified tuberculosis of central nervous system, tubercle bacilli not found by bacteriological examination, but tuberculosis confirmed histologically
013.96	Unspecified tuberculosis of central nervous system, tubercle bacilli not found by bacteriological or histological examination, but tuberculosis confirmed by other methods [inoculation of animals]
014.00	Tuberculous peritonitis, unspecified
014.01	Tuberculous peritonitis, bacteriological or histological examination not done
014.02	Tuberculous peritonitis, bacteriological or histological examination unknown (at present)
014.03	Tuberculous peritonitis, tubercle bacilli found (in sputum) by microscopy
014.04	Tuberculous peritonitis, tubercle bacilli not found (in sputum) by microscopy, but found by bacterial culture
014.05	Tuberculous peritonitis, tubercle bacilli not found by bacteriological examination, but tuberculosis confirmed histologically
014.06	Tuberculous peritonitis, tubercle bacilli not found by bacteriological or histological examination, but tuberculosis confirmed by other methods [inoculation of animals]
018.00	Acute miliary tuberculosis, unspecified
018.01	Acute miliary tuberculosis, bacteriological or histological examination not done
018.02	Acute miliary tuberculosis, bacteriological or histological examination unknown (at present)
018.03	Acute miliary tuberculosis, tubercle bacilli found (in sputum) by microscopy
018.04	Acute miliary tuberculosis, tubercle bacilli not found (in sputum) by microscopy, but found by bacterial culture
018.05	Acute miliary tuberculosis, tubercle bacilli not found by bacteriological examination, but tuberculosis confirmed histologically
018.06	Acute miliary tuberculosis, tubercle bacilli not found by bacteriological or histological examination, but tuberculosis confirmed by other methods [inoculation of animals]
018.80	Other specified miliary tuberculosis, unspecified
018.81	Other specified miliary tuberculosis, bacteriological or histological examination not done
018.82	Other specified miliary tuberculosis, bacteriological or histological examination unknown (at present)
018.83	Other specified miliary tuberculosis, tubercle bacilli found (in sputum) by microscopy

018.84	Other specified miliary tuberculosis, tubercle bacilli not found (in sputum) by microscopy, but found by bacterial culture
018.85	Other specified miliary tuberculosis, tubercle bacilli not found by bacteriological examination, but tuberculosis confirmed histologically
018.86	Other specified miliary tuberculosis, tubercle bacilli not found by bacteriological or histological examination, but tuberculosis confirmed by other methods [inoculation of animals]
018.90	Miliary tuberculosis, unspecified, unspecified
018.91	Miliary tuberculosis, unspecified, bacteriological or histological examination not done
018.92	Miliary tuberculosis, unspecified, bacteriological or histological examination unknown (at present)
018.93	Miliary tuberculosis, unspecified, tubercle bacilli found (in sputum) by microscopy
018.94	Miliary tuberculosis, unspecified, tubercle bacilli not found (in sputum) by microscopy, but found by bacterial culture
018.95	Miliary tuberculosis, unspecified, tubercle bacilli not found by bacteriological examination, but tuberculosis confirmed histologically
018.96	Miliary tuberculosis, unspecified, tubercle bacilli not found by bacteriological or histological examination, but tuberculosis confirmed by other methods [inoculation of animals]
020.0	Bubonic plague
020.1	Cellulocutaneous plague
020.2	Septicemic plague
020.3	Primary pneumonic plague
020.4	Secondary pneumonic plague
020.5	Pneumonic plague, unspecified
020.8	Other specified types of plague
020.9	Plague, unspecified
022.1	Pulmonary anthrax
022.3	Anthrax septicemia
036.0	Meningococcal meningitis
036.1	Meningococcal encephalitis
036.2	Meningococcemia
036.3	Waterhouse-Friderichsen syndrome, meningococcal
036.40	Meningococcal carditis, unspecified
036.41	Meningococcal pericarditis
036.42	Meningococcal endocarditis
036.43	Meningococcal myocarditis
037	Tetanus
038.0	Streptococcal septicemia
038.10	Staphylococcal septicemia, unspecified
038.11	Methicillin susceptible Staphylococcus aureus septicemia
038.12	Methicillin resistant Staphylococcus aureus septicemia
038.19	Other staphylococcal septicemia
038.2	Pneumococcal septicemia [Streptococcus pneumoniae septicemia]
038.3	Septicemia due to anaerobes
038.40	Septicemia due to gram-negative organism, unspecified
038.41	Septicemia due to hemophilus influenzae [H. influenzae]
038.42	Septicemia due to escherichia coli [E. coli]
038.43	Septicemia due to pseudomonas
038.44	Septicemia due to serratia
038.49	Other septicemia due to gram-negative organisms
038.8	Other specified septicemias
038.9	Unspecified septicemia
040.0	Gas gangrene
040.82	Toxic shock syndrome
042	Human immunodeficiency virus [HIV] disease
045.00	Acute paralytic poliomyelitis specified as bulbar, poliovirus, unspecified type

045.01	Acute paralytic poliomyelitis specified as bulbar, poliovirus type I
045.02	Acute paralytic poliomyelitis specified as bulbar, poliovirus type II
045.03	Acute paralytic poliomyelitis specified as bulbar, poliovirus type III
045.10	Acute poliomyelitis with other paralysis, poliovirus, unspecified type
045.11	Acute poliomyelitis with other paralysis, poliovirus type I
045.12	Acute poliomyelitis with other paralysis, poliovirus type II
045.13	Acute poliomyelitis with other paralysis, poliovirus type III
052.0	Postvaricella encephalitis
052.1	Varicella (hemorrhagic) pneumonitis
052.2	Postvaricella myelitis
053.0	Herpes zoster with meningitis
053.14	Herpes zoster myelitis
054.3	Herpetic meningoencephalitis
054.5	Herpetic septicemia
054.72	Herpes simplex meningitis
054.74	Herpes simplex myelitis
055.0	Postmeasles encephalitis
055.1	Postmeasles pneumonia
056.01	Encephalomyelitis due to rubella
058.21	Human herpesvirus 6 encephalitis
058.29	Other human herpesvirus encephalitis
062.0	Japanese encephalitis
062.1	Western equine encephalitis
062.2	Eastern equine encephalitis
062.3	St. Louis encephalitis
062.4	Australian encephalitis
062.5	California virus encephalitis
062.8	Other specified mosquito-borne viral encephalitis
062.9	Mosquito-borne viral encephalitis, unspecified
063.0	Russian spring-summer [taiga] encephalitis
063.1	Louping ill
063.2	Central european encephalitis
063.8	Other specified tick-borne viral encephalitis
063.9	Tick-borne viral encephalitis, unspecified
064	Viral encephalitis transmitted by other and unspecified arthropods
066.40	West Nile Fever, unspecified
066.41	West Nile Fever with encephalitis
066.42	West Nile Fever with other neurologic manifestation
066.49	West Nile Fever with other complications
070.0	Viral hepatitis A with hepatic coma
070.20	Viral hepatitis B with hepatic coma, acute or unspecified, without mention of hepatitis delta
070.21	Viral hepatitis B with hepatic coma, acute or unspecified, with hepatitis delta
070.22	Chronic viral hepatitis B with hepatic coma without hepatitis delta
070.23	Chronic viral hepatitis B with hepatic coma with hepatitis delta
070.41	Acute hepatitis C with hepatic coma
070.42	Hepatitis delta without mention of active hepatitis B disease with hepatic coma
070.43	Hepatitis E with hepatic coma
070.44	Chronic hepatitis C with hepatic coma
070.49	Other specified viral hepatitis with hepatic coma
070.6	Unspecified viral hepatitis with hepatic coma
070.71	Unspecified viral hepatitis C with hepatic coma
072.1	Mumps meningitis
072.2	Mumps encephalitis
073.0	Ornithosis with pneumonia
084.0	Falciparum malaria [malignant tertian]
090.41	Congenital syphilitic encephalitis

090.42	Congenital syphilitic meningitis
091.81	Acute syphilitic meningitis (secondary)
094.2	Syphilitic meningitis
094.81	Syphilitic encephalitis
094.87	Syphilitic ruptured cerebral aneurysm
098.82	Gonococcal meningitis
098.83	Gonococcal pericarditis
098.84	Gonococcal endocarditis
100.81	Leptospiral meningitis (aseptic)
112.4	Candidiasis of lung
112.5	Disseminated candidiasis
112.81	Candidal endocarditis
112.83	Candidal meningitis
114.2	Coccidioidal meningitis
115.01	Infection by Histoplasma capsulatum, meningitis
115.03	Infection by Histoplasma capsulatum, pericarditis
115.04	Infection by Histoplasma capsulatum, endocarditis
115.05	Infection by Histoplasma capsulatum, pneumonia
115.11	Infection by Histoplasma duboisii, meningitis
115.13	Infection by Histoplasma duboisii, pericarditis
115.14	Infection by Histoplasma duboisii, endocarditis
115.15	Infection by Histoplasma duboisii, pneumonia
115.91	Histoplasmosis, unspecified, meningitis
115.93	Histoplasmosis, unspecified, pericarditis
115.94	Histoplasmosis, unspecified, endocarditis
115.95	Histoplasmosis, unspecified, pneumonia
117.7	Zygomycosis [Phycomycosis or Mucormycosis]
130.0	Meningoencephalitis due to toxoplasmosis
130.3	Myocarditis due to toxoplasmosis
130.4	Pneumonitis due to toxoplasmosis
130.8	Multisystemic disseminated toxoplasmosis
136.3	Pneumocystosis
242.01	Toxic diffuse goiter with mention of thyrotoxic crisis or storm
242.11	Toxic uninodular goiter with mention of thyrotoxic crisis or storm
242.21	Toxic multinodular goiter with mention of thyrotoxic crisis or storm
242.31	Toxic nodular goiter, unspecified type, with mention of thyrotoxic crisis or storm
242.41	Thyrotoxicosis from ectopic thyroid nodule with mention of thyrotoxic crisis or storm
242.81	Thyrotoxicosis of other specified origin with mention of thyrotoxic crisis or storm
242.91	Thyrotoxicosis without mention of goiter or other cause, with mention of thyrotoxic crisis or storm
249.10	Secondary diabetes mellitus with ketoacidosis, not stated as uncontrolled, or unspecified
249.11	Secondary diabetes mellitus with ketoacidosis, uncontrolled
249.20	Secondary diabetes mellitus with hyperosmolarity, not stated as uncontrolled, or unspecified
249.21	Secondary diabetes mellitus with hyperosmolarity, uncontrolled
249.30	Secondary diabetes mellitus with other coma, not stated as uncontrolled, or unspecified
249.31	Secondary diabetes mellitus with other coma, uncontrolled
250.10	Diabetes with ketoacidosis, type II or unspecified type, not stated as uncontrolled
250.11	Diabetes with ketoacidosis, type I [juvenile type], not stated as uncontrolled
250.12	Diabetes with ketoacidosis, type II or unspecified type, uncontrolled
250.13	Diabetes with ketoacidosis, type I [juvenile type], uncontrolled
250.20	Diabetes with hyperosmolarity, type II or unspecified type, not stated as uncontrolled

250.21	Diabetes with hyperosmolarity, type I [juvenile type], not stated as uncontrolled
250.22	Diabetes with hyperosmolarity, type II or unspecified type, uncontrolled
250.23	Diabetes with hyperosmolarity, type I [juvenile type], uncontrolled
250.30	Diabetes with other coma, type II or unspecified type, not stated as uncontrolled
250.31	Diabetes with other coma, type I [juvenile type], not stated as uncontrolled
250.32	Diabetes with other coma, type II or unspecified type, uncontrolled
250.33	Diabetes with other coma, type I [juvenile type], uncontrolled
260	Kwashiorkor
261	Nutritional marasmus
262	Other severe protein-calorie malnutrition
277.01	Cystic fibrosis with meconium ileus
277.02	Cystic fibrosis with pulmonary manifestations
277.88	Tumor lysis syndrome
282.42	Sickle-cell thalassemia with crisis
282.62	Hb-SS disease with crisis
282.64	Sickle-cell/Hb-C disease with crisis
282.69	Other sickle-cell disease with crisis
283.11	Hemolytic-uremic syndrome
284.11	Antineoplastic chemotherapy induced pancytopenia
284.12	Other drug-induced pancytopenia
284.81	Red cell aplasia (acquired)(adult)(with thymoma)
284.89	Other specified aplastic anemias
286.0	Congenital factor VIII disorder
286.1	Congenital factor IX disorder
286.6	Defibrination syndrome
320.0	Hemophilus meningitis
320.1	Pneumococcal meningitis
320.2	Streptococcal meningitis
320.3	Staphylococcal meningitis
320.7	Meningitis in other bacterial diseases classified elsewhere
320.81	Anaerobic meningitis
320.82	Meningitis due to gram-negative bacteria, not elsewhere classified
320.89	Meningitis due to other specified bacteria
320.9	Meningitis due to unspecified bacterium
321.0	Cryptococcal meningitis
321.1	Meningitis in other fungal diseases
321.2	Meningitis due to viruses not elsewhere classified
321.3	Meningitis due to trypanosomiasis
321.4	Meningitis in sarcoidosis
321.8	Meningitis due to other nonbacterial organisms classified elsewhere
322.0	Nonpyogenic meningitis
322.1	Eosinophilic meningitis
322.9	Meningitis, unspecified
323.01	Encephalitis and encephalomyelitis in viral diseases classified elsewhere
323.02	Myelitis in viral diseases classified elsewhere
323.1	Encephalitis, myelitis, and encephalomyelitis in rickettsial diseases classified elsewhere
323.2	Encephalitis, myelitis, and encephalomyelitis in protozoal diseases classified elsewhere
323.41	Other encephalitis and encephalomyelitis due to other infections classified elsewhere
323.42	Other myelitis due to other infections classified elsewhere
323.51	Encephalitis and encephalomyelitis following immunization procedures
323.52	Myelitis following immunization procedures

323.61	Infectious acute disseminated encephalomyelitis (ADEM)
323.62	Other postinfectious encephalitis and encephalomyelitis
323.63	Postinfectious myelitis
323.71	Toxic encephalitis and encephalomyelitis
323.72	Toxic myelitis
323.81	Other causes of encephalitis and encephalomyelitis
323.82	Other causes of myelitis
323.9	Unspecified causes of encephalitis, myelitis, and encephalomyelitis
324.0	Intracranial abscess
324.1	Intraspinal abscess
324.9	Intracranial and intraspinal abscess of unspecified site
325	Phlebitis and thrombophlebitis of intracranial venous sinuses
331.81	Reye's syndrome
333.92	Neuroleptic malignant syndrome
336.1	Vascular myelopathies
343.2	Congenital quadriplegia
344.00	Quadriplegia, unspecified
344.01	Quadriplegia, C1-C4, complete
344.02	Quadriplegia, C1-C4, incomplete
344.03	Quadriplegia, C5-C7, complete
344.04	Quadriplegia, C5-C7, incomplete
344.09	Other quadriplegia
344.81	Locked-in state
345.2	Petit mal status
345.3	Grand mal status
345.71	Epilepsia partialis continua, with intractable epilepsy
348.30	Encephalopathy, unspecified
348.31	Metabolic encephalopathy
348.39	Other encephalopathy
348.4	Compression of brain
348.5	Cerebral edema
348.82	Brain death
349.82	Toxic encephalopathy
358.01	Myasthenia gravis with (acute) exacerbation
410.01	Acute myocardial infarction of anterolateral wall, initial episode of care
410.11	Acute myocardial infarction of other anterior wall, initial episode of care
410.21	Acute myocardial infarction of inferolateral wall, initial episode of care
410.31	Acute myocardial infarction of inferoposterior wall, initial episode of care
410.41	Acute myocardial infarction of other inferior wall, initial episode of care
410.51	Acute myocardial infarction of other lateral wall, initial episode of care
410.61	True posterior wall infarction, initial episode of care
410.71	Subendocardial infarction, initial episode of care
410.81	Acute myocardial infarction of other specified sites, initial episode of care
410.91	Acute myocardial infarction of unspecified site, initial episode of care
414.12	Dissection of coronary artery
415.0	Acute cor pulmonale
415.11	Iatrogenic pulmonary embolism and infarction
415.12	Septic pulmonary embolism
415.13	Saddle embolus of pulmonary artery
415.19	Other pulmonary embolism and infarction
421.0	Acute and subacute bacterial endocarditis
421.1	Acute and subacute infective endocarditis in diseases classified elsewhere

421.9	Acute endocarditis, unspecified
422.0	Acute myocarditis in diseases classified elsewhere
422.90	Acute myocarditis, unspecified
422.91	Idiopathic myocarditis
422.92	Septic myocarditis
422.93	Toxic myocarditis
422.99	Other acute myocarditis
427.41	Ventricular fibrillation
427.42	Ventricular flutter
427.5	Cardiac arrest
428.21	Acute systolic heart failure
428.23	Acute on chronic systolic heart failure
428.31	Acute diastolic heart failure
428.33	Acute on chronic diastolic heart failure
428.41	Acute combined systolic and diastolic heart failure
428.43	Acute on chronic combined systolic and diastolic heart failure
429.5	Rupture of chordae tendineae
429.6	Rupture of papillary muscle
430	Subarachnoid hemorrhage
431	Intracerebral hemorrhage
432.0	Nontraumatic extradural hemorrhage
432.1	Subdural hemorrhage
433.01	Occlusion and stenosis of basilar artery with cerebral infarction
433.11	Occlusion and stenosis of carotid artery with cerebral infarction
433.21	Occlusion and stenosis of vertebral artery with cerebral infarction
433.31	Occlusion and stenosis of multiple and bilateral precerebral arteries with cerebral infarction
433.81	Occlusion and stenosis of other specified precerebral artery with cerebral infarction
433.91	Occlusion and stenosis of unspecified precerebral artery with cerebral infarction
434.01	Cerebral thrombosis with cerebral infarction
434.11	Cerebral embolism with cerebral infarction
434.91	Cerebral artery occlusion, unspecified with cerebral infarction
441.00	Dissection of aorta, unspecified site
441.01	Dissection of aorta, thoracic
441.02	Dissection of aorta, abdominal
441.03	Dissection of aorta, thoracoabdominal
441.1	Thoracic aneurysm, ruptured
441.3	Abdominal aneurysm, ruptured
441.5	Aortic aneurysm of unspecified site, ruptured
441.6	Thoracoabdominal aneurysm, ruptured
443.21	Dissection of carotid artery
443.22	Dissection of iliac artery
443.23	Dissection of renal artery
443.24	Dissection of vertebral artery
443.29	Dissection of other artery
444.01	Saddle embolus of abdominal aorta
446.6	Thrombotic microangiopathy
452	Portal vein thrombosis
453.0	Budd-chiari syndrome
453.2	Other venous embolism and thrombosis of inferior vena cava
456.0	Esophageal varices with bleeding
456.20	Esophageal varices in diseases classified elsewhere, with bleeding
464.01	Acute laryngitis with obstruction
464.11	Acute tracheitis with obstruction
464.21	Acute laryngotracheitis with obstruction
464.31	Acute epiglottitis with obstruction
464.51	Supraglottitis unspecified, with obstruction

480.0	Pneumonia due to adenovirus
480.1	Pneumonia due to respiratory syncytial virus
480.2	Pneumonia due to parainfluenza virus
480.3	Pneumonia due to SARS-associated coronavirus
480.8	Pneumonia due to other virus not elsewhere classified
480.9	Viral pneumonia, unspecified
481	Pneumococcal pneumonia [Streptococcus pneumoniae pneumonia]
482.0	Pneumonia due to Klebsiella pneumoniae
482.1	Pneumonia due to Pseudomonas
482.2	Pneumonia due to Hemophilus influenzae [H. influenzae]
482.30	Pneumonia due to Streptococcus, unspecified
482.31	Pneumonia due to Streptococcus, group A
482.32	Pneumonia due to Streptococcus, group B
482.39	Pneumonia due to other Streptococcus
482.40	Pneumonia due to Staphylococcus, unspecified
482.41	Methicillin susceptible pneumonia due to Staphylococcus aureus
482.42	Methicillin resistant pneumonia due to Staphylococcus aureus
482.49	Other Staphylococcus pneumonia
482.81	Pneumonia due to anaerobes
482.82	Pneumonia due to escherichia coli [E. coli]
482.83	Pneumonia due to other gram-negative bacteria
482.84	Pneumonia due to Legionnaires' disease
482.89	Pneumonia due to other specified bacteria
482.9	Bacterial pneumonia, unspecified
483.0	Pneumonia due to mycoplasma pneumoniae
483.1	Pneumonia due to chlamydia
483.8	Pneumonia due to other specified organism
484.1	Pneumonia in cytomegalic inclusion disease
484.3	Pneumonia in whooping cough
484.5	Pneumonia in anthrax
484.6	Pneumonia in aspergillosis
484.7	Pneumonia in other systemic mycoses
484.8	Pneumonia in other infectious diseases classified elsewhere
485	Bronchopneumonia, organism unspecified
486	Pneumonia, organism unspecified
487.0	Influenza with pneumonia
488.01	Influenza due to identified avian influenza virus with pneumonia
488.11	Influenza due to identified 2009 H1N1 influenza virus with pneumonia
488.81	Influenza due to identified novel influenza A virus with pneumonia
506.1	Acute pulmonary edema due to fumes and vapors
507.0	Pneumonitis due to inhalation of food or vomitus
507.1	Pneumonitis due to inhalation of oils and essences
507.8	Pneumonitis due to other solids and liquids
510.0	Empyema with fistula
510.9	Empyema without mention of fistula
511.1	Pleurisy with effusion, with mention of a bacterial cause other than tuberculosis
512.0	Spontaneous tension pneumothorax
513.0	Abscess of lung
513.1	Abscess of mediastinum
516.4	Lymphangioleiomyomatosis
516.61	Neuroendocrine cell hyperplasia of infancy
516.62	Pulmonary interstitial glycogenosis
516.63	Surfactant mutations of the lung
516.64	Alveolar capillary dysplasia with vein misalignment
516.69	Other interstitial lung diseases of childhood
518.4	Acute edema of lung, unspecified

518.51	Acute respiratory failure following trauma and surgery
518.52	Other pulmonary insufficiency, not elsewhere classified, following trauma and surgery
518.53	Acute and chronic respiratory failure following trauma and surgery
518.81	Acute respiratory failure
518.84	Acute and chronic respiratory failure
519.2	Mediastinitis
530.21	Ulcer of esophagus with bleeding
530.4	Perforation of esophagus
530.7	Gastroesophageal laceration-hemorrhage syndrome
530.82	Esophageal hemorrhage
530.84	Tracheoesophageal fistula
531.00	Acute gastric ulcer with hemorrhage, without mention of obstruction
531.01	Acute gastric ulcer with hemorrhage, with obstruction
531.10	Acute gastric ulcer with perforation, without mention of obstruction
531.11	Acute gastric ulcer with perforation, with obstruction
531.20	Acute gastric ulcer with hemorrhage and perforation, without mention of obstruction
531.21	Acute gastric ulcer with hemorrhage and perforation, with obstruction
531.31	Acute gastric ulcer without mention of hemorrhage or perforation, with obstruction
531.40	Chronic or unspecified gastric ulcer with hemorrhage, without mention of obstruction
531.41	Chronic or unspecified gastric ulcer with hemorrhage, with obstruction
531.50	Chronic or unspecified gastric ulcer with perforation, without mention of obstruction
531.51	Chronic or unspecified gastric ulcer with perforation, with obstruction
531.60	Chronic or unspecified gastric ulcer with hemorrhage and perforation, without mention of obstruction
531.61	Chronic or unspecified gastric ulcer with hemorrhage and perforation, with obstruction
531.71	Chronic gastric ulcer without mention of hemorrhage or perforation, with obstruction
531.91	Gastric ulcer, unspecified as acute or chronic, without mention of hemorrhage or perforation, with obstruction
532.00	Acute duodenal ulcer with hemorrhage, without mention of obstruction
532.01	Acute duodenal ulcer with hemorrhage, with obstruction
532.10	Acute duodenal ulcer with perforation, without mention of obstruction
532.11	Acute duodenal ulcer with perforation, with obstruction
532.20	Acute duodenal ulcer with hemorrhage and perforation, without mention of obstruction
532.21	Acute duodenal ulcer with hemorrhage and perforation, with obstruction
532.31	Acute duodenal ulcer without mention of hemorrhage or perforation, with obstruction
532.40	Chronic or unspecified duodenal ulcer with hemorrhage, without mention of obstruction
532.41	Chronic or unspecified duodenal ulcer with hemorrhage, with obstruction
532.50	Chronic or unspecified duodenal ulcer with perforation, without mention of obstruction
532.51	Chronic or unspecified duodenal ulcer with perforation, with obstruction
532.60	Chronic or unspecified duodenal ulcer with hemorrhage and perforation, without mention of obstruction
532.61	Chronic or unspecified duodenal ulcer with hemorrhage and perforation, with obstruction
532.71	Chronic duodenal ulcer without mention of hemorrhage or perforation, with obstruction
532.91	Duodenal ulcer, unspecified as acute or chronic, without mention of hemorrhage or perforation, with obstruction
533.00	Acute peptic ulcer of unspecified site with hemorrhage, without mention of obstruction
533.01	Acute peptic ulcer of unspecified site with hemorrhage, with obstruction
533.10	Acute peptic ulcer of unspecified site with perforation, without mention of obstruction
533.11	Acute peptic ulcer of unspecified site with perforation, with obstruction
533.20	Acute peptic ulcer of unspecified site with hemorrhage and perforation, without mention of obstruction
533.21	Acute peptic ulcer of unspecified site with hemorrhage and perforation, with obstruction
533.31	Acute peptic ulcer of unspecified site without mention of hemorrhage and perforation, with obstruction
533.40	Chronic or unspecified peptic ulcer of unspecified site with hemorrhage, without mention of obstruction
533.41	Chronic or unspecified peptic ulcer of unspecified site with hemorrhage, with obstruction
533.50	Chronic or unspecified peptic ulcer of unspecified site with perforation, without mention of obstruction
533.51	Chronic or unspecified peptic ulcer of unspecified site with perforation, with obstruction
533.60	Chronic or unspecified peptic ulcer of unspecified site with hemorrhage and perforation, without mention of obstruction
533.61	Chronic or unspecified peptic ulcer of unspecified site with hemorrhage and perforation, with obstruction
533.71	Chronic peptic ulcer of unspecified site without mention of hemorrhage or perforation, with obstruction
533.91	Peptic ulcer of unspecified site, unspecified as acute or chronic, without mention of hemorrhage or perforation, with obstruction
534.00	Acute gastrojejunal ulcer with hemorrhage, without mention of obstruction
534.01	Acute gastrojejunal ulcer, with hemorrhage, with obstruction
534.10	Acute gastrojejunal ulcer with perforation, without mention of obstruction
534.11	Acute gastrojejunal ulcer with perforation, with obstruction
534.20	Acute gastrojejunal ulcer with hemorrhage and perforation, without mention of obstruction
534.21	Acute gastrojejunal ulcer with hemorrhage and perforation, with obstruction
534.31	Acute gastrojejunal ulcer without mention of hemorrhage or perforation, with obstruction
534.40	Chronic or unspecified gastrojejunal ulcer with hemorrhage, without mention of obstruction
534.41	Chronic or unspecified gastrojejunal ulcer, with hemorrhage, with obstruction
534.50	Chronic or unspecified gastrojejunal ulcer with perforation, without mention of obstruction
534.51	Chronic or unspecified gastrojejunal ulcer with perforation, with obstruction
534.60	Chronic or unspecified gastrojejunal ulcer with hemorrhage and perforation, without mention of obstruction
534.61	Chronic or unspecified gastrojejunal ulcer with hemorrhage and perforation, with obstruction
534.71	Chronic gastrojejunal ulcer without mention of hemorrhage or perforation, with obstruction
534.91	Gastrojejunal ulcer, unspecified as acute or chronic, without mention of hemorrhage or perforation, with obstruction
535.01	Acute gastritis, with hemorrhage
535.11	Atrophic gastritis, with hemorrhage
535.21	Gastric mucosal hypertrophy, with hemorrhage

535.31	Alcoholic gastritis, with hemorrhage
535.41	Other specified gastritis, with hemorrhage
535.51	Unspecified gastritis and gastroduodenitis, with hemorrhage
535.61	Duodenitis, with hemorrhage
535.71	Eosinophilic gastritis, with hemorrhage
537.83	Angiodysplasia of stomach and duodenum with hemorrhage
537.84	Dieulafoy lesion (hemorrhagic) of stomach and duodenum
540.0	Acute appendicitis with generalized peritonitis
540.1	Acute appendicitis with peritoneal abscess
550.00	Inguinal hernia, with gangrene, unilateral or unspecified (not specified as recurrent)
550.01	Inguinal hernia, with gangrene, unilateral or unspecified, recurrent
550.02	Inguinal hernia, with gangrene, bilateral (not specified as recurrent)
550.03	Inguinal hernia, with gangrene, bilateral, recurrent
551.00	Femoral hernia with gangrene, unilateral or unspecified (not specified as recurrent)
551.01	Femoral hernia with gangrene, unilateral or unspecified, recurrent
551.02	Femoral hernia with gangrene, bilateral (not specified as recurrent)
551.03	Femoral hernia with gangrene, bilateral, recurrent
551.1	Umbilical hernia with gangrene
551.20	Ventral hernia, unspecified, with gangrene
551.21	Incisional ventral hernia, with gangrene
551.29	Other ventral hernia with gangrene
551.3	Diaphragmatic hernia with gangrene
551.8	Hernia of other specified sites, with gangrene
551.9	Hernia of unspecified site, with gangrene
557.0	Acute vascular insufficiency of intestine
560.2	Volvulus
562.02	Diverticulosis of small intestine with hemorrhage
562.03	Diverticulitis of small intestine with hemorrhage
562.12	Diverticulosis of colon with hemorrhage
562.13	Diverticulitis of colon with hemorrhage
567.0	Peritonitis in infectious diseases classified elsewhere
567.1	Pneumococcal peritonitis
567.21	Peritonitis (acute) generalized
567.22	Peritoneal abscess
567.23	Spontaneous bacterial peritonitis
567.29	Other suppurative peritonitis
567.31	Psoas muscle abscess
567.38	Other retroperitoneal abscess
567.39	Other retroperitoneal infections
567.81	Choleperitonitis
567.89	Other specified peritonitis
567.9	Unspecified peritonitis
568.81	Hemoperitoneum (nontraumatic)
569.83	Perforation of intestine
569.85	Angiodysplasia of intestine with hemorrhage
569.86	Dieulafoy lesion (hemorrhagic) of intestine
570	Acute and subacute necrosis of liver
572.0	Abscess of liver
572.1	Portal pyemia
572.2	Hepatic encephalopathy
572.4	Hepatorenal syndrome
573.4	Hepatic infarction
574.81	Calculus of gallbladder and bile duct with acute and chronic cholecystitis, with obstruction
575.4	Perforation of gallbladder
576.2	Obstruction of bile duct
576.3	Perforation of bile duct

577.0	Acute pancreatitis
580.0	Acute glomerulonephritis with lesion of proliferative glomerulonephritis
580.4	Acute glomerulonephritis with lesion of rapidly progressive glomerulonephritis
580.81	Acute glomerulonephritis in diseases classified elsewhere
580.89	Acute glomerulonephritis with other specified pathological lesion in kidney
580.9	Acute glomerulonephritis with unspecified pathological lesion in kidney
583.4	Nephritis and nephropathy, not specified as acute or chronic, with lesion of rapidly progressive glomerulonephritis
583.6	Nephritis and nephropathy, not specified as acute or chronic, with lesion of renal cortical necrosis
584.5	Acute kidney failure with lesion of tubular necrosis
584.6	Acute kidney failure with lesion of renal cortical necrosis
584.7	Acute kidney failure with lesion of renal medullary [papillary] necrosis
585.6	End stage renal disease
590.11	Acute pyelonephritis with lesion of renal medullary necrosis
590.2	Renal and perinephric abscess
596.6	Rupture of bladder, nontraumatic
614.5	Acute or unspecified pelvic peritonitis, female
634.30	Spontaneous abortion, complicated by renal failure, unspecified
634.31	Spontaneous abortion, complicated by renal failure, incomplete
634.32	Spontaneous abortion, complicated by renal failure, complete
634.50	Spontaneous abortion, complicated by shock, unspecified
634.51	Spontaneous abortion, complicated by shock, incomplete
634.52	Spontaneous abortion, complicated by shock, complete
634.61	Spontaneous abortion, complicated by embolism, incomplete
634.62	Spontaneous abortion, complicated by embolism, complete
635.30	Legally induced abortion, complicated by renal failure,unspecified
635.31	Legally induced abortion, complicated by renal failure, incomplete
635.32	Legally induced abortion, complicated by renal failure, complete
635.50	Legally induced abortion, complicated by shock, unspecified
635.51	Legally induced abortion, complicated by shock, incomplete
635.52	Legally induced abortion, complicated by shock, complete
635.60	Legally induced abortion, complicated by embolism, unspecified
635.61	Legally induced abortion, complicated by embolism, incomplete
635.62	Legally induced abortion, complicated by embolism, complete
636.30	Illegally induced abortion, complicated by renal failure, unspecified
636.31	Illegally induced abortion, complicated by renal failure, incomplete
636.32	Illegally induced abortion, complicated by renal failure, complete
636.50	Illegally induced abortion, complicated by shock, unspecified
636.51	Illegally induced abortion, complicated by shock, incomplete
636.52	Illegally induced abortion, complicated by shock, complete
636.60	Illegally induced abortion, complicated by embolism, unspecified
636.61	Illegally induced abortion, complicated by embolism, incomplete
636.62	Illegally induced abortion, complicated by embolism, complete
637.30	Unspecified abortion, complicated by renal failure, unspecified
637.31	Unspecified abortion, complicated by renal failure, incomplete
637.32	Unspecified abortion, complicated by renal failure, complete
637.50	Unspecified abortion, complicated by shock, unspecified
637.51	Unspecified abortion, complicated by shock, incomplete
637.52	Unspecified abortion, complicated by shock, complete
637.60	Unspecified abortion, complicated by embolism, unspecified
637.61	Unspecified abortion, complicated by embolism, incomplete
637.62	Unspecified abortion, complicated by embolism, complete
638.3	Failed attempted abortion complicated by renal failure

638.5	Failed attempted abortion complicated by shock
638.6	Failed attempted abortion complicated by embolism
639.3	Kidney failure following abortion and ectopic and molar pregnancies
639.5	Shock following abortion or ectopic and molar pregnancies
639.6	Embolism following abortion or ectopic and molar pregnancies
641.11	Hemorrhage from placenta previa, delivered, with or without mention of antepartum condition
641.13	Hemorrhage from placenta previa, antepartum condition or complication
641.21	Premature separation of placenta, delivered, with or without mention of antepartum condition
641.31	Antepartum hemorrhage associated with coagulation defects, delivered, with or without mention of antepartum condition
641.33	Antepartum hemorrhage associated with coagulation defects, antepartum condition or complication
642.11	Hypertension secondary to renal disease, complicating pregnancy, childbirth, and the puerperium, delivered, with or without mention of antepartum condition
642.12	Hypertension secondary to renal disease, complicating pregnancy, childbirth, and the puerperium, delivered, with mention of postpartum complication
642.42	Mild or unspecified pre-eclampsia, delivered, with mention of postpartum complication
642.51	Severe pre-eclampsia, delivered, with or without mention of antepartum condition
642.52	Severe pre-eclampsia, delivered, with mention of postpartum complication
642.53	Severe pre-eclampsia, antepartum condition or complication
642.54	Severe pre-eclampsia, postpartum condition or complication
642.61	Eclampsia, delivered, with or without mention of antepartum condition
642.62	Eclampsia, delivered, with mention of postpartum complication
642.63	Eclampsia, antepartum condition or complication
642.64	Eclampsia, postpartum condition or complication
642.71	Pre-eclampsia or eclampsia superimposed on pre-existing hypertension, delivered, with or without mention of antepartum condition
642.72	Pre-eclampsia or eclampsia superimposed on pre-existing hypertension, delivered, with mention of postpartum complication
642.73	Pre-eclampsia or eclampsia superimposed on pre-existing hypertension, antepartum condition or complication
642.74	Pre-eclampsia or eclampsia superimposed on pre-existing hypertension, postpartum condition or complication
644.03	Threatened premature labor, antepartum condition or complication
644.21	Early onset of delivery, delivered, with or without mention of antepartum condition
648.01	Diabetes mellitus of mother, complicating pregnancy, childbirth, or the puerperium, delivered, with or without mention of antepartum condition
648.02	Diabetes mellitus of mother, complicating pregnancy, childbirth, or the puerperium, delivered, with mention of postpartum complication
654.51	Cervical incompetence, delivered, with or without mention of antepartum condition
654.52	Cervical incompetence, delivered, with mention of postpartum complication
654.53	Cervical incompetence, antepartum condition or complication
654.54	Cervical incompetence, postpartum condition or complication
658.41	Infection of amniotic cavity, delivered, with or without mention of antepartum condition
658.43	Infection of amniotic cavity, antepartum condition or complication
659.31	Generalized infection during labor, delivered, with or without mention of antepartum condition
659.33	Generalized infection during labor, antepartum condition or complication
665.01	Rupture of uterus before onset of labor, delivered, with or without mention of antepartum condition
665.03	Rupture of uterus before onset of labor, antepartum condition or complication
665.11	Rupture of uterus during labor, delivered, with or without mention of antepartum condition
669.11	Shock during or following labor and delivery, delivered, with or without mention of antepartum condition
669.12	Shock during or following labor and delivery, delivered, with mention of postpartum complication
669.13	Shock during or following labor and delivery, antepartum condition or complication
669.14	Shock during or following labor and delivery, postpartum condition or complication
669.21	Maternal hypotension syndrome, delivered, with or without mention of antepartum condition
669.22	Maternal hypotension syndrome, delivered, with mention of postpartum complication
669.32	Acute kidney failure following labor and delivery, delivered, with mention of postpartum complication
669.34	Acute kidney failure following labor and delivery, postpartum condition or complication
670.02	Major puerperal infection, delivered, with mention of postpartum complication
670.04	Major puerperal infection, postpartum condition or complication
670.22	Puerperal sepsis, delivered, with mention of postpartum complication
670.24	Puerperal sepsis, postpartum condition or complication
670.32	Puerperal septic thrombophlebitis, delivered, with mention of postpartum complication
670.34	Puerperal septic thrombophlebitis, postpartum condition or complication
670.80	Other major puerperal infection, unspecified as to episode of care or not applicable
670.82	Other major puerperal infection, delivered, with mention of postpartum complication
670.84	Other major puerperal infection, postpartum condition or complication
671.31	Deep phlebothrombosis, antepartum, delivered, with or without mention of antepartum condition
671.33	Deep phlebothrombosis, antepartum, antepartum condition or complication
671.42	Deep phlebothrombosis, postpartum, delivered, with mention of postpartum complication
671.44	Deep phlebothrombosis, postpartum, postpartum condition or complication
673.01	Obstetrical air embolism, delivered, with or without mention of antepartum condition
673.02	Obstetrical air embolism, delivered, with mention of postpartum complication
673.03	Obstetrical air embolism, antepartum condition or complication
673.04	Obstetrical air embolism, postpartum condition or complication
673.11	Amniotic fluid embolism, delivered, with or without mention of antepartum condition
673.12	Amniotic fluid embolism, delivered, with mention of postpartum complication
673.13	Amniotic fluid embolism, antepartum condition or complication
673.14	Amniotic fluid embolism, postpartum condition or complication
673.21	Obstetrical blood-clot embolism, delivered, with or without mention of antepartum condition
673.22	Obstetrical blood-clot embolism, delivered, with mention of postpartum complication

673.23	Obstetrical blood-clot embolism, antepartum condition or complication
673.24	Obstetrical blood-clot embolism, postpartum condition or complication
673.31	Obstetrical pyemic and septic embolism, delivered, with or without mention of antepartum condition
673.32	Obstetrical pyemic and septic embolism, delivered, with mention of postpartum complication
673.33	Obstetrical pyemic and septic embolism, antepartum condition or complication
673.34	Obstetrical pyemic and septic embolism, postpartum condition or complication
673.81	Other obstetrical pulmonary embolism, delivered, with or without mention of antepartum condition
673.82	Other obstetrical pulmonary embolism, delivered, with mention of postpartum complication
673.83	Other obstetrical pulmonary embolism, antepartum condition or complication
673.84	Other obstetrical pulmonary embolism, postpartum condition or complication
674.01	Cerebrovascular disorders in the puerperium, delivered, with or without mention of antepartum condition
674.50	Peripartum cardiomyopathy, unspecified as to episode of care or not applicable
674.51	Peripartum cardiomyopathy, delivered, with or without mention of antepartum condition
674.52	Peripartum cardiomyopathy, delivered, with mention of postpartum condition
674.53	Peripartum cardiomyopathy, antepartum condition or complication
674.54	Peripartum cardiomyopathy, postpartum condition or complication
707.23	Pressure ulcer, stage III
707.24	Pressure ulcer, stage IV
728.86	Necrotizing fasciitis
740.0	Anencephalus
740.1	Craniorachischisis
740.2	Iniencephaly
742.2	Congenital reduction deformities of brain
745.0	Common truncus
745.10	Complete transposition of great vessels
745.11	Double outlet right ventricle
745.19	Other transposition of great vessels
745.2	Tetralogy of fallot
745.3	Common ventricle
745.7	Cor biloculare
746.01	Atresia of pulmonary valve, congenital
746.1	Tricuspid atresia and stenosis, congenital
746.2	Ebstein's anomaly
746.7	Hypoplastic left heart syndrome
746.81	Subaortic stenosis
746.82	Cor triatriatum
746.84	Obstructive anomalies of heart, not elsewhere classified
746.86	Congenital heart block
747.11	Interruption of aortic arch
747.31	Pulmonary artery coarctation and atresia
747.32	Pulmonary arteriovenous malformation
747.39	Other anomalies of pulmonary artery and pulmonary circulation
747.81	Anomalies of cerebrovascular system
747.83	Persistent fetal circulation
748.5	Agenesis, hypoplasia, and dysplasia of lung
750.3	Tracheoesophageal fistula, esophageal atresia and stenosis

751.61	Biliary atresia
755.55	Acrocephalosyndactyly
756.6	Anomalies of diaphragm
756.70	Anomaly of abdominal wall, unspecified
756.71	Prune belly syndrome
756.72	Omphalocele
756.73	Gastroschisis
756.79	Other congenital anomalies of abdominal wall
758.32	Velo-cardio-facial syndrome
759.4	Conjoined twins
767.0	Subdural and cerebral hemorrhage
768.5	Severe birth asphyxia
768.73	Severe hypoxic-ischemic encephalopathy
769	Respiratory distress syndrome in newborn
770.0	Congenital pneumonia
770.12	Meconium aspiration with respiratory symptoms
770.14	Aspiration of clear amniotic fluid with respiratory symptoms
770.16	Aspiration of blood with respiratory symptoms
770.18	Other fetal and newborn aspiration with respiratory symptoms
770.2	Interstitial emphysema and related conditions
770.3	Pulmonary hemorrhage
770.7	Chronic respiratory disease arising in the perinatal period
770.84	Respiratory failure of newborn
770.86	Aspiration of postnatal stomach contents with respiratory symptoms
770.87	Respiratory arrest of newborn
771.1	Congenital cytomegalovirus infection
771.2	Other congenital infections specific to the perinatal period
771.3	Tetanus neonatorum
771.81	Septicemia [sepsis] of newborn
772.13	Intraventricular hemorrhage, grade III
772.14	Intraventricular hemorrhage, grade IV
772.2	Subarachnoid hemorrhage of fetus or newborn
772.4	Gastrointestinal hemorrhage of fetus or newborn
773.3	Hydrops fetalis due to isoimmunization
773.4	Kernicterus of fetus or newborn due to isoimmunization
774.4	Perinatal jaundice due to hepatocellular damage
774.7	Kernicterus of fetus or newborn not due to isoimmunization
775.7	Late metabolic acidosis of newborn
776.1	Transient neonatal thrombocytopenia
776.2	Disseminated intravascular coagulation in newborn
776.7	Transient neonatal neutropenia
777.50	Necrotizing enterocolitis in newborn, unspecified
777.51	Stage I necrotizing enterocolitis in newborn
777.52	Stage II necrotizing enterocolitis in newborn
777.53	Stage III necrotizing enterocolitis in newborn
777.6	Perinatal intestinal perforation
778.0	Hydrops fetalis not due to isoimmunization
779.0	Convulsions in newborn
779.2	Cerebral depression, coma, and other abnormal cerebral signs in fetus or newborn
779.32	Bilious vomiting in newborn
779.7	Periventricular leukomalacia
779.85	Cardiac arrest of newborn
780.01	Coma
780.72	Functional quadriplegia
785.51	Cardiogenic shock
785.52	Septic shock
785.59	Other shock without mention of trauma

Appendix A — Numeric MCC List

799.1   Respiratory arrest

800.03   Closed fracture of vault of skull without mention of intracranial injury, with moderate [1-24 hours] loss of consciousness

800.04   Closed fracture of vault of skull without mention of intracranial injury, with prolonged [more than 24 hours] loss of consciousness and return to pre-existing conscious level

800.05   Closed fracture of vault of skull without mention of intracranial injury, with prolonged [more than 24 hours] loss of consciousness, without return to pre-existing conscious level

800.10   Closed fracture of vault of skull with cerebral laceration and contusion, unspecified state of consciousness

800.11   Closed fracture of vault of skull with cerebral laceration and contusion, with no loss of consciousness

800.12   Closed fracture of vault of skull with cerebral laceration and contusion, with brief [less than one hour] loss of consciousness

800.13   Closed fracture of vault of skull with cerebral laceration and contusion, with moderate [1-24 hours] loss of consciousness

800.14   Closed fracture of vault of skull with cerebral laceration and contusion, with prolonged [more than 24 hours] loss of consciousness and return to pre-existing conscious level

800.15   Closed fracture of vault of skull with cerebral laceration and contusion, with prolonged [more than 24 hours] loss of consciousness, without return to pre-existing conscious level

800.16   Closed fracture of vault of skull with cerebral laceration and contusion, with loss of consciousness of unspecified duration

800.19   Closed fracture of vault of skull with cerebral laceration and contusion, with concussion, unspecified

800.20   Closed fracture of vault of skull with subarachnoid, subdural, and extradural hemorrhage, unspecified state of consciousness

800.21   Closed fracture of vault of skull with subarachnoid, subdural, and extradural hemorrhage, with no loss of consciousness

800.22   Closed fracture of vault of skull with subarachnoid, subdural, and extradural hemorrhage, with brief [less than one hour] loss of consciousness

800.23   Closed fracture of vault of skull with subarachnoid, subdural, and extradural hemorrhage, with moderate [1-24 hours] loss of consciousness

800.24   Closed fracture of vault of skull with subarachnoid, subdural, and extradural hemorrhage, with prolonged [more than 24 hours] loss of consciousness and return to pre-existing conscious level

800.25   Closed fracture of vault of skull with subarachnoid, subdural, and extradural hemorrhage, with prolonged [more than 24 hours] loss of consciousness, without return to pre-existing conscious level

800.26   Closed fracture of vault of skull with subarachnoid, subdural, and extradural hemorrhage, with loss of consciousness of unspecified duration

800.29   Closed fracture of vault of skull with subarachnoid, subdural, and extradural hemorrhage, with concussion, unspecified

800.30   Closed fracture of vault of skull with other and unspecified intracranial hemorrhage, unspecified state of consciousness

800.31   Closed fracture of vault of skull with other and unspecified intracranial hemorrhage, with no loss of consciousness

800.32   Closed fracture of vault of skull with other and unspecified intracranial hemorrhage, with brief [less than one hour] loss of consciousness

800.33   Closed fracture of vault of skull with other and unspecified intracranial hemorrhage, with moderate [1-24 hours] loss of consciousness

800.34   Closed fracture of vault of skull with other and unspecified intracranial hemorrhage, with prolonged [more than 24 hours] loss of consciousness and return to pre-existing conscious level

800.35   Closed fracture of vault of skull with other and unspecified intracranial hemorrhage, with prolonged [more than 24 hours] loss of consciousness, without return to pre-existing conscious level

800.36   Closed fracture of vault of skull with other and unspecified intracranial hemorrhage, with loss of consciousness of unspecified duration

800.39   Closed fracture of vault of skull with other and unspecified intracranial hemorrhage, with concussion, unspecified

800.43   Closed fracture of vault of skull with intracranial injury of other and unspecified nature, with moderate [1-24 hours] loss of consciousness

800.44   Closed fracture of vault of skull with intracranial injury of other and unspecified nature, with prolonged [more than 24 hours] loss of consciousness and return to pre-existing conscious level

800.45   Closed fracture of vault of skull with intracranial injury of other and unspecified nature, with prolonged [more than 24 hours] loss of consciousness, without return to pre-existing conscious level

800.50   Open fracture of vault of skull without mention of intracranial injury, unspecified state of consciousness

800.51   Open fracture of vault of skull without mention of intracranial injury, with no loss of consciousness

800.52   Open fracture of vault of skull without mention of intracranial injury, with brief [less than one hour] loss of consciousness

800.53   Open fracture of vault of skull without mention of intracranial injury, with moderate [1-24 hours] loss of consciousness

800.54   Open fracture of vault of skull without mention of intracranial injury, with prolonged [more than 24 hours] loss of consciousness and return to pre-existing conscious level

800.55   Open fracture of vault of skull without mention of intracranial injury, with prolonged [more than 24 hours] loss of consciousness, without return to pre-existing conscious level

800.56   Open fracture of vault of skull without mention of intracranial injury, with loss of consciousness of unspecified duration

800.59   Open fracture of vault of skull without mention of intracranial injury, with concussion, unspecified

800.60   Open fracture of vault of skull with cerebral laceration and contusion, unspecified state of consciousness

800.61   Open fracture of vault of skull with cerebral laceration and contusion, with no loss of consciousness

800.62   Open fracture of vault of skull with cerebral laceration and contusion, with brief [less than one hour] loss of consciousness

800.63   Open fracture of vault of skull with cerebral laceration and contusion, with moderate [1-24 hours] loss of consciousness

800.64   Open fracture of vault of skull with cerebral laceration and contusion, with prolonged [more than 24 hours] loss of consciousness and return to pre-existing conscious level

800.65   Open fracture of vault of skull with cerebral laceration and contusion, with prolonged [more than 24 hours] loss of consciousness, without return to pre-existing conscious level

800.66   Open fracture of vault of skull with cerebral laceration and contusion, with loss of consciousness of unspecified duration

800.69   Open fracture of vault of skull with cerebral laceration and contusion, with concussion, unspecified

800.70   Open fracture of vault of skull with subarachnoid, subdural, and extradural hemorrhage, unspecified state of consciousness

800.71   Open fracture of vault of skull with subarachnoid, subdural, and extradural hemorrhage, with no loss of consciousness

800.72   Open fracture of vault of skull with subarachnoid, subdural, and extradural hemorrhage, with brief [less than one hour] loss of consciousness

800.73   Open fracture of vault of skull with subarachnoid, subdural, and extradural hemorrhage, with moderate [1-24 hours] loss of consciousness

800.74   Open fracture of vault of skull with subarachnoid, subdural, and extradural hemorrhage, with prolonged [more than 24 hours] loss of consciousness and return to pre-existing conscious level

800.75   Open fracture of vault of skull with subarachnoid, subdural, and extradural hemorrhage, with prolonged [more than 24 hours] loss of consciousness, without return to pre-existing conscious level

800.76   Open fracture of vault of skull with subarachnoid, subdural, and extradural hemorrhage, with loss of consciousness of unspecified duration

800.79	Open fracture of vault of skull with subarachnoid, subdural, and extradural hemorrhage, with concussion, unspecified
800.80	Open fracture of vault of skull with other and unspecified intracranial hemorrhage, unspecified state of consciousness
800.81	Open fracture of vault of skull with other and unspecified intracranial hemorrhage, with no loss of consciousness
800.82	Open fracture of vault of skull with other and unspecified intracranial hemorrhage, with brief [less than one hour] loss of consciousness
800.83	Open fracture of vault of skull with other and unspecified intracranial hemorrhage, with moderate [1-24 hours] loss of consciousness
800.84	Open fracture of vault of skull with other and unspecified intracranial hemorrhage, with prolonged [more than 24 hours] loss of consciousness and return to pre-existing conscious level
800.85	Open fracture of vault of skull with other and unspecified intracranial hemorrhage, with prolonged [more than 24 hours] loss of consciousness, without return to pre-existing conscious level
800.86	Open fracture of vault of skull with other and unspecified intracranial hemorrhage, with loss of consciousness of unspecified duration
800.89	Open fracture of vault of skull with other and unspecified intracranial hemorrhage, with concussion, unspecified
800.90	Open fracture of vault of skull with intracranial injury of other and unspecified nature, unspecified state of consciousness
800.91	Open fracture of vault of skull with intracranial injury of other and unspecified nature, with no loss of consciousness
800.92	Open fracture of vault of skull with intracranial injury of other and unspecified nature, with brief [less than one hour] loss of consciousness
800.93	Open fracture of vault of skull with intracranial injury of other and unspecified nature, with moderate [1-24 hours] loss of consciousness
800.94	Open fracture of vault of skull with intracranial injury of other and unspecified nature, with prolonged [more than 24 hours] loss of consciousness and return to pre-existing conscious level
800.95	Open fracture of vault of skull with intracranial injury of other and unspecified nature, with prolonged [more than 24 hours] loss of consciousness, without return to pre-existing conscious level
800.96	Open fracture of vault of skull with intracranial injury of other and unspecified nature, with loss of consciousness of unspecified duration
800.99	Open fracture of vault of skull with intracranial injury of other and unspecified nature, with concussion, unspecified
801.03	Closed fracture of base of skull without mention of intra cranial injury, with moderate [1-24 hours] loss of consciousness
801.04	Closed fracture of base of skull without mention of intra cranial injury, with prolonged [more than 24 hours] loss of consciousness and return to pre-existing conscious level
801.05	Closed fracture of base of skull without mention of intra cranial injury, with prolonged [more than 24 hours] loss of consciousness, without return to pre-existing conscious level
801.10	Closed fracture of base of skull with cerebral laceration and contusion, unspecified state of consciousness
801.11	Closed fracture of base of skull with cerebral laceration and contusion, with no loss of consciousness
801.12	Closed fracture of base of skull with cerebral laceration and contusion, with brief [less than one hour] loss of consciousness
801.13	Closed fracture of base of skull with cerebral laceration and contusion, with moderate [1-24 hours] loss of consciousness
801.14	Closed fracture of base of skull with cerebral laceration and contusion, with prolonged [more than 24 hours] loss of consciousness and return to pre-existing conscious level
801.15	Closed fracture of base of skull with cerebral laceration and contusion, with prolonged [more than 24 hours] loss of consciousness, without return to pre-existing conscious level
801.16	Closed fracture of base of skull with cerebral laceration and contusion, with loss of consciousness of unspecified duration
801.19	Closed fracture of base of skull with cerebral laceration and contusion, with concussion, unspecified
801.20	Closed fracture of base of skull with subarachnoid, subdural, and extradural hemorrhage, unspecified state of consciousness
801.21	Closed fracture of base of skull with subarachnoid, subdural, and extradural hemorrhage, with no loss of consciousness
801.22	Closed fracture of base of skull with subarachnoid, subdural, and extradural hemorrhage, with brief [less than one hour] loss of consciousness
801.23	Closed fracture of base of skull with subarachnoid, subdural, and extradural hemorrhage, with moderate [1-24 hours] loss of consciousness
801.24	Closed fracture of base of skull with subarachnoid, subdural, and extradural hemorrhage, with prolonged [more than 24 hours] loss of consciousness and return to pre-existing conscious level
801.25	Closed fracture of base of skull with subarachnoid, subdural, and extradural hemorrhage, with prolonged [more than 24 hours] loss of consciousness, without return to pre-existing conscious level
801.26	Closed fracture of base of skull with subarachnoid, subdural, and extradural hemorrhage, with loss of consciousness of unspecified duration
801.29	Closed fracture of base of skull with subarachnoid, subdural, and extradural hemorrhage, with concussion, unspecified
801.30	Closed fracture of base of skull with other and unspecified intracranial hemorrhage, unspecified state of consciousness
801.31	Closed fracture of base of skull with other and unspecified intracranial hemorrhage, with no loss of consciousness
801.32	Closed fracture of base of skull with other and unspecified intracranial hemorrhage, with brief [less than one hour] loss of consciousness
801.33	Closed fracture of base of skull with other and unspecified intracranial hemorrhage, with moderate [1-24 hours] loss of consciousness
801.34	Closed fracture of base of skull with other and unspecified intracranial hemorrhage, with prolonged [more than 24 hours] loss of consciousness and return to pre-existing conscious level
801.35	Closed fracture of base of skull with other and unspecified intracranial hemorrhage, with prolonged [more than 24 hours] loss of consciousness, without return to pre-existing conscious level
801.36	Closed fracture of base of skull with other and unspecified intracranial hemorrhage, with loss of consciousness of unspecified duration
801.39	Closed fracture of base of skull with other and unspecified intracranial hemorrhage, with concussion, unspecified
801.43	Closed fracture of base of skull with intracranial injury of other and unspecified nature, with moderate [1-24 hours] loss of consciousness
801.44	Closed fracture of base of skull with intracranial injury of other and unspecified nature, with prolonged [more than 24 hours) loss of consciousness and return to pre-existing conscious level
801.45	Closed fracture of base of skull with intracranial injury of other and unspecified nature, with prolonged [more than 24 hours] loss of consciousness, without return to pre-existing conscious level
801.50	Open fracture of base of skull without mention of intracranial injury, unspecified state of consciousness
801.51	Open fracture of base of skull without mention of intracranial injury, with no loss of consciousness
801.52	Open fracture of base of skull without mention of intracranial injury, with brief [less than one hour] loss of consciousness
801.53	Open fracture of base of skull without mention of intracranial injury, with moderate [1-24 hours] loss of consciousness
801.54	Open fracture of base of skull without mention of intracranial injury, with prolonged [more than 24 hours] loss of consciousness and return to pre-existing conscious level
801.55	Open fracture of base of skull without mention of intracranial injury, with prolonged [more than 24 hours] loss of consciousness, without return to pre-existing conscious level

801.56 Open fracture of base of skull without mention of intracranial injury, with loss of consciousness of unspecified duration

801.59 Open fracture of base of skull without mention of intracranial injury, with concussion, unspecified

801.60 Open fracture of base of skull with cerebral laceration and contusion, unspecified state of consciousness

801.61 Open fracture of base of skull with cerebral laceration and contusion, with no loss of consciousness

801.62 Open fracture of base of skull with cerebral laceration and contusion, with brief [less than one hour] loss of consciousness

801.63 Open fracture of base of skull with cerebral laceration and contusion, with moderate [1-24 hours] loss of consciousness

801.64 Open fracture of base of skull with cerebral laceration and contusion, with prolonged [more than 24 hours] loss of consciousness and return to pre-existing conscious level

801.65 Open fracture of base of skull with cerebral laceration and contusion, with prolonged [more than 24 hours] loss of consciousness, without return to pre-existing conscious level

801.66 Open fracture of base of skull with cerebral laceration and contusion, with loss of consciousness of unspecified duration

801.69 Open fracture of base of skull with cerebral laceration and contusion, with concussion, unspecified

801.70 Open fracture of base of skull with subarachnoid, subdural, and extradural hemorrhage, unspecified state of consciousness

801.71 Open fracture of base of skull with subarachnoid, subdural, and extradural hemorrhage, with no loss of consciousness

801.72 Open fracture of base of skull with subarachnoid, subdural, and extradural hemorrhage, with brief [less than one hour] loss of consciousness

801.73 Open fracture of base of skull with subarachnoid, subdural, and extradural hemorrhage, with moderate [1-24 hours] loss of consciousness

801.74 Open fracture of base of skull with subarachnoid, subdural, and extradural hemorrhage, with prolonged [more than 24 hours] loss of consciousness and return to pre-existing conscious level

801.75 Open fracture of base of skull with subarachnoid, subdural, and extradural hemorrhage, with prolonged [more than 24 hours] loss of consciousness, without return to pre-existing conscious level

801.76 Open fracture of base of skull with subarachnoid, subdural, and extradural hemorrhage, with loss of consciousness of unspecified duration

801.79 Open fracture of base of skull with subarachnoid, subdural, and extradural hemorrhage, with concussion, unspecified

801.80 Open fracture of base of skull with other and unspecified intracranial hemorrhage, unspecified state of consciousness

801.81 Open fracture of base of skull with other and unspecified intracranial hemorrhage, with no loss of consciousness

801.82 Open fracture of base of skull with other and unspecified intracranial hemorrhage, with brief [less than one hour] loss of consciousness

801.83 Open fracture of base of skull with other and unspecified intracranial hemorrhage, with moderate [1-24 hours] loss of consciousness

801.84 Open fracture of base of skull with other and unspecified intracranial hemorrhage, with prolonged [more than 24 hours] loss of consciousness and return to pre-existing conscious level

801.85 Open fracture of base of skull with other and unspecified intracranial hemorrhage, with prolonged [more than 24 hours] loss of consciousness, without return to pre-existing conscious level

801.86 Open fracture of base of skull with other and unspecified intracranial hemorrhage, with loss of consciousness of unspecified duration

801.89 Open fracture of base of skull with other and unspecified intracranial hemorrhage, with concussion, unspecified

801.90 Open fracture of base of skull with intracranial injury of other and unspecified nature, unspecified state of consciousness

801.91 Open fracture of base of skull with intracranial injury of other and unspecified nature, with no loss of consciousness

801.92 Open fracture of base of skull with intracranial injury of other and unspecified nature, with brief [less than one hour] loss of consciousness

801.93 Open fracture of base of skull with intracranial injury of other and unspecified nature, with moderate [1-24 hours] loss of consciousness

801.94 Open fracture of base of skull with intracranial injury of other and unspecified nature, with prolonged [more than 24 hours] loss of consciousness and return to pre-existing conscious level

801.95 Open fracture of base of skull with intracranial injury of other and unspecified nature, with prolonged [more than 24 hours] loss of consciousness, without return to pre-existing conscious level

801.96 Open fracture of base of skull with intracranial injury of other and unspecified nature, with loss of consciousness of unspecified duration

801.99 Open fracture of base of skull with intracranial injury of other and unspecified nature, with concussion, unspecified

803.03 Other closed skull fracture without mention of intracranial injury, with moderate [1-24 hours] loss of consciousness

803.04 Other closed skull fracture without mention of intracranial injury, with prolonged [more than 24 hours] loss of consciousness and return to pre-existing conscious level

803.05 Other closed skull fracture without mention of intracranial injury, with prolonged [more than 24 hours] loss of consciousness, without return to pre-existing conscious level

803.10 Other closed skull fracture with cerebral laceration and contusion, unspecified state of consciousness

803.11 Other closed skull fracture with cerebral laceration and contusion, with no loss of consciousness

803.12 Other closed skull fracture with cerebral laceration and contusion, with brief [less than one hour] loss of consciousness

803.13 Other closed skull fracture with cerebral laceration and contusion, with moderate [1-24 hours] loss of consciousness

803.14 Other closed skull fracture with cerebral laceration and contusion, with prolonged [more than 24 hours] loss of consciousness and return to pre-existing conscious level

803.15 Other closed skull fracture with cerebral laceration and contusion, with prolonged [more than 24 hours] loss of consciousness, without return to pre-existing conscious level

803.16 Other closed skull fracture with cerebral laceration and contusion, with loss of consciousness of unspecified duration

803.19 Other closed skull fracture with cerebral laceration and contusion, with concussion, unspecified

803.20 Other closed skull fracture with subarachnoid, subdural, and extradural hemorrhage, unspecified state of consciousness

803.21 Other closed skull fracture with subarachnoid, subdural, and extradural hemorrhage, with no loss of consciousness

803.22 Other closed skull fracture with subarachnoid, subdural, and extradural hemorrhage, with brief [less than one hour] loss of consciousness

803.23 Other closed skull fracture with subarachnoid, subdural, and extradural hemorrhage, with moderate [1-24 hours] loss of consciousness

803.24 Other closed skull fracture with subarachnoid, subdural, and extradural hemorrhage, with prolonged [more than 24 hours] loss of consciousness and return to pre-existing conscious level

803.25 Other closed skull fracture with subarachnoid, subdural, and extradural hemorrhage, with prolonged [more than 24 hours] loss of consciousness, without return to pre-existing conscious level

803.26 Other closed skull fracture with subarachnoid, subdural, and extradural hemorrhage, with loss of consciousness of unspecified duration

803.29 Other closed skull fracture with subarachnoid, subdural, and extradural hemorrhage, with concussion, unspecified

803.30 Other closed skull fracture with other and unspecified intracranial hemorrhage, unspecified state of unconsciousness

803.31   Other closed skull fracture with other and unspecified intracranial hemorrhage, with no loss of consciousness

803.32   Other closed skull fracture with other and unspecified intracranial hemorrhage, with brief [less than one hour] loss of consciousness

803.33   Other closed skull fracture with other and unspecified intracranial hemorrhage, with moderate [1-24 hours] loss of consciousness

803.34   Other closed skull fracture with other and unspecified intracranial hemorrhage, with prolonged [more than 24 hours] loss of consciousness and return to pre-existing conscious level

803.35   Other closed skull fracture with other and unspecified intracranial hemorrhage, with prolonged [more than 24 hours] loss of consciousness, without return to pre-existing conscious level

803.36   Other closed skull fracture with other and unspecified intracranial hemorrhage, with loss of consciousness of unspecified duration

803.39   Other closed skull fracture with other and unspecified intracranial hemorrhage, with concussion, unspecified

803.43   Other closed skull fracture with intracranial injury of other and unspecified nature, with moderate [1-24 hours] loss of consciousness

803.44   Other closed skull fracture with intracranial injury of other and unspecified nature, with prolonged [more than 24 hours] loss of consciousness and return to pre-existing conscious level

803.45   Other closed skull fracture with intracranial injury of other and unspecified nature, with prolonged [more than 24 hours] loss of consciousness, without return to pre-existing conscious level

803.50   Other open skull fracture without mention of injury, unspecified state of consciousness

803.51   Other open skull fracture without mention of intracranial injury, with no loss of consciousness

803.52   Other open skull fracture without mention of intracranial injury, with brief [less than one hour] loss of consciousness

803.53   Other open skull fracture without mention of intracranial injury, with moderate [1-24 hours] loss of consciousness

803.54   Other open skull fracture without mention of intracranial injury, with prolonged [more than 24 hours] loss of consciousness and return to pre-existing conscious level

803.55   Other open skull fracture without mention of intracranial injury, with prolonged [more than 24 hours] loss of consciousness, without return to pre-existing conscious level

803.56   Other open skull fracture without mention of intracranial injury, with loss of consciousness of unspecified duration

803.59   Other open skull fracture without mention of intracranial injury, with concussion, unspecified

803.60   Other open skull fracture with cerebral laceration and contusion, unspecified state of consciousness

803.61   Other open skull fracture with cerebral laceration and contusion, with no loss of consciousness

803.62   Other open skull fracture with cerebral laceration and contusion, with brief [less than one hour] loss of consciousness

803.63   Other open skull fracture with cerebral laceration and contusion, with moderate [1-24 hours] loss of consciousness

803.64   Other open skull fracture with cerebral laceration and contusion, with prolonged [more than 24 hours] loss of consciousness and return to pre-existing conscious level

803.65   Other open skull fracture with cerebral laceration and contusion, with prolonged [more than 24 hours] loss of consciousness, without return to pre-existing conscious level

803.66   Other open skull fracture with cerebral laceration and contusion, with loss of consciousness of unspecified duration

803.69   Other open skull fracture with cerebral laceration and contusion, with concussion, unspecified

803.70   Other open skull fracture with subarachnoid, subdural, and extradural hemorrhage, unspecified state of consciousness

803.71   Other open skull fracture with subarachnoid, subdural, and extradural hemorrhage, with no loss of consciousness

803.72   Other open skull fracture with subarachnoid, subdural, and extradural hemorrhage, with brief [less than one hour] loss of consciousness

803.73   Other open skull fracture with subarachnoid, subdural, and extradural hemorrhage, with moderate [1-24 hours] loss of consciousness

803.74   Other open skull fracture with subarachnoid, subdural, and extradural hemorrhage, with prolonged [more than 24 hours] loss of consciousness and return to pre-existing conscious level

803.75   Other open skull fracture with subarachnoid, subdural, and extradural hemorrhage, with prolonged [more than 24 hours] loss of consciousness, without return to pre-existing conscious level

803.76   Other open skull fracture with subarachnoid, subdural, and extradural hemorrhage, with loss of consciousness of unspecified duration

803.79   Other open skull fracture with subarachnoid, subdural, and extradural hemorrhage, with concussion, unspecified

803.80   Other open skull fracture with other and unspecified intracranial hemorrhage, unspecified state of consciousness

803.81   Other open skull fracture with other and unspecified intracranial hemorrhage, with no loss of consciousness

803.82   Other open skull fracture with other and unspecified intracranial hemorrhage, with brief [less than one hour] loss of consciousness

803.83   Other open skull fracture with other and unspecified intracranial hemorrhage, with moderate [1-24 hours] loss of consciousness

803.84   Other open skull fracture with other and unspecified intracranial hemorrhage, with prolonged [more than 24 hours] loss of consciousness and return to pre-existing conscious level

803.85   Other open skull fracture with other and unspecified intracranial hemorrhage, with prolonged [more than 24 hours] loss of consciousness, without return to pre-existing conscious level

803.86   Other open skull fracture with other and unspecified intracranial hemorrhage, with loss of consciousness of unspecified duration

803.89   Other open skull fracture with other and unspecified intracranial hemorrhage, with concussion, unspecified

803.90   Other open skull fracture with intracranial injury of other and unspecified nature, unspecified state of consciousness

803.91   Other open skull fracture with intracranial injury of other and unspecified nature, with no loss of consciousness

803.92   Other open skull fracture with intracranial injury of other and unspecified nature, with brief [less than one hour] loss of consciousness

803.93   Other open skull fracture with intracranial injury of other and unspecified nature, with moderate [1-24 hours] loss of consciousness

803.94   Other open skull fracture with intracranial injury of other and unspecified nature, with prolonged [more than 24 hours] loss of consciousness and return to pre-existing conscious level

803.95   Other open skull fracture with intracranial injury of other and unspecified nature, with prolonged [more than 24 hours] loss of consciousness, without return to pre-existing conscious level

803.96   Other open skull fracture with intracranial injury of other and unspecified nature, with loss of consciousness of unspecified duration

803.99   Other open skull fracture with intracranial injury of other and unspecified nature, with concussion, unspecified

804.03   Closed fractures involving skull or face with other bones, without mention of intracranial injury, with moderate [1-24 hours] loss of consciousness

804.04   Closed fractures involving skull or face with other bones, without mention or intracranial injury, with prolonged [more than 24 hours] loss of consciousness and return to pre-existing conscious level

804.05   Closed fractures involving skull of face with other bones, without mention of intracranial injury, with prolonged [more than 24 hours] loss of consciousness, without return to pre-existing conscious level

804.10 Closed fractures involving skull or face with other bones, with cerebral laceration and contusion, unspecified state of consciousness

804.11 Closed fractures involving skull or face with other bones, with cerebral laceration and contusion, with no loss of consciousness

804.12 Closed fractures involving skull or face with other bones, with cerebral laceration and contusion, with brief [less than one hour] loss of consciousness

804.13 Closed fractures involving skull or face with other bones, with cerebral laceration and contusion, with moderate [1-24 hours] loss of consciousness

804.14 Closed fractures involving skull or face with other bones, with cerebral laceration and contusion, with prolonged [more than 24 hours] loss of consciousness and return to pre-existing conscious level

804.15 Closed fractures involving skull or face with other bones, with cerebral laceration and contusion, with prolonged [more than 24 hours] loss of consciousness, without return to pre-existing conscious level

804.16 Closed fractures involving skull or face with other bones, with cerebral laceration and contusion, with loss of consciousness of unspecified duration

804.19 Closed fractures involving skull or face with other bones, with cerebral laceration and contusion, with concussion, unspecified

804.20 Closed fractures involving skull or face with other bones with subarachnoid, subdural, and extradural hemorrhage, unspecified state of consciousness

804.21 Closed fractures involving skull or face with other bones with subarachnoid, subdural, and extradural hemorrhage, with no loss of consciousness

804.22 Closed fractures involving skull or face with other bones with subarachnoid, subdural, and extradural hemorrhage, with brief [less than one hour] loss of consciousness

804.23 Closed fractures involving skull or face with other bones with subarachnoid, subdural, and extradural hemorrhage, with moderate [1-24 hours] loss of consciousness

804.24 Closed fractures involving skull or face with other bones with subarachnoid, subdural, and extradural hemorrhage, with prolonged [more than 24 hours] loss of consciousness and return to pre-existing conscious level

804.25 Closed fractures involving skull or face with other bones with subarachnoid, subdural, and extradural hemorrhage, with prolonged [more than 24 hours] loss of consciousness, without return to pre-existing conscious level

804.26 Closed fractures involving skull or face with other bones with subarachnoid, subdural, and extradural hemorrhage, with loss of consciousness of unspecified duration

804.29 Closed fractures involving skull or face with other bones with subarachnoid, subdural, and extradural hemorrhage, with concussion, unspecified

804.30 Closed fractures involving skull or face with other bones, with other and unspecified intracranial hemorrhage, unspecified state of consciousness

804.31 Closed fractures involving skull or face with other bones, with other and unspecified intracranial hemorrhage, with no loss of consciousness

804.32 Closed fractures involving skull or face with other bones, with other and unspecified intracranial hemorrhage, with brief [less than one hour] loss of consciousness

804.33 Closed fractures involving skull or face with other bones, with other and unspecified intracranial hemorrhage, with moderate [1-24 hours] loss of consciousness

804.34 Closed fractures involving skull or face with other bones, with other and unspecified intracranial hemorrhage, with prolonged [more than 24 hours] loss of consciousness and return to pre-existing conscious level

804.35 Closed fractures involving skull or face with other bones, with other and unspecified intracranial hemorrhage, with prolonged [more than 24 hours] loss of consciousness, without return to pre-existing conscious level

804.36 Closed fractures involving skull or face with other bones, with other and unspecified intracranial hemorrhage, with loss of consciousness of unspecified duration

804.39 Closed fractures involving skull or face with other bones, with other and unspecified intracranial hemorrhage, with concussion, unspecified

804.43 Closed fractures involving skull or face with other bones, with intracranial injury of other and unspecified nature, with moderate [1-24 hours] loss of consciousness

804.44 Closed fractures involving skull or face with other bones, with intracranial injury of other and unspecified nature, with prolonged [more than 24 hours] loss of consciousness and return to pre-existing conscious level

804.45 Closed fractures involving skull or face with other bones, with intracranial injury of other and unspecified nature, with prolonged [more than 24 hours] loss of consciousness, without return to pre-existing conscious level

804.53 Open fractures involving skull or face with other bones, without mention of intracranial injury, with moderate [1-24 hours] loss of consciousness

804.54 Open fractures involving skull or face with other bones, without mention of intracranial injury, with prolonged [more than 24 hours] loss of consciousness and return to pre-existing conscious level

804.55 Open fractures involving skull or face with other bones, without mention of intracranial injury, with prolonged [more than 24 hours] loss of consciousness, without return to pre-existing conscious level

804.60 Open fractures involving skull or face with other bones, with cerebral laceration and contusion, unspecified state of consciousness

804.61 Open fractures involving skull or face with other bones, with cerebral laceration and contusion, with no loss of consciousness

804.62 Open fractures involving skull or face with other bones, with cerebral laceration and contusion, with brief [less than one hour] loss of consciousness

804.63 Open fractures involving skull or face with other bones, with cerebral laceration and contusion, with moderate [1-24 hours] loss of consciousness

804.64 Open fractures involving skull or face with other bones, with cerebral laceration and contusion, with prolonged [more than 24 hours] loss of consciousness and return to pre-existing conscious level

804.65 Open fractures involving skull or face with other bones, with cerebral laceration and contusion, with prolonged [more than 24 hours] loss of consciousness, without return to pre-existing conscious level

804.66 Open fractures involving skull or face with other bones, with cerebral laceration and contusion, with loss of consciousness of unspecified duration

804.69 Open fractures involving skull or face with other bones, with cerebral laceration and contusion, with concussion, unspecified

804.70 Open fractures involving skull or face with other bones with subarachnoid, subdural, and extradural hemorrhage, unspecified state of consciousness

804.71 Open fractures involving skull or face with other bones with subarachnoid, subdural, and extradural hemorrhage, with no loss of consciousness

804.72 Open fractures involving skull or face with other bones with subarachnoid, subdural, and extradural hemorrhage, with brief [less than one hour] loss of consciousness

804.73 Open fractures involving skull or face with other bones with subarachnoid, subdural, and extradural hemorrhage, with moderate [1-24 hours] loss of consciousness

Appendix A — Numeric MCC List

804.74	Open fractures involving skull or face with other bones with subarachnoid, subdural, and extradural hemorrhage, with prolonged [more than 24 hours] loss of consciousness and return to pre-existing conscious level
804.75	Open fractures involving skull or face with other bones with subarachnoid, subdural, and extradural hemorrhage, with prolonged [more than 24 hours] loss of consciousness, without return to pre-existing conscious level
804.76	Open fractures involving skull or face with other bones with subarachnoid, subdural, and extradural hemorrhage, with loss of consciousness of unspecified duration
804.79	Open fractures involving skull or face with other bones with subarachnoid, subdural, and extradural hemorrhage, with concussion, unspecified
804.80	Open fractures involving skull or face with other bones, with other and unspecified intracranial hemorrhage, unspecified state of consciousness
804.81	Open fractures involving skull or face with other bones, with other and unspecified intracranial hemorrhage, with no loss of consciousness
804.82	Open fractures involving skull or face with other bones, with other and unspecified intracranial hemorrhage, with brief [less than one hour] loss of consciousness
804.83	Open fractures involving skull or face with other bones, with other and unspecified intracranial hemorrhage, with moderate [1-24 hours] loss of consciousness
804.84	Open fractures involving skull or face with other bones, with other and unspecified intracranial hemorrhage, with prolonged [more than 24 hours] loss of consciousness and return to pre-existing conscious level
804.85	Open fractures involving skull or face with other bones, with other and unspecified intracranial hemorrhage, with prolonged [more than 24 hours] loss consciousness, without return to pre-existing conscious level
804.86	Open fractures involving skull or face with other bones, with other and unspecified intracranial hemorrhage, with loss of consciousness of unspecified duration
804.89	Open fractures involving skull or face with other bones, with other and unspecified intracranial hemorrhage, with concussion, unspecified
804.93	Open fractures involving skull or face with other bones, with intracranial injury of other and unspecified nature, with moderate [1-24 hours] loss of consciousness
804.94	Open fractures involving skull or face with other bones, with intracranial injury of other and unspecified nature, with prolonged [more than 24 hours] loss of consciousness and return to pre-existing conscious level
804.95	Open fractures involving skull or face with other bones, with intracranial injury of other and unspecified nature, with prolonged [more than 24 hours] loss of consciousness without return to pre-existing conscious level
805.10	Open fracture of cervical vertebra, unspecified level
805.11	Open fracture of first cervical vertebra
805.12	Open fracture of second cervical vertebra
805.13	Open fracture of third cervical vertebra
805.14	Open fracture of fourth cervical vertebra
805.15	Open fracture of fifth cervical vertebra
805.16	Open fracture of sixth cervical vertebra
805.17	Open fracture of seventh cervical vertebra
805.18	Open fracture of multiple cervical vertebrae
805.3	Open fracture of dorsal [thoracic] vertebra without mention of spinal cord injury
805.5	Open fracture of lumbar vertebra without mention of spinal cord injury
805.7	Open fracture of sacrum and coccyx without mention of spinal cord injury
805.9	Open fracture of unspecified vertebral column without mention of spinal cord injury
806.00	Closed fracture of C1-C4 level with unspecified spinal cord injury
806.01	Closed fracture of C1-C4 level with complete lesion of cord
806.02	Closed fracture of C1-C4 level with anterior cord syndrome
806.03	Closed fracture of C1-C4 level with central cord syndrome
806.04	Closed fracture of C1-C4 level with other specified spinal cord injury
806.05	Closed fracture of C5-C7 level with unspecified spinal cord injury
806.06	Closed fracture of C5-C7 level with complete lesion of cord
806.07	Closed fracture of C5-C7 level with anterior cord syndrome
806.08	Closed fracture of C5-C7 level with central cord syndrome
806.09	Closed fracture of C5-C7 level with other specified spinal cord injury
806.10	Open fracture of C1-C4 level with unspecified spinal cord injury
806.11	Open fracture of C1-C4 level with complete lesion of cord
806.12	Open fracture of C1-C4 level with anterior cord syndrome
806.13	Open fracture of C1-C4 level with central cord syndrome
806.14	Open fracture of C1-C4 level with other specified spinal cord injury
806.15	Open fracture of C5-C7 level with unspecified spinal cord injury
806.16	Open fracture of C5-C7 level with complete lesion of cord
806.17	Open fracture of C5-C7 level with anterior cord syndrome
806.18	Open fracture of C5-C7 level with central cord syndrome
806.19	Open fracture of C5-C7 level with other specified spinal cord injury
806.20	Closed fracture of T1-T6 level with unspecified spinal cord injury
806.21	Closed fracture of T1-T6 level with complete lesion of cord
806.22	Closed fracture of T1-T6 level with anterior cord syndrome
806.23	Closed fracture of T1-T6 level with central cord syndrome
806.24	Closed fracture of T1-T6 level with other specified spinal cord injury
806.25	Closed fracture of T7-T12 level with unspecified spinal cord injury
806.26	Closed fracture of T7-T12 level with complete lesion of cord
806.27	Closed fracture of T7-T12 level with anterior cord syndrome
806.28	Closed fracture of T7-T12 level with central cord syndrome
806.29	Closed fracture of T7-T12 level with other specified spinal cord injury
806.30	Open fracture of T1-T6 level with unspecified spinal cord injury
806.31	Open fracture of T1-T6 level with complete lesion of cord
806.32	Open fracture of T1-T6 level with anterior cord syndrome
806.33	Open fracture of T1-T6 level with central cord syndrome
806.34	Open fracture of T1-T6 level with other specified spinal cord injury
806.35	Open fracture of T7-T12 level with unspecified spinal cord injury
806.36	Open fracture of T7-T12 level with complete lesion of cord
806.37	Open fracture of T7-T12 level with anterior cord syndrome
806.38	Open fracture of T7-T12 level with central cord syndrome
806.39	Open fracture of T7-T12 level with other specified spinal cord injury
806.4	Closed fracture of lumbar spine with spinal cord injury
806.5	Open fracture of lumbar spine with spinal cord injury
806.60	Closed fracture of sacrum and coccyx with unspecified spinal cord injury
806.61	Closed fracture of sacrum and coccyx with complete cauda equina lesion
806.62	Closed fracture of sacrum and coccyx with other cauda equina injury
806.69	Closed fracture of sacrum and coccyx with other spinal cord injury
806.70	Open fracture of sacrum and coccyx with unspecified spinal cord injury
806.71	Open fracture of sacrum and coccyx with complete cauda equina lesion
806.72	Open fracture of sacrum and coccyx with other cauda equina injury
806.79	Open fracture of sacrum and coccyx with other spinal cord injury

806.8	Closed fracture of unspecified vertebral column with spinal cord injury
806.9	Open fracture of unspecified vertebral column with spinal cord injury
807.10	Open fracture of rib(s), unspecified
807.11	Open fracture of one rib
807.12	Open fracture of two ribs
807.13	Open fracture of three ribs
807.14	Open fracture of four ribs
807.15	Open fracture of five ribs
807.16	Open fracture of six ribs
807.17	Open fracture of seven ribs
807.18	Open fracture of eight or more ribs
807.19	Open fracture of multiple ribs, unspecified
807.3	Open fracture of sternum
807.4	Flail chest
807.5	Closed fracture of larynx and trachea
807.6	Open fracture of larynx and trachea
808.0	Closed fracture of acetabulum
808.1	Open fracture of acetabulum
808.3	Open fracture of pubis
808.51	Open fracture of ilium
808.52	Open fracture of ischium
808.53	Multiple open pelvic fractures with disruption of pelvic circle
808.54	Multiple open pelvic fractures without disruption of pelvic circle
808.59	Open fracture of other specified part of pelvis
808.9	Open unspecified fracture of pelvis
809.1	Fracture of bones of trunk, open
812.10	Open fracture of unspecified part of upper end of humerus
812.11	Open fracture of surgical neck of humerus
812.12	Open fracture of anatomical neck of humerus
812.13	Open fracture of greater tuberosity of humerus
812.19	Other open fracture of upper end of humerus
812.30	Open fracture of unspecified part of humerus
812.31	Open fracture of shaft of humerus
812.50	Open fracture of unspecified part of lower end of humerus
812.51	Open supracondylar fracture of humerus
812.52	Open fracture of lateral condyle of humerus
812.53	Open fracture of medial condyle of humerus
812.54	Open fracture of unspecified condyle(s) of humerus
812.59	Other open fracture of lower end of humerus
813.10	Open fracture of upper end of forearm, unspecified
813.11	Open fracture of olecranon process of ulna
813.12	Open fracture of coronoid process of ulna
813.13	Open Monteggia's fracture
813.14	Other and unspecified open fractures of proximal end of ulna (alone)
813.15	Open fracture of head of radius
813.16	Open fracture of neck of radius
813.17	Other and unspecified open fractures of proximal end of radius (alone)
813.18	Open fracture of radius with ulna, upper end (any part)
813.30	Open fracture of shaft of radius or ulna, unspecified
813.31	Open fracture of shaft of radius (alone)
813.32	Open fracture of shaft of ulna (alone)
813.33	Open fracture of shaft of radius with ulna
813.50	Open fracture of lower end of forearm, unspecified
813.51	Open Colles' fracture
813.52	Other open fractures of distal end of radius (alone)
813.53	Open fracture of distal end of ulna (alone)
813.54	Open fracture of lower end of radius with ulna
813.90	Open fracture of unspecified part of forearm
813.91	Open fracture of unspecified part of radius (alone)
813.92	Open fracture of unspecified part of ulna (alone)
813.93	Open fracture of unspecified part of radius with ulna
820.00	Closed fracture of intracapsular section of neck of femur, unspecified
820.01	Closed fracture of epiphysis (separation) (upper) of neck of femur
820.02	Closed fracture of midcervical section of neck of femur
820.03	Closed fracture of base of neck of femur
820.09	Other closed transcervical fracture of neck of femur
820.10	Open fracture of intracapsular section of neck of femur, unspecified
820.11	Open fracture of epiphysis (separation) (upper) of neck of femur
820.12	Open fracture of midcervical section of neck of femur
820.13	Open fracture of base of neck of femur
820.19	Other open transcervical fracture of neck of femur
820.20	Closed fracture of trochanteric section of neck of femur
820.21	Closed fracture of intertrochanteric section of neck of femur
820.22	Closed fracture of subtrochanteric section of neck of femur
820.30	Open fracture of trochanteric section of neck of femur, unspecified
820.31	Open fracture of intertrochanteric section of neck of femur
820.32	Open fracture of subtrochanteric section of neck of femur
820.8	Closed fracture of unspecified part of neck of femur
820.9	Open fracture of unspecified part of neck of femur
821.00	Closed fracture of unspecified part of femur
821.01	Closed fracture of shaft of femur
821.10	Open fracture of unspecified part of femur
821.11	Open fracture of shaft of femur
821.30	Open fracture of lower end of femur, unspecified part
821.31	Open fracture of condyle, femoral
821.32	Open fracture of epiphysis. Lower (separation) of femur
821.33	Open supracondylar fracture of femur
821.39	Other open fracture of lower end of femur
823.10	Open fracture of upper end of tibia alone
823.11	Open fracture of upper end of fibula alone
823.12	Open fracture of upper end of fibula with tibia
823.30	Open fracture of shaft of tibia alone
823.31	Open fracture of shaft of fibula alone
823.32	Open fracture of shaft of fibula with tibia
823.90	Open fracture of unspecified part of tibia alone
823.91	Open fracture of unspecified part of fibula alone
823.92	Open fracture of unspecified part of fibula with tibia
828.0	Closed multiple fractures involving both lower limbs, lower with upper limb, and lower limb(s) with rib(s) and sternum
828.1	Open multiple fractures involving both lower limbs, lower with upper limb, and lower limb(s) with rib(s) and sternum
835.10	Open dislocation of hip, unspecified site
835.11	Open posterior dislocation of hip
835.12	Open obturator dislocation of hip
835.13	Other open anterior dislocation of hip
839.10	Open dislocation, cervical vertebra, unspecified
839.11	Open dislocation, first cervical vertebra
839.12	Open dislocation, second cervical vertebra
839.13	Open dislocation, third cervical vertebra
839.14	Open dislocation, fourth cervical vertebra
839.15	Open dislocation, fifth cervical vertebra
839.16	Open dislocation, sixth cervical vertebra
839.17	Open dislocation, seventh cervical vertebra
839.18	Open dislocation, multiple cervical vertebrae

© 2013 OptumInsight, Inc.

839.30   Open dislocation, lumbar vertebra

839.31   Open dislocation, thoracic vertebra

839.50   Open dislocation, vertebra, unspecified site

839.59   Open dislocation, vertebra, other

839.71   Open dislocation, sternum

850.4   Concussion with prolonged loss of consciousness, without return to pre-existing conscious level

851.05   Cortex (cerebral) contusion without mention of open intracranial wound, with prolonged [more than 24 hours] loss of consciousness without return to pre-existing conscious level

851.10   Cortex (cerebral) contusion with open intracranial wound, unspecified state of consciousness

851.11   Cortex (cerebral) contusion with open intracranial wound, with no loss of consciousness

851.12   Cortex (cerebral) contusion with open intracranial wound, with brief [less than one hour] loss of consciousness

851.13   Cortex (cerebral) contusion with open intracranial wound, with moderate [1-24 hours] loss of consciousness

851.14   Cortex (cerebral) contusion with open intracranial wound, with prolonged [more than 24 hours] loss of consciousness and return to pre-existing conscious level

851.15   Cortex (cerebral) contusion with open intracranial wound, with prolonged [more than 24 hours] loss of consciousness without return to pre-existing conscious level

851.16   Cortex (cerebral) contusion with open intracranial wound, with loss of consciousness of unspecified duration

851.19   Cortex (cerebral) contusion with open intracranial wound, with concussion, unspecified

851.20   Cortex (cerebral) laceration without mention of open intracranial wound, unspecified state of consciousness

851.21   Cortex (cerebral) laceration without mention of open intracranial wound, with no loss of consciousness

851.22   Cortex (cerebral) laceration without mention of open intracranial wound, with brief [less than one hour] loss of consciousness

851.23   Cortex (cerebral) laceration without mention of open intracranial wound, with moderate [1-24 hours] loss of consciousness

851.24   Cortex (cerebral) laceration without mention of open intracranial wound, with prolonged [more than 24 hours] loss of consciousness and return to pre-existing conscious level

851.25   Cortex (cerebral) laceration without mention of open intracranial wound, with prolonged [more than 24 hours] loss of consciousness without return to pre-existing conscious level

851.26   Cortex (cerebral) laceration without mention of open intracranial wound, with loss of consciousness of unspecified duration

851.29   Cortex (cerebral) laceration without mention of open intracranial wound, with concussion, unspecified

851.30   Cortex (cerebral) laceration with open intracranial wound, unspecified state of consciousness

851.31   Cortex (cerebral) laceration with open intracranial wound, with no loss of consciousness

851.32   Cortex (cerebral) laceration with open intracranial wound, with brief [less than one hour] loss of consciousness

851.33   Cortex (cerebral) laceration with open intracranial wound, with moderate [1-24 hours] loss of consciousness

851.34   Cortex (cerebral) laceration with open intracranial wound, with prolonged [more than 24 hours] loss of consciousness and return to pre-existing conscious level

851.35   Cortex (cerebral) laceration with open intracranial wound, with prolonged [more than 24 hours] loss of consciousness without return to pre-existing conscious level

851.36   Cortex (cerebral) laceration with open intracranial wound, with loss of consciousness of unspecified duration

851.39   Cortex (cerebral) laceration with open intracranial wound, with concussion, unspecified

851.45   Cerebellar or brain stem contusion without mention of open intracranial wound, with prolonged [more than 24 hours] loss of consciousness without return to pre-existing conscious level

851.50   Cerebellar or brain stem contusion with open intracranial wound, unspecified state of consciousness

851.51   Cerebellar or brain stem contusion with open intracranial wound, with no loss of consciousness

851.52   Cerebellar or brain stem contusion with open intracranial wound, with brief [less than one hour] loss of consciousness

851.53   Cerebellar or brain stem contusion with open intracranial wound, with moderate [1-24 hours] loss of consciousness

851.54   Cerebellar or brain stem contusion with open intracranial wound, with prolonged [more than 24 hours] loss of consciousness and return to pre-existing conscious level

851.55   Cerebellar or brain stem contusion with open intracranial wound, with prolonged [more than 24 hours] loss of consciousness without return to pre-existing conscious level

851.56   Cerebellar or brain stem contusion with open intracranial wound, with loss of consciousness of unspecified duration

851.59   Cerebellar or brain stem contusion with open intracranial wound, with concussion, unspecified

851.60   Cerebellar or brain stem laceration without mention of open intracranial wound, unspecified state of consciousness

851.61   Cerebellar or brain stem laceration without mention of open intracranial wound, with no loss of consciousness

851.62   Cerebellar or brain stem laceration without mention of open intracranial wound, with brief [less than 1 hour] loss of consciousness

851.63   Cerebellar or brain stem laceration without mention of open intracranial wound, with moderate [1-24 hours] loss of consciousness

851.64   Cerebellar or brain stem laceration without mention of open intracranial wound, with prolonged [more than 24 hours] loss of consciousness and return to pre-existing conscious level

851.65   Cerebellar or brain stem laceration without mention of open intracranial wound, with prolonged [more than 24 hours] loss of consciousness without return to pre-existing conscious level

851.66   Cerebellar or brain stem laceration without mention of open intracranial wound, with loss of consciousness of unspecified duration

851.69   Cerebellar or brain stem laceration without mention of open intracranial wound, with concussion, unspecified

851.70   Cerebellar or brain stem laceration with open intracranial wound, unspecified state of consciousness

851.71   Cerebellar or brain stem laceration with open intracranial wound, with no loss of consciousness

851.72   Cerebellar or brain stem laceration with open intracranial wound, with brief [less than one hour] loss of consciousness

851.73   Cerebellar or brain stem laceration with open intracranial wound, with moderate [1-24 hours] loss of consciousness

851.74   Cerebellar or brain stem laceration with open intracranial wound, with prolonged [more than 24 hours] loss of consciousness and return to pre-existing conscious level

851.75   Cerebellar or brain stem laceration with open intracranial wound, with prolonged [more than 24 hours] loss of consciousness without return to pre-existing conscious level

851.76   Cerebellar or brain stem laceration with open intracranial wound, with loss of consciousness of unspecified duration

851.79   Cerebellar or brain stem laceration with open intracranial wound, with concussion, unspecified

851.80   Other and unspecified cerebral laceration and contusion, without mention of open intracranial wound, unspecified state of consciousness

851.81   Other and unspecified cerebral laceration and contusion, without mention of open intracranial wound, with no loss of consciousness

851.82 Other and unspecified cerebral laceration and contusion, without mention of open intracranial wound, with brief [less than one hour] loss of consciousness

851.83 Other and unspecified cerebral laceration and contusion, without mention of open intracranial wound, with moderate [1-24 hours] loss of consciousness

851.84 Other and unspecified cerebral laceration and contusion, without mention of open intracranial wound, with prolonged [more than 24 hours] loss of consciousness and return to pre- existing conscious level

851.85 Other and unspecified cerebral laceration and contusion, without mention of open intracranial wound, with prolonged [more than 24 hours] loss of consciousness without return to pre-existing conscious level

851.86 Other and unspecified cerebral laceration and contusion, without mention of open intracranial wound, with loss of consciousness of unspecified duration

851.89 Other and unspecified cerebral laceration and contusion, without mention of open intracranial wound, with concussion, unspecified

851.90 Other and unspecified cerebral laceration and contusion, with open intracranial wound, unspecified state of consciousness

851.91 Other and unspecified cerebral laceration and contusion, with open intracranial wound, with no loss of consciousness

851.92 Other and unspecified cerebral laceration and contusion, with open intracranial wound, with brief [less than one hour] loss of consciousness

851.93 Other and unspecified cerebral laceration and contusion, with open intracranial wound, with moderate [1-24 hours] loss of consciousness

851.94 Other and unspecified cerebral laceration and contusion, with open intracranial wound, with prolonged [more than 24 hours] loss of consciousness and return to pre-existing conscious level

851.95 Other and unspecified cerebral laceration and contusion, with open intracranial wound, with prolonged [more than 24 hours] loss of consciousness without return to pre-existing conscious level

851.96 Other and unspecified cerebral laceration and contusion, with open intracranial wound, with loss of consciousness of unspecified duration

851.99 Other and unspecified cerebral laceration and contusion, with open intracranial wound, with concussion, unspecified

852.00 Subarachnoid hemorrhage following injury without mention of open intracranial wound, unspecified state of consciousness

852.01 Subarachnoid hemorrhage following injury without mention of open intracranial wound, with no loss of consciousness

852.02 Subarachnoid hemorrhage following injury without mention of open intracranial wound, with brief [less than one hour] loss of consciousness

852.03 Subarachnoid hemorrhage following injury without mention of open intracranial wound, with moderate [1-24 hours] loss of consciousness

852.04 Subarachnoid hemorrhage following injury without mention of open intracranial wound, with prolonged [more than 24 hours] loss of consciousness and return to pre-existing conscious level

852.05 Subarachnoid hemorrhage following injury without mention of open intracranial wound, with prolonged [more than 24 hours] loss of consciousness without return to pre-existing conscious level

852.06 Subarachnoid hemorrhage following injury without mention of open intracranial wound, with loss of consciousness of unspecified duration

852.09 Subarachnoid hemorrhage following injury without mention of open intracranial wound, with concussion, unspecified

852.10 Subarachnoid hemorrhage following injury with open intracranial wound, unspecified state of consciousness

852.11 Subarachnoid hemorrhage following injury with open intracranial wound, with no loss of consciousness

852.12 Subarachnoid hemorrhage following injury with open intracranial wound, with brief [less than one hour] loss of consciousness

852.13 Subarachnoid hemorrhage following injury with open intracranial wound, with moderate [1-24 hours] loss of consciousness

852.14 Subarachnoid hemorrhage following injury with open intracranial wound, with prolonged [more than 24 hours) loss of consciousness and return to pre-existing conscious level

852.15 Subarachnoid hemorrhage following injury with open intracranial wound, with prolonged [more than 24 hours] loss of consciousness without return to pre-existing conscious level

852.16 Subarachnoid hemorrhage following injury with open intracranial wound, with loss of consciousness of unspecified duration

852.19 Subarachnoid hemorrhage following injury with open intracranial wound, with concussion, unspecified

852.20 Subdural hemorrhage following injury without mention of open intracranial wound, unspecified state of consciousness

852.21 Subdural hemorrhage following injury without mention of open intracranial wound, with no loss of consciousness

852.22 Subdural hemorrhage following injury without mention of open intracranial wound, with brief [less than one hour] loss of consciousness

852.23 Subdural hemorrhage following injury without mention of open intracranial wound, with moderate [1-24 hours] loss of consciousness

852.24 Subdural hemorrhage following injury without mention of open intracranial wound, with prolonged [more than 24 hours] loss of consciousness and return to pre-existing conscious level

852.25 Subdural hemorrhage following injury without mention of open intracranial wound, with prolonged [more than 24 hours] loss of consciousness without return to pre-existing conscious level

852.26 Subdural hemorrhage following injury without mention of open intracranial wound, with loss of consciousness of unspecified duration

852.29 Subdural hemorrhage following injury without mention of open intracranial wound, with concussion, unspecified

852.30 Subdural hemorrhage following injury with open intracranial wound, unspecified state of consciousness

852.31 Subdural hemorrhage following injury with open intracranial wound, with no loss of consciousness

852.32 Subdural hemorrhage following injury with open intracranial wound, with brief [less than one hour] loss of consciousness

852.33 Subdural hemorrhage following injury with open intracranial wound, with moderate [1-24 hours] loss of consciousness

852.34 Subdural hemorrhage following injury with open intracranial wound, with prolonged [more than 24 hours] loss of consciousness and return to pre-existing conscious level

852.35 Subdural hemorrhage following injury with open intracranial wound, with prolonged [more than 24 hours] loss of consciousness without return to pre-existing conscious level

852.36 Subdural hemorrhage following injury with open intracranial wound, with loss of consciousness of unspecified duration

852.39 Subdural hemorrhage following injury with open intracranial wound, with concussion, unspecified

852.40 Extradural hemorrhage following injury without mention of open intracranial wound, unspecified state of consciousness

852.41 Extradural hemorrhage following injury without mention of open intracranial wound, with no loss of consciousness

852.42 Extradural hemorrhage following injury without mention of open intracranial wound, with brief [less than 1 hour] loss of consciousness

852.43 Extradural hemorrhage following injury without mention of open intracranial wound, with moderate [1-24 hours] loss of consciousness

852.44 Extradural hemorrhage following injury without mention of open intracranial wound, with prolonged [more than 24 hours] loss of consciousness and return to pre-existing conscious level

852.45 Extradural hemorrhage following injury without mention of open intracranial wound, with prolonged [more than 24 hours] loss of consciousness without return to pre-existing conscious level

852.46   Extradural hemorrhage following injury without mention of open intracranial wound, with loss of consciousness of unspecified duration

852.49   Extradural hemorrhage following injury without mention of open intracranial wound, with concussion, unspecified

852.50   Extradural hemorrhage following injury with open intracranial wound, unspecified state of consciousness

852.51   Extradural hemorrhage following injury with open intracranial wound, with no loss of consciousness

852.52   Extradural hemorrhage following injury with open intracranial wound, with brief [less than one hour] loss of consciousness

852.53   Extradural hemorrhage following injury with open intracranial wound, with moderate [1-24 hours] loss of consciousness

852.54   Extradural hemorrhage following injury with open intracranial wound, with prolonged [more than 24 hours] loss of consciousness and return to pre-existing conscious level

852.55   Extradural hemorrhage following injury with open intracranial wound, with prolonged [more than 24 hours] loss of consciousness without return to pre-existing conscious level

852.56   Extradural hemorrhage following injury with open intracranial wound, with loss of consciousness of unspecified duration

852.59   Extradural hemorrhage following injury with open intracranial wound, with concussion, unspecified

853.00   Other and unspecified intracranial hemorrhage following injury without mention of open intracranial wound, unspecified state of consciousness

853.01   Other and unspecified intracranial hemorrhage following injury without mention of open intracranial wound, with no loss of consciousness

853.02   Other and unspecified intracranial hemorrhage following injury without mention of open intracranial wound, with brief [less than one hour] loss of consciousness

853.03   Other and unspecified intracranial hemorrhage following injury without mention of open intracranial wound, with moderate [1-24 hours] loss of consciousness

853.04   Other and unspecified intracranial hemorrhage following injury without mention of open intracranial wound, with prolonged [more than 24 hours] loss of consciousness and return to pre-existing conscious level

853.05   Other and unspecified intracranial hemorrhage following injury without mention of open intracranial wound, with prolonged [more than 24 hours] loss of consciousness without return to pre-existing conscious level

853.06   Other and unspecified intracranial hemorrhage following injury without mention of open intracranial wound, with loss of consciousness of unspecified duration

853.09   Other and unspecified intracranial hemorrhage following injury without mention of open intracranial wound, with concussion, unspecified

853.10   Other and unspecified intracranial hemorrhage following injury with open intracranial wound, unspecified state of consciousness

853.11   Other and unspecified intracranial hemorrhage following injury with open intracranial wound, with no loss of consciousness

853.12   Other and unspecified intracranial hemorrhage following injury with open intracranial wound, with brief [less than one hour] loss of consciousness

853.13   Other and unspecified intracranial hemorrhage following injury with open intracranial wound, with moderate [1-24 hours] loss of consciousness

853.14   Other and unspecified intracranial hemorrhage following injury with open intracranial wound, with prolonged [more than 24 hours] loss of consciousness and return to pre-existing conscious level

853.15   Other and unspecified intracranial hemorrhage following injury with open intracranial wound, with prolonged [more than 24 hours] loss of consciousness without return to pre-existing conscious level

853.16   Other and unspecified intracranial hemorrhage following injury with open intracranial wound, with loss of consciousness of unspecified duration

853.19   Other and unspecified intracranial hemorrhage following injury with open intracranial wound, with concussion, unspecified

854.05   Intracranial injury of other and unspecified nature without mention of open intracranial wound, with prolonged [more than 24 hours] loss of consciousness without return to pre-existing conscious level

854.10   Intracranial injury of other and unspecified nature with open intracranial wound, unspecified state of consciousness

854.11   Intracranial injury of other and unspecified nature with open intracranial wound, with no loss of consciousness

854.12   Intracranial injury of other and unspecified nature with open intracranial wound, with brief [less than one hour] loss of consciousness

854.13   Intracranial injury of other and unspecified nature with open intracranial wound, with moderate [1-24 hours] loss of consciousness

854.14   Intracranial injury of other and unspecified nature with open intracranial wound, with prolonged [more than 24 hours] loss of consciousness and return to pre-existing conscious level

854.15   Intracranial injury of other and unspecified nature with open intracranial wound, with prolonged [more than 24 hours] loss of consciousness without return to pre-existing conscious level

854.16   Intracranial injury of other and unspecified nature with open intracranial wound, with loss of consciousness of unspecified duration

854.19   Intracranial injury of other and unspecified nature with open intracranial wound, with concussion, unspecified

860.1   Traumatic pneumothorax with open wound into thorax

860.2   Traumatic hemothorax without mention of open wound into thorax

860.3   Traumatic hemothorax with open wound into thorax

860.4   Traumatic pneumohemothorax without mention of open wound into thorax

860.5   Traumatic pneumohemothorax with open wound into thorax

861.02   Laceration of heart without penetration of heart chambers or without mention of open wound into thorax

861.03   Laceration of heart with penetration of heart chambers without mention of open wound into thorax

861.10   Unspecified injury of heart with open wound into thorax

861.11   Contusion of heart with open wound into thorax

861.12   Laceration of heart without penetration of heart chambers, with open wound into thorax

861.13   Laceration of heart with penetration of heart chambers with open wound into thorax

861.22   Laceration of lung without mention of open wound into thorax

861.30   Unspecified injury of lung with open wound into thorax

861.31   Contusion of lung with open wound into thorax

861.32   Laceration of lung with open wound into thorax

862.1   Injury to diaphragm, with open wound into cavity

862.21   Injury to bronchus without mention of open wound into cavity

862.22   Injury to esophagus without mention of open wound into cavity

862.31   Injury to bronchus with open wound into cavity

862.32   Injury to esophagus with open wound into cavity

862.39   Injury to other specified intrathoracic organs with open wound into cavity

862.9   Injury to multiple and unspecified intrathoracic organs, with open wound into cavity

863.1   Injury to stomach, with open wound into cavity

863.30   Injury to small intestine, unspecified site, with open wound into cavity

863.31   Injury to duodenum, with open wound into cavity

863.39   Other injury to small intestine, with open wound into cavity

863.50	Injury to colon, unspecified site, with open wound into cavity
863.51	Injury to ascending [right] colon, with open wound into cavity
863.52	Injury to transverse colon, with open wound into cavity
863.53	Injury to descending [left] colon, with open wound into cavity
863.54	Injury to sigmoid colon, with open wound into cavity
863.55	Injury to rectum, with open wound into cavity
863.56	Injury to multiple sites in colon and rectum, with open wound into cavity
863.59	Other injury to colon or rectum, with open wound into cavity
863.90	Injury to gastrointestinal tract, unspecified site, with open wound into cavity
863.91	Injury to pancreas, head, with open wound into cavity
863.92	Injury to pancreas, body, with open wound into cavity
863.93	Injury to pancreas, tail, with open wound into cavity
863.94	Injury to pancreas, multiple and unspecified sites, with open wound into cavity
863.95	Injury to appendix, with open wound into cavity
863.99	Injury to other gastrointestinal sites, with open wound into cavity
864.03	Injury to liver without mention of open wound into cavity, laceration, moderate
864.04	Injury to liver without mention of open wound into cavity, laceration, major
864.10	Injury to liver with open wound into cavity, unspecified injury
864.11	Injury to liver with open wound into cavity, hematoma and contusion
864.12	Injury to liver with open wound into cavity, laceration, minor
864.13	Injury to liver with open wound into cavity, laceration, moderate
864.14	Injury to liver with open wound into cavity, laceration, major
864.15	Injury to liver with open wound into cavity, laceration, unspecified
864.19	Other injury to liver with open wound into cavity
865.03	Injury to spleen without mention of open wound into cavity, laceration extending into parenchyma
865.04	Injury to spleen without mention of open wound into cavity, massive parenchymal disruption
865.10	Injury to spleen with open wound into cavity, unspecified injury
865.11	Injury to spleen with open wound into cavity, hematoma without rupture of capsule
865.12	Injury to spleen with open wound into cavity, capsular tears, without major disruption of parenchyma
865.13	Injury to spleen with open wound into cavity, laceration extending into parenchyma
865.14	Injury to spleen with open wound into cavity, massive parenchyma disruption
865.19	Other injury to spleen with open wound into cavity
866.03	Injury to kidney without mention of open wound into cavity, complete disruption of kidney parenchyma
866.10	Injury to kidney with open wound into cavity, unspecified injury
866.11	Injury to kidney with open wound into cavity, hematoma without rupture of capsule
866.12	Injury to kidney with open wound into cavity, laceration
866.13	Injury to kidney with open wound into cavity, complete disruption of kidney parenchyma
867.1	Injury to bladder and urethra, with open wound into cavity
867.3	Injury to ureter, with open wound into cavity
867.5	Injury to uterus, with open wound into cavity
867.7	Injury to other specified pelvic organs, with open wound into cavity
867.9	Injury to unspecified pelvic organ, with open wound into cavity
868.10	Injury to other intra-abdominal organs with open wound into cavity, unspecified intra-abdominal organ
868.11	Injury to other intra-abdominal organs with open wound into cavity, adrenal gland
868.12	Injury to other intra-abdominal organs with open wound into cavity, bile duct and gallbladder
868.13	Injury to other intra-abdominal organs with open wound into cavity, peritoneum
868.14	Injury to other intra-abdominal organs with open wound into cavity, retroperitoneum
868.19	Injury to other and multiple intra-abdominal organs, with open wound into cavity
869.1	Internal injury to unspecified or ill-defined organs with open wound into cavity
874.00	Open wound of larynx with trachea, without mention of complication
874.01	Open wound of larynx, without mention of complication
874.02	Open wound of trachea, without mention of complication
874.10	Open wound of larynx with trachea, complicated
874.11	Open wound of larynx, complicated
874.12	Open wound of trachea, complicated
887.6	Traumatic amputation of arm and hand (complete) (partial), bilateral [any level], without mention of complication
887.7	Traumatic amputation of arm and hand (complete) (partial), bilateral [any level], complicated
896.2	Traumatic amputation of foot (complete) (partial), bilateral, without mention of complication
896.3	Traumatic amputation of foot (complete) (partial), bilateral, complicated
897.6	Traumatic amputation of leg(s) (complete) (partial), bilateral [any level]), without mention of complication
897.7	Traumatic amputation of leg(s) (complete) (partial), bilateral [any level], complicated
901.0	Injury to thoracic aorta
901.1	Injury to innominate and subclavian arteries
901.2	Injury to superior vena cava
901.3	Injury to innominate and subclavian veins
901.40	Injury to pulmonary vessel(s), unspecified
901.41	Injury to pulmonary artery
901.42	Injury to pulmonary vein
901.83	Injury to multiple blood vessels of thorax
902.0	Injury to abdominal aorta
902.10	Injury to inferior vena cava, unspecified
902.11	Injury to hepatic veins
902.19	Injury to inferior vena cava, other
902.20	Injury to celiac and mesenteric arteries, unspecified
902.21	Injury to gastric artery
902.22	Injury to hepatic artery
902.23	Injury to splenic artery
902.24	Injury to other specified branches of celiac axis
902.25	Injury to superior mesenteric artery (trunk)
902.26	Injury to primary branches of superior mesenteric artery
902.27	Injury to inferior mesenteric artery
902.29	Injury to celiac and mesenteric arteries, other
902.31	Injury to superior mesenteric vein and primary subdivisions
902.32	Injury to inferior mesenteric vein
902.33	Injury to portal vein
902.34	Injury to splenic vein
902.39	Injury to portal and splenic veins, other
902.40	Injury to renal vessel(s), unspecified
902.41	Injury to renal artery
902.42	Injury to renal vein
902.49	Injury to renal blood vessels, other
902.50	Injury to iliac vessel(s), unspecified
902.51	Injury to hypogastric artery

Appendix A — Numeric MCC List

902.52	Injury to hypogastric vein
902.53	Injury to iliac artery
902.54	Injury to iliac vein
902.59	Injury to iliac blood vessels, other
902.87	Injury to multiple blood vessels of abdomen and pelvis
903.00	Injury to axillary vessel(s), unspecified
903.01	Injury to axillary artery
903.02	Injury to axillary vein
904.0	Injury to common femoral artery
904.1	Injury to superficial femoral artery
904.2	Injury to femoral veins
904.40	Injury to popliteal vessel(s), unspecified
904.41	Injury to popliteal artery
904.42	Injury to popliteal vein
948.21	Burn [any degree] involving 20-29 percent of body surface with third degree burn, 10-19%
948.22	Burn [any degree] involving 20-29 percent of body surface with third degree burn, 20-29%
948.31	Burn [any degree] involving 30-39 percent of body surface with third degree burn, 10-19%
948.32	Burn [any degree] involving 30-39 percent of body surface with third degree burn, 20-29%
948.33	Burn [any degree] involving 30-39 percent of body surface with third degree burn, 30-39%
948.41	Burn [any degree] involving 40-49 percent of body surface with third degree burn, 10-19%
948.42	Burn [any degree] involving 40-49 percent of body surface with third degree burn, 20-29%
948.43	Burn [any degree] involving 40-49 percent of body surface with third degree burn, 30-39%
948.44	Burn [any degree] involving 40-49 percent of body surface with third degree burn, 40-49%
948.51	Burn [any degree] involving 50-59 percent of body surface with third degree burn, 10-19%
948.52	Burn [any degree] involving 50-59 percent of body surface with third degree burn, 20-29%
948.53	Burn [any degree] involving 50-59 percent of body surface with third degree burn, 30-39%
948.54	Burn [any degree] involving 50-59 percent of body surface with third degree burn, 40-49%
948.55	Burn [any degree] involving 50-59 percent of body surface with third degree burn, 50-59%
948.61	Burn [any degree] involving 60-69 percent of body surface with third degree burn, 10-19%
948.62	Burn [any degree] involving 60-69 percent of body surface with third degree burn, 20-29%
948.63	Burn [any degree] involving 60-69 percent of body surface with third degree burn, 30-39%
948.64	Burn [any degree] involving 60-69 percent of body surface with third degree burn, 40-49%
948.65	Burn (any degree) involving 60-69 percent of body surface with third degree burn, 50-59%
948.66	Burn [any degree] involving 60-69 percent of body surface with third degree burn, 60-69%
948.71	Burn [any degree] involving 70-79 percent of body surface with third degree burn, 10-19%
948.72	Burn [any degree] involving 70-79 percent of body surface with third degree burn, 20-29%
948.73	Burn [any degree] involving 70-79 percent of body surface with third degree burn, 30-39%
948.74	Burn [any degree] involving 70-79 percent of body surface with third degree burn, 40-49%
948.75	Burn [any degree] involving 70-79 percent of body surface with third degree burn, 50-59%
948.76	Burn [any degree] involving 70-79 percent of body surface with third degree burn, 60-69%
948.77	Burn [any degree] involving 70-79 percent of body surface with third degree burn, 70-79%
948.81	Burn [any degree] involving 80-89 percent of body surface with third degree burn, 10-19%
948.82	Burn [any degree] involving 80-89 percent of body surface with third degree burn, 20-29%
948.83	Burn [any degree] involving 80-89 percent of body surface with third degree burn, 30-39%
948.84	Burn [any degree] involving 80-89 percent of body surface with third degree burn, 40-49%
948.85	Burn [any degree] involving 80-89 percent of body surface with third degree burn, 50-59%
948.86	Burn [any degree] involving 80-89 percent of body surface with third degree burn, 60-69%
948.87	Burn [any degree] involving 80-89 percent of body surface with third degree burn, 70-79%
948.88	Burn [any degree] involving 80-89 percent of body surface with third degree burn, 80-89%
948.91	Burn [any degree] involving 90 percent or more of body surface with third degree burn, 10-19%
948.92	Burn [any degree] involving 90 percent or more of body surface with third degree burn, 20-29%
948.93	Burn [any degree] involving 90 percent or more of body surface with third degree burn, 30-39%
948.94	Burn [any degree] involving 90 percent or more of body surface with third degree burn, 40-49%
948.95	Burn [any degree] involving 90 percent or more of body surface with third degree burn, 50-59%
948.96	Burn [any degree] involving 90 percent or more of body surface with third degree burn, 60-69%
948.97	Burn [any degree] involving 90 percent or more of body surface with third degree burn, 70-79%
948.98	Burn [any degree] involving 90 percent or more of body surface with third degree burn, 80-89%
948.99	Burn [any degree] involving 90 percent or more of body surface with third degree burn, 90% or more of body surface
952.00	C1-C4 level with unspecified spinal cord injury
952.01	C1-C4 level with complete lesion of spinal cord
952.02	C1-C4 level with anterior cord syndrome
952.03	C1-C4 level with central cord syndrome
952.04	C1-C4 level with other specified spinal cord injury
952.05	C5-C7 level with unspecified spinal cord injury
952.06	C5-C7 level with complete lesion of spinal cord
952.07	C5-C7 level with anterior cord syndrome
952.08	C5-C7 level with central cord syndrome
952.09	C5-C7 level with other specified spinal cord injury
952.10	T1-T6 level with unspecified spinal cord injury
952.11	T1-T6 level with complete lesion of spinal cord
952.12	T1-T6 level with anterior cord syndrome
952.13	T1-T6 level with central cord syndrome
952.14	T1-T6 level with other specified spinal cord injury
952.15	T7-T12 level with unspecified spinal cord injury
952.16	T7-T12 level with complete lesion of spinal cord
952.17	T7-T12 level with anterior cord syndrome
952.18	T7-T12 level with central cord syndrome
952.19	T7-T12 level with other specified spinal cord injury
952.2	Lumbar spinal cord injury without evidence of spinal bone injury
952.3	Sacral spinal cord injury without evidence of spinal bone injury
952.4	Cauda equina spinal cord injury without evidence of spinal bone injury

952.8	Multiple sites of spinal cord injury without evidence of spinal bone injury
958.0	Air embolism
958.1	Fat embolism
958.4	Traumatic shock
958.5	Traumatic anuria
995.91	Sepsis
995.92	Severe sepsis
995.94	Systemic inflammatory response syndrome due to noninfectious process with acute organ dysfunction
998.01	Postoperative shock, cardiogenic
998.02	Postoperative shock, septic
998.09	Postoperative shock, other
999.1	Air embolism as a complication of medical care, not elsewhere classified

Alphabetic MCC List

441.3	Abdominal aneurysm, ruptured
572.0	Abscess of liver
513.0	Abscess of lung
513.1	Abscess of mediastinum
755.55	Acrocephalosyndactyly
518.84	Acute and chronic respiratory failure
518.53	Acute and chronic respiratory failure following trauma and surgery
421.0	Acute and subacute bacterial endocarditis
421.1	Acute and subacute infective endocarditis in diseases classified elsewhere
570	Acute and subacute necrosis of liver
540.0	Acute appendicitis with generalized peritonitis
540.1	Acute appendicitis with peritoneal abscess
428.41	Acute combined systolic and diastolic heart failure
415.0	Acute cor pulmonale
428.31	Acute diastolic heart failure
532.21	Acute duodenal ulcer with hemorrhage and perforation, with obstruction
532.20	Acute duodenal ulcer with hemorrhage and perforation, without mention of obstruction
532.01	Acute duodenal ulcer with hemorrhage, with obstruction
532.00	Acute duodenal ulcer with hemorrhage, without mention of obstruction
532.11	Acute duodenal ulcer with perforation, with obstruction
532.10	Acute duodenal ulcer with perforation, without mention of obstruction
532.31	Acute duodenal ulcer without mention of hemorrhage or perforation, with obstruction
518.4	Acute edema of lung, unspecified
421.9	Acute endocarditis, unspecified
464.31	Acute epiglottitis with obstruction
531.21	Acute gastric ulcer with hemorrhage and perforation, with obstruction
531.20	Acute gastric ulcer with hemorrhage and perforation, without mention of obstruction
531.01	Acute gastric ulcer with hemorrhage, with obstruction
531.00	Acute gastric ulcer with hemorrhage, without mention of obstruction
531.11	Acute gastric ulcer with perforation, with obstruction
531.10	Acute gastric ulcer with perforation, without mention of obstruction
531.31	Acute gastric ulcer without mention of hemorrhage or perforation, with obstruction
535.01	Acute gastritis, with hemorrhage
534.21	Acute gastrojejunal ulcer with hemorrhage and perforation, with obstruction
534.20	Acute gastrojejunal ulcer with hemorrhage and perforation, without mention of obstruction
534.00	Acute gastrojejunal ulcer with hemorrhage, without mention of obstruction
534.11	Acute gastrojejunal ulcer with perforation, with obstruction
534.10	Acute gastrojejunal ulcer with perforation, without mention of obstruction
534.31	Acute gastrojejunal ulcer without mention of hemorrhage or perforation, with obstruction
534.01	Acute gastrojejunal ulcer, with hemorrhage, with obstruction
580.81	Acute glomerulonephritis in diseases classified elsewhere
580.0	Acute glomerulonephritis with lesion of proliferative glomerulonephritis
580.4	Acute glomerulonephritis with lesion of rapidly progressive glomerulonephritis
580.89	Acute glomerulonephritis with other specified pathological lesion in kidney
580.9	Acute glomerulonephritis with unspecified pathological lesion in kidney
070.41	Acute hepatitis C with hepatic coma
669.32	Acute kidney failure following labor and delivery, delivered, with mention of postpartum complication
669.34	Acute kidney failure following labor and delivery, postpartum condition or complication
584.6	Acute kidney failure with lesion of renal cortical necrosis
584.7	Acute kidney failure with lesion of renal medullary [papillary] necrosis
584.5	Acute kidney failure with lesion of tubular necrosis
464.01	Acute laryngitis with obstruction
464.21	Acute laryngotracheitis with obstruction
018.01	Acute miliary tuberculosis, bacteriological or histological examination not done
018.02	Acute miliary tuberculosis, bacteriological or histological examination unknown (at present)
018.03	Acute miliary tuberculosis, tubercle bacilli found (in sputum) by microscopy
018.04	Acute miliary tuberculosis, tubercle bacilli not found (in sputum) by microscopy, but found by bacterial culture
018.05	Acute miliary tuberculosis, tubercle bacilli not found by bacteriological examination, but tuberculosis confirmed histologically
018.06	Acute miliary tuberculosis, tubercle bacilli not found by bacteriological or histological examination, but tuberculosis confirmed by other methods [inoculation of animals]
018.00	Acute miliary tuberculosis, unspecified
410.01	Acute myocardial infarction of anterolateral wall, initial episode of care
410.21	Acute myocardial infarction of inferolateral wall, initial episode of care
410.31	Acute myocardial infarction of inferoposterior wall, initial episode of care
410.11	Acute myocardial infarction of other anterior wall, initial episode of care
410.41	Acute myocardial infarction of other inferior wall, initial episode of care
410.51	Acute myocardial infarction of other lateral wall, initial episode of care
410.81	Acute myocardial infarction of other specified sites, initial episode of care
410.91	Acute myocardial infarction of unspecified site, initial episode of care
422.0	Acute myocarditis in diseases classified elsewhere
422.90	Acute myocarditis, unspecified
428.43	Acute on chronic combined systolic and diastolic heart failure
428.33	Acute on chronic diastolic heart failure
428.23	Acute on chronic systolic heart failure
614.5	Acute or unspecified pelvic peritonitis, female
577.0	Acute pancreatitis
045.01	Acute paralytic poliomyelitis specified as bulbar, poliovirus type I
045.02	Acute paralytic poliomyelitis specified as bulbar, poliovirus type II
045.03	Acute paralytic poliomyelitis specified as bulbar, poliovirus type III
045.00	Acute paralytic poliomyelitis specified as bulbar, poliovirus, unspecified type
533.21	Acute peptic ulcer of unspecified site with hemorrhage and perforation, with obstruction
533.20	Acute peptic ulcer of unspecified site with hemorrhage and perforation, without mention of obstruction
533.01	Acute peptic ulcer of unspecified site with hemorrhage, with obstruction

533.00	Acute peptic ulcer of unspecified site with hemorrhage, without mention of obstruction
533.11	Acute peptic ulcer of unspecified site with perforation, with obstruction
533.10	Acute peptic ulcer of unspecified site with perforation, without mention of obstruction
533.31	Acute peptic ulcer of unspecified site without mention of hemorrhage and perforation, with obstruction
045.11	Acute poliomyelitis with other paralysis, poliovirus type I
045.12	Acute poliomyelitis with other paralysis, poliovirus type II
045.13	Acute poliomyelitis with other paralysis, poliovirus type III
045.10	Acute poliomyelitis with other paralysis, poliovirus, unspecified type
506.1	Acute pulmonary edema due to fumes and vapors
590.11	Acute pyelonephritis with lesion of renal medullary necrosis
518.81	Acute respiratory failure
518.51	Acute respiratory failure following trauma and surgery
091.81	Acute syphilitic meningitis (secondary)
428.21	Acute systolic heart failure
464.11	Acute tracheitis with obstruction
557.0	Acute vascular insufficiency of intestine
748.5	Agenesis, hypoplasia, and dysplasia of lung
958.0	Air embolism
999.1	Air embolism as a complication of medical care, not elsewhere classified
535.31	Alcoholic gastritis, with hemorrhage
516.64	Alveolar capillary dysplasia with vein misalignment
006.5	Amebic brain abscess
006.3	Amebic liver abscess
006.4	Amebic lung abscess
673.13	Amniotic fluid embolism, antepartum condition or complication
673.12	Amniotic fluid embolism, delivered, with mention of postpartum complication
673.11	Amniotic fluid embolism, delivered, with or without mention of antepartum condition
673.14	Amniotic fluid embolism, postpartum condition or complication
320.81	Anaerobic meningitis
740.0	Anencephalus
569.85	Angiodysplasia of intestine with hemorrhage
537.83	Angiodysplasia of stomach and duodenum with hemorrhage
747.81	Anomalies of cerebrovascular system
756.6	Anomalies of diaphragm
756.70	Anomaly of abdominal wall, unspecified
641.33	Antepartum hemorrhage associated with coagulation defects, antepartum condition or complication
641.31	Antepartum hemorrhage associated with coagulation defects, delivered, with or without mention of antepartum condition
022.3	Anthrax septicemia
284.11	Antineoplastic chemotherapy induced pancytopenia
441.5	Aortic aneurysm of unspecified site, ruptured
770.16	Aspiration of blood with respiratory symptoms
770.14	Aspiration of clear amniotic fluid with respiratory symptoms
770.86	Aspiration of postnatal stomach contents with respiratory symptoms
746.01	Atresia of pulmonary valve, congenital
535.11	Atrophic gastritis, with hemorrhage
062.4	Australian encephalitis
482.9	Bacterial pneumonia, unspecified
751.61	Biliary atresia
779.32	Bilious vomiting in newborn
348.82	Brain death

485	Bronchopneumonia, organism unspecified
020.0	Bubonic plague
453.0	Budd-chiari syndrome
948.65	Burn (any degree) involving 60-69 percent of body surface with third degree burn, 50-59%
948.21	Burn [any degree] involving 20-29 percent of body surface with third degree burn, 10-19%
948.22	Burn [any degree] involving 20-29 percent of body surface with third degree burn, 20-29%
948.31	Burn [any degree] involving 30-39 percent of body surface with third degree burn, 10-19%
948.32	Burn [any degree] involving 30-39 percent of body surface with third degree burn, 20-29%
948.33	Burn [any degree] involving 30-39 percent of body surface with third degree burn, 30-39%
948.41	Burn [any degree] involving 40-49 percent of body surface with third degree burn, 10-19%
948.42	Burn [any degree] involving 40-49 percent of body surface with third degree burn, 20-29%
948.43	Burn [any degree] involving 40-49 percent of body surface with third degree burn, 30-39%
948.44	Burn [any degree] involving 40-49 percent of body surface with third degree burn, 40-49%
948.51	Burn [any degree] involving 50-59 percent of body surface with third degree burn, 10-19%
948.52	Burn [any degree] involving 50-59 percent of body surface with third degree burn, 20-29%
948.53	Burn [any degree] involving 50-59 percent of body surface with third degree burn, 30-39%
948.54	Burn [any degree] involving 50-59 percent of body surface with third degree burn, 40-49%
948.55	Burn [any degree] involving 50-59 percent of body surface with third degree burn, 50-59%
948.61	Burn [any degree] involving 60-69 percent of body surface with third degree burn, 10-19%
948.62	Burn [any degree] involving 60-69 percent of body surface with third degree burn, 20-29%
948.63	Burn [any degree] involving 60-69 percent of body surface with third degree burn, 30-39%
948.64	Burn [any degree] involving 60-69 percent of body surface with third degree burn, 40-49%
948.66	Burn [any degree] involving 60-69 percent of body surface with third degree burn, 60-69%
948.71	Burn [any degree] involving 70-79 percent of body surface with third degree burn, 10-19%
948.72	Burn [any degree] involving 70-79 percent of body surface with third degree burn, 20-29%
948.73	Burn [any degree] involving 70-79 percent of body surface with third degree burn, 30-39%
948.74	Burn [any degree] involving 70-79 percent of body surface with third degree burn, 40-49%
948.75	Burn [any degree] involving 70-79 percent of body surface with third degree burn, 50-59%
948.76	Burn [any degree] involving 70-79 percent of body surface with third degree burn, 60-69%
948.77	Burn [any degree] involving 70-79 percent of body surface with third degree burn, 70-79%
948.81	Burn [any degree] involving 80-89 percent of body surface with third degree burn, 10-19%
948.82	Burn [any degree] involving 80-89 percent of body surface with third degree burn, 20-29%
948.83	Burn [any degree] involving 80-89 percent of body surface with third degree burn, 30-39%
948.84	Burn [any degree] involving 80-89 percent of body surface with third degree burn, 40-49%

948.85	Burn [any degree] involving 80-89 percent of body surface with third degree burn, 50-59%
948.86	Burn [any degree] involving 80-89 percent of body surface with third degree burn, 60-69%
948.87	Burn [any degree] involving 80-89 percent of body surface with third degree burn, 70-79%
948.88	Burn [any degree] involving 80-89 percent of body surface with third degree burn, 80-89%
948.91	Burn [any degree] involving 90 percent or more of body surface with third degree burn, 10-19%
948.92	Burn [any degree] involving 90 percent or more of body surface with third degree burn, 20-29%
948.93	Burn [any degree] involving 90 percent or more of body surface with third degree burn, 30-39%
948.94	Burn [any degree] involving 90 percent or more of body surface with third degree burn, 40-49%
948.95	Burn [any degree] involving 90 percent or more of body surface with third degree burn, 50-59%
948.96	Burn [any degree] involving 90 percent or more of body surface with third degree burn, 60-69%
948.97	Burn [any degree] involving 90 percent or more of body surface with third degree burn, 70-79%
948.98	Burn [any degree] involving 90 percent or more of body surface with third degree burn, 80-89%
948.99	Burn [any degree] involving 90 percent or more of body surface with third degree burn, 90% or more of body surface
952.02	C1-C4 level with anterior cord syndrome
952.03	C1-C4 level with central cord syndrome
952.01	C1-C4 level with complete lesion of spinal cord
952.04	C1-C4 level with other specified spinal cord injury
952.00	C1-C4 level with unspecified spinal cord injury
952.07	C5-C7 level with anterior cord syndrome
952.08	C5-C7 level with central cord syndrome
952.06	C5-C7 level with complete lesion of spinal cord
952.09	C5-C7 level with other specified spinal cord injury
952.05	C5-C7 level with unspecified spinal cord injury
574.81	Calculus of gallbladder and bile duct with acute and chronic cholecystitis, with obstruction
062.5	California virus encephalitis
112.81	Candidal endocarditis
112.83	Candidal meningitis
112.4	Candidiasis of lung
427.5	Cardiac arrest
779.85	Cardiac arrest of newborn
785.51	Cardiogenic shock
952.4	Cauda equina spinal cord injury without evidence of spinal bone injury
020.1	Cellulocutaneous plague
063.2	Central european encephalitis
851.50	Cerebellar or brain stem contusion with open intracranial wound, unspecified state of consciousness
851.52	Cerebellar or brain stem contusion with open intracranial wound, with brief [less than one hour] loss of consciousness
851.59	Cerebellar or brain stem contusion with open intracranial wound, with concussion, unspecified
851.56	Cerebellar or brain stem contusion with open intracranial wound, with loss of consciousness of unspecified duration
851.53	Cerebellar or brain stem contusion with open intracranial wound, with moderate [1-24 hours] loss of consciousness
851.51	Cerebellar or brain stem contusion with open intracranial wound, with no loss of consciousness
851.54	Cerebellar or brain stem contusion with open intracranial wound, with prolonged [more than 24 hours] loss of consciousness and return to pre-existing conscious level

851.55	Cerebellar or brain stem contusion with open intracranial wound, with prolonged [more than 24 hours] loss of consciousness without return to pre-existing conscious level
851.45	Cerebellar or brain stem contusion without mention of open intracranial wound, with prolonged [more than 24 hours] loss of consciousness without return to pre-existing conscious level
851.70	Cerebellar or brain stem laceration with open intracranial wound, unspecified state of consciousness
851.72	Cerebellar or brain stem laceration with open intracranial wound, with brief [less than one hour] loss of consciousness
851.79	Cerebellar or brain stem laceration with open intracranial wound, with concussion, unspecified
851.76	Cerebellar or brain stem laceration with open intracranial wound, with loss of consciousness of unspecified duration
851.73	Cerebellar or brain stem laceration with open intracranial wound, with moderate [1-24 hours] loss of consciousness
851.71	Cerebellar or brain stem laceration with open intracranial wound, with no loss of consciousness
851.74	Cerebellar or brain stem laceration with open intracranial wound, with prolonged [more than 24 hours] loss of consciousness and return to pre-existing conscious level
851.75	Cerebellar or brain stem laceration with open intracranial wound, with prolonged [more than 24 hours] loss of consciousness without return to pre-existing conscious level
851.60	Cerebellar or brain stem laceration without mention of open intracranial wound, unspecified state of consciousness
851.62	Cerebellar or brain stem laceration without mention of open intracranial wound, with brief [less than 1 hour] loss of consciousness
851.69	Cerebellar or brain stem laceration without mention of open intracranial wound, with concussion, unspecified
851.66	Cerebellar or brain stem laceration without mention of open intracranial wound, with loss of consciousness of unspecified duration
851.63	Cerebellar or brain stem laceration without mention of open intracranial wound, with moderate [1-24 hours] loss of consciousness
851.61	Cerebellar or brain stem laceration without mention of open intracranial wound, with no loss of consciousness
851.64	Cerebellar or brain stem laceration without mention of open intracranial wound, with prolonged [more than 24 hours] loss of consciousness and return to pre-existing conscious level
851.65	Cerebellar or brain stem laceration without mention of open intracranial wound, with prolonged [more than 24 hours] loss of consciousness without return to pre-existing conscious level
434.91	Cerebral artery occlusion, unspecified with cerebral infarction
779.2	Cerebral depression, coma, and other abnormal cerebral signs in fetus or newborn
348.5	Cerebral edema
434.11	Cerebral embolism with cerebral infarction
434.01	Cerebral thrombosis with cerebral infarction
674.01	Cerebrovascular disorders in the puerperium, delivered, with or without mention of antepartum condition
654.53	Cervical incompetence, antepartum condition or complication
654.52	Cervical incompetence, delivered, with mention of postpartum complication
654.51	Cervical incompetence, delivered, with or without mention of antepartum condition
654.54	Cervical incompetence, postpartum condition or complication
567.81	Choleperitonitis
532.71	Chronic duodenal ulcer without mention of hemorrhage or perforation, with obstruction
531.71	Chronic gastric ulcer without mention of hemorrhage or perforation, with obstruction
534.71	Chronic gastrojejunal ulcer without mention of hemorrhage or perforation, with obstruction

070.44	Chronic hepatitis C with hepatic coma
532.61	Chronic or unspecified duodenal ulcer with hemorrhage and perforation, with obstruction
532.60	Chronic or unspecified duodenal ulcer with hemorrhage and perforation, without mention of obstruction
532.41	Chronic or unspecified duodenal ulcer with hemorrhage, with obstruction
532.40	Chronic or unspecified duodenal ulcer with hemorrhage, without mention of obstruction
532.51	Chronic or unspecified duodenal ulcer with perforation, with obstruction
532.50	Chronic or unspecified duodenal ulcer with perforation, without mention of obstruction
531.61	Chronic or unspecified gastric ulcer with hemorrhage and perforation, with obstruction
531.60	Chronic or unspecified gastric ulcer with hemorrhage and perforation, without mention of obstruction
531.41	Chronic or unspecified gastric ulcer with hemorrhage, with obstruction
531.40	Chronic or unspecified gastric ulcer with hemorrhage, without mention of obstruction
531.51	Chronic or unspecified gastric ulcer with perforation, with obstruction
531.50	Chronic or unspecified gastric ulcer with perforation, without mention of obstruction
534.61	Chronic or unspecified gastrojejunal ulcer with hemorrhage and perforation, with obstruction
534.60	Chronic or unspecified gastrojejunal ulcer with hemorrhage and perforation, without mention of obstruction
534.40	Chronic or unspecified gastrojejunal ulcer with hemorrhage, without mention of obstruction
534.51	Chronic or unspecified gastrojejunal ulcer with perforation, with obstruction
534.50	Chronic or unspecified gastrojejunal ulcer with perforation, without mention of obstruction
534.41	Chronic or unspecified gastrojejunal ulcer, with hemorrhage, with obstruction
533.61	Chronic or unspecified peptic ulcer of unspecified site with hemorrhage and perforation, with obstruction
533.60	Chronic or unspecified peptic ulcer of unspecified site with hemorrhage and perforation, without mention of obstruction
533.41	Chronic or unspecified peptic ulcer of unspecified site with hemorrhage, with obstruction
533.40	Chronic or unspecified peptic ulcer of unspecified site with hemorrhage, without mention of obstruction
533.51	Chronic or unspecified peptic ulcer of unspecified site with perforation, with obstruction
533.50	Chronic or unspecified peptic ulcer of unspecified site with perforation, without mention of obstruction
533.71	Chronic peptic ulcer of unspecified site without mention of hemorrhage or perforation, with obstruction
770.7	Chronic respiratory disease arising in the perinatal period
070.23	Chronic viral hepatitis B with hepatic coma with hepatitis delta
070.22	Chronic viral hepatitis B with hepatic coma without hepatitis delta
808.0	Closed fracture of acetabulum
820.03	Closed fracture of base of neck of femur
801.10	Closed fracture of base of skull with cerebral laceration and contusion, unspecified state of consciousness
801.12	Closed fracture of base of skull with cerebral laceration and contusion, with brief [less than one hour] loss of consciousness
801.19	Closed fracture of base of skull with cerebral laceration and contusion, with concussion, unspecified
801.16	Closed fracture of base of skull with cerebral laceration and contusion, with loss of consciousness of unspecified duration
801.13	Closed fracture of base of skull with cerebral laceration and contusion, with moderate [1-24 hours] loss of consciousness
801.11	Closed fracture of base of skull with cerebral laceration and contusion, with no loss of consciousness
801.14	Closed fracture of base of skull with cerebral laceration and contusion, with prolonged [more than 24 hours] loss of consciousness and return to pre-existing conscious level
801.15	Closed fracture of base of skull with cerebral laceration and contusion, with prolonged [more than 24 hours] loss of consciousness, without return to pre-existing conscious level
801.43	Closed fracture of base of skull with intracranial injury of other and unspecified nature, with moderate [1-24 hours] loss of consciousness
801.44	Closed fracture of base of skull with intracranial injury of other and unspecified nature, with prolonged [more than 24 hours) loss of consciousness and return to pre-existing conscious level
801.45	Closed fracture of base of skull with intracranial injury of other and unspecified nature, with prolonged [more than 24 hours] loss of consciousness, without return to pre-existing conscious level
801.30	Closed fracture of base of skull with other and unspecified intracranial hemorrhage, unspecified state of consciousness
801.32	Closed fracture of base of skull with other and unspecified intracranial hemorrhage, with brief [less than one hour] loss of consciousness
801.39	Closed fracture of base of skull with other and unspecified intracranial hemorrhage, with concussion, unspecified
801.36	Closed fracture of base of skull with other and unspecified intracranial hemorrhage, with loss of consciousness of unspecified duration
801.33	Closed fracture of base of skull with other and unspecified intracranial hemorrhage, with moderate [1-24 hours] loss of consciousness
801.31	Closed fracture of base of skull with other and unspecified intracranial hemorrhage, with no loss of consciousness
801.34	Closed fracture of base of skull with other and unspecified intracranial hemorrhage, with prolonged [more than 24 hours] loss of consciousness and return to pre-existing conscious level
801.35	Closed fracture of base of skull with other and unspecified intracranial hemorrhage, with prolonged [more than 24 hours] loss of consciousness, without return to pre-existing conscious level
801.20	Closed fracture of base of skull with subarachnoid, subdural, and extradural hemorrhage, unspecified state of consciousness
801.22	Closed fracture of base of skull with subarachnoid, subdural, and extradural hemorrhage, with brief [less than one hour] loss of consciousness
801.29	Closed fracture of base of skull with subarachnoid, subdural, and extradural hemorrhage, with concussion, unspecified
801.26	Closed fracture of base of skull with subarachnoid, subdural, and extradural hemorrhage, with loss of consciousness of unspecified duration
801.23	Closed fracture of base of skull with subarachnoid, subdural, and extradural hemorrhage, with moderate [1-24 hours] loss of consciousness
801.21	Closed fracture of base of skull with subarachnoid, subdural, and extradural hemorrhage, with no loss of consciousness
801.24	Closed fracture of base of skull with subarachnoid, subdural, and extradural hemorrhage, with prolonged [more than 24 hours] loss of consciousness and return to pre-existing conscious level
801.25	Closed fracture of base of skull with subarachnoid, subdural, and extradural hemorrhage, with prolonged [more than 24 hours] loss of consciousness, without return to pre-existing conscious level
801.03	Closed fracture of base of skull without mention of intra cranial injury, with moderate [1-24 hours] loss of consciousness
801.04	Closed fracture of base of skull without mention of intra cranial injury, with prolonged [more than 24 hours] loss of consciousness and return to pre-existing conscious level

801.05	Closed fracture of base of skull without mention of intra cranial injury, with prolonged [more than 24 hours] loss of consciousness, without return to pre-existing conscious level
806.02	Closed fracture of C1-C4 level with anterior cord syndrome
806.03	Closed fracture of C1-C4 level with central cord syndrome
806.01	Closed fracture of C1-C4 level with complete lesion of cord
806.04	Closed fracture of C1-C4 level with other specified spinal cord injury
806.00	Closed fracture of C1-C4 level with unspecified spinal cord injury
806.07	Closed fracture of C5-C7 level with anterior cord syndrome
806.08	Closed fracture of C5-C7 level with central cord syndrome
806.06	Closed fracture of C5-C7 level with complete lesion of cord
806.09	Closed fracture of C5-C7 level with other specified spinal cord injury
806.05	Closed fracture of C5-C7 level with unspecified spinal cord injury
820.01	Closed fracture of epiphysis (separation) (upper) of neck of femur
820.21	Closed fracture of intertrochanteric section of neck of femur
820.00	Closed fracture of intracapsular section of neck of femur, unspecified
807.5	Closed fracture of larynx and trachea
806.4	Closed fracture of lumbar spine with spinal cord injury
820.02	Closed fracture of midcervical section of neck of femur
806.61	Closed fracture of sacrum and coccyx with complete cauda equina lesion
806.62	Closed fracture of sacrum and coccyx with other cauda equina injury
806.69	Closed fracture of sacrum and coccyx with other spinal cord injury
806.60	Closed fracture of sacrum and coccyx with unspecified spinal cord injury
821.01	Closed fracture of shaft of femur
820.22	Closed fracture of subtrochanteric section of neck of femur
806.22	Closed fracture of T1-T6 level with anterior cord syndrome
806.23	Closed fracture of T1-T6 level with central cord syndrome
806.21	Closed fracture of T1-T6 level with complete lesion of cord
806.24	Closed fracture of T1-T6 level with other specified spinal cord injury
806.20	Closed fracture of T1-T6 level with unspecified spinal cord injury
806.27	Closed fracture of T7-T12 level with anterior cord syndrome
806.28	Closed fracture of T7-T12 level with central cord syndrome
806.26	Closed fracture of T7-T12 level with complete lesion of cord
806.29	Closed fracture of T7-T12 level with other specified spinal cord injury
806.25	Closed fracture of T7-T12 level with unspecified spinal cord injury
820.20	Closed fracture of trochanteric section of neck of femur
821.00	Closed fracture of unspecified part of femur
820.8	Closed fracture of unspecified part of neck of femur
806.8	Closed fracture of unspecified vertebral column with spinal cord injury
800.10	Closed fracture of vault of skull with cerebral laceration and contusion, unspecified state of consciousness
800.12	Closed fracture of vault of skull with cerebral laceration and contusion, with brief [less than one hour] loss of consciousness
800.19	Closed fracture of vault of skull with cerebral laceration and contusion, with concussion, unspecified
800.16	Closed fracture of vault of skull with cerebral laceration and contusion, with loss of consciousness of unspecified duration
800.13	Closed fracture of vault of skull with cerebral laceration and contusion, with moderate [1-24 hours] loss of consciousness
800.11	Closed fracture of vault of skull with cerebral laceration and contusion, with no loss of consciousness
800.14	Closed fracture of vault of skull with cerebral laceration and contusion, with prolonged [more than 24 hours] loss of consciousness and return to pre-existing conscious level

800.15	Closed fracture of vault of skull with cerebral laceration and contusion, with prolonged [more than 24 hours] loss of consciousness, without return to pre-existing conscious level
800.43	Closed fracture of vault of skull with intracranial injury of other and unspecified nature, with moderate [1-24 hours] loss of consciousness
800.44	Closed fracture of vault of skull with intracranial injury of other and unspecified nature, with prolonged [more than 24 hours] loss of consciousness and return to pre-existing conscious level
800.45	Closed fracture of vault of skull with intracranial injury of other and unspecified nature, with prolonged [more than 24 hours] loss of consciousness, without return to pre-existing conscious level
800.30	Closed fracture of vault of skull with other and unspecified intracranial hemorrhage, unspecified state of consciousness
800.32	Closed fracture of vault of skull with other and unspecified intracranial hemorrhage, with brief [less than one hour] loss of consciousness
800.39	Closed fracture of vault of skull with other and unspecified intracranial hemorrhage, with concussion, unspecified
800.36	Closed fractures of vault of skull with other and unspecified intracranial hemorrhage, with loss of consciousness of unspecified duration
800.33	Closed fracture of vault of skull with other and unspecified intracranial hemorrhage, with moderate [1-24 hours] loss of consciousness
800.31	Closed fracture of vault of skull with other and unspecified intracranial hemorrhage, with no loss of consciousness
800.34	Closed fracture of vault of skull with other and unspecified intracranial hemorrhage, with prolonged [more than 24 hours] loss of consciousness and return to pre-existing conscious level
800.35	Closed fracture of vault of skull with other and unspecified intracranial hemorrhage, with prolonged [more than 24 hours] loss of consciousness, without return to pre-existing conscious level
800.20	Closed fracture of vault of skull with subarachnoid, subdural, and extradural hemorrhage, unspecified state of consciousness
800.22	Closed fracture of vault of skull with subarachnoid, subdural, and extradural hemorrhage, with brief [less than one hour] loss of consciousness
800.29	Closed fracture of vault of skull with subarachnoid, subdural, and extradural hemorrhage, with concussion, unspecified
800.26	Closed fracture of vault of skull with subarachnoid, subdural, and extradural hemorrhage, with loss of consciousness of unspecified duration
800.23	Closed fracture of vault of skull with subarachnoid, subdural, and extradural hemorrhage, with moderate [1-24 hours] loss of consciousness
800.21	Closed fracture of vault of skull with subarachnoid, subdural, and extradural hemorrhage, with no loss of consciousness
800.24	Closed fracture of vault of skull with subarachnoid, subdural, and extradural hemorrhage, with prolonged [more than 24 hours] loss of consciousness and return to pre-existing conscious level
800.25	Closed fracture of vault of skull with subarachnoid, subdural, and extradural hemorrhage, with prolonged [more than 24 hours] loss of consciousness, without return to pre-existing conscious level
800.03	Closed fracture of vault of skull without mention of intracranial injury, with moderate [1-24 hours] loss of consciousness
800.04	Closed fracture of vault of skull without mention of intracranial injury, with prolonged [more than 24 hours] loss of consciousness and return to pre-existing conscious level
800.05	Closed fracture of vault of skull without mention of intracranial injury, with prolonged [more than 24 hours] loss of consciousness, without return to pre-existing conscious level
804.05	Closed fractures involving skull of face with other bones, without mention of intracranial injury, with prolonged [more than 24 hours] loss of consciousness, without return to pre-existing conscious level

804.20	Closed fractures involving skull or face with other bones with subarachnoid, subdural, and extradural hemorrhage, unspecified state of consciousness
804.22	Closed fractures involving skull or face with other bones with subarachnoid, subdural, and extradural hemorrhage, with brief [less than one hour] loss of consciousness
804.29	Closed fractures involving skull or face with other bones with subarachnoid, subdural, and extradural hemorrhage, with concussion, unspecified
804.26	Closed fractures involving skull or face with other bones with subarachnoid, subdural, and extradural hemorrhage, with loss of consciousness of unspecified duration
804.23	Closed fractures involving skull or face with other bones with subarachnoid, subdural, and extradural hemorrhage, with moderate [1-24 hours] loss of consciousness
804.21	Closed fractures involving skull or face with other bones with subarachnoid, subdural, and extradural hemorrhage, with no loss of consciousness
804.24	Closed fractures involving skull or face with other bones with subarachnoid, subdural, and extradural hemorrhage, with prolonged [more than 24 hours] loss of consciousness and return to pre-existing conscious level
804.25	Closed fractures involving skull or face with other bones with subarachnoid, subdural, and extradural hemorrhage, with prolonged [more than 24 hours] loss of consciousness, without return to pre-existing conscious level
804.10	Closed fractures involving skull or face with other bones, with cerebral laceration and contusion, unspecified state of consciousness
804.12	Closed fractures involving skull or face with other bones, with cerebral laceration and contusion, with brief [less than one hour] loss of consciousness
804.19	Closed fractures involving skull or face with other bones, with cerebral laceration and contusion, with concussion, unspecified
804.16	Closed fractures involving skull or face with other bones, with cerebral laceration and contusion, with loss of consciousness of unspecified duration
804.13	Closed fractures involving skull or face with other bones, with cerebral laceration and contusion, with moderate [1-24 hours] loss of consciousness
804.11	Closed fractures involving skull or face with other bones, with cerebral laceration and contusion, with no loss of consciousness
804.14	Closed fractures involving skull or face with other bones, with cerebral laceration and contusion, with prolonged [more than 24 hours] loss of consciousness and return to pre-existing conscious level
804.15	Closed fractures involving skull or face with other bones, with cerebral laceration and contusion, with prolonged [more than 24 hours] loss of consciousness, without return to pre-existing conscious level
804.43	Closed fractures involving skull or face with other bones, with intracranial injury of other and unspecified nature, with moderate [1-24 hours] loss of consciousness
804.44	Closed fractures involving skull or face with other bones, with intracranial injury of other and unspecified nature, with prolonged [more than 24 hours] loss of consciousness and return to pre-existing conscious level
804.45	Closed fractures involving skull or face with other bones, with intracranial injury of other and unspecified nature, with prolonged [more than 24 hours] loss of consciousness, without return to pre-existing conscious level
804.30	Closed fractures involving skull or face with other bones, with other and unspecified intracranial hemorrhage, unspecified state of consciousness
804.32	Closed fractures involving skull or face with other bones, with other and unspecified intracranial hemorrhage, with brief [less than one hour] loss of consciousness
804.39	Closed fractures involving skull or face with other bones, with other and unspecified intracranial hemorrhage, with concussion, unspecified
804.36	Closed fractures involving skull or face with other bones, with other and unspecified intracranial hemorrhage, with loss of consciousness of unspecified duration
804.33	Closed fractures involving skull or face with other bones, with other and unspecified intracranial hemorrhage, with moderate [1-24 hours] loss of consciousness
804.31	Closed fractures involving skull or face with other bones, with other and unspecified intracranial hemorrhage, with no loss of consciousness
804.34	Closed fractures involving skull or face with other bones, with other and unspecified intracranial hemorrhage, with prolonged [more than 24 hours] loss of consciousness and return to pre-existing conscious level
804.35	Closed fractures involving skull or face with other bones, with other and unspecified intracranial hemorrhage, with prolonged [more than 24 hours] loss of consciousness, without return to pre-existing conscious level
804.03	Closed fractures involving skull or face with other bones, without mention of intracranial injury, with moderate [1-24 hours] loss of consciousness
804.04	Closed fractures involving skull or face with other bones, without mention or intracranial injury, with prolonged [more than 24 hours] loss of consciousness and return to pre-existing conscious level
828.0	Closed multiple fractures involving both lower limbs, lower with upper limb, and lower limb(s) with rib(s) and sternum
114.2	Coccidioidal meningitis
780.01	Coma
745.0	Common truncus
745.3	Common ventricle
745.10	Complete transposition of great vessels
348.4	Compression of brain
850.4	Concussion with prolonged loss of consciousness, without return to pre-existing conscious level
771.1	Congenital cytomegalovirus infection
286.1	Congenital factor IX disorder
286.0	Congenital factor VIII disorder
746.86	Congenital heart block
770.0	Congenital pneumonia
343.2	Congenital quadriplegia
742.2	Congenital reduction deformities of brain
090.41	Congenital syphilitic encephalitis
090.42	Congenital syphilitic meningitis
759.4	Conjoined twins
861.11	Contusion of heart with open wound into thorax
861.31	Contusion of lung with open wound into thorax
779.0	Convulsions in newborn
745.7	Cor biloculare
746.82	Cor triatriatum
851.10	Cortex (cerebral) contusion with open intracranial wound, unspecified state of consciousness
851.12	Cortex (cerebral) contusion with open intracranial wound, with brief [less than one hour] loss of consciousness
851.19	Cortex (cerebral) contusion with open intracranial wound, with concussion, unspecified
851.16	Cortex (cerebral) contusion with open intracranial wound, with loss of consciousness of unspecified duration
851.13	Cortex (cerebral) contusion with open intracranial wound, with moderate [1-24 hours] loss of consciousness
851.11	Cortex (cerebral) contusion with open intracranial wound, with no loss of consciousness

851.14	Cortex (cerebral) contusion with open intracranial wound, with prolonged [more than 24 hours] loss of consciousness and return to pre-existing conscious level
851.15	Cortex (cerebral) contusion with open intracranial wound, with prolonged [more than 24 hours] loss of consciousness without return to pre-existing conscious level
851.05	Cortex (cerebral) contusion without mention of open intracranial wound, with prolonged [more than 24 hours] loss of consciousness without return to pre-existing conscious level
851.30	Cortex (cerebral) laceration with open intracranial wound, unspecified state of consciousness
851.32	Cortex (cerebral) laceration with open intracranial wound, with brief [less than one hour] loss of consciousness
851.39	Cortex (cerebral) laceration with open intracranial wound, with concussion, unspecified
851.36	Cortex (cerebral) laceration with open intracranial wound, with loss of consciousness of unspecified duration
851.33	Cortex (cerebral) laceration with open intracranial wound, with moderate [1-24 hours] loss of consciousness
851.31	Cortex (cerebral) laceration with open intracranial wound, with no loss of consciousness
851.34	Cortex (cerebral) laceration with open intracranial wound, with prolonged [more than 24 hours] loss of consciousness and return to pre-existing conscious level
851.35	Cortex (cerebral) laceration with open intracranial wound, with prolonged [more than 24 hours] loss of consciousness without return to pre-existing conscious level
851.20	Cortex (cerebral) laceration without mention of open intracranial wound, unspecified state of consciousness
851.22	Cortex (cerebral) laceration without mention of open intracranial wound, with brief [less than one hour] loss of consciousness
851.29	Cortex (cerebral) laceration without mention of open intracranial wound, with concussion, unspecified
851.26	Cortex (cerebral) laceration without mention of open intracranial wound, with loss of consciousness of unspecified duration
851.23	Cortex (cerebral) laceration without mention of open intracranial wound, with moderate [1-24 hours] loss of consciousness
851.21	Cortex (cerebral) laceration without mention of open intracranial wound, with no loss of consciousness
851.24	Cortex (cerebral) laceration without mention of open intracranial wound, with prolonged [more than 24 hours] loss of consciousness and return to pre-existing conscious level
851.25	Cortex (cerebral) laceration without mention of open intracranial wound, with prolonged [more than 24 hours] loss of consciousness without return to pre-existing conscious level
740.1	Craniorachischisis
321.0	Cryptococcal meningitis
277.01	Cystic fibrosis with meconium ileus
277.02	Cystic fibrosis with pulmonary manifestations
671.33	Deep phlebothrombosis, antepartum, antepartum condition or complication
671.31	Deep phlebothrombosis, antepartum, delivered, with or without mention of antepartum condition
671.42	Deep phlebothrombosis, postpartum, delivered, with mention of postpartum complication
671.44	Deep phlebothrombosis, postpartum, postpartum condition or complication
286.6	Defibrination syndrome
648.02	Diabetes mellitus of mother, complicating pregnancy, childbirth, or the puerperium, delivered, with mention of postpartum complication
648.01	Diabetes mellitus of mother, complicating pregnancy, childbirth, or the puerperium, delivered, with or without mention of antepartum condition
250.21	Diabetes with hyperosmolarity, type I [juvenile type], not stated as uncontrolled

250.23	Diabetes with hyperosmolarity, type I [juvenile type], uncontrolled
250.20	Diabetes with hyperosmolarity, type II or unspecified type, not stated as uncontrolled
250.22	Diabetes with hyperosmolarity, type II or unspecified type, uncontrolled
250.11	Diabetes with ketoacidosis, type I [juvenile type], not stated as uncontrolled
250.13	Diabetes with ketoacidosis, type I [juvenile type], uncontrolled
250.10	Diabetes with ketoacidosis, type II or unspecified type, not stated as uncontrolled
250.12	Diabetes with ketoacidosis, type II or unspecified type, uncontrolled
250.31	Diabetes with other coma, type I [juvenile type], not stated as uncontrolled
250.33	Diabetes with other coma, type I [juvenile type], uncontrolled
250.30	Diabetes with other coma, type II or unspecified type, not stated as uncontrolled
250.32	Diabetes with other coma, type II or unspecified type, uncontrolled
551.3	Diaphragmatic hernia with gangrene
569.86	Dieulafoy lesion (hemorrhagic) of intestine
537.84	Dieulafoy lesion (hemorrhagic) of stomach and duodenum
441.02	Dissection of aorta, abdominal
441.01	Dissection of aorta, thoracic
441.03	Dissection of aorta, thoracoabdominal
441.00	Dissection of aorta, unspecified site
443.21	Dissection of carotid artery
414.12	Dissection of coronary artery
443.22	Dissection of iliac artery
443.29	Dissection of other artery
443.23	Dissection of renal artery
443.24	Dissection of vertebral artery
112.5	Disseminated candidiasis
776.2	Disseminated intravascular coagulation in newborn
562.13	Diverticulitis of colon with hemorrhage
562.03	Diverticulitis of small intestine with hemorrhage
562.12	Diverticulosis of colon with hemorrhage
562.02	Diverticulosis of small intestine with hemorrhage
745.11	Double outlet right ventricle
532.91	Duodenal ulcer, unspecified as acute or chronic, without mention of hemorrhage or perforation, with obstruction
535.61	Duodenitis, with hemorrhage
644.21	Early onset of delivery, delivered, with or without mention of antepartum condition
062.2	Eastern equine encephalitis
746.2	Ebstein's anomaly
642.63	Eclampsia, antepartum condition or complication
642.62	Eclampsia, delivered, with mention of postpartum complication
642.61	Eclampsia, delivered, with or without mention of antepartum condition
642.64	Eclampsia, postpartum condition or complication
639.6	Embolism following abortion or ectopic and molar pregnancies
510.0	Empyema with fistula
510.9	Empyema without mention of fistula
323.51	Encephalitis and encephalomyelitis following immunization procedures
323.01	Encephalitis and encephalomyelitis in viral diseases classified elsewhere
323.2	Encephalitis, myelitis, and encephalomyelitis in protozoal diseases classified elsewhere
323.1	Encephalitis, myelitis, and encephalomyelitis in rickettsial diseases classified elsewhere
056.01	Encephalomyelitis due to rubella

348.30	Encephalopathy, unspecified
585.6	End stage renal disease
535.71	Eosinophilic gastritis, with hemorrhage
322.1	Eosinophilic meningitis
345.71	Epilepsia partialis continua, with intractable epilepsy
530.82	Esophageal hemorrhage
456.20	Esophageal varices in diseases classified elsewhere, with bleeding
456.0	Esophageal varices with bleeding
852.50	Extradural hemorrhage following injury with open intracranial wound, unspecified state of consciousness
852.52	Extradural hemorrhage following injury with open intracranial wound, with brief [less than one hour] loss of consciousness
852.59	Extradural hemorrhage following injury with open intracranial wound, with concussion, unspecified
852.56	Extradural hemorrhage following injury with open intracranial wound, with loss of consciousness of unspecified duration
852.53	Extradural hemorrhage following injury with open intracranial wound, with moderate [1-24 hours] loss of consciousness
852.51	Extradural hemorrhage following injury with open intracranial wound, with no loss of consciousness
852.54	Extradural hemorrhage following injury with open intracranial wound, with prolonged [more than 24 hours] loss of consciousness and return to pre-existing conscious level
852.55	Extradural hemorrhage following injury with open intracranial wound, with prolonged [more than 24 hours] loss of consciousness without return to pre-existing conscious level
852.40	Extradural hemorrhage following injury without mention of open intracranial wound, unspecified state of consciousness
852.42	Extradural hemorrhage following injury without mention of open intracranial wound, with brief [less than 1 hour] loss of consciousness
852.49	Extradural hemorrhage following injury without mention of open intracranial wound, with concussion, unspecified
852.46	Extradural hemorrhage following injury without mention of open intracranial wound, with loss of consciousness of unspecified duration
852.43	Extradural hemorrhage following injury without mention of open intracranial wound, with moderate [1-24 hours] loss of consciousness
852.41	Extradural hemorrhage following injury without mention of open intracranial wound, with no loss of consciousness
852.44	Extradural hemorrhage following injury without mention of open intracranial wound, with prolonged [more than 24 hours] loss of consciousness and return to pre-existing conscious level
852.45	Extradural hemorrhage following injury without mention of open intracranial wound, with prolonged [more than 24 hours] loss of consciousness without return to pre-existing conscious level
638.6	Failed attempted abortion complicated by embolism
638.3	Failed attempted abortion complicated by renal failure
638.5	Failed attempted abortion complicated by shock
084.0	Falciparum malaria [malignant tertian]
958.1	Fat embolism
551.02	Femoral hernia with gangrene, bilateral (not specified as recurrent)
551.03	Femoral hernia with gangrene, bilateral, recurrent
551.00	Femoral hernia with gangrene, unilateral or unspecified (not specified as recurrent)
551.01	Femoral hernia with gangrene, unilateral or unspecified, recurrent
807.4	Flail chest
809.1	Fracture of bones of trunk, open
780.72	Functional quadriplegia
040.0	Gas gangrene
535.21	Gastric mucosal hypertrophy, with hemorrhage
531.91	Gastric ulcer, unspecified as acute or chronic, without mention of hemorrhage or perforation, with obstruction
530.7	Gastroesophageal laceration-hemorrhage syndrome
772.4	Gastrointestinal hemorrhage of fetus or newborn
534.91	Gastrojejunal ulcer, unspecified as acute or chronic, without mention of hemorrhage or perforation, with obstruction
756.73	Gastroschisis
659.33	Generalized infection during labor, antepartum condition or complication
659.31	Generalized infection during labor, delivered, with or without mention of antepartum condition
098.84	Gonococcal endocarditis
098.82	Gonococcal meningitis
098.83	Gonococcal pericarditis
345.3	Grand mal status
282.62	Hb-SS disease with crisis
283.11	Hemolytic-uremic syndrome
568.81	Hemoperitoneum (nontraumatic)
320.0	Hemophilus meningitis
641.13	Hemorrhage from placenta previa, antepartum condition or complication
641.11	Hemorrhage from placenta previa, delivered, with or without mention of antepartum condition
572.2	Hepatic encephalopathy
573.4	Hepatic infarction
070.42	Hepatitis delta without mention of active hepatitis B disease with hepatic coma
070.43	Hepatitis E with hepatic coma
572.4	Hepatorenal syndrome
551.8	Hernia of other specified sites, with gangrene
551.9	Hernia of unspecified site, with gangrene
054.72	Herpes simplex meningitis
054.74	Herpes simplex myelitis
053.14	Herpes zoster myelitis
053.0	Herpes zoster with meningitis
054.3	Herpetic meningoencephalitis
054.5	Herpetic septicemia
115.94	Histoplasmosis, unspecified, endocarditis
115.91	Histoplasmosis, unspecified, meningitis
115.93	Histoplasmosis, unspecified, pericarditis
115.95	Histoplasmosis, unspecified, pneumonia
058.21	Human herpesvirus 6 encephalitis
042	Human immunodeficiency virus [HIV] disease
773.3	Hydrops fetalis due to isoimmunization
778.0	Hydrops fetalis not due to isoimmunization
642.12	Hypertension secondary to renal disease, complicating pregnancy, childbirth, and the puerperium, delivered, with mention of postpartum complication
642.11	Hypertension secondary to renal disease, complicating pregnancy, childbirth, and the puerperium, delivered, with or without mention of antepartum condition
746.7	Hypoplastic left heart syndrome
415.11	Iatrogenic pulmonary embolism and infarction
422.91	Idiopathic myocarditis
636.62	Illegally induced abortion, complicated by embolism, complete
636.61	Illegally induced abortion, complicated by embolism, incomplete
636.60	Illegally induced abortion, complicated by embolism, unspecified
636.32	Illegally induced abortion, complicated by renal failure, complete
636.31	Illegally induced abortion, complicated by renal failure, incomplete
636.30	Illegally induced abortion, complicated by renal failure, unspecified
636.52	Illegally induced abortion, complicated by shock, complete
636.51	Illegally induced abortion, complicated by shock, incomplete

636.50	Illegally induced abortion, complicated by shock, unspecified
551.21	Incisional ventral hernia, with gangrene
115.04	Infection by Histoplasma capsulatum, endocarditis
115.01	Infection by Histoplasma capsulatum, meningitis
115.03	Infection by Histoplasma capsulatum, pericarditis
115.05	Infection by Histoplasma capsulatum, pneumonia
115.14	Infection by Histoplasma duboisii, endocarditis
115.11	Infection by Histoplasma duboisii, meningitis
115.13	Infection by Histoplasma duboisii, pericarditis
115.15	Infection by Histoplasma duboisii, pneumonia
658.43	Infection of amniotic cavity, antepartum condition or complication
658.41	Infection of amniotic cavity, delivered, with or without mention of antepartum condition
323.61	Infectious acute disseminated encephalomyelitis (ADEM)
488.11	Influenza due to identified 2009 H1N1 influenza virus with pneumonia
488.01	Influenza due to identified avian influenza virus with pneumonia
488.81	Influenza due to identified novel influenza A virus with pneumonia
487.0	Influenza with pneumonia
550.02	Inguinal hernia, with gangrene, bilateral (not specified as recurrent)
550.03	Inguinal hernia, with gangrene, bilateral, recurrent
550.00	Inguinal hernia, with gangrene, unilateral or unspecified (not specified as recurrent)
550.01	Inguinal hernia, with gangrene, unilateral or unspecified, recurrent
740.2	Iniencephaly
902.0	Injury to abdominal aorta
863.95	Injury to appendix, with open wound into cavity
863.51	Injury to ascending [right] colon, with open wound into cavity
903.01	Injury to axillary artery
903.02	Injury to axillary vein
903.00	Injury to axillary vessel(s), unspecified
867.1	Injury to bladder and urethra, with open wound into cavity
862.31	Injury to bronchus with open wound into cavity
862.21	Injury to bronchus without mention of open wound into cavity
902.29	Injury to celiac and mesenteric arteries, other
902.20	Injury to celiac and mesenteric arteries, unspecified
863.50	Injury to colon, unspecified site, with open wound into cavity
904.0	Injury to common femoral artery
863.53	Injury to descending [left] colon, with open wound into cavity
862.1	Injury to diaphragm, with open wound into cavity
863.31	Injury to duodenum, with open wound into cavity
862.32	Injury to esophagus with open wound into cavity
862.22	Injury to esophagus without mention of open wound into cavity
904.2	Injury to femoral veins
902.21	Injury to gastric artery
863.90	Injury to gastrointestinal tract, unspecified site, with open wound into cavity
902.22	Injury to hepatic artery
902.11	Injury to hepatic veins
902.51	Injury to hypogastric artery
902.52	Injury to hypogastric vein
902.53	Injury to iliac artery
902.59	Injury to iliac blood vessels, other
902.54	Injury to iliac vein
902.50	Injury to iliac vessel(s), unspecified
902.27	Injury to inferior mesenteric artery
902.32	Injury to inferior mesenteric vein
902.19	Injury to inferior vena cava, other
902.10	Injury to inferior vena cava, unspecified

901.1	Injury to innominate and subclavian arteries
901.3	Injury to innominate and subclavian veins
866.13	Injury to kidney with open wound into cavity, complete disruption of kidney parenchyma
866.11	Injury to kidney with open wound into cavity, hematoma without rupture of capsule
866.12	Injury to kidney with open wound into cavity, laceration
866.10	Injury to kidney with open wound into cavity, unspecified injury
866.03	Injury to kidney without mention of open wound into cavity, complete disruption of kidney parenchyma
864.11	Injury to liver with open wound into cavity, hematoma and contusion
864.14	Injury to liver with open wound into cavity, laceration, major
864.12	Injury to liver with open wound into cavity, laceration, minor
864.13	Injury to liver with open wound into cavity, laceration, moderate
864.15	Injury to liver with open wound into cavity, laceration, unspecified
864.10	Injury to liver with open wound into cavity, unspecified injury
864.04	Injury to liver without mention of open wound into cavity, laceration, major
864.03	Injury to liver without mention of open wound into cavity, laceration, moderate
862.9	Injury to multiple and unspecified intrathoracic organs, with open wound into cavity
902.87	Injury to multiple blood vessels of abdomen and pelvis
901.83	Injury to multiple blood vessels of thorax
863.56	Injury to multiple sites in colon and rectum, with open wound into cavity
868.19	Injury to other and multiple intra-abdominal organs, with open wound into cavity
863.99	Injury to other gastrointestinal sites, with open wound into cavity
868.11	Injury to other intra-abdominal organs with open wound into cavity, adrenal gland
868.12	Injury to other intra-abdominal organs with open wound into cavity, bile duct and gallbladder
868.13	Injury to other intra-abdominal organs with open wound into cavity, peritoneum
868.14	Injury to other intra-abdominal organs with open wound into cavity, retroperitoneum
868.10	Injury to other intra-abdominal organs with open wound into cavity, unspecified intra-abdominal organ
902.24	Injury to other specified branches of celiac axis
862.39	Injury to other specified intrathoracic organs with open wound into cavity
867.7	Injury to other specified pelvic organs, with open wound into cavity
863.92	Injury to pancreas, body, with open wound into cavity
863.91	Injury to pancreas, head, with open wound into cavity
863.94	Injury to pancreas, multiple and unspecified sites, with open wound into cavity
863.93	Injury to pancreas, tail, with open wound into cavity
904.41	Injury to popliteal artery
904.42	Injury to popliteal vein
904.40	Injury to popliteal vessel(s), unspecified
902.39	Injury to portal and splenic veins, other
902.33	Injury to portal vein
902.26	Injury to primary branches of superior mesenteric artery
901.41	Injury to pulmonary artery
901.42	Injury to pulmonary vein
901.40	Injury to pulmonary vessel(s), unspecified
863.55	Injury to rectum, with open wound into cavity
902.41	Injury to renal artery
902.49	Injury to renal blood vessels, other

902.42	Injury to renal vein
902.40	Injury to renal vessel(s), unspecified
863.54	Injury to sigmoid colon, with open wound into cavity
863.30	Injury to small intestine, unspecified site, with open wound into cavity
865.12	Injury to spleen with open wound into cavity, capsular tears, without major disruption of parenchyma
865.11	Injury to spleen with open wound into cavity, hematoma without rupture of capsule
865.13	Injury to spleen with open wound into cavity, laceration extending into parenchyma
865.14	Injury to spleen with open wound into cavity, massive parenchyma disruption
865.10	Injury to spleen with open wound into cavity, unspecified injury
865.03	Injury to spleen without mention of open wound into cavity, laceration extending into parenchyma
865.04	Injury to spleen without mention of open wound into cavity, massive parenchymal disruption
902.23	Injury to splenic artery
902.34	Injury to splenic vein
863.1	Injury to stomach, with open wound into cavity
904.1	Injury to superficial femoral artery
902.25	Injury to superior mesenteric artery (trunk)
902.31	Injury to superior mesenteric vein and primary subdivisions
901.2	Injury to superior vena cava
901.0	Injury to thoracic aorta
863.52	Injury to transverse colon, with open wound into cavity
867.9	Injury to unspecified pelvic organ, with open wound into cavity
867.3	Injury to ureter, with open wound into cavity
867.5	Injury to uterus, with open wound into cavity
869.1	Internal injury to unspecified or ill-defined organs with open wound into cavity
747.11	Interruption of aortic arch
770.2	Interstitial emphysema and related conditions
431	Intracerebral hemorrhage
324.0	Intracranial abscess
324.9	Intracranial and intraspinal abscess of unspecified site
854.10	Intracranial injury of other and unspecified nature with open intracranial wound, unspecified state of consciousness
854.12	Intracranial injury of other and unspecified nature with open intracranial wound, with brief [less than one hour] loss of consciousness
854.19	Intracranial injury of other and unspecified nature with open intracranial wound, with concussion, unspecified
854.16	Intracranial injury of other and unspecified nature with open intracranial wound, with loss of consciousness of unspecified duration
854.13	Intracranial injury of other and unspecified nature with open intracranial wound, with moderate [1-24 hours] loss of consciousness
854.11	Intracranial injury of other and unspecified nature with open intracranial wound, with no loss of consciousness
854.14	Intracranial injury of other and unspecified nature with open intracranial wound, with prolonged [more than 24 hours] loss of consciousness and return to pre-existing conscious level
854.15	Intracranial injury of other and unspecified nature with open intracranial wound, with prolonged [more than 24 hours] loss of consciousness without return to pre-existing conscious level
854.05	Intracranial injury of other and unspecified nature without mention of open intracranial wound, with prolonged [more than 24 hours] loss of consciousness without return to pre-existing conscious level
324.1	Intraspinal abscess
772.13	Intraventricular hemorrhage, grade III

772.14	Intraventricular hemorrhage, grade IV
062.0	Japanese encephalitis
773.4	Kernicterus of fetus or newborn due to isoimmunization
774.7	Kernicterus of fetus or newborn not due to isoimmunization
639.3	Kidney failure following abortion and ectopic and molar pregnancies
260	Kwashiorkor
861.13	Laceration of heart with penetration of heart chambers with open wound into thorax
861.03	Laceration of heart with penetration of heart chambers without mention of open wound into thorax
861.02	Laceration of heart without penetration of heart chambers or without mention of open wound into thorax
861.12	Laceration of heart without penetration of heart chambers, with open wound into thorax
861.32	Laceration of lung with open wound into thorax
861.22	Laceration of lung without mention of open wound into thorax
775.7	Late metabolic acidosis of newborn
635.62	Legally induced abortion, complicated by embolism, complete
635.61	Legally induced abortion, complicated by embolism, incomplete
635.60	Legally induced abortion, complicated by embolism, unspecified
635.32	Legally induced abortion, complicated by renal failure, complete
635.31	Legally induced abortion, complicated by renal failure, incomplete
635.30	Legally induced abortion, complicated by renal failure,unspecified
635.52	Legally induced abortion, complicated by shock, complete
635.51	Legally induced abortion, complicated by shock, incomplete
635.50	Legally induced abortion, complicated by shock, unspecified
100.81	Leptospiral meningitis (aseptic)
344.81	Locked-in state
063.1	Louping ill
952.2	Lumbar spinal cord injury without evidence of spinal bone injury
516.4	Lymphangioleiomyomatosis
670.02	Major puerperal infection, delivered, with mention of postpartum complication
670.04	Major puerperal infection, postpartum condition or complication
669.22	Maternal hypotension syndrome, delivered, with mention of postpartum complication
669.21	Maternal hypotension syndrome, delivered, with or without mention of antepartum condition
770.12	Meconium aspiration with respiratory symptoms
519.2	Mediastinitis
320.82	Meningitis due to gram-negative bacteria, not elsewhere classified
321.8	Meningitis due to other nonbacterial organisms classified elsewhere
320.89	Meningitis due to other specified bacteria
321.3	Meningitis due to trypanosomiasis
320.9	Meningitis due to unspecified bacterium
321.2	Meningitis due to viruses not elsewhere classified
320.7	Meningitis in other bacterial diseases classified elsewhere
321.1	Meningitis in other fungal diseases
321.4	Meningitis in sarcoidosis
322.9	Meningitis, unspecified
036.40	Meningococcal carditis, unspecified
036.1	Meningococcal encephalitis
036.42	Meningococcal endocarditis
036.0	Meningococcal meningitis
036.43	Meningococcal myocarditis
036.41	Meningococcal pericarditis
036.2	Meningococcemia
130.0	Meningoencephalitis due to toxoplasmosis
348.31	Metabolic encephalopathy

482.42	Methicillin resistant pneumonia due to Staphylococcus aureus
038.12	Methicillin resistant Staphylococcus aureus septicemia
482.41	Methicillin susceptible pneumonia due to Staphylococcus aureus
038.11	Methicillin susceptible Staphylococcus aureus septicemia
642.42	Mild or unspecified pre-eclampsia, delivered, with mention of postpartum complication
018.91	Miliary tuberculosis, unspecified, bacteriological or histological examination not done
018.92	Miliary tuberculosis, unspecified, bacteriological or histological examination unknown (at present)
018.93	Miliary tuberculosis, unspecified, tubercle bacilli found (in sputum) by microscopy
018.94	Miliary tuberculosis, unspecified, tubercle bacilli not found (in sputum) by microscopy, but found by bacterial culture
018.95	Miliary tuberculosis, unspecified, tubercle bacilli not found by bacteriological examination, but tuberculosis confirmed histologically
018.96	Miliary tuberculosis, unspecified, tubercle bacilli not found by bacteriological or histological examination, but tuberculosis confirmed by other methods [inoculation of animals]
018.90	Miliary tuberculosis, unspecified, unspecified
062.9	Mosquito-borne viral encephalitis, unspecified
808.53	Multiple open pelvic fractures with disruption of pelvic circle
808.54	Multiple open pelvic fractures without disruption of pelvic circle
952.8	Multiple sites of spinal cord injury without evidence of spinal bone injury
130.8	Multisystemic disseminated toxoplasmosis
072.2	Mumps encephalitis
072.1	Mumps meningitis
358.01	Myasthenia gravis with (acute) exacerbation
323.52	Myelitis following immunization procedures
323.02	Myelitis in viral diseases classified elsewhere
130.3	Myocarditis due to toxoplasmosis
777.50	Necrotizing enterocolitis in newborn, unspecified
728.86	Necrotizing fasciitis
583.4	Nephritis and nephropathy, not specified as acute or chronic, with lesion of rapidly progressive glomerulonephritis
583.6	Nephritis and nephropathy, not specified as acute or chronic, with lesion of renal cortical necrosis
516.61	Neuroendocrine cell hyperplasia of infancy
333.92	Neuroleptic malignant syndrome
322.0	Nonpyogenic meningitis
432.0	Nontraumatic extradural hemorrhage
261	Nutritional marasmus
673.03	Obstetrical air embolism, antepartum condition or complication
673.02	Obstetrical air embolism, delivered, with mention of postpartum complication
673.01	Obstetrical air embolism, delivered, with or without mention of antepartum condition
673.04	Obstetrical air embolism, postpartum condition or complication
673.23	Obstetrical blood-clot embolism, antepartum condition or complication
673.22	Obstetrical blood-clot embolism, delivered, with mention of postpartum complication
673.21	Obstetrical blood-clot embolism, delivered, with or without mention of antepartum condition
673.24	Obstetrical blood-clot embolism, postpartum condition or complication
673.33	Obstetrical pyemic and septic embolism, antepartum condition or complication
673.32	Obstetrical pyemic and septic embolism, delivered, with mention of postpartum complication

673.31	Obstetrical pyemic and septic embolism, delivered, with or without mention of antepartum condition
673.34	Obstetrical pyemic and septic embolism, postpartum condition or complication
576.2	Obstruction of bile duct
746.84	Obstructive anomalies of heart, not elsewhere classified
433.01	Occlusion and stenosis of basilar artery with cerebral infarction
433.11	Occlusion and stenosis of carotid artery with cerebral infarction
433.31	Occlusion and stenosis of multiple and bilateral precerebral arteries with cerebral infarction
433.81	Occlusion and stenosis of other specified precerebral artery with cerebral infarction
433.91	Occlusion and stenosis of unspecified precerebral artery with cerebral infarction
433.21	Occlusion and stenosis of vertebral artery with cerebral infarction
756.72	Omphalocele
813.51	Open Colles' fracture
835.10	Open dislocation of hip, unspecified site
839.10	Open dislocation, cervical vertebra, unspecified
839.15	Open dislocation, fifth cervical vertebra
839.11	Open dislocation, first cervical vertebra
839.14	Open dislocation, fourth cervical vertebra
839.30	Open dislocation, lumbar vertebra
839.18	Open dislocation, multiple cervical vertebrae
839.12	Open dislocation, second cervical vertebra
839.17	Open dislocation, seventh cervical vertebra
839.16	Open dislocation, sixth cervical vertebra
839.71	Open dislocation, sternum
839.13	Open dislocation, third cervical vertebra
839.31	Open dislocation, thoracic vertebra
839.50	Open dislocation, vertebra, unspecified site
839.59	Open dislocation, vertebra, other
808.1	Open fracture of acetabulum
812.12	Open fracture of anatomical neck of humerus
820.13	Open fracture of base of neck of femur
801.60	Open fracture of base of skull with cerebral laceration and contusion, unspecified state of consciousness
801.62	Open fracture of base of skull with cerebral laceration and contusion, with brief [less than one hour] loss of consciousness
801.69	Open fracture of base of skull with cerebral laceration and contusion, with concussion, unspecified
801.66	Open fracture of base of skull with cerebral laceration and contusion, with loss of consciousness of unspecified duration
801.63	Open fracture of base of skull with cerebral laceration and contusion, with moderate [1-24 hours] loss of consciousness
801.61	Open fracture of base of skull with cerebral laceration and contusion, with no loss of consciousness
801.64	Open fracture of base of skull with cerebral laceration and contusion, with prolonged [more than 24 hours] loss of consciousness and return to pre-existing conscious level
801.65	Open fracture of base of skull with cerebral laceration and contusion, with prolonged [more than 24 hours] loss of consciousness, without return to pre-existing conscious level
801.90	Open fracture of base of skull with intracranial injury of other and unspecified nature, unspecified state of consciousness
801.92	Open fracture of base of skull with intracranial injury of other and unspecified nature, with brief [less than one hour] loss of consciousness
801.99	Open fracture of base of skull with intracranial injury of other and unspecified nature, with concussion, unspecified
801.96	Open fracture of base of skull with intracranial injury of other and unspecified nature, with loss of consciousness of unspecified duration

Appendix A — Alphabetic MCC List

801.93	Open fracture of base of skull with intracranial injury of other and unspecified nature, with moderate [1-24 hours] loss of consciousness
801.91	Open fracture of base of skull with intracranial injury of other and unspecified nature, with no loss of consciousness
801.94	Open fracture of base of skull with intracranial injury of other and unspecified nature, with prolonged [more than 24 hours] loss of consciousness and return to pre-existing conscious level
801.95	Open fracture of base of skull with intracranial injury of other and unspecified nature, with prolonged [more than 24 hours] loss of consciousness, without return to pre-existing conscious level
801.80	Open fracture of base of skull with other and unspecified intracranial hemorrhage, unspecified state of consciousness
801.82	Open fracture of base of skull with other and unspecified intracranial hemorrhage, with brief [less than one hour] loss of consciousness
801.89	Open fracture of base of skull with other and unspecified intracranial hemorrhage, with concussion, unspecified
801.86	Open fracture of base of skull with other and unspecified intracranial hemorrhage, with loss of consciousness of unspecified duration
801.83	Open fracture of base of skull with other and unspecified intracranial hemorrhage, with moderate [1-24 hours] loss of consciousness
801.81	Open fracture of base of skull with other and unspecified intracranial hemorrhage, with no loss of consciousness
801.84	Open fracture of base of skull with other and unspecified intracranial hemorrhage, with prolonged [more than 24 hours] loss of consciousness and return to pre-existing conscious level
801.85	Open fracture of base of skull with other and unspecified intracranial hemorrhage, with prolonged [more than 24 hours] loss of consciousness, without return to pre-existing conscious level
801.70	Open fracture of base of skull with subarachnoid, subdural, and extradural hemorrhage, unspecified state of consciousness
801.72	Open fracture of base of skull with subarachnoid, subdural, and extradural hemorrhage, with brief [less than one hour] loss of consciousness
801.79	Open fracture of base of skull with subarachnoid, subdural, and extradural hemorrhage, with concussion, unspecified
801.76	Open fracture of base of skull with subarachnoid, subdural, and extradural hemorrhage, with loss of consciousness of unspecified duration
801.73	Open fracture of base of skull with subarachnoid, subdural, and extradural hemorrhage, with moderate [1-24 hours] loss of consciousness
801.71	Open fracture of base of skull with subarachnoid, subdural, and extradural hemorrhage, with no loss of consciousness
801.74	Open fracture of base of skull with subarachnoid, subdural, and extradural hemorrhage, with prolonged [more than 24 hours] loss of consciousness and return to pre-existing conscious level
801.75	Open fracture of base of skull with subarachnoid, subdural, and extradural hemorrhage, with prolonged [more than 24 hours] loss of consciousness, without return to pre-existing conscious level
801.50	Open fracture of base of skull without mention of intracranial injury, unspecified state of consciousness
801.52	Open fracture of base of skull without mention of intracranial injury, with brief [less than one hour] loss of consciousness
801.59	Open fracture of base of skull without mention of intracranial injury, with concussion, unspecified
801.56	Open fracture of base of skull without mention of intracranial injury, with loss of consciousness of unspecified duration
801.53	Open fracture of base of skull without mention of intracranial injury, with moderate [1-24 hours] loss of consciousness
801.51	Open fracture of base of skull without mention of intracranial injury, with no loss of consciousness
801.54	Open fracture of base of skull without mention of intracranial injury, with prolonged [more than 24 hours] loss of consciousness and return to pre-existing conscious level
801.55	Open fracture of base of skull without mention of intracranial injury, with prolonged [more than 24 hours] loss of consciousness, without return to pre-existing conscious level
806.12	Open fracture of C1-C4 level with anterior cord syndrome
806.13	Open fracture of C1-C4 level with central cord syndrome
806.11	Open fracture of C1-C4 level with complete lesion of cord
806.14	Open fracture of C1-C4 level with other specified spinal cord injury
806.10	Open fracture of C1-C4 level with unspecified spinal cord injury
806.17	Open fracture of C5-C7 level with anterior cord syndrome
806.18	Open fracture of C5-C7 level with central cord syndrome
806.16	Open fracture of C5-C7 level with complete lesion of cord
806.19	Open fracture of C5-C7 level with other specified spinal cord injury
806.15	Open fracture of C5-C7 level with unspecified spinal cord injury
805.10	Open fracture of cervical vertebra, unspecified level
821.31	Open fracture of condyle, femoral
813.12	Open fracture of coronoid process of ulna
813.53	Open fracture of distal end of ulna (alone)
805.3	Open fracture of dorsal [thoracic] vertebra without mention of spinal cord injury
807.18	Open fracture of eight or more ribs
820.11	Open fracture of epiphysis (separation) (upper) of neck of femur
821.32	Open fracture of epiphysis. Lower (separation) of femur
805.15	Open fracture of fifth cervical vertebra
805.11	Open fracture of first cervical vertebra
807.15	Open fracture of five ribs
807.14	Open fracture of four ribs
805.14	Open fracture of fourth cervical vertebra
812.13	Open fracture of greater tuberosity of humerus
813.15	Open fracture of head of radius
808.51	Open fracture of ilium
820.31	Open fracture of intertrochanteric section of neck of femur
820.10	Open fracture of intracapsular section of neck of femur, unspecified
808.52	Open fracture of ischium
807.6	Open fracture of larynx and trachea
812.52	Open fracture of lateral condyle of humerus
821.30	Open fracture of lower end of femur, unspecified part
813.50	Open fracture of lower end of forearm, unspecified
813.54	Open fracture of lower end of radius with ulna
806.5	Open fracture of lumbar spine with spinal cord injury
805.5	Open fracture of lumbar vertebra without mention of spinal cord injury
812.53	Open fracture of medial condyle of humerus
820.12	Open fracture of midcervical section of neck of femur
805.18	Open fracture of multiple cervical vertebrae
807.19	Open fracture of multiple ribs, unspecified
813.16	Open fracture of neck of radius
813.11	Open fracture of olecranon process of ulna
807.11	Open fracture of one rib
808.59	Open fracture of other specified part of pelvis
808.3	Open fracture of pubis
813.18	Open fracture of radius with ulna, upper end (any part)
807.10	Open fracture of rib(s), unspecified
806.71	Open fracture of sacrum and coccyx with complete cauda equina lesion
806.72	Open fracture of sacrum and coccyx with other cauda equina injury
806.79	Open fracture of sacrum and coccyx with other spinal cord injury
806.70	Open fracture of sacrum and coccyx with unspecified spinal cord injury
805.7	Open fracture of sacrum and coccyx without mention of spinal cord injury

805.12	Open fracture of second cervical vertebra
807.17	Open fracture of seven ribs
805.17	Open fracture of seventh cervical vertebra
821.11	Open fracture of shaft of femur
823.31	Open fracture of shaft of fibula alone
823.32	Open fracture of shaft of fibula with tibia
812.31	Open fracture of shaft of humerus
813.31	Open fracture of shaft of radius (alone)
813.30	Open fracture of shaft of radius or ulna, unspecified
813.33	Open fracture of shaft of radius with ulna
823.30	Open fracture of shaft of tibia alone
813.32	Open fracture of shaft of ulna (alone)
807.16	Open fracture of six ribs
805.16	Open fracture of sixth cervical vertebra
807.3	Open fracture of sternum
820.32	Open fracture of subtrochanteric section of neck of femur
812.11	Open fracture of surgical neck of humerus
806.32	Open fracture of T1-T6 level with anterior cord syndrome
806.33	Open fracture of T1-T6 level with central cord syndrome
806.31	Open fracture of T1-T6 level with complete lesion of cord
806.34	Open fracture of T1-T6 level with other specified spinal cord injury
806.30	Open fracture of T1-T6 level with unspecified spinal cord injury
806.37	Open fracture of T7-T12 level with anterior cord syndrome
806.38	Open fracture of T7-T12 level with central cord syndrome
806.36	Open fracture of T7-T12 level with complete lesion of cord
806.39	Open fracture of T7-T12 level with other specified spinal cord injury
806.35	Open fracture of T7-T12 level with unspecified spinal cord injury
805.13	Open fracture of third cervical vertebra
807.13	Open fracture of three ribs
820.30	Open fracture of trochanteric section of neck of femur, unspecified
807.12	Open fracture of two ribs
812.54	Open fracture of unspecified condyle(s) of humerus
821.10	Open fracture of unspecified part of femur
823.91	Open fracture of unspecified part of fibula alone
823.92	Open fracture of unspecified part of fibula with tibia
813.90	Open fracture of unspecified part of forearm
812.30	Open fracture of unspecified part of humerus
812.50	Open fracture of unspecified part of lower end of humerus
820.9	Open fracture of unspecified part of neck of femur
813.91	Open fracture of unspecified part of radius (alone)
813.93	Open fracture of unspecified part of radius with ulna
823.90	Open fracture of unspecified part of tibia alone
813.92	Open fracture of unspecified part of ulna (alone)
812.10	Open fracture of unspecified part of upper end of humerus
806.9	Open fracture of unspecified vertebral column with spinal cord injury
805.9	Open fracture of unspecified vertebral column without mention of spinal cord injury
823.11	Open fracture of upper end of fibula alone
823.12	Open fracture of upper end of fibula with tibia
813.10	Open fracture of upper end of forearm, unspecified
823.10	Open fracture of upper end of tibia alone
800.60	Open fracture of vault of skull with cerebral laceration and contusion, unspecified state of consciousness
800.62	Open fracture of vault of skull with cerebral laceration and contusion, with brief [less than one hour] loss of consciousness
800.69	Open fracture of vault of skull with cerebral laceration and contusion, with concussion, unspecified
800.66	Open fracture of vault of skull with cerebral laceration and contusion, with loss of consciousness of unspecified duration

800.63	Open fracture of vault of skull with cerebral laceration and contusion, with moderate [1-24 hours] loss of consciousness
800.61	Open fracture of vault of skull with cerebral laceration and contusion, with no loss of consciousness
800.64	Open fracture of vault of skull with cerebral laceration and contusion, with prolonged [more than 24 hours] loss of consciousness and return to pre-existing conscious level
800.65	Open fracture of vault of skull with cerebral laceration and contusion, with prolonged [more than 24 hours] loss of consciousness, without return to pre-existing conscious level
800.90	Open fracture of vault of skull with intracranial injury of other and unspecified nature, unspecified state of consciousness
800.92	Open fracture of vault of skull with intracranial injury of other and unspecified nature, with brief [less than one hour] loss of consciousness
800.99	Open fracture of vault of skull with intracranial injury of other and unspecified nature, with concussion, unspecified
800.96	Open fracture of vault of skull with intracranial injury of other and unspecified nature, with loss of consciousness of unspecified duration
800.93	Open fracture of vault of skull with intracranial injury of other and unspecified nature, with moderate [1-24 hours] loss of consciousness
800.91	Open fracture of vault of skull with intracranial injury of other and unspecified nature, with no loss of consciousness
800.94	Open fracture of vault of skull with intracranial injury of other and unspecified nature, with prolonged [more than 24 hours] loss of consciousness and return to pre-existing conscious level
800.95	Open fracture of vault of skull with intracranial injury of other and unspecified nature, with prolonged [more than 24 hours] loss of consciousness, without return to pre-existing conscious level
800.80	Open fracture of vault of skull with other and unspecified intracranial hemorrhage, unspecified state of consciousness
800.82	Open fracture of vault of skull with other and unspecified intracranial hemorrhage, with brief [less than one hour] loss of consciousness
800.89	Open fracture of vault of skull with other and unspecified intracranial hemorrhage, with concussion, unspecified
800.86	Open fracture of vault of skull with other and unspecified intracranial hemorrhage, with loss of consciousness of unspecified duration
800.83	Open fracture of vault of skull with other and unspecified intracranial hemorrhage, with moderate [1-24 hours] loss of consciousness
800.81	Open fracture of vault of skull with other and unspecified intracranial hemorrhage, with no loss of consciousness
800.84	Open fracture of vault of skull with other and unspecified intracranial hemorrhage, with prolonged [more than 24 hours] loss of consciousness and return to pre-existing conscious level
800.85	Open fracture of vault of skull with other and unspecified intracranial hemorrhage, with prolonged [more than 24 hours] loss of consciousness, without return to pre-existing conscious level
800.70	Open fracture of vault of skull with subarachnoid, subdural, and extradural hemorrhage, unspecified state of consciousness
800.72	Open fracture of vault of skull with subarachnoid, subdural, and extradural hemorrhage, with brief [less than one hour] loss of consciousness
800.79	Open fracture of vault of skull with subarachnoid, subdural, and extradural hemorrhage, with concussion, unspecified
800.76	Open fracture of vault of skull with subarachnoid, subdural, and extradural hemorrhage, with loss of consciousness of unspecified duration
800.73	Open fracture of vault of skull with subarachnoid, subdural, and extradural hemorrhage, with moderate [1-24 hours] loss of consciousness
800.71	Open fracture of vault of skull with subarachnoid, subdural, and extradural hemorrhage, with no loss of consciousness

800.74 Open fracture of vault of skull with subarachnoid, subdural, and extradural hemorrhage, with prolonged [more than 24 hours] loss of consciousness and return to pre-existing conscious level

800.75 Open fracture of vault of skull with subarachnoid, subdural, and extradural hemorrhage, with prolonged [more than 24 hours] loss of consciousness, without return to pre-existing conscious level

800.50 Open fracture of vault of skull without mention of intracranial injury, unspecified state of consciousness

800.52 Open fracture of vault of skull without mention of intracranial injury, with brief [less than one hour] loss of consciousness

800.59 Open fracture of vault of skull without mention of intracranial injury, with concussion, unspecified

800.56 Open fracture of vault of skull without mention of intracranial injury, with loss of consciousness of unspecified duration

800.53 Open fracture of vault of skull without mention of intracranial injury, with moderate [1-24 hours] loss of consciousness

800.51 Open fracture of vault of skull without mention of intracranial injury, with no loss of consciousness

800.54 Open fracture of vault of skull without mention of intracranial injury, with prolonged [more than 24 hours] loss of consciousness and return to pre-existing conscious level

800.55 Open fracture of vault of skull without mention of intracranial injury, with prolonged [more than 24 hours] loss of consciousness, without return to pre-existing conscious level

804.70 Open fractures involving skull or face with other bones with subarachnoid, subdural, and extradural hemorrhage, unspecified state of consciousness

804.72 Open fractures involving skull or face with other bones with subarachnoid, subdural, and extradural hemorrhage, with brief [less than one hour] loss of consciousness

804.79 Open fractures involving skull or face with other bones with subarachnoid, subdural, and extradural hemorrhage, with concussion, unspecified

804.76 Open fractures involving skull or face with other bones with subarachnoid, subdural, and extradural hemorrhage, with loss of consciousness of unspecified duration

804.73 Open fractures involving skull or face with other bones with subarachnoid, subdural, and extradural hemorrhage, with moderate [1-24 hours] loss of consciousness

804.71 Open fractures involving skull or face with other bones with subarachnoid, subdural, and extradural hemorrhage, with no loss of consciousness

804.74 Open fractures involving skull or face with other bones with subarachnoid, subdural, and extradural hemorrhage, with prolonged [more than 24 hours] loss of consciousness and return to pre-existing conscious level

804.75 Open fractures involving skull or face with other bones with subarachnoid, subdural, and extradural hemorrhage, with prolonged [more than 24 hours] loss of consciousness, without return to pre-existing conscious level

804.60 Open fractures involving skull or face with other bones, with cerebral laceration and contusion, unspecified state of consciousness

804.62 Open fractures involving skull or face with other bones, with cerebral laceration and contusion, with brief [less than one hour] loss of consciousness

804.69 Open fractures involving skull or face with other bones, with cerebral laceration and contusion, with concussion, unspecified

804.66 Open fractures involving skull or face with other bones, with cerebral laceration and contusion, with loss of consciousness of unspecified duration

804.63 Open fractures involving skull or face with other bones, with cerebral laceration and contusion, with moderate [1-24 hours] loss of consciousness

804.61 Open fractures involving skull or face with other bones, with cerebral laceration and contusion, with no loss of consciousness

804.64 Open fractures involving skull or face with other bones, with cerebral laceration and contusion, with prolonged [more than 24 hours] loss of consciousness and return to pre-existing conscious level

804.65 Open fractures involving skull or face with other bones, with cerebral laceration and contusion, with prolonged [more than 24 hours] loss of consciousness, without return to pre-existing conscious level

804.93 Open fractures involving skull or face with other bones, with intracranial injury of other and unspecified nature, with moderate [1-24 hours] loss of consciousness

804.94 Open fractures involving skull or face with other bones, with intracranial injury of other and unspecified nature, with prolonged [more than 24 hours] loss of consciousness and return to pre-existing conscious level

804.95 Open fractures involving skull or face with other bones, with intracranial injury of other and unspecified nature, with prolonged [more than 24 hours] loss of consciousness without return to pre-existing conscious level

804.80 Open fractures involving skull or face with other bones, with other and unspecified intracranial hemorrhage, unspecified state of consciousness

804.82 Open fractures involving skull or face with other bones, with other and unspecified intracranial hemorrhage, with brief [less than one hour] loss of consciousness

804.89 Open fractures involving skull or face with other bones, with other and unspecified intracranial hemorrhage, with concussion, unspecified

804.86 Open fractures involving skull or face with other bones, with other and unspecified intracranial hemorrhage, with loss of consciousness of unspecified duration

804.83 Open fractures involving skull or face with other bones, with other and unspecified intracranial hemorrhage, with moderate [1-24 hours] loss of consciousness

804.81 Open fractures involving skull or face with other bones, with other and unspecified intracranial hemorrhage, with no loss of consciousness

804.85 Open fractures involving skull or face with other bones, with other and unspecified intracranial hemorrhage, with prolonged [more than 24 hours] loss consciousness, without return to pre-existing conscious level

804.84 Open fractures involving skull or face with other bones, with other and unspecified intracranial hemorrhage, with prolonged [more than 24 hours] loss of consciousness and return to pre-existing conscious level

804.53 Open fractures involving skull or face with other bones, without mention of intracranial injury, with moderate [1-24 hours] loss of consciousness

804.54 Open fractures involving skull or face with other bones, without mention of intracranial injury, with prolonged [more than 24 hours] loss of consciousness and return to pre-existing conscious level

804.55 Open fractures involving skull or face with other bones, without mention of intracranial injury, with prolonged [more than 24 hours] loss of consciousness, without return to pre-existing conscious level

813.13 Open Monteggia's fracture

828.1 Open multiple fractures involving both lower limbs, lower with upper limb, and lower limb(s) with rib(s) and sternum

835.12 Open obturator dislocation of hip

835.11 Open posterior dislocation of hip

821.33 Open supracondylar fracture of femur

812.51 Open supracondylar fracture of humerus

808.9 Open unspecified fracture of pelvis

874.10 Open wound of larynx with trachea, complicated

874.00 Open wound of larynx with trachea, without mention of complication

874.11 Open wound of larynx, complicated

874.01 Open wound of larynx, without mention of complication

874.12 Open wound of trachea, complicated

874.02 Open wound of trachea, without mention of complication

073.0 Ornithosis with pneumonia

422.99 Other acute myocarditis

851.90 Other and unspecified cerebral laceration and contusion, with open intracranial wound, unspecified state of consciousness

851.92 Other and unspecified cerebral laceration and contusion, with open intracranial wound, with brief [less than one hour] loss of consciousness

851.99 Other and unspecified cerebral laceration and contusion, with open intracranial wound, with concussion, unspecified

851.96 Other and unspecified cerebral laceration and contusion, with open intracranial wound, with loss of consciousness of unspecified duration

851.93 Other and unspecified cerebral laceration and contusion, with open intracranial wound, with moderate [1-24 hours] loss of consciousness

851.91 Other and unspecified cerebral laceration and contusion, with open intracranial wound, with no loss of consciousness

851.94 Other and unspecified cerebral laceration and contusion, with open intracranial wound, with prolonged [more than 24 hours] loss of consciousness and return to pre-existing conscious level

851.95 Other and unspecified cerebral laceration and contusion, with open intracranial wound, with prolonged [more than 24 hours] loss of consciousness without return to pre-existing conscious level

851.80 Other and unspecified cerebral laceration and contusion, without mention of open intracranial wound, unspecified state of consciousness

851.82 Other and unspecified cerebral laceration and contusion, without mention of open intracranial wound, with brief [less than one hour] loss of consciousness

851.89 Other and unspecified cerebral laceration and contusion, without mention of open intracranial wound, with concussion, unspecified

851.86 Other and unspecified cerebral laceration and contusion, without mention of open intracranial wound, with loss of consciousness of unspecified duration

851.83 Other and unspecified cerebral laceration and contusion, without mention of open intracranial wound, with moderate [1-24 hours] loss of consciousness

851.81 Other and unspecified cerebral laceration and contusion, without mention of open intracranial wound, with no loss of consciousness

851.84 Other and unspecified cerebral laceration and contusion, without mention of open intracranial wound, with prolonged [more than 24 hours] loss of consciousness and return to pre- existing conscious level

851.85 Other and unspecified cerebral laceration and contusion, without mention of open intracranial wound, with prolonged [more than 24 hours] loss of consciousness without return to pre-existing conscious level

853.10 Other and unspecified intracranial hemorrhage following injury with open intracranial wound, unspecified state of consciousness

853.12 Other and unspecified intracranial hemorrhage following injury with open intracranial wound, with brief [less than one hour] loss of consciousness

853.19 Other and unspecified intracranial hemorrhage following injury with open intracranial wound, with concussion, unspecified

853.16 Other and unspecified intracranial hemorrhage following injury with open intracranial wound, with loss of consciousness of unspecified duration

853.13 Other and unspecified intracranial hemorrhage following injury with open intracranial wound, with moderate [1-24 hours] loss of consciousness

853.11 Other and unspecified intracranial hemorrhage following injury with open intracranial wound, with no loss of consciousness

853.14 Other and unspecified intracranial hemorrhage following injury with open intracranial wound, with prolonged [more than 24 hours] loss of consciousness and return to pre-existing conscious level

853.15 Other and unspecified intracranial hemorrhage following injury with open intracranial wound, with prolonged [more than 24 hours] loss of consciousness without return to pre-existing conscious level

853.00 Other and unspecified intracranial hemorrhage following injury without mention of open intracranial wound, unspecified state of consciousness

853.02 Other and unspecified intracranial hemorrhage following injury without mention of open intracranial wound, with brief [less than one hour] loss of consciousness

853.09 Other and unspecified intracranial hemorrhage following injury without mention of open intracranial wound, with concussion, unspecified

853.06 Other and unspecified intracranial hemorrhage following injury without mention of open intracranial wound, with loss of consciousness of unspecified duration

853.03 Other and unspecified intracranial hemorrhage following injury without mention of open intracranial wound, with moderate [1-24 hours] loss of consciousness

853.01 Other and unspecified intracranial hemorrhage following injury without mention of open intracranial wound, with no loss of consciousness

853.04 Other and unspecified intracranial hemorrhage following injury without mention of open intracranial wound, with prolonged [more than 24 hours] loss of consciousness and return to pre-existing conscious level

853.05 Other and unspecified intracranial hemorrhage following injury without mention of open intracranial wound, with prolonged [more than 24 hours] loss of consciousness without return to pre-existing conscious level

813.17 Other and unspecified open fractures of proximal end of radius (alone)

813.14 Other and unspecified open fractures of proximal end of ulna (alone)

747.39 Other anomalies of pulmonary artery and pulmonary circulation

323.81 Other causes of encephalitis and encephalomyelitis

323.82 Other causes of myelitis

803.10 Other closed skull fracture with cerebral laceration and contusion, unspecified state of consciousness

803.12 Other closed skull fracture with cerebral laceration and contusion, with brief [less than one hour] loss of consciousness

803.19 Other closed skull fracture with cerebral laceration and contusion, with concussion, unspecified

803.16 Other closed skull fracture with cerebral laceration and contusion, with loss of consciousness of unspecified duration

803.13 Other closed skull fracture with cerebral laceration and contusion, with moderate [1-24 hours] loss of consciousness

803.11 Other closed skull fracture with cerebral laceration and contusion, with no loss of consciousness

803.14 Other closed skull fracture with cerebral laceration and contusion, with prolonged [more than 24 hours] loss of consciousness and return to pre-existing conscious level

803.15 Other closed skull fracture with cerebral laceration and contusion, with prolonged [more than 24 hours] loss of consciousness, without return to pre-existing conscious level

803.43 Other closed skull fracture with intracranial injury of other and unspecified nature, with moderate [1-24 hours] loss of consciousness

803.44 Other closed skull fracture with intracranial injury of other and unspecified nature, with prolonged [more than 24 hours] loss of consciousness and return to pre-existing conscious level

803.45 Other closed skull fracture with intracranial injury of other and unspecified nature, with prolonged [more than 24 hours] loss of consciousness, without return to pre-existing conscious level

803.30	Other closed skull fracture with other and unspecified intracranial hemorrhage, unspecified state of unconsciousness
803.32	Other closed skull fracture with other and unspecified intracranial hemorrhage, with brief [less than one hour] loss of consciousness
803.39	Other closed skull fracture with other and unspecified intracranial hemorrhage, with concussion, unspecified
803.36	Other closed skull fracture with other and unspecified intracranial hemorrhage, with loss of consciousness of unspecified duration
803.33	Other closed skull fracture with other and unspecified intracranial hemorrhage, with moderate [1-24 hours] loss of consciousness
803.31	Other closed skull fracture with other and unspecified intracranial hemorrhage, with no loss of consciousness
803.34	Other closed skull fracture with other and unspecified intracranial hemorrhage, with prolonged [more than 24 hours] loss of consciousness and return to pre-existing conscious level
803.35	Other closed skull fracture with other and unspecified intracranial hemorrhage, with prolonged [more than 24 hours] loss of consciousness, without return to pre-existing conscious level
803.20	Other closed skull fracture with subarachnoid, subdural, and extradural hemorrhage, unspecified state of consciousness
803.22	Other closed skull fracture with subarachnoid, subdural, and extradural hemorrhage, with brief [less than one hour] loss of consciousness
803.29	Other closed skull fracture with subarachnoid, subdural, and extradural hemorrhage, with concussion, unspecified
803.26	Other closed skull fracture with subarachnoid, subdural, and extradural hemorrhage, with loss of consciousness of unspecified duration
803.23	Other closed skull fracture with subarachnoid, subdural, and extradural hemorrhage, with moderate [1-24 hours] loss of consciousness
803.21	Other closed skull fracture with subarachnoid, subdural, and extradural hemorrhage, with no loss of consciousness
803.24	Other closed skull fracture with subarachnoid, subdural, and extradural hemorrhage, with prolonged [more than 24 hours] loss of consciousness and return to pre-existing conscious level
803.25	Other closed skull fracture with subarachnoid, subdural, and extradural hemorrhage, with prolonged [more than 24 hours] loss of consciousness, without return to pre-existing conscious level
803.03	Other closed skull fracture without mention of intracranial injury, with moderate [1-24 hours] loss of consciousness
803.04	Other closed skull fracture without mention of intracranial injury, with prolonged [more than 24 hours] loss of consciousness and return to pre-existing conscious level
803.05	Other closed skull fracture without mention of intracranial injury, with prolonged [more than 24 hours] loss of consciousness, without return to pre-existing conscious level
820.09	Other closed transcervical fracture of neck of femur
756.79	Other congenital anomalies of abdominal wall
771.2	Other congenital infections specific to the perinatal period
284.12	Other drug-induced pancytopenia
323.41	Other encephalitis and encephalomyelitis due to other infections classified elsewhere
348.39	Other encephalopathy
770.18	Other fetal and newborn aspiration with respiratory symptoms
058.29	Other human herpesvirus encephalitis
863.59	Other injury to colon or rectum, with open wound into cavity
864.19	Other injury to liver with open wound into cavity
863.39	Other injury to small intestine, with open wound into cavity
865.19	Other injury to spleen with open wound into cavity
516.69	Other interstitial lung diseases of childhood
670.82	Other major puerperal infection, delivered, with mention of postpartum complication
670.84	Other major puerperal infection, postpartum condition or complication
670.80	Other major puerperal infection, unspecified as to episode of care or not applicable
323.42	Other myelitis due to other infections classified elsewhere
673.83	Other obstetrical pulmonary embolism, antepartum condition or complication
673.82	Other obstetrical pulmonary embolism, delivered, with mention of postpartum complication
673.81	Other obstetrical pulmonary embolism, delivered, with or without mention of antepartum condition
673.84	Other obstetrical pulmonary embolism, postpartum condition or complication
835.13	Other open anterior dislocation of hip
821.39	Other open fracture of lower end of femur
812.59	Other open fracture of lower end of humerus
812.19	Other open fracture of upper end of humerus
813.52	Other open fractures of distal end of radius (alone)
803.60	Other open skull fracture with cerebral laceration and contusion, unspecified state of consciousness
803.62	Other open skull fracture with cerebral laceration and contusion, with brief [less than one hour] loss of consciousness
803.69	Other open skull fracture with cerebral laceration and contusion, with concussion, unspecified
803.66	Other open skull fracture with cerebral laceration and contusion, with loss of consciousness of unspecified duration
803.63	Other open skull fracture with cerebral laceration and contusion, with moderate [1-24 hours] loss of consciousness
803.61	Other open skull fracture with cerebral laceration and contusion, with no loss of consciousness
803.64	Other open skull fracture with cerebral laceration and contusion, with prolonged [more than 24 hours] loss of consciousness and return to pre-existing conscious level
803.65	Other open skull fracture with cerebral laceration and contusion, with prolonged [more than 24 hours] loss of consciousness, without return to pre-existing conscious level
803.90	Other open skull fracture with intracranial injury of other and unspecified nature, unspecified state of consciousness
803.92	Other open skull fracture with intracranial injury of other and unspecified nature, with brief [less than one hour] loss of consciousness
803.99	Other open skull fracture with intracranial injury of other and unspecified nature, with concussion, unspecified
803.96	Other open skull fracture with intracranial injury of other and unspecified nature, with loss of consciousness of unspecified duration
803.93	Other open skull fracture with intracranial injury of other and unspecified nature, with moderate [1-24 hours] loss of consciousness
803.91	Other open skull fracture with intracranial injury of other and unspecified nature, with no loss of consciousness
803.94	Other open skull fracture with intracranial injury of other and unspecified nature, with prolonged [more than 24 hours] loss of consciousness and return to pre-existing conscious level
803.95	Other open skull fracture with intracranial injury of other and unspecified nature, with prolonged [more than 24 hours] loss of consciousness, without return to pre-existing conscious level
803.80	Other open skull fracture with other and unspecified intracranial hemorrhage, unspecified state of consciousness
803.82	Other open skull fracture with other and unspecified intracranial hemorrhage, with brief [less than one hour] loss of consciousness
803.89	Other open skull fracture with other and unspecified intracranial hemorrhage, with concussion, unspecified
803.86	Other open skull fracture with other and unspecified intracranial hemorrhage, with loss of consciousness of unspecified duration
803.83	Other open skull fracture with other and unspecified intracranial hemorrhage, with moderate [1-24 hours] loss of consciousness

803.81	Other open skull fracture with other and unspecified intracranial hemorrhage, with no loss of consciousness
803.84	Other open skull fracture with other and unspecified intracranial hemorrhage, with prolonged [more than 24 hours] loss of consciousness and return to pre-existing conscious level
803.85	Other open skull fracture with other and unspecified intracranial hemorrhage, with prolonged [more than 24 hours] loss of consciousness, without return to pre-existing conscious level
803.70	Other open skull fracture with subarachnoid, subdural, and extradural hemorrhage, unspecified state of consciousness
803.72	Other open skull fracture with subarachnoid, subdural, and extradural hemorrhage, with brief [less than one hour] loss of consciousness
803.79	Other open skull fracture with subarachnoid, subdural, and extradural hemorrhage, with concussion, unspecified
803.76	Other open skull fracture with subarachnoid, subdural, and extradural hemorrhage, with loss of consciousness of unspecified duration
803.73	Other open skull fracture with subarachnoid, subdural, and extradural hemorrhage, with moderate [1-24 hours] loss of consciousness
803.71	Other open skull fracture with subarachnoid, subdural, and extradural hemorrhage, with no loss of consciousness
803.74	Other open skull fracture with subarachnoid, subdural, and extradural hemorrhage, with prolonged [more than 24 hours] loss of consciousness and return to pre-existing conscious level
803.75	Other open skull fracture with subarachnoid, subdural, and extradural hemorrhage, with prolonged [more than 24 hours] loss of consciousness, without return to pre-existing conscious level
803.50	Other open skull fracture without mention of injury, unspecified state of consciousness
803.52	Other open skull fracture without mention of intracranial injury, with brief [less than one hour] loss of consciousness
803.59	Other open skull fracture without mention of intracranial injury, with concussion, unspecified
803.56	Other open skull fracture without mention of intracranial injury, with loss of consciousness of unspecified duration
803.53	Other open skull fracture without mention of intracranial injury, with moderate [1-24 hours] loss of consciousness
803.51	Other open skull fracture without mention of intracranial injury, with no loss of consciousness
803.54	Other open skull fracture without mention of intracranial injury, with prolonged [more than 24 hours] loss of consciousness and return to pre-existing conscious level
803.55	Other open skull fracture without mention of intracranial injury, with prolonged [more than 24 hours] loss of consciousness, without return to pre-existing conscious level
820.19	Other open transcervical fracture of neck of femur
323.62	Other postinfectious encephalitis and encephalomyelitis
415.19	Other pulmonary embolism and infarction
518.52	Other pulmonary insufficiency, not elsewhere classified, following trauma and surgery
344.09	Other quadriplegia
567.38	Other retroperitoneal abscess
567.39	Other retroperitoneal infections
038.49	Other septicemia due to gram-negative organisms
262	Other severe protein-calorie malnutrition
785.59	Other shock without mention of trauma
282.69	Other sickle-cell disease with crisis
284.89	Other specified aplastic anemias
535.41	Other specified gastritis, with hemorrhage
018.81	Other specified miliary tuberculosis, bacteriological or histological examination not done
018.82	Other specified miliary tuberculosis, bacteriological or histological examination unknown (at present)
018.83	Other specified miliary tuberculosis, tubercle bacilli found (in sputum) by microscopy
018.84	Other specified miliary tuberculosis, tubercle bacilli not found (in sputum) by microscopy, but found by bacterial culture
018.85	Other specified miliary tuberculosis, tubercle bacilli not found by bacteriological examination, but tuberculosis confirmed histologically
018.86	Other specified miliary tuberculosis, tubercle bacilli not found by bacteriological or histological examination, but tuberculosis confirmed by other methods [inoculation of animals]
018.80	Other specified miliary tuberculosis, unspecified
062.8	Other specified mosquito-borne viral encephalitis
567.89	Other specified peritonitis
038.8	Other specified septicemias
063.8	Other specified tick-borne viral encephalitis
013.81	Other specified tuberculosis of central nervous system, bacteriological or histological examination not done
013.82	Other specified tuberculosis of central nervous system, bacteriological or histological examination unknown (at present)
013.83	Other specified tuberculosis of central nervous system, tubercle bacilli found (in sputum) by microscopy
013.84	Other specified tuberculosis of central nervous system, tubercle bacilli not found (in sputum) by microscopy, but found by bacterial culture
013.85	Other specified tuberculosis of central nervous system, tubercle bacilli not found by bacteriological examination, but tuberculosis confirmed histologically
013.86	Other specified tuberculosis of central nervous system, tubercle bacilli not found by bacteriological or histological examination, but tuberculosis confirmed by other methods [inoculation of animals]
013.80	Other specified tuberculosis of central nervous system, unspecified
020.8	Other specified types of plague
070.49	Other specified viral hepatitis with hepatic coma
038.19	Other staphylococcal septicemia
482.49	Other Staphylococcus pneumonia
567.29	Other suppurative peritonitis
745.19	Other transposition of great vessels
453.2	Other venous embolism and thrombosis of inferior vena cava
551.29	Other ventral hernia with gangrene
533.91	Peptic ulcer of unspecified site, unspecified as acute or chronic, without mention of hemorrhage or perforation, with obstruction
576.3	Perforation of bile duct
530.4	Perforation of esophagus
575.4	Perforation of gallbladder
569.83	Perforation of intestine
777.6	Perinatal intestinal perforation
774.4	Perinatal jaundice due to hepatocellular damage
674.53	Peripartum cardiomyopathy, antepartum condition or complication
674.52	Peripartum cardiomyopathy, delivered, with mention of postpartum condition
674.51	Peripartum cardiomyopathy, delivered, with or without mention of antepartum condition
674.54	Peripartum cardiomyopathy, postpartum condition or complication
674.50	Peripartum cardiomyopathy, unspecified as to episode of care or not applicable
567.22	Peritoneal abscess
567.21	Peritonitis (acute) generalized
567.0	Peritonitis in infectious diseases classified elsewhere
779.7	Periventricular leukomalacia
747.83	Persistent fetal circulation
345.2	Petit mal status

325	Phlebitis and thrombophlebitis of intracranial venous sinuses
020.9	Plague, unspecified
511.1	Pleurisy with effusion, with mention of a bacterial cause other than tuberculosis
320.1	Pneumococcal meningitis
567.1	Pneumococcal peritonitis
481	Pneumococcal pneumonia [Streptococcus pneumoniae pneumonia]
038.2	Pneumococcal septicemia [Streptococcus pneumoniae septicemia]
136.3	Pneumocystosis
480.0	Pneumonia due to adenovirus
482.81	Pneumonia due to anaerobes
483.1	Pneumonia due to chlamydia
482.82	Pneumonia due to escherichia coli [E. coli]
482.2	Pneumonia due to Hemophilus influenzae [H. influenzae]
482.0	Pneumonia due to Klebsiella pneumoniae
482.84	Pneumonia due to Legionnaires' disease
483.0	Pneumonia due to mycoplasma pneumoniae
482.83	Pneumonia due to other gram-negative bacteria
482.89	Pneumonia due to other specified bacteria
483.8	Pneumonia due to other specified organism
482.39	Pneumonia due to other Streptococcus
480.8	Pneumonia due to other virus not elsewhere classified
480.2	Pneumonia due to parainfluenza virus
482.1	Pneumonia due to Pseudomonas
480.1	Pneumonia due to respiratory syncytial virus
480.3	Pneumonia due to SARS-associated coronavirus
482.40	Pneumonia due to Staphylococcus, unspecified
482.31	Pneumonia due to Streptococcus, group A
482.32	Pneumonia due to Streptococcus, group B
482.30	Pneumonia due to Streptococcus, unspecified
484.5	Pneumonia in anthrax
484.6	Pneumonia in aspergillosis
484.1	Pneumonia in cytomegalic inclusion disease
484.8	Pneumonia in other infectious diseases classified elsewhere
484.7	Pneumonia in other systemic mycoses
484.3	Pneumonia in whooping cough
486	Pneumonia, organism unspecified
020.5	Pneumonic plague, unspecified
507.0	Pneumonitis due to inhalation of food or vomitus
507.1	Pneumonitis due to inhalation of oils and essences
507.8	Pneumonitis due to other solids and liquids
130.4	Pneumonitis due to toxoplasmosis
572.1	Portal pyemia
452	Portal vein thrombosis
323.63	Postinfectious myelitis
055.0	Postmeasles encephalitis
055.1	Postmeasles pneumonia
998.01	Postoperative shock, cardiogenic
998.09	Postoperative shock, other
998.02	Postoperative shock, septic
052.0	Postvaricella encephalitis
052.2	Postvaricella myelitis
642.73	Pre-eclampsia or eclampsia superimposed on pre-existing hypertension, antepartum condition or complication
642.72	Pre-eclampsia or eclampsia superimposed on pre-existing hypertension, delivered, with mention of postpartum complication
642.71	Pre-eclampsia or eclampsia superimposed on pre-existing hypertension, delivered, with or without mention of antepartum condition

642.74	Pre-eclampsia or eclampsia superimposed on pre-existing hypertension, postpartum condition or complication
641.21	Premature separation of placenta, delivered, with or without mention of antepartum condition
707.23	Pressure ulcer, stage III
707.24	Pressure ulcer, stage IV
020.3	Primary pneumonic plague
756.71	Prune belly syndrome
567.31	Psoas muscle abscess
670.22	Puerperal sepsis, delivered, with mention of postpartum complication
670.24	Puerperal sepsis, postpartum condition or complication
670.32	Puerperal septic thrombophlebitis, delivered, with mention of postpartum complication
670.34	Puerperal septic thrombophlebitis, postpartum condition or complication
022.1	Pulmonary anthrax
747.32	Pulmonary arteriovenous malformation
747.31	Pulmonary artery coarctation and atresia
770.3	Pulmonary hemorrhage
516.62	Pulmonary interstitial glycogenosis
344.01	Quadriplegia, C1-C4, complete
344.02	Quadriplegia, C1-C4, incomplete
344.03	Quadriplegia, C5-C7, complete
344.04	Quadriplegia, C5-C7, incomplete
344.00	Quadriplegia, unspecified
284.81	Red cell aplasia (acquired)(adult)(with thymoma)
590.2	Renal and perinephric abscess
799.1	Respiratory arrest
770.87	Respiratory arrest of newborn
769	Respiratory distress syndrome in newborn
770.84	Respiratory failure of newborn
331.81	Reye's syndrome
596.6	Rupture of bladder, nontraumatic
429.5	Rupture of chordae tendineae
429.6	Rupture of papillary muscle
665.03	Rupture of uterus before onset of labor, antepartum condition or complication
665.01	Rupture of uterus before onset of labor, delivered, with or without mention of antepartum condition
665.11	Rupture of uterus during labor, delivered, with or without mention of antepartum condition
063.0	Russian spring-summer [taiga] encephalitis
952.3	Sacral spinal cord injury without evidence of spinal bone injury
444.01	Saddle embolus of abdominal aorta
415.13	Saddle embolus of pulmonary artery
003.21	Salmonella meningitis
003.22	Salmonella pneumonia
003.1	Salmonella septicemia
249.20	Secondary diabetes mellitus with hyperosmolarity, not stated as uncontrolled, or unspecified
249.21	Secondary diabetes mellitus with hyperosmolarity, uncontrolled
249.10	Secondary diabetes mellitus with ketoacidosis, not stated as uncontrolled, or unspecified
249.11	Secondary diabetes mellitus with ketoacidosis, uncontrolled
249.30	Secondary diabetes mellitus with other coma, not stated as uncontrolled, or unspecified
249.31	Secondary diabetes mellitus with other coma, uncontrolled
020.4	Secondary pneumonic plague
995.91	Sepsis
422.92	Septic myocarditis

415.12	Septic pulmonary embolism
785.52	Septic shock
771.81	Septicemia [sepsis] of newborn
038.3	Septicemia due to anaerobes
038.42	Septicemia due to escherichia coli [E. coli]
038.40	Septicemia due to gram-negative organism, unspecified
038.41	Septicemia due to hemophilus influenzae [H. influenzae]
038.43	Septicemia due to pseudomonas
038.44	Septicemia due to serratia
020.2	Septicemic plague
768.5	Severe birth asphyxia
768.73	Severe hypoxic-ischemic encephalopathy
642.53	Severe pre-eclampsia, antepartum condition or complication
642.52	Severe pre-eclampsia, delivered, with mention of postpartum complication
642.51	Severe pre-eclampsia, delivered, with or without mention of antepartum condition
642.54	Severe pre-eclampsia, postpartum condition or complication
995.92	Severe sepsis
669.13	Shock during or following labor and delivery, antepartum condition or complication
669.12	Shock during or following labor and delivery, delivered, with mention of postpartum complication
669.11	Shock during or following labor and delivery, delivered, with or without mention of antepartum condition
669.14	Shock during or following labor and delivery, postpartum condition or complication
639.5	Shock following abortion or ectopic and molar pregnancies
282.42	Sickle-cell thalassemia with crisis
282.64	Sickle-cell/Hb-C disease with crisis
634.62	Spontaneous abortion, complicated by embolism, complete
634.61	Spontaneous abortion, complicated by embolism, incomplete
634.32	Spontaneous abortion, complicated by renal failure, complete
634.31	Spontaneous abortion, complicated by renal failure, incomplete
634.30	Spontaneous abortion, complicated by renal failure, unspecified
634.52	Spontaneous abortion, complicated by shock, complete
634.51	Spontaneous abortion, complicated by shock, incomplete
634.50	Spontaneous abortion, complicated by shock, unspecified
567.23	Spontaneous bacterial peritonitis
512.0	Spontaneous tension pneumothorax
062.3	St. Louis encephalitis
777.51	Stage I necrotizing enterocolitis in newborn
777.52	Stage II necrotizing enterocolitis in newborn
777.53	Stage III necrotizing enterocolitis in newborn
320.3	Staphylococcal meningitis
038.10	Staphylococcal septicemia, unspecified
320.2	Streptococcal meningitis
038.0	Streptococcal septicemia
746.81	Subaortic stenosis
430	Subarachnoid hemorrhage
852.10	Subarachnoid hemorrhage following injury with open intracranial wound, unspecified state of consciousness
852.12	Subarachnoid hemorrhage following injury with open intracranial wound, with brief [less than one hour] loss of consciousness
852.19	Subarachnoid hemorrhage following injury with open intracranial wound, with concussion, unspecified
852.16	Subarachnoid hemorrhage following injury with open intracranial wound, with loss of consciousness of unspecified duration
852.13	Subarachnoid hemorrhage following injury with open intracranial wound, with moderate [1-24 hours] loss of consciousness
852.11	Subarachnoid hemorrhage following injury with open intracranial wound, with no loss of consciousness
852.14	Subarachnoid hemorrhage following injury with open intracranial wound, with prolonged [more than 24 hours) loss of consciousness and return to pre-existing conscious level
852.15	Subarachnoid hemorrhage following injury with open intracranial wound, with prolonged [more than 24 hours] loss of consciousness without return to pre-existing conscious level
852.00	Subarachnoid hemorrhage following injury without mention of open intracranial wound, unspecified state of consciousness
852.02	Subarachnoid hemorrhage following injury without mention of open intracranial wound, with brief [less than one hour] loss of consciousness
852.09	Subarachnoid hemorrhage following injury without mention of open intracranial wound, with concussion, unspecified
852.06	Subarachnoid hemorrhage following injury without mention of open intracranial wound, with loss of consciousness of unspecified duration
852.03	Subarachnoid hemorrhage following injury without mention of open intracranial wound, with moderate [1-24 hours] loss of consciousness
852.01	Subarachnoid hemorrhage following injury without mention of open intracranial wound, with no loss of consciousness
852.04	Subarachnoid hemorrhage following injury without mention of open intracranial wound, with prolonged [more than 24 hours] loss of consciousness and return to pre-existing conscious level
852.05	Subarachnoid hemorrhage following injury without mention of open intracranial wound, with prolonged [more than 24 hours] loss of consciousness without return to pre-existing conscious level
772.2	Subarachnoid hemorrhage of fetus or newborn
767.0	Subdural and cerebral hemorrhage
432.1	Subdural hemorrhage
852.30	Subdural hemorrhage following injury with open intracranial wound, unspecified state of consciousness
852.32	Subdural hemorrhage following injury with open intracranial wound, with brief [less than one hour] loss of consciousness
852.39	Subdural hemorrhage following injury with open intracranial wound, with concussion, unspecified
852.36	Subdural hemorrhage following injury with open intracranial wound, with loss of consciousness of unspecified duration
852.33	Subdural hemorrhage following injury with open intracranial wound, with moderate [1-24 hours] loss of consciousness
852.31	Subdural hemorrhage following injury with open intracranial wound, with no loss of consciousness
852.34	Subdural hemorrhage following injury with open intracranial wound, with prolonged [more than 24 hours] loss of consciousness and return to pre-existing conscious level
852.35	Subdural hemorrhage following injury with open intracranial wound, with prolonged [more than 24 hours] loss of consciousness without return to pre-existing conscious level
852.20	Subdural hemorrhage following injury without mention of open intracranial wound, unspecified state of consciousness
852.22	Subdural hemorrhage following injury without mention of open intracranial wound, with brief [less than one hour] loss of consciousness
852.29	Subdural hemorrhage following injury without mention of open intracranial wound, with concussion, unspecified
852.26	Subdural hemorrhage following injury without mention of open intracranial wound, with loss of consciousness of unspecified duration
852.23	Subdural hemorrhage following injury without mention of open intracranial wound, with moderate [1-24 hours] loss of consciousness
852.21	Subdural hemorrhage following injury without mention of open intracranial wound, with no loss of consciousness

852.24	Subdural hemorrhage following injury without mention of open intracranial wound, with prolonged [more than 24 hours] loss of consciousness and return to pre-existing conscious level
852.25	Subdural hemorrhage following injury without mention of open intracranial wound, with prolonged [more than 24 hours] loss of consciousness without return to pre-existing conscious level
410.71	Subendocardial infarction, initial episode of care
464.51	Supraglottitis unspecified, with obstruction
516.63	Surfactant mutations of the lung
094.81	Syphilitic encephalitis
094.2	Syphilitic meningitis
094.87	Syphilitic ruptured cerebral aneurysm
995.94	Systemic inflammatory response syndrome due to noninfectious process with acute organ dysfunction
952.12	T1-T6 level with anterior cord syndrome
952.13	T1-T6 level with central cord syndrome
952.11	T1-T6 level with complete lesion of spinal cord
952.14	T1-T6 level with other specified spinal cord injury
952.10	T1-T6 level with unspecified spinal cord injury
952.17	T7-T12 level with anterior cord syndrome
952.18	T7-T12 level with central cord syndrome
952.16	T7-T12 level with complete lesion of spinal cord
952.19	T7-T12 level with other specified spinal cord injury
952.15	T7-T12 level with unspecified spinal cord injury
037	Tetanus
771.3	Tetanus neonatorum
745.2	Tetralogy of fallot
441.1	Thoracic aneurysm, ruptured
441.6	Thoracoabdominal aneurysm, ruptured
644.03	Threatened premature labor, antepartum condition or complication
446.6	Thrombotic microangiopathy
242.41	Thyrotoxicosis from ectopic thyroid nodule with mention of thyrotoxic crisis or storm
242.81	Thyrotoxicosis of other specified origin with mention of thyrotoxic crisis or storm
242.91	Thyrotoxicosis without mention of goiter or other cause, with mention of thyrotoxic crisis or storm
063.9	Tick-borne viral encephalitis, unspecified
242.01	Toxic diffuse goiter with mention of thyrotoxic crisis or storm
323.71	Toxic encephalitis and encephalomyelitis
349.82	Toxic encephalopathy
242.21	Toxic multinodular goiter with mention of thyrotoxic crisis or storm
323.72	Toxic myelitis
422.93	Toxic myocarditis
242.31	Toxic nodular goiter, unspecified type, with mention of thyrotoxic crisis or storm
040.82	Toxic shock syndrome
242.11	Toxic uninodular goiter with mention of thyrotoxic crisis or storm
530.84	Tracheoesophageal fistula
750.3	Tracheoesophageal fistula, esophageal atresia and stenosis
776.7	Transient neonatal neutropenia
776.1	Transient neonatal thrombocytopenia
887.7	Traumatic amputation of arm and hand (complete) (partial), bilateral [any level], complicated
887.6	Traumatic amputation of arm and hand (complete) (partial), bilateral [any level], without mention of complication
896.3	Traumatic amputation of foot (complete) (partial), bilateral, complicated
896.2	Traumatic amputation of foot (complete) (partial), bilateral, without mention of complication

897.7	Traumatic amputation of leg(s) (complete) (partial), bilateral [any level], complicated
897.6	Traumatic amputation of leg(s) (complete) (partial), bilateral [any level]), without mention of complication
958.5	Traumatic anuria
860.3	Traumatic hemothorax with open wound into thorax
860.2	Traumatic hemothorax without mention of open wound into thorax
860.5	Traumatic pneumohemothorax with open wound into thorax
860.4	Traumatic pneumohemothorax without mention of open wound into thorax
860.1	Traumatic pneumothorax with open wound into thorax
958.4	Traumatic shock
746.1	Tricuspid atresia and stenosis, congenital
410.61	True posterior wall infarction, initial episode of care
013.21	Tuberculoma of brain, bacteriological or histological examination not done
013.22	Tuberculoma of brain, bacteriological or histological examination unknown (at present)
013.23	Tuberculoma of brain, tubercle bacilli found (in sputum) by microscopy
013.24	Tuberculoma of brain, tubercle bacilli not found (in sputum) by microscopy, but found by bacterial culture
013.25	Tuberculoma of brain, tubercle bacilli not found by bacteriological examination, but tuberculosis confirmed histologically
013.26	Tuberculoma of brain, tubercle bacilli not found by bacteriological or histological examination, but tuberculosis confirmed by other methods [inoculation of animals]
013.20	Tuberculoma of brain, unspecified
013.11	Tuberculoma of meninges, bacteriological or histological examination not done
013.12	Tuberculoma of meninges, bacteriological or histological examination unknown (at present)
013.13	Tuberculoma of meninges, tubercle bacilli found (in sputum) by microscopy
013.14	Tuberculoma of meninges, tubercle bacilli not found (in sputum) by microscopy, but found by bacterial culture
013.15	Tuberculoma of meninges, tubercle bacilli not found by bacteriological examination, but tuberculosis confirmed histologically
013.16	Tuberculoma of meninges, tubercle bacilli not found by bacteriological or histological examination, but tuberculosis confirmed by other methods [inoculation of animals]
013.10	Tuberculoma of meninges, unspecified
013.41	Tuberculoma of spinal cord, bacteriological or histological examination not done
013.42	Tuberculoma of spinal cord, bacteriological or histological examination unknown (at present)
013.43	Tuberculoma of spinal cord, tubercle bacilli found (in sputum) by microscopy
013.44	Tuberculoma of spinal cord, tubercle bacilli not found (in sputum) by microscopy, but found by bacterial culture
013.45	Tuberculoma of spinal cord, tubercle bacilli not found by bacteriological examination, but tuberculosis confirmed histologically
013.46	Tuberculoma of spinal cord, tubercle bacilli not found by bacteriological or histological examination, but tuberculosis confirmed by other methods [inoculation of animals]
013.40	Tuberculoma of spinal cord, unspecified
013.31	Tuberculous abscess of brain, bacteriological or histological examination not done
013.32	Tuberculous abscess of brain, bacteriological or histological examination unknown (at present)
013.33	Tuberculous abscess of brain, tubercle bacilli found (in sputum) by microscopy

Appendix A — Alphabetic MCC List

013.34	Tuberculous abscess of brain, tubercle bacilli not found (in sputum) by microscopy, but found by bacterial culture
013.35	Tuberculous abscess of brain, tubercle bacilli not found by bacteriological examination, but tuberculosis confirmed histologically
013.36	Tuberculous abscess of brain, tubercle bacilli not found by bacteriological or histological examination, but tuberculosis confirmed by other methods [inoculation of animals]
013.30	Tuberculous abscess of brain, unspecified
013.51	Tuberculous abscess of spinal cord, bacteriological or histological examination not done
013.52	Tuberculous abscess of spinal cord, bacteriological or histological examination unknown (at present)
013.53	Tuberculous abscess of spinal cord, tubercle bacilli found (in sputum) by microscopy
013.54	Tuberculous abscess of spinal cord, tubercle bacilli not found (in sputum) by microscopy, but found by bacterial culture
013.55	Tuberculous abscess of spinal cord, tubercle bacilli not found by bacteriological examination, but tuberculosis confirmed histologically
013.56	Tuberculous abscess of spinal cord, tubercle bacilli not found by bacteriological or histological examination, but tuberculosis confirmed by other methods [inoculation of animals]
013.50	Tuberculous abscess of spinal cord, unspecified
013.61	Tuberculous encephalitis or myelitis, bacteriological or histological examination not done
013.62	Tuberculous encephalitis or myelitis, bacteriological or histological examination unknown (at present)
013.63	Tuberculous encephalitis or myelitis, tubercle bacilli found (in sputum) by microscopy
013.64	Tuberculous encephalitis or myelitis, tubercle bacilli not found (in sputum) by microscopy, but found by bacterial culture
013.65	Tuberculous encephalitis or myelitis, tubercle bacilli not found by bacteriological examination, but tuberculosis confirmed histologically
013.66	Tuberculous encephalitis or myelitis, tubercle bacilli not found by bacteriological or histological examination, but tuberculosis confirmed by other methods [inoculation of animals]
013.60	Tuberculous encephalitis or myelitis, unspecified
013.01	Tuberculous meningitis, bacteriological or histological examination not done
013.02	Tuberculous meningitis, bacteriological or histological examination unknown (at present)
013.03	Tuberculous meningitis, tubercle bacilli found (in sputum) by microscopy
013.04	Tuberculous meningitis, tubercle bacilli not found (in sputum) by microscopy, but found by bacterial culture
013.05	Tuberculous meningitis, tubercle bacilli not found by bacteriological examination, but tuberculosis confirmed histologically
013.06	Tuberculous meningitis, tubercle bacilli not found by bacteriological or histological examination, but tuberculosis confirmed by other methods [inoculation of animals]
013.00	Tuberculous meningitis, unspecified
014.01	Tuberculous peritonitis, bacteriological or histological examination not done
014.02	Tuberculous peritonitis, bacteriological or histological examination unknown (at present)
014.03	Tuberculous peritonitis, tubercle bacilli found (in sputum) by microscopy
014.04	Tuberculous peritonitis, tubercle bacilli not found (in sputum) by microscopy, but found by bacterial culture
014.05	Tuberculous peritonitis, tubercle bacilli not found by bacteriological examination, but tuberculosis confirmed histologically

014.06	Tuberculous peritonitis, tubercle bacilli not found by bacteriological or histological examination, but tuberculosis confirmed by other methods [inoculation of animals]
014.00	Tuberculous peritonitis, unspecified
011.61	Tuberculous pneumonia [any form], bacteriological or histological examination not done
011.62	Tuberculous pneumonia [any form], bacteriological or histological examination unknown (at present)
011.63	Tuberculous pneumonia [any form], tubercle bacilli found (in sputum) by microscopy
011.64	Tuberculous pneumonia [any form], tubercle bacilli not found (in sputum) by microscopy, but found by bacterial culture
011.65	Tuberculous pneumonia [any form], tubercle bacilli not found by bacteriological examination, but tuberculosis confirmed histologically
011.66	Tuberculous pneumonia [any form], tubercle bacilli not found by bacteriological or histological examination, but tuberculosis confirmed by other methods [inoculation of animals]
011.60	Tuberculous pneumonia [any form], unspecified
277.88	Tumor lysis syndrome
530.21	Ulcer of esophagus with bleeding
551.1	Umbilical hernia with gangrene
637.62	Unspecified abortion, complicated by embolism, complete
637.61	Unspecified abortion, complicated by embolism, incomplete
637.60	Unspecified abortion, complicated by embolism, unspecified
637.32	Unspecified abortion, complicated by renal failure, complete
637.31	Unspecified abortion, complicated by renal failure, incomplete
637.30	Unspecified abortion, complicated by renal failure, unspecified
637.52	Unspecified abortion, complicated by shock, complete
637.51	Unspecified abortion, complicated by shock, incomplete
637.50	Unspecified abortion, complicated by shock, unspecified
323.9	Unspecified causes of encephalitis, myelitis, and encephalomyelitis
535.51	Unspecified gastritis and gastroduodenitis, with hemorrhage
861.10	Unspecified injury of heart with open wound into thorax
861.30	Unspecified injury of lung with open wound into thorax
567.9	Unspecified peritonitis
038.9	Unspecified septicemia
013.91	Unspecified tuberculosis of central nervous system, bacteriological or histological examination not done
013.92	Unspecified tuberculosis of central nervous system, bacteriological or histological examination unknown (at present)
013.93	Unspecified tuberculosis of central nervous system, tubercle bacilli found (in sputum) by microscopy
013.94	Unspecified tuberculosis of central nervous system, tubercle bacilli not found (in sputum) by microscopy, but found by bacterial culture
013.95	Unspecified tuberculosis of central nervous system, tubercle bacilli not found by bacteriological examination, but tuberculosis confirmed histologically
013.96	Unspecified tuberculosis of central nervous system, tubercle bacilli not found by bacteriological or histological examination, but tuberculosis confirmed by other methods [inoculation of animals]
013.90	Unspecified tuberculosis of central nervous system, unspecified
070.71	Unspecified viral hepatitis C with hepatic coma
070.6	Unspecified viral hepatitis with hepatic coma
052.1	Varicella (hemorrhagic) pneumonitis
336.1	Vascular myelopathies
758.32	Velo-cardio-facial syndrome
551.20	Ventral hernia, unspecified, with gangrene
427.41	Ventricular fibrillation
427.42	Ventricular flutter
064	Viral encephalitis transmitted by other and unspecified arthropods
070.0	Viral hepatitis A with hepatic coma

070.21	Viral hepatitis B with hepatic coma, acute or unspecified, with hepatitis delta
070.20	Viral hepatitis B with hepatic coma, acute or unspecified, without mention of hepatitis delta
480.9	Viral pneumonia, unspecified
560.2	Volvulus
036.3	Waterhouse-Friderichsen syndrome, meningococcal
066.41	West Nile Fever with encephalitis
066.49	West Nile Fever with other complications
066.42	West Nile Fever with other neurologic manifestation
066.40	West Nile Fever, unspecified
062.1	Western equine encephalitis
117.7	Zygomycosis [Phycomycosis or Mucormycosis]

Appendix B — MS-DRG Surgical Hierarchy Table

The surgical hierarchy reflects the relative resources requirement of the various surgical procedures of each major diagnostic category (MDC). The hierarchy is based upon variables such as principal diagnosis, surgical class, complications and comorbidities.

Arranging the surgical DRGs in this manner allows for the assignment of patients with multiple procedures related to the principal diagnosis to a surgical DRG that best reflects the resources used in the care of that patient. Since patients can be assigned to only one surgical class for each inpatient stay, patients with multiple procedures related to the principal diagnosis are assigned to the DRG associated with the most resource-intensive surgical class.

Pre MDC

Heart transplant or implant of heart assist system w MCC; w/o MCC	001–002
ECMO or trach w MV 96+ hrs or PDX exc face, mouth & neck w maj O.R.; w/o maj O.R.	003–004
Liver transplant w MCC; w/o MCC or intestinal transplant	005–006
Allogeneic bone marrow transplant	014
Lung transplant	007
Simultaneous pancreas/kidney transplant	008
Autologous bone marrow transplant w CC/MCC; w/o CC/MCC	016–017
Pancreas transplant	010
Tracheostomy for face, mouth & neck diagnoses w MCC; w CC; w/o CC/MCC	011–013
Multiple Significant Trauma	955-959
HIV Infections	969-970

MDC 1   DISEASES & DISORDERS OF THE NERVOUS SYSTEM

Intracranial vascular procedures w PDX hemorrhage w MCC; w CC; w/o CC/MCC	020–022
Cranio w major dev impl/acute complex CNS PDX w MCC or chemo implant	023
Cranio w major dev impl/acute complex CNS PDX w/o MCC	024
Craniotomy & endovascular intracranial procedures w MCC; w CC; w/o CC/MCC	025–027
Spinal procedures w MCC; w CC or spinal neurostimulators; w/o CC/MCC	028–030
Ventricular shunt procedures w MCC; w CC; w/o CC/MCC	031–033
Carotid artery stent procedure w MCC; w CC; w/o CC/MCC	034–036
Extracranial procedures w MCC; w CC; w/o CC/MCC	037–039
Periph/cranial nerve & other nerv syst proc w MCC; w CC or periph neurostim; w/o CC/MCC	040–042

MDC 2   DISEASES & DISORDERS OF THE EYE

Orbital procedures w CC/MCC; w/o CC/MCC	113–114
Extraocular procedures except orbit	115
Intraocular procedures w CC/MCC; w/o CC/MCC	116–117

MDC 3   DISEASES & DISORDERS OF THE EAR, NOSE, MOUTH & THROAT

Major head & neck procedures w CC/MCC or major device; w/o CC/MCC	129–130
Cranial/facial procedures w CC/MCC; w/o CC/MCC	131–132
Other ear, nose, mouth & throat O.R. procedures w CC/MCC; w/o CC/MCC	133–134
Sinus & mastoid procedures w CC/MCC; w/o CC/MCC	135–136
Mouth procedures w CC/MCC; w/o CC/MCC	137–138
Salivary gland procedures	139

MDC 4   DISEASES & DISORDERS OF THE RESPIRATORY SYSTEM

Major chest procedures w MCC; w CC; w/o CC/MCC	163–165
Other resp system O.R. procedures w MCC; w CC; w/o CC/MCC	166–168

MDC 5   DISEASES & DISORDERS OF THE CIRCULATORY SYSTEM

Other heart assist system implant	215
Cardiac valve & oth maj cardiothoracic proc w or w/o card cath w MCC; w CC; w/o CC/MCC	216–221
Cardiac defib implant w cardiac cath w; w/o AMI/HF/shock w MCC; w/o MCC	222–225
Cardiac defibrillator implant w/o cardiac cath w MCC; w/o MCC	226–227
Other cardiothoracic procedures w MCC; w CC; w/o CC/MCC	228–230
Coronary bypass w PTCA w MCC; w/o MCC	231–232
Coronary bypass w cardiac cath w MCC; w/o MCC	233–234
Coronary bypass w/o cardiac cath w MCC; w/o MCC	235–236
Major cardiovasc procedures w MCC	237
Major cardiovasc procedures w/o MCC	238
Amputation for circ sys disorders exc upper limb & toe w MCC; w CC; w/o CC/MCC	239–241
Permanent cardiac pacemaker implant w MCC; w CC; w/o CC/MCC	242–244
AICD generator procedures	245
AICD lead procedures	265
Perc cardiovasc proc w drug-eluting stent w MCC or 4+ vessels/stents	246
Perc cardiovasc proc w drug-eluting stent w/o MCC	247
Perc cardiovasc proc w non-drug-eluting stent w MCC or 4+ vessels/stents	248
Perc cardiovasc proc w non-drug-eluting stent w/o MCC	249
Perc cardiovasc proc w/o coronary artery stent w MCC; w/o MCC	250–251
Other vascular procedures w MCC; w CC; w/o CC/MCC	252–254
Upper limb & toe amputation for circ system disorders w MCC; w CC; w/o CC/MCC	255–257
Cardiac pacemaker device replacement w MCC; w/o MCC	258–259
Cardiac pacemaker revision except device replacement w MCC; w CC; w/o CC/MCC	260–262
Vein ligation & stripping	263
Other circulatory system O.R. procedures	264

MDC 6 DISEASES & DISORDERS OF THE DIGESTIVE SYSTEM

Stomach, esophageal & duodenal proc w MCC; w CC; w/o CC/MCC	326–328
Major small & large bowel procedures w MCC; w CC; w/o CC/MCC	329–331
Rectal resection w MCC; w CC; w/o CC/MCC	332–334
Peritoneal adhesiolysis w MCC; w CC; w/o CC/MCC	335–337
Appendectomy w; w/o complicated principal diag w MCC; w CC; w/o CC/MCC	338–343
Minor small & large bowel procedures w MCC; w CC; w/o CC/MCC	344–346
Anal & stomal procedures w MCC; w CC; w/o CC/MCC	347–349
Inguinal & femoral hernia procedures w MCC; w CC; w/o CC/MCC	350–352
Hernia procedures except inguinal & femoral w MCC; w CC; w/o CC/MCC	353–355
Other digestive system O.R. procedures w MCC; w CC; w/o CC/MCC	356–358

MDC 7 DISEASES & DISORDERS OF THE HEPATOBILIARY SYSTEM & PANCREAS

Pancreas, liver & shunt procedures w MCC; w CC; w/o CC/MCC	405–407
Biliary tract proc except only cholecyst w or w/o c.d.e. w MCC; w CC; w/o CC/MCC	408–410
Cholecystectomy w c.d.e. w MCC; w CC; w/o CC/MCC	411–413
Cholecystectomy except by laparoscope w/o c.d.e. w MCC; w CC; w/o CC/MCC	414–416
Laparoscopic cholecystectomy w/o c.d.e. w MCC; w CC; w/o CC/MCC	417–419
Hepatobiliary diagnostic procedures w MCC; w CC; w/o CC/MCC	420–422
Other hepatobiliary or pancreas O.R. procedures w MCC; w CC; w/o CC/MCC	423–425

MDC 8 DISEASES & DISORDERS OF THE MUSCULOSKELETAL SYSTEM & CONNECTIVE TISSUE

Combined anterior/posterior spinal fusion w MCC; w CC; w/o CC/MCC	453–455
Spinal fus exc cerv w spinal curv/malig/infec or 9+ fus w MCC; w CC; w/o CC/MCC	456–458
Spinal fusion except cervical w MCC; w/o MCC	459–460
Bilateral or multiple major joint procs of lower extremity w MCC; w/o MCC	461–462
Wnd debrid & skn graft exc hand, for musculo-conn tiss dis w MCC; w CC; w/o CC/MCC	463–465
Revision of hip or knee replacement w MCC; w CC; w/o CC/MCC	466–468
Major joint replacement or reattachment of lower extremity w MCC; w/o MCC	469–470
Cervical spinal fusion w MCC; w CC; w/o CC/MCC	471–473
Amputation for musculoskeletal sys & conn tissue dis w CC; w/o CC/MCC	474–476
Biopsies of musculoskeletal system & connective tissue w MCC; w CC; w/o CC/MCC	477–479
Hip & femur procedures except major joint w MCC; w CC; w/o CC/MCC	480–482
Major joint & limb reattachment proc of upper extremity w CC/MCC; w/o CC/MCC	483–484
Knee procedures w pdx of infection w MCC; w CC; w/o CC/MCC	485–487
Knee procedures w/o pdx of infection w CC/MCC; w/o CC/MCC	488–489
Back & neck proc exc spinal fusion w CC/MCC; w/o CC/MCC or disc device/neurostim	490–491

MDC 8— Continued

Lower extrem & humer proc except hip,foot,femur w MCC; w CC; w/o CC/MCC	492–494
Local excision & removal int fix devices exc hip & femur w MCC; w CC; w/o CC/MCC	495–497
Local excision & removal int fix devices of hip & femur w CC/MCC; w/o CC/MCC	498–499
Soft tissue procedures w MCC; w CC; w/o CC/MCC	500–502
Foot procedures w MCC; w CC; w/o CC/MCC	503–505
Major thumb or joint procedures	506
Major shoulder or elbow joint procedures w CC/MCC; w/o CC/MCC	507–508
Arthroscopy	509
Shoulder,elbow or forearm proc,exc major joint proc w MCC; w CC; w/o CC/MCC	510–512
Hand or wrist proc, except major thumb or joint proc w CC/MCC; w/o CC/MCC	513–514
Other musculoskelet sys & conn tiss O.R. proc w MCC; w CC; w/o CC/MCC	515–517

MDC 9 DISEASES & DISORDERS OF THE SKIN, SUBCUTANEOUS TISSUE, & BREAST

Skin graft for skin ulcer or cellulitis w MCC; w CC; w/o CC/MCC	573–575
Skin graft exc for skin ulcer or cellulitis w MCC; w CC; w/o CC/MCC	576–578
Skin debridement w MCC; w CC; w/o MCC/CC	570–572
Other skin, subcut tiss & breast proc w MCC; w CC; w/o CC/MCC	579–581
Mastectomy for malignancy w CC/MCC; w/o CC/MCC	582–583
Breast biopsy, local excision & other breast procedures w CC/MCC; w/o CC/MCC	584–585

MDC 10 ENDOCRINE, NUTRITIONAL, & METABOLIC DISEASES & DISORDERS

Amputat of lower limb for endocrine, nutrit, & metabol dis w MCC; w CC; w/o CC/MCC	616–618
O.R. procedures for obesity w MCC; w CC; w/o CC/MCC	619–621
Skin grafts & wound debrid for endoc, nutrit & metab dis w MCC; w CC; w/o CC/MCC	622–624
Adrenal & pituitary procedures w CC/MCC; w/o CC/MCC	614–615
Thyroid, parathyroid & thyroglossal procedures w MCC; w CC; w/o CC/MCC	625–627
Other endocrine, nutrit & metab O.R. proc w MCC; w CC; w/o CC/MCC	628–630

MDC 11 DISEASES AND DISORDERS OF THE KIDNEY & URINARY TRACT

Kidney transplant	652
Major bladder procedures w MCC; w CC; w/o CC/MCC	653–655
Kidney & ureter procedures for neoplasm or non-neoplasm w MCC; w CC; w/o CC/MCC	656–661
Minor bladder procedures w MCC; w CC; w/o CC/MCC	662–664
Prostatectomy w MCC; w CC; w/o CC/MCC	665–667
Transurethral procedures w MCC; w CC; w/o CC/MCC	668–670
Urethral procedures w CC/MCC; w/o CC/MCC	671–672
Other kidney & urinary tract procedures w MCC; w CC; w/o CC/MCC	673–675

MDC 12   DISEASES & DISORDERS OF THE MALE REPRODUCTIVE SYSTEM

Major male pelvic procedures w CC/MCC; w/o CC/MCC	707–708
Penis procedures w CC/MCC; w/o CC/MCC	709–710
Testes procedures w CC/MCC; w/o CC/MCC	711–712
Transurethral prostatectomy w CC/MCC; w/o CC/MCC	713–714
Other male reproductive system O.R. proc for malignancy w CC/MCC; w/o CC/MCC	715–716
Other male reproductive system O.R. proc exc malignancy w CC/MCC; w/o CC/MCC	717–718

MDC 13   DISEASES & DISORDERS OF THE FEMALE REPRODUCTIVE SYSTEM

Pelvic evisceration, rad hysterectomy & rad vulvectomy w CC/MCC; w/o CC/MCC	734–735
Uterine & adnexa proc for ovarian or adnexal malignancy w MCC; w CC; w/o CC/MCC	736–738
Uterine,adnexa proc for non-ovarian/adnexal malig w MCC; w CC; w/o CC/MCC	739–741
Uterine & adnexa proc for non-malignancy w CC/MCC; w/o CC/MCC	742–743
D&C, conization, laparoscopy & tubal interruption w CC/MCC; w/o CC/MCC	744–745
Vagina, cervix & vulva procedures w CC/MCC; w/o CC/MCC	746–747
Female reproductive system reconstructive procedures	748
Other female reproductive system O.R. procedures w CC/MCC; w/o CC/MCC	749–750

MDC 14   PREGNANCY, CHILDBIRTH, & THE PUERPERIUM

Cesarean section w CC/MCC; w/o CC/MCC	765–766
Vaginal delivery w sterilization &/or D&C	767
Vaginal delivery w O.R. proc except steril &/or D&C	768
Postpartum & post abortion diagnoses w O.R. procedure	769
Abortion w D&C, aspiration curettage or hysterotomy	770

MDC 15   NEWBORNS & OTHER NEONATES W CONDITIONS ORIGINATING IN THE PERINATAL PERIOD

None	

MDC 16   DISEASES & DISORDERS OF THE BLOOD AND BLOOD FORMING ORGANS & IMMUNOLOGICAL DISORDERS

Splenectomy w MCC; w CC; w/o CC/MCC	799–801
Other O.R. proc of the blood & blood forming organs w MCC; w CC; w/o CC/MCC	802–804

MDC 17   MYELOPROLIFERATIVE DISEASES & DISORDERS, POORLY DIFFERENTIATED NEOPLASM

Lymphoma & leukemia w major O.R. procedure w MCC; w CC; w/o CC/MCC	820–822
Lymphoma & non-acute leukemia w other O.R. proc w MCC; w CC; w/o CC/MCC	823–825
Myeloprolif disord or poorly diff neopl w maj O.R. proc w MCC; w CC; w/o CC/MCC	826–828
Myeloprolif disord or poorly diff neopl w other O.R. proc w CC/MCC; w/o CC/MCC	829–830

MDC 18   INFECTIOUS & PARASITIC DISEASES, SYSTEMIC OR UNSPECIFIED SITES

Postoperative or posttraumatic infections w O.R. proc w MCC; w CC; w/o CC/MCC	856–858
Infectious & parasitic diseases w O.R. procedure w MCC; w CC; w/o CC/MCC	853–855

MDC 19   MENTAL DISEASES & DISORDERS

O.R. procedure w principal diagnoses of mental illness	876

MDC 20   ALCOHOL/DRUG USE & ALCOHOL/DRUG INDUCED ORGANIC MENTAL DISORDERS

None	

MDC 21   INJURIES, POISONINGS, & TOXIC EFFECTS OF DRUGS

Wound debridements for injuries w MCC; w CC; w/o CC/MCC	901–903
Skin grafts for injuries w CC/MCC; w/o CC/MCC	904–905
Hand procedures for injuries	906
Other O.R. procedures for injuries w MCC; w CC; w/o CC/MCC	907–909

MDC 22   BURNS

Extensive burns or full thickness burns w MV 96+ hrs w skin graft	927
Full thickness burn w skin graft or inhal inj w CC/MCC; w/o CC/MCC	928–929

MDC 23   FACTORS INFLUENCING HEALTH STATUS & OTHER CONTACTS WITH HEALTH SERVICES

O.R. proc w diagnoses of other contact w health services w MCC; w CC; w/o CC/MCC	939–941

MDC 24   MULTIPLE SIGNIFICANT TRAUMA

Craniotomy for multiple significant trauma	955
Limb reattachment, hip & femur proc for multiple significant trauma	956
Other O.R. procedures for multiple significant trauma w MCC; w CC; w/o CC/MCC	957–959

MDC 25   HUMAN IMMUNODEFICIENCY VIRUS INFECTIONS

HIV w extensive O.R. procedure w MCC; w/o MCC	969–970

Appendix C — MS-LTC-DRG Crosswalk

1. The SSO threshold is calculated as 5/6th of the geometric average length of stay of the MS-LTC-DRG (as specified in §412.529(a) in conjunction with §412.503).

* In determining the MS-LTC-DRG relative weights for FY 2014, these MS-LTC-DRGs were adjusted for nonmonotonicity as discussed in section VII.B.3.g. (step 6) of the preamble of the FY 2014 IPPS/LTCH PPS final rule.

MS-LTC-DRG	MS-LTC-DRG Title	FY 2012 LTCH Cases	Relative Weight	Geometric Avg Length of Stay	Short-Stay Outlier (SSO) Threshold[1]
001	Heart transplant or implant of heart assist system w MCC	0	0.0000	0.0	0.0
002	Heart transplant or implant of heart assist system w/o MCC	0	0.0000	0.0	0.0
003	ECMO or trach w MV 96+ hrs or PDX exc face, mouth & neck w maj O.R.	350	4.1277	61.2	51.0
004	Trach w MV 96+ hrs or PDX exc face, mouth & neck w/o maj O.R.	1,819	2.9345	43.5	36.3
005	Liver transplant w MCC or intestinal transplant	0	0.0000	0.0	0.0
006	Liver transplant w/o MCC	0	0.0000	0.0	0.0
007	Lung transplant	0	0.0000	0.0	0.0
008	Simultaneous pancreas/kidney transplant	0	0.0000	0.0	0.0
010	Pancreas transplant	0	0.0000	0.0	0.0
011	Tracheostomy for face,mouth & neck diagnoses w MCC	0	0.9152	23.1	19.3
012	Tracheostomy for face,mouth & neck diagnoses w CC	0	0.7689	22.3	18.6
013	Tracheostomy for face,mouth & neck diagnoses w/o CC/MCC	0	0.4572	17.4	14.5
014	Allogeneic bone marrow transplant	0	0.5574	19.7	16.4
016	Autologous bone marrow transplant w CC/MCC	0	0.5574	19.7	16.4
017	Autologous bone marrow transplant w/o CC/MCC	0	0.5574	19.7	16.4
020	Intracranial vascular procedures w PDX hemorrhage w MCC	0	0.8622	22.7	18.9
021	Intracranial vascular procedures w PDX hemorrhage w CC	0	0.5540	19.6	16.3
022	Intracranial vascular procedures w PDX hemorrhage w/o CC/MCC	0	0.5540	19.6	16.3
023	Craniotomy w major device implant or acute complex CNS PDX w MCC	1	1.6227	34.5	28.8
024	Craniotomy w major device implant or acute complex CNS PDX w/o MCC	0	0.7689	22.3	18.6
025	Craniotomy & endovascular intracranial procedures w MCC	3	1.6227	34.5	28.8
026	Craniotomy & endovascular intracranial procedures w CC	1	0.7689	22.3	18.6
027	Craniotomy & endovascular intracranial procedures w/o CC/MCC	0	0.7689	22.3	18.6
028	Spinal procedures w MCC	17	1.6227	34.5	28.8
029	Spinal procedures w CC	12	1.1259	27.4	22.8
030	Spinal procedures w/o CC/MCC	0	0.6037	20.3	16.9
031	Ventricular shunt procedures w MCC	3	1.6227	34.5	28.8
032	Ventricular shunt procedures w CC	0	0.6037	20.3	16.9
033	Ventricular shunt procedures w/o CC/MCC	0	0.6037	20.3	16.9
034	Carotid artery stent procedure w MCC	0	1.1259	27.4	22.8
035	Carotid artery stent procedurew CC	0	1.1259	27.4	22.8
036	Carotid artery stent procedure w/o CC/MCC	0	1.1259	27.4	22.8
037	Extracranial procedures w MCC	15	1.6227	34.5	28.8
038	Extracranial procedures w CC	3	1.1259	27.4	22.8
039	Extracranial procedures w/o CC/MCC	0	0.4572	17.4	14.5
040	Periph & cranial nerve & other nerv syst proc w MCC	173	1.4450	35.9	29.9

MS-LTC-DRG	MS-LTC-DRG Title	FY 2012 LTCH Cases	Relative Weight	Geometric Avg Length of Stay	Short-Stay Outlier (SSO) Threshold[1]
041	Periph & cranial nerve & other nerv syst proc w CC	59	0.9264	28.6	23.8
042	Periph & cranial nerve & other nerv syst proc w/o CC/MCC	2	0.6003	19.8	16.5
052	Spinal disorders & injuries w CC/MCC*	58	1.2035	35.7	29.8
053	Spinal disorders & injuries w/o CC/MCC*	3	1.2035	35.7	29.8
054	Nervous system neoplasms w MCC	36	0.7479	21.1	17.6
055	Nervous system neoplasms w/o MCC	12	0.4572	17.4	14.5
056	Degenerative nervous system disorders w MCC	815	0.7914	25.0	20.8
057	Degenerative nervous system disorders w/o MCC	705	0.5655	23.3	19.4
058	Multiple sclerosis & cerebellar ataxia w MCC	9	0.7689	22.3	18.6
059	Multiple sclerosis & cerebellar ataxia w CC	11	0.6003	19.8	16.5
060	Multiple sclerosis & cerebellar ataxia w/o CC/MCC	1	0.4572	17.4	14.5
061	Acute ischemic stroke w use of thrombolytic agent w MCC	0	0.8212	24.6	20.5
062	Acute ischemic stroke w use of thrombolytic agent w CC	0	0.6898	25.5	21.3
063	Acute ischemic stroke w use of thrombolytic agent w/o CC/MCC	0	0.4572	17.4	14.5
064	Intracranial hemorrhage or cerebral infarction w MCC	98	0.8622	22.7	18.9
065	Intracranial hemorrhage or cerebral infarction w CC or tPA in 24 hours*	37	0.5540	19.6	16.3
066	Intracranial hemorrhage or cerebral infarction w/o CC/MCC*	2	0.5540	19.6	16.3
067	Nonspecific cva & precerebral occlusion w/o infarct w MCC	4	0.7689	22.3	18.6
068	Nonspecific cva & precerebral occlusion w/o infarct w/o MCC	1	0.4572	17.4	14.5
069	Transient ischemia	8	0.7689	22.3	18.6
070	Nonspecific cerebrovascular disorders w MCC	239	0.8212	24.6	20.5
071	Nonspecific cerebrovascular disorders w CC	244	0.6898	25.5	21.3
072	Nonspecific cerebrovascular disorders w/o CC/MCC	6	0.4572	17.4	14.5
073	Cranial & peripheral nerve disorders w MCC	139	0.8555	23.3	19.4
074	Cranial & peripheral nerve disorders w/o MCC	133	0.6037	20.3	16.9
075	Viral meningitis w CC/MCC	12	0.6003	19.8	16.5
076	Viral meningitis w/o CC/MCC	1	0.4572	17.4	14.5
077	Hypertensive encephalopathy w MCC	7	1.1259	27.4	22.8
078	Hypertensive encephalopathy w CC	1	0.4572	17.4	14.5
079	Hypertensive encephalopathy w/o CC/MCC	0	0.4572	17.4	14.5
080	Nontraumatic stupor & coma w MCC	7	0.7689	22.3	18.6
081	Nontraumatic stupor & coma w/o MCC	1	0.6003	19.8	16.5
082	Traumatic stupor & coma, coma >1 hr w MCC	15	1.1259	27.4	22.8
083	Traumatic stupor & coma, coma >1 hr w CC	5	0.7689	22.3	18.6
084	Traumatic stupor & coma, coma >1 hr w/o CC/MCC	0	0.4572	17.4	14.5
085	Traumatic stupor & coma, coma <1 hr w MCC	105	0.8906	24.9	20.8
086	Traumatic stupor & coma, coma <1 hr w CC	38	0.6367	22.1	18.4
087	Traumatic stupor & coma, coma <1 hr w/o CC/MCC	6	0.4572	17.4	14.5
088	Concussion w MCC	1	1.1259	27.4	22.8
089	Concussion w CC	1	0.7689	22.3	18.6
090	Concussion w/o CC/MCC	0	0.7689	22.3	18.6
091	Other disorders of nervous system w MCC	244	1.0084	24.7	20.6
092	Other disorders of nervous system w CC	98	0.6157	21.2	17.7

MS-LTC-DRG	MS-LTC-DRG Title	FY 2012 LTCH Cases	Relative Weight	Geometric Avg Length of Stay	Short-Stay Outlier (SSO) Threshold[1]
093	Other disorders of nervous system w/o CC/MCC	11	0.6003	19.8	16.5
094	Bacterial & tuberculous infections of nervous system w MCC	260	1.1051	28.1	23.4
095	Bacterial & tuberculous infections of nervous system w CC*	102	0.8131	23.7	19.8
096	Bacterial & tuberculous infections of nervous system w/o CC/MCC*	7	0.8131	23.7	19.8
097	Non-bacterial infect of nervous sys exc viral meningitis w MCC	64	0.8147	20.5	17.1
098	Non-bacterial infect of nervous sys exc viral meningitis w CC	24	0.6003	19.8	16.5
099	Non-bacterial infect of nervous sys exc viral meningitis w/o CC/MCC	4	0.4572	17.4	14.5
100	Seizures w MCC	61	0.6855	20.7	17.3
101	Seizures w/o MCC	13	0.4572	17.4	14.5
102	Headaches w MCC	4	1.1259	27.4	22.8
103	Headaches w/o MCC	0	0.4572	17.4	14.5
113	Orbital procedures w CC/MCC	2	1.6227	34.5	28.8
114	Orbital procedures w/o CC/MCC	0	0.6003	19.8	16.5
115	Extraocular procedures except orbit	0	0.6003	19.8	16.5
116	Intraocular procedures w CC/MCC	0	1.6227	34.5	28.8
117	Intraocular procedures w/o CC/MCC	0	0.6003	19.8	16.5
121	Acute major eye infections w CC/MCC	22	0.7689	22.3	18.6
122	Acute major eye infections w/o CC/MCC	0	0.6003	19.8	16.5
123	Neurological eye disorders	0	0.6003	19.8	16.5
124	Other disorders of the eye w MCC	6	1.6227	34.5	28.8
125	Other disorders of the eye w/o MCC	7	0.6003	19.8	16.5
129	Major head & neck procedures w CC/MCC or major device	0	1.2591	26.7	22.3
130	Major head & neck procedures w/o CC/MCC	0	1.2591	26.7	22.3
131	Cranial/facial procedures w CC/MCC	0	0.7689	22.3	18.6
132	Cranial/facial procedures w/o CC/MCC	0	0.4572	17.4	14.5
133	Other ear, nose, mouth & throat O.R. procedures w CC/MCC	5	0.7689	22.3	18.6
134	Other ear, nose, mouth & throat O.R. procedures w/o CC/MCC	0	0.4572	17.4	14.5
135	Sinus & mastoid procedures w CC/MCC	0	0.7689	22.3	18.6
136	Sinus & mastoid procedures w/o CC/MCC	0	0.4572	17.4	14.5
137	Mouth procedures w CC/MCC	0	0.7689	22.3	18.6
138	Mouth procedures w/o CC/MCC	0	0.4572	17.4	14.5
139	Salivary gland procedures	0	0.7037	24.6	20.5
146	Ear, nose, mouth & throat malignancy w MCC*	39	1.2591	26.7	22.3
147	Ear, nose, mouth & throat malignancy w CC*	6	1.2591	26.7	22.3
148	Ear, nose, mouth & throat malignancy w/o CC/MCC	0	0.7037	24.6	20.5
149	Dysequilibrium	1	0.4572	17.4	14.5
150	Epistaxis w MCC	0	0.8062	21.8	18.2
151	Epistaxis w/o MCC	0	0.4572	17.4	14.5
152	Otitis media & URI w MCC	32	0.8062	21.8	18.2
153	Otitis media & URI w/o MCC	16	0.4572	17.4	14.5
154	Nasal trauma & deformity w MCC	30	0.9152	23.1	19.3
155	Nasal trauma & deformity w CC	24	0.7689	22.3	18.6
156	Nasal trauma & deformity w/o CC/MCC	2	0.4572	17.4	14.5

MS-LTC-DRG	MS-LTC-DRG Title	FY 2012 LTCH Cases	Relative Weight	Geometric Avg Length of Stay	Short-Stay Outlier (SSO) Threshold[1]
157	Dental & Oral Diseases w MCC	40	1.1941	26.9	22.4
158	Dental & Oral Diseases w CC*	35	0.7037	24.6	20.5
159	Dental & Oral Diseases w/o CC/MCC*	6	0.7037	24.6	20.5
163	Major chest procedures w MCC	37	2.2646	38.5	32.1
164	Major chest procedures w CC	6	1.6227	34.5	28.8
165	Major chest procedures w/o CC/MCC	0	1.6227	34.5	28.8
166	Other resp system O.R. procedures w MCC	1,886	2.4308	40.0	33.3
167	Other resp system O.R. procedures w CC	128	1.2768	29.8	24.8
168	Other resp system O.R. procedures w/o CC/MCC	2	0.7689	22.3	18.6
175	Pulmonary embolism w MCC	101	0.7085	20.2	16.8
176	Pulmonary embolism w/o MCC	47	0.5324	17.9	14.9
177	Respiratory infections & inflammations w MCC	4,266	0.8803	22.2	18.5
178	Respiratory infections & inflammations w CC	1,261	0.6960	19.7	16.4
179	Respiratory infections & inflammations w/o CC/MCC	89	0.5521	17.4	14.5
180	Respiratory neoplasms w MCC	88	0.7067	17.9	14.9
181	Respiratory neoplasms w CC	31	0.6457	17.1	14.3
182	Respiratory neoplasms w/o CC/MCC	0	0.4572	17.4	14.5
183	Major chest trauma w MCC	2	0.6003	19.8	16.5
184	Major chest trauma w CC	3	0.6003	19.8	16.5
185	Major chest trauma w/o CC/MCC	0	0.6003	19.8	16.5
186	Pleural effusion w MCC	176	0.8346	20.6	17.2
187	Pleural effusion w CC	35	0.6621	17.7	14.8
188	Pleural effusion w/o CC/MCC	2	0.4572	17.4	14.5
189	Pulmonary edema & respiratory failure	12,549	0.9161	21.6	18.0
190	Chronic obstructive pulmonary disease w MCC	2,279	0.7377	19.5	16.3
191	Chronic obstructive pulmonary disease w CC	745	0.6285	18.2	15.2
192	Chronic obstructive pulmonary disease w/o CC/MCC	154	0.4956	15.6	13.0
193	Simple pneumonia & pleurisy w MCC	2,036	0.7693	20.2	16.8
194	Simple pneumonia & pleurisy w CC	962	0.6001	17.7	14.8
195	Simple pneumonia & pleurisy w/o CC/MCC	81	0.4829	15.3	12.8
196	Interstitial lung disease w MCC	128	0.7216	18.5	15.4
197	Interstitial lung disease w CC	51	0.6394	18.9	15.8
198	Interstitial lung disease w/o CC/MCC	12	0.6003	19.8	16.5
199	Pneumothorax w MCC	75	0.7866	20.3	16.9
200	Pneumothorax w CC	14	0.4572	17.4	14.5
201	Pneumothorax w/o CC/MCC	5	0.4572	17.4	14.5
202	Bronchitis & asthma w CC/MCC	95	0.6541	18.5	15.4
203	Bronchitis & asthma w/o CC/MCC	3	0.6003	19.8	16.5
204	Respiratory signs & symptoms	88	0.7664	21.3	17.8
205	Other respiratory system diagnoses w MCC	290	0.8812	21.6	18.0
206	Other respiratory system diagnoses w/o MCC	73	0.6314	18.0	15.0
207	Respiratory system diagnosis w ventilator support 96+ hours	15,306	1.9725	32.2	26.8
208	Respiratory system diagnosis w ventilator support <96 hours	2,123	1.1066	21.8	18.2

MS-LTC-DRG	MS-LTC-DRG Title	FY 2012 LTCH Cases	Relative Weight	Geometric Avg Length of Stay	Short-Stay Outlier (SSO) Threshold[1]
215	Other heart assist system implant	0	0.4572	17.4	14.5
216	Cardiac valve & oth maj cardiothoracic proc w card cath w MCC	1	0.4572	17.4	14.5
217	Cardiac valve & oth maj cardiothoracic proc w card cath w CC	0	0.4572	17.4	14.5
218	Cardiac valve & oth maj cardiothoracic proc w card cath w/o CC/MCC	0	0.4572	17.4	14.5
219	Cardiac valve & oth maj cardiothoracic proc w/o card cath w MCC	0	1.6227	34.5	28.8
220	Cardiac valve & oth maj cardiothoracic proc w/o card cath w CC	0	1.6227	34.5	28.8
221	Cardiac valve & oth maj cardiothoracic proc w/o card cath w/o CC/MCC	0	1.1259	27.4	22.8
222	Cardiac defib implant w cardiac cath w AMI/HF/shock w MCC	0	1.6227	34.5	28.8
223	Cardiac defib implant w cardiac cath w AMI/HF/shock w/o MCC	0	1.1259	27.4	22.8
224	Cardiac defib implant w cardiac cath w/o AMI/HF/shock w MCC	0	1.6227	34.5	28.8
225	Cardiac defib implant w cardiac cath w/o AMI/HF/shock w/o MCC	0	0.7689	22.3	18.6
226	Cardiac defibrillator implant w/o cardiac cath w MCC	10	1.6227	34.5	28.8
227	Cardiac defibrillator implant w/o cardiac cath w/o MCC	5	1.1259	27.4	22.8
228	Other cardiothoracic procedures w MCC	0	1.5434	33.1	27.6
229	Other cardiothoracic procedures w CC	0	1.1975	30.9	25.8
230	Other cardiothoracic procedures w/o CC/MCC	0	1.1259	27.4	22.8
231	Coronary bypass w PTCA w MCC	0	1.6227	34.5	28.8
232	Coronary bypass w PTCA w/o MCC	0	1.1259	27.4	22.8
233	Coronary bypass w cardiac cath w MCC	1	1.1259	27.4	22.8
234	Coronary bypass w cardiac cath w/o MCC	0	1.1259	27.4	22.8
235	Coronary bypass w/o cardiac cath w MCC	0	1.6227	34.5	28.8
236	Coronary bypass w/o cardiac cath w/o MCC	0	1.1259	27.4	22.8
237	Major cardiovascular procedures w MCC	6	1.6227	34.5	28.8
238	Major cardiovascular procedures w/o MCC	2	1.1259	27.4	22.8
239	Amputation for circ sys disorders exc upper limb & toe w MCC	167	1.5092	37.3	31.1
240	Amputation for circ sys disorders exc upper limb & toe w CC	50	1.1138	30.7	25.6
241	Amputation for circ sys disorders exc upper limb & toe w/o CC/MCC	1	0.7689	22.3	18.6
242	Permanent cardiac pacemaker implant w MCC	13	1.6227	34.5	28.8
243	Permanent cardiac pacemaker implant w CC	5	1.1259	27.4	22.8
244	Permanent cardiac pacemaker implant w/o CC/MCC	0	1.1259	27.4	22.8
245	AICD generator procedures	2	0.7689	22.3	18.6
246	Percutaneous cardiovascular proc w drug-eluting stent w MCC	1	1.6227	34.5	28.8
247	Percutaneous cardiovascular proc w drug-eluting stent w/o MCC	0	1.1259	27.4	22.8
248	Percutaneous cardiovasc proc w non-drug-eluting stent w MCC	2	1.1259	27.4	22.8
249	Percutaneous cardiovasc proc w non-drug-eluting stent w/o MCC	0	1.1259	27.4	22.8
250	Perc cardiovasc proc w/o coronary artery stent or AMI w MCC	3	1.6227	34.5	28.8
251	Perc cardiovasc proc w/o coronary artery stent or AMI w/o MCC	0	1.1259	27.4	22.8
252	Other vascular procedures w MCC	172	1.5434	33.1	27.6
253	Other vascular procedures w CC	60	1.1975	30.9	25.8
254	Other vascular procedures w/o CC/MCC	1	0.4572	17.4	14.5
255	Upper limb & toe amputation for circ system disorders w MCC	51	1.2972	33.0	27.5
256	Upper limb & toe amputation for circ system disorders w CC	32	1.1068	30.8	25.7
257	Upper limb & toe amputation for circ system disorders w/o CC/MCC	1	0.6003	19.8	16.5

MS-LTC-DRG	MS-LTC-DRG Title	FY 2012 LTCH Cases	Relative Weight	Geometric Avg Length of Stay	Short-Stay Outlier (SSO) Threshold[1]
258	Cardiac pacemaker device replacement w MCC	1	1.1259	27.4	22.8
259	Cardiac pacemaker device replacement w/o MCC	0	1.1259	27.4	22.8
260	Cardiac pacemaker revision except device replacement w MCC	7	1.6227	34.5	28.8
261	Cardiac pacemaker revision except device replacement w CC	1	0.4572	17.4	14.5
262	Cardiac pacemaker revision except device replacement w/o CC/MCC	0	0.4572	17.4	14.5
263	Vein ligation & stripping	2	1.1259	27.4	22.8
264	Other circulatory system O.R. procedures	727	1.0857	29.8	24.8
265	AICD lead procedures	0	1.6227	34.5	28.8
280	Circulatory disorders w AMI, discharged alive w MCC	276	0.8032	22.5	18.8
281	Circulatory disorders w AMI, discharged alive w CC	54	0.6318	20.4	17.0
282	Circulatory disorders w AMI, discharged alive w/o CC/MCC	4	0.4572	17.4	14.5
283	Circulatory disorders w AMI, expired w MCC	50	0.8051	16.5	13.8
284	Circulatory disorders w AMI, expired w CC	6	0.7689	22.3	18.6
285	Circulatory disorders w AMI, expired w/o CC/MCC	0	0.7689	22.3	18.6
286	Circulatory disorders except AMI, w card cath w MCC	4	1.6227	34.5	28.8
287	Circulatory disorders except AMI, w card cath w/o MCC	2	0.6003	19.8	16.5
288	Acute & subacute endocarditis w MCC	699	1.0103	25.7	21.4
289	Acute & subacute endocarditis w CC	168	0.8201	25.4	21.2
290	Acute & subacute endocarditis w/o CC/MCC	12	0.7689	22.3	18.6
291	Heart failure & shock w MCC	1,609	0.8158	21.3	17.8
292	Heart failure & shock w CC	683	0.6105	19.2	16.0
293	Heart failure & shock w/o CC/MCC	40	0.4754	16.9	14.1
294	Deep vein thrombophlebitis w CC/MCC	0	0.5819	20.3	16.9
295	Deep vein thrombophlebitis w/o CC/MCC	0	0.4572	17.4	14.5
296	Cardiac arrest, unexplained w MCC	0	0.8158	21.3	17.8
297	Cardiac arrest, unexplained w CC	0	0.6105	19.2	16.0
298	Cardiac arrest, unexplained w/o CC/MCC	0	0.4754	16.9	14.1
299	Peripheral vascular disorders w MCC	903	0.7990	22.8	19.0
300	Peripheral vascular disorders w CC	736	0.5819	20.3	16.9
301	Peripheral vascular disorders w/o CC/MCC	22	0.4572	17.4	14.5
302	Atherosclerosis w MCC	61	0.7201	19.5	16.3
303	Atherosclerosis w/o MCC	28	0.6990	22.6	18.8
304	Hypertension w MCC	5	0.7689	22.3	18.6
305	Hypertension w/o MCC	3	0.4572	17.4	14.5
306	Cardiac congenital & valvular disorders w MCC*	44	0.8344	22.4	18.7
307	Cardiac congenital & valvular disorders w/o MCC*	11	0.8344	22.4	18.7
308	Cardiac arrhythmia & conduction disorders w MCC	103	0.7635	21.2	17.7
309	Cardiac arrhythmia & conduction disorders w CC	45	0.5149	17.2	14.3
310	Cardiac arrhythmia & conduction disorders w/o CC/MCC	9	0.4572	17.4	14.5
311	Angina pectoris	3	0.6003	19.8	16.5
312	Syncope & collapse	40	0.5624	20.7	17.3
313	Chest pain	1	0.7689	22.3	18.6
314	Other circulatory system diagnoses w MCC	1,929	0.9337	23.3	19.4

MS-LTC-DRG	MS-LTC-DRG Title	FY 2012 LTCH Cases	Relative Weight	Geometric Avg Length of Stay	Short-Stay Outlier (SSO) Threshold[1]
315	Other circulatory system diagnoses w CC	228	0.6717	20.4	17.0
316	Other circulatory system diagnoses w/o CC/MCC	15	0.6003	19.8	16.5
326	Stomach, esophageal & duodenal proc w MCC	25	2.0651	38.7	32.3
327	Stomach, esophageal & duodenal proc w CC	1	1.6227	34.5	28.8
328	Stomach, esophageal & duodenal proc w/o CC/MCC	0	0.4572	17.4	14.5
329	Major small & large bowel procedures w MCC	33	1.7996	37.9	31.6
330	Major small & large bowel procedures w CC	7	1.1259	27.4	22.8
331	Major small & large bowel procedures w/o CC/MCC	0	0.4572	17.4	14.5
332	Rectal resection w MCC	0	1.1259	27.4	22.8
333	Rectal resection w CC	0	0.6003	19.8	16.5
334	Rectal resection w/o CC/MCC	0	0.4572	17.4	14.5
335	Peritoneal adhesiolysis w MCC	8	1.6227	34.5	28.8
336	Peritoneal adhesiolysis w CC	1	1.6227	34.5	28.8
337	Peritoneal adhesiolysis w/o CC/MCC	0	0.4572	17.4	14.5
338	Appendectomy w complicated principal diag w MCC	0	0.9365	24.0	20.0
339	Appendectomy w complicated principal diag w CC	0	0.6934	20.5	17.1
340	Appendectomy w complicated principal diag w/o CC/MCC	0	0.6003	19.8	16.5
341	Appendectomy w/o complicated principal diag w MCC	0	0.9365	24.0	20.0
342	Appendectomy w/o complicated principal diag w CC	0	0.6934	20.5	17.1
343	Appendectomy w/o complicated principal diag w/o CC/MCC	0	0.6003	19.8	16.5
344	Minor small & large bowel procedures w MCC	2	1.6227	34.5	28.8
345	Minor small & large bowel procedures w CC	0	0.6934	20.5	17.1
346	Minor small & large bowel procedures w/o CC/MCC	0	0.6003	19.8	16.5
347	Anal & stomal procedures w MCC	9	1.1259	27.4	22.8
348	Anal & stomal procedures w CC	1	0.6003	19.8	16.5
349	Anal & stomal procedures w/o CC/MCC	0	0.6003	19.8	16.5
350	Inguinal & femoral hernia procedures w MCC	0	0.4572	17.4	14.5
351	Inguinal & femoral hernia procedures w CC	2	0.4572	17.4	14.5
352	Inguinal & femoral hernia procedures w/o CC/MCC	0	0.4572	17.4	14.5
353	Hernia procedures except inguinal & femoral w MCC	2	1.6227	34.5	28.8
354	Hernia procedures except inguinal & femoral w CC	0	0.6934	20.5	17.1
355	Hernia procedures except inguinal & femoral w/o CC/MCC	0	0.6003	19.8	16.5
356	Other digestive system O.R. procedures w MCC	195	1.4422	34.0	28.3
357	Other digestive system O.R. procedures w CC	31	0.9556	27.7	23.1
358	Other digestive system O.R. procedures w/o CC/MCC	1	0.4572	17.4	14.5
368	Major esophageal disorders w MCC	43	1.0092	24.8	20.7
369	Major esophageal disorders w CC	5	0.6003	19.8	16.5
370	Major esophageal disorders w/o CC/MCC	0	0.6003	19.8	16.5
371	Major gastrointestinal disorders & peritoneal infections w MCC	1,331	0.9365	24.0	20.0
372	Major gastrointestinal disorders & peritoneal infections w CC	344	0.6934	20.5	17.1
373	Major gastrointestinal disorders & peritoneal infections w/o CC/MCC	15	0.6003	19.8	16.5
374	Digestive malignancy w MCC	70	0.9421	22.1	18.4
375	Digestive malignancy w CC	28	0.6534	19.8	16.5

MS-LTC-DRG	MS-LTC-DRG Title	FY 2012 LTCH Cases	Relative Weight	Geometric Avg Length of Stay	Short-Stay Outlier (SSO) Threshold[1]
376	Digestive malignancy w/o CC/MCC	2	0.4572	17.4	14.5
377	G.I. hemorrhage w MCC	121	0.8923	23.5	19.6
378	G.I. hemorrhage w CC	28	0.5798	19.8	16.5
379	G.I. hemorrhage w/o CC/MCC	5	0.4572	17.4	14.5
380	Complicated peptic ulcer w MCC	39	1.0345	24.8	20.7
381	Complicated peptic ulcer w CC*	12	0.6003	19.8	16.5
382	Complicated peptic ulcer w/o CC/MCC*	1	0.6003	19.8	16.5
383	Uncomplicated peptic ulcer w MCC	15	0.7689	22.3	18.6
384	Uncomplicated peptic ulcer w/o MCC	6	0.6003	19.8	16.5
385	Inflammatory bowel disease w MCC	61	0.8777	22.3	18.6
386	Inflammatory bowel disease w CC*	27	0.5879	19.4	16.2
387	Inflammatory bowel disease w/o CC/MCC*	2	0.5879	19.4	16.2
388	G.I. obstruction w MCC	281	0.9924	23.1	19.3
389	G.I. obstruction w CC	87	0.6572	19.0	15.8
390	G.I. obstruction w/o CC/MCC	3	0.4572	17.4	14.5
391	Esophagitis, gastroent & misc digest disorders w MCC	449	0.8485	23.2	19.3
392	Esophagitis, gastroent & misc digest disorders w/o MCC	212	0.6264	19.9	16.6
393	Other digestive system diagnoses w MCC	1,120	1.0609	25.5	21.3
394	Other digestive system diagnoses w CC	313	0.7160	21.8	18.2
395	Other digestive system diagnoses w/o CC/MCC	15	0.6003	19.8	16.5
405	Pancreas, liver & shunt procedures w MCC	10	1.6227	34.5	28.8
406	Pancreas, liver & shunt procedures w CC	3	1.6227	34.5	28.8
407	Pancreas, liver & shunt procedures w/o CC/MCC	0	1.6227	34.5	28.8
408	Biliary tract proc except only cholecyst w or w/o c.d.e. w MCC	0	0.6003	19.8	16.5
409	Biliary tract proc except only cholecyst w or w/o c.d.e. w CC	1	0.6003	19.8	16.5
410	Biliary tract proc except only cholecyst w or w/o c.d.e. w/o CC/MCC	0	0.6003	19.8	16.5
411	Cholecystectomy w c.d.e. w MCC	1	1.1259	27.4	22.8
412	Cholecystectomy w c.d.e. w CC	0	1.1259	27.4	22.8
413	Cholecystectomy w c.d.e. w/o CC/MCC	0	1.1259	27.4	22.8
414	Cholecystectomy except by laparoscope w/o c.d.e. w MCC	0	1.1259	27.4	22.8
415	Cholecystectomy except by laparoscope w/o c.d.e. w CC	0	1.1259	27.4	22.8
416	Cholecystectomy except by laparoscope w/o c.d.e. w/o CC/MCC	0	0.6003	19.8	16.5
417	Laparoscopic cholecystectomy w/o c.d.e. w MCC	10	1.1259	27.4	22.8
418	Laparoscopic cholecystectomy w/o c.d.e. w CC	3	0.6003	19.8	16.5
419	Laparoscopic cholecystectomy w/o c.d.e. w/o CC/MCC	0	0.6003	19.8	16.5
420	Hepatobiliary diagnostic procedures w MCC	1	0.7689	22.3	18.6
421	Hepatobiliary diagnostic procedures w CC	0	0.7689	22.3	18.6
422	Hepatobiliary diagnostic procedures w/o CC/MCC	0	0.7689	22.3	18.6
423	Other hepatobiliary or pancreas O.R. procedures w MCC	15	1.6227	34.5	28.8
424	Other hepatobiliary or pancreas O.R. procedures w CC	4	1.6227	34.5	28.8
425	Other hepatobiliary or pancreas O.R. procedures w/o CC/MCC	0	1.6227	34.5	28.8
432	Cirrhosis & alcoholic hepatitis w MCC	84	0.7193	20.0	16.7
433	Cirrhosis & alcoholic hepatitis w CC	6	0.4572	17.4	14.5

MS-LTC-DRG	MS-LTC-DRG Title	FY 2012 LTCH Cases	Relative Weight	Geometric Avg Length of Stay	Short-Stay Outlier (SSO) Threshold[1]
434	Cirrhosis & alcoholic hepatitis w/o CC/MCC	0	0.4572	17.4	14.5
435	Malignancy of hepatobiliary system or pancreas w MCC	40	0.8701	21.7	18.1
436	Malignancy of hepatobiliary system or pancreas w CC	12	0.7689	22.3	18.6
437	Malignancy of hepatobiliary system or pancreas w/o CC/MCC	0	0.7689	22.3	18.6
438	Disorders of pancreas except malignancy w MCC	376	1.0750	25.1	20.9
439	Disorders of pancreas except malignancy w CC	84	0.6931	19.5	16.3
440	Disorders of pancreas except malignancy w/o CC/MCC	6	0.4572	17.4	14.5
441	Disorders of liver except malig,cirr,alc hepa w MCC	225	0.8231	20.6	17.2
442	Disorders of liver except malig,cirr,alc hepa w CC	76	0.5894	20.2	16.8
443	Disorders of liver except malig,cirr,alc hepa w/o CC/MCC	4	0.4572	17.4	14.5
444	Disorders of the biliary tract w MCC	208	0.8617	23.1	19.3
445	Disorders of the biliary tract w CC	40	0.5561	18.7	15.6
446	Disorders of the biliary tract w/o CC/MCC	4	0.4572	17.4	14.5
453	Combined anterior/posterior spinal fusion w MCC	0	1.6227	34.5	28.8
454	Combined anterior/posterior spinal fusion w CC	2	1.6227	34.5	28.8
455	Combined anterior/posterior spinal fusion w/o CC/MCC	0	1.6227	34.5	28.8
456	Spinal fusion exc cerv w spinal curv, malig or 9+ fusions w MCC	2	1.6227	34.5	28.8
457	Spinal fusion exc cerv w spinal curv, malig or 9+ fusions w CC	1	1.6227	34.5	28.8
458	Spinal fusion exc cerv w spinal curv, malig or 9+ fusions w/o CC/MCC	1	1.6227	34.5	28.8
459	Spinal fusion except cervical w MCC	4	1.6227	34.5	28.8
460	Spinal fusion except cervical w/o MCC	1	1.6227	34.5	28.8
461	Bilateral or multiple major joint procs of lower extremity w MCC	0	1.6227	34.5	28.8
462	Bilateral or multiple major joint procs of lower extremity w/o MCC	0	1.6227	34.5	28.8
463	Wnd debrid & skn grft exc hand, for musculo-conn tiss dis w MCC	1,198	1.4039	37.8	31.5
464	Wnd debrid & skn grft exc hand, for musculo-conn tiss dis w CC*	353	1.0917	33.1	27.6
465	Wnd debrid & skn grft exc hand, for musculo-conn tiss dis w/o CC/MCC*	18	1.0917	33.1	27.6
466	Revision of hip or knee replacement w MCC	3	1.6227	34.5	28.8
467	Revision of hip or knee replacement w CC	9	1.6227	34.5	28.8
468	Revision of hip or knee replacement w/o CC/MCC	0	1.6227	34.5	28.8
469	Major joint replacement or reattachment of lower extremity w MCC	2	1.6227	34.5	28.8
470	Major joint replacement or reattachment of lower extremity w/o MCC	3	1.6227	34.5	28.8
471	Cervical spinal fusion w MCC	4	1.1259	27.4	22.8
472	Cervical spinal fusion w CC	1	1.1259	27.4	22.8
473	Cervical spinal fusion w/o CC/MCC	1	0.7689	22.3	18.6
474	Amputation for musculoskeletal sys & conn tissue dis w MCC	136	1.5854	37.9	31.6
475	Amputation for musculoskeletal sys & conn tissue dis w CC	42	1.2516	33.0	27.5
476	Amputation for musculoskeletal sys & conn tissue dis w/o CC/MCC	3	0.6003	19.8	16.5
477	Biopsies of musculoskeletal system & connective tissue w MCC	49	1.4716	38.8	32.3
478	Biopsies of musculoskeletal system & connective tissue w CC	10	1.1259	27.4	22.8
479	Biopsies of musculoskeletal system & connective tissue w/o CC/MCC	0	0.6003	19.8	16.5
480	Hip & femur procedures except major joint w MCC	13	1.6227	34.5	28.8
481	Hip & femur procedures except major joint w CC*	4	1.6227	34.5	28.8
482	Hip & femur procedures except major joint w/o CC/MCC*	1	1.6227	34.5	28.8

MS-LTC-DRG	MS-LTC-DRG Title	FY 2012 LTCH Cases	Relative Weight	Geometric Avg Length of Stay	Short-Stay Outlier (SSO) Threshold[1]
483	Major joint & limb reattachment proc of upper extremity w CC/MCC	0	1.6227	34.5	28.8
484	Major joint & limb reattachment proc of upper extremity w/o CC/MCC	0	1.6227	34.5	28.8
485	Knee procedures w pdx of infection w MCC	16	1.1259	27.4	22.8
486	Knee procedures w pdx of infection w CC	8	1.1259	27.4	22.8
487	Knee procedures w pdx of infection w/o CC/MCC	1	0.7689	22.3	18.6
488	Knee procedures w/o pdx of infection w CC/MCC	1	1.6227	34.5	28.8
489	Knee procedures w/o pdx of infection w/o CC/MCC	0	1.6227	34.5	28.8
490	Back & neck procedures except spinal fusion w CC/MCC or disc devices	7	1.6227	34.5	28.8
491	Back & neck procedures except spinal fusion w/o CC/MCC	0	1.6227	34.5	28.8
492	Lower extrem & humer proc except hip,foot,femur w MCC	13	1.6227	34.5	28.8
493	Lower extrem & humer proc except hip,foot,femur w CC*	14	1.1259	27.4	22.8
494	Lower extrem & humer proc except hip,foot,femur w/o CC/MCC*	1	1.1259	27.4	22.8
495	Local excision & removal int fix devices exc hip & femur w MCC	145	1.4748	38.5	32.1
496	Local excision & removal int fix devices exc hip & femur w CC	27	1.0858	35.9	29.9
497	Local excision & removal int fix devices exc hip & femur w/o CC/MCC	3	0.7689	22.3	18.6
498	Local excision & removal int fix devices of hip & femur w CC/MCC	13	1.1259	27.4	22.8
499	Local excision & removal int fix devices of hip & femur w/o CC/MCC	0	0.7689	22.3	18.6
500	Soft tissue procedures w MCC	319	1.3737	35.4	29.5
501	Soft tissue procedures w CC	51	0.9006	31.0	25.8
502	Soft tissue procedures w/o CC/MCC	7	0.6003	19.8	16.5
503	Foot procedures w MCC	55	1.2520	30.7	25.6
504	Foot procedures w CC*	33	0.8879	23.6	19.7
505	Foot procedures w/o CC/MCC*	3	0.8879	23.6	19.7
506	Major thumb or joint procedures	0	0.4572	17.4	14.5
507	Major shoulder or elbow joint procedures w CC/MCC	4	1.6227	34.5	28.8
508	Major shoulder or elbow joint procedures w/o CC/MCC	0	1.6227	34.5	28.8
509	Arthroscopy	0	0.6003	19.8	16.5
510	Shoulder,elbow or forearm proc,exc major joint proc w MCC	0	1.3737	35.4	29.5
511	Shoulder,elbow or forearm proc,exc major joint proc w CC	0	0.9006	31.0	25.8
512	Shoulder,elbow or forearm proc,exc major joint proc w/o CC/MCC	0	0.6003	19.8	16.5
513	Hand or wrist proc, except major thumb or joint proc w CC/MCC	9	1.1259	27.4	22.8
514	Hand or wrist proc, except major thumb or joint proc w/o CC/MCC	2	0.4572	17.4	14.5
515	Other musculoskelet sys & conn tiss O.R. proc w MCC	87	1.2796	30.8	25.7
516	Other musculoskelet sys & conn tiss O.R. proc w CC	22	1.1259	27.4	22.8
517	Other musculoskelet sys & conn tiss O.R. proc w/o CC/MCC	0	0.6003	19.8	16.5
533	Fractures of femur w MCC	0	0.6003	19.8	16.5
534	Fractures of femur w/o MCC	1	0.6003	19.8	16.5
535	Fractures of hip & pelvis w MCC	8	0.6003	19.8	16.5
536	Fractures of hip & pelvis w/o MCC	8	0.4572	17.4	14.5
537	Sprains, strains, & dislocations of hip, pelvis & thigh w CC/MCC	1	0.6003	19.8	16.5
538	Sprains, strains, & dislocations of hip, pelvis & thigh w/o CC/MCC	0	0.6003	19.8	16.5
539	Osteomyelitis w MCC	2,522	1.0324	29.7	24.8
540	Osteomyelitis w CC	896	0.8221	27.4	22.8

MS-LTC-DRG	MS-LTC-DRG Title	FY 2012 LTCH Cases	Relative Weight	Geometric Avg Length of Stay	Short-Stay Outlier (SSO) Threshold[1]
541	Osteomyelitis w/o CC/MCC	90	0.7533	25.5	21.3
542	Pathological fractures & musculoskelet & conn tiss malig w MCC	35	0.8898	22.1	18.4
543	Pathological fractures & musculoskelet & conn tiss malig w CC*	11	0.6003	19.8	16.5
544	Pathological fractures & musculoskelet & conn tiss malig w/o CC/MCC*	1	0.6003	19.8	16.5
545	Connective tissue disorders w MCC	59	0.8594	22.2	18.5
546	Connective tissue disorders w CC	27	0.7053	18.2	15.2
547	Connective tissue disorders w/o CC/MCC	3	0.4572	17.4	14.5
548	Septic arthritis w MCC	308	0.9411	26.1	21.8
549	Septic arthritis w CC	197	0.7462	25.1	20.9
550	Septic arthritis w/o CC/MCC	27	0.5514	22.8	19.0
551	Medical back problems w MCC	177	1.0231	28.9	24.1
552	Medical back problems w/o MCC	110	0.7015	23.9	19.9
553	Bone diseases & arthropathies w MCC	11	1.1259	27.4	22.8
554	Bone diseases & arthropathies w/o MCC	6	0.4572	17.4	14.5
555	Signs & symptoms of musculoskeletal system & conn tissue w MCC	16	0.6003	19.8	16.5
556	Signs & symptoms of musculoskeletal system & conn tissue w/o MCC	17	0.6003	19.8	16.5
557	Tendonitis, myositis & bursitis w MCC	177	0.8180	23.8	19.8
558	Tendonitis, myositis & bursitis w/o MCC	101	0.6243	20.3	16.9
559	Aftercare, musculoskeletal system & connective tissue w MCC	2,081	0.8915	26.0	21.7
560	Aftercare, musculoskeletal system & connective tissue w CC	1,344	0.7481	25.1	20.9
561	Aftercare, musculoskeletal system & connective tissue w/o CC/MCC	154	0.6102	21.9	18.3
562	Fx, sprn, strn & disl except femur, hip, pelvis & thigh w MCC	8	0.7689	22.3	18.6
563	Fx, sprn, strn & disl except femur, hip, pelvis & thigh w/o MCC	7	0.4572	17.4	14.5
564	Other musculoskeletal sys & connective tissue diagnoses w MCC	456	0.8881	23.8	19.8
565	Other musculoskeletal sys & connective tissue diagnoses w CC	276	0.7325	23.4	19.5
566	Other musculoskeletal sys & connective tissue diagnoses w/o CC/MCC	23	0.6003	19.8	16.5
570	Skin debridement w MCC	1,954	1.1692	33.2	27.7
571	Skin debridement w CC	247	0.8739	27.1	22.6
572	Skin debridement w/o CC/MCC	29	0.6753	25.7	21.4
573	Skin graft &/or debrid for skn ulcer or cellulitis w MCC	665	1.5234	42.6	35.5
574	Skin graft &/or debrid for skn ulcer or cellulitis w CC	59	0.9253	31.3	26.1
575	Skin graft &/or debrid for skn ulcer or cellulitis w/o CC/MCC	7	0.7689	22.3	18.6
576	Skin graft &/or debrid exc for skin ulcer or cellulitis w MCC	17	1.6227	34.5	28.8
577	Skin graft &/or debrid exc for skin ulcer or cellulitis w CC	13	1.6227	34.5	28.8
578	Skin graft &/or debrid exc for skin ulcer or cellulitis w/o CC/MCC	2	0.7689	22.3	18.6
579	Other skin, subcut tiss & breast proc w MCC	1,071	1.2015	33.8	28.2
580	Other skin, subcut tiss & breast proc w CC	100	0.9640	27.3	22.8
581	Other skin, subcut tiss & breast proc w/o CC/MCC	7	0.6003	19.8	16.5
582	Mastectomy for malignancy w CC/MCC	0	0.9640	27.3	22.8
583	Mastectomy for malignancy w/o CC/MCC	0	0.6003	19.8	16.5
584	Breast biopsy, local excision & other breast procedures w CC/MCC	2	1.6227	34.5	28.8
585	Breast biopsy, local excision & other breast procedures w/o CC/MCC	0	0.5770	20.0	16.7
592	Skin ulcers w MCC	3,760	0.8301	25.2	21.0

MS-LTC-DRG	MS-LTC-DRG Title	FY 2012 LTCH Cases	Relative Weight	Geometric Avg Length of Stay	Short-Stay Outlier (SSO) Threshold[1]
593	Skin ulcers w CC	487	0.6411	22.3	18.6
594	Skin ulcers w/o CC/MCC	34	0.5539	20.0	16.7
595	Major skin disorders w MCC	36	0.8981	23.8	19.8
596	Major skin disorders w/o MCC	39	0.5977	21.2	17.7
597	Malignant breast disorders w MCC	6	1.1259	27.4	22.8
598	Malignant breast disorders w CC	5	0.6003	19.8	16.5
599	Malignant breast disorders w/o CC/MCC	2	0.4572	17.4	14.5
600	Non-malignant breast disorders w CC/MCC	24	1.1259	27.4	22.8
601	Non-malignant breast disorders w/o CC/MCC	0	0.4572	17.4	14.5
602	Cellulitis w MCC	1,451	0.7391	21.5	17.9
603	Cellulitis w/o MCC	1,399	0.5298	18.5	15.4
604	Trauma to the skin, subcut tiss & breast w MCC	54	0.8867	24.0	20.0
605	Trauma to the skin, subcut tiss & breast w/o MCC	42	0.6566	22.5	18.8
606	Minor skin disorders w MCC	124	0.8694	23.4	19.5
607	Minor skin disorders w/o MCC	127	0.5770	20.0	16.7
614	Adrenal & pituitary procedures w CC/MCC	0	1.0720	28.9	24.1
615	Adrenal & pituitary procedures w/o CC/MCC	0	1.0720	28.9	24.1
616	Amputat of lower limb for endocrine,nutrit,& metabol dis w MCC	133	1.5272	38.7	32.3
617	Amputat of lower limb for endocrine,nutrit,& metabol dis w CC	139	1.0659	30.8	25.7
618	Amputat of lower limb for endocrine,nutrit,& metabol dis w/o CC/MCC	2	0.7689	22.3	18.6
619	O.R. procedures for obesity w MCC	0	1.4422	34.0	28.3
620	O.R. procedures for obesity w CC	0	0.9556	27.7	23.1
621	O.R. procedures for obesity w/o CC/MCC	0	0.4572	17.4	14.5
622	Skin grafts & wound debrid for endoc, nutrit & metab dis w MCC	418	1.2699	34.5	28.8
623	Skin grafts & wound debrid for endoc, nutrit & metab dis w CC	442	0.9836	29.9	24.9
624	Skin grafts & wound debrid for endoc, nutrit & metab dis w/o CC/MCC	6	0.6003	19.8	16.5
625	Thyroid, parathyroid & thyroglossal procedures w MCC	2	1.6227	34.5	28.8
626	Thyroid, parathyroid & thyroglossal procedures w CC	0	1.0720	28.9	24.1
627	Thyroid, parathyroid & thyroglossal procedures w/o CC/MCC	0	1.0720	28.9	24.1
628	Other endocrine, nutrit & metab O.R. proc w MCC	150	1.3607	34.9	29.1
629	Other endocrine, nutrit & metab O.R. proc w CC*	144	1.0720	28.9	24.1
630	Other endocrine, nutrit & metab O.R. proc w/o CC/MCC*	2	1.0720	28.9	24.1
637	Diabetes w MCC	931	0.9351	26.4	22.0
638	Diabetes w CC	1,339	0.7452	23.7	19.8
639	Diabetes w/o CC/MCC	18	0.6003	19.8	16.5
640	Nutritional & misc metabolic disorders w MCC	809	0.8181	22.5	18.8
641	Nutritional & misc metabolic disorders w/o MCC	336	0.6120	20.1	16.8
642	Inborn errors of metabolism	1	0.6003	19.8	16.5
643	Endocrine disorders w MCC	49	0.9617	24.2	20.2
644	Endocrine disorders w CC	16	0.6003	19.8	16.5
645	Endocrine disorders w/o CC/MCC	1	0.4572	17.4	14.5
652	Kidney transplant	0	0.0000	0.0	0.0
653	Major bladder procedures w MCC	1	1.6227	34.5	28.8

MS-LTC-DRG	MS-LTC-DRG Title	FY 2012 LTCH Cases	Relative Weight	Geometric Avg Length of Stay	Short-Stay Outlier (SSO) Threshold[1]
654	Major bladder procedures w CC	1	0.7689	22.3	18.6
655	Major bladder procedures w/o CC/MCC	0	0.7689	22.3	18.6
656	Kidney & ureter procedures for neoplasm w MCC	0	1.1259	27.4	22.8
657	Kidney & ureter procedures forneoplasm w CC	0	0.6003	19.8	16.5
658	Kidney & ureter procedures for neoplasm w/o CC/MCC	0	0.4572	17.4	14.5
659	Kidney & ureter procedures for non-neoplasm w MCC	11	1.6227	34.5	28.8
660	Kidney & ureter procedures for non-neoplasm w CC	4	0.7689	22.3	18.6
661	Kidney & ureter procedures for non-neoplasm w/o CC/MCC	0	0.7689	22.3	18.6
662	Minor bladder procedures w MCC*	1	0.7689	22.3	18.6
663	Minor bladder procedures w CC*	2	0.7689	22.3	18.6
664	Minor bladder procedures w/o CC/MCC	0	0.4572	17.4	14.5
665	Prostatectomy w MCC	2	1.1259	27.4	22.8
666	Prostatectomy w CC	0	0.9678	24.5	20.4
667	Prostatectomy w/o CC/MCC	0	0.7689	22.3	18.6
668	Transurethral procedures w MCC	6	1.6227	34.5	28.8
669	Transurethral procedures w CC	5	1.1259	27.4	22.8
670	Transurethral procedures w/o CC/MCC	0	1.1259	27.4	22.8
671	Urethral procedures w CC/MCC	1	0.7689	22.3	18.6
672	Urethral procedures w/o CC/MCC	0	0.7689	22.3	18.6
673	Other kidney & urinary tract procedures w MCC	266	1.3664	31.9	26.6
674	Other kidney & urinary tract procedures w CC	45	0.9678	24.5	20.4
675	Other kidney & urinary tract procedures w/o CC/MCC	2	0.7689	22.3	18.6
682	Renal failure w MCC	1,964	0.9173	23.1	19.3
683	Renal failure w CC	553	0.6882	20.5	17.1
684	Renal failure w/o CC/MCC	22	0.4572	17.4	14.5
685	Admit for renal dialysis	13	1.1259	27.4	22.8
686	Kidney & urinary tract neoplasms w MCC	16	1.1259	27.4	22.8
687	Kidney & urinary tract neoplasms w CC	9	0.6003	19.8	16.5
688	Kidney & urinary tract neoplasms w/o CC/MCC	1	0.4572	17.4	14.5
689	Kidney & urinary tract infections w MCC	1,137	0.6876	21.5	17.9
690	Kidney & urinary tract infections w/o MCC	655	0.5097	18.2	15.2
691	Urinary stones w esw lithotripsy w CC/MCC	0	1.1259	27.4	22.8
692	Urinary stones w esw lithotripsy w/o CC/MCC	0	0.6003	19.8	16.5
693	Urinary stones w/o esw lithotripsy w MCC	14	1.1259	27.4	22.8
694	Urinary stones w/ot esw lithotripsy w/o MCC	2	0.6003	19.8	16.5
695	Kidney & urinary tract signs & symptoms w MCC	7	1.1259	27.4	22.8
696	Kidney & urinary tract signs & symptoms w/o MCC	2	0.4572	17.4	14.5
697	Urethral stricture	0	0.4572	17.4	14.5
698	Other kidney & urinary tract diagnoses w MCC	391	0.8596	23.2	19.3
699	Other kidney & urinary tract diagnoses w CC*	115	0.6416	20.5	17.1
700	Other kidney & urinary tract diagnoses w/o CC/MCC*	2	0.6416	20.5	17.1
707	Major male pelvic procedures w CC/MCC	0	0.9678	24.5	20.4
708	Major male pelvic procedures w/o CC/MCC	0	0.7689	22.3	18.6

MS-LTC-DRG	MS-LTC-DRG Title	FY 2012 LTCH Cases	Relative Weight	Geometric Avg Length of Stay	Short-Stay Outlier (SSO)[1] Threshold
709	Penis procedures w CC/MCC	7	1.1259	27.4	22.8
710	Penis procedures w/o CC/MCC	0	1.1259	27.4	22.8
711	Testes procedures w CC/MCC	14	1.6227	34.5	28.8
712	Testes procedures w/o CC/MCC	0	1.6227	34.5	28.8
713	Transurethral prostatectomy w CC/MCC	0	0.9678	24.5	20.4
714	Transurethral prostatectomy w/o CC/MCC	0	0.7689	22.3	18.6
715	Other male reproductive system O.R. proc for malignancy w CC/MCC	0	0.6003	19.8	16.5
716	Other male reproductive system O.R. proc for malignancy w/o CC/MCC	0	0.4572	17.4	14.5
717	Other male reproductive system O.R. proc exc malignancy w CC/MCC	24	1.1259	27.4	22.8
718	Other male reproductive system O.R. proc exc malignancy w/o CC/MCC	0	0.7689	22.3	18.6
722	Malignancy, male reproductive system w MCC	3	0.6003	19.8	16.5
723	Malignancy, male reproductive system w CC	3	0.6003	19.8	16.5
724	Malignancy, male reproductive system w/o CC/MCC	0	0.6003	19.8	16.5
725	Benign prostatic hypertrophy w MCC*	3	0.6003	19.8	16.5
726	Benign prostatic hypertrophy w/o MCC*	2	0.6003	19.8	16.5
727	Inflammation of the male reproductive system w MCC	85	0.8121	21.9	18.3
728	Inflammation of the male reproductive system w/o MCC	50	0.6016	20.3	16.9
729	Other male reproductive system diagnoses w CC/MCC	93	0.7820	22.8	19.0
730	Other male reproductive system diagnoses w/o CC/MCC	2	0.6003	19.8	16.5
734	Pelvic evisceration, rad hysterectomy & rad vulvectomy w CC/MCC	0	0.7689	22.3	18.6
735	Pelvic evisceration, rad hysterectomy & rad vulvectomy w/o CC/MCC	0	0.7689	22.3	18.6
736	Uterine & adnexa proc for ovarian or adnexal malignancy w MCC	0	0.7689	22.3	18.6
737	Uterine & adnexa proc for ovarian or adnexal malignancy w CC	0	0.7689	22.3	18.6
738	Uterine & adnexa proc for ovarian or adnexal malignancy w/o CC/MCC	0	0.7689	22.3	18.6
739	Uterine,adnexa proc for non-ovarian/adnexal malig w MCC	0	1.3607	34.9	29.1
740	Uterine,adnexa proc for non-ovarian/adnexal malig w CC	0	1.0720	28.9	24.1
741	Uterine,adnexa proc for non-ovarian/adnexal malig w/o CC/MCC	0	1.0720	28.9	24.1
742	Uterine & adnexa proc for non-malignancy w CC/MCC	0	0.7689	22.3	18.6
743	Uterine & adnexa proc for non-malignancy w/o CC/MCC	0	0.7689	22.3	18.6
744	D&C, conization, laparascopy & tubal interruption w CC/MCC	0	0.7689	22.3	18.6
745	D&C, conization, laparascopy & tubal interruption w/o CC/MCC	0	0.7689	22.3	18.6
746	Vagina, cervix & vulva procedures w CC/MCC	6	1.1259	27.4	22.8
747	Vagina, cervix & vulva procedures w/o CC/MCC	0	0.7689	22.3	18.6
748	Female reproductive system reconstructive procedures	0	0.7689	22.3	18.6
749	Other female reproductive system O.R. procedures w CC/MCC	3	0.7689	22.3	18.6
750	Other female reproductive system O.R. procedures w/o CC/MCC	0	0.7689	22.3	18.6
754	Malignancy, female reproductive system w MCC	24	1.1259	27.4	22.8
755	Malignancy, female reproductive system w CC	12	0.7689	22.3	18.6
756	Malignancy, female reproductive system w/o CC/MCC	1	0.4572	17.4	14.5
757	Infections, female reproductive system w MCC	98	0.7039	21.8	18.2
758	Infections, female reproductive system w CC*	45	0.7033	22.8	19.0
759	Infections, female reproductive system w/o CC/MCC*	1	0.7033	22.8	19.0
760	Menstrual & other female reproductive system disorders w CC/MCC	1	1.6227	34.5	28.8

MS-LTC-DRG	MS-LTC-DRG Title	FY 2012 LTCH Cases	Relative Weight	Geometric Avg Length of Stay	Short-Stay Outlier (SSO) Threshold[1]
761	Menstrual & other female reproductive system disorders w/o CC/MCC	0	1.6227	34.5	28.8
765	Cesarean section w CC/MCC	0	0.7689	22.3	18.6
766	Cesarean section w/o CC/MCC	0	0.7689	22.3	18.6
767	Vaginal delivery w sterilization &/or D&C	0	0.7689	22.3	18.6
768	Vaginal delivery w O.R. proc except steril &/or D&C	0	0.7689	22.3	18.6
769	Postpartum & post abortion diagnoses w O.R. procedure	0	0.7689	22.3	18.6
770	Abortion w D&C, aspiration curettage or hysterotomy	0	0.7689	22.3	18.6
774	Vaginal delivery w complicating diagnoses	0	0.7689	22.3	18.6
775	Vaginal delivery w/o complicating diagnoses	0	0.7689	22.3	18.6
776	Postpartum & post abortion diagnoses w/o O.R. procedure	3	1.1259	27.4	22.8
777	Ectopic pregnancy	0	1.1259	27.4	22.8
778	Threatened abortion	0	1.1259	27.4	22.8
779	Abortion w/o D&C	0	1.1259	27.4	22.8
780	False labor	0	1.1259	27.4	22.8
781	Other antepartum diagnoses w medical complications	2	0.4572	17.4	14.5
782	Other antepartum diagnoses w/o medical complications	0	1.1259	27.4	22.8
789	Neonates, died or transferred to another acute care facility	0	1.1259	27.4	22.8
790	Extreme immaturity or respiratory distress syndrome, neonate	0	1.1259	27.4	22.8
791	Prematurity w major problems	0	1.1259	27.4	22.8
792	Prematurity w/o major problems	0	1.1259	27.4	22.8
793	Full term neonate w major problems	0	1.1259	27.4	22.8
794	Neonate w other significant problems	0	1.1259	27.4	22.8
795	Normal newborn	0	1.1259	27.4	22.8
799	Splenectomy w MCC	0	1.4422	34.0	28.3
800	Splenectomy w CC	0	0.9556	27.7	23.1
801	Splenectomy w/o CC/MCC	0	0.4572	17.4	14.5
802	Other O.R. proc of the blood & blood forming organs w MCC	5	1.1259	27.4	22.8
803	Other O.R. proc of the blood & blood forming organs w CC	5	0.7689	22.3	18.6
804	Other O.R. proc of the blood & blood forming organs w/o CC/MCC	0	0.7689	22.3	18.6
808	Major hematol/immun diag exc sickle cell crisis & coagul w MCC	42	0.8766	20.5	17.1
809	Major hematol/immun diag exc sickle cell crisis & coagul w CC	17	0.6003	19.8	16.5
810	Major hematol/immun diag exc sickle cell crisis & coagul w/o CC/MCC	0	0.5574	19.7	16.4
811	Red blood cell disorders w MCC	57	0.8231	21.8	18.2
812	Red blood cell disorders w/o MCC	26	0.5574	19.7	16.4
813	Coagulation disorders	27	0.7607	19.1	15.9
814	Reticuloendothelial & immunity disorders w MCC	22	0.7689	22.3	18.6
815	Reticuloendothelial & immunity disorders w CC	7	0.4572	17.4	14.5
816	Reticuloendothelial & immunity disorders w/o CC/MCC	1	0.4572	17.4	14.5
820	Lymphoma & leukemia w major O.R. procedure w MCC	0	0.7689	22.3	18.6
821	Lymphoma & leukemia w major O.R. procedure w CC	0	0.7689	22.3	18.6
822	Lymphoma & leukemia w major O.R. procedure w/o CC/MCC	1	0.4572	17.4	14.5
823	Lymphoma & non-acute leukemia w other O.R. proc w MCC	7	1.1259	27.4	22.8
824	Lymphoma & non-acute leukemia w other O.R. proc w CC	1	0.7689	22.3	18.6

MS-LTC-DRG	MS-LTC-DRG Title	FY 2012 LTCH Cases	Relative Weight	Geometric Avg Length of Stay	Short-Stay Outlier (SSO) Threshold[1]
825	Lymphoma & non-acute leukemia w other O.R. proc w/o CC/MCC	0	0.7689	22.3	18.6
826	Myeloprolif disord or poorly diff neopl w maj O.R. proc w MCC	0	1.1259	27.4	22.8
827	Myeloprolif disord or poorly diff neopl w maj O.R. proc w CC	0	0.7689	22.3	18.6
828	Myeloprolif disord or poorly diff neopl w maj O.R. proc w/o CC/MCC	0	0.7689	22.3	18.6
829	Myeloprolif disord or poorly diff neopl w other O.R. proc w CC/MCC	6	1.1259	27.4	22.8
830	Myeloprolif disord or poorly diff neopl w other O.R. proc w/o CC/MCC	0	0.7689	22.3	18.6
834	Acute leukemia w/o major O.R. procedure w MCC	21	0.7689	22.3	18.6
835	Acute leukemia w/o major O.R. procedure w CC	7	0.6003	19.8	16.5
836	Acute leukemia w/o major O.R. procedure w/o CC/MCC	1	0.6003	19.8	16.5
837	Chemo w acute leukemia as sdx or w high dose chemo agent w MCC*	1	1.6227	34.5	28.8
838	Chemo w acute leukemia as sdx or w high dose chemo agent w CC*	1	1.6227	34.5	28.8
839	Chemo w acute leukemia as sdx or w high dose chemo agent w/o CC/MCC	0	0.6003	19.8	16.5
840	Lymphoma & non-acute leukemia w MCC	72	0.9793	20.8	17.3
841	Lymphoma & non-acute leukemia w CC	22	0.6003	19.8	16.5
842	Lymphoma & non-acute leukemia w/o CC/MCC	1	0.4572	17.4	14.5
843	Other myeloprolif dis or poorly diff neopl diag w MCC	7	0.7689	22.3	18.6
844	Other myeloprolif dis or poorly diff neopl diag w CC	4	0.4572	17.4	14.5
845	Other myeloprolif dis or poorly diff neopl diag w/o CC/MCC	1	0.4572	17.4	14.5
846	Chemotherapy w/o acute leukemia as secondary diagnosis w MCC	43	1.2444	26.6	22.2
847	Chemotherapy w/o acute leukemia as secondary diagnosis w CC	39	1.1006	26.0	21.7
848	Chemotherapy w/o acute leukemia as secondary diagnosis w/o CC/MCC	1	0.7689	22.3	18.6
849	Radiotherapy	53	0.9153	22.0	18.3
853	Infectious & parasitic diseases w O.R. procedure w MCC	1,547	1.7613	37.3	31.1
854	Infectious & parasitic diseases w O.R. procedure w CC	85	0.9197	27.8	23.2
855	Infectious & parasitic diseases w O.R. procedure w/o CC/MCC	2	0.6003	19.8	16.5
856	Postoperative or post-traumatic infections w O.R. proc w MCC	458	1.5460	35.3	29.4
857	Postoperative or post-traumatic infections w O.R. proc w CC	135	1.0334	30.1	25.1
858	Postoperative or post-traumatic infections w O.R. proc w/o CC/MCC	7	0.7689	22.3	18.6
862	Postoperative & post-traumatic infections w MCC	1,939	1.0078	25.3	21.1
863	Postoperative & post-traumatic infections w/o MCC	830	0.7292	23.1	19.3
864	Fever of unknown origin	11	0.6003	19.8	16.5
865	Viral illness w MCC*	72	0.7306	20.3	16.9
866	Viral illness w/o MCC*	12	0.7306	20.3	16.9
867	Other infectious & parasitic diseases diagnoses w MCC	443	1.0704	23.4	19.5
868	Other infectious & parasitic diseases diagnoses w CC*	56	0.7114	21.0	17.5
869	Other infectious & parasitic diseases diagnoses w/o CC/MCC*	2	0.7114	21.0	17.5
870	Septicemia w MV 96+ hours	1,828	2.1254	30.7	25.6
871	Septicemia w/o MV 96+ hours w MCC	8,102	0.8813	22.8	19.0
872	Septicemia w/o MV 96+ hours w/o MCC	1,073	0.5951	19.6	16.3
876	O.R. procedure w principal diagnoses of mental illness	6	1.1259	27.4	22.8
880	Acute adjustment reaction & psychosocial dysfunction	9	0.4572	17.4	14.5
881	Depressive neuroses	12	0.4572	17.4	14.5
882	Neuroses except depressive	71	0.3942	22.9	19.1

MS-LTC-DRG	MS-LTC-DRG Title	FY 2012 LTCH Cases	Relative Weight	Geometric Avg Length of Stay	Short-Stay Outlier (SSO) Threshold[1]
883	Disorders of personality & impulse control	62	0.4463	24.3	20.3
884	Organic disturbances & mental retardation	74	0.4043	22.3	18.6
885	Psychoses	695	0.4735	22.6	18.8
886	Behavioral & developmental disorders	11	0.4572	17.4	14.5
887	Other mental disorder diagnoses	0	0.4572	17.4	14.5
894	Alcohol/drug abuse or dependence, left ama	4	0.4572	17.4	14.5
895	Alcohol/drug abuse or dependence w rehabilitation therapy	259	0.4389	25.6	21.3
896	Alcohol/drug abuse or dependence w/o rehabilitation therapy w MCC	21	0.6003	19.8	16.5
897	Alcohol/drug abuse or dependence w/o rehabilitation therapy w/o MCC	40	0.4080	23.6	19.7
901	Wound debridements for injuries w MCC	353	1.4460	34.3	28.6
902	Wound debridements for injuries w CC	203	0.9891	30.2	25.2
903	Wound debridements for injuries w/o CC/MCC	10	0.4572	17.4	14.5
904	Skin grafts for injuries w CC/MCC*	97	1.3786	35.0	29.2
905	Skin grafts for injuries w/o CC/MCC*	2	1.3786	35.0	29.2
906	Hand procedures for injuries	0	0.4572	17.4	14.5
907	Other O.R. procedures for injuries w MCC	196	1.5215	34.2	28.5
908	Other O.R. procedures for injuries w CC	72	0.9603	28.5	23.8
909	Other O.R. procedures for injuries w/o CC/MCC	0	0.5847	20.2	16.8
913	Traumatic injury w MCC	63	0.8593	22.8	19.0
914	Traumatic injury w/o MCC	70	0.5847	20.2	16.8
915	Allergic reactions w MCC	0	0.4572	17.4	14.5
916	Allergic reactions w/o MCC	1	0.4572	17.4	14.5
917	Poisoning & toxic effects of drugs w MCC	18	0.7689	22.3	18.6
918	Poisoning & toxic effects of drugs w/o MCC	9	0.4572	17.4	14.5
919	Complications of treatment w MCC	2,074	1.1362	26.9	22.4
920	Complications of treatment w CC	846	0.7497	22.6	18.8
921	Complications of treatment w/o CC/MCC	28	0.5000	17.6	14.7
922	Other injury, poisoning & toxic effect diag w MCC	16	0.7689	22.3	18.6
923	Other injury, poisoning & toxic effect diag w/o MCC	14	0.7689	22.3	18.6
927	Extensive burns or full thickness burns w MV 96+ hrs w skin graft	0	1.1259	27.4	22.8
928	Full thickness burn w skin graft or inhal inj w CC/MCC	7	1.1259	27.4	22.8
929	Full thickness burn w skin graft or inhal inj w/o CC/MCC	0	1.1259	27.4	22.8
933	Extensive burns or full thickness burns w MV 96+ hrs w/o skin graft	6	0.7689	22.3	18.6
934	Full thickness burn w/o skin grft or inhal inj	44	0.7185	23.6	19.7
935	Non-extensive burns	41	0.7214	23.1	19.3
939	O.R. proc w diagnoses of other contact w health services w MCC	248	1.3118	32.1	26.8
940	O.R. proc w diagnoses of other contact w health services w CC	97	0.8701	28.4	23.7
941	O.R. proc w diagnoses of other contact w health services w/o CC/MCC	5	0.6003	19.8	16.5
945	Rehabilitation w CC/MCC	991	0.6292	20.8	17.3
946	Rehabilitation w/o CC/MCC	61	0.3925	18.2	15.2
947	Signs & symptoms w MCC	61	0.7903	21.4	17.8
948	Signs & symptoms w/o MCC	26	0.4915	20.0	16.7
949	Aftercare w CC/MCC	2,832	0.7286	22.0	18.3

MS-LTC-DRG	MS-LTC-DRG Title	FY 2012 LTCH Cases	Relative Weight	Geometric Avg Length of Stay	Short-Stay Outlier (SSO) Threshold[1]
950	Aftercare w/o CC/MCC	93	0.4010	16.1	13.4
951	Other factors influencing health status	59	1.1807	29.6	24.7
955	Craniotomy for multiple significant trauma	0	1.6227	34.5	28.8
956	Limb reattachment, hip & femur proc for multiple significant trauma	0	1.6227	34.5	28.8
957	Other O.R. procedures for multiple significant trauma w MCC	1	1.6227	34.5	28.8
958	Other O.R. procedures for multiple significant trauma w CC	0	0.7689	22.3	18.6
959	Other O.R. procedures for multiple significant trauma w/o CC/MCC	0	0.7689	22.3	18.6
963	Other multiple significant trauma w MCC	17	1.1259	27.4	22.8
964	Other multiple significant trauma w CC*	4	0.7689	22.3	18.6
965	Other multiple significant trauma w/o CC/MCC*	1	0.7689	22.3	18.6
969	HIV w extensive O.R. procedure w MCC	29	1.6502	32.9	27.4
970	HIV w extensive O.R. procedure w/o MCC	1	0.7689	22.3	18.6
974	HIV w major related condition w MCC	246	1.0267	22.3	18.6
975	HIV w major related condition w CC*	51	0.5376	16.9	14.1
976	HIV w major related condition w/o CC/MCC*	6	0.5376	16.9	14.1
977	HIV w or w/o other related condition	30	0.6255	21.1	17.6
981	Extensive O.R. procedure unrelated to principal diagnosis w MCC	1,455	2.1297	38.9	32.4
982	Extensive O.R. procedure unrelated to principal diagnosis w CC	183	1.0691	30.7	25.6
983	Extensive O.R. procedure unrelated to principal diagnosis w/o CC/MCC	2	0.7689	22.3	18.6
984	Prostatic O.R. procedure unrelated to principal diagnosis w MCC	15	1.6227	34.5	28.8
985	Prostatic O.R. procedure unrelated to principal diagnosis w CC	3	0.7689	22.3	18.6
986	Prostatic O.R. procedure unrelated to principal diagnosis w/o CC/MCC	1	0.7689	22.3	18.6
987	Non-extensive O.R. proc unrelated to principal diagnosis w MCC	687	1.6516	36.6	30.5
988	Non-extensive O.R. proc unrelated to principal diagnosis w CC	111	1.0781	29.3	24.4
989	Non-extensive O.R. proc unrelated to principal diagnosis w/o CC/MCC	3	0.6003	19.8	16.5
998	Principal Diagnosis Invalid as Discharge Diagnosis	0	0.0000	0.0	0.0
999	Ungroupable	0	0.0000	0.0	0.0

Appendix D — National Average Payment Table

The national average payment for each DRG is calculated by multiplying the current relative weight of the DRG by the national average hospital Medic_ base rate. The national average hospital Medicare base rate is the sum of the full update labor-related and nonlabor-related amounts published in the *Fe_ Register*, FY 2014 Final Rule, Table 1A. National Adjusted Operating Standardized Amounts; Labor/Nonlabor (if wage index greater than 1) or Table 1B. National Adjusted Operating Standardized Amounts; Labor/Nonlabor (if wage index less than or equal to 1). This information is provided as a benchmark reference only. There is no official publication of the average hospital base rate; therefore the national average payments provided in this table are approximate.

DRG		Description	GMLOS	AMLOS	Relative Weight	National Payment Rate
	001	HEART TRANSPLANT OR IMPLANT OF HEART ASSIST SYSTEM W MCC	28.3	35.9	25.3518	$136,146.26
	002	HEART TRANSPLANT OR IMPLANT OF HEART ASSIST SYSTEM W/O MCC	15.9	18.6	15.2738	$82,024.58
T	003	ECMO OR TRACH W MV 96+ HRS OR PDX EXC FACE, MOUTH & NECK W MAJ O.R.	27.2	33.2	17.6369	$94,715.09
T	004	TRACH W MV 96+ HRS OR PDX EXC FACE, MOUTH & NECK W/O MAJ O.R.	20.3	24.7	10.9288	$58,690.72
	005	LIVER TRANSPLANT W MCC OR INTESTINAL TRANSPLANT	15.1	20.1	10.4214	$55,965.84
	006	LIVER TRANSPLANT W/O MCC	7.9	9.0	4.7639	$25,583.48
	007	LUNG TRANSPLANT	15.4	17.9	9.1929	$49,368.45
	008	SIMULTANEOUS PANCREAS/KIDNEY TRANSPLANT	9.5	11.0	5.1527	$27,671.44
	010	PANCREAS TRANSPLANT	8.8	10.3	4.1554	$22,315.66
	011	TRACHEOSTOMY FOR FACE,MOUTH & NECK DIAGNOSES W MCC	11.4	14.0	4.7246	$25,372.42
	012	TRACHEOSTOMY FOR FACE,MOUTH & NECK DIAGNOSES W CC	8.3	9.8	3.2291	$17,341.17
	013	TRACHEOSTOMY FOR FACE,MOUTH & NECK DIAGNOSES W/O CC/MCC	5.7	6.5	2.1647	$11,625.05
	014	ALLOGENEIC BONE MARROW TRANSPLANT	20.7	26.2	10.6157	$57,009.28
	016	AUTOLOGOUS BONE MARROW TRANSPLANT W CC/MCC	18.1	19.5	6.0304	$32,384.94
	017	AUTOLOGOUS BONE MARROW TRANSPLANT W/O CC/MCC	9.9	13.2	4.2906	$23,041.72
	020	INTRACRANIAL VASCULAR PROCEDURES W PDX HEMORRHAGE W MCC	14.3	17.4	9.3897	$50,425.32
	021	INTRACRANIAL VASCULAR PROCEDURES W PDX HEMORRHAGE W CC	11.9	13.4	6.4458	$34,615.75
	022	INTRACRANIAL VASCULAR PROCEDURES W PDX HEMORRHAGE W/O CC/MCC	5.5	7.3	4.7113	$25,301.00
T	023	CRANIO W MAJOR DEV IMPL/ACUTE COMPLEX CNS PDX W MCC OR CHEMO IMPLANT	8.0	11.2	5.1587	$27,703.66
T	024	CRANIO W MAJOR DEV IMPL/ACUTE COMPLEX CNS PDX W/O MCC	4.5	6.6	3.7121	$19,935.02
T	025	CRANIOTOMY & ENDOVASCULAR INTRACRANIAL PROCEDURES W MCC	7.8	10.1	4.4422	$23,855.86
T	026	CRANIOTOMY & ENDOVASCULAR INTRACRANIAL PROCEDURES W CC	5.0	6.5	2.9842	$16,025.99
T	027	CRANIOTOMY & ENDOVASCULAR INTRACRANIAL PROCEDURES W/O CC/MCC	2.6	3.4	2.2505	$12,085.82
SP	028	SPINAL PROCEDURES W MCC	9.6	12.3	5.4339	$29,181.56
SP	029	SPINAL PROCEDURES W CC OR SPINAL NEUROSTIMULATORS	4.6	6.2	3.0782	$16,530.80
SP	030	SPINAL PROCEDURES W/O CC/MCC	2.5	3.3	1.8091	$9,715.37
T	031	VENTRICULAR SHUNT PROCEDURES W MCC	7.7	11.0	3.9460	$21,191.12
T	032	VENTRICULAR SHUNT PROCEDURES W CC	3.4	4.9	1.9780	$10,622.41
T	033	VENTRICULAR SHUNT PROCEDURES W/O CC/MCC	2.0	2.5	1.5226	$8,176.79

Calculated with an average hospital Medicare base rate of $5,370.28. Each hospital's base rate and corresponding payment will vary. The national average hospital Medicare base rate is the sum of the full update labor-related and nonlabor-related amounts published in the Federal Register, FY 2014 Final Rule, Table 1A. National Adjusted Operating Standardized Amounts; Labor/Nonlabor (if wage index greater than 1) or Table 1B. National Adjusted Operating Standardized Amounts; Labor/Nonlabor (if wage index less than or equal to 1).

MS-DRGs 998 and 999 contain cases that could not be assigned to valid DRGs.

Note: If there is no value in either the geometric mean length of stay or the arithmetic mean length of stay columns, the volume of cases is insufficient to determine a meaningful computation of these statistics.

			GMLOS	AMLOS	Relative Weight	National Payment Rate
		...T PROCEDURE W MCC	4.7	6.9	3.4145	$18,336.82
		...STENT PROCEDURE W CC	2.1	3.1	2.1781	$11,697.01
		...ARTERY STENT PROCEDURE W/O CC/MCC	1.3	1.5	1.7224	$9,249.77
		...EXTRACRANIAL PROCEDURES W MCC	5.5	7.9	3.0641	$16,455.07
		EXTRACRANIAL PROCEDURES W CC	2.4	3.5	1.5958	$8,569.89
	039	EXTRACRANIAL PROCEDURES W/O CC/MCC	1.4	1.6	1.0452	$5,613.02
SP	040	PERIPH/CRANIAL NERVE & OTHER NERV SYST PROC W MCC	8.3	11.0	3.7851	$20,327.05
SP	041	PERIPH/CRANIAL NERVE & OTHER NERV SYST PROC W CC OR PERIPH NEUROSTIM	5.0	6.4	2.1731	$11,670.16
SP	042	PERIPH/CRANIAL NERVE & OTHER NERV SYST PROC W/O CC/MCC	2.6	3.4	1.8616	$9,997.31
	052	SPINAL DISORDERS & INJURIES W CC/MCC	4.0	5.3	1.4102	$7,573.17
	053	SPINAL DISORDERS & INJURIES W/O CC/MCC	2.7	3.3	0.8746	$4,696.85
T	054	NERVOUS SYSTEM NEOPLASMS W MCC	4.1	5.5	1.3195	$7,086.08
T	055	NERVOUS SYSTEM NEOPLASMS W/O MCC	3.1	4.2	1.0100	$5,423.98
T	056	DEGENERATIVE NERVOUS SYSTEM DISORDERS W MCC	5.3	7.1	1.7368	$9,327.10
T	057	DEGENERATIVE NERVOUS SYSTEM DISORDERS W/O MCC	3.6	4.7	0.9841	$5,284.89
	058	MULTIPLE SCLEROSIS & CEREBELLAR ATAXIA W MCC	5.4	7.1	1.6027	$8,606.95
	059	MULTIPLE SCLEROSIS & CEREBELLAR ATAXIA W CC	4.0	4.9	1.0399	$5,584.55
	060	MULTIPLE SCLEROSIS & CEREBELLAR ATAXIA W/O CC/MCC	3.1	3.7	0.7899	$4,241.98
	061	ACUTE ISCHEMIC STROKE W USE OF THROMBOLYTIC AGENT W MCC	5.8	7.5	2.7316	$14,669.46
	062	ACUTE ISCHEMIC STROKE W USE OF THROMBOLYTIC AGENT W CC	4.2	4.9	1.8561	$9,967.78
	063	ACUTE ISCHEMIC STROKE W USE OF THROMBOLYTIC AGENT W/O CC/MCC	3.0	3.4	1.4685	$7,886.26
T	064	INTRACRANIAL HEMORRHAGE OR CEREBRAL INFARCTION W MCC	4.7	6.3	1.7417	$9,353.42
T	065	INTRACRANIAL HEMORRHAGE OR CEREBRAL INFARCTION W CC OR TPA IN 24 HRS	3.5	4.3	1.0776	$5,787.01
T	066	INTRACRANIAL HEMORRHAGE OR CEREBRAL INFARCTION W/O CC/MCC	2.5	2.9	0.7566	$4,063.15
	067	NONSPECIFIC CVA & PRECEREBRAL OCCLUSION W/O INFARCT W MCC	4.1	5.3	1.4172	$7,610.76
	068	NONSPECIFIC CVA & PRECEREBRAL OCCLUSION W/O INFARCT W/O MCC	2.5	3.1	0.8582	$4,608.77
	069	TRANSIENT ISCHEMIA	2.2	2.6	0.6948	$3,731.27
T	070	NONSPECIFIC CEREBROVASCULAR DISORDERS W MCC	4.9	6.6	1.6593	$8,910.91
T	071	NONSPECIFIC CEREBROVASCULAR DISORDERS W CC	3.6	4.6	0.9796	$5,260.73
T	072	NONSPECIFIC CEREBROVASCULAR DISORDERS W/O CC/MCC	2.3	2.9	0.6919	$3,715.70
	073	CRANIAL & PERIPHERAL NERVE DISORDERS W MCC	3.9	5.3	1.3014	$6,988.88
	074	CRANIAL & PERIPHERAL NERVE DISORDERS W/O MCC	3.1	3.9	0.8786	$4,718.33
	075	VIRAL MENINGITIS W CC/MCC	5.2	6.5	1.5918	$8,548.41
	076	VIRAL MENINGITIS W/O CC/MCC	3.2	3.7	0.8425	$4,524.46
	077	HYPERTENSIVE ENCEPHALOPATHY W MCC	4.6	6.0	1.6290	$8,748.19
	078	HYPERTENSIVE ENCEPHALOPATHY W CC	3.1	3.9	0.9467	$5,084.04
	079	HYPERTENSIVE ENCEPHALOPATHY W/O CC/MCC	2.3	2.8	0.7118	$3,822.57
	080	NONTRAUMATIC STUPOR & COMA W MCC	3.7	5.1	1.2252	$6,579.67

Calculated with an average hospital Medicare base rate of $5,370.28. Each hospital's base rate and corresponding payment will vary. The national average hospital Medicare base rate is the sum of the full update labor-related and nonlabor-related amounts published in the Federal Register, FY 2014 Final Rule, Table 1A. National Adjusted Operating Standardized Amounts; Labor/Nonlabor (if wage index greater than 1) or Table 1B. National Adjusted Operating Standardized Amounts; Labor/Nonlabor (if wage index less than or equal to 1).

MS-DRGs 998 and 999 contain cases that could not be assigned to valid DRGs.

Note: If there is no value in either the geometric mean length of stay or the arithmetic mean length of stay columns, the volume of cases is insufficient to determine a meaningful computation of these statistics.

DRG		Description	GMLOS	AMLOS	Relative Weight	National Payment Rate
	081	NONTRAUMATIC STUPOR & COMA W/O MCC	2.6	3.4	0.7455	$4,003.54
	082	TRAUMATIC STUPOR & COMA, COMA >1 HR W MCC	3.4	5.7	1.9463	$10,452.18
	083	TRAUMATIC STUPOR & COMA, COMA >1 HR W CC	3.4	4.4	1.2643	$6,789.65
	084	TRAUMATIC STUPOR & COMA, COMA >1 HR W/O CC/MCC	2.1	2.7	0.8491	$4,559.90
T	085	TRAUMATIC STUPOR & COMA, COMA <1 HR W MCC	4.9	6.7	1.9733	$10,597.17
T	086	TRAUMATIC STUPOR & COMA, COMA <1 HR W CC	3.3	4.2	1.1105	$5,963.70
T	087	TRAUMATIC STUPOR & COMA, COMA <1 HR W/O CC/MCC	2.2	2.7	0.7345	$3,944.47
	088	CONCUSSION W MCC	3.9	5.1	1.5029	$8,070.99
	089	CONCUSSION W CC	2.7	3.3	0.9406	$5,051.29
	090	CONCUSSION W/O CC/MCC	1.9	2.3	0.7140	$3,834.38
T	091	OTHER DISORDERS OF NERVOUS SYSTEM W MCC	4.3	5.9	1.5851	$8,512.43
T	092	OTHER DISORDERS OF NERVOUS SYSTEM W CC	3.1	3.9	0.8918	$4,789.22
T	093	OTHER DISORDERS OF NERVOUS SYSTEM W/O CC/MCC	2.2	2.7	0.6614	$3,551.90
	094	BACTERIAL & TUBERCULOUS INFECTIONS OF NERVOUS SYSTEM W MCC	8.3	10.8	3.4974	$18,782.02
	095	BACTERIAL & TUBERCULOUS INFECTIONS OF NERVOUS SYSTEM W CC	6.2	7.7	2.2787	$12,237.26
	096	BACTERIAL & TUBERCULOUS INFECTIONS OF NERVOUS SYSTEM W/O CC/MCC	4.5	5.4	1.9694	$10,576.23
	097	NON-BACTERIAL INFECT OF NERVOUS SYS EXC VIRAL MENINGITIS W MCC	8.5	11.0	3.1963	$17,165.03
	098	NON-BACTERIAL INFECT OF NERVOUS SYS EXC VIRAL MENINGITIS W CC	5.8	7.4	1.7657	$9,482.30
	099	NON-BACTERIAL INFECT OF NERVOUS SYS EXC VIRAL MENINGITIS W/O CC/MCC	4.1	5.0	1.1835	$6,355.73
T	100	SEIZURES W MCC	4.2	5.7	1.5185	$8,154.77
T	101	SEIZURES W/O MCC	2.6	3.3	0.7569	$4,064.76
	102	HEADACHES W MCC	3.1	4.2	1.0430	$5,601.20
	103	HEADACHES W/O MCC	2.3	2.9	0.6663	$3,578.22
	113	ORBITAL PROCEDURES W CC/MCC	4.0	5.6	1.8998	$10,202.46
	114	ORBITAL PROCEDURES W/O CC/MCC	2.3	2.9	1.0216	$5,486.28
	115	EXTRAOCULAR PROCEDURES EXCEPT ORBIT	3.2	4.3	1.2543	$6,735.94
	116	INTRAOCULAR PROCEDURES W CC/MCC	3.2	4.8	1.4806	$7,951.24
	117	INTRAOCULAR PROCEDURES W/O CC/MCC	1.8	2.4	0.8211	$4,409.54
	121	ACUTE MAJOR EYE INFECTIONS W CC/MCC	3.9	4.8	1.0215	$5,485.74
	122	ACUTE MAJOR EYE INFECTIONS W/O CC/MCC	2.9	3.5	0.6147	$3,301.11
	123	NEUROLOGICAL EYE DISORDERS	2.2	2.7	0.6963	$3,739.33
	124	OTHER DISORDERS OF THE EYE W MCC	3.7	5.1	1.1990	$6,438.97
	125	OTHER DISORDERS OF THE EYE W/O MCC	2.5	3.1	0.6812	$3,658.23
	129	MAJOR HEAD & NECK PROCEDURES W CC/MCC OR MAJOR DEVICE	3.6	5.1	2.1925	$11,774.34
	130	MAJOR HEAD & NECK PROCEDURES W/O CC/MCC	2.1	2.6	1.2687	$6,813.27
	131	CRANIAL/FACIAL PROCEDURES W CC/MCC	3.9	5.4	2.2038	$11,835.02
	132	CRANIAL/FACIAL PROCEDURES W/O CC/MCC	2.0	2.6	1.2855	$6,903.49
	133	OTHER EAR, NOSE, MOUTH & THROAT O.R. PROCEDURES W CC/MCC	3.6	5.3	1.7824	$9,571.99

Calculated with an average hospital Medicare base rate of $5,370.28. Each hospital's base rate and corresponding payment will vary. The national average hospital Medicare base rate is the sum of the full update labor-related and nonlabor-related amounts published in the Federal Register, FY 2014 Final Rule, Table 1A. National Adjusted Operating Standardized Amounts; Labor/Nonlabor (if wage index greater than 1) or Table 1B. National Adjusted Operating Standardized Amounts; Labor/Nonlabor (if wage index less than or equal to 1).

MS-DRGs 998 and 999 contain cases that could not be assigned to valid DRGs.

Note: If there is no value in either the geometric mean length of stay or the arithmetic mean length of stay columns, the volume of cases is insufficient to determine a meaningful computation of these statistics.

Appendix D — National Average Payment Table

DRG		Description	GMLOS	AMLOS	Relative Weight	National Payment Rate
	134	OTHER EAR, NOSE, MOUTH & THROAT O.R. PROCEDURES W/O CC/MCC	1.8	2.4	0.9584	$5,146.88
	135	SINUS & MASTOID PROCEDURES W CC/MCC	4.1	5.9	2.0110	$10,799.63
	136	SINUS & MASTOID PROCEDURES W/O CC/MCC	1.8	2.4	0.9709	$5,214.00
	137	MOUTH PROCEDURES W CC/MCC	3.7	5.0	1.3477	$7,237.53
	138	MOUTH PROCEDURES W/O CC/MCC	2.0	2.5	0.8304	$4,459.48
	139	SALIVARY GLAND PROCEDURES	1.5	2.0	0.9169	$4,924.01
	146	EAR, NOSE, MOUTH & THROAT MALIGNANCY W MCC	5.6	8.2	2.0402	$10,956.45
	147	EAR, NOSE, MOUTH & THROAT MALIGNANCY W CC	3.9	5.4	1.2317	$6,614.57
	148	EAR, NOSE, MOUTH & THROAT MALIGNANCY W/O CC/MCC	2.3	3.0	0.7688	$4,128.67
	149	DYSEQUILIBRIUM	2.1	2.5	0.6184	$3,320.98
	150	EPISTAXIS W MCC	3.7	4.9	1.3298	$7,141.40
	151	EPISTAXIS W/O MCC	2.2	2.8	0.6557	$3,521.29
	152	OTITIS MEDIA & URI W MCC	3.3	4.3	1.0042	$5,392.84
	153	OTITIS MEDIA & URI W/O MCC	2.4	2.9	0.6439	$3,457.92
	154	OTHER EAR, NOSE, MOUTH & THROAT DIAGNOSES W MCC	4.1	5.5	1.3785	$7,402.93
	155	OTHER EAR, NOSE, MOUTH & THROAT DIAGNOSES W CC	3.1	3.9	0.8610	$4,623.81
	156	OTHER EAR, NOSE, MOUTH & THROAT DIAGNOSES W/O CC/MCC	2.3	2.8	0.6160	$3,308.09
	157	DENTAL & ORAL DISEASES W MCC	4.5	6.1	1.5380	$8,259.49
	158	DENTAL & ORAL DISEASES W CC	3.1	3.9	0.8525	$4,578.16
	159	DENTAL & ORAL DISEASES W/O CC/MCC	2.1	2.6	0.6100	$3,275.87
T	163	MAJOR CHEST PROCEDURES W MCC	11.0	13.4	5.0952	$27,362.65
T	164	MAJOR CHEST PROCEDURES W CC	5.6	6.7	2.6086	$14,008.91
T	165	MAJOR CHEST PROCEDURES W/O CC/MCC	3.3	4.0	1.7943	$9,635.89
T	166	OTHER RESP SYSTEM O.R. PROCEDURES W MCC	8.8	11.2	3.6741	$19,730.95
T	167	OTHER RESP SYSTEM O.R. PROCEDURES W CC	5.2	6.6	1.9860	$10,665.38
T	168	OTHER RESP SYSTEM O.R. PROCEDURES W/O CC/MCC	3.0	3.9	1.3101	$7,035.60
T	175	PULMONARY EMBOLISM W MCC	5.3	6.4	1.5346	$8,241.23
T	176	PULMONARY EMBOLISM W/O MCC	3.7	4.4	0.9891	$5,311.74
T	177	RESPIRATORY INFECTIONS & INFLAMMATIONS W MCC	6.4	7.9	1.9934	$10,705.12
T	178	RESPIRATORY INFECTIONS & INFLAMMATIONS W CC	5.1	6.1	1.3955	$7,494.23
T	179	RESPIRATORY INFECTIONS & INFLAMMATIONS W/O CC/MCC	3.7	4.5	0.9741	$5,231.19
	180	RESPIRATORY NEOPLASMS W MCC	5.4	7.1	1.7026	$9,143.44
	181	RESPIRATORY NEOPLASMS W CC	3.8	5.0	1.1725	$6,296.65
	182	RESPIRATORY NEOPLASMS W/O CC/MCC	2.6	3.3	0.7905	$4,245.21
	183	MAJOR CHEST TRAUMA W MCC	4.8	5.9	1.4649	$7,866.92
	184	MAJOR CHEST TRAUMA W CC	3.4	4.1	0.9832	$5,280.06
	185	MAJOR CHEST TRAUMA W/O CC/MCC	2.5	2.9	0.6907	$3,709.25
T	186	PLEURAL EFFUSION W MCC	4.9	6.3	1.5727	$8,445.84

Calculated with an average hospital Medicare base rate of $5,370.28. Each hospital's base rate and corresponding payment will vary. The national average hospital Medicare base rate is the sum of the full update labor-related and nonlabor-related amounts published in the Federal Register, FY 2014 Final Rule, Table 1A. National Adjusted Operating Standardized Amounts; Labor/Nonlabor (if wage index greater than 1) or Table 1B. National Adjusted Operating Standardized Amounts; Labor/Nonlabor (if wage index less than or equal to 1).

MS-DRGs 998 and 999 contain cases that could not be assigned to valid DRGs.

Note: If there is no value in either the geometric mean length of stay or the arithmetic mean length of stay columns, the volume of cases is insufficient to determine a meaningful computation of these statistics.

T *Transfer DRG*   SP *Special Payment*

© 2013 OptumInsight, Inc.

DRG		Description	GMLOS	AMLOS	Relative Weight	National Payment Rate
T	187	PLEURAL EFFUSION W CC	3.6	4.5	1.0808	$5,804.20
T	188	PLEURAL EFFUSION W/O CC/MCC	2.6	3.3	0.7468	$4,010.53
	189	PULMONARY EDEMA & RESPIRATORY FAILURE	3.9	5.0	1.2184	$6,543.15
T	190	CHRONIC OBSTRUCTIVE PULMONARY DISEASE W MCC	4.2	5.1	1.1708	$6,287.52
T	191	CHRONIC OBSTRUCTIVE PULMONARY DISEASE W CC	3.5	4.2	0.9343	$5,017.45
T	192	CHRONIC OBSTRUCTIVE PULMONARY DISEASE W/O CC/MCC	2.8	3.3	0.7120	$3,823.64
T	193	SIMPLE PNEUMONIA & PLEURISY W MCC	5.0	6.1	1.4550	$7,813.76
T	194	SIMPLE PNEUMONIA & PLEURISY W CC	3.8	4.6	0.9771	$5,247.30
T	195	SIMPLE PNEUMONIA & PLEURISY W/O CC/MCC	2.9	3.4	0.6997	$3,757.58
T	196	INTERSTITIAL LUNG DISEASE W MCC	5.4	6.8	1.6686	$8,960.85
T	197	INTERSTITIAL LUNG DISEASE W CC	3.8	4.7	1.0627	$5,707.00
T	198	INTERSTITIAL LUNG DISEASE W/O CC/MCC	2.9	3.6	0.7958	$4,273.67
	199	PNEUMOTHORAX W MCC	5.9	7.6	1.8127	$9,734.71
	200	PNEUMOTHORAX W CC	3.3	4.3	0.9692	$5,204.88
	201	PNEUMOTHORAX W/O CC/MCC	2.6	3.3	0.7053	$3,787.66
	202	BRONCHITIS & ASTHMA W CC/MCC	3.2	3.9	0.8678	$4,660.33
	203	BRONCHITIS & ASTHMA W/O CC/MCC	2.5	3.0	0.6391	$3,432.15
	204	RESPIRATORY SIGNS & SYMPTOMS	2.1	2.7	0.6780	$3,641.05
T	205	OTHER RESPIRATORY SYSTEM DIAGNOSES W MCC	4.0	5.4	1.3935	$7,483.49
T	206	OTHER RESPIRATORY SYSTEM DIAGNOSES W/O MCC	2.5	3.2	0.7911	$4,248.43
T	207	RESPIRATORY SYSTEM DIAGNOSIS W VENTILATOR SUPPORT 96+ HOURS	12.1	14.1	5.2556	$28,224.04
	208	RESPIRATORY SYSTEM DIAGNOSIS W VENTILATOR SUPPORT <96 HOURS	5.0	6.8	2.2871	$12,282.37
	215	OTHER HEART ASSIST SYSTEM IMPLANT	10.0	16.7	14.7790	$79,367.37
SP	216	CARDIAC VALVE & OTH MAJ CARDIOTHORACIC PROC W CARD CATH W MCC	13.1	15.8	9.4801	$50,910.79
SP	217	CARDIAC VALVE & OTH MAJ CARDIOTHORACIC PROC W CARD CATH W CC	8.4	9.7	6.2835	$33,744.15
SP	218	CARDIAC VALVE & OTH MAJ CARDIOTHORACIC PROC W CARD CATH W/O CC/MCC	6.1	7.2	5.4262	$29,140.21
SP	219	CARDIAC VALVE & OTH MAJ CARDIOTHORACIC PROC W/O CARD CATH W MCC	10.0	12.1	7.9191	$42,527.78
SP	220	CARDIAC VALVE & OTH MAJ CARDIOTHORACIC PROC W/O CARD CATH W CC	6.6	7.3	5.2917	$28,417.91
SP	221	CARDIAC VALVE & OTH MAJ CARDIOTHORACIC PROC W/O CARD CATH W/O CC/MCC	4.9	5.5	4.6424	$24,930.99
	222	CARDIAC DEFIB IMPLANT W CARDIAC CATH W AMI/HF/SHOCK W MCC	9.6	11.9	8.8167	$47,348.15
	223	CARDIAC DEFIB IMPLANT W CARDIAC CATH W AMI/HF/SHOCK W/O MCC	4.6	6.2	6.4257	$34,507.81
	224	CARDIAC DEFIB IMPLANT W CARDIAC CATH W/O AMI/HF/SHOCK W MCC	8.1	10.0	7.7224	$41,471.45
	225	CARDIAC DEFIB IMPLANT W CARDIAC CATH W/O AMI/HF/SHOCK W/O MCC	4.1	4.9	5.9206	$31,795.28
	226	CARDIAC DEFIBRILLATOR IMPLANT W/O CARDIAC CATH W MCC	6.0	8.4	7.0099	$37,645.13
	227	CARDIAC DEFIBRILLATOR IMPLANT W/O CARDIAC CATH W/O MCC	2.2	3.2	5.5397	$29,749.74
	228	OTHER CARDIOTHORACIC PROCEDURES W MCC	11.1	13.2	6.8682	$36,884.16
	229	OTHER CARDIOTHORACIC PROCEDURES W CC	6.9	7.8	4.4413	$23,851.02

Calculated with an average hospital Medicare base rate of $5,370.28. Each hospital's base rate and corresponding payment will vary. The national average hospital Medicare base rate is the sum of the full update labor-related and nonlabor-related amounts published in the Federal Register, FY 2014 Final Rule, Table 1A. National Adjusted Operating Standardized Amounts; Labor/Nonlabor (if wage index greater than 1) or Table 1B. National Adjusted Operating Standardized Amounts; Labor/Nonlabor (if wage index less than or equal to 1).

MS-DRGs 998 and 999 contain cases that could not be assigned to valid DRGs.

Note: If there is no value in either the geometric mean length of stay or the arithmetic mean length of stay columns, the volume of cases is insufficient to determine a meaningful computation of these statistics.

	DRG	Description	GMLOS	AMLOS	Relative Weight	National Payment Rate
	230	OTHER CARDIOTHORACIC PROCEDURES W/O CC/MCC	4.4	5.1	3.6669	$19,692.28
	231	CORONARY BYPASS W PTCA W MCC	10.7	12.4	7.8158	$41,973.03
	232	CORONARY BYPASS W PTCA W/O MCC	8.1	8.9	5.6145	$30,151.44
T	233	CORONARY BYPASS W CARDIAC CATH W MCC	11.9	13.4	7.3887	$39,679.39
T	234	CORONARY BYPASS W CARDIAC CATH W/O MCC	8.0	8.6	4.8270	$25,922.34
T	235	CORONARY BYPASS W/O CARDIAC CATH W MCC	9.2	10.6	5.8478	$31,404.32
T	236	CORONARY BYPASS W/O CARDIAC CATH W/O MCC	6.0	6.5	3.8011	$20,412.97
	237	MAJOR CARDIOVASC PROCEDURES W MCC	6.9	9.8	5.0962	$27,368.02
	238	MAJOR CARDIOVASC PROCEDURES W/O MCC	2.6	3.8	3.3576	$18,031.25
T	239	AMPUTATION FOR CIRC SYS DISORDERS EXC UPPER LIMB & TOE W MCC	10.9	13.9	4.8601	$26,100.10
T	240	AMPUTATION FOR CIRC SYS DISORDERS EXC UPPER LIMB & TOE W CC	7.2	8.8	2.6789	$14,386.44
T	241	AMPUTATION FOR CIRC SYS DISORDERS EXC UPPER LIMB & TOE W/O CC/MCC	4.6	5.5	1.4226	$7,639.76
T	242	PERMANENT CARDIAC PACEMAKER IMPLANT W MCC	5.9	7.6	3.7491	$20,133.72
T	243	PERMANENT CARDIAC PACEMAKER IMPLANT W CC	3.7	4.6	2.6716	$14,347.24
T	244	PERMANENT CARDIAC PACEMAKER IMPLANT W/O CC/MCC	2.4	2.9	2.1608	$11,604.10
	245	AICD GENERATOR PROCEDURES	3.3	4.7	4.7022	$25,252.13
	246	PERC CARDIOVASC PROC W DRUG-ELUTING STENT W MCC OR 4+ VESSELS/STENTS	3.9	5.2	3.1830	$17,093.60
	247	PERC CARDIOVASC PROC W DRUG-ELUTING STENT W/O MCC	2.1	2.5	2.0408	$10,959.67
	248	PERC CARDIOVASC PROC W NON-DRUG-ELUTING STENT W MCC OR 4+ VES/STENTS	4.6	6.2	2.9479	$15,831.05
	249	PERC CARDIOVASC PROC W NON-DRUG-ELUTING STENT W/O MCC	2.4	3.0	1.8245	$9,798.08
	250	PERC CARDIOVASC PROC W/O CORONARY ARTERY STENT W MCC	5.1	7.0	2.9881	$16,046.93
	251	PERC CARDIOVASC PROC W/O CORONARY ARTERY STENT W/O MCC	2.4	3.1	1.9737	$10,599.32
	252	OTHER VASCULAR PROCEDURES W MCC	5.3	7.7	3.1477	$16,904.03
	253	OTHER VASCULAR PROCEDURES W CC	4.1	5.5	2.5172	$13,518.07
	254	OTHER VASCULAR PROCEDURES W/O CC/MCC	2.2	2.9	1.7012	$9,135.92
T	255	UPPER LIMB & TOE AMPUTATION FOR CIRC SYSTEM DISORDERS W MCC	6.8	8.8	2.6404	$14,179.69
T	256	UPPER LIMB & TOE AMPUTATION FOR CIRC SYSTEM DISORDERS W CC	5.3	6.5	1.5973	$8,577.95
T	257	UPPER LIMB & TOE AMPUTATION FOR CIRC SYSTEM DISORDERS W/O CC/MCC	3.0	3.7	0.9017	$4,842.38
	258	CARDIAC PACEMAKER DEVICE REPLACEMENT W MCC	4.9	6.2	2.7229	$14,622.74
	259	CARDIAC PACEMAKER DEVICE REPLACEMENT W/O MCC	2.7	3.4	1.9462	$10,451.64
	260	CARDIAC PACEMAKER REVISION EXCEPT DEVICE REPLACEMENT W MCC	7.7	10.5	3.7238	$19,997.85
	261	CARDIAC PACEMAKER REVISION EXCEPT DEVICE REPLACEMENT W CC	3.2	4.3	1.7284	$9,281.99
	262	CARDIAC PACEMAKER REVISION EXCEPT DEVICE REPLACEMENT W/O CC/MCC	2.3	2.9	1.3866	$7,446.43
	263	VEIN LIGATION & STRIPPING	3.6	5.2	1.8888	$10,143.38
T	264	OTHER CIRCULATORY SYSTEM O.R. PROCEDURES	5.6	8.2	2.7138	$14,573.87
	265	AICD LEAD PROCEDURES	2.5	3.6	2.6890	$14,440.68
T	280	ACUTE MYOCARDIAL INFARCTION, DISCHARGED ALIVE W MCC	4.7	6.0	1.7431	$9,360.94

Calculated with an average hospital Medicare base rate of $5,370.28. Each hospital's base rate and corresponding payment will vary. The national average hospital Medicare base rate is the sum of the full update labor-related and nonlabor-related amounts published in the Federal Register, FY 2014 Final Rule, Table 1A. National Adjusted Operating Standardized Amounts; Labor/Nonlabor (if wage index greater than 1) or Table 1B. National Adjusted Operating Standardized Amounts; Labor/Nonlabor (if wage index less than or equal to 1).

MS-DRGs 998 and 999 contain cases that could not be assigned to valid DRGs.

Note: If there is no value in either the geometric mean length of stay or the arithmetic mean length of stay columns, the volume of cases is insufficient to determine a meaningful computation of these statistics.

DRG		Description	GMLOS	AMLOS	Relative Weight	National Payment Rate
T	281	ACUTE MYOCARDIAL INFARCTION, DISCHARGED ALIVE W CC	3.1	3.8	1.0568	$5,675.31
T	282	ACUTE MYOCARDIAL INFARCTION, DISCHARGED ALIVE W/O CC/MCC	2.1	2.5	0.7551	$4,055.10
	283	ACUTE MYOCARDIAL INFARCTION, EXPIRED W MCC	3.0	4.7	1.6885	$9,067.72
	284	ACUTE MYOCARDIAL INFARCTION, EXPIRED W CC	1.8	2.5	0.7614	$4,088.93
	285	ACUTE MYOCARDIAL INFARCTION, EXPIRED W/O CC/MCC	1.4	1.7	0.5227	$2,807.05
	286	CIRCULATORY DISORDERS EXCEPT AMI, W CARD CATH W MCC	4.9	6.7	2.1058	$11,308.74
	287	CIRCULATORY DISORDERS EXCEPT AMI, W CARD CATH W/O MCC	2.4	3.1	1.0866	$5,835.35
T	288	ACUTE & SUBACUTE ENDOCARDITIS W MCC	7.8	9.9	2.7956	$15,013.15
T	289	ACUTE & SUBACUTE ENDOCARDITIS W CC	5.7	7.0	1.7891	$9,607.97
T	290	ACUTE & SUBACUTE ENDOCARDITIS W/O CC/MCC	3.9	4.8	1.2359	$6,637.13
T	291	HEART FAILURE & SHOCK W MCC	4.6	5.9	1.5031	$8,072.07
T	292	HEART FAILURE & SHOCK W CC	3.7	4.5	0.9938	$5,336.98
T	293	HEART FAILURE & SHOCK W/O CC/MCC	2.6	3.1	0.6723	$3,610.44
	294	DEEP VEIN THROMBOPHLEBITIS W CC/MCC	4.0	4.9	0.9439	$5,069.01
	295	DEEP VEIN THROMBOPHLEBITIS W/O CC/MCC	3.1	3.6	0.6287	$3,376.30
	296	CARDIAC ARREST, UNEXPLAINED W MCC	1.9	2.9	1.3013	$6,988.35
	297	CARDIAC ARREST, UNEXPLAINED W CC	1.2	1.5	0.6063	$3,256.00
	298	CARDIAC ARREST, UNEXPLAINED W/O CC/MCC	1.0	1.1	0.4260	$2,287.74
T	299	PERIPHERAL VASCULAR DISORDERS W MCC	4.4	5.6	1.3647	$7,328.82
T	300	PERIPHERAL VASCULAR DISORDERS W CC	3.6	4.5	0.9666	$5,190.91
T	301	PERIPHERAL VASCULAR DISORDERS W/O CC/MCC	2.7	3.3	0.6681	$3,587.88
	302	ATHEROSCLEROSIS W MCC	2.9	3.9	1.0287	$5,524.41
	303	ATHEROSCLEROSIS W/O MCC	1.9	2.3	0.6034	$3,240.43
	304	HYPERTENSION W MCC	3.3	4.4	1.0268	$5,514.20
	305	HYPERTENSION W/O MCC	2.1	2.6	0.6176	$3,316.68
	306	CARDIAC CONGENITAL & VALVULAR DISORDERS W MCC	3.9	5.3	1.3659	$7,335.27
	307	CARDIAC CONGENITAL & VALVULAR DISORDERS W/O MCC	2.6	3.3	0.7917	$4,251.65
	308	CARDIAC ARRHYTHMIA & CONDUCTION DISORDERS W MCC	3.8	4.9	1.2088	$6,491.59
	309	CARDIAC ARRHYTHMIA & CONDUCTION DISORDERS W CC	2.7	3.3	0.7867	$4,224.80
	310	CARDIAC ARRHYTHMIA & CONDUCTION DISORDERS W/O CC/MCC	1.9	2.3	0.5512	$2,960.10
	311	ANGINA PECTORIS	1.8	2.2	0.5649	$3,033.67
	312	SYNCOPE & COLLAPSE	2.4	3.0	0.7228	$3,881.64
	313	CHEST PAIN	1.8	2.1	0.5992	$3,217.87
T	314	OTHER CIRCULATORY SYSTEM DIAGNOSES W MCC	4.9	6.7	1.8941	$10,171.85
T	315	OTHER CIRCULATORY SYSTEM DIAGNOSES W CC	3.1	4.0	0.9534	$5,120.02
T	316	OTHER CIRCULATORY SYSTEM DIAGNOSES W/O CC/MCC	2.0	2.5	0.6358	$3,414.42
T	326	STOMACH, ESOPHAGEAL & DUODENAL PROC W MCC	11.6	14.9	5.6013	$30,080.55
T	327	STOMACH, ESOPHAGEAL & DUODENAL PROC W CC	6.1	8.0	2.6598	$14,283.87

Calculated with an average hospital Medicare base rate of $5,370.28. Each hospital's base rate and corresponding payment will vary. The national average hospital Medicare base rate is the sum of the full update labor-related and nonlabor-related amounts published in the Federal Register, FY 2014 Final Rule, Table 1A. National Adjusted Operating Standardized Amounts; Labor/Nonlabor (if wage index greater than 1) or Table 1B. National Adjusted Operating Standardized Amounts; Labor/Nonlabor (if wage index less than or equal to 1).

MS-DRGs 998 and 999 contain cases that could not be assigned to valid DRGs.

Note: If there is no value in either the geometric mean length of stay or the arithmetic mean length of stay columns, the volume of cases is insufficient to determine a meaningful computation of these statistics.

DRG		Description	GMLOS	AMLOS	Relative Weight	National Payment Rate
T	328	STOMACH, ESOPHAGEAL & DUODENAL PROC W/O CC/MCC	2.6	3.4	1.4765	$7,929.22
T	329	MAJOR SMALL & LARGE BOWEL PROCEDURES W MCC	11.9	14.6	5.1272	$27,534.50
T	330	MAJOR SMALL & LARGE BOWEL PROCEDURES W CC	7.3	8.5	2.5609	$13,752.75
T	331	MAJOR SMALL & LARGE BOWEL PROCEDURES W/O CC/MCC	4.4	4.9	1.6380	$8,796.52
T	332	RECTAL RESECTION W MCC	10.9	13.2	4.7072	$25,278.98
T	333	RECTAL RESECTION W CC	6.4	7.4	2.4466	$13,138.93
T	334	RECTAL RESECTION W/O CC/MCC	3.7	4.3	1.5849	$8,511.36
T	335	PERITONEAL ADHESIOLYSIS W MCC	10.7	13.0	4.1615	$22,348.42
T	336	PERITONEAL ADHESIOLYSIS W CC	7.0	8.4	2.3513	$12,627.14
T	337	PERITONEAL ADHESIOLYSIS W/O CC/MCC	4.1	5.0	1.5742	$8,453.89
	338	APPENDECTOMY W COMPLICATED PRINCIPAL DIAG W MCC	7.8	9.5	3.1217	$16,764.40
	339	APPENDECTOMY W COMPLICATED PRINCIPAL DIAG W CC	5.1	6.0	1.7117	$9,192.31
	340	APPENDECTOMY W COMPLICATED PRINCIPAL DIAG W/O CC/MCC	3.0	3.5	1.1741	$6,305.25
	341	APPENDECTOMY W/O COMPLICATED PRINCIPAL DIAG W MCC	4.6	6.3	2.1821	$11,718.49
	342	APPENDECTOMY W/O COMPLICATED PRINCIPAL DIAG W CC	2.8	3.5	1.2968	$6,964.18
	343	APPENDECTOMY W/O COMPLICATED PRINCIPAL DIAG W/O CC/MCC	1.6	1.9	0.9358	$5,025.51
	344	MINOR SMALL & LARGE BOWEL PROCEDURES W MCC	8.9	11.3	3.5966	$19,314.75
	345	MINOR SMALL & LARGE BOWEL PROCEDURES W CC	5.5	6.5	1.6865	$9,056.98
	346	MINOR SMALL & LARGE BOWEL PROCEDURES W/O CC/MCC	4.0	4.4	1.2174	$6,537.78
	347	ANAL & STOMAL PROCEDURES W MCC	6.3	8.5	2.5182	$13,523.44
	348	ANAL & STOMAL PROCEDURES W CC	4.0	5.1	1.3585	$7,295.53
	349	ANAL & STOMAL PROCEDURES W/O CC/MCC	2.4	3.0	0.8834	$4,744.11
	350	INGUINAL & FEMORAL HERNIA PROCEDURES W MCC	5.8	7.8	2.4598	$13,209.81
	351	INGUINAL & FEMORAL HERNIA PROCEDURES W CC	3.5	4.5	1.3761	$7,390.04
	352	INGUINAL & FEMORAL HERNIA PROCEDURES W/O CC/MCC	2.0	2.5	0.9239	$4,961.60
	353	HERNIA PROCEDURES EXCEPT INGUINAL & FEMORAL W MCC	6.2	8.0	2.7885	$14,975.03
	354	HERNIA PROCEDURES EXCEPT INGUINAL & FEMORAL W CC	4.0	5.0	1.6401	$8,807.80
	355	HERNIA PROCEDURES EXCEPT INGUINAL & FEMORAL W/O CC/MCC	2.5	3.0	1.1783	$6,327.80
T	356	OTHER DIGESTIVE SYSTEM O.R. PROCEDURES W MCC	8.6	11.5	3.8388	$20,615.43
T	357	OTHER DIGESTIVE SYSTEM O.R. PROCEDURES W CC	5.4	6.9	2.1448	$11,518.18
T	358	OTHER DIGESTIVE SYSTEM O.R. PROCEDURES W/O CC/MCC	3.2	4.1	1.3942	$7,487.24
	368	MAJOR ESOPHAGEAL DISORDERS W MCC	5.0	6.6	1.8779	$10,084.85
	369	MAJOR ESOPHAGEAL DISORDERS W CC	3.5	4.2	1.0660	$5,724.72
	370	MAJOR ESOPHAGEAL DISORDERS W/O CC/MCC	2.5	3.0	0.7486	$4,020.19
T	371	MAJOR GASTROINTESTINAL DISORDERS & PERITONEAL INFECTIONS W MCC	6.2	7.9	1.9027	$10,218.03
T	372	MAJOR GASTROINTESTINAL DISORDERS & PERITONEAL INFECTIONS W CC	4.8	5.8	1.1733	$6,300.95
T	373	MAJOR GASTROINTESTINAL DISORDERS & PERITONEAL INFECTIONS W/O CC/MCC	3.6	4.2	0.8103	$4,351.54

Calculated with an average hospital Medicare base rate of $5,370.28. Each hospital's base rate and corresponding payment will vary. The national average hospital Medicare base rate is the sum of the full update labor-related and nonlabor-related amounts published in the Federal Register, FY 2014 Final Rule, Table 1A. National Adjusted Operating Standardized Amounts; Labor/Nonlabor (if wage index greater than 1) or Table 1B. National Adjusted Operating Standardized Amounts; Labor/Nonlabor (if wage index less than or equal to 1).

MS-DRGs 998 and 999 contain cases that could not be assigned to valid DRGs.

Note: If there is no value in either the geometric mean length of stay or the arithmetic mean length of stay columns, the volume of cases is insufficient to determine a meaningful computation of these statistics.

DRG		Description	GMLOS	AMLOS	Relative Weight	National Payment Rate
T	374	DIGESTIVE MALIGNANCY W MCC	6.2	8.4	2.1051	$11,304.98
T	375	DIGESTIVE MALIGNANCY W CC	4.2	5.4	1.2561	$6,745.61
T	376	DIGESTIVE MALIGNANCY W/O CC/MCC	2.7	3.5	0.8738	$4,692.55
T	377	G.I. HEMORRHAGE W MCC	4.8	6.1	1.7629	$9,467.27
T	378	G.I. HEMORRHAGE W CC	3.3	3.9	1.0029	$5,385.85
T	379	G.I. HEMORRHAGE W/O CC/MCC	2.4	2.8	0.6937	$3,725.36
T	380	COMPLICATED PEPTIC ULCER W MCC	5.5	7.2	1.9223	$10,323.29
T	381	COMPLICATED PEPTIC ULCER W CC	3.8	4.6	1.1199	$6,014.18
T	382	COMPLICATED PEPTIC ULCER W/O CC/MCC	2.7	3.3	0.7784	$4,180.23
	383	UNCOMPLICATED PEPTIC ULCER W MCC	4.4	5.5	1.3850	$7,437.84
	384	UNCOMPLICATED PEPTIC ULCER W/O MCC	3.0	3.6	0.8501	$4,565.28
	385	INFLAMMATORY BOWEL DISEASE W MCC	6.0	7.8	1.7973	$9,652.00
	386	INFLAMMATORY BOWEL DISEASE W CC	4.0	5.0	1.0097	$5,422.37
	387	INFLAMMATORY BOWEL DISEASE W/O CC/MCC	3.1	3.8	0.7533	$4,045.43
T	388	G.I. OBSTRUCTION W MCC	5.3	7.0	1.6170	$8,683.74
T	389	G.I. OBSTRUCTION W CC	3.6	4.5	0.8853	$4,754.31
T	390	G.I. OBSTRUCTION W/O CC/MCC	2.7	3.2	0.6046	$3,246.87
	391	ESOPHAGITIS, GASTROENT & MISC DIGEST DISORDERS W MCC	3.9	5.1	1.1903	$6,392.24
	392	ESOPHAGITIS, GASTROENT & MISC DIGEST DISORDERS W/O MCC	2.9	3.5	0.7395	$3,971.32
	393	OTHER DIGESTIVE SYSTEM DIAGNOSES W MCC	4.7	6.5	1.6563	$8,894.79
	394	OTHER DIGESTIVE SYSTEM DIAGNOSES W CC	3.5	4.4	0.9653	$5,183.93
	395	OTHER DIGESTIVE SYSTEM DIAGNOSES W/O CC/MCC	2.4	3.0	0.6669	$3,581.44
T	405	PANCREAS, LIVER & SHUNT PROCEDURES W MCC	11.0	14.5	5.4333	$29,178.34
T	406	PANCREAS, LIVER & SHUNT PROCEDURES W CC	6.0	7.6	2.7667	$14,857.95
T	407	PANCREAS, LIVER & SHUNT PROCEDURES W/O CC/MCC	4.2	5.1	1.9139	$10,278.18
	408	BILIARY TRACT PROC EXCEPT ONLY CHOLECYST W OR W/O C.D.E. W MCC	10.6	13.2	4.1182	$22,115.89
	409	BILIARY TRACT PROC EXCEPT ONLY CHOLECYST W OR W/O C.D.E. W CC	6.7	7.9	2.4337	$13,069.65
	410	BILIARY TRACT PROC EXCEPT ONLY CHOLECYST W OR W/O C.D.E. W/O CC/MCC	4.3	5.0	1.5123	$8,121.47
	411	CHOLECYSTECTOMY W C.D.E. W MCC	9.3	11.3	3.5968	$19,315.82
	412	CHOLECYSTECTOMY W C.D.E. W CC	6.5	7.6	2.3659	$12,705.55
	413	CHOLECYSTECTOMY W C.D.E. W/O CC/MCC	4.2	5.0	1.7220	$9,247.62
T	414	CHOLECYSTECTOMY EXCEPT BY LAPAROSCOPE W/O C.D.E. W MCC	8.8	10.6	3.6208	$19,444.71
T	415	CHOLECYSTECTOMY EXCEPT BY LAPAROSCOPE W/O C.D.E. W CC	5.8	6.7	2.0173	$10,833.47
T	416	CHOLECYSTECTOMY EXCEPT BY LAPAROSCOPE W/O C.D.E. W/O CC/MCC	3.5	4.1	1.3268	$7,125.29
	417	LAPAROSCOPIC CHOLECYSTECTOMY W/O C.D.E. W MCC	6.0	7.5	2.4784	$13,309.70
	418	LAPAROSCOPIC CHOLECYSTECTOMY W/O C.D.E. W CC	4.1	5.0	1.6536	$8,880.30
	419	LAPAROSCOPIC CHOLECYSTECTOMY W/O C.D.E. W/O CC/MCC	2.6	3.1	1.2239	$6,572.69
	420	HEPATOBILIARY DIAGNOSTIC PROCEDURES W MCC	8.7	12.3	3.6786	$19,755.11

Calculated with an average hospital Medicare base rate of $5,370.28. Each hospital's base rate and corresponding payment will vary. The national average hospital Medicare base rate is the sum of the full update labor-related and nonlabor-related amounts published in the Federal Register, FY 2014 Final Rule, Table 1A. National Adjusted Operating Standardized Amounts; Labor/Nonlabor (if wage index greater than 1) or Table 1B. National Adjusted Operating Standardized Amounts; Labor/Nonlabor (if wage index less than or equal to 1).

MS-DRGs 998 and 999 contain cases that could not be assigned to valid DRGs.

Note: If there is no value in either the geometric mean length of stay or the arithmetic mean length of stay columns, the volume of cases is insufficient to determine a meaningful computation of these statistics.

DRG		Description	GMLOS	AMLOS	Relative Weight	National Payment Rate
	421	HEPATOBILIARY DIAGNOSTIC PROCEDURES W CC	4.6	6.3	1.7714	$9,512.91
	422	HEPATOBILIARY DIAGNOSTIC PROCEDURES W/O CC/MCC	3.1	3.9	1.2175	$6,538.32
	423	OTHER HEPATOBILIARY OR PANCREAS O.R. PROCEDURES W MCC	9.6	13.0	4.2183	$22,653.45
	424	OTHER HEPATOBILIARY OR PANCREAS O.R. PROCEDURES W CC	6.3	8.2	2.3149	$12,431.66
	425	OTHER HEPATOBILIARY OR PANCREAS O.R. PROCEDURES W/O CC/MCC	3.8	4.9	1.6396	$8,805.11
	432	CIRRHOSIS & ALCOHOLIC HEPATITIS W MCC	4.7	6.3	1.7150	$9,210.03
	433	CIRRHOSIS & ALCOHOLIC HEPATITIS W CC	3.3	4.1	0.9249	$4,966.97
	434	CIRRHOSIS & ALCOHOLIC HEPATITIS W/O CC/MCC	2.4	3.0	0.6156	$3,305.94
	435	MALIGNANCY OF HEPATOBILIARY SYSTEM OR PANCREAS W MCC	5.2	6.9	1.7356	$9,320.66
	436	MALIGNANCY OF HEPATOBILIARY SYSTEM OR PANCREAS W CC	3.9	5.0	1.1548	$6,201.60
	437	MALIGNANCY OF HEPATOBILIARY SYSTEM OR PANCREAS W/O CC/MCC	2.8	3.6	0.9282	$4,984.69
	438	DISORDERS OF PANCREAS EXCEPT MALIGNANCY W MCC	5.1	7.0	1.7210	$9,242.25
	439	DISORDERS OF PANCREAS EXCEPT MALIGNANCY W CC	3.6	4.5	0.9162	$4,920.25
	440	DISORDERS OF PANCREAS EXCEPT MALIGNANCY W/O CC/MCC	2.7	3.2	0.6452	$3,464.90
T	441	DISORDERS OF LIVER EXCEPT MALIG,CIRR,ALC HEPA W MCC	5.0	6.8	1.8534	$9,953.28
T	442	DISORDERS OF LIVER EXCEPT MALIG,CIRR,ALC HEPA W CC	3.4	4.3	0.9280	$4,983.62
T	443	DISORDERS OF LIVER EXCEPT MALIG,CIRR,ALC HEPA W/O CC/MCC	2.6	3.2	0.6418	$3,446.65
	444	DISORDERS OF THE BILIARY TRACT W MCC	4.7	6.1	1.6060	$8,624.67
	445	DISORDERS OF THE BILIARY TRACT W CC	3.4	4.2	1.0476	$5,625.91
	446	DISORDERS OF THE BILIARY TRACT W/O CC/MCC	2.4	2.9	0.7499	$4,027.17
	453	COMBINED ANTERIOR/POSTERIOR SPINAL FUSION W MCC	9.7	12.2	11.7453	$63,075.55
	454	COMBINED ANTERIOR/POSTERIOR SPINAL FUSION W CC	5.1	6.1	8.0200	$43,069.65
	455	COMBINED ANTERIOR/POSTERIOR SPINAL FUSION W/O CC/MCC	3.1	3.6	6.2882	$33,769.39
	456	SPINAL FUS EXC CERV W SPINAL CURV/MALIG/INFEC OR 9+ FUS W MCC	10.2	12.5	9.5871	$51,485.41
	457	SPINAL FUS EXC CERV W SPINAL CURV/MALIG/INFEC OR 9+ FUS W CC	5.6	6.5	6.8188	$36,618.87
	458	SPINAL FUS EXC CERV W SPINAL CURV/MALIG/INFEC OR 9+ FUS W/O CC/MCC	3.3	3.8	5.1378	$27,591.42
T	459	SPINAL FUSION EXCEPT CERVICAL W MCC	7.1	8.7	6.8163	$36,605.44
T	460	SPINAL FUSION EXCEPT CERVICAL W/O MCC	3.1	3.6	4.0221	$21,599.80
	461	BILATERAL OR MULTIPLE MAJOR JOINT PROCS OF LOWER EXTREMITY W MCC	6.1	7.5	5.0254	$26,987.81
	462	BILATERAL OR MULTIPLE MAJOR JOINT PROCS OF LOWER EXTREMITY W/O MCC	3.5	3.8	3.5190	$18,898.02
T	463	WND DEBRID & SKN GRFT EXC HAND, FOR MUSCULO-CONN TISS DIS W MCC	10.4	14.0	5.1152	$27,470.06
T	464	WND DEBRID & SKN GRFT EXC HAND, FOR MUSCULO-CONN TISS DIS W CC	6.2	8.0	3.0243	$16,241.34
T	465	WND DEBRID & SKN GRFT EXC HAND, FOR MUSCULO-CONN TISS DIS W/O CC/MCC	3.8	4.8	1.9199	$10,310.40
T	466	REVISION OF HIP OR KNEE REPLACEMENT W MCC	7.0	8.6	5.2748	$28,327.15
T	467	REVISION OF HIP OR KNEE REPLACEMENT W CC	3.9	4.5	3.4140	$18,334.14
T	468	REVISION OF HIP OR KNEE REPLACEMENT W/O CC/MCC	3.0	3.2	2.7624	$14,834.86
T	469	MAJOR JOINT REPLACEMENT OR REATTACHMENT OF LOWER EXTREMITY W MCC	6.2	7.4	3.4377	$18,461.41

Calculated with an average hospital Medicare base rate of $5,370.28. Each hospital's base rate and corresponding payment will vary. The national average hospital Medicare base rate is the sum of the full update labor-related and nonlabor-related amounts published in the Federal Register, FY 2014 Final Rule, Table 1A. National Adjusted Operating Standardized Amounts; Labor/Nonlabor (if wage index greater than 1) or Table 1B. National Adjusted Operating Standardized Amounts; Labor/Nonlabor (if wage index less than or equal to 1).

MS-DRGs 998 and 999 contain cases that could not be assigned to valid DRGs.

Note: If there is no value in either the geometric mean length of stay or the arithmetic mean length of stay columns, the volume of cases is insufficient to determine a meaningful computation of these statistics.

	DRG	Description	GMLOS	AMLOS	Relative Weight	National Payment Rate
T	470	MAJOR JOINT REPLACEMENT OR REATTACHMENT OF LOWER EXTREMITY W/O MCC	3.1	3.4	2.1463	$11,526.23
	471	CERVICAL SPINAL FUSION W MCC	6.4	8.9	4.9444	$26,552.81
	472	CERVICAL SPINAL FUSION W CC	2.5	3.5	2.9288	$15,728.48
	473	CERVICAL SPINAL FUSION W/O CC/MCC	1.5	1.8	2.2458	$12,060.57
T	474	AMPUTATION FOR MUSCULOSKELETAL SYS & CONN TISSUE DIS W MCC	8.8	11.2	3.6884	$19,807.74
T	475	AMPUTATION FOR MUSCULOSKELETAL SYS & CONN TISSUE DIS W CC	5.7	7.1	2.0488	$11,002.63
T	476	AMPUTATION FOR MUSCULOSKELETAL SYS & CONN TISSUE DIS W/O CC/MCC	3.1	3.9	1.0717	$5,755.33
SP	477	BIOPSIES OF MUSCULOSKELETAL SYSTEM & CONNECTIVE TISSUE W MCC	8.6	10.8	3.2827	$17,629.02
SP	478	BIOPSIES OF MUSCULOSKELETAL SYSTEM & CONNECTIVE TISSUE W CC	5.4	6.7	2.2115	$11,876.37
SP	479	BIOPSIES OF MUSCULOSKELETAL SYSTEM & CONNECTIVE TISSUE W/O CC/MCC	3.3	4.2	1.7340	$9,312.07
SP	480	HIP & FEMUR PROCEDURES EXCEPT MAJOR JOINT W MCC	7.1	8.3	3.0694	$16,483.54
SP	481	HIP & FEMUR PROCEDURES EXCEPT MAJOR JOINT W CC	4.8	5.2	1.9721	$10,590.73
SP	482	HIP & FEMUR PROCEDURES EXCEPT MAJOR JOINT W/O CC/MCC	3.9	4.2	1.6305	$8,756.24
T	483	MAJOR JOINT & LIMB REATTACHMENT PROC OF UPPER EXTREMITY W CC/MCC	2.8	3.4	2.6488	$14,224.80
T	484	MAJOR JOINT & LIMB REATTACHMENT PROC OF UPPER EXTREMITY W/O CC/MCC	1.8	2.0	2.2298	$11,974.65
	485	KNEE PROCEDURES W PDX OF INFECTION W MCC	8.4	10.3	3.2719	$17,571.02
	486	KNEE PROCEDURES W PDX OF INFECTION W CC	5.6	6.5	2.0199	$10,847.43
	487	KNEE PROCEDURES W PDX OF INFECTION W/O CC/MCC	4.1	4.6	1.5215	$8,170.88
T	488	KNEE PROCEDURES W/O PDX OF INFECTION W CC/MCC	3.5	4.3	1.7379	$9,333.01
T	489	KNEE PROCEDURES W/O PDX OF INFECTION W/O CC/MCC	2.5	2.8	1.2799	$6,873.42
	490	BACK & NECK PROC EXC SPINAL FUSION W CC/MCC OR DISC DEVICE/NEUROSTIM	3.4	4.6	1.8845	$10,120.29
	491	BACK & NECK PROC EXC SPINAL FUSION W/O CC/MCC	1.9	2.3	1.0893	$5,849.85
SP	492	LOWER EXTREM & HUMER PROC EXCEPT HIP,FOOT,FEMUR W MCC	6.4	8.0	3.1831	$17,094.14
SP	493	LOWER EXTREM & HUMER PROC EXCEPT HIP,FOOT,FEMUR W CC	4.0	4.8	1.9971	$10,724.99
SP	494	LOWER EXTREM & HUMER PROC EXCEPT HIP,FOOT,FEMUR W/O CC/MCC	2.7	3.2	1.5073	$8,094.62
SP	495	LOCAL EXCISION & REMOVAL INT FIX DEVICES EXC HIP & FEMUR W MCC	7.2	9.6	2.9110	$15,632.89
SP	496	LOCAL EXCISION & REMOVAL INT FIX DEVICES EXC HIP & FEMUR W CC	4.0	5.2	1.7290	$9,285.21
SP	497	LOCAL EXCISION & REMOVAL INT FIX DEVICES EXC HIP & FEMUR W/O CC/MCC	2.1	2.6	1.1731	$6,299.88
	498	LOCAL EXCISION & REMOVAL INT FIX DEVICES OF HIP & FEMUR W CC/MCC	5.3	7.2	2.1924	$11,773.80
	499	LOCAL EXCISION & REMOVAL INT FIX DEVICES OF HIP & FEMUR W/O CC/MCC	2.1	2.6	0.9577	$5,143.12
SP	500	SOFT TISSUE PROCEDURES W MCC	7.3	9.8	3.0116	$16,173.14
SP	501	SOFT TISSUE PROCEDURES W CC	4.4	5.5	1.5804	$8,487.19
SP	502	SOFT TISSUE PROCEDURES W/O CC/MCC	2.4	2.9	1.1277	$6,056.06
	503	FOOT PROCEDURES W MCC	6.3	7.8	2.2584	$12,128.24
	504	FOOT PROCEDURES W CC	4.9	5.9	1.6133	$8,663.87
	505	FOOT PROCEDURES W/O CC/MCC	2.7	3.3	1.2072	$6,483.00
	506	MAJOR THUMB OR JOINT PROCEDURES	2.9	3.8	1.2041	$6,466.35

Calculated with an average hospital Medicare base rate of $5,370.28. Each hospital's base rate and corresponding payment will vary. The national average hospital Medicare base rate is the sum of the full update labor-related and nonlabor-related amounts published in the Federal Register, FY 2014 Final Rule, Table 1A. National Adjusted Operating Standardized Amounts; Labor/Nonlabor (if wage index greater than 1) or Table 1B. National Adjusted Operating Standardized Amounts; Labor/Nonlabor (if wage index less than or equal to 1).

MS-DRGs 998 and 999 contain cases that could not be assigned to valid DRGs.

Note: If there is no value in either the geometric mean length of stay or the arithmetic mean length of stay columns, the volume of cases is insufficient to determine a meaningful computation of these statistics.

DRG		Description	GMLOS	AMLOS	Relative Weight	National Payment Rate
	507	MAJOR SHOULDER OR ELBOW JOINT PROCEDURES W CC/MCC	4.1	5.6	1.9667	$10,561.73
	508	MAJOR SHOULDER OR ELBOW JOINT PROCEDURES W/O CC/MCC	2.0	2.4	1.3190	$7,083.40
	509	ARTHROSCOPY	2.7	3.5	1.3245	$7,112.94
T	510	SHOULDER,ELBOW OR FOREARM PROC,EXC MAJOR JOINT PROC W MCC	4.8	6.0	2.2717	$12,199.67
T	511	SHOULDER,ELBOW OR FOREARM PROC,EXC MAJOR JOINT PROC W CC	3.2	3.8	1.5894	$8,535.52
T	512	SHOULDER,ELBOW OR FOREARM PROC,EXC MAJOR JOINT PROC W/O CC/MCC	2.0	2.3	1.2266	$6,587.19
	513	HAND OR WRIST PROC, EXCEPT MAJOR THUMB OR JOINT PROC W CC/MCC	3.7	4.9	1.4122	$7,583.91
	514	HAND OR WRIST PROC, EXCEPT MAJOR THUMB OR JOINT PROC W/O CC/MCC	2.2	2.7	0.8781	$4,715.64
SP	515	OTHER MUSCULOSKELET SYS & CONN TISS O.R. PROC W MCC	7.5	9.6	3.3340	$17,904.51
SP	516	OTHER MUSCULOSKELET SYS & CONN TISS O.R. PROC W CC	4.5	5.5	2.0160	$10,826.48
SP	517	OTHER MUSCULOSKELET SYS & CONN TISS O.R. PROC W/O CC/MCC	2.8	3.4	1.6777	$9,009.72
T	533	FRACTURES OF FEMUR W MCC	4.3	5.6	1.3759	$7,388.97
T	534	FRACTURES OF FEMUR W/O MCC	2.9	3.6	0.7364	$3,954.67
T	535	FRACTURES OF HIP & PELVIS W MCC	4.2	5.4	1.3085	$7,027.01
T	536	FRACTURES OF HIP & PELVIS W/O MCC	3.0	3.5	0.7091	$3,808.07
	537	SPRAINS, STRAINS, & DISLOCATIONS OF HIP, PELVIS & THIGH W CC/MCC	3.4	4.0	0.8604	$4,620.59
	538	SPRAINS, STRAINS, & DISLOCATIONS OF HIP, PELVIS & THIGH W/O CC/MCC	2.4	2.8	0.6870	$3,689.38
T	539	OSTEOMYELITIS W MCC	6.2	8.1	1.8631	$10,005.37
T	540	OSTEOMYELITIS W CC	4.9	6.1	1.3063	$7,015.20
T	541	OSTEOMYELITIS W/O CC/MCC	3.6	4.7	0.9743	$5,232.26
T	542	PATHOLOGICAL FRACTURES & MUSCULOSKELET & CONN TISS MALIG W MCC	6.0	7.9	1.9451	$10,445.73
T	543	PATHOLOGICAL FRACTURES & MUSCULOSKELET & CONN TISS MALIG W CC	4.2	5.2	1.1267	$6,050.69
T	544	PATHOLOGICAL FRACTURES & MUSCULOSKELET & CONN TISS MALIG W/O CC/MCC	3.2	3.7	0.7736	$4,154.45
T	545	CONNECTIVE TISSUE DISORDERS W MCC	6.0	8.5	2.4445	$13,127.65
T	546	CONNECTIVE TISSUE DISORDERS W CC	4.0	5.0	1.1711	$6,289.13
T	547	CONNECTIVE TISSUE DISORDERS W/O CC/MCC	2.9	3.6	0.8061	$4,328.98
	548	SEPTIC ARTHRITIS W MCC	5.9	7.6	1.7811	$9,565.01
	549	SEPTIC ARTHRITIS W CC	4.3	5.2	1.1101	$5,961.55
	550	SEPTIC ARTHRITIS W/O CC/MCC	3.1	3.8	0.8149	$4,376.24
T	551	MEDICAL BACK PROBLEMS W MCC	5.0	6.4	1.6317	$8,762.69
T	552	MEDICAL BACK PROBLEMS W/O MCC	3.2	3.9	0.8467	$4,547.02
	553	BONE DISEASES & ARTHROPATHIES W MCC	4.4	5.6	1.2370	$6,643.04
	554	BONE DISEASES & ARTHROPATHIES W/O MCC	2.9	3.6	0.7181	$3,856.40
	555	SIGNS & SYMPTOMS OF MUSCULOSKELETAL SYSTEM & CONN TISSUE W MCC	3.7	5.0	1.1974	$6,430.37
	556	SIGNS & SYMPTOMS OF MUSCULOSKELETAL SYSTEM & CONN TISSUE W/O MCC	2.6	3.2	0.7066	$3,794.64
T	557	TENDONITIS, MYOSITIS & BURSITIS W MCC	5.1	6.4	1.4756	$7,924.39
T	558	TENDONITIS, MYOSITIS & BURSITIS W/O MCC	3.4	4.0	0.8337	$4,477.20

Calculated with an average hospital Medicare base rate of $5,370.28. Each hospital's base rate and corresponding payment will vary. The national average hospital Medicare base rate is the sum of the full update labor-related and nonlabor-related amounts published in the Federal Register, FY 2014 Final Rule, Table 1A. National Adjusted Operating Standardized Amounts; Labor/Nonlabor (if wage index greater than 1) or Table 1B. National Adjusted Operating Standardized Amounts; Labor/Nonlabor (if wage index less than or equal to 1).

MS-DRGs 998 and 999 contain cases that could not be assigned to valid DRGs.

Note: If there is no value in either the geometric mean length of stay or the arithmetic mean length of stay columns, the volume of cases is insufficient to determine a meaningful computation of these statistics.

T *Transfer DRG*   SP *Special Payment*

DRG		Description	GMLOS	AMLOS	Relative Weight	National Payment Rate
T	559	AFTERCARE, MUSCULOSKELETAL SYSTEM & CONNECTIVE TISSUE W MCC	5.0	6.9	1.8639	$10,009.66
T	560	AFTERCARE, MUSCULOSKELETAL SYSTEM & CONNECTIVE TISSUE W CC	3.4	4.4	1.0260	$5,509.91
T	561	AFTERCARE, MUSCULOSKELETAL SYSTEM & CONNECTIVE TISSUE W/O CC/MCC	2.0	2.5	0.6408	$3,441.28
T	562	FX, SPRN, STRN & DISL EXCEPT FEMUR, HIP, PELVIS & THIGH W MCC	4.4	5.5	1.3528	$7,264.91
T	563	FX, SPRN, STRN & DISL EXCEPT FEMUR, HIP, PELVIS & THIGH W/O MCC	3.0	3.5	0.7535	$4,046.51
	564	OTHER MUSCULOSKELETAL SYS & CONNECTIVE TISSUE DIAGNOSES W MCC	4.5	6.1	1.4855	$7,977.55
	565	OTHER MUSCULOSKELETAL SYS & CONNECTIVE TISSUE DIAGNOSES W CC	3.6	4.4	0.9281	$4,984.16
	566	OTHER MUSCULOSKELETAL SYS & CONNECTIVE TISSUE DIAGNOSES W/O CC/MCC	2.6	3.3	0.6642	$3,566.94
T	570	SKIN DEBRIDEMENT W MCC	7.2	9.4	2.4154	$12,971.37
T	571	SKIN DEBRIDEMENT W CC	5.4	6.5	1.4906	$8,004.94
T	572	SKIN DEBRIDEMENT W/O CC/MCC	3.8	4.6	1.0077	$5,411.63
T	573	SKIN GRAFT FOR SKIN ULCER OR CELLULITIS W MCC	8.2	12.3	3.4623	$18,593.52
T	574	SKIN GRAFT FOR SKIN ULCER OR CELLULITIS W CC	7.1	9.6	2.6883	$14,436.92
T	575	SKIN GRAFT FOR SKIN ULCER OR CELLULITIS W/O CC/MCC	4.2	5.4	1.4376	$7,720.31
	576	SKIN GRAFT EXC FOR SKIN ULCER OR CELLULITIS W MCC	7.9	12.3	4.2927	$23,053.00
	577	SKIN GRAFT EXC FOR SKIN ULCER OR CELLULITIS W CC	4.0	5.9	2.0212	$10,854.41
	578	SKIN GRAFT EXC FOR SKIN ULCER OR CELLULITIS W/O CC/MCC	2.4	3.3	1.2617	$6,775.68
T	579	OTHER SKIN, SUBCUT TISS & BREAST PROC W MCC	7.0	9.2	2.6106	$14,019.65
T	580	OTHER SKIN, SUBCUT TISS & BREAST PROC W CC	3.8	5.1	1.5398	$8,269.16
T	581	OTHER SKIN, SUBCUT TISS & BREAST PROC W/O CC/MCC	2.0	2.6	1.0605	$5,695.18
	582	MASTECTOMY FOR MALIGNANCY W CC/MCC	2.0	2.7	1.1913	$6,397.61
	583	MASTECTOMY FOR MALIGNANCY W/O CC/MCC	1.5	1.7	0.9711	$5,215.08
	584	BREAST BIOPSY, LOCAL EXCISION & OTHER BREAST PROCEDURES W CC/MCC	3.5	4.8	1.6998	$9,128.40
	585	BREAST BIOPSY, LOCAL EXCISION & OTHER BREAST PROCEDURES W/O CC/MCC	2.0	2.6	1.3162	$7,068.36
T	592	SKIN ULCERS W MCC	5.1	6.6	1.4131	$7,588.74
T	593	SKIN ULCERS W CC	4.2	5.1	1.0094	$5,420.76
T	594	SKIN ULCERS W/O CC/MCC	3.1	3.9	0.6814	$3,659.31
	595	MAJOR SKIN DISORDERS W MCC	5.7	7.8	1.9464	$10,452.71
	596	MAJOR SKIN DISORDERS W/O MCC	3.6	4.6	0.9284	$4,985.77
	597	MALIGNANT BREAST DISORDERS W MCC	5.2	7.1	1.7064	$9,163.85
	598	MALIGNANT BREAST DISORDERS W CC	3.9	5.1	1.0817	$5,809.03
	599	MALIGNANT BREAST DISORDERS W/O CC/MCC	2.5	3.1	0.6547	$3,515.92
	600	NON-MALIGNANT BREAST DISORDERS W CC/MCC	3.8	4.7	0.9963	$5,350.41
	601	NON-MALIGNANT BREAST DISORDERS W/O CC/MCC	2.8	3.4	0.6445	$3,461.15
T	602	CELLULITIS W MCC	5.0	6.3	1.4607	$7,844.37
T	603	CELLULITIS W/O MCC	3.6	4.2	0.8402	$4,512.11
	604	TRAUMA TO THE SKIN, SUBCUT TISS & BREAST W MCC	3.9	5.1	1.3223	$7,101.12
	605	TRAUMA TO THE SKIN, SUBCUT TISS & BREAST W/O MCC	2.6	3.2	0.7372	$3,958.97

Calculated with an average hospital Medicare base rate of $5,370.28. Each hospital's base rate and corresponding payment will vary. The national average hospital Medicare base rate is the sum of the full update labor-related and nonlabor-related amounts published in the Federal Register, FY 2014 Final Rule, Table 1A. National Adjusted Operating Standardized Amounts; Labor/Nonlabor (if wage index greater than 1) or Table 1B. National Adjusted Operating Standardized Amounts; Labor/Nonlabor (if wage index less than or equal to 1).

MS-DRGs 998 and 999 contain cases that could not be assigned to valid DRGs.

Note: If there is no value in either the geometric mean length of stay or the arithmetic mean length of stay columns, the volume of cases is insufficient to determine a meaningful computation of these statistics.

DRG		Description	GMLOS	AMLOS	Relative Weight	National Payment Rate
	606	MINOR SKIN DISORDERS W MCC	4.3	6.0	1.3594	$7,300.36
	607	MINOR SKIN DISORDERS W/O MCC	2.8	3.6	0.7043	$3,782.29
	614	ADRENAL & PITUITARY PROCEDURES W CC/MCC	4.3	5.9	2.5455	$13,670.05
	615	ADRENAL & PITUITARY PROCEDURES W/O CC/MCC	2.3	2.7	1.4579	$7,829.33
T	616	AMPUTAT OF LOWER LIMB FOR ENDOCRINE,NUTRIT,& METABOL DIS W MCC	10.9	13.1	4.0773	$21,896.24
T	617	AMPUTAT OF LOWER LIMB FOR ENDOCRINE,NUTRIT,& METABOL DIS W CC	6.1	7.4	2.0071	$10,778.69
T	618	AMPUTAT OF LOWER LIMB FOR ENDOCRINE,NUTRIT,& METABOL DIS W/O CC/MCC	4.3	5.2	1.2489	$6,706.94
	619	O.R. PROCEDURES FOR OBESITY W MCC	4.8	7.7	3.6200	$19,440.41
	620	O.R. PROCEDURES FOR OBESITY W CC	2.7	3.2	1.9399	$10,417.81
	621	O.R. PROCEDURES FOR OBESITY W/O CC/MCC	1.8	2.0	1.5772	$8,470.01
T	622	SKIN GRAFTS & WOUND DEBRID FOR ENDOC, NUTRIT & METAB DIS W MCC	9.1	12.2	3.3505	$17,993.12
T	623	SKIN GRAFTS & WOUND DEBRID FOR ENDOC, NUTRIT & METAB DIS W CC	5.7	7.1	1.8239	$9,794.85
T	624	SKIN GRAFTS & WOUND DEBRID FOR ENDOC, NUTRIT & METAB DIS W/O CC/MCC	3.5	4.2	0.9635	$5,174.26
	625	THYROID, PARATHYROID & THYROGLOSSAL PROCEDURES W MCC	4.4	7.3	2.4009	$12,893.51
	626	THYROID, PARATHYROID & THYROGLOSSAL PROCEDURES W CC	2.0	2.8	1.2459	$6,690.83
	627	THYROID, PARATHYROID & THYROGLOSSAL PROCEDURES W/O CC/MCC	1.3	1.4	0.8458	$4,542.18
T	628	OTHER ENDOCRINE, NUTRIT & METAB O.R. PROC W MCC	6.6	9.6	3.3515	$17,998.49
T	629	OTHER ENDOCRINE, NUTRIT & METAB O.R. PROC W CC	6.0	7.2	2.1292	$11,434.40
T	630	OTHER ENDOCRINE, NUTRIT & METAB O.R. PROC W/O CC/MCC	3.0	3.8	1.3444	$7,219.80
T	637	DIABETES W MCC	4.2	5.5	1.3888	$7,458.24
T	638	DIABETES W CC	3.0	3.7	0.8252	$4,431.56
T	639	DIABETES W/O CC/MCC	2.2	2.6	0.5708	$3,065.36
T	640	MISC DISORDERS OF NUTRITION,METABOLISM,FLUIDS/ELECTROLYTES W MCC	3.3	4.6	1.1111	$5,966.92
T	641	MISC DISORDERS OF NUTRITION,METABOLISM,FLUIDS/ELECTROLYTES W/O MCC	2.8	3.4	0.6992	$3,754.90
	642	INBORN AND OTHER DISORDERS OF METABOLISM	3.2	4.2	1.0674	$5,732.24
T	643	ENDOCRINE DISORDERS W MCC	5.5	6.9	1.6693	$8,964.61
T	644	ENDOCRINE DISORDERS W CC	3.9	4.7	1.0194	$5,474.46
T	645	ENDOCRINE DISORDERS W/O CC/MCC	2.8	3.4	0.7041	$3,781.21
	652	KIDNEY TRANSPLANT	5.8	6.8	3.1530	$16,932.49
T	653	MAJOR BLADDER PROCEDURES W MCC	12.7	15.4	5.9558	$31,984.31
T	654	MAJOR BLADDER PROCEDURES W CC	7.8	8.9	3.0944	$16,617.79
T	655	MAJOR BLADDER PROCEDURES W/O CC/MCC	4.7	5.5	2.1671	$11,637.93
	656	KIDNEY & URETER PROCEDURES FOR NEOPLASM W MCC	7.2	9.3	3.5221	$18,914.66
	657	KIDNEY & URETER PROCEDURES FOR NEOPLASM W CC	4.5	5.4	2.0261	$10,880.72
	658	KIDNEY & URETER PROCEDURES FOR NEOPLASM W/O CC/MCC	2.8	3.1	1.5074	$8,095.16
T	659	KIDNEY & URETER PROCEDURES FOR NON-NEOPLASM W MCC	7.6	10.3	3.4051	$18,286.34
T	660	KIDNEY & URETER PROCEDURES FOR NON-NEOPLASM W CC	4.3	5.6	1.8827	$10,110.63
T	661	KIDNEY & URETER PROCEDURES FOR NON-NEOPLASM W/O CC/MCC	2.3	2.8	1.3435	$7,214.97

Calculated with an average hospital Medicare base rate of $5,370.28. Each hospital's base rate and corresponding payment will vary. The national average hospital Medicare base rate is the sum of the full update labor-related and nonlabor-related amounts published in the Federal Register, FY 2014 Final Rule, Table 1A. National Adjusted Operating Standardized Amounts; Labor/Nonlabor (if wage index greater than 1) or Table 1B. National Adjusted Operating Standardized Amounts; Labor/Nonlabor (if wage index less than or equal to 1).

MS-DRGs 998 and 999 contain cases that could not be assigned to valid DRGs.

Note: If there is no value in either the geometric mean length of stay or the arithmetic mean length of stay columns, the volume of cases is insufficient to determine a meaningful computation of these statistics.

DRG		Description	GMLOS	AMLOS	Relative Weight	National Payment Rate
	662	MINOR BLADDER PROCEDURES W MCC	7.7	10.2	2.9801	$16,003.97
	663	MINOR BLADDER PROCEDURES W CC	3.9	5.3	1.5666	$8,413.08
	664	MINOR BLADDER PROCEDURES W/O CC/MCC	1.7	2.2	1.2208	$6,556.04
	665	PROSTATECTOMY W MCC	9.2	11.7	3.1414	$16,870.20
	666	PROSTATECTOMY W CC	4.5	6.2	1.7042	$9,152.03
	667	PROSTATECTOMY W/O CC/MCC	2.0	2.6	0.8949	$4,805.86
	668	TRANSURETHRAL PROCEDURES W MCC	6.6	8.8	2.5573	$13,733.42
	669	TRANSURETHRAL PROCEDURES W CC	3.0	4.1	1.2693	$6,816.50
	670	TRANSURETHRAL PROCEDURES W/O CC/MCC	1.9	2.4	0.8354	$4,486.33
	671	URETHRAL PROCEDURES W CC/MCC	4.3	5.7	1.5887	$8,531.76
	672	URETHRAL PROCEDURES W/O CC/MCC	1.9	2.3	0.8835	$4,744.64
	673	OTHER KIDNEY & URINARY TRACT PROCEDURES W MCC	6.5	9.7	3.1150	$16,728.42
	674	OTHER KIDNEY & URINARY TRACT PROCEDURES W CC	5.1	6.9	2.2378	$12,017.61
	675	OTHER KIDNEY & URINARY TRACT PROCEDURES W/O CC/MCC	1.9	2.7	1.3807	$7,414.75
T	682	RENAL FAILURE W MCC	4.7	6.2	1.5401	$8,270.77
T	683	RENAL FAILURE W CC	3.7	4.5	0.9655	$5,185.01
T	684	RENAL FAILURE W/O CC/MCC	2.5	3.0	0.6213	$3,336.55
	685	ADMIT FOR RENAL DIALYSIS	2.6	3.4	0.9282	$4,984.69
	686	KIDNEY & URINARY TRACT NEOPLASMS W MCC	5.4	7.2	1.7237	$9,256.75
	687	KIDNEY & URINARY TRACT NEOPLASMS W CC	3.7	4.8	1.0441	$5,607.11
	688	KIDNEY & URINARY TRACT NEOPLASMS W/O CC/MCC	2.2	2.7	0.6867	$3,687.77
T	689	KIDNEY & URINARY TRACT INFECTIONS W MCC	4.3	5.3	1.1300	$6,068.42
T	690	KIDNEY & URINARY TRACT INFECTIONS W/O MCC	3.2	3.8	0.7693	$4,131.36
	691	URINARY STONES W ESW LITHOTRIPSY W CC/MCC	3.0	3.8	1.5454	$8,299.23
	692	URINARY STONES W ESW LITHOTRIPSY W/O CC/MCC	1.7	2.0	1.0690	$5,740.83
	693	URINARY STONES W/O ESW LITHOTRIPSY W MCC	4.1	5.3	1.4186	$7,618.28
	694	URINARY STONES W/O ESW LITHOTRIPSY W/O MCC	2.0	2.4	0.6879	$3,694.22
	695	KIDNEY & URINARY TRACT SIGNS & SYMPTOMS W MCC	4.2	5.5	1.2773	$6,859.46
	696	KIDNEY & URINARY TRACT SIGNS & SYMPTOMS W/O MCC	2.5	3.1	0.6615	$3,552.44
	697	URETHRAL STRICTURE	2.5	3.2	0.8225	$4,417.06
T	698	OTHER KIDNEY & URINARY TRACT DIAGNOSES W MCC	5.1	6.4	1.5681	$8,421.14
T	699	OTHER KIDNEY & URINARY TRACT DIAGNOSES W CC	3.5	4.4	0.9890	$5,311.21
T	700	OTHER KIDNEY & URINARY TRACT DIAGNOSES W/O CC/MCC	2.6	3.2	0.7026	$3,773.16
	707	MAJOR MALE PELVIC PROCEDURES W CC/MCC	3.0	4.1	1.8265	$9,808.82
	708	MAJOR MALE PELVIC PROCEDURES W/O CC/MCC	1.4	1.6	1.2928	$6,942.70
	709	PENIS PROCEDURES W CC/MCC	4.0	6.2	2.1038	$11,298.00
	710	PENIS PROCEDURES W/O CC/MCC	1.5	1.9	1.3429	$7,211.75
	711	TESTES PROCEDURES W CC/MCC	5.5	7.6	2.0316	$10,910.26

Calculated with an average hospital Medicare base rate of $5,370.28. Each hospital's base rate and corresponding payment will vary. The national average hospital Medicare base rate is the sum of the full update labor-related and nonlabor-related amounts published in the Federal Register, FY 2014 Final Rule, Table 1A. National Adjusted Operating Standardized Amounts; Labor/Nonlabor (if wage index greater than 1) or Table 1B. National Adjusted Operating Standardized Amounts; Labor/Nonlabor (if wage index less than or equal to 1).

MS-DRGs 998 and 999 contain cases that could not be assigned to valid DRGs.

Note: If there is no value in either the geometric mean length of stay or the arithmetic mean length of stay columns, the volume of cases is insufficient to determine a meaningful computation of these statistics.

DRG	Description	GMLOS	AMLOS	Relative Weight	National Payment Rate
712	TESTES PROCEDURES W/O CC/MCC	2.3	3.0	0.9580	$5,144.73
713	TRANSURETHRAL PROSTATECTOMY W CC/MCC	3.3	4.5	1.3814	$7,418.50
714	TRANSURETHRAL PROSTATECTOMY W/O CC/MCC	1.7	2.0	0.7402	$3,975.08
715	OTHER MALE REPRODUCTIVE SYSTEM O.R. PROC FOR MALIGNANCY W CC/MCC	5.5	7.8	2.2268	$11,958.54
716	OTHER MALE REPRODUCTIVE SYSTEM O.R. PROC FOR MALIGNANCY W/O CC/MCC	1.5	1.8	0.9629	$5,171.04
717	OTHER MALE REPRODUCTIVE SYSTEM O.R. PROC EXC MALIGNANCY W CC/MCC	4.9	6.7	1.7495	$9,395.30
718	OTHER MALE REPRODUCTIVE SYSTEM O.R. PROC EXC MALIGNANCY W/O CC/MCC	2.3	2.9	0.8786	$4,718.33
722	MALIGNANCY, MALE REPRODUCTIVE SYSTEM W MCC	5.3	7.1	1.6031	$8,609.10
723	MALIGNANCY, MALE REPRODUCTIVE SYSTEM W CC	3.9	5.0	1.0532	$5,655.98
724	MALIGNANCY, MALE REPRODUCTIVE SYSTEM W/O CC/MCC	1.8	2.4	0.5501	$2,954.19
725	BENIGN PROSTATIC HYPERTROPHY W MCC	4.4	5.6	1.2644	$6,790.18
726	BENIGN PROSTATIC HYPERTROPHY W/O MCC	2.8	3.4	0.7159	$3,844.58
727	INFLAMMATION OF THE MALE REPRODUCTIVE SYSTEM W MCC	4.8	6.2	1.4106	$7,575.32
728	INFLAMMATION OF THE MALE REPRODUCTIVE SYSTEM W/O MCC	3.2	3.9	0.7821	$4,200.10
729	OTHER MALE REPRODUCTIVE SYSTEM DIAGNOSES W CC/MCC	3.7	5.0	1.1196	$6,012.57
730	OTHER MALE REPRODUCTIVE SYSTEM DIAGNOSES W/O CC/MCC	2.2	2.8	0.6266	$3,365.02
734	PELVIC EVISCERATION, RAD HYSTERECTOMY & RAD VULVECTOMY W CC/MCC	4.6	6.7	2.5547	$13,719.45
735	PELVIC EVISCERATION, RAD HYSTERECTOMY & RAD VULVECTOMY W/O CC/MCC	1.9	2.3	1.1910	$6,396.00
736	UTERINE & ADNEXA PROC FOR OVARIAN OR ADNEXAL MALIGNANCY W MCC	10.1	12.4	4.2211	$22,668.49
737	UTERINE & ADNEXA PROC FOR OVARIAN OR ADNEXAL MALIGNANCY W CC	5.3	6.2	2.0310	$10,907.04
738	UTERINE & ADNEXA PROC FOR OVARIAN OR ADNEXAL MALIGNANCY W/O CC/MCC	2.9	3.3	1.2602	$6,767.63
739	UTERINE,ADNEXA PROC FOR NON-OVARIAN/ADNEXAL MALIG W MCC	6.5	8.7	3.1647	$16,995.33
740	UTERINE,ADNEXA PROC FOR NON-OVARIAN/ADNEXAL MALIG W CC	3.1	4.1	1.5819	$8,495.25
741	UTERINE,ADNEXA PROC FOR NON-OVARIAN/ADNEXAL MALIG W/O CC/MCC	1.8	2.1	1.1470	$6,159.71
742	UTERINE & ADNEXA PROC FOR NON-MALIGNANCY W CC/MCC	3.0	4.0	1.4972	$8,040.38
743	UTERINE & ADNEXA PROC FOR NON-MALIGNANCY W/O CC/MCC	1.7	1.9	0.9903	$5,318.19
744	D&C, CONIZATION, LAPAROSCOPY & TUBAL INTERRUPTION W CC/MCC	3.9	5.5	1.5084	$8,100.53
745	D&C, CONIZATION, LAPAROSCOPY & TUBAL INTERRUPTION W/O CC/MCC	1.9	2.4	0.8514	$4,572.26
746	VAGINA, CERVIX & VULVA PROCEDURES W CC/MCC	3.0	4.3	1.3694	$7,354.06
747	VAGINA, CERVIX & VULVA PROCEDURES W/O CC/MCC	1.6	1.8	0.8814	$4,733.36
748	FEMALE REPRODUCTIVE SYSTEM RECONSTRUCTIVE PROCEDURES	1.5	1.8	1.0096	$5,421.83
749	OTHER FEMALE REPRODUCTIVE SYSTEM O.R. PROCEDURES W CC/MCC	6.1	8.4	2.6239	$14,091.08
750	OTHER FEMALE REPRODUCTIVE SYSTEM O.R. PROCEDURES W/O CC/MCC	2.2	2.8	1.0854	$5,828.90
754	MALIGNANCY, FEMALE REPRODUCTIVE SYSTEM W MCC	5.8	8.4	1.9784	$10,624.56
755	MALIGNANCY, FEMALE REPRODUCTIVE SYSTEM W CC	3.7	5.0	1.0880	$5,842.86
756	MALIGNANCY, FEMALE REPRODUCTIVE SYSTEM W/O CC/MCC	2.1	2.6	0.6334	$3,401.54
757	INFECTIONS, FEMALE REPRODUCTIVE SYSTEM W MCC	5.7	7.2	1.5292	$8,212.23

Calculated with an average hospital Medicare base rate of $5,370.28. Each hospital's base rate and corresponding payment will vary. The national average hospital Medicare base rate is the sum of the full update labor-related and nonlabor-related amounts published in the Federal Register, FY 2014 Final Rule, Table 1A. National Adjusted Operating Standardized Amounts; Labor/Nonlabor (if wage index greater than 1) or Table 1B. National Adjusted Operating Standardized Amounts; Labor/Nonlabor (if wage index less than or equal to 1).

MS-DRGs 998 and 999 contain cases that could not be assigned to valid DRGs.

Note: If there is no value in either the geometric mean length of stay or the arithmetic mean length of stay columns, the volume of cases is insufficient to determine a meaningful computation of these statistics.

Ⓣ *Transfer DRG*   ⓈⓅ *Special Payment*

© 2013 OptumInsight, Inc.

DRG	Description	GMLOS	AMLOS	Relative Weight	National Payment Rate
758	INFECTIONS, FEMALE REPRODUCTIVE SYSTEM W CC	4.2	5.2	1.0452	$5,613.02
759	INFECTIONS, FEMALE REPRODUCTIVE SYSTEM W/O CC/MCC	3.2	3.8	0.6995	$3,756.51
760	MENSTRUAL & OTHER FEMALE REPRODUCTIVE SYSTEM DISORDERS W CC/MCC	2.8	3.6	0.8063	$4,330.06
761	MENSTRUAL & OTHER FEMALE REPRODUCTIVE SYSTEM DISORDERS W/O CC/MCC	1.8	2.2	0.4904	$2,633.59
765	CESAREAN SECTION W CC/MCC	3.9	4.8	1.1125	$5,974.44
766	CESAREAN SECTION W/O CC/MCC	2.9	3.1	0.7766	$4,170.56
767	VAGINAL DELIVERY W STERILIZATION &/OR D&C	2.7	3.6	0.9235	$4,959.45
768	VAGINAL DELIVERY W O.R. PROC EXCEPT STERIL &/OR D&C	3.1	3.2	1.0976	$5,894.42
769	POSTPARTUM & POST ABORTION DIAGNOSES W O.R. PROCEDURE	4.3	6.4	2.1785	$11,699.15
770	ABORTION W D&C, ASPIRATION CURETTAGE OR HYSTEROTOMY	1.6	2.1	0.7070	$3,796.79
774	VAGINAL DELIVERY W COMPLICATING DIAGNOSES	2.5	3.0	0.7137	$3,832.77
775	VAGINAL DELIVERY W/O COMPLICATING DIAGNOSES	2.1	2.3	0.5625	$3,020.78
776	POSTPARTUM & POST ABORTION DIAGNOSES W/O O.R. PROCEDURE	2.5	3.4	0.7075	$3,799.47
777	ECTOPIC PREGNANCY	1.6	2.1	0.9550	$5,128.62
778	THREATENED ABORTION	1.9	2.9	0.5247	$2,817.79
779	ABORTION W/O D&C	1.5	1.8	0.4843	$2,600.83
780	FALSE LABOR	1.2	1.4	0.2515	$1,350.63
781	OTHER ANTEPARTUM DIAGNOSES W MEDICAL COMPLICATIONS	2.7	3.9	0.7568	$4,064.23
782	OTHER ANTEPARTUM DIAGNOSES W/O MEDICAL COMPLICATIONS	1.6	2.3	0.4463	$2,396.76
789	NEONATES, DIED OR TRANSFERRED TO ANOTHER ACUTE CARE FACILITY	1.8	1.8	1.5258	$8,193.97
790	EXTREME IMMATURITY OR RESPIRATORY DISTRESS SYNDROME, NEONATE	17.9	17.9	5.0315	$27,020.56
791	PREMATURITY W MAJOR PROBLEMS	13.3	13.3	3.4363	$18,453.89
792	PREMATURITY W/O MAJOR PROBLEMS	8.6	8.6	2.0734	$11,134.74
793	FULL TERM NEONATE W MAJOR PROBLEMS	4.7	4.7	3.5299	$18,956.55
794	NEONATE W OTHER SIGNIFICANT PROBLEMS	3.4	3.4	1.2494	$6,709.63
795	NORMAL NEWBORN	3.1	3.1	0.1692	$908.65
799	SPLENECTOMY W MCC	9.9	12.9	5.0639	$27,194.56
800	SPLENECTOMY W CC	5.2	6.8	2.5234	$13,551.36
801	SPLENECTOMY W/O CC/MCC	2.8	3.5	1.5980	$8,581.71
802	OTHER O.R. PROC OF THE BLOOD & BLOOD FORMING ORGANS W MCC	7.7	10.4	3.1642	$16,992.64
803	OTHER O.R. PROC OF THE BLOOD & BLOOD FORMING ORGANS W CC	4.7	6.3	1.8831	$10,112.77
804	OTHER O.R. PROC OF THE BLOOD & BLOOD FORMING ORGANS W/O CC/MCC	2.3	3.0	1.1558	$6,206.97
808	MAJOR HEMATOL/IMMUN DIAG EXC SICKLE CELL CRISIS & COAGUL W MCC	6.1	8.1	2.2217	$11,931.15
809	MAJOR HEMATOL/IMMUN DIAG EXC SICKLE CELL CRISIS & COAGUL W CC	3.8	4.8	1.1901	$6,391.17
810	MAJOR HEMATOL/IMMUN DIAG EXC SICKLE CELL CRISIS & COAGUL W/O CC/MCC	2.7	3.3	0.8226	$4,417.59
811	RED BLOOD CELL DISORDERS W MCC	3.6	4.8	1.2488	$6,706.41
812	RED BLOOD CELL DISORDERS W/O MCC	2.6	3.4	0.7985	$4,288.17
813	COAGULATION DISORDERS	3.6	5.0	1.6433	$8,824.98

Calculated with an average hospital Medicare base rate of $5,370.28. Each hospital's base rate and corresponding payment will vary. The national average hospital Medicare base rate is the sum of the full update labor-related and nonlabor-related amounts published in the Federal Register, FY 2014 Final Rule, Table 1A. National Adjusted Operating Standardized Amounts; Labor/Nonlabor (if wage index greater than 1) or Table 1B. National Adjusted Operating Standardized Amounts; Labor/Nonlabor (if wage index less than or equal to 1).

MS-DRGs 998 and 999 contain cases that could not be assigned to valid DRGs.

Note: If there is no value in either the geometric mean length of stay or the arithmetic mean length of stay columns, the volume of cases is insufficient to determine a meaningful computation of these statistics.

DRG		Description	GMLOS	AMLOS	Relative Weight	National Payment Rate
	814	RETICULOENDOTHELIAL & IMMUNITY DISORDERS W MCC	4.9	6.8	1.6910	$9,081.14
	815	RETICULOENDOTHELIAL & IMMUNITY DISORDERS W CC	3.3	4.2	0.9844	$5,286.50
	816	RETICULOENDOTHELIAL & IMMUNITY DISORDERS W/O CC/MCC	2.4	2.9	0.6655	$3,573.92
	820	LYMPHOMA & LEUKEMIA W MAJOR O.R. PROCEDURE W MCC	13.0	17.1	5.8779	$31,565.97
	821	LYMPHOMA & LEUKEMIA W MAJOR O.R. PROCEDURE W CC	4.8	6.9	2.4025	$12,902.10
	822	LYMPHOMA & LEUKEMIA W MAJOR O.R. PROCEDURE W/O CC/MCC	2.2	2.8	1.2336	$6,624.78
	823	LYMPHOMA & NON-ACUTE LEUKEMIA W OTHER O.R. PROC W MCC	11.3	14.7	4.4850	$24,085.71
	824	LYMPHOMA & NON-ACUTE LEUKEMIA W OTHER O.R. PROC W CC	5.9	7.7	2.1684	$11,644.92
	825	LYMPHOMA & NON-ACUTE LEUKEMIA W OTHER O.R. PROC W/O CC/MCC	2.9	4.0	1.2935	$6,946.46
	826	MYELOPROLIF DISORD OR POORLY DIFF NEOPL W MAJ O.R. PROC W MCC	10.8	14.0	4.9280	$26,464.74
	827	MYELOPROLIF DISORD OR POORLY DIFF NEOPL W MAJ O.R. PROC W CC	5.3	6.8	2.2746	$12,215.24
	828	MYELOPROLIF DISORD OR POORLY DIFF NEOPL W MAJ O.R. PROC W/O CC/MCC	2.7	3.3	1.3642	$7,326.14
	829	MYELOPROLIF DISORD OR POORLY DIFF NEOPL W OTHER O.R. PROC W CC/MCC	6.7	10.2	3.1769	$17,060.84
	830	MYELOPROLIF DISORD OR POORLY DIFF NEOPL W OTHER O.R. PROC W/O CC/MCC	2.4	3.1	1.2781	$6,863.75
	834	ACUTE LEUKEMIA W/O MAJOR O.R. PROCEDURE W MCC	10.3	16.8	5.3828	$28,907.14
	835	ACUTE LEUKEMIA W/O MAJOR O.R. PROCEDURE W CC	4.6	7.5	2.1606	$11,603.03
	836	ACUTE LEUKEMIA W/O MAJOR O.R. PROCEDURE W/O CC/MCC	2.9	4.3	1.2240	$6,573.22
	837	CHEMO W ACUTE LEUKEMIA AS SDX OR W HIGH DOSE CHEMO AGENT W MCC	15.6	21.2	6.0485	$32,482.14
	838	CHEMO W ACUTE LEUKEMIA AS SDX W CC OR HIGH DOSE CHEMO AGENT	6.7	9.7	2.8181	$15,133.99
	839	CHEMO W ACUTE LEUKEMIA AS SDX W/O CC/MCC	4.8	5.5	1.3175	$7,075.34
T	840	LYMPHOMA & NON-ACUTE LEUKEMIA W MCC	7.5	10.5	3.0843	$16,563.55
T	841	LYMPHOMA & NON-ACUTE LEUKEMIA W CC	4.8	6.3	1.6167	$8,682.13
T	842	LYMPHOMA & NON-ACUTE LEUKEMIA W/O CC/MCC	3.1	4.1	1.0830	$5,816.01
	843	OTHER MYELOPROLIF DIS OR POORLY DIFF NEOPL DIAG W MCC	5.3	7.2	1.7768	$9,541.91
	844	OTHER MYELOPROLIF DIS OR POORLY DIFF NEOPL DIAG W CC	4.1	5.3	1.1701	$6,283.76
	845	OTHER MYELOPROLIF DIS OR POORLY DIFF NEOPL DIAG W/O CC/MCC	2.8	3.7	0.7830	$4,204.93
	846	CHEMOTHERAPY W/O ACUTE LEUKEMIA AS SECONDARY DIAGNOSIS W MCC	5.7	8.2	2.4337	$13,069.65
	847	CHEMOTHERAPY W/O ACUTE LEUKEMIA AS SECONDARY DIAGNOSIS W CC	3.0	3.6	1.1062	$5,940.60
	848	CHEMOTHERAPY W/O ACUTE LEUKEMIA AS SECONDARY DIAGNOSIS W/O CC/MCC	2.5	3.0	0.8635	$4,637.24
	849	RADIOTHERAPY	4.6	6.0	1.4239	$7,646.74
T	853	INFECTIOUS & PARASITIC DISEASES W O.R. PROCEDURE W MCC	11.1	14.3	5.3491	$28,726.16
T	854	INFECTIOUS & PARASITIC DISEASES W O.R. PROCEDURE W CC	7.0	8.5	2.4891	$13,367.16
T	855	INFECTIOUS & PARASITIC DISEASES W O.R. PROCEDURE W/O CC/MCC	3.6	4.9	1.5849	$8,511.36
T	856	POSTOPERATIVE OR POST-TRAUMATIC INFECTIONS W O.R. PROC W MCC	10.1	13.4	4.7874	$25,709.68
T	857	POSTOPERATIVE OR POST-TRAUMATIC INFECTIONS W O.R. PROC W CC	5.7	7.1	2.0412	$10,961.82
T	858	POSTOPERATIVE OR POST-TRAUMATIC INFECTIONS W O.R. PROC W/O CC/MCC	3.9	4.8	1.3115	$7,043.12
T	862	POSTOPERATIVE & POST-TRAUMATIC INFECTIONS W MCC	5.6	7.4	1.8903	$10,151.44

Calculated with an average hospital Medicare base rate of $5,370.28. Each hospital's base rate and corresponding payment will vary. The national average hospital Medicare base rate is the sum of the full update labor-related and nonlabor-related amounts published in the Federal Register, FY 2014 Final Rule, Table 1A. National Adjusted Operating Standardized Amounts; Labor/Nonlabor (if wage index greater than 1) or Table 1B. National Adjusted Operating Standardized Amounts; Labor/Nonlabor (if wage index less than or equal to 1).

MS-DRGs 998 and 999 contain cases that could not be assigned to valid DRGs.

Note: If there is no value in either the geometric mean length of stay or the arithmetic mean length of stay columns, the volume of cases is insufficient to determine a meaningful computation of these statistics.

T *Transfer DRG*   SP *Special Payment*

DRG		Description	GMLOS	AMLOS	Relative Weight	National Payment Rate
T	863	POSTOPERATIVE & POST-TRAUMATIC INFECTIONS W/O MCC	3.8	4.6	0.9845	$5,287.04
	864	FEVER	2.9	3.6	0.8441	$4,533.05
	865	VIRAL ILLNESS W MCC	4.9	6.8	1.7351	$9,317.97
	866	VIRAL ILLNESS W/O MCC	2.9	3.5	0.7855	$4,218.35
T	867	OTHER INFECTIOUS & PARASITIC DISEASES DIAGNOSES W MCC	6.8	9.2	2.6139	$14,037.37
T	868	OTHER INFECTIOUS & PARASITIC DISEASES DIAGNOSES W CC	4.0	5.0	1.0775	$5,786.48
T	869	OTHER INFECTIOUS & PARASITIC DISEASES DIAGNOSES W/O CC/MCC	2.9	3.5	0.7406	$3,977.23
T	870	SEPTICEMIA OR SEVERE SEPSIS W MV 96+ HOURS	12.5	14.6	5.9187	$31,785.08
T	871	SEPTICEMIA OR SEVERE SEPSIS W/O MV 96+ HOURS W MCC	5.1	6.7	1.8527	$9,949.52
T	872	SEPTICEMIA OR SEVERE SEPSIS W/O MV 96+ HOURS W/O MCC	4.1	4.9	1.0687	$5,739.22
	876	O.R. PROCEDURE W PRINCIPAL DIAGNOSES OF MENTAL ILLNESS	7.5	12.3	2.8172	$15,129.15
	880	ACUTE ADJUSTMENT REACTION & PSYCHOSOCIAL DYSFUNCTION	2.2	2.9	0.6388	$3,430.53
	881	DEPRESSIVE NEUROSES	3.2	4.4	0.6541	$3,512.70
	882	NEUROSES EXCEPT DEPRESSIVE	3.2	4.4	0.6953	$3,733.96
	883	DISORDERS OF PERSONALITY & IMPULSE CONTROL	4.7	7.7	1.2682	$6,810.59
T	884	ORGANIC DISTURBANCES & MENTAL RETARDATION	4.0	5.7	1.0060	$5,402.50
	885	PSYCHOSES	5.4	7.3	1.0048	$5,396.06
	886	BEHAVIORAL & DEVELOPMENTAL DISORDERS	4.2	7.1	0.9173	$4,926.16
	887	OTHER MENTAL DISORDER DIAGNOSES	2.9	4.5	0.9795	$5,260.19
	894	ALCOHOL/DRUG ABUSE OR DEPENDENCE, LEFT AMA	2.1	2.9	0.4509	$2,421.46
	895	ALCOHOL/DRUG ABUSE OR DEPENDENCE W REHABILITATION THERAPY	9.1	11.7	1.1939	$6,411.58
T	896	ALCOHOL/DRUG ABUSE OR DEPENDENCE W/O REHABILITATION THERAPY W MCC	4.7	6.5	1.5146	$8,133.83
T	897	ALCOHOL/DRUG ABUSE OR DEPENDENCE W/O REHABILITATION THERAPY W/O MCC	3.2	4.0	0.6824	$3,664.68
	901	WOUND DEBRIDEMENTS FOR INJURIES W MCC	9.3	13.9	4.0316	$21,650.82
	902	WOUND DEBRIDEMENTS FOR INJURIES W CC	4.9	6.6	1.7077	$9,170.83
	903	WOUND DEBRIDEMENTS FOR INJURIES W/O CC/MCC	3.1	4.2	1.0527	$5,653.29
	904	SKIN GRAFTS FOR INJURIES W CC/MCC	7.2	10.7	3.1738	$17,044.19
	905	SKIN GRAFTS FOR INJURIES W/O CC/MCC	3.2	4.3	1.2475	$6,699.42
	906	HAND PROCEDURES FOR INJURIES	2.4	3.5	1.2228	$6,566.78
T	907	OTHER O.R. PROCEDURES FOR INJURIES W MCC	7.7	10.7	3.9235	$21,070.29
T	908	OTHER O.R. PROCEDURES FOR INJURIES W CC	4.4	5.8	1.9485	$10,463.99
T	909	OTHER O.R. PROCEDURES FOR INJURIES W/O CC/MCC	2.5	3.2	1.2150	$6,524.89
	913	TRAUMATIC INJURY W MCC	3.7	5.0	1.1683	$6,274.10
	914	TRAUMATIC INJURY W/O MCC	2.5	3.1	0.7110	$3,818.27
	915	ALLERGIC REACTIONS W MCC	3.6	4.9	1.4721	$7,905.59
	916	ALLERGIC REACTIONS W/O MCC	1.7	2.1	0.5139	$2,759.79
T	917	POISONING & TOXIC EFFECTS OF DRUGS W MCC	3.5	4.8	1.4093	$7,568.34

Calculated with an average hospital Medicare base rate of $5,370.28. Each hospital's base rate and corresponding payment will vary. The national average hospital Medicare base rate is the sum of the full update labor-related and nonlabor-related amounts published in the Federal Register, FY 2014 Final Rule, Table 1A. National Adjusted Operating Standardized Amounts; Labor/Nonlabor (if wage index greater than 1) or Table 1B. National Adjusted Operating Standardized Amounts; Labor/Nonlabor (if wage index less than or equal to 1).

MS-DRGs 998 and 999 contain cases that could not be assigned to valid DRGs.

Note: If there is no value in either the geometric mean length of stay or the arithmetic mean length of stay columns, the volume of cases is insufficient to determine a meaningful computation of these statistics.

DRG		Description	GMLOS	AMLOS	Relative Weight	National Payment Rate
T	918	POISONING & TOXIC EFFECTS OF DRUGS W/O MCC	2.1	2.7	0.6346	$3,407.98
	919	COMPLICATIONS OF TREATMENT W MCC	4.4	6.1	1.7206	$9,240.10
	920	COMPLICATIONS OF TREATMENT W CC	3.1	4.0	0.9779	$5,251.60
	921	COMPLICATIONS OF TREATMENT W/O CC/MCC	2.2	2.8	0.6522	$3,502.50
	922	OTHER INJURY, POISONING & TOXIC EFFECT DIAG W MCC	4.0	5.6	1.5088	$8,102.68
	923	OTHER INJURY, POISONING & TOXIC EFFECT DIAG W/O MCC	2.2	2.9	0.6620	$3,555.13
	927	EXTENSIVE BURNS OR FULL THICKNESS BURNS W MV 96+ HRS W SKIN GRAFT	22.3	30.7	16.4534	$88,359.36
	928	FULL THICKNESS BURN W SKIN GRAFT OR INHAL INJ W CC/MCC	11.9	16.1	5.7744	$31,010.14
	929	FULL THICKNESS BURN W SKIN GRAFT OR INHAL INJ W/O CC/MCC	5.1	7.2	2.2090	$11,862.95
	933	EXTENSIVE BURNS OR FULL THICKNESS BURNS W MV 96+ HRS W/O SKIN GRAFT	2.6	8.2	3.2785	$17,606.46
	934	FULL THICKNESS BURN W/O SKIN GRFT OR INHAL INJ	4.2	6.1	1.6045	$8,616.61
	935	NON-EXTENSIVE BURNS	3.2	4.8	1.3909	$7,469.52
	939	O.R. PROC W DIAGNOSES OF OTHER CONTACT W HEALTH SERVICES W MCC	6.6	9.8	3.1182	$16,745.61
	940	O.R. PROC W DIAGNOSES OF OTHER CONTACT W HEALTH SERVICES W CC	3.7	5.3	1.7675	$9,491.97
	941	O.R. PROC W DIAGNOSES OF OTHER CONTACT W HEALTH SERVICES W/O CC/MCC	2.2	2.8	1.3403	$7,197.79
T	945	REHABILITATION W CC/MCC	8.3	10.1	1.3804	$7,413.13
T	946	REHABILITATION W/O CC/MCC	6.5	7.4	1.2037	$6,464.21
T	947	SIGNS & SYMPTOMS W MCC	3.6	4.8	1.1324	$6,081.31
T	948	SIGNS & SYMPTOMS W/O MCC	2.6	3.3	0.6897	$3,703.88
	949	AFTERCARE W CC/MCC	2.8	4.1	1.0038	$5,390.69
	950	AFTERCARE W/O CC/MCC	2.3	3.5	0.6005	$3,224.85
	951	OTHER FACTORS INFLUENCING HEALTH STATUS	2.4	5.5	0.8578	$4,606.63
	955	CRANIOTOMY FOR MULTIPLE SIGNIFICANT TRAUMA	7.2	10.6	5.4056	$29,029.59
T	956	LIMB REATTACHMENT, HIP & FEMUR PROC FOR MULTIPLE SIGNIFICANT TRAUMA	6.8	8.3	3.8321	$20,579.45
	957	OTHER O.R. PROCEDURES FOR MULTIPLE SIGNIFICANT TRAUMA W MCC	9.7	13.9	6.7306	$36,145.21
	958	OTHER O.R. PROCEDURES FOR MULTIPLE SIGNIFICANT TRAUMA W CC	7.3	8.9	3.8734	$20,801.24
	959	OTHER O.R. PROCEDURES FOR MULTIPLE SIGNIFICANT TRAUMA W/O CC/MCC	4.3	5.4	2.5391	$13,635.68
	963	OTHER MULTIPLE SIGNIFICANT TRAUMA W MCC	5.5	8.1	2.6733	$14,356.37
	964	OTHER MULTIPLE SIGNIFICANT TRAUMA W CC	4.1	5.0	1.3904	$7,466.84
	965	OTHER MULTIPLE SIGNIFICANT TRAUMA W/O CC/MCC	3.0	3.6	0.9824	$5,275.76
	969	HIV W EXTENSIVE O.R. PROCEDURE W MCC	12.0	16.7	5.4896	$29,480.69
	970	HIV W EXTENSIVE O.R. PROCEDURE W/O MCC	4.9	7.1	2.2785	$12,236.18
	974	HIV W MAJOR RELATED CONDITION W MCC	6.7	9.3	2.6335	$14,142.63
	975	HIV W MAJOR RELATED CONDITION W CC	4.7	6.1	1.3383	$7,187.05
	976	HIV W MAJOR RELATED CONDITION W/O CC/MCC	3.3	4.2	0.8627	$4,632.94
	977	HIV W OR W/O OTHER RELATED CONDITION	3.6	4.8	1.1194	$6,011.49
T	981	EXTENSIVE O.R. PROCEDURE UNRELATED TO PRINCIPAL DIAGNOSIS W MCC	10.1	13.1	4.9319	$26,485.68
T	982	EXTENSIVE O.R. PROCEDURE UNRELATED TO PRINCIPAL DIAGNOSIS W CC	5.9	7.6	2.8504	$15,307.45

Calculated with an average hospital Medicare base rate of $5,370.28. Each hospital's base rate and corresponding payment will vary. The national average hospital Medicare base rate is the sum of the full update labor-related and nonlabor-related amounts published in the Federal Register, FY 2014 Final Rule, Table 1A. National Adjusted Operating Standardized Amounts; Labor/Nonlabor (if wage index greater than 1) or Table 1B. National Adjusted Operating Standardized Amounts; Labor/Nonlabor (if wage index less than or equal to 1).

MS-DRGs 998 and 999 contain cases that could not be assigned to valid DRGs.

Note: If there is no value in either the geometric mean length of stay or the arithmetic mean length of stay columns, the volume of cases is insufficient to determine a meaningful computation of these statistics.

T *Transfer DRG*   SP *Special Payment*   © 2013 OptumInsight, Inc.

DRG		Description	GMLOS	AMLOS	Relative Weight	National Payment Rate
T	983	EXTENSIVE O.R. PROCEDURE UNRELATED TO PRINCIPAL DIAGNOSIS W/O CC/MCC	2.8	3.8	1.7462	$9,377.58
	984	PROSTATIC O.R. PROCEDURE UNRELATED TO PRINCIPAL DIAGNOSIS W MCC	9.3	12.5	3.4143	$18,335.75
	985	PROSTATIC O.R. PROCEDURE UNRELATED TO PRINCIPAL DIAGNOSIS W CC	5.1	7.2	1.8859	$10,127.81
	986	PROSTATIC O.R. PROCEDURE UNRELATED TO PRINCIPAL DIAGNOSIS W/O CC/MCC	2.1	3.0	1.0389	$5,579.18
T	987	NON-EXTENSIVE O.R. PROC UNRELATED TO PRINCIPAL DIAGNOSIS W MCC	8.4	11.2	3.3422	$17,948.55
T	988	NON-EXTENSIVE O.R. PROC UNRELATED TO PRINCIPAL DIAGNOSIS W CC	4.8	6.4	1.7554	$9,426.99
T	989	NON-EXTENSIVE O.R. PROC UNRELATED TO PRINCIPAL DIAGNOSIS W/O CC/MCC	2.3	3.0	1.0430	$5,601.20
	998	PRINCIPAL DIAGNOSIS INVALID AS DISCHARGE DIAGNOSIS	0.0	0.0	0.0000	$0.00
	999	UNGROUPABLE	0.0	0.0	0.0000	$0.00

Calculated with an average hospital Medicare base rate of $5,370.28. Each hospital's base rate and corresponding payment will vary. The national average hospital Medicare base rate is the sum of the full update labor-related and nonlabor-related amounts published in the Federal Register, FY 2014 Final Rule, Table 1A. National Adjusted Operating Standardized Amounts; Labor/Nonlabor (if wage index greater than 1) or Table 1B. National Adjusted Operating Standardized Amounts; Labor/Nonlabor (if wage index less than or equal to 1).

MS-DRGs 998 and 999 contain cases that could not be assigned to valid DRGs.

Note: If there is no value in either the geometric mean length of stay or the arithmetic mean length of stay columns, the volume of cases is insufficient to determine a meaningful computation of these statistics.

Peer Grouping	MS-DRG	Description	Discharges	Average Age	Average Length of Stay	Average Total Charge	Average Allowed
National	001	HEART TRANSPLANT OR IMPLANT OF HEART ASSIST SYSTEM W MCC	1921	61	36.1	$816,777	$179,428
National	002	HEART TRANSPLANT OR IMPLANT OF HEART ASSIST SYSTEM W/O MCC	410	60	19.0	$517,457	$102,957
National	003	ECMO OR TRACH W MV 96+ HRS OR PDX EXC FACE, MOUTH & NECK W MAJ O.R.	23237	70	34.2	$476,659	$105,718
National	004	TRACH W MV 96+ HRS OR PDX EXC FACE, MOUTH & NECK W/O MAJ O.R.	25488	69	27.0	$287,944	$65,550
National	005	LIVER TRANSPLANT W MCC OR INTESTINAL TRANSPLANT	1252	58	20.7	$467,344	$82,540
National	006	LIVER TRANSPLANT W/O MCC	414	60	9.1	$269,025	$34,191
National	007	LUNG TRANSPLANT	676	60	18.1	$440,526	$74,698
National	008	SIMULTANEOUS PANCREAS/KIDNEY TRANSPLANT	512	43	11.1	$334,909	$38,834
National	010	PANCREAS TRANSPLANT	94	44	10.3	$237,325	$35,033
National	011	TRACHEOSTOMY FOR FACE,MOUTH & NECK DIAGNOSES W MCC	2178	69	14.0	$144,990	$32,841
National	012	TRACHEOSTOMY FOR FACE,MOUTH & NECK DIAGNOSES W CC	2596	69	10.0	$106,025	$20,272
National	013	TRACHEOSTOMY FOR FACE,MOUTH & NECK DIAGNOSES W/O CC/MCC	1172	69	6.6	$68,168	$11,613
National	014	ALLOGENEIC BONE MARROW TRANSPLANT	932	61	26.2	$334,471	$78,439
National	016	AUTOLOGOUS BONE MARROW TRANSPLANT W CC/MCC	2090	66	19.6	$185,084	$45,626
National	017	AUTOLOGOUS BONE MARROW TRANSPLANT W/O CC/MCC	341	67	14.0	$137,054	$31,200
National	020	INTRACRANIAL VASCULAR PROCEDURES W PDX HEMORRHAGE W MCC	1598	70	17.3	$290,894	$56,593
National	021	INTRACRANIAL VASCULAR PROCEDURES W PDX HEMORRHAGE W CC	600	68	13.6	$192,896	$41,215
National	022	INTRACRANIAL VASCULAR PROCEDURES W PDX HEMORRHAGE W/O CC/MCC	162	68	7.3	$141,888	$26,242
National	023	CRANIO W MAJOR DEV IMPL/ACUTE COMPLEX CNS PDX W MCC OR CHEMO IMPLANT	6718	72	11.2	$155,403	$31,583
National	024	CRANIO W MAJOR DEV IMPL/ACUTE COMPLEX CNS PDX W/O MCC	2311	72	6.7	$109,374	$20,123
National	025	CRANIOTOMY & ENDOVASCULAR INTRACRANIAL PROCEDURES W MCC	19406	72	10.2	$129,443	$27,250
National	026	CRANIOTOMY & ENDOVASCULAR INTRACRANIAL PROCEDURES W CC	12419	71	6.5	$86,945	$16,438
National	027	CRANIOTOMY & ENDOVASCULAR INTRACRANIAL PROCEDURES W/O CC/MCC	14308	69	3.4	$68,657	$11,815
National	028	SPINAL PROCEDURES W MCC	2528	68	12.6	$151,892	$34,575
National	029	SPINAL PROCEDURES W CC OR SPINAL NEUROSTIMULATORS	4891	66	6.3	$84,687	$16,421
National	030	SPINAL PROCEDURES W/O CC/MCC	4023	66	3.3	$49,130	$9,038
National	031	VENTRICULAR SHUNT PROCEDURES W MCC	1416	66	10.9	$105,696	$24,491
National	032	VENTRICULAR SHUNT PROCEDURES W CC	3087	64	4.9	$56,101	$10,910
National	033	VENTRICULAR SHUNT PROCEDURES W/O CC/MCC	3625	72	2.6	$42,155	$7,414
National	034	CAROTID ARTERY STENT PROCEDURE W MCC	1095	74	7.2	$102,936	$18,779
National	035	CAROTID ARTERY STENT PROCEDURE W CC	2958	74	3.2	$61,789	$11,215
National	036	CAROTID ARTERY STENT PROCEDURE W/O CC/MCC	6687	74	1.6	$47,327	$8,143

Peer Grouping	MS-DRG	Description	Discharges	Average Age	Average Length of Stay	Average Total Charge	Average Allowed
National	037	EXTRACRANIAL PROCEDURES W MCC	5840	71	8.2	$89,520	$17,500
National	038	EXTRACRANIAL PROCEDURES W CC	15480	74	3.5	$47,330	$7,881
National	039	EXTRACRANIAL PROCEDURES W/O CC/MCC	43123	74	1.6	$31,014	$4,661
National	040	PERIPH/CRANIAL NERVE & OTHER NERV SYST PROC W MCC	6077	70	12.1	$107,630	$24,192
National	041	PERIPH/CRANIAL NERVE & OTHER NERV SYST PROC W CC OR PERIPH NEUROSTIM	8394	68	6.5	$59,275	$11,721
National	042	PERIPH/CRANIAL NERVE & OTHER NERV SYST PROC W/O CC/MCC	3438	67	3.3	$52,484	$8,598
National	052	SPINAL DISORDERS & INJURIES W CC/MCC	1854	72	9.5	$47,737	$12,769
National	053	SPINAL DISORDERS & INJURIES W/O CC/MCC	596	72	12.1	$33,788	$5,180
National	054	NERVOUS SYSTEM NEOPLASMS W MCC	13365	73	5.7	$40,313	$8,172
National	055	NERVOUS SYSTEM NEOPLASMS W/O MCC	11696	72	4.5	$31,210	$5,877
National	056	DEGENERATIVE NERVOUS SYSTEM DISORDERS W MCC	15125	77	10.2	$45,873	$11,446
National	057	DEGENERATIVE NERVOUS SYSTEM DISORDERS W/O MCC	78780	79	9.5	$28,098	$7,983
National	058	MULTIPLE SCLEROSIS & CEREBELLAR ATAXIA W MCC	1152	57	10.0	$61,773	$9,531
National	059	MULTIPLE SCLEROSIS & CEREBELLAR ATAXIA W CC	4269	55	5.3	$30,124	$5,629
National	060	MULTIPLE SCLEROSIS & CEREBELLAR ATAXIA W/O CC/MCC	4250	52	3.9	$23,791	$3,925
National	061	ACUTE ISCHEMIC STROKE W USE OF THROMBOLYTIC AGENT W MCC	4634	79	7.7	$85,096	$15,972
National	062	ACUTE ISCHEMIC STROKE W USE OF THROMBOLYTIC AGENT W CC	7109	78	5.0	$58,606	$10,157
National	063	ACUTE ISCHEMIC STROKE W USE OF THROMBOLYTIC AGENT W/O CC/MCC	2302	75	3.5	$49,587	$7,567
National	064	INTRACRANIAL HEMORRHAGE OR CEREBRAL INFARCTION W MCC	86066	78	6.6	$49,871	$10,289
National	065	INTRACRANIAL HEMORRHAGE OR CEREBRAL INFARCTION W CC	137666	78	4.6	$31,545	$5,921
National	066	INTRACRANIAL HEMORRHAGE OR CEREBRAL INFARCTION W/O CC/MCC	78636	77	3.1	$23,894	$3,861
National	067	NONSPECIFIC CVA & PRECEREBRAL OCCLUSION W/O INFARCT W MCC	1488	75	5.5	$42,447	$8,298
National	068	NONSPECIFIC CVA & PRECEREBRAL OCCLUSION W/O INFARCT W/O MCC	10108	77	3.1	$26,639	$4,187
National	069	TRANSIENT ISCHEMIA	109875	77	2.5	$21,629	$3,026
National	070	NONSPECIFIC CEREBROVASCULAR DISORDERS W MCC	16106	72	7.0	$45,746	$10,325
National	071	NONSPECIFIC CEREBROVASCULAR DISORDERS W CC	20033	76	5.3	$27,681	$5,823
National	072	NONSPECIFIC CEREBROVASCULAR DISORDERS W/O CC/MCC	6806	75	3.0	$21,430	$3,298
National	073	CRANIAL & PERIPHERAL NERVE DISORDERS W MCC	10761	57	5.7	$37,198	$7,778
National	074	CRANIAL & PERIPHERAL NERVE DISORDERS W/O MCC	35861	65	3.9	$25,118	$4,375
National	075	VIRAL MENINGITIS W CC/MCC	1891	67	6.6	$49,982	$9,804
National	076	VIRAL MENINGITIS W/O CC/MCC	842	62	3.7	$25,744	$4,047
National	077	HYPERTENSIVE ENCEPHALOPATHY W MCC	2163	66	6.2	$46,900	$9,615
National	078	HYPERTENSIVE ENCEPHALOPATHY W CC	3519	76	4.0	$28,084	$5,041
National	079	HYPERTENSIVE ENCEPHALOPATHY W/O CC/MCC	1105	77	2.8	$21,916	$3,345
National	080	NONTRAUMATIC STUPOR & COMA W MCC	2115	72	5.2	$33,510	$7,127
National	081	NONTRAUMATIC STUPOR & COMA W/O MCC	7553	75	3.6	$20,473	$4,013
National	082	TRAUMATIC STUPOR & COMA, COMA >1 HR W MCC	3796	77	6.3	$61,686	$12,538

Peer Grouping	MS-DRG	Description	Discharges	Average Age	Average Length of Stay	Average Total Charge	Average Allowed
National	083	TRAUMATIC STUPOR & COMA, COMA >1 HR W CC	3558	76	5.1	$40,070	$7,668
National	084	TRAUMATIC STUPOR & COMA, COMA >1 HR W/O CC/MCC	3295	76	2.8	$28,227	$4,202
National	085	TRAUMATIC STUPOR & COMA, COMA <1 HR W MCC	12345	78	7.2	$56,825	$12,366
National	086	TRAUMATIC STUPOR & COMA, COMA <1 HR W CC	21001	80	4.5	$32,779	$6,224
National	087	TRAUMATIC STUPOR & COMA, COMA <1 HR W/O CC/MCC	17300	80	2.8	$22,775	$3,807
National	088	CONCUSSION W MCC	1124	75	5.1	$44,855	$9,216
National	089	CONCUSSION W CC	3600	76	3.4	$29,324	$4,810
National	090	CONCUSSION W/O CC/MCC	2685	74	2.2	$23,469	$3,201
National	091	OTHER DISORDERS OF NERVOUS SYSTEM W MCC	13628	70	6.8	$45,521	$9,977
National	092	OTHER DISORDERS OF NERVOUS SYSTEM W CC	25177	72	4.3	$26,002	$4,944
National	093	OTHER DISORDERS OF NERVOUS SYSTEM W/O CC/MCC	14469	71	3.0	$20,558	$3,125
National	094	BACTERIAL & TUBERCULOUS INFECTIONS OF NERVOUS SYSTEM W MCC	1959	69	13.9	$103,717	$23,043
National	095	BACTERIAL & TUBERCULOUS INFECTIONS OF NERVOUS SYSTEM W CC	1503	68	9.5	$69,170	$14,778
National	096	BACTERIAL & TUBERCULOUS INFECTIONS OF NERVOUS SYSTEM W/O CC/MCC	651	69	5.8	$58,507	$10,316
National	097	NON-BACTERIAL INFECT OF NERVOUS SYS EXC VIRAL MENINGITIS W MCC	1757	71	11.7	$93,090	$19,719
National	098	NON-BACTERIAL INFECT OF NERVOUS SYS EXC VIRAL MENINGITIS W CC	1412	69	7.9	$53,136	$10,320
National	099	NON-BACTERIAL INFECT OF NERVOUS SYS EXC VIRAL MENINGITIS W/O CC/MCC	623	68	5.3	$36,572	$6,608
National	100	SEIZURES W MCC	26882	66	5.8	$43,839	$8,922
National	101	SEIZURES W/O MCC	64772	64	3.3	$22,914	$3,847
National	102	HEADACHES W MCC	1789	59	4.3	$32,177	$5,598
National	103	HEADACHES W/O MCC	16167	62	2.8	$20,932	$2,915
National	113	ORBITAL PROCEDURES W CC/MCC	811	74	5.6	$59,751	$11,836
National	114	ORBITAL PROCEDURES W/O CC/MCC	485	73	2.9	$34,004	$4,894
National	115	EXTRAOCULAR PROCEDURES EXCEPT ORBIT	1074	74	4.2	$40,100	·$6,934
National	116	INTRAOCULAR PROCEDURES W CC/MCC	573	71	4.8	$45,944	$8,091
National	117	INTRAOCULAR PROCEDURES W/O CC/MCC	476	72	2.5	$26,258	$3,847
National	121	ACUTE MAJOR EYE INFECTIONS W CC/MCC	963	69	5.2	$28,900	$6,152
National	122	ACUTE MAJOR EYE INFECTIONS W/O CC/MCC	513	69	3.6	$16,111	$3,054
National	123	NEUROLOGICAL EYE DISORDERS	3841	72	2.6	$23,533	$3,125
National	124	OTHER DISORDERS OF THE EYE W MCC	1045	69	5.2	$34,622	$7,040
National	125	OTHER DISORDERS OF THE EYE W/O MCC	5498	74	3.2	$20,086	$3,371
National	129	MAJOR HEAD & NECK PROCEDURES W CC/MCC OR MAJOR DEVICE	2043	72	5.1	$70,160	$13,986
National	130	MAJOR HEAD & NECK PROCEDURES W/O CC/MCC	1372	73	2.7	$43,600	$6,430
National	131	CRANIAL/FACIAL PROCEDURES W CC/MCC	1520	67	5.5	$73,846	$14,946
National	132	CRANIAL/FACIAL PROCEDURES W/O CC/MCC	923	64	2.5	$41,527	$6,410
National	133	OTHER EAR, NOSE, MOUTH & THROAT O.R. PROCEDURES W CC/MCC	2930	68	5.4	$54,044	$10,272
National	134	OTHER EAR, NOSE, MOUTH & THROAT O.R. PROCEDURES W/O CC/MCC	2804	68	2.2	$30,622	$4,118
National	135	SINUS & MASTOID PROCEDURES W CC/MCC	486	65	6.0	$63,764	$12,121

Peer Grouping	MS-DRG	Description	Discharges	Average Age	Average Length of Stay	Average Total Charge	Average Allowed
National	136	SINUS & MASTOID PROCEDURES W/O CC/MCC	339	70	2.3	$32,687	$4,911
National	137	MOUTH PROCEDURES W CC/MCC	1237	66	4.9	$39,398	$7,298
National	138	MOUTH PROCEDURES W/O CC/MCC	962	71	2.5	$25,530	$3,544
National	139	SALIVARY GLAND PROCEDURES	1229	70	1.8	$29,295	$4,092
National	146	EAR, NOSE, MOUTH & THROAT MALIGNANCY W MCC	951	70	9.6	$62,531	$14,577
National	147	EAR, NOSE, MOUTH & THROAT MALIGNANCY W CC	1600	71	5.8	$36,355	$7,304
National	148	EAR, NOSE, MOUTH & THROAT MALIGNANCY W/O CC/MCC	571	71	3.4	$23,717	$3,895
National	149	DYSEQUILIBRIUM	36598	77	2.4	$19,078	$2,662
National	150	EPISTAXIS W MCC	1555	71	5.0	$36,021	$7,462
National	151	EPISTAXIS W/O MCC	6572	77	2.8	$16,762	$3,072
National	152	OTITIS MEDIA & URI W MCC	2664	66	4.5	$28,806	$5,642
National	153	OTITIS MEDIA & URI W/O MCC	13080	72	2.9	$17,855	$2,949
National	154	OTHER EAR, NOSE, MOUTH & THROAT DIAGNOSES W MCC	3126	72	5.7	$39,526	$8,246
National	155	OTHER EAR, NOSE, MOUTH & THROAT DIAGNOSES W CC	7344	74	3.9	$24,786	$4,597
National	156	OTHER EAR, NOSE, MOUTH & THROAT DIAGNOSES W/O CC/MCC	3719	73	2.8	$17,575	$2,813
National	157	DENTAL & ORAL DISEASES W MCC	1958	69	6.7	$45,431	$10,339
National	158	DENTAL & ORAL DISEASES W CC	4578	70	4.1	$24,485	$4,875
National	159	DENTAL & ORAL DISEASES W/O CC/MCC	1810	69	2.6	$17,604	$2,620
National	163	MAJOR CHEST PROCEDURES W MCC	15197	70	13.4	$136,540	$28,558
National	164	MAJOR CHEST PROCEDURES W CC	22473	72	6.7	$72,171	$13,792
National	165	MAJOR CHEST PROCEDURES W/O CC/MCC	13056	71	4.0	$52,079	$9,201
National	166	OTHER RESP SYSTEM O.R. PROCEDURES W MCC	25967	72	14.1	$117,917	$25,371
National	167	OTHER RESP SYSTEM O.R. PROCEDURES W CC	19005	73	6.8	$55,780	$10,910
National	168	OTHER RESP SYSTEM O.R. PROCEDURES W/O CC/MCC	4366	72	3.9	$37,598	$6,180
National	175	PULMONARY EMBOLISM W MCC	21343	74	6.4	$41,368	$8,515
National	176	PULMONARY EMBOLISM W/O MCC	50857	73	4.4	$26,739	$5,097
National	177	RESPIRATORY INFECTIONS & INFLAMMATIONS W MCC	84417	77	8.8	$54,668	$12,431
National	178	RESPIRATORY INFECTIONS & INFLAMMATIONS W CC	68352	77	6.4	$36,279	$8,264
National	179	RESPIRATORY INFECTIONS & INFLAMMATIONS W/O CC/MCC	16983	78	4.6	$24,378	$5,470
National	180	RESPIRATORY NEOPLASMS W MCC	25078	74	7.1	$48,617	$9,722
National	181	RESPIRATORY NEOPLASMS W CC	26309	75	5.1	$34,017	$6,490
National	182	RESPIRATORY NEOPLASMS W/O CC/MCC	2906	75	3.4	$23,123	$4,138
National	183	MAJOR CHEST TRAUMA W MCC	3833	78	5.9	$40,808	$7,720
National	184	MAJOR CHEST TRAUMA W CC	8705	78	4.1	$28,954	$4,895
National	185	MAJOR CHEST TRAUMA W/O CC/MCC	2841	80	2.9	$20,306	$3,100
National	186	PLEURAL EFFUSION W MCC	12619	73	6.5	$42,232	$8,896
National	187	PLEURAL EFFUSION W CC	12194	76	4.5	$29,849	$5,790
National	188	PLEURAL EFFUSION W/O CC/MCC	3585	78	3.3	$20,698	$3,811
National	189	PULMONARY EDEMA & RESPIRATORY FAILURE	136169	72	7.1	$41,122	$9,209
National	190	CHRONIC OBSTRUCTIVE PULMONARY DISEASE W MCC	173847	73	5.3	$31,295	$6,303
National	191	CHRONIC OBSTRUCTIVE PULMONARY DISEASE W CC	170717	72	4.2	$24,609	$4,893
National	192	CHRONIC OBSTRUCTIVE PULMONARY DISEASE W/O CC/MCC	132517	71	3.3	$17,978	$3,433
National	193	SIMPLE PNEUMONIA & PLEURISY W MCC	155696	75	6.3	$38,576	$8,203

Peer Grouping	MS-DRG	Description	Discharges	Average Age	Average Length of Stay	Average Total Charge	Average Allowed
National	194	SIMPLE PNEUMONIA & PLEURISY W CC	232435	77	4.6	$25,050	$5,338
National	195	SIMPLE PNEUMONIA & PLEURISY W/O CC/MCC	102158	77	3.5	$17,321	$3,659
National	196	INTERSTITIAL LUNG DISEASE W MCC	9034	74	7.0	$45,365	$9,408
National	197	INTERSTITIAL LUNG DISEASE W CC	6775	73	4.8	$29,752	$5,820
National	198	INTERSTITIAL LUNG DISEASE W/O CC/MCC	2880	74	3.6	$22,313	$4,044
National	199	PNEUMOTHORAX W MCC	4937	75	7.8	$49,075	$10,067
National	200	PNEUMOTHORAX W CC	10033	74	4.3	$26,568	$4,977
National	201	PNEUMOTHORAX W/O CC/MCC	3520	72	3.3	$18,931	$3,407
National	202	BRONCHITIS & ASTHMA W CC/MCC	45561	71	3.9	$23,418	$4,274
National	203	BRONCHITIS & ASTHMA W/O CC/MCC	29520	70	3.0	$16,303	$2,750
National	204	RESPIRATORY SIGNS & SYMPTOMS	25035	73	2.7	$19,832	$3,225
National	205	OTHER RESPIRATORY SYSTEM DIAGNOSES W MCC	9916	70	5.9	$41,157	$8,311
National	206	OTHER RESPIRATORY SYSTEM DIAGNOSES W/O MCC	22808	74	3.2	$22,606	$3,778
National	207	RESPIRATORY SYSTEM DIAGNOSIS W VENTILATOR SUPPORT 96+ HOURS	53113	70	21.4	$169,794	$41,589
National	208	RESPIRATORY SYSTEM DIAGNOSIS W VENTILATOR SUPPORT <96 HOURS	86193	71	7.3	$65,746	$13,427
National	215	OTHER HEART ASSIST SYSTEM IMPLANT	314	66	16.8	$406,796	$95,963
National	216	CARDIAC VALVE & OTH MAJ CARDIOTHORACIC PROC W CARD CATH W MCC	13266	74	15.9	$269,941	$58,728
National	217	CARDIAC VALVE & OTH MAJ CARDIOTHORACIC PROC W CARD CATH W CC	7593	76	9.8	$180,525	$37,168
National	218	CARDIAC VALVE & OTH MAJ CARDIOTHORACIC PROC W CARD CATH W/O CC/MCC	1301	76	7.3	$155,071	$28,341
National	219	CARDIAC VALVE & OTH MAJ CARDIOTHORACIC PROC W/O CARD CATH W MCC	21522	74	12.3	$226,220	$48,550
National	220	CARDIAC VALVE & OTH MAJ CARDIOTHORACIC PROC W/O CARD CATH W CC	26488	75	7.3	$148,719	$28,948
National	221	CARDIAC VALVE & OTH MAJ CARDIOTHORACIC PROC W/O CARD CATH W/O CC/MCC	6254	75	5.5	$126,093	$22,706
National	222	CARDIAC DEFIB IMPLANT W CARDIAC CATH W AMI/HF/SHOCK W MCC	2152	71	12.1	$238,150	$51,031
National	223	CARDIAC DEFIB IMPLANT W CARDIAC CATH W AMI/HF/SHOCK W/O MCC	2408	72	6.3	$168,672	$34,575
National	224	CARDIAC DEFIB IMPLANT W CARDIAC CATH W/O AMI/HF/SHOCK W MCC	2948	71	10.0	$208,312	$44,510
National	225	CARDIAC DEFIB IMPLANT W CARDIAC CATH W/O AMI/HF/SHOCK W/O MCC	3717	73	5.0	$154,649	$31,868
National	226	CARDIAC DEFIBRILLATOR IMPLANT W/O CARDIAC CATH W MCC	6226	71	8.5	$179,043	$39,869
National	227	CARDIAC DEFIBRILLATOR IMPLANT W/O CARDIAC CATH W/O MCC	23426	73	3.2	$136,030	$26,419
National	228	OTHER CARDIOTHORACIC PROCEDURES W MCC	2175	70	13.3	$204,924	$44,304
National	229	OTHER CARDIOTHORACIC PROCEDURES W CC	2541	70	7.9	$130,965	$24,944
National	230	OTHER CARDIOTHORACIC PROCEDURES W/O CC/MCC	690	69	5.2	$107,409	$18,785
National	231	CORONARY BYPASS W PTCA W MCC	1469	71	12.3	$231,416	$45,466
National	232	CORONARY BYPASS W PTCA W/O MCC	1237	71	9.0	$165,893	$29,654
National	233	CORONARY BYPASS W CARDIAC CATH W MCC	16048	71	13.5	$204,099	$37,808
National	234	CORONARY BYPASS W CARDIAC CATH W/O MCC	25843	72	8.7	$136,446	$23,706

Peer Grouping	MS-DRG	Description	Discharges	Average Age	Average Length of Stay	Average Total Charge	Average Allowed
National	235	CORONARY BYPASS W/O CARDIAC CATH W MCC	10133	70	10.7	$160,312	$32,057
National	236	CORONARY BYPASS W/O CARDIAC CATH W/O MCC	24824	71	6.5	$107,633	$19,031
National	237	MAJOR CARDIOVASC PROCEDURES W MCC	24004	72	9.9	$146,742	$30,937
National	238	MAJOR CARDIOVASC PROCEDURES W/O MCC	44203	74	3.9	$86,967	$16,519
National	239	AMPUTATION FOR CIRC SYS DISORDERS EXC UPPER LIMB & TOE W MCC	11422	68	14.6	$118,399	$26,742
National	240	AMPUTATION FOR CIRC SYS DISORDERS EXC UPPER LIMB & TOE W CC	11413	74	9.2	$66,600	$13,718
National	241	AMPUTATION FOR CIRC SYS DISORDERS EXC UPPER LIMB & TOE W/O CC/MCC	1670	75	5.9	$37,675	$7,262
National	242	PERMANENT CARDIAC PACEMAKER IMPLANT W MCC	21164	80	7.7	$96,015	$20,477
National	243	PERMANENT CARDIAC PACEMAKER IMPLANT W CC	39767	80	4.6	$68,721	$13,724
National	244	PERMANENT CARDIAC PACEMAKER IMPLANT W/O CC/MCC	36568	80	2.9	$54,918	$9,900
National	245	AICD GENERATOR PROCEDURES	2925	73	4.4	$119,479	$21,141
National	246	PERC CARDIOVASC PROC W DRUG-ELUTING STENT W MCC OR 4+ VESSELS/STENTS	37835	71	5.2	$96,195	$17,388
National	247	PERC CARDIOVASC PROC W DRUG-ELUTING STENT W/O MCC	140760	72	2.4	$64,207	$8,852
National	248	PERC CARDIOVASC PROC W NON-DRUG-ELUTING STENT W MCC OR 4+ VES/STENTS	15402	73	6.3	$91,308	$16,751
National	249	PERC CARDIOVASC PROC W NON-DRUG-ELUTING STENT W/O MCC	37267	74	2.9	$59,521	$8,691
National	250	PERC CARDIOVASC PROC W/O CORONARY ARTERY STENT W MCC	11360	72	7.1	$96,837	$17,573
National	251	PERC CARDIOVASC PROC W/O CORONARY ARTERY STENT W/O MCC	39033	72	2.9	$69,058	$8,939
National	252	OTHER VASCULAR PROCEDURES W MCC	43223	66	7.9	$89,194	$18,795
National	253	OTHER VASCULAR PROCEDURES W CC	49808	74	5.8	$72,156	$13,343
National	254	OTHER VASCULAR PROCEDURES W/O CC/MCC	37621	73	2.7	$50,517	$7,845
National	255	UPPER LIMB & TOE AMPUTATION FOR CIRC SYSTEM DISORDERS W MCC	2681	63	9.5	$67,482	$15,004
National	256	UPPER LIMB & TOE AMPUTATION FOR CIRC SYSTEM DISORDERS W CC	3710	71	6.8	$41,577	$8,402
National	257	UPPER LIMB & TOE AMPUTATION FOR CIRC SYSTEM DISORDERS W/O CC/MCC	418	74	4.0	$24,513	$4,638
National	258	CARDIAC PACEMAKER DEVICE REPLACEMENT W MCC	777	83	6.3	$73,641	$17,178
National	259	CARDIAC PACEMAKER DEVICE REPLACEMENT W/O MCC	3485	82	3.3	$50,433	$9,235
National	260	CARDIAC PACEMAKER REVISION EXCEPT DEVICE REPLACEMENT W MCC	2267	71	10.9	$107,837	$22,686
National	261	CARDIAC PACEMAKER REVISION EXCEPT DEVICE REPLACEMENT W CC	4240	74	4.3	$49,037	$9,135
National	262	CARDIAC PACEMAKER REVISION EXCEPT DEVICE REPLACEMENT W/O CC/MCC	2119	76	2.8	$37,338	$5,692
National	263	VEIN LIGATION & STRIPPING	528	69	5.0	$49,096	$9,209
National	264	OTHER CIRCULATORY SYSTEM O.R. PROCEDURES	22910	64	8.9	$73,246	$16,001
National	265	AICD LEAD PROCEDURES	1432	71	3.7	$74,628	$12,651
National	280	ACUTE MYOCARDIAL INFARCTION, DISCHARGED ALIVE W MCC	80400	78	6.1	$46,468	$9,553
National	281	ACUTE MYOCARDIAL INFARCTION, DISCHARGED ALIVE W CC	58858	78	3.8	$30,171	$5,628
National	282	ACUTE MYOCARDIAL INFARCTION, DISCHARGED ALIVE W/O CC/MCC	37102	77	2.5	$22,663	$3,592

Peer Grouping	MS-DRG	Description	Discharges	Average Age	Average Length of Stay	Average Total Charge	Average Allowed
National	283	ACUTE MYOCARDIAL INFARCTION, EXPIRED W MCC	13325	80	4.8	$49,751	$9,984
National	284	ACUTE MYOCARDIAL INFARCTION, EXPIRED W CC	3126	84	2.5	$22,189	$4,215
National	285	ACUTE MYOCARDIAL INFARCTION, EXPIRED W/O CC/MCC	1223	85	1.7	$14,613	$2,349
National	286	CIRCULATORY DISORDERS EXCEPT AMI, W CARD CATH W MCC	32813	69	6.8	$64,538	$11,826
National	287	CIRCULATORY DISORDERS EXCEPT AMI, W CARD CATH W/O MCC	137653	71	3.1	$35,691	$4,901
National	288	ACUTE & SUBACUTE ENDOCARDITIS W MCC	3207	68	14.1	$81,873	$20,186
National	289	ACUTE & SUBACUTE ENDOCARDITIS W CC	1416	73	9.7	$52,401	$12,074
National	290	ACUTE & SUBACUTE ENDOCARDITIS W/O CC/MCC	254	72	6.2	$34,686	$6,728
National	291	HEART FAILURE & SHOCK W MCC	222886	76	6.0	$39,230	$8,332
National	292	HEART FAILURE & SHOCK W CC	261027	78	4.5	$25,444	$5,203
National	293	HEART FAILURE & SHOCK W/O CC/MCC	107302	80	3.1	$17,170	$3,279
National	294	DEEP VEIN THROMBOPHLEBITIS W CC/MCC	1000	73	4.9	$23,711	$5,150
National	295	DEEP VEIN THROMBOPHLEBITIS W/O CC/MCC	353	77	3.6	$13,106	$3,241
National	296	CARDIAC ARREST, UNEXPLAINED W MCC	2960	72	3.0	$40,923	$7,317
National	297	CARDIAC ARREST, UNEXPLAINED W CC	809	77	1.6	$17,876	$3,363
National	298	CARDIAC ARREST, UNEXPLAINED W/O CC/MCC	429	80	1.1	$13,019	$1,862
National	299	PERIPHERAL VASCULAR DISORDERS W MCC	25776	72	6.4	$38,228	$8,206
National	300	PERIPHERAL VASCULAR DISORDERS W CC	55218	75	4.8	$25,195	$5,230
National	301	PERIPHERAL VASCULAR DISORDERS W/O CC/MCC	30327	76	3.3	$17,032	$3,152
National	302	ATHEROSCLEROSIS W MCC	7123	70	4.2	$28,232	$5,900
National	303	ATHEROSCLEROSIS W/O MCC	42420	74	2.5	$17,216	$2,716
National	304	HYPERTENSION W MCC	3600	74	4.4	$28,858	$5,189
National	305	HYPERTENSION W/O MCC	42286	74	2.6	$17,924	$2,703
National	306	CARDIAC CONGENITAL & VALVULAR DISORDERS W MCC	4085	79	5.6	$38,165	$8,243
National	307	CARDIAC CONGENITAL & VALVULAR DISORDERS W/O MCC	6923	82	3.6	$22,255	$4,506
National	308	CARDIAC ARRHYTHMIA & CONDUCTION DISORDERS W MCC	81190	77	5.0	$32,774	$6,604
National	309	CARDIAC ARRHYTHMIA & CONDUCTION DISORDERS W CC	132261	77	3.3	$21,703	$3,973
National	310	CARDIAC ARRHYTHMIA & CONDUCTION DISORDERS W/O CC/MCC	141941	77	2.3	$15,436	$2,330
National	311	ANGINA PECTORIS	14667	73	2.2	$15,213	$2,169
National	312	SYNCOPE & COLLAPSE	170855	77	2.8	$20,656	$3,072
National	313	CHEST PAIN	159856	70	2.0	$17,574	$2,025
National	314	OTHER CIRCULATORY SYSTEM DIAGNOSES W MCC	64873	63	7.3	$52,433	$11,344
National	315	OTHER CIRCULATORY SYSTEM DIAGNOSES W CC	32802	71	4.1	$26,735	$5,093
National	316	OTHER CIRCULATORY SYSTEM DIAGNOSES W/O CC/MCC	10322	73	2.5	$18,082	$2,873
National	326	STOMACH, ESOPHAGEAL & DUODENAL PROC W MCC	13264	73	15.1	$154,931	$33,675
National	327	STOMACH, ESOPHAGEAL & DUODENAL PROC W CC	12991	71	8.0	$76,411	$15,125
National	328	STOMACH, ESOPHAGEAL & DUODENAL PROC W/O CC/MCC	12782	70	3.4	$43,355	$6,866
National	329	MAJOR SMALL & LARGE BOWEL PROCEDURES W MCC	50897	75	14.7	$135,916	$30,315
National	330	MAJOR SMALL & LARGE BOWEL PROCEDURES W CC	68884	73	8.5	$68,128	$13,715
National	331	MAJOR SMALL & LARGE BOWEL PROCEDURES W/O CC/MCC	31337	72	4.9	$43,917	$7,939
National	332	RECTAL RESECTION W MCC	1703	75	13.2	$123,926	$27,032
National	333	RECTAL RESECTION W CC	5462	74	7.5	$66,190	$13,016

Peer Grouping	MS-DRG	Description	Discharges	Average Age	Average Length of Stay	Average Total Charge	Average Allowed
National	334	RECTAL RESECTION W/O CC/MCC	3875	75	4.4	$43,861	$7,903
National	335	PERITONEAL ADHESIOLYSIS W MCC	8472	73	13.1	$112,371	$24,497
National	336	PERITONEAL ADHESIOLYSIS W CC	15905	71	8.3	$63,535	$12,662
National	337	PERITONEAL ADHESIOLYSIS W/O CC/MCC	9251	69	4.9	$43,075	$7,251
National	338	APPENDECTOMY W COMPLICATED PRINCIPAL DIAG W MCC	1475	71	9.6	$88,806	$19,018
National	339	APPENDECTOMY W COMPLICATED PRINCIPAL DIAG W CC	3726	71	6.0	$48,777	$9,342
National	340	APPENDECTOMY W COMPLICATED PRINCIPAL DIAG W/O CC/MCC	3678	70	3.6	$34,092	$5,770
National	341	APPENDECTOMY W/O COMPLICATED PRINCIPAL DIAG W MCC	1101	67	6.4	$64,697	$13,376
National	342	APPENDECTOMY W/O COMPLICATED PRINCIPAL DIAG W CC	3428	68	3.5	$38,860	$6,595
National	343	APPENDECTOMY W/O COMPLICATED PRINCIPAL DIAG W/O CC/MCC	7072	67	1.9	$28,839	$4,219
National	344	MINOR SMALL & LARGE BOWEL PROCEDURES W MCC	1140	70	11.4	$99,815	$20,719
National	345	MINOR SMALL & LARGE BOWEL PROCEDURES W CC	4132	70	6.5	$45,582	$9,204
National	346	MINOR SMALL & LARGE BOWEL PROCEDURES W/O CC/MCC	3281	70	4.4	$32,503	$5,714
National	347	ANAL & STOMAL PROCEDURES W MCC	1841	67	8.9	$74,562	$15,721
National	348	ANAL & STOMAL PROCEDURES W CC	5203	68	5.1	$37,504	$7,340
National	349	ANAL & STOMAL PROCEDURES W/O CC/MCC	4007	69	2.8	$24,277	$3,424
National	350	INGUINAL & FEMORAL HERNIA PROCEDURES W MCC	2050	76	7.8	$68,623	$14,506
National	351	INGUINAL & FEMORAL HERNIA PROCEDURES W CC	5152	78	4.4	$38,899	$7,036
National	352	INGUINAL & FEMORAL HERNIA PROCEDURES W/O CC/MCC	6510	77	2.4	$26,287	$3,711
National	353	HERNIA PROCEDURES EXCEPT INGUINAL & FEMORAL W MCC	4237	67	8.1	$78,864	$16,764
National	354	HERNIA PROCEDURES EXCEPT INGUINAL & FEMORAL W CC	11851	68	4.9	$44,628	$7,911
National	355	HERNIA PROCEDURES EXCEPT INGUINAL & FEMORAL W/O CC/MCC	13585	69	2.8	$31,475	$4,578
National	356	OTHER DIGESTIVE SYSTEM O.R. PROCEDURES W MCC	9243	71	12.2	$106,467	$23,805
National	357	OTHER DIGESTIVE SYSTEM O.R. PROCEDURES W CC	9101	73	7.0	$59,356	$11,712
National	358	OTHER DIGESTIVE SYSTEM O.R. PROCEDURES W/O CC/MCC	2400	69	4.0	$40,168	$6,455
National	368	MAJOR ESOPHAGEAL DISORDERS W MCC	4222	69	6.9	$52,565	$11,276
National	369	MAJOR ESOPHAGEAL DISORDERS W CC	6519	72	4.2	$29,412	$5,497
National	370	MAJOR ESOPHAGEAL DISORDERS W/O CC/MCC	1832	72	2.9	$21,410	$3,432
National	371	MAJOR GASTROINTESTINAL DISORDERS & PERITONEAL INFECTIONS W MCC	29148	71	8.9	$52,655	$12,341
National	372	MAJOR GASTROINTESTINAL DISORDERS & PERITONEAL INFECTIONS W CC	45250	76	5.9	$30,556	$6,907
National	373	MAJOR GASTROINTESTINAL DISORDERS & PERITONEAL INFECTIONS W/O CC/MCC	14374	75	4.2	$20,955	$4,257
National	374	DIGESTIVE MALIGNANCY W MCC	10726	75	8.7	$58,385	$12,626
National	375	DIGESTIVE MALIGNANCY W CC	20948	76	5.6	$35,386	$7,040
National	376	DIGESTIVE MALIGNANCY W/O CC/MCC	2680	76	3.7	$25,323	$4,246
National	377	G.I. HEMORRHAGE W MCC	65840	74	6.1	$46,915	$9,986
National	378	G.I. HEMORRHAGE W CC	174524	78	3.9	$26,720	$5,054
National	379	G.I. HEMORRHAGE W/O CC/MCC	49112	78	2.8	$18,420	$3,157
National	380	COMPLICATED PEPTIC ULCER W MCC	3566	72	7.4	$53,433	$11,128
National	381	COMPLICATED PEPTIC ULCER W CC	7133	74	4.6	$31,415	$5,811
National	382	COMPLICATED PEPTIC ULCER W/O CC/MCC	2571	71	3.2	$22,614	$3,690

Peer Grouping	MS-DRG	Description	Discharges	Average Age	Average Length of Stay	Average Total Charge	Average Allowed
National	383	UNCOMPLICATED PEPTIC ULCER W MCC	1340	69	5.7	$39,838	$7,430
National	384	UNCOMPLICATED PEPTIC ULCER W/O MCC	8122	72	3.5	$24,857	$3,833
National	385	INFLAMMATORY BOWEL DISEASE W MCC	2649	65	8.3	$52,639	$11,309
National	386	INFLAMMATORY BOWEL DISEASE W CC	10585	63	4.9	$28,383	$5,384
National	387	INFLAMMATORY BOWEL DISEASE W/O CC/MCC	5052	60	3.7	$21,385	$3,620
National	388	G.I. OBSTRUCTION W MCC	22632	74	7.2	$44,287	$9,623
National	389	G.I. OBSTRUCTION W CC	67071	74	4.5	$24,389	$4,717
National	390	G.I. OBSTRUCTION W/O CC/MCC	50131	74	3.2	$17,203	$2,888
National	391	ESOPHAGITIS, GASTROENT & MISC DIGEST DISORDERS W MCC	59633	68	5.2	$33,456	$6,666
National	392	ESOPHAGITIS, GASTROENT & MISC DIGEST DISORDERS W/O MCC	301838	72	3.3	$20,533	$3,185
National	393	OTHER DIGESTIVE SYSTEM DIAGNOSES W MCC	28864	72	7.4	$49,796	$10,876
National	394	OTHER DIGESTIVE SYSTEM DIAGNOSES W CC	59300	74	4.4	$27,180	$5,134
National	395	OTHER DIGESTIVE SYSTEM DIAGNOSES W/O CC/MCC	23330	74	3.0	$19,169	$2,921
National	405	PANCREAS, LIVER & SHUNT PROCEDURES W MCC	5655	70	14.7	$161,064	$35,302
National	406	PANCREAS, LIVER & SHUNT PROCEDURES W CC	6879	70	7.8	$85,648	$15,875
National	407	PANCREAS, LIVER & SHUNT PROCEDURES W/O CC/MCC	2762	71	5.0	$60,188	$10,438
National	408	BILIARY TRACT PROC EXCEPT ONLY CHOLECYST W OR W/O C.D.E. W MCC	1348	74	13.4	$121,131	$25,103
National	409	BILIARY TRACT PROC EXCEPT ONLY CHOLECYST W OR W/O C.D.E. W CC	1301	73	8.0	$70,103	$13,221
National	410	BILIARY TRACT PROC EXCEPT ONLY CHOLECYST W OR W/O C.D.E. W/O CC/MCC	437	73	5.1	$44,648	$7,777
National	411	CHOLECYSTECTOMY W C.D.E. W MCC	598	75	11.4	$101,414	$20,437
National	412	CHOLECYSTECTOMY W C.D.E. W CC	653	74	7.8	$67,590	$13,153
National	413	CHOLECYSTECTOMY W C.D.E. W/O CC/MCC	413	73	5.1	$48,305	$8,648
National	414	CHOLECYSTECTOMY EXCEPT BY LAPAROSCOPE W/O C.D.E. W MCC	4426	73	10.6	$97,617	$20,673
National	415	CHOLECYSTECTOMY EXCEPT BY LAPAROSCOPE W/O C.D.E. W CC	5899	72	6.7	$55,669	$10,659
National	416	CHOLECYSTECTOMY EXCEPT BY LAPAROSCOPE W/O C.D.E. W/O CC/MCC	3933	70	4.1	$37,399	$6,633
National	417	LAPAROSCOPIC CHOLECYSTECTOMY W/O C.D.E. W MCC	20690	72	7.5	$70,935	$13,992
National	418	LAPAROSCOPIC CHOLECYSTECTOMY W/O C.D.E. W CC	32374	72	4.9	$47,810	$8,387
National	419	LAPAROSCOPIC CHOLECYSTECTOMY W/O C.D.E. W/O CC/MCC	30298	70	3.0	$35,555	$5,203
National	420	HEPATOBILIARY DIAGNOSTIC PROCEDURES W MCC	758	70	12.3	$108,333	$24,134
National	421	HEPATOBILIARY DIAGNOSTIC PROCEDURES W CC	1030	72	6.2	$53,078	$10,598
National	422	HEPATOBILIARY DIAGNOSTIC PROCEDURES W/O CC/MCC	247	71	4.0	$39,220	$6,191
National	423	OTHER HEPATOBILIARY OR PANCREAS O.R. PROCEDURES W MCC	1696	68	13.3	$124,590	$27,507
National	424	OTHER HEPATOBILIARY OR PANCREAS O.R. PROCEDURES W CC	925	70	8.3	$67,701	$13,498
National	425	OTHER HEPATOBILIARY OR PANCREAS O.R. PROCEDURES W/O CC/MCC	114	67	4.9	$49,810	$8,876
National	432	CIRRHOSIS & ALCOHOLIC HEPATITIS W MCC	14130	64	6.4	$48,618	$9,996
National	433	CIRRHOSIS & ALCOHOLIC HEPATITIS W CC	9251	65	4.1	$26,445	$4,952
National	434	CIRRHOSIS & ALCOHOLIC HEPATITIS W/O CC/MCC	360	63	2.9	$17,247	$2,790

Peer Grouping	MS-DRG	Description	Discharges	Average Age	Average Length of Stay	Average Total Charge	Average Allowed
National	435	MALIGNANCY OF HEPATOBILIARY SYSTEM OR PANCREAS W MCC	15578	75	7.0	$51,057	$10,241
National	436	MALIGNANCY OF HEPATOBILIARY SYSTEM OR PANCREAS W CC	14114	75	5.1	$33,864	$6,313
National	437	MALIGNANCY OF HEPATOBILIARY SYSTEM OR PANCREAS W/O CC/MCC	2282	75	3.6	$28,072	$4,610
National	438	DISORDERS OF PANCREAS EXCEPT MALIGNANCY W MCC	18172	65	7.5	$50,832	$11,002
National	439	DISORDERS OF PANCREAS EXCEPT MALIGNANCY W CC	34708	67	4.5	$26,521	$5,046
National	440	DISORDERS OF PANCREAS EXCEPT MALIGNANCY W/O CC/MCC	25203	66	3.2	$18,840	$3,158
National	441	DISORDERS OF LIVER EXCEPT MALIG,CIRR,ALC HEPA W MCC	23767	64	7.1	$53,872	$11,527
National	442	DISORDERS OF LIVER EXCEPT MALIG,CIRR,ALC HEPA W CC	25985	65	4.3	$26,448	$5,165
National	443	DISORDERS OF LIVER EXCEPT MALIG,CIRR,ALC HEPA W/O CC/MCC	5769	65	3.2	$18,633	$3,285
National	444	DISORDERS OF THE BILIARY TRACT W MCC	15624	75	6.3	$46,553	$9,420
National	445	DISORDERS OF THE BILIARY TRACT W CC	23692	76	4.2	$30,759	$5,500
National	446	DISORDERS OF THE BILIARY TRACT W/O CC/MCC	13776	75	2.9	$22,072	$3,274
National	453	COMBINED ANTERIOR/POSTERIOR SPINAL FUSION W MCC	1756	68	12.5	$312,038	$70,531
National	454	COMBINED ANTERIOR/POSTERIOR SPINAL FUSION W CC	4568	67	6.1	$204,453	$44,513
National	455	COMBINED ANTERIOR/POSTERIOR SPINAL FUSION W/O CC/MCC	3959	65	3.6	$153,544	$32,571
National	456	SPINAL FUS EXC CERV W SPINAL CURV/MALIG/INFEC OR 9+ FUS W MCC	1656	69	12.8	$261,207	$63,649
National	457	SPINAL FUS EXC CERV W SPINAL CURV/MALIG/INFEC OR 9+ FUS W CC	4480	70	6.6	$174,758	$39,175
National	458	SPINAL FUS EXC CERV W SPINAL CURV/MALIG/INFEC OR 9+ FUS W/O CC/MCC	2088	70	3.8	$124,094	$28,708
National	459	SPINAL FUSION EXCEPT CERVICAL W MCC	5344	70	8.8	$163,057	$35,922
National	460	SPINAL FUSION EXCEPT CERVICAL W/O MCC	85656	68	3.6	$95,291	$20,134
National	461	BILATERAL OR MULTIPLE MAJOR JOINT PROCS OF LOWER EXTREMITY W MCC	624	71	7.4	$124,052	$27,934
National	462	BILATERAL OR MULTIPLE MAJOR JOINT PROCS OF LOWER EXTREMITY W/O MCC	11591	70	3.8	$83,121	$17,007
National	463	WND DEBRID & SKN GRFT EXC HAND, FOR MUSCULO-CONN TISS DIS W MCC	6967	67	19.0	$136,454	$32,487
National	464	WND DEBRID & SKN GRFT EXC HAND, FOR MUSCULO-CONN TISS DIS W CC	10851	69	9.0	$79,154	$16,440
National	465	WND DEBRID & SKN GRFT EXC HAND, FOR MUSCULO-CONN TISS DIS W/O CC/MCC	2905	69	5.0	$52,142	$9,768
National	466	REVISION OF HIP OR KNEE REPLACEMENT W MCC	4974	74	8.6	$124,854	$27,004
National	467	REVISION OF HIP OR KNEE REPLACEMENT W CC	28032	72	4.5	$83,031	$17,026
National	468	REVISION OF HIP OR KNEE REPLACEMENT W/O CC/MCC	20180	70	3.2	$67,425	$13,294
National	469	MAJOR JOINT REPLACEMENT OR REATTACHMENT OF LOWER EXTREMITY W MCC	33131	78	7.4	$82,010	$17,490
National	470	MAJOR JOINT REPLACEMENT OR REATTACHMENT OF LOWER EXTREMITY W/O MCC	526210	73	3.4	$51,396	$10,063
National	471	CERVICAL SPINAL FUSION W MCC	4043	69	9.0	$134,568	$27,947
National	472	CERVICAL SPINAL FUSION W CC	13157	66	3.6	$77,589	$15,139
National	473	CERVICAL SPINAL FUSION W/O CC/MCC	34607	64	1.8	$56,600	$10,321

Peer Grouping	MS-DRG	Description	Discharges	Average Age	Average Length of Stay	Average Total Charge	Average Allowed
National	474	AMPUTATION FOR MUSCULOSKELETAL SYS & CONN TISSUE DIS W MCC	3731	64	12.7	$97,269	$21,680
National	475	AMPUTATION FOR MUSCULOSKELETAL SYS & CONN TISSUE DIS W CC	4721	67	7.5	$53,122	$10,533
National	476	AMPUTATION FOR MUSCULOSKELETAL SYS & CONN TISSUE DIS W/O CC/MCC	1377	65	4.0	$29,848	$5,602
National	477	BIOPSIES OF MUSCULOSKELETAL SYSTEM & CONNECTIVE TISSUE W MCC	3178	73	11.5	$91,307	$20,311
National	478	BIOPSIES OF MUSCULOSKELETAL SYSTEM & CONNECTIVE TISSUE W CC	8814	76	6.8	$61,226	$11,877
National	479	BIOPSIES OF MUSCULOSKELETAL SYSTEM & CONNECTIVE TISSUE W/O CC/MCC	3703	78	4.2	$47,299	$8,252
National	480	HIP & FEMUR PROCEDURES EXCEPT MAJOR JOINT W MCC	30122	80	8.4	$78,935	$17,062
National	481	HIP & FEMUR PROCEDURES EXCEPT MAJOR JOINT W CC	96275	82	5.2	$50,443	$10,024
National	482	HIP & FEMUR PROCEDURES EXCEPT MAJOR JOINT W/O CC/MCC	32645	80	4.2	$41,638	$7,998
National	483	MAJOR JOINT & LIMB REATTACHMENT PROC OF UPPER EXTREMITY W CC/MCC	16871	74	3.3	$64,741	$12,545
National	484	MAJOR JOINT & LIMB REATTACHMENT PROC OF UPPER EXTREMITY W/O CC/MCC	27595	73	2.0	$53,513	$9,918
National	485	KNEE PROCEDURES W PDX OF INFECTION W MCC	1472	70	10.6	$90,593	$19,296
National	486	KNEE PROCEDURES W PDX OF INFECTION W CC	3310	71	6.6	$55,499	$11,060
National	487	KNEE PROCEDURES W PDX OF INFECTION W/O CC/MCC	1315	70	4.7	$40,681	$7,591
National	488	KNEE PROCEDURES W/O PDX OF INFECTION W CC/MCC	4238	69	4.3	$46,217	$8,877
National	489	KNEE PROCEDURES W/O PDX OF INFECTION W/O CC/MCC	5322	69	2.7	$33,409	$5,435
National	490	BACK & NECK PROC EXC SPINAL FUSION W CC/MCC OR DISC DEVICE/NEUROSTIM	23444	72	4.5	$53,177	$9,190
National	491	BACK & NECK PROC EXC SPINAL FUSION W/O CC/MCC	44798	71	2.1	$31,437	$4,029
National	492	LOWER EXTREM & HUMER PROC EXCEPT HIP,FOOT,FEMUR W MCC	6719	69	8.2	$84,461	$17,478
National	493	LOWER EXTREM & HUMER PROC EXCEPT HIP,FOOT,FEMUR W CC	25209	71	4.8	$53,394	$9,639
National	494	LOWER EXTREM & HUMER PROC EXCEPT HIP,FOOT,FEMUR W/O CC/MCC	26028	70	3.0	$39,341	$6,192
National	495	LOCAL EXCISION & REMOVAL INT FIX DEVICES EXC HIP & FEMUR W MCC	2269	65	11.9	$85,952	$19,259
National	496	LOCAL EXCISION & REMOVAL INT FIX DEVICES EXC HIP & FEMUR W CC	6163	67	5.4	$48,585	$9,058
National	497	LOCAL EXCISION & REMOVAL INT FIX DEVICES EXC HIP & FEMUR W/O CC/MCC	5312	67	2.5	$33,073	$5,296
National	498	LOCAL EXCISION & REMOVAL INT FIX DEVICES OF HIP & FEMUR W CC/MCC	1622	69	7.5	$61,916	$12,396
National	499	LOCAL EXCISION & REMOVAL INT FIX DEVICES OF HIP & FEMUR W/O CC/MCC	799	70	2.5	$27,141	$4,420
National	500	SOFT TISSUE PROCEDURES W MCC	2708	65	13.5	$96,399	$22,514
National	501	SOFT TISSUE PROCEDURES W CC	6533	69	5.7	$43,867	$8,407
National	502	SOFT TISSUE PROCEDURES W/O CC/MCC	5548	70	2.8	$31,161	$4,820
National	503	FOOT PROCEDURES W MCC	1265	67	9.1	$65,934	$14,340
National	504	FOOT PROCEDURES W CC	3830	70	6.1	$44,239	$8,211
National	505	FOOT PROCEDURES W/O CC/MCC	2505	68	3.2	$32,365	$5,312

Peer Grouping	MS-DRG	Description	Discharges	Average Age	Average Length of Stay	Average Total Charge	Average Allowed
National	506	MAJOR THUMB OR JOINT PROCEDURES	768	70	3.7	$33,903	$5,708
National	507	MAJOR SHOULDER OR ELBOW JOINT PROCEDURES W CC/MCC	777	69	5.8	$55,209	$10,383
National	508	MAJOR SHOULDER OR ELBOW JOINT PROCEDURES W/O CC/MCC	802	69	2.2	$34,221	$5,082
National	509	ARTHROSCOPY	253	71	3.5	$37,369	$6,681
National	510	SHOULDER,ELBOW OR FOREARM PROC,EXC MAJOR JOINT PROC W MCC	1266	74	6.2	$62,466	$11,773
National	511	SHOULDER,ELBOW OR FOREARM PROC,EXC MAJOR JOINT PROC W CC	4762	76	3.8	$43,431	$7,305
National	512	SHOULDER,ELBOW OR FOREARM PROC,EXC MAJOR JOINT PROC W/O CC/MCC	6714	74	2.2	$32,944	$4,715
National	513	HAND OR WRIST PROC, EXCEPT MAJOR THUMB OR JOINT PROC W CC/MCC	1785	67	4.9	$40,561	$7,042
National	514	HAND OR WRIST PROC, EXCEPT MAJOR THUMB OR JOINT PROC W/O CC/MCC	1067	68	2.7	$24,969	$3,874
National	515	OTHER MUSCULOSKELET SYS & CONN TISS O.R. PROC W MCC	4613	75	10.1	$92,195	$19,227
National	516	OTHER MUSCULOSKELET SYS & CONN TISS O.R. PROC W CC	11724	78	5.6	$55,261	$10,356
National	517	OTHER MUSCULOSKELET SYS & CONN TISS O.R. PROC W/O CC/MCC	8822	76	3.3	$44,735	$7,601
National	533	FRACTURES OF FEMUR W MCC	1003	75	5.8	$35,553	$8,913
National	534	FRACTURES OF FEMUR W/O MCC	4065	81	4.0	$18,465	$4,251
National	535	FRACTURES OF HIP & PELVIS W MCC	9186	82	5.7	$33,886	$7,410
National	536	FRACTURES OF HIP & PELVIS W/O MCC	38890	84	4.1	$18,374	$4,329
National	537	SPRAINS, STRAINS, & DISLOCATIONS OF HIP, PELVIS & THIGH W CC/MCC	938	80	4.0	$23,851	$4,420
National	538	SPRAINS, STRAINS, & DISLOCATIONS OF HIP, PELVIS & THIGH W/O CC/MCC	596	80	3.0	$18,302	$3,017
National	539	OSTEOMYELITIS W MCC	6040	66	18.9	$80,196	$21,271
National	540	OSTEOMYELITIS W CC	5637	70	10.1	$43,579	$10,492
National	541	OSTEOMYELITIS W/O CC/MCC	1460	70	6.7	$28,506	$6,345
National	542	PATHOLOGICAL FRACTURES & MUSCULOSKELET & CONN TISS MALIG W MCC	6399	75	8.1	$52,070	$11,454
National	543	PATHOLOGICAL FRACTURES & MUSCULOSKELET & CONN TISS MALIG W CC	17482	78	5.3	$31,217	$6,266
National	544	PATHOLOGICAL FRACTURES & MUSCULOSKELET & CONN TISS MALIG W/O CC/MCC	5649	81	3.8	$20,122	$3,877
National	545	CONNECTIVE TISSUE DISORDERS W MCC	4580	64	8.8	$67,808	$15,719
National	546	CONNECTIVE TISSUE DISORDERS W CC	7015	67	5.2	$32,967	$6,522
National	547	CONNECTIVE TISSUE DISORDERS W/O CC/MCC	3386	68	3.6	$21,936	$3,806
National	548	SEPTIC ARTHRITIS W MCC	954	69	14.5	$67,996	$17,557
National	549	SEPTIC ARTHRITIS W CC	1811	71	7.6	$34,678	$8,903
National	550	SEPTIC ARTHRITIS W/O CC/MCC	712	73	4.8	$22,468	$4,641
National	551	MEDICAL BACK PROBLEMS W MCC	15111	76	6.8	$44,134	$9,246
National	552	MEDICAL BACK PROBLEMS W/O MCC	84385	77	3.9	$23,137	$4,076
National	553	BONE DISEASES & ARTHROPATHIES W MCC	3097	72	5.9	$37,484	$8,290
National	554	BONE DISEASES & ARTHROPATHIES W/O MCC	23414	76	4.4	$18,310	$4,807
National	555	SIGNS & SYMPTOMS OF MUSCULOSKELETAL SYSTEM & CONN TISSUE W MCC	4062	70	5.0	$33,630	$6,989

Peer Grouping	MS-DRG	Description	Discharges	Average Age	Average Length of Stay	Average Total Charge	Average Allowed
National	556	SIGNS & SYMPTOMS OF MUSCULOSKELETAL SYSTEM & CONN TISSUE W/O MCC	21698	75	3.2	$19,362	$3,223
National	557	TENDONITIS, MYOSITIS & BURSITIS W MCC	5443	74	7.2	$41,107	$8,936
National	558	TENDONITIS, MYOSITIS & BURSITIS W/O MCC	20950	75	4.2	$22,685	$4,553
National	559	AFTERCARE, MUSCULOSKELETAL SYSTEM & CONNECTIVE TISSUE W MCC	4768	73	16.5	$72,392	$19,503
National	560	AFTERCARE, MUSCULOSKELETAL SYSTEM & CONNECTIVE TISSUE W CC	8236	73	8.8	$36,439	$9,248
National	561	AFTERCARE, MUSCULOSKELETAL SYSTEM & CONNECTIVE TISSUE W/O CC/MCC	5470	74	3.8	$18,779	$4,153
National	562	FX, SPRN, STRN & DISL EXCEPT FEMUR, HIP, PELVIS & THIGH W MCC	7213	76	5.6	$35,302	$7,619
National	563	FX, SPRN, STRN & DISL EXCEPT FEMUR, HIP, PELVIS & THIGH W/O MCC	36228	79	3.6	$19,661	$3,629
National	564	OTHER MUSCULOSKELETAL SYS & CONNECTIVE TISSUE DIAGNOSES W MCC	2887	65	9.5	$51,292	$11,938
National	565	OTHER MUSCULOSKELETAL SYS & CONNECTIVE TISSUE DIAGNOSES W CC	5476	70	5.7	$28,603	$6,204
National	566	OTHER MUSCULOSKELETAL SYS & CONNECTIVE TISSUE DIAGNOSES W/O CC/MCC	1746	72	4.0	$19,124	$3,962
National	570	SKIN DEBRIDEMENT W MCC	7095	70	16.8	$79,290	$21,432
National	571	SKIN DEBRIDEMENT W CC	6422	69	7.4	$38,653	$8,622
National	572	SKIN DEBRIDEMENT W/O CC/MCC	2871	68	4.9	$25,151	$4,875
National	573	SKIN GRAFT FOR SKIN ULCER OR CELLULITIS W MCC	3661	61	18.9	$104,337	$26,399
National	574	SKIN GRAFT FOR SKIN ULCER OR CELLULITIS W CC	1560	67	10.6	$68,206	$15,184
National	575	SKIN GRAFT FOR SKIN ULCER OR CELLULITIS W/O CC/MCC	598	70	5.8	$38,039	$7,002
National	576	SKIN GRAFT EXC FOR SKIN ULCER OR CELLULITIS W MCC	580	71	13.1	$131,102	$26,185
National	577	SKIN GRAFT EXC FOR SKIN ULCER OR CELLULITIS W CC	2270	74	6.0	$61,506	$11,208
National	578	SKIN GRAFT EXC FOR SKIN ULCER OR CELLULITIS W/O CC/MCC	2481	73	3.1	$37,186	$5,470
National	579	OTHER SKIN, SUBCUT TISS & BREAST PROC W MCC	7888	68	13.3	$77,823	$18,741
National	580	OTHER SKIN, SUBCUT TISS & BREAST PROC W CC	12655	69	5.2	$41,721	$7,554
National	581	OTHER SKIN, SUBCUT TISS & BREAST PROC W/O CC/MCC	11453	70	2.5	$30,470	$4,092
National	582	MASTECTOMY FOR MALIGNANCY W CC/MCC	4456	73	2.6	$34,340	$5,530
National	583	MASTECTOMY FOR MALIGNANCY W/O CC/MCC	6486	74	1.7	$28,556	$3,927
National	584	BREAST BIOPSY, LOCAL EXCISION & OTHER BREAST PROCEDURES W CC/MCC	966	64	4.8	$50,033	$8,515
National	585	BREAST BIOPSY, LOCAL EXCISION & OTHER BREAST PROCEDURES W/O CC/MCC	1631	65	2.4	$36,751	$4,816
National	592	SKIN ULCERS W MCC	11758	70	13.9	$56,306	$14,516
National	593	SKIN ULCERS W CC	7980	73	6.5	$27,339	$6,431
National	594	SKIN ULCERS W/O CC/MCC	1194	73	4.6	$16,633	$4,282
National	595	MAJOR SKIN DISORDERS W MCC	1507	73	8.4	$56,080	$13,004
National	596	MAJOR SKIN DISORDERS W/O MCC	5640	74	4.7	$24,317	$4,840
National	597	MALIGNANT BREAST DISORDERS W MCC	895	72	7.8	$48,070	$9,805
National	598	MALIGNANT BREAST DISORDERS W CC	2015	73	5.7	$30,211	$6,743
National	599	MALIGNANT BREAST DISORDERS W/O CC/MCC	226	75	3.1	$17,113	$3,316
National	600	NON-MALIGNANT BREAST DISORDERS W CC/MCC	1473	64	5.0	$27,000	$5,552
National	601	NON-MALIGNANT BREAST DISORDERS W/O CC/MCC	927	64	3.4	$16,326	$2,803

Peer Grouping	MS-DRG	Description	Discharges	Average Age	Average Length of Stay	Average Total Charge	Average Allowed
National	602	CELLULITIS W MCC	33323	70	7.1	$39,179	$8,797
National	603	CELLULITIS W/O MCC	180086	71	4.3	$20,665	$4,301
National	604	TRAUMA TO THE SKIN, SUBCUT TISS & BREAST W MCC	3511	76	5.4	$37,646	$7,742
National	605	TRAUMA TO THE SKIN, SUBCUT TISS & BREAST W/O MCC	21381	80	3.2	$20,907	$3,600
National	606	MINOR SKIN DISORDERS W MCC	2156	66	7.3	$41,555	$9,725
National	607	MINOR SKIN DISORDERS W/O MCC	8913	70	3.8	$19,242	$3,772
National	614	ADRENAL & PITUITARY PROCEDURES W CC/MCC	2109	68	6.1	$82,473	$15,199
National	615	ADRENAL & PITUITARY PROCEDURES W/O CC/MCC	1735	69	2.7	$46,780	$7,393
National	616	AMPUTAT OF LOWER LIMB FOR ENDOCRINE,NUTRIT,& METABOL DIS W MCC	2136	66	15.2	$108,925	$24,854
National	617	AMPUTAT OF LOWER LIMB FOR ENDOCRINE,NUTRIT,& METABOL DIS W CC	10805	65	7.8	$52,901	$10,636
National	618	AMPUTAT OF LOWER LIMB FOR ENDOCRINE,NUTRIT,& METABOL DIS W/O CC/MCC	136	67	5.6	$32,089	$6,694
National	619	O.R. PROCEDURES FOR OBESITY W MCC	1009	55	7.9	$104,338	$21,676
National	620	O.R. PROCEDURES FOR OBESITY W CC	4011	55	3.2	$56,826	$9,281
National	621	O.R. PROCEDURES FOR OBESITY W/O CC/MCC	12511	55	2.0	$44,818	$6,741
National	622	SKIN GRAFTS & WOUND DEBRID FOR ENDOC, NUTRIT & METAB DIS W MCC	1620	67	18.8	$102,792	$28,075
National	623	SKIN GRAFTS & WOUND DEBRID FOR ENDOC, NUTRIT & METAB DIS W CC	3828	63	10.1	$54,556	$12,920
National	624	SKIN GRAFTS & WOUND DEBRID FOR ENDOC, NUTRIT & METAB DIS W/O CC/MCC	261	64	5.0	$26,029	$5,781
National	625	THYROID, PARATHYROID & THYROGLOSSAL PROCEDURES W MCC	1335	60	7.3	$72,740	$14,857
National	626	THYROID, PARATHYROID & THYROGLOSSAL PROCEDURES W CC	3300	68	2.8	$38,828	$5,854
National	627	THYROID, PARATHYROID & THYROGLOSSAL PROCEDURES W/O CC/MCC	11089	70	1.4	$26,360	$3,156
National	628	OTHER ENDOCRINE, NUTRIT & METAB O.R. PROC W MCC	4418	64	10.8	$93,427	$20,978
National	629	OTHER ENDOCRINE, NUTRIT & METAB O.R. PROC W CC	6462	66	7.9	$57,500	$12,095
National	630	OTHER ENDOCRINE, NUTRIT & METAB O.R. PROC W/O CC/MCC	416	69	4.1	$40,133	$7,226
National	637	DIABETES W MCC	27172	65	6.4	$40,011	$8,586
National	638	DIABETES W CC	67382	65	4.2	$23,307	$4,548
National	639	DIABETES W/O CC/MCC	25829	66	2.7	$15,287	$2,565
National	640	MISC DISORDERS OF NUTRITION,METABOLISM,FLUIDS/ELECTROLYTES W MCC	73793	68	4.9	$30,006	$6,556
National	641	MISC DISORDERS OF NUTRITION,METABOLISM,FLUIDS/ELECTROLYTES W/O MCC	181417	76	3.4	$18,146	$3,439
National	642	INBORN AND OTHER DISORDERS OF METABOLISM	2200	57	4.4	$30,815	$6,338
National	643	ENDOCRINE DISORDERS W MCC	8447	75	7.1	$45,045	$9,679
National	644	ENDOCRINE DISORDERS W CC	16245	74	4.7	$27,826	$5,585
National	645	ENDOCRINE DISORDERS W/O CC/MCC	7500	74	3.4	$19,939	$3,415
National	652	KIDNEY TRANSPLANT	11041	51	6.8	$191,388	$24,078
National	653	MAJOR BLADDER PROCEDURES W MCC	2225	73	15.7	$163,898	$34,310
National	654	MAJOR BLADDER PROCEDURES W CC	5009	73	8.9	$89,754	$16,912
National	655	MAJOR BLADDER PROCEDURES W/O CC/MCC	1802	73	5.6	$67,846	$11,328
National	656	KIDNEY & URETER PROCEDURES FOR NEOPLASM W MCC	4324	71	9.4	$102,844	$21,684

Peer Grouping	MS-DRG	Description	Discharges	Average Age	Average Length of Stay	Average Total Charge	Average Allowed
National	657	KIDNEY & URETER PROCEDURES FOR NEOPLASM W CC	10771	73	5.3	$58,672	$10,643
National	658	KIDNEY & URETER PROCEDURES FOR NEOPLASM W/O CC/MCC	9010	72	3.1	$44,241	$7,166
National	659	KIDNEY & URETER PROCEDURES FOR NON-NEOPLASM W MCC	4948	64	10.6	$95,777	$22,074
National	660	KIDNEY & URETER PROCEDURES FOR NON-NEOPLASM W CC	10890	69	5.6	$53,355	$10,177
National	661	KIDNEY & URETER PROCEDURES FOR NON-NEOPLASM W/O CC/MCC	5101	69	2.7	$39,862	$6,193
National	662	MINOR BLADDER PROCEDURES W MCC	880	73	10.0	$80,727	$17,924
National	663	MINOR BLADDER PROCEDURES W CC	2044	75	5.2	$41,990	$7,978
National	664	MINOR BLADDER PROCEDURES W/O CC/MCC	2262	73	2.0	$33,704	$4,914
National	665	PROSTATECTOMY W MCC	666	78	11.6	$82,751	$20,118
National	666	PROSTATECTOMY W CC	2044	79	6.2	$45,752	$8,536
National	667	PROSTATECTOMY W/O CC/MCC	1884	78	2.5	$24,455	$3,484
National	668	TRANSURETHRAL PROCEDURES W MCC	4204	74	8.9	$71,926	$14,962
National	669	TRANSURETHRAL PROCEDURES W CC	18435	74	4.1	$35,925	$6,274
National	670	TRANSURETHRAL PROCEDURES W/O CC/MCC	7490	76	2.3	$23,567	$3,308
National	671	URETHRAL PROCEDURES W CC/MCC	905	72	5.5	$44,942	$8,359
National	672	URETHRAL PROCEDURES W/O CC/MCC	656	72	2.3	$28,144	$3,967
National	673	OTHER KIDNEY & URINARY TRACT PROCEDURES W MCC	13235	66	10.3	$86,071	$18,645
National	674	OTHER KIDNEY & URINARY TRACT PROCEDURES W CC	9635	67	7.2	$61,905	$11,973
National	675	OTHER KIDNEY & URINARY TRACT PROCEDURES W/O CC/MCC	2044	70	2.6	$39,417	$6,427
National	682	RENAL FAILURE W MCC	129507	72	6.6	$41,506	$9,419
National	683	RENAL FAILURE W CC	190795	75	4.5	$25,611	$5,176
National	684	RENAL FAILURE W/O CC/MCC	36237	76	3.0	$16,715	$2,986
National	685	ADMIT FOR RENAL DIALYSIS	3296	63	3.3	$21,945	$4,563
National	686	KIDNEY & URINARY TRACT NEOPLASMS W MCC	1648	75	7.6	$49,496	$10,773
National	687	KIDNEY & URINARY TRACT NEOPLASMS W CC	3846	77	4.9	$29,566	$5,801
National	688	KIDNEY & URINARY TRACT NEOPLASMS W/O CC/MCC	629	77	3.1	$20,375	$3,191
National	689	KIDNEY & URINARY TRACT INFECTIONS W MCC	89235	78	5.5	$29,767	$6,549
National	690	KIDNEY & URINARY TRACT INFECTIONS W/O MCC	250306	79	3.8	$19,913	$3,980
National	691	URINARY STONES W ESW LITHOTRIPSY W CC/MCC	1172	68	3.8	$39,664	$7,478
National	692	URINARY STONES W ESW LITHOTRIPSY W/O CC/MCC	317	67	2.0	$27,056	$4,319
National	693	URINARY STONES W/O ESW LITHOTRIPSY W MCC	2741	71	5.6	$40,653	$7,383
National	694	URINARY STONES W/O ESW LITHOTRIPSY W/O MCC	22318	70	2.4	$20,658	$3,059
National	695	KIDNEY & URINARY TRACT SIGNS & SYMPTOMS W MCC	1862	76	5.5	$34,161	$7,286
National	696	KIDNEY & URINARY TRACT SIGNS & SYMPTOMS W/O MCC	13006	78	3.1	$17,268	$3,066
National	697	URETHRAL STRICTURE	691	74	3.2	$23,082	$3,846
National	698	OTHER KIDNEY & URINARY TRACT DIAGNOSES W MCC	37016	69	6.7	$42,309	$9,428
National	699	OTHER KIDNEY & URINARY TRACT DIAGNOSES W CC	38241	69	4.4	$27,484	$5,655
National	700	OTHER KIDNEY & URINARY TRACT DIAGNOSES W/O CC/MCC	8724	73	3.2	$19,054	$3,487
National	707	MAJOR MALE PELVIC PROCEDURES W CC/MCC	5944	69	4.0	$54,124	$8,930
National	708	MAJOR MALE PELVIC PROCEDURES W/O CC/MCC	19172	69	1.6	$40,708	$5,633
National	709	PENIS PROCEDURES W CC/MCC	883	66	6.0	$58,193	$12,027
National	710	PENIS PROCEDURES W/O CC/MCC	1220	69	1.7	$37,830	$5,277

Peer Grouping	MS-DRG	Description	Discharges	Average Age	Average Length of Stay	Average Total Charge	Average Allowed
National	711	TESTES PROCEDURES W CC/MCC	780	69	8.1	$59,153	$12,055
National	712	TESTES PROCEDURES W/O CC/MCC	351	68	2.9	$25,798	$3,660
National	713	TRANSURETHRAL PROSTATECTOMY W CC/MCC	8362	77	4.3	$36,735	$5,868
National	714	TRANSURETHRAL PROSTATECTOMY W/O CC/MCC	14292	76	1.8	$20,536	$2,273
National	715	OTHER MALE REPRODUCTIVE SYSTEM O.R. PROC FOR MALIGNANCY W CC/MCC	521	77	7.5	$61,312	$10,339
National	716	OTHER MALE REPRODUCTIVE SYSTEM O.R. PROC FOR MALIGNANCY W/O CC/MCC	340	71	1.7	$33,343	$3,681
National	717	OTHER MALE REPRODUCTIVE SYSTEM O.R. PROC EXC MALIGNANCY W CC/MCC	937	75	7.4	$48,468	$10,343
National	718	OTHER MALE REPRODUCTIVE SYSTEM O.R. PROC EXC MALIGNANCY W/O CC/MCC	410	75	2.8	$24,517	$3,826
National	722	MALIGNANCY, MALE REPRODUCTIVE SYSTEM W MCC	641	77	7.7	$45,660	$9,389
National	723	MALIGNANCY, MALE REPRODUCTIVE SYSTEM W CC	1947	78	5.6	$29,449	$5,932
National	724	MALIGNANCY, MALE REPRODUCTIVE SYSTEM W/O CC/MCC	252	76	3.2	$15,722	$3,865
National	725	BENIGN PROSTATIC HYPERTROPHY W MCC	753	78	5.7	$34,965	$7,132
National	726	BENIGN PROSTATIC HYPERTROPHY W/O MCC	4837	79	3.4	$19,148	$3,507
National	727	INFLAMMATION OF THE MALE REPRODUCTIVE SYSTEM W MCC	2024	69	7.1	$41,032	$8,803
National	728	INFLAMMATION OF THE MALE REPRODUCTIVE SYSTEM W/O MCC	7568	70	4.0	$20,920	$3,949
National	729	OTHER MALE REPRODUCTIVE SYSTEM DIAGNOSES W CC/MCC	1108	67	6.5	$34,188	$7,685
National	730	OTHER MALE REPRODUCTIVE SYSTEM DIAGNOSES W/O CC/MCC	347	66	2.9	$17,588	$3,044
National	734	PELVIC EVISCERATION, RAD HYSTERECTOMY & RAD VULVECTOMY W CC/MCC	1905	71	6.7	$78,362	$14,625
National	735	PELVIC EVISCERATION, RAD HYSTERECTOMY & RAD VULVECTOMY W/O CC/MCC	1458	72	2.3	$37,273	$5,559
National	736	UTERINE & ADNEXA PROC FOR OVARIAN OR ADNEXAL MALIGNANCY W MCC	1034	73	12.7	$124,010	$27,007
National	737	UTERINE & ADNEXA PROC FOR OVARIAN OR ADNEXAL MALIGNANCY W CC	3990	72	6.2	$59,902	$10,823
National	738	UTERINE & ADNEXA PROC FOR OVARIAN OR ADNEXAL MALIGNANCY W/O CC/MCC	866	71	3.4	$38,831	$5,689
National	739	UTERINE,ADNEXA PROC FOR NON-OVARIAN/ADNEXAL MALIG W MCC	1058	71	8.8	$94,122	$20,154
National	740	UTERINE,ADNEXA PROC FOR NON-OVARIAN/ADNEXAL MALIG W CC	5272	71	4.0	$48,693	$7,918
National	741	UTERINE,ADNEXA PROC FOR NON-OVARIAN/ADNEXAL MALIG W/O CC/MCC	5900	72	2.1	$36,935	$5,106
National	742	UTERINE & ADNEXA PROC FOR NON-MALIGNANCY W CC/MCC	11013	62	3.9	$43,991	$7,466
National	743	UTERINE & ADNEXA PROC FOR NON-MALIGNANCY W/O CC/MCC	24998	64	1.9	$29,465	$3,925
National	744	D&C, CONIZATION, LAPAROSCOPY & TUBAL INTERRUPTION W CC/MCC	1963	69	5.5	$44,719	$8,767
National	745	D&C, CONIZATION, LAPAROSCOPY & TUBAL INTERRUPTION W/O CC/MCC	1057	69	2.4	$26,615	$3,904
National	746	VAGINA, CERVIX & VULVA PROCEDURES W CC/MCC	2586	71	4.3	$40,112	$7,038
National	747	VAGINA, CERVIX & VULVA PROCEDURES W/O CC/MCC	5442	72	1.7	$25,725	$3,465
National	748	FEMALE REPRODUCTIVE SYSTEM RECONSTRUCTIVE PROCEDURES	11140	72	1.7	$28,101	$3,716

Peer Grouping	MS-DRG	Description	Discharges	Average Age	Average Length of Stay	Average Total Charge	Average Allowed
National	749	OTHER FEMALE REPRODUCTIVE SYSTEM O.R. PROCEDURES W CC/MCC	1352	69	8.3	$73,803	$15,178
National	750	OTHER FEMALE REPRODUCTIVE SYSTEM O.R. PROCEDURES W/O CC/MCC	390	63	2.7	$32,267	$5,320
National	754	MALIGNANCY, FEMALE REPRODUCTIVE SYSTEM W MCC	1582	74	9.1	$56,790	$13,341
National	755	MALIGNANCY, FEMALE REPRODUCTIVE SYSTEM W CC	4127	74	5.4	$31,122	$6,543
National	756	MALIGNANCY, FEMALE REPRODUCTIVE SYSTEM W/O CC/MCC	434	72	3.1	$19,515	$3,552
National	757	INFECTIONS, FEMALE REPRODUCTIVE SYSTEM W MCC	1692	73	8.1	$43,605	$10,228
National	758	INFECTIONS, FEMALE REPRODUCTIVE SYSTEM W CC	2548	72	5.5	$29,186	$6,262
National	759	INFECTIONS, FEMALE REPRODUCTIVE SYSTEM W/O CC/MCC	1076	67	3.9	$19,043	$3,810
National	760	MENSTRUAL & OTHER FEMALE REPRODUCTIVE SYSTEM DISORDERS W CC/MCC	2523	66	3.6	$22,829	$4,216
National	761	MENSTRUAL & OTHER FEMALE REPRODUCTIVE SYSTEM DISORDERS W/O CC/MCC	1112	64	2.2	$13,917	$2,137
National	765	CESAREAN SECTION W CC/MCC	4516	33	4.8	$28,294	$7,235
National	766	CESAREAN SECTION W/O CC/MCC	3229	31	3.1	$18,201	$4,337
National	767	VAGINAL DELIVERY W STERILIZATION &/OR D&C	180	33	3.8	$17,136	$2,213
National	768	VAGINAL DELIVERY W O.R. PROC EXCEPT STERIL &/OR D&C	14	33	3.3	$28,598	$11,060
National	769	POSTPARTUM & POST ABORTION DIAGNOSES W O.R. PROCEDURE	115	33	6.5	$64,189	$13,104
National	770	ABORTION W D&C, ASPIRATION CURETTAGE OR HYSTEROTOMY	183	34	2.3	$21,897	$3,221
National	774	VAGINAL DELIVERY W COMPLICATING DIAGNOSES	2314	32	3.2	$16,253	$4,031
National	775	VAGINAL DELIVERY W/O COMPLICATING DIAGNOSES	7206	31	2.3	$11,602	$2,494
National	776	POSTPARTUM & POST ABORTION DIAGNOSES W/O O.R. PROCEDURE	870	33	4.3	$20,951	$4,381
National	777	ECTOPIC PREGNANCY	259	33	2.1	$29,580	$4,896
National	778	THREATENED ABORTION	544	31	2.8	$11,713	$2,387
National	779	ABORTION W/O D&C	116	32	2.0	$14,496	$2,043
National	780	FALSE LABOR	50	33	1.4	$5,644	$697
National	781	OTHER ANTEPARTUM DIAGNOSES W MEDICAL COMPLICATIONS	4351	32	4.7	$19,851	$4,236
National	782	OTHER ANTEPARTUM DIAGNOSES W/O MEDICAL COMPLICATIONS	202	32	2.2	$10,144	$1,380
National	799	SPLENECTOMY W MCC	571	68	12.8	$148,820	$32,400
National	800	SPLENECTOMY W CC	644	69	6.7	$73,178	$15,288
National	801	SPLENECTOMY W/O CC/MCC	413	68	3.7	$45,760	$7,827
National	802	OTHER O.R. PROC OF THE BLOOD & BLOOD FORMING ORGANS W MCC	1014	71	10.7	$92,789	$21,538
National	803	OTHER O.R. PROC OF THE BLOOD & BLOOD FORMING ORGANS W CC	1280	71	6.4	$53,324	$9,895
National	804	OTHER O.R. PROC OF THE BLOOD & BLOOD FORMING ORGANS W/O CC/MCC	741	69	2.9	$35,889	$4,934
National	808	MAJOR HEMATOL/IMMUN DIAG EXC SICKLE CELL CRISIS & COAGUL W MCC	10241	71	8.2	$63,282	$13,409
National	809	MAJOR HEMATOL/IMMUN DIAG EXC SICKLE CELL CRISIS & COAGUL W CC	24226	71	4.8	$32,865	$6,781
National	810	MAJOR HEMATOL/IMMUN DIAG EXC SICKLE CELL CRISIS & COAGUL W/O CC/MCC	4017	72	3.3	$23,174	$4,406

Peer Grouping	MS-DRG	Description	Discharges	Average Age	Average Length of Stay	Average Total Charge	Average Allowed
National	811	RED BLOOD CELL DISORDERS W MCC	39507	70	4.9	$33,328	$6,863
National	812	RED BLOOD CELL DISORDERS W/O MCC	116601	70	3.4	$21,112	$3,910
National	813	COAGULATION DISORDERS	11632	73	5.0	$57,141	$11,831
National	814	RETICULOENDOTHELIAL & IMMUNITY DISORDERS W MCC	1881	69	7.0	$49,484	$10,779
National	815	RETICULOENDOTHELIAL & IMMUNITY DISORDERS W CC	4086	71	4.2	$28,389	$5,259
National	816	RETICULOENDOTHELIAL & IMMUNITY DISORDERS W/O CC/MCC	1700	72	2.9	$18,527	$3,538
National	820	LYMPHOMA & LEUKEMIA W MAJOR O.R. PROCEDURE W MCC	1469	72	17.0	$178,020	$39,261
National	821	LYMPHOMA & LEUKEMIA W MAJOR O.R. PROCEDURE W CC	2221	72	6.7	$70,989	$13,682
National	822	LYMPHOMA & LEUKEMIA W MAJOR O.R. PROCEDURE W/O CC/MCC	2045	72	2.8	$39,479	$6,136
National	823	LYMPHOMA & NON-ACUTE LEUKEMIA W OTHER O.R. PROC W MCC	2211	74	15.2	$137,105	$28,439
National	824	LYMPHOMA & NON-ACUTE LEUKEMIA W OTHER O.R. PROC W CC	3347	74	7.8	$67,142	$13,110
National	825	LYMPHOMA & NON-ACUTE LEUKEMIA W OTHER O.R. PROC W/O CC/MCC	1370	74	3.8	$40,434	$6,621
National	826	MYELOPROLIF DISORD OR POORLY DIFF NEOPL W MAJ O.R. PROC W MCC	777	71	14.0	$149,512	$34,160
National	827	MYELOPROLIF DISORD OR POORLY DIFF NEOPL W MAJ O.R. PROC W CC	1840	72	6.9	$68,780	$13,611
National	828	MYELOPROLIF DISORD OR POORLY DIFF NEOPL W MAJ O.R. PROC W/O CC/MCC	1179	71	3.4	$43,737	$7,210
National	829	MYELOPROLIF DISORD OR POORLY DIFF NEOPL W OTHER O.R. PROC W CC/MCC	1554	71	10.1	$93,125	$19,608
National	830	MYELOPROLIF DISORD OR POORLY DIFF NEOPL W OTHER O.R. PROC W/O CC/MCC	431	72	3.1	$40,687	$6,399
National	834	ACUTE LEUKEMIA W/O MAJOR O.R. PROCEDURE W MCC	4848	73	17.3	$160,628	$37,982
National	835	ACUTE LEUKEMIA W/O MAJOR O.R. PROCEDURE W CC	3469	75	8.2	$64,641	$15,814
National	836	ACUTE LEUKEMIA W/O MAJOR O.R. PROCEDURE W/O CC/MCC	1237	76	4.6	$35,539	$7,265
National	837	CHEMO W ACUTE LEUKEMIA AS SDX OR W HIGH DOSE CHEMO AGENT W MCC	2268	68	21.1	$178,434	$45,691
National	838	CHEMO W ACUTE LEUKEMIA AS SDX W CC OR HIGH DOSE CHEMO AGENT	1966	67	9.8	$88,842	$22,968
National	839	CHEMO W ACUTE LEUKEMIA AS SDX W/O CC/MCC	1736	67	5.5	$37,654	$8,092
National	840	LYMPHOMA & NON-ACUTE LEUKEMIA W MCC	9541	74	10.8	$89,296	$19,631
National	841	LYMPHOMA & NON-ACUTE LEUKEMIA W CC	11647	75	6.5	$46,974	$9,549
National	842	LYMPHOMA & NON-ACUTE LEUKEMIA W/O CC/MCC	3706	74	4.1	$32,257	$5,510
National	843	OTHER MYELOPROLIF DIS OR POORLY DIFF NEOPL DIAG W MCC	2103	73	7.5	$52,075	$11,594
National	844	OTHER MYELOPROLIF DIS OR POORLY DIFF NEOPL DIAG W CC	3463	74	5.4	$34,199	$6,610
National	845	OTHER MYELOPROLIF DIS OR POORLY DIFF NEOPL DIAG W/O CC/MCC	740	74	3.8	$22,923	$4,166
National	846	CHEMOTHERAPY W/O ACUTE LEUKEMIA AS SECONDARY DIAGNOSIS W MCC	3393	67	8.5	$74,094	$16,521
National	847	CHEMOTHERAPY W/O ACUTE LEUKEMIA AS SECONDARY DIAGNOSIS W CC	25511	69	3.6	$34,337	$6,238
National	848	CHEMOTHERAPY W/O ACUTE LEUKEMIA AS SECONDARY DIAGNOSIS W/O CC/MCC	1233	68	3.0	$25,315	$4,737
National	849	RADIOTHERAPY	1039	70	6.9	$46,984	$9,091

Peer Grouping	MS-DRG	Description	Discharges	Average Age	Average Length of Stay	Average Total Charge	Average Allowed
National	853	INFECTIOUS & PARASITIC DISEASES W O.R. PROCEDURE W MCC	58778	71	15.3	$146,986	$33,091
National	854	INFECTIOUS & PARASITIC DISEASES W O.R. PROCEDURE W CC	12508	71	8.6	$66,729	$13,995
National	855	INFECTIOUS & PARASITIC DISEASES W O.R. PROCEDURE W/O CC/MCC	387	71	5.3	$45,706	$9,069
National	856	POSTOPERATIVE OR POST-TRAUMATIC INFECTIONS W O.R. PROC W MCC	7602	67	15.2	$127,884	$29,356
National	857	POSTOPERATIVE OR POST-TRAUMATIC INFECTIONS W O.R. PROC W CC	11558	68	7.5	$54,112	$11,274
National	858	POSTOPERATIVE OR POST-TRAUMATIC INFECTIONS W O.R. PROC W/O CC/MCC	2360	68	4.9	$35,220	$6,806
National	862	POSTOPERATIVE & POST-TRAUMATIC INFECTIONS W MCC	14115	68	10.2	$60,543	$13,933
National	863	POSTOPERATIVE & POST-TRAUMATIC INFECTIONS W/O MCC	25204	68	5.3	$27,484	$5,902
National	864	FEVER	22242	71	3.6	$23,488	$4,376
National	865	VIRAL ILLNESS W MCC	2958	68	7.3	$51,950	$10,497
National	866	VIRAL ILLNESS W/O MCC	8131	72	3.5	$21,976	$3,511
National	867	OTHER INFECTIOUS & PARASITIC DISEASES DIAGNOSES W MCC	6497	69	10.6	$79,112	$17,800
National	868	OTHER INFECTIOUS & PARASITIC DISEASES DIAGNOSES W CC	3106	72	5.3	$29,440	$6,295
National	869	OTHER INFECTIOUS & PARASITIC DISEASES DIAGNOSES W/O CC/MCC	839	72	3.7	$18,608	$3,617
National	870	SEPTICEMIA OR SEVERE SEPSIS W MV 96+ HOURS	38236	71	15.9	$170,731	$37,306
National	871	SEPTICEMIA OR SEVERE SEPSIS W/O MV 96+ HOURS W MCC	419268	75	7.1	$51,588	$11,122
National	872	SEPTICEMIA OR SEVERE SEPSIS W/O MV 96+ HOURS W/O MCC	151823	76	5.0	$28,630	$5,890
National	876	O.R. PROCEDURE W PRINCIPAL DIAGNOSES OF MENTAL ILLNESS	1191	65	21.9	$79,001	$18,645
National	880	ACUTE ADJUSTMENT REACTION & PSYCHOSOCIAL DYSFUNCTION	12788	65	4.6	$18,369	$3,928
National	881	DEPRESSIVE NEUROSES	22973	56	6.7	$15,352	$4,275
National	882	NEUROSES EXCEPT DEPRESSIVE	8254	51	8.8	$17,052	$4,817
National	883	DISORDERS OF PERSONALITY & IMPULSE CONTROL	3136	46	12.7	$27,445	$8,025
National	884	ORGANIC DISTURBANCES & MENTAL RETARDATION	54793	80	10.9	$27,746	$8,125
National	885	PSYCHOSES	473087	52	13.1	$25,326	$7,430
National	886	BEHAVIORAL & DEVELOPMENTAL DISORDERS	2473	57	11.7	$23,980	$7,220
National	887	OTHER MENTAL DISORDER DIAGNOSES	1048	56	17.4	$30,731	$7,001
National	894	ALCOHOL/DRUG ABUSE OR DEPENDENCE, LEFT AMA	7672	49	3.1	$9,915	$2,399
National	895	ALCOHOL/DRUG ABUSE OR DEPENDENCE W REHABILITATION THERAPY	15023	51	12.1	$18,764	$8,183
National	896	ALCOHOL/DRUG ABUSE OR DEPENDENCE W/O REHABILITATION THERAPY W MCC	10330	62	6.9	$38,445	$8,246
National	897	ALCOHOL/DRUG ABUSE OR DEPENDENCE W/O REHABILITATION THERAPY W/O MCC	71639	56	5.4	$15,601	$3,893
National	901	WOUND DEBRIDEMENTS FOR INJURIES W MCC	1240	65	21.5	$130,954	$33,810
National	902	WOUND DEBRIDEMENTS FOR INJURIES W CC	2252	69	9.0	$51,359	$12,917
National	903	WOUND DEBRIDEMENTS FOR INJURIES W/O CC/MCC	933	69	4.6	$28,656	$6,118
National	904	SKIN GRAFTS FOR INJURIES W CC/MCC	2585	67	11.9	$94,054	$21,356
National	905	SKIN GRAFTS FOR INJURIES W/O CC/MCC	958	68	4.4	$36,974	$6,932
National	906	HAND PROCEDURES FOR INJURIES	950	67	3.4	$36,042	$5,416

Peer Grouping	MS-DRG	Description	Discharges	Average Age	Average Length of Stay	Average Total Charge	Average Allowed
National	907	OTHER O.R. PROCEDURES FOR INJURIES W MCC	10751	64	11.5	$110,214	$25,110
National	908	OTHER O.R. PROCEDURES FOR INJURIES W CC	11353	69	6.0	$53,198	$10,586
National	909	OTHER O.R. PROCEDURES FOR INJURIES W/O CC/MCC	5528	68	3.2	$34,281	$5,861
National	913	TRAUMATIC INJURY W MCC	1221	75	6.2	$36,834	$9,108
National	914	TRAUMATIC INJURY W/O MCC	6981	77	3.5	$20,348	$4,023
National	915	ALLERGIC REACTIONS W MCC	2334	68	5.0	$41,831	$7,929
National	916	ALLERGIC REACTIONS W/O MCC	7696	70	2.1	$14,018	$2,000
National	917	POISONING & TOXIC EFFECTS OF DRUGS W MCC	31427	59	4.9	$39,865	$8,313
National	918	POISONING & TOXIC EFFECTS OF DRUGS W/O MCC	43465	60	2.8	$17,981	$3,043
National	919	COMPLICATIONS OF TREATMENT W MCC	15996	65	9.6	$61,620	$13,913
National	920	COMPLICATIONS OF TREATMENT W CC	19702	71	5.0	$29,891	$6,136
National	921	COMPLICATIONS OF TREATMENT W/O CC/MCC	7645	70	2.8	$17,963	$3,121
National	922	OTHER INJURY, POISONING & TOXIC EFFECT DIAG W MCC	1412	72	5.9	$44,485	$9,276
National	923	OTHER INJURY, POISONING & TOXIC EFFECT DIAG W/O MCC	3522	74	3.1	$19,824	$3,481
National	927	EXTENSIVE BURNS OR FULL THICKNESS BURNS W MV 96+ HRS W SKIN GRAFT	205	66	31.0	$470,096	$110,580
National	928	FULL THICKNESS BURN W SKIN GRAFT OR INHAL INJ W CC/MCC	1253	66	16.8	$163,798	$38,084
National	929	FULL THICKNESS BURN W SKIN GRAFT OR INHAL INJ W/O CC/MCC	444	66	7.6	$63,400	$14,030
National	933	EXTENSIVE BURNS OR FULL THICKNESS BURNS W MV 96+ HRS W/O SKIN GRAFT	185	73	8.0	$91,264	$23,396
National	934	FULL THICKNESS BURN W/O SKIN GRFT OR INHAL INJ	770	67	7.2	$43,777	$9,586
National	935	NON-EXTENSIVE BURNS	2771	66	5.1	$37,111	$8,506
National	939	O.R. PROC W DIAGNOSES OF OTHER CONTACT W HEALTH SERVICES W MCC	2529	68	17.4	$94,735	$24,878
National	940	O.R. PROC W DIAGNOSES OF OTHER CONTACT W HEALTH SERVICES W CC	3487	72	10.9	$60,083	$15,278
National	941	O.R. PROC W DIAGNOSES OF OTHER CONTACT W HEALTH SERVICES W/O CC/MCC	1504	69	3.8	$38,519	$7,173
National	945	REHABILITATION W CC/MCC	308568	75	13.2	$39,644	$17,139
National	946	REHABILITATION W/O CC/MCC	68648	76	10.6	$28,763	$13,521
National	947	SIGNS & SYMPTOMS W MCC	17327	70	5.0	$30,559	$6,468
National	948	SIGNS & SYMPTOMS W/O MCC	70807	75	3.3	$18,648	$3,577
National	949	AFTERCARE W CC/MCC	4060	70	19.2	$64,644	$19,412
National	950	AFTERCARE W/O CC/MCC	487	72	8.1	$22,952	$6,321
National	951	OTHER FACTORS INFLUENCING HEALTH STATUS	1957	71	12.5	$25,428	$8,682
National	955	CRANIOTOMY FOR MULTIPLE SIGNIFICANT TRAUMA	568	73	10.5	$175,409	$37,284
National	956	LIMB REATTACHMENT, HIP & FEMUR PROC FOR MULTIPLE SIGNIFICANT TRAUMA	5652	80	8.5	$100,916	$20,925
National	957	OTHER O.R. PROCEDURES FOR MULTIPLE SIGNIFICANT TRAUMA W MCC	2259	68	14.1	$206,007	$43,829
National	958	OTHER O.R. PROCEDURES FOR MULTIPLE SIGNIFICANT TRAUMA W CC	1628	69	9.1	$120,216	$22,660
National	959	OTHER O.R. PROCEDURES FOR MULTIPLE SIGNIFICANT TRAUMA W/O CC/MCC	228	69	5.4	$77,566	$13,246
National	963	OTHER MULTIPLE SIGNIFICANT TRAUMA W MCC	2657	76	8.6	$81,866	$17,075
National	964	OTHER MULTIPLE SIGNIFICANT TRAUMA W CC	4138	77	5.5	$42,693	$8,194

Peer Grouping	MS-DRG	Description	Discharges	Average Age	Average Length of Stay	Average Total Charge	Average Allowed
National	965	OTHER MULTIPLE SIGNIFICANT TRAUMA W/O CC/MCC	1131	78	3.9	$29,865	$5,343
National	969	HIV W EXTENSIVE O.R. PROCEDURE W MCC	645	51	17.6	$169,439	$45,152
National	970	HIV W EXTENSIVE O.R. PROCEDURE W/O MCC	84	51	7.3	$66,424	$14,698
National	974	HIV W MAJOR RELATED CONDITION W MCC	6072	52	10.3	$81,064	$20,208
National	975	HIV W MAJOR RELATED CONDITION W CC	4121	51	7.6	$42,855	$9,121
National	976	HIV W MAJOR RELATED CONDITION W/O CC/MCC	1363	49	6.3	$31,914	$5,781
National	977	HIV W OR W/O OTHER RELATED CONDITION	3216	51	6.7	$35,913	$7,209
National	981	EXTENSIVE O.R. PROCEDURE UNRELATED TO PRINCIPAL DIAGNOSIS W MCC	29524	71	15.0	$139,540	$31,318
National	982	EXTENSIVE O.R. PROCEDURE UNRELATED TO PRINCIPAL DIAGNOSIS W CC	20514	73	7.9	$76,761	$16,134
National	983	EXTENSIVE O.R. PROCEDURE UNRELATED TO PRINCIPAL DIAGNOSIS W/O CC/MCC	4957	71	3.8	$48,493	$8,965
National	984	PROSTATIC O.R. PROCEDURE UNRELATED TO PRINCIPAL DIAGNOSIS W MCC	539	78	13.3	$93,462	$21,730
National	985	PROSTATIC O.R. PROCEDURE UNRELATED TO PRINCIPAL DIAGNOSIS W CC	975	79	7.3	$51,528	$11,678
National	986	PROSTATIC O.R. PROCEDURE UNRELATED TO PRINCIPAL DIAGNOSIS W/O CC/MCC	483	77	3.1	$29,204	$5,534
National	987	NON-EXTENSIVE O.R. PROC UNRELATED TO PRINCIPAL DIAGNOSIS W MCC	9530	69	13.7	$97,437	$22,449
National	988	NON-EXTENSIVE O.R. PROC UNRELATED TO PRINCIPAL DIAGNOSIS W CC	10781	71	6.8	$49,852	$10,055
National	989	NON-EXTENSIVE O.R. PROC UNRELATED TO PRINCIPAL DIAGNOSIS W/O CC/MCC	3634	70	3.0	$31,327	$5,108

Appendix F — Medicare Case Mix Index Data

2014 IPPS Impact File

State	Average Daily Census	Average Number of Beds	Average CMI V31
AK	56	118	1.47098
AL	75	146	1.28783
AR	79	151	1.40953
AZ	111	196	1.65517
CA	120	207	1.59860
CO	92	159	1.63679
CT	145	212	1.44530
DC	222	328	1.66951
DE	208	302	1.56149
FL	173	289	1.50929
GA	100	172	1.45260
HI	102	156	1.59915
IA	87	168	1.49949
ID	74	151	1.89242
IL	122	211	1.45445
IN	92	166	1.51461
KS	55	110	1.62823
KY	103	184	1.33950
LA	66	131	1.49427
MA	144	217	1.38617
MD	176	249	1.46829
ME	72	130	1.37744
MI	136	220	1.48864
MN	99	169	1.46213
MO	108	201	1.46329
MS	65	142	1.25379
MT	61	120	1.64110
NC	138	215	1.48030
ND	114	180	1.70448
NE	79	150	1.80430
NH	89	153	1.53183
NJ	191	289	1.52804
NM	60	116	1.28473
NV	129	199	1.60073
NY	190	255	1.42348
OH	112	187	1.50445
OK	57	108	1.39290
OR	100	168	1.59773

For acute care hospitals where case mix index (CMI) > 0

No critical access hospital (CAH)

State	Average Daily Census	Average Number of Beds	Average CMI V31
PA	124	199	1.49004
PR	115	155	1.38827
RI	137	209	1.45488
SC	110	186	1.45728
SD	48	92	1.62051
TN	100	176	1.40877
TX	88	162	1.53645
UT	60	125	1.59940
VA	114	198	1.39952
VT	77	126	1.47225
WA	121	201	1.60100
WI	83	154	1.54925
WV	96	178	1.36367
WY	29	79	1.46731

For acute care hospitals where case mix index (CMI) > 0

No critical access hospital (CAH)

Glossary of DRG Terms

against medical advice: Discharge status of patients who leave the hospital after signing a form that releases the hospital from responsibility, or those who leave the hospital premises without notifying hospital personnel.

arithmetic mean length of stay: Average number of days within a given DRG-stay in the hospital, also referred to as the average length of stay. The AMLOS is used to determine payment for outlier cases.

base rate: Payment weight assigned to hospitals to calculate diagnosis-related group (DRG) reimbursement. The base payment rate is divided into labor-related and nonlabor shares. The labor-related share is adjusted by the wage index applicable to the area where the hospital is located, and if the hospital is located in Alaska or Hawaii, the nonlabor share is adjusted by a cost of living adjustment factor. This base payment rate is multiplied by the DRG relative weight to calculate DRG reimbursement.

case mix index: Sum of all DRG relative weights for cases over a given period of time, divided by the number of Medicare cases.

charges: Dollar amount assigned to a service or procedure by a provider and reported to a payer.

complication/comorbidity (CC): Condition that, when present, leads to substantially increased hospital resource use, such as intensive monitoring, expensive and technically complex services, and extensive care requiring a greater number of caregivers. Significant acute disease, acute exacerbations of significant chronic diseases, advanced or end stage chronic diseases, and chronic diseases associated with extensive debility are representative of CC conditions.

discharge: Situation in which the patient leaves an acute care (prospective payment) hospital after receiving complete acute care treatment.

discharge status: Disposition of the patient at discharge (e.g., left against medical advice, discharged home, transferred to an acute care hospital, expired).

geometric mean length of stay: Statistically adjusted value for all cases for a given diagnosis-related group, allowing for the outliers, transfer cases, and negative outlier cases that would normally skew the data. The GMLOS is used to determine payment only for transfer cases (i.e., the per diem rate).

grouper: Software program that assigns diagnosis-related groups (DRGs).

homogeneous: Group of patients consuming similar types and amounts of hospital resources.

hospital-acquired condition (HAC): A significant, reasonably preventable condition determined to have occurred during a hospital visit, identified via the assignment of certain present on admission (POA) indicators. The MCC or CC status for the code for the HAC condition is invalidated when the POA indicator is N or U, thus potentially affecting DRG reimbursement.

major complication/comorbidity (MCC): Diagnosis codes that reflect the highest level of severity and have potential to increase reimbursement. *See also* complications/comorbidity.

major diagnostic category: Broad classification of diagnoses typically grouped by body system.

Medicare severity-adjusted diagnosis-related group (MS-DRG): Group of 751 classifications of diagnoses in which patients demonstrate similar resource consumption and length-of-stay patterns. MS-DRGs are a modification of the prior system that more accurately reflect the severity of a patient's illness and resources used.

nonoperating room procedure: Procedure that does not normally require the use of the operating room and that can affect MS-DRG assignment.

operating room (OR) procedure: Defined group of procedures that normally require the use of an operating room.

other diagnosis: All conditions (secondary) that exist at the time of admission or that develop subsequently that affect the treatment received and/or the length of stay. Diagnoses that relate to an earlier episode and that have no bearing on the current hospital stay are not to be reported.

outliers: There are two types of outliers: cost and day outliers. A cost outlier is a case in which the costs for treating the patient are extraordinarily high compared with other cases classified to the same MS-DRG. A cost outlier is paid an amount in excess of the cut-off threshold for a given MS-DRG. Payment for day outliers was eliminated with discharges occurring on or after October 1, 1997.

per diem rate: Payment made to the hospital from which a patient is transferred for each day of stay. It is determined by dividing the full MS-DRG payment by the GMLOS for the MS-DRG. The payment rate for the first day of stay is twice the per diem rate, and subsequent days are paid at the per diem rate up to the full DRG amount.

PMDC (Pre-major diagnostic category): Fifteen MS-DRGs to which cases are directly assigned based upon procedure codes before classification to an MDC, including MS-DRGs for the heart, liver, bone marrow transplants, simultaneous pancreas/kidney transplant, pancreas transplant, lung transplant, and five MS-DRGs for tracheostomies.

present on admission (POA): CMS-mandated assignment of indicators Y (Yes), N (No), U (Unknown), W (Clinically undetermined), or 1 (Exempt) to identify each condition as present or not present at the time the order for inpatient admission occurs for Medicare patients. A POA indicator should be listed for the principal diagnosis as well as secondary diagnoses and external cause of injury codes, unless present on the exempt list found in the ICD-9-CM Official Guidelines for Coding and Reporting.

principal diagnosis: Condition established after study to be chiefly responsible for occasioning the admission of the patient to the hospital for care.

principal procedure: Procedure performed for definitive treatment rather than for diagnostic or exploratory purposes, or that was necessary to treat a complication. Usually related to the principal diagnosis.

relative weight: Assigned weight that is intended to reflect the relative resource consumption associated with each MS-DRG. The higher the relative weight, the greater the payment to the hospital. The relative weights are calculated by CMS and published in the final prospective payment system rule.

surgical hierarchy: Ordering of surgical cases from most to least resource intensive. Application of this decision rule is necessary when patient stays involve multiple surgical procedures, each of which, occurring by itself, could result in assignment to a different MS-DRG. All patients must be assigned to only one MS-DRG per admission.

transfer: A situation in which the patient is transferred to another acute care hospital for related care.